Surgical Oncology

Theory and Multidisciplinary Practice

SECOND EDITION

Surgical Oncology

Theory and Multidisciplinary Practice

Edited by

Graeme Poston, DSc MS MBBS FRCS(Eng) FRCS(Ed)
Professor of Surgery, University of Liverpool and Consultant
Hepatobiliary Surgeon, Aintree University Hospital
Liverpool, UK

Lynda Wyld, BMedSci MBChB, PhD, FRCS(Gen Surg)
Reader in Surgical Oncology, University of Sheffield, UK and
Honorary Consultant Oncoplastic Breast Surgeon, Doncaster Royal Infirmary
Doncaster, UK

Riccardo A Audisio, MD FRCS(Eng)
Professor of Surgery, University of Liverpool and Consultant
Breast Surrgeon, Whiston and St Helen's Hospital, St Helens
Liverpool, UK

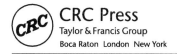

CRC Press
Taylor & Francis Group
Boca Raton London New York

CRC Press is an imprint of the
Taylor & Francis Group, an **informa** business

CRC Press
Taylor & Francis Group
6000 Broken Sound Parkway NW, Suite 300
Boca Raton, FL 33487-2742

First issued in paperback 2020

© 2017 by Taylor & Francis Group, LLC
CRC Press is an imprint of Taylor & Francis Group, an Informa business

No claim to original U.S. Government works

Version Date: 20160128

ISBN 13: 978-0-367-57439-0 (pbk)
ISBN 13: 978-1-4987-0199-0 (hbk)

This book contains information obtained from authentic and highly regarded sources. While all reasonable efforts have been made to publish reliable data and information, neither the author[s] nor the publisher can accept any legal responsibility or liability for any errors or omissions that may be made. The publishers wish to make clear that any views or opinions expressed in this book by individual editors, authors or contributors are personal to them and do not necessarily reflect the views/opinions of the publishers. The information or guidance contained in this book is intended for use by medical, scientific or health-care professionals and is provided strictly as a supplement to the medical or other professional's own judgement, their knowledge of the patient's medical history, relevant manufacturer's instructions and the appropriate best practice guidelines. Because of the rapid advances in medical science, any information or advice on dosages, procedures or diagnoses should be independently verified. The reader is strongly urged to consult the relevant national drug formulary and the drug companies' and device or material manufacturers' printed instructions, and their websites, before administering or utilizing any of the drugs, devices or materials mentioned in this book. This book does not indicate whether a particular treatment is appropriate or suitable for a particular individual. Ultimately it is the sole responsibility of the medical professional to make his or her own professional judgements, so as to advise and treat patients appropriately. The authors and publishers have also attempted to trace the copyright holders of all material reproduced in this publication and apologize to copyright holders if permission to publish in this form has not been obtained. If any copyright material has not been acknowledged please write and let us know so we may rectify in any future reprint.

Library of Congress Cataloging-in-Publication Data

Names: Poston, Graeme J., editor. | Wyld, Lynda, editor. | Audisio, Riccardo
A., editor.
Title: Surgical oncology : theory and multidisciplinary practice / [edited
by] Graeme J. Poston, Lynda Wyld, Riccardo A. Audisio.
Other titles: Textbook of surgical oncology (Poston)
Description: Second edition. | Boca Raton : CRC Press/Taylor & Francis, 2016.
| Preceded by Textbook of surgical oncology / edited by Graeme J. Poston,
R. Daniel Beauchamp, Theo J.M. Ruers. 2007. | Includes bibliographical
references and index.
Identifiers: LCCN 2016003701 (print) | LCCN 2016003999 (ebook) | ISBN
9781498701990 (hardcover : alk. paper) | ISBN 9781498702003 (e-book) |
ISBN 9781498715980 (vital book)
Subjects: | MESH: Neoplasms--surgery | Medical Oncology
Classification: LCC RD651 (print) | LCC RD651 (ebook) | NLM QZ 268 | DDC
616.99/4059--dc23
LC record available at http://lccn.loc.gov/2016003701

Visit the Taylor & Francis Web site at
http://www.taylorandfrancis.com

and the CRC Press Web site at
http://www.crcpress.com

Dedication

Surgical Oncology: Theory and Multidisciplinary Practice, Second Edition, is dedicated to our patients across Europe in the hope that we will not fail them. This textbook has been written by a global multidisciplinary team of cancer experts from across Europe and beyond in the hope that it will inspire a new generation of surgeons to strive toward best practice and outcomes in cancer surgery.

Contents

Foreword

THE MULTIDISCIPLINARY CANCER CARE TEAM

It is timely that the European Society of Surgical Oncology (ESSO) gathers highly recognized cancer care professionals to write this outstanding book on surgical oncology with a focus on multidisciplinary practice. Personalized cancer care does involve several different disciplines, and surgery has a central role in both curative and palliative treatment. At early stages of a cancer disease curative surgery is often enough, but at later stages multimodality treatments are mostly preferred and must be considered.

A prerequisite for optimal decision making at the multidisciplinary tumour board is high-quality pretreatment diagnostics. Here as well as for optimal treatment the competence by different cancer specialities is crucial. The radiologists and pathologists have important roles to provide relevant diagnostic information. The surgeon must understand the strengths of other treatment options, and radiation oncologists, medical oncologists and interventionists must know the strengths and weaknesses of the surgical procedures. Only then can a multidisciplinary team deliver quality decisions to benefit patients.

Surgical Oncology: Theory and Multidisciplinary Practice, Second Edition, provides not only residents and specialists in surgery but also other cancer specialities and professions the fundamental knowledge necessary for optimal cancer care.

Peter Naredi
ECCO President

I was delighted to be invited, as a medical oncologist, to provide a foreword to *Surgical Oncology: Theory and Multidisciplinary Practice,* Second Edition, as this reinforces the true spirit of collaboration and multidisciplinarity that is now the cornerstone of excellent cancer care across Europe.

As the treatment and care of cancer patients becomes more complex, their optimal management requires the expertise of specialists from many different disciplines, including, but not limited to, surgery, radiation therapy, medical oncology, cancer nursing, pathology and imaging.

This has inevitably led to the development of both a multidisciplinary approach and multidisciplinary teams (MDTs). The advantages of working in an MDT environment include management consistency, coordination and communication, educational opportunities and, potentially, improved outcomes. Despite the fact that cancer treatment given through an MDT is logical and has become the 'standard of care' in many leading cancer centres in the world, it is disappointing to find only scarce evidence showing that such an approach is imperative [1,2].

One of the first studies that clearly showed that the MDT may improve patient outcome was a retrospective study from Scotland [3]. This study was performed following the observation of large differences in the survival outcome of patients with ovarian cancer and showed that management by an MDT at a joint clinic improved patient survival, even after adjustment for other clinical and pathological parameters ($p < 0.001$).

Later, other studies suggested that there is an outcome and survival advantage across the various settings of different cancer sub-specialities, ranging from primary surgery to the palliative treatment of stage IV cancers. However, most of these studies were observational and retrospective in nature [4–8]. In reality, the practical implementation of the MDT demonstrates a paradox in cancer treatment: we demand evidence-based medicine for the individual, but not for general cancer care platforms [6]. Prospective studies demonstrating the already broadly accepted added value of the MDT are desirable, especially in a challenging economic environment.

Breast cancer is one example where the MDT has become imperative, especially for primary early stage treatment. Since the time when the 'Halsted procedure' – involving removal of the entire breast, axillary nodes and chest muscles – was considered the standard and the only treatment modality for breast cancer, major advances have been made.

First, it was shown that adding radiation therapy (RT) to lumpectomy was as effective as a mastectomy and far less disfiguring [9]. Later, the sentinel node biopsy (SNB) procedure, which can spare patients without nodal involvement from axillary lymph node dissection (ALND), was introduced [10]. Recently it has even been shown that patients with a positive SNB can – in some clinical situations – be spared ALND, as long as they receive radiation [11,12].

Radiation treatment has also evolved over time. While post-lumpectomy radiation is standard, the exact indications of post-mastectomy RT are still a matter of controversy. Given the emergence of new RT techniques, current efforts focus on minimizing RT. New techniques such as intense modulation radiotherapy (IMRT), partial breast irradiation (PBI) and intraoperative RT or brachytherapy have become available. However, it is crucial to select the right patients for these modern treatments [13,14].

Systemic treatment decisions for breast cancer are clearly influenced by data gathered from pathology, imaging and surgical procedures. Hormonal therapy is generally provided to treat estrogen receptor (ER) positive tumours, while trastuzumab is given only for HER2 positive tumours [15,17]. Neoadjuvant or adjuvant chemotherapy treatment decisions are also directly influenced by clinical and pathological data gathered by MDT.

Because the various treatment modalities are influenced by each other in the treatment of breast cancer, it is undisputed that all personnel involved in the care of one specific individual should discuss and treat the person in an MDT setting. For example, if the surgeon considers sparing ALND in a patient whose SNB is positive, this will result in a lack of formal nodal staging, which may in turn impact decisions on hormonal and chemotherapy treatment. Moreover, it will require post-surgical RT, which may lead to changes in the timing or modality of reconstructive plastic surgeries.

After MDT discussions, the treating physician can go back to the patient with more solid options to discuss, leading to more confidence in the patient–doctor relationship. Interestingly, in a recent survey, 63% of the investigators from western Europe declared that the MDT was a mandatory part of breast cancer care in their country [18]. Similar conclusions are likely to be reached for the treatment and care of all other cancer types.

Lastly, the MDT is likely to expand in the following years, given the gradual implementation in the clinic of powerful diagnostic technologies such as next-generation sequencing designed to move from 'precision medicine' to 'personalized medicine'. These technologies will call for additional experts – such as geneticists and bioinformaticians – to enrich the MDT. The human being residing within the patient will need to be remembered in all treatment decisions.

Marine Piccart
ECCO Past-President

REFERENCES

1. Fleissig A, Jenkins V, Catt S, Fallowfield L. Multidisciplinary teams in cancer care: are they effective in the UK? *Lancet Oncol* 2006;7(11):935–43.

2. Fennell ML, Das IP, Clauser S, Petrelli N, Salner A. The organization of multidisciplinary care teams: modeling internal and external influences on cancer care quality. *J Natl Cancer Inst Monogr* 2010;2010(40):72–80.

3. Junor EJ, Hole DJ, Gillis CR. Management of ovarian cancer: referral to a multidisciplinary team matters. *Br J Cancer* 1994;70(2):363–70.

4. Forrest LM, McMillan DC, McArdle CS, Dunlop DJ. An evaluation of the impact of a multidisciplinary team, in a single centre, on treatment and survival in patients with inoperable non-small-cell lung cancer. *Br J Cancer* 2005;93(9):977–8.

5. Stephens MR, Lewis WG, Brewster AE, Lord I, Blackshaw GRJC, Hodzovic I, et al. Multidisciplinary team management is associated with improved outcomes after surgery for esophageal cancer. *Dis Esophagus Off J Int Soc Dis Esophagus ISDE* 2006;19(3):164–71.

6. Taylor C, Munro AJ, Glynne-Jones R, Griffith C, Trevatt P, Richards M, et al. Multidisciplinary team working in cancer: what is the evidence? *BMJ* 2010;340:c951.

7. Coory M, Gkolia P, Yang IA, Bowman RV, Fong KM. Systematic review of multidisciplinary teams in the management of lung cancer. *Lung Cancer Amst Neth* 2008;60(1):14–21.

8. Morris E, Haward RA, Gilthorpe MS, Craigs C, Forman D. The impact of the Calman-Hine report on the processes and outcomes of care for Yorkshire's colorectal cancer patients. *Br J Cancer* 2006;95(8):979–85.

9. Fisher B, Slack NH, Cavanaugh PJ, Gardner B, Ravdin RG. Postoperative radiotherapy in the treatment of breast cancer: results of the NSABP clinical trial. *Ann Surg* 1970;172(4):711–32.

10. Veronesi U, Paganelli G, Galimberti V, Viale G, Zurrida S, Bedoni M, et al. Sentinel-node biopsy to avoid axillary dissection in breast cancer with clinically negative lymph-nodes. *Lancet* 1997;349(9069):1864–7.

11. Donker M, van Tienhoven G, Straver ME, Meijnen P, van de Velde CJH, Mansel RE, et al. Radiotherapy or surgery of the axilla after a positive sentinel node in breast cancer (EORTC 10981-22023 AMAROS): a randomised, multicentre, open-label, phase 3 non-inferiority trial. *Lancet Oncol* 2014;15(12):1303–10.

12. Giuliano AE, Hunt KK, Ballman KV, Beitsch PD, Whitworth PW, Blumencranz PW, et al. Axillary dissection vs no axillary dissection in women with invasive breast cancer and sentinel node metastasis: a randomized clinical trial. *JAMA J Am Med Assoc* 2011;305(6):569–75.

13. Veronesi U, Orecchia R, Maisonneuve P, Viale G, Rotmensz N, Sangalli C, et al. Intraoperative radiotherapy versus external radiotherapy for early breast cancer (ELIOT): a randomised controlled equivalence trial. *Lancet Oncol* 2013;14(13):1269–77.

14. Smith GL, Xu Y, Buchholz TA, Giordano SH, Jiang J, Shih Y-CT, et al. Association between treatment with brachytherapy vs whole-breast irradiation and

subsequent mastectomy, complications, and survival among older women with invasive breast cancer. *J Am Med Assoc* 2012;307(17):1827–37.

15. Slamon D, Eiermann W, Robert N, Pienkowski T, Martin M, Press M, et al. Adjuvant trastuzumab in HER2-positive breast cancer. *N Engl J Med* 2011;365(14):1273–83.

16. Piccart-Gebhart MJ, Procter M, Leyland-Jones B, Goldhirsch A, Untch M, Smith I, et al. Trastuzumab after adjuvant chemotherapy in HER2-positive breast cancer. *N Engl J Med* 2005;353(16):1659–72.

17. Romond EH, Perez EA, Bryant J, Suman VJ, Geyer CE Jr, Davidson NE, et al. Trastuzumab plus adjuvant chemotherapy for operable HER2-positive breast cancer. *N Engl J Med* 2005;353(16):1673–84.

18. Saini KS, Taylor C, Ramirez A-J, Palmieri C, Gunnarsson U, Schmoll HJ, et al. Role of the multidisciplinary team in breast cancer management: results from a large international survey involving 39 countries. *Ann Oncol Off J Eur Soc Med Oncol ESMO* 2012;23(4):853–9.

UNION EUROPÉENNE DES MÉDECINS SPÉCIALISTES
EUROPEAN UNION OF MEDICAL SPECIALISTS-UEMS

THE UEMS Section of Surgery

EUROPEAN SOCIETY OF SURGICAL ONCOLOGY

It is with great pleasure that I have agreed to write a foreword for this textbook, which is the work of the most prestigious group of authors in the field with experience and expertise which are second to none.

This textbook is a must read for any colleague involved in the field of surgical oncology for the following reasons:

- The entire width and depth of the field are covered comprehensively; each chapter has a wealth of scientific and clinical information provided in a clear, robust and fluent way.
- Each topic is covered holistically from the relevant elements of basic science to complex and innovative clinical practice, always enriched with most helpful examples reflecting the experience of the authors and aiming to stimulate the critical thinking of the readers.
- The textbook really focuses on a sound multidisciplinary approach reflecting the overall philosophy of the authors regarding the character of modern practice in surgical oncology. I am confident that the educationally superb way with which this approach is presented in the book will be 'game changing' even for those who still believe that they can practice within the narrow boundaries of their own specialty.
- The authors give emphasis to patient-centred care; this is of course of paramount importance for all patients, but even more so for cancer patients. A thorough

analysis of issues related to quality of care, quality of outcomes, and above all, quality of life is clearly evident in the whole book.

- The overall content of the book mirrors the syllabus and core curriculum of the European training requirements in surgical oncology as they have been developed by the Division of Surgical Oncology of the Section of Surgery of the European Union of Medical Specialists (UEMS) and the European Society of Surgical Oncology (ESSO). The textbook is an invaluable tool for the preparation of the relevant European exam in surgical oncology.

As president of the UEMS Section of Surgery, I feel particularly proud that this truly excellent textbook reflects the superb work that has been done over the last few years by the executive and all the members of the UEMS Division of Surgical Oncology in collaboration with ESSO; they have our grateful thanks and most sincere congratulations.

I am sure that all colleagues who are involved in the truly challenging and ever-changing field of surgical oncology will find this textbook a most helpful companion and powerful ally in their day-to-day practice.

Enjoy reading it!

Vassilios Papalois
Imperial College Healthcare NHS Trust
European Union of Medical Specialists

Preface

Surgery is the oldest form of effective cancer treatment and 60% of people cured of cancer are cured by surgery alone [1]. The diagnosis and treatment of cancer has rapidly evolved over the past quarter of a century, with advances in screening and surveillance, diagnostic accuracy, effective systemic therapies and accuracy of radiation therapies, in addition to those in surgical oncology. Furthermore, for those whose cancer remains incurable, these advances significantly contribute to prolonged good quality of life that can now be frequently measured in years, rather than months. Lastly, the morbidity and mortality risks of these treatments have markedly improved, in particular those associated with the more complex cancer operations.

The advances in cancer surgery over the last 25 years (minimal access surgery, enhanced recovery, anaesthesia and intensive care), associated with better use of perioperative (neoadjuvant, adjuvant and conversion) therapies (systemic and radiation), have led to ever-improving outcomes in terms of both disease-free and overall survival. Furthermore, other medical disciplines allied to surgery, such as interventional radiology and nuclear medicine, now allow us to effectively treat patients previously thought beyond the scope of standard care [2]. This observation is especially true for the elderly, a group in which the majority of cancers occur in western society.

These advances are encapsulated in the application of multidisciplinarity: the principle that all disciplines are now essential in the management of patients suffering from cancer. All are equally important, and none pre-eminent. Multidisciplinary team working is now the standard of care in most countries, and a legal requirement in many.

Clinical trials in surgical oncology remain challenging [3]. However, advances in cancer surgery need surgeons who can conduct careful prospective evaluations of new operative techniques and technologies, in addition to the application of new adjunctive therapies to improve operative outcomes. It is, however, essential that surgeons pay meticulous attention to quality assurance, in particular operative technique, when conducting such studies.

Lastly, the most significant recent advances relate to greater understanding of molecular medicine, in particular the genetic mutational markers of better or worse prognosis, so allowing more appropriate uses of increasingly scarcer resources targeted at those whose potential benefit is greater: the age of precision medicine. We would hope that the next 10 years will see the application of precision surgery to the ever-increasing benefit of our cancer patients.

Lynda Wyld
University of Sheffield Medical School
Sheffield, UK

Riccardo A Audisio
University of Liverpool
St Helens, UK

Graeme J Poston
University of Liverpool
Liverpool, UK

REFERENCES

1. Wyld L, Audisio RA, Poston GJ. The evolution of cancer surgery and future perspectives. *Nat Rev Clin Oncol* 2015;12(2):115–24.
2. Franklin JM, Gebski V, Poston GJ, Sharma RA. Clinical trials of interventional oncology-moving from efficacy to outcomes. *Nat Rev Clin Oncol* 2015;12(2):93–104.
3. Evrard S, McKelvie-Sibareu P, van de Velde C, Nordlinger B, Poston G. What can we learn from oncology surgical trials? *Nat Rev Clin Oncol* 2016;13(1):55–62.

Contributors

Andy Adam
Department of Radiology
London, UK

Akash Agarwal
Department of Surgical Oncology
Dr Ram Manohar Lohia Institute of Medical Sciences
Lucknow, India

William H Allum
Department of Surgery
Royal Marsden NHS Foundation Trust
London, UK

Oscar Alonso-Casado
Department of Surgical Oncology
MD Anderson Cancer Center
Madrid, Spain

Robert U Ashford
East Midlands Sarcoma Service
Department of Orthopaedic Surgery
University Hospitals of Leicester, UK

Celine P E Asselbergs
Department of Urology
Academic Medical Center
Amsterdam, The Netherlands

Riccardo A Audisio
University of Liverpool
St Helens Teaching Hospital
St Helens, UK

Atul Bagul
St George's Hospital
London, UK

Saba Balasubramanian
Sheffield Teaching Hospitals
Sheffield, UK

Charles Balch
Department of Surgery
Division of Surgical Oncology
University of Texas Southwestern Medical Center
Dallas, Texas, USA

Alberto Biondi
Department of Surgery
'A. Gemelli' Hospital
Università Cattolica del Sacro Cuore
Rome, Italy

Petra G Boelens
Department of Surgery
Leiden University Medical Center
Leiden, The Netherlands

Leonora S F Boogerd
Department of Surgery
Leiden University Medical Center
Leiden, The Netherlands

Martin C Boonstra
Department of Surgery
Leiden University Medical Center
Leiden, The Netherlands

Inne H M Borel Rinkes
Department of Surgery
University Medical Center Utrecht
Utrecht, The Netherlands

Marco Braga
Department of Surgery
San Raffaele Hospital
Milan, Italy

Gina Brown
Royal Marsden NHS Foundation Trust
and
Department of Radiology
Imperial College London
London, UK

Johan Bussink
Department of Radiation Oncology
Radboud University Medical Centre
Nijmegen, The Netherlands

Clare Byrne
University Hospital Aintree
Liverpool, UK

Juan Miguel Cejalvo
Department of Hematology and Medical Oncology
Biomedical Research Institute INCLIVA
University of Valencia
Valencia, Spain

Andrés Cervantes
Department of Hematology and Medical Oncology
Biomedical Research Institute INCLIVA
University of Valencia
Valencia, Spain

Arun Chaturvedi
Department of Surgical Oncology
Dr Ram Manohar Lohia Institute of Medical Sciences
Lucknow, India

Sarah C Darby
Clinical Trial Service Unit
Nuffield Department of Population Health
University of Oxford
Oxford, UK

Marcello Deraco
Colorectal Unit, Responsible, Peritoneal Malignancies
Fondazione IRCCS Istituto Nazionale dei Tumori
Milan, Italy

Theo M de Reijke
Department of Urology
Academic Medical Center
Amsterdam, The Netherlands

Domenico D'Ugo
Department of Surgery
'A. Gemelli' Hospital
Università Cattolica del Sacro Cuore
Rome, Italy

Nicholas C Eastley
East Midlands Sarcoma Service
Department of Orthopaedic Surgery
University Hospitals of Leicester, UK

Ibrahim Edhemović
Department of Surgical Oncology
Institute of Oncology Ljubljana
Ljubljana, Slovenia

Dominique Elias
Department of Surgical Oncology
Institut Gustave Roussy
Villejuif, France

Bang Wool Eom
Center for Gastric Cancer and Department of Surgery
Research institute and Hospital
National Cancer Centre
Goyang, Republic of Korea

Laura Esposito
Visceral Sarcoma Unit
Department of Surgery
San Giovanni Battista Hospital
University of Turin
Torino, Italy

David Evans
Department of Radiology
King's College Hospital
London, UK

Serge Evrard
Department of Surgery
Bergonie Institute
Bordeaux, France

Gabriella Ferrandina
Department of Gynecology/Obstetrics
Catholic University
Rome, Italy

Elisa Fontana
Department of Medicine
Royal Marsden NHS Foundation Trust
London, UK

Sheila Fraser
Royal North Shore Hospital
Sydney, Australia

Valentina Gambardella
Department of Hematology and Medical Oncology
Biomedical Research Institute INCLIVA
University of Valencia
Valencia, Spain

D Gareth Evans
Department of Genomic Medicine
Institute of Human Development
St Mary's Hospital
University of Manchester
Manchester, UK

Paula Ghaneh
Department of Molecular and Clinical Cancer Medicine
University of Liverpool
Liverpool, UK

Timothy Gilbert
Department of Molecular and Clinical Cancer Medicine
University of Liverpool
Liverpool, UK

Santiago González-Moreno
Peritoneal Surface Oncology Program
Department of Surgical Oncology
MD Anderson Cancer Center
Madrid, Spain

Amit Goyal
Department of Otorhinolaryngology
All India Institute of Medical Sciences
Jodhpur, India

Robert J Grimer
Royal Orthopaedic Hospital
Birmingham, UK

Alessandro Gronchi
Sarcoma Unit
Department of Surgery
Fondazione IRCCS Istituto Nazionale dei Tumori
Milan, Italy

Rachel Grossman
Department of Neurosurgery
Tel Aviv Medical Center
Sackler Faculty of Medicine
Tel Aviv University
Tel Aviv, Israel

Birgit Gruenberger
Department of Internal Medicine
Hospital of St John of God
Vienna, Austria

Thomas Gruenberger
Department of Surgery
Rudolfstiftung Hospital
Vienna, Austria

Sameer Gupta
Department of Surgical Oncology
King George's Medical University
Lucknow, India

Henricus J M Handgraaf
Department of Surgery
Leiden University Medical Center
Leiden, The Netherlands

Andrew J Hayes
Department of Surgical Oncology
The Royal Marsden NHS Foundation Trust
London, UK

Päivi Heikkilä
Department of Pathology
Helsinki University Hospital
Helsinki, Finland

Shahzad Ilyas
Department of Radiology
Consultant Interventional Radiologist
Guy's and St Thomas' Hospital Trust
London, UK

Robert P Jones
School of Cancer Studies
Institute of Translational Medicine
University of Liverpool
and
Liverpool Hepatobiliary Centre
Aintree University Hospital
Liverpool, UK

Karsten Juhl Jørgensen
The Nordic Cochrane Centre
Rigshospitalet
Copenhagen, Denmark

Electron Kebebew
Endocrine Oncology Branch
National Cancer Institute
National Institutes of Health
Bethesda, Maryland, USA

Xavier M Keutgen
Endocrine Oncology Branch
National Cancer Institute
National Institutes of Health
Bethesda, Maryland, USA

Young-Woo Kim
Center for Gastric Cancer and Department of Surgery
Research Institute and Hospital
National Cancer Centre
Goyang, Republic of Korea

Tibor Kovacs
Guy's and St Thomas' NHS Foundation Trust
London, UK

Koert F D Kuhlmann
Department of Surgical Oncology
Antoni van Leeuwenhoek – Netherlands Cancer Institute
Amsterdam, The Netherlands

Anneke C M Kusters
Department of Urology
Academic Medical Center
Amsterdam, The Netherlands

Konstantinos Lasithiotakis
Department of General Surgery
York Teaching Hospital
NHS Foundation Trust
London, UK

Iain Lawrie
Consultant and Honorary Clinical Senior Lecturer in Palliative Medicine
The Pennine Acute Hospitals NHS Trust
The University of Manchester, UK

Marjut Leidenius
Department of Breast Surgery
Comprehensive Cancer Centre
Helsinki University Hospital
Helsinki, Finland

Maria Carmen Lirosi
Department of Surgery
'A. Gemelli' Hospital
Università Cattolica del Sacro Cuore
Rome, Italy

Mari Lloyd-Williams
Professor and Honorary Consultant in Palliative Medicine
Academic Palliative and Supportive Care Studies Group (APSCSG)
Institute Psychology, Health and Society University of Liverpool, UK

Tanveer Abdul Majeed
Department of Surgical Oncology
Asian Cancer Institute
Mumbai, India

Hassan Z Malik
Liverpool Hepatobiliary Centre
Aintree University Hospital
Liverpool, UK

Kulbir Mann
Department of Molecular and Clinical Cancer Medicine
University of Liverpool
Liverpool, UK

Gurdeep S Mannu
Clinical Trial Service Unit
Nuffield Department of Population Health
University of Oxford
Oxford, UK

Daniele Marrelli
Department of Human Pathology and Oncology Unit of Surgical Oncology
University of Siena
Siena, Italy

Johanna Mattson
Department of Solid Tumours
Comprehensive Cancer Centre
Helsinki University Hospital
Helsinki, Finland

Pippa McKelvie-Sebileau
Institut Bergonie
Bordeaux, France

Tuomo Meretoja
Comprehensive Cancer Centre
Helsinki University Hospital
Helsinki, Finland

Sanjeev Misra
Department of Surgical Oncology
All India Institute of Medical Sciences
Jodhpur, India

David A L Morgan
Department of Clinical Oncology (Retd.)
Nottingham University Hospitals
Nottingham, UK

Per J Nilsson
Division of Coloproctology
Center for Digestive Diseases
Karolinska University Hospital
Stockholm, Sweden

Sarah T O'Dwyer
Consultant Surgeon
The Colorectal and Peritoneal Oncology Centre
The Christie Hospital NHSFT
Manchester, UK

Frances Oldfield
Department of Molecular and Clinical Cancer Medicine
University of Liverpool
Liverpool, UK

Gloria Ortega-Pérez
Department of Surgical Oncology
Peritoneal Surface Oncology Program
MD Anderson Cancer Center
Madrid, Spain

Daniel H Palmer
School of Cancer Studies
Institute of Translational Medicine
University of Liverpool
and
Liverpool Hepatobiliary Centre
Aintree University Hospital
Liverpool, UK

Puneet Pareek
Department of Radiation Oncology
All India Institute of Medical Sciences
Jodhpur, India

Ji Yeon Park
Center for Gastric Cancer and Department of Surgery
Research Institute and Hospital
National Cancer Center
Goyang, Republic of Korea

Michael Parry
Royal Orthopaedic Hospital
Birmingham, UK

Nicholas Pavlidis
Department of Medical Oncology
Medical School
University of Ioannina
Ioannina, Greece

Pompiliu Piso
Department of Surgery
Klinik für Allgemein- und Viszeralchirurgie
Krankenhaus Barmherzige Brüder Regensburg
Regensburg, Germany

Wojciech P Polkowski
Department of Surgical Oncology
Medical University of Lublin
Lublin, Poland

Karol Polom
Department of Human Pathology and Oncology
Unit of Surgical Oncology
University of Siena
Siena, Italy

Philip Poortmans
Department of Radiation Oncology
Radboud University Medical Center
Nijmegen, The Netherlands

Graeme J Poston
School of Cancer Studies
University of Liverpool
University Hospital Aintree
Liverpool, UK

Saskia Rademakers
Department of Radiation Oncology
Radboud University Medical Center
Nijmegen, The Netherlands

Zvi Ram
Department of Neurosurgery
Tel Aviv Medical Center
Sackler Faculty of Medicine
Tel Aviv University
Tel Aviv, Israel

Michel Rivoire
Department of Surgery
Leon Berard Cancer Center
Lyon, France

Derek J Rosario
University of Sheffield
Royal Hallamshire Hospital
Sheffield, UK

Susana Roselló
Department of Hematology and Medical Oncology
Biomedical Research Institute INCLIVA
University of Valencia
Valencia, Spain

Franco Roviello
Department of Human Pathology and Oncology
Unit of Surgical Oncology
University of Siena
Siena, Italy

Isabel T Rubio
Breast Cancer Centre
Hospital Universitari Vall d'Hebron
Barcelona, Spain

Theo J M Ruers
Netherlands Cancer Institute
Amsterdam, The Netherlands

Harm J T Rutten
School of Oncology and Developmental Biology
University of Maastricht, Maastricht
and

Catharina Hospital Eindhoven
Eindhoven, The Netherlands

Tarun Sabharwal
Department of Radiology
Consultant Interventional Radiologist
Guy's and St Thomas' Hospital Trust
London, UK

Samira M Sadowski
Endocrine Oncology Branch
National Cancer Institute
National Institutes of Health
Bethesda, Maryland, USA
and
Thoracic and Endocrine Surgery
University Hospitals of Geneva
Geneva, Switzerland

Sergio Sandrucci
Visceral Sarcoma Unit
Department of Surgery
San Giovanni Battista Hospital
University of Turin Cso Dogliortti
Torino, Italy

Dhairyasheel Savant
Department of Surgical Oncology
Asian Cancer Institute
Mumbai, India

Giovanni Scambia
Department of Gynecology/Obstetrics
Catholic University
Rome, Italy

Wolfgang Schima
Department of Diagnostic and Interventional Radiology
Krankenhaus Göttlicher Heiland
Krankenhaus der Barmherzigen Schwestern
and
Sankt Josef-Krankenhaus
Vienna, Austria

Michael Shackcloth
Liverpool Heart and Chest Hospital
Liverpool, UK

Stan Sidhu
University of Sydney Endocrine Surgical Unit
Royal North Shore Hospital
Sydney, Australia

Ponnandai S Somasundar
Department of Surgery
Roger Williams Medical Center
Boston University
Providence, Rhode Island, USA

Silvia Stacchiotti
Sarcoma Unit
Department of Cancer Medicine
Fondazione IRCCS Istituto Nazionale Tumori
Milan, Italy

Naureen Starling
Department of Medicine
Royal Marsden NHS Foundation Trust
London, UK

Paul H Sugarbaker
Program in Peritoneal Surface Oncology
Center for Gastrointestinal Malignancies
MedStar Washington Hospital Center
Washington, DC, USA

Pieter J Tanis
Department of Surgery
Academic Medical Centre
Amsterdam, The Netherlands

Alexander L Vahrmeijer
Department of Surgery
Leiden University Medical Center
Leiden, The Netherlands

Kurt van der Speeten
Department of Surgical Oncology
Ziekenhuis Oost-Limburg
Universiteit Hasselt
and
Department of Life Sciences
BIOMED Research Institute
Oncology Research Cluster
Genk, Belgium

Cornelis J H van de Velde
Department of Surgical Oncology
Leiden University Medical Center
Leiden, The Netherlands

Rogier K van der Vijgh
Department of Urology
Academic Medical Center
Amsterdam, The Netherlands

Menno R Vriens
Department of Surgery
University Medical Center Utrecht
Utrecht, The Netherlands

Lona Vyas
Department of Urology
Royal Hallamshire Hospital
Sheffield, UK

Nicholas P West
Pathology and Tumour Biology
Leeds Institute of Cancer and Pathology
St James's University Hospital
Leeds, UK

Michel W J M Wouters
Department of Surgical Oncology
Netherlands Cancer Institute- Antoni van Leeuwenhoek
Amsterdam, The Netherlands

Lynda Wyld
University of Sheffield Medical School
Sheffield, UK

Odysseas Zoras
Department of Surgical Oncology
University Hospital of Heraklion
Crete, Greece

PART 1

Basic principles of oncology

Cancer epidemiology

GURDEEP S MANNU AND SARAH C DARBY

INTRODUCTION

Epidemiology is the branch of medicine that studies how and why different groups of people have different risks of developing disease and the factors that are responsible for these differences. It is the cornerstone of public health and, by identifying risk factors and targets for disease prevention, it provides the basis for policy decisions and evidence-based disease control and prevention. Epidemiological data on changes in disease rates over time can also be used to monitor the impact of primary prevention strategies.

CANCER IN THE UK

More than 327,000 people in the UK were newly diagnosed with cancer of one type or another in 2012, and more than 157,000 died of the disease [1]. The most common cancers to be diagnosed are breast cancer in women and prostate cancer in men (see Figure 1.1) [1], while the most common type of cancer to cause death is lung cancer in both men and women. The different types of cancer that predominate vary with age. Leukaemia and brain cancer are by far the most common in both boys and girls (see Figure 1.2). Among teenagers and young adults, lymphomas continue to be common in both sexes, while testicular cancer and other germ-cell tumours are relatively common in young men, and breast cancer and other carcinomas in young women. Among men aged 25–49, testicular cancer is the most common cancer, while at older ages prostate, lung and

bowel cancer predominate. Breast cancer is the most common cancer in women in all age groups beyond 25, while at ages 50 and above lung and bowel cancers also contribute substantially to the numbers of new cases of cancer. Further information on the numbers of cancers diagnosed in the UK is given in [2].

Overall, cancer is much rarer in childhood than in adults and, after childhood, the numbers of new cases of cancer diagnosed annually increase with age up to about 60 in women and 70 in men (see Figure 1.3). Beyond these ages the numbers level off in women and start to decrease in men. This reflects the decreasing number of people in the population at older ages, due principally to the effect of mortality, but also to changes in migration and the birth rate. The effect of variation in the numbers of people in different age groups in a population on the number of cancer cases diagnosed in each age group can be taken into account by considering annual incidence rates, i.e. the number of cases occurring each year divided by the number of people in the relevant age group of the population. Incidence rates for all types of cancer combined continue to increase throughout life in both men and women. When comparing cancer levels in different populations, and within the same population at different time periods, it is usually more appropriate to consider rates rather than numbers of cancers. It is also necessary to take into account the different age structures of different populations by using an appropriate form of age standardization (see 'Cancer Worldwide' section on page 6).

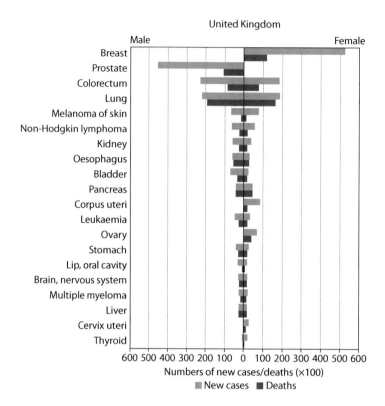

Figure 1.1 Numbers of new cases of cancer and deaths occurring each year in the UK in 2012. (Reproduced from Ferlay J, et al., GLOBOCAN 2012 v1.0, Cancer Incidence and Mortality Worldwide: IARC CancerBase No. 11 [Internet]. Lyon, France: International Agency for Research on Cancer; 2013, available from: http://globocan.iarc.fr, accessed 16 October 2014.)

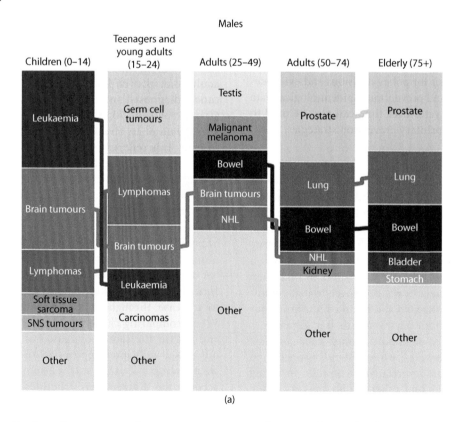

Figure 1.2 The distribution of cancer types by age group among males (a) in the UK for the years 2009–2011. (Reproduced from Cancer Research UK, Cancer incidence by age, London: Cancer Research UK; 2014, available from http://www. cancerresearchuk.org/cancer-info/cancerstats/incidence/age, accessed March 2016.) *(Continued)*

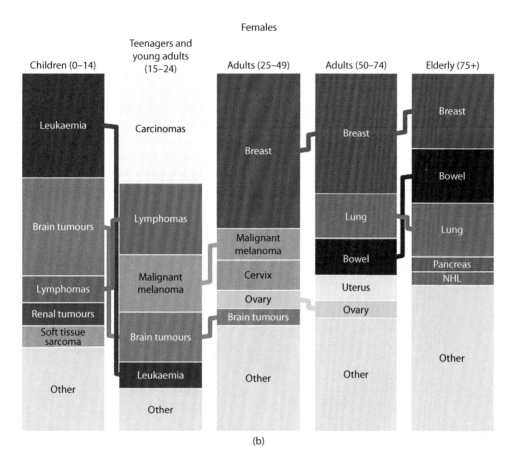

(b)

Figure 1.2 (Continued) The distribution of cancer types by age group among females **(b)** in the UK for the years 2009–2011. (Reproduced from Cancer Research UK, Cancer incidence by age, London: Cancer Research UK; 2014, available from http://www.cancerresearchuk.org/cancer-info/cancerstats/incidence/age, accessed March 2016).

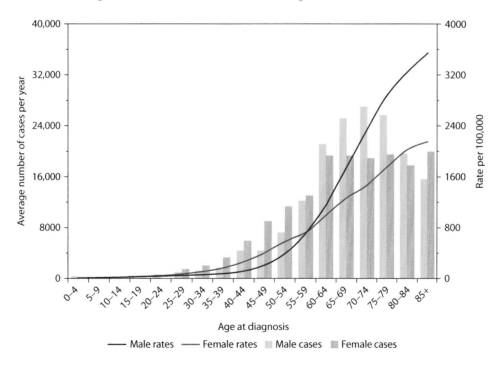

Figure 1.3 Numbers of new cases of cancer of all types occurring each year in the UK by age, and annual age-specific incidence rates per 100,000 population, for males and females in 2009–2011. (Reproduced from Cancer Research UK, Cancer incidence by age, London: Cancer Research UK; 2014, available from http://www.cancerresearchuk.org/cancer-info/cancerstats/incidence/age, accessed 5 January 2014.)

CANCER WORLDWIDE

At present, more than 14 million new cases of cancer occur each year worldwide and more than 8 million deaths are attributable to cancer annually [1]. For some cancers incidence rates are increasing, and for others they are decreasing. The number of new cases occurring overall is, however, increasing year on year, due mainly to increases in population size and longevity but also to the increasing effect of tobacco consumption in middle- and low-income countries (see below). If current trends continue, then there will be around 22 million new cancer cases globally in 2030 [3].

Cancer imposes a substantial burden of morbidity and mortality in every country worldwide, but the types of cancer that are common differ between countries (Figure 1.4). In men, lung cancer is the most important fatal cancer in much of the world, although prostate cancer predominates in sub-Saharan Africa and parts of Latin America. Leukaemia, Kaposi's sarcoma and cancers of the liver, oesophagus, lip and oral cavity are each the most common fatal cancer in men in a few countries.

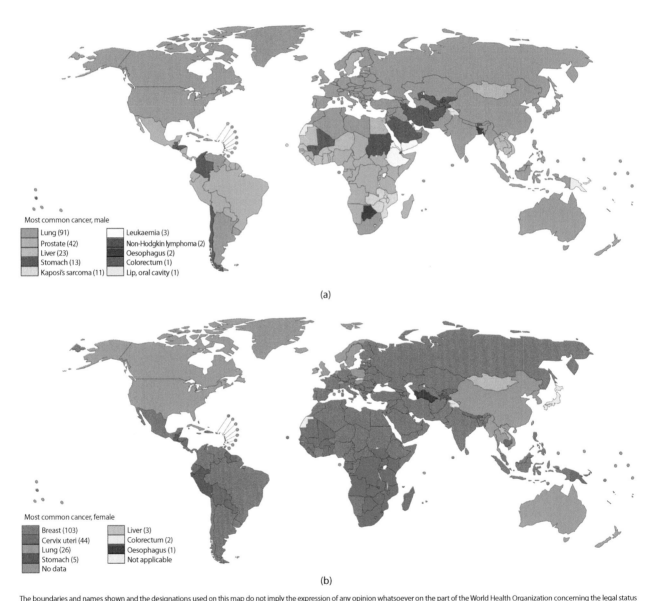

The boundaries and names shown and the designations used on this map do not imply the expression of any opinion whatsoever on the part of the World Health Organization concerning the legal status of any country, territory, city or area or of its authorities, or concerning the delimitation of its frontiers or boundaries. Dotted and dashed lines on maps represent approximate border lines for which there may not yet be full agreement.

Figure 1.4 Most common fatal cancer by country in males (a) and females (b). Values shown are age-standardized rates, i.e. summary measures of the rates that would have occurred if the population in each country had the same standard age structure. (Reproduced from Ferlay J, et al., GLOBOCAN 2012 v1.0, Cancer Incidence and Mortality Worldwide: IARC CancerBase No. 11 [Internet]. Lyon, France: International Agency for Research on Cancer 2013.)

In women, lung cancer is the most common fatal cancer in North America, northern Europe, China and Australia. Breast cancer mortality exceeds that of lung cancer in North Africa, southern Europe, Russia, the Middle East, much of Latin America and parts of Australasia, while cervical cancer predominates in sub-Saharan Africa and parts of Latin America. Further information on the numbers of cancers in different countries around the world is given in [1].

For many types of cancer, incidence rates vary by more than a factor of 10 between different countries. In some cases, substantial differences also occur between populations with similar ethnic and genetic compositions, and between men and women in the same population, even for cancers of organs that are common to both men and women. These observations suggest that the environment plays a major role in the causation of cancer and also that different cancers may well have different causes. Confirmation of the role of the environment in cancer causation has come from studies of migrant populations, among whom cancer rates tend to change from those of the country that they have left toward those of the country to which they have migrated [4,5].

EPIDEMIOLOGICAL STUDIES

Studies comparing cancer rates in different populations are termed 'descriptive studies'. Although such studies have been useful in suggesting that different environmental causes predominate in different places, their role in identifying specific causes of cancer is usually limited. Other types of descriptive study focus on individuals and include case reports and case series. Studies such as these may provide the initial pointers as to the specific factors involved in causing a particular type of cancer, but the strength of the evidence that they provide is usually weak, in that it is not usually possible to rule out other explanations for the observations.

More detailed studies, known as 'analytical studies', in which the extent to which different individuals within a population have been differently exposed to specific factors is documented and then related to the subsequent rate at which the cancer in question occurs, can provide stronger evidence. The design of such studies usually falls into one of two basic categories: a 'cohort study' or a 'case-control study'. In a cohort study, a population of individuals who have not yet developed the disease in question is identified, and the extent to which each individual has been exposed to the agent in question is ascertained. The individuals in the population are then followed up over time, occurrences of the disease in question are identified and the association between the disease rates in those with different levels of exposure to the putative cause is studied. Where the follow-up starts from the time the study is initiated and is carried out prospectively, it is clear that the study may take many years to complete. Sometimes, however, a cohort study can make use of information that has already been collected, such as employment or medical records, in which case the study may be carried out within a shorter timescale.

In a case-control study, individuals in a population who have already developed the disease in question – the cases – are identified, as are individuals who have not yet developed the disease – the controls. The extent to which both cases and controls had previously been exposed to the agent in question is then ascertained and, once again, the association between disease rates and exposure levels studied. By sampling only a proportion of the individuals who are eligible to be controls, case-control studies involve studying a smaller number of individuals than cohort studies, which may result in a cheaper study. However, if the exposure histories are collected retrospectively, for example by administering questionnaires to the study participants, care must be taken to avoid recall bias arising from the fact that the cases may be more likely than the controls to remember exposures to factors thought to be harmful.

Irrespective of the study design, it is clear that the associations revealed in the data will be informative only if the study has been able to take into account all the other variables that are strongly associated with both the disease under study and the exposure of interest. Otherwise the association will be distorted or 'confounded'. In a cohort study, the effect of potential confounders is often removed during the analysis using statistical techniques such as regression or stratification. These techniques may also be used in the analysis of case-control studies, but in such studies there is the additional possibility of removing at least some of the potential confounders during the design phase of the study, by choosing controls whose distribution across the potential confounding variables is matched to that of the cases. Further information about different types of epidemiological study is given in [6,7].

ASSESSMENT OF CAUSATION

Irrespective of the excellence of the design, data collection and statistical analysis, or the striking nature of the results, a single epidemiological study is unlikely to provide conclusive evidence as to whether or not an association between exposure and disease is causal. This is because such studies are observational in nature, and the investigator has not determined the allocation of the study subjects to putative risk factors. Rather it is determined by a variety of factors, many of which may be unknown to the investigator and which cannot, therefore, be taken into account. This is in contrast to trials and other experimental studies, where the investigator can use randomization to ensure that individuals allocated to different exposure levels are unlikely to differ systematically from each other, and where single studies can often provide strong evidence of causality.

Determining causation from observational studies is a crucial component of epidemiology. In 1965, Austin Bradford Hill proposed nine criteria to help assess the causality of associations between environmental exposures and diseases such as cancer [8]. These criteria are listed in Table 1.1, together with an illustration of how they could be used in considering the information on smoking and lung cancer available at the time. As Bradford Hill pointed out, the criteria are guidelines, rather than hard and fast rules.

In fact, one criterion – that of specificity – does not apply in the case of smoking and lung cancer. Reaching a consensus as to whether the evidence regarding causality is conclusive can be difficult. Although by 1965 many people judged the evidence of a causal relation to be overwhelming, several eminent scientists still did not find the relationship biologically plausible (see Table 1.1).

The International Agency for Research on Cancer (IARC) has a process to facilitate the reaching of a consensus as to

Table 1.1 Bradford Hill criteria

Criterion	Description	Example from lung cancer and smoking, based on evidence in 1965
1. Strength	The larger the impact of the exposure on the outcome, the stronger is the evidence for a causal link.	Tobacco smoking was associated with a more than tenfold increase in lung cancer mortality.
2. Consistency	There is strong evidence for causality when similar results are found in studies that use different designs.	In 1964, the US Surgeon General found 29 retrospective and 7 prospective studies reporting a positive association between smoking and lung cancer.
3. Specificity	There is stronger evidence for causality if a particular exposure is associated just with a specific type of cancer.	Tobacco smoking increased the risk of lung cancer, but it also increased the risks of many other cancers and many non-neoplastic diseases. Thus lung cancer and smoking did not – and still do not – meet this criterion.
4. Temporality	The exposure needs to come before the disease for it to be a causal agent.	The increase in lung cancer mortality in men in the UK came several decades after an increase in cigarette smoking by men in the armed services in World War I.
5. Biological gradient	A dose–response relationship between the exposure and the outcome suggests causality.	The lung cancer death rate rose linearly with number of cigarettes smoked per day in the studies available to Bradford Hill in 1965. In some more recent studies this linear relationship has been less clear, as many smokers have smoked variable numbers of cigarettes at different time periods.
6. Plausibility	It is helpful if the causal association is biologically plausible, according to contemporary scientific knowledge.	What is biologically plausible depends on the biological knowledge of the day. In 1965, several eminent scientists, including J Berkson, J Neyman and RA Fisher, were still not convinced that the relationship between cigarette smoking and lung cancer was causal [47]. They did not find such a relationship plausible.
7. Coherence	The cause-and-effect interpretation of the data should not conflict with the generally known facts of the biology and natural history of the disease.	Factors carcinogenic to the skin of animals had been identified in cigarette smoke.
8. Experiment	Experimental evidence, when available, strongly suggests causality.	True experimental evidence on the relationship between smoking and lung cancer in humans is unlikely ever to become available. However, the fact that cessation of tobacco smoking had a clear effect on lung cancer-related mortality provided 'semi-experimental' evidence.
9. Analogy	If inhaling one substance can be shown to cause lung cancer, then it is easier to believe that inhaling another substance may do so as well.	The fact that inhaling cigarette smoke caused lung cancer made it easier to believe that inhaling asbestos fibres or the progeny of radon gas also caused lung cancer.

Note: Nine criteria proposed in 1965 by Bradford Hill to help assess whether associations between environmental exposures and diseases such as cancer are causal [8], together with examples as to how they could be used in considering the information available on smoking and lung cancer that was available in 1965.

whether an agent is a human carcinogen [9]. It assembles groups of expert scientists from a variety of disciplines to examine the evidence relating to various factors. The factors include chemicals, complex mixtures, occupational exposures, physical agents, biological agents and lifestyle factors. Since 1971, more than 900 agents have been evaluated, of which more than 400 have been identified either as carcinogenic or as probably or possibly carcinogenic. The IARC reviews provide an authoritative and up-to-date resource for environmental causes of cancer, and many national health agencies use them as scientific support for strategies to prevent exposure to factors that cause cancer. Some of these factors are discussed below. More detailed information is given in [10].

CAUSES OF CANCER

Tobacco

Tobacco smoke contains a multitude of harmful substances, including more than 70 different carcinogens. Lung cancer is the cancer most often caused by tobacco, but it also causes cancers of the oral cavity, naso-, oro- and hypopharynx, nasal cavity and paranasal sinuses, larynx, oesophagus, stomach, pancreas, liver, colorectum, kidney (body and pelvis), ureter, urinary bladder, uterine cervix, ovary (mucinous) and myeloid leukaemia [11]. Parental tobacco smoking is also an established cause of hepatoblastoma in children, while tobacco chewing causes cancers of the mouth, oesophagus, pancreas and bladder [12,13].

Tobacco is by far the most important preventable cause of cancer and accounts for around 20% of cancer deaths worldwide, as well as causing large numbers of deaths from many other diseases [14,15]. There are more than 1.3 billion smokers worldwide, and tobacco use is currently responsible for the death of approximately 6 million people annually [16]. Use is still increasing in many places, especially in low- and middle-income countries, and if current trends continue, then tobacco use may be responsible for an estimated 1 billion deaths during the twenty-first century.

Preventive measures can reduce tobacco-related mortality, and a striking example is provided by data from the UK (Figure 1.5). The causal relationship between tobacco and lung cancer was established in the 1960s, at which time mortality from tobacco-related cancer was increasing rapidly among men in the UK. Following the introduction of preventive strategies, particularly by encouraging current smokers to quit, smoking-related mortality started to decrease from about 1970. By 2010 tobacco-related cancer mortality in men was down to around one-third of its value in 1970. Among women, tobacco-related cancer mortality has been lower than in men but continued to increase until around 1990.

Hormonal and reproductive factors

Reproductive and menstrual factors are important in the aetiology of breast, endometrial and ovarian cancers [17]. Their role was suspected as early as the eighteenth century

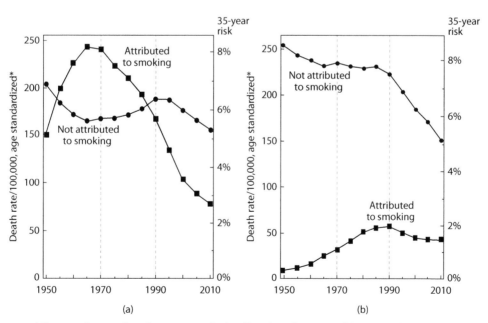

* The mortality rates have been age standardized by taking the means of the 7 annual death rates in the component 5-year age ranges.

Figure 1.5 Total cancer mortality rates at ages 35–69 in the United Kingdom and 35-year cumulative risks of death, subdivided into the contributions attributable and not attributable to smoking in males (a) and females (b). (Reproduced from Peto R, et al., in Stewart BW, Wild CP, eds., *World Cancer Report 2014*, Lyon, France: International Agency for Research on Cancer, World Health Organization; 2014, pp. 839–51.)

by the Italian physician Bernardino Ramazzini, who noted, 'Cancerous tumours are very often generated in women's breasts, and tumours of this sort are found in nuns more than in any other women' [18]. It is now accepted that multiparous women have a lower risk of developing breast cancer than their nulliparous counterparts. However, other hormonal factors are also associated with an increased risk of breast cancer, including early age of menarche, late age of first full-term pregnancy, late age of menopause and use of hormone replacement therapy [17]. Breast feeding, on the other hand, is a protective factor and is associated with a reduced risk of breast cancer. Although these associations are thought to be causal, the hormonal mechanisms underlying them are not yet fully understood. It is clear, however, that increased exposure to endogenous oestrogen levels increases the risk of breast cancer and can also drive disease progression. The principal sources of endogenous oestrogen in premenopausal women are the ovaries. Consequently, clinicians used surgical, radiotherapeutic and medical ovarian ablative and suppressive techniques as an adjuvant treatment in breast cancer for many years prior to the development of modern chemotherapy, radiotherapy and endocrine treatments.

The reproductive risk factors for endometrial and ovarian cancer are similar to those for breast cancer. Obesity (see below) is another factor that increases the risk of both endometrial and ovarian cancer [17], and its role is thought to be mediated through hormonal mechanisms. Obesity also influences breast cancer risk, and here the relationship is complicated, as it is associated with a small reduction in risk in premenopausal women but, following menopause, this relationship reverses and obesity increases breast cancer risk. The role of the combined oestrogen–progestogen contraceptive pill also differs between breast cancer and the other reproductive cancers, conferring a slightly higher risk of breast cancer but a substantially lower long-term risk of endometrial and ovarian cancers. The fact that the same exogenous hormone exerts such a variety of effects suggests independent and complex mechanisms underlying these types of cancers.

Cervical cancer differs from the other main female reproductive cancers in that the vast majority of cervical cancers are due to human papillomavirus infection (see below), but there is also some evidence for a role of hormonal factors in cervical cancer [19]. The role of hormonal factors in the aetiology of testicular, prostate and some other cancers in men is being revealed, although clear risk relationships remain to be identified [17,20].

Alcohol

The link between the consumption of alcohol and the risk of cancer has been established since the beginning of the twentieth century [21]. Alcohol causes cancer of the liver, oral cavity, pharynx, larynx, oesophagus, colorectum and female breast [22,23]. Alcohol consumption is increasing in many countries worldwide, and alcohol-related cancers were estimated to be the cause of 337,400 deaths globally in 2010 [10,24]. Most of these deaths were from liver cancer in men. The process underlying the carcinogenic properties of alcohol consumption is multifaceted and not fully understood, but is likely to involve different mechanisms for different cancers. For instance, prolonged alcohol consumption results in liver cirrhosis, and this is likely the primary reason for the increased risk of liver cancer from alcohol abuse [25].

The main metabolite of alcohol is acetaldehyde, which is highly toxic and mutagenic. A large body of evidence from laboratory, animal and genetic linkage studies supports the finding that acetaldehyde is the major factor responsible for alcohol-related cancers in the gastrointestinal tract [21]. Alcohol also acts as a solvent for tobacco carcinogens, which may partly explain the very large risks of cancers of the mouth, pharynx, oesophagus and larynx cancer when alcohol consumption is combined with smoking, compared to the risk from alcohol consumption in lifelong non-smokers [14,24]. Alcohol has a role in folate metabolism and in the production of reactive oxygen and nitrogen species which may also play a role in carcinogenic pathways [24]. Alcohol also increases endogenous oestrogen levels, and this may explain why the risk of breast cancer is increased in women with high alcohol consumption [26]. It is clear that heavy alcohol consumption has a complex role in cancer induction, and also that even light alcohol consumption contributes to the burden of cancer in many countries worldwide.

Obesity, diet and physical activity

In 2012, approximately 3.6% (481,000 persons) of all cancers diagnosed in adults aged at least 30 years were attributable to high body mass index [26]. Obesity increases the risk of cancers of the kidney, oesophagus, pancreas, colon and female reproductive system, as well as postmenopausal breast cancer (see above) [10]. The underlying mechanism between obesity and the increased risk of reproductive cancers is uncertain; it may result from the increased conversion of androgens into circulating oestrogens in adipose tissue. Other endocrine factors from increased adiposity may also have synergistic effects in increasing this risk, but these are poorly understood at present [27]. It is clear, however, that regular exercise and limiting caloric intake help to reduce the risk of many cancers, both by preventing obesity and by more complex processes.

The impact of specific dietary and related lifestyle factors has been notoriously difficult to determine. There are problems with recall bias in case-control studies, while cohort studies often suffer from short-term follow-up as well as imperfect quantification of dietary intake and exercise [28]. High consumption of red meat, especially processed meat, is associated with an increased risk of colorectal cancer, while high salt intake increases the risk of gastric cancer [29,30]. There is also evidence that regular physical activity reduces the risks of multiple cancers by contributing to weight control and may reduce the risks of colorectal and breast cancer by additional mechanisms. Higher intakes of fruit, vegetables and dietary fibre may be protective against various cancers, with the strongest evidence for a protective role of dietary fibre in relation to colorectal cancer.

Overall, trials of vitamin and mineral supplementation to prevent cancer have been largely null, with evidence of benefit in cancer risk reduction only in populations with dietary deficiencies, and evidence for adverse effect of some supplements in generally well-nourished populations [10,31]. Although recommendations about specific dietary factors to reduce cancer risk are unlikely to do much harm, this is not true of all dietary factors related to cancer [14]. For instance, calcium is required for bone growth and many other processes and it is beneficial in reducing the risk of colorectal cancer. However, high calcium intake, and to a lesser degree high consumption of dairy products, has been associated with prostate cancer [32]. This illustrates the intricate mechanisms underlying dietary correlations with disease, which can make clinically meaningful guidance difficult to formulate.

Occupation, radiation and pollution

Epidemiological studies of workers in specific occupations have played a major role in cancer epidemiology and have enabled the identification of a number of carcinogens. Examples include bladder cancer in workers in dye factories, lung cancer in metal workers, mesothelioma in craftsmen working with asbestos and scrotal cancer in chimney sweeps. To date, 32 occupational agents have been definitively identified as carcinogenic to humans [33]. Exposure to many other occupational factors is thought to increase the risk of cancer, but at present sufficient evidence to confirm or refute a causal relationship is lacking.

Exposure to ionizing radiation is an established cause of most types of cancer [34] and, as the dose–response relationship is approximately linear at low doses, exposures even at low levels are likely to incur some risk. Until recently, the largest source of exposure to ionizing radiation in the general population both in the UK and in many other countries was the natural radioactive gas radon, which emanates from the ground and can reach appreciable concentrations in houses and other small buildings. Exposure to ionizing radiation from diagnostic medical procedures – especially computerized-tomography scans – has increased rapidly in many countries and now exceeds exposure from radon in several countries.

Ultraviolet radiation, whether from direct sunlight in the absence of sun protection or from tanning machines, is established as the main cause of cutaneous malignant melanoma, basal cell carcinoma and squamous cell carcinoma [35,36]. Some studies have suggested that exposure to radiofrequency electromagnetic radiation from mobile phones may cause glioma or acoustic neuromas, and these are at present classified by IARC as possibly carcinogenic.

Many known, probable and possible carcinogens pollute the environment. Air pollution from vehicle emissions, power generation, household combustion of solid fuels and a range of industries contain known carcinogens including diesel emissions, polycyclic aromatic hydrocarbons, benzene and 1,3-butadiene, together with inorganic carcinogens such as asbestos, arsenic and chromium compounds. Exposure to particulate matter in outdoor air pollution causes lung cancer. In drinking water, inorganic arsenic is a recognized carcinogen [37].

Exposure to occupational carcinogens, to ionizing and ultraviolet radiation and to environmental pollutants is regulated in many countries [38]. Unfortunately, however, exposures in many low- and middle-income countries are often poorly controlled, and substantial exposure levels continue to occur in many parts of the world.

Infections

Infection with certain viruses, bacteria or parasites can cause cancer. A list of the infectious agents classified as carcinogenic by the IARC is given in Table 1.2 [39,40]. Most of these agents increase the risk for an infected individual by more than a factor of 10. It has been estimated that, in 2008, a few chronic infections were responsible for more than 2 million new cancer cases worldwide, i.e. 16% of all new cancer cases [40]. This percentage varies substantially by continent and country. The fraction of cancer attributable to infections is largest in sub-Saharan Africa (33%) and smallest in Australia, New Zealand and North America (≤4%), while for Europe it was estimated to be 7%. Table 1.2 includes only agents with sufficient data for a definitive causative link to be established. There are many more infectious agents which may be carcinogenic, but there are limited or only correlational data at present [41].

GENETIC EPIDEMIOLOGY

In recent years there have been rapid advances in genetic techniques and molecular analysis allowing the identification of genetic causes of cancer. An example is the discovery that mutations in *BRCA1* and *BRCA2* genes are associated with an increased lifetime risk of breast and ovarian cancers [42]. This field is discussed further in Chapter 2. By assessing the genetic and molecular profiles in large-scale populations and combining them with exposure data, the field of genetic cancer epidemiology

Table 1.2 Major cancer sites where infections are an established cause and estimated number of attributable cases in 2008

Cancer site	Pathogen (type of pathogen)	Number[b]
Stomach	*Helicobacter pylori* (Gram-negative bacterium)	650,000
Liver	Hepatitis B virus (DNA virus), hepatitis C virus (HCV) (RNA virus), Southeast Asian liver fluke: *Opisthorchis viverrini* (Trematode), Chinese liver fluke: *Clonorchis sinensis* (Trematode)	580,000
Cervix uteri	Human papillomavirus (HPV) (DNA virus) with or without HIV[a]	530,000
Anogenital (penis, vulva, vagina, anus)	HPV with or without HIV[a]	56,000
Nasopharynx	Epstein–Barr virus (EBV) (human herpes virus 4)	72,000
Oropharynx	HPV with or without tobacco or alcohol consumption	22,000
Kaposi's sarcoma	Human herpes virus type 8 with or without HIV[a]	43,000
Non-Hodgkin lymphoma	*Helicobacter pylori*, EBV with or without HIV,[a] HCV, human T-cell lymphotropic virus type 1	49,000
Hodgkin lymphoma	EBV with or without HIV[a]	33,000
Bladder	*Schistosoma haematobium* (Trematode)	6000
Total number of cancers attributable worldwide to infectious agents in 2008		**2,000,000 (i.e. 16% of all new cancer cases worldwide)**

Source: Adapted from de Martel C, et al., *Lancet Oncol* 2012;13(6):607–15.
[a] Infection with human immunodeficiency virus (HIV) type 1 (RNA retrovirus) greatly increases the risk.
[b] Number of new cases attributable each year to infection (% of total cancers caused by infective agents).

is also beginning to increase knowledge of why the same exposure causes some people to develop cancer and not others.

MONITORING AND PREVENTING CANCER IN THE UK

In most populations, the rates of many cancers have varied over time in response to changes to exposures to the relevant carcinogens and also to preventive measures. In the UK, both incidence and mortality rates for liver cancer and malignant melanoma have been increasing in recent years in both males and females, as a result of increases in alcohol consumption and exposure to sunlight, respectively (Figure 1.6). In contrast, stomach cancer incidence and mortality rates have been decreasing in both males and females, due to a reduction in the prevalence of *Helicobacter pylori* infection and from changes in diet. For lung cancer, incidence and mortality rates are currently decreasing in men, following the implementation of measures to reduce smoking (see above), although preventive measures have not yet resulted in a clear reduction in lung cancer rates for women in the UK. For some cancers incidence rates have increased recently, while mortality rates have decreased over the same time period. For myeloma and non-Hodgkin lymphoma, this is likely to be due principally to more effective treatment, while for others, such as cancers of the breast, bowel and cervix, nationwide screening programmes are likely to have played a role by increasing the number of cases

diagnosed. This has the effect of making incidence rates appear to have increased. At the same time screening leads to cases being diagnosed at an earlier stage, resulting in longer survival and lower mortality rates.

In order to estimate the extent to which cancer could, in principle, be prevented, Parkin et al. have estimated the fraction of cancers occurring in the UK in 2010 that can be attributed to suboptimal past exposures of 14 major lifestyle and environmental risk factors: tobacco, alcohol, four elements of diet (consumption of meat, fruit and vegetables, fibre and salt), overweight, lack of physical exercise, occupation, infections, ionizing and solar radiation, use of exogenous hormones and breast feeding (Table 1.3) [43]. Exposure to each of these factors is potentially modifiable. Tobacco smoking was by far the most important factor, responsible for 60,000 cases (19.4% of all new cancer cases) in 2010. The relative importance of other exposures differed by sex. In men, deficient intake of fruits and vegetables (6.1%), occupational exposures (4.9%) and alcohol consumption (4.6%) were next in importance, while in women, overweight and obesity were responsible for 6.9% of cancers, through their effect on breast cancer, followed by infectious agents (3.7%). Overall, exposure to less than optimum levels of the 14 factors considered was responsible for 42.7% of cancers in the UK – a total of about 134,000 cases in 2010. Calculations such as these illustrate the extent to which cancer could, in principle, be prevented. They are also helpful in prioritizing cancer control strategies, including the formulation of realistically achievable targets.

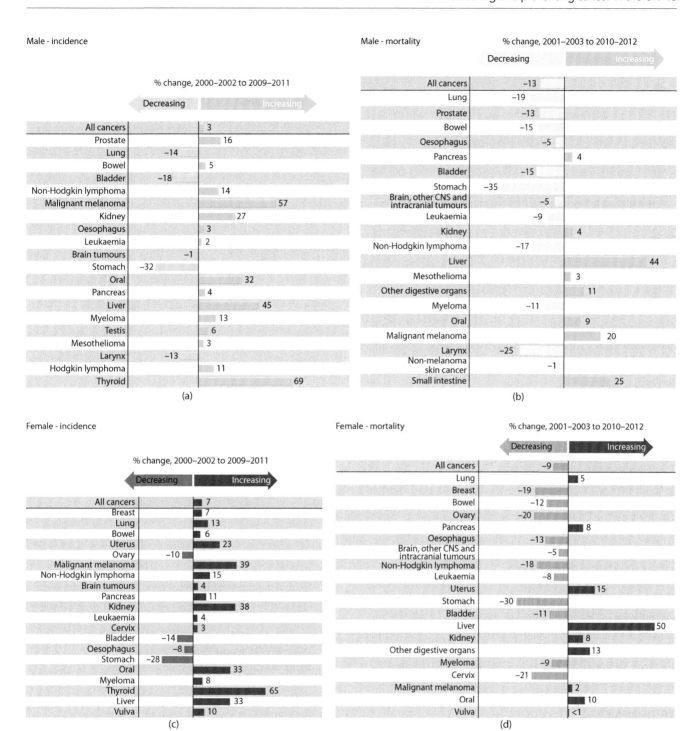

Figure 1.6 Recent changes in incidence and mortality rates of the 20 most common cancers in the UK for males (a, b) and females (c, d). In each panel cancers are listed in descending order of incidence (or mortality) rate. Percentages are changes in the age-standardized rate, using the European standard population. (Reproduced from Cancer Research UK, Cancer stats report – Cancer incidence for common cancers 2014, London: Cancer Research UK, available from http://www.cancerresearchuk.org/cancer-info/cancerstats/incidence/commoncancers/uk-cancer-incidence-statistics-for-common-cancers, accessed March 2016.)

Table 1.3 Percentages and numbers of cases of cancer in the United Kingdom in 2010 attributable to suboptimal past exposure to preventable factors

| Factor | Optimal exposure | Percentage of all new cancer cases | | | Total number of cases (males and females combined) |
		Males	Females	Persons	
Tobacco	Nil	23.0	15.6	19.4	60,837
Diet					
Fruit and vegetables	≥5 servings per day	6.1	3.4	4.7	14,902
Red and preserved meat	Nil	3.5	1.9	2.7	8411
Fibre	≥23 g per day	1.4	1.7	1.5	4856
Salt	≤6 g per day	0.9	0.2	0.5	1694
Overweight and obesity	Body mass index ≤25 kg m^{-2}	4.1	6.9	5.5	17,294
Alcohol	Nil	4.6	3.3	4.0	12,458
Occupational exposures	Nil	4.9	2.4	3.7	11,494
Ultraviolet solar radiation	As in 1903 cohort	3.5	3.6	3.5	11,097
Infections	Nil	2.5	3.7	3.1	9745
Ionizing radiation	Nil	1.7	2.0	1.8	5807
Physical exercise	≥30 min 5 times per week	0.4	1.7	1.0	3275
Breast feeding	Minimum of 6 months	—	1.7	0.9	2699
Postmenopausal hormones	Nil	—	1.1	0.5	1675
Total due to suboptimal past exposures		**45.3**	**40.1**	**42.7**	**134,000**

Source: Data from Parkin DM, et al., *Br J Cancer* 2011;105(Suppl 2):S77–81.

ACKNOWLEDGEMENTS

Freddie Bray and Mathieu Laversanne, Section of Cancer Surveillance at the International Agency for Research on Cancer (IARC), for their help in providing Figures 1.1 and 1.4. GSM is funded by the National Institute for Health Research Biomedical Research Centre. SCD is funded by Cancer Research UK.

REFERENCES

1. Ferlay J, Soerjomataram I, Ervik M, Dikshit R, Eser S, Mathers C, Rebelo M, Parkin DM, Forman D, Bray F. GLOBOCAN 2012 v1.0, Cancer incidence and mortality worldwide: IARC Cancer Base no. 11. Lyon, France: International Agency for Research on Cancer; 2013. Available from http://globocan.iarc.fr (accessed 16 October 2014).

2. Cancer Research UK. Cancer stats report – Cancer incidence for common cancers 2014. London: Cancer Research UK. Available from http://www.cancer-researchuk.org/cancer-info/cancerstats/incidence/commoncancers/uk-cancer-incidence-statistics-for-common-cancers (accessed 5 January 2014).

3. Bray F, Jemal A, Grey N, Ferlay J, Forman D. Global cancer transitions according to the Human Development Index (2008–2030): a population-based study. *Lancet Oncol* 2012;13(8):790–801.

4. Le GM, Gomez SL, Clarke CA, Glaser SL, West DW. Cancer incidence patterns among Vietnamese in the United States and Ha Noi, Vietnam. *Int J Cancer* 2002;102(4):412–7.

5. Ziegler RG, Hoover RN, Pike MC, Hildesheim A, Nomura AM, West DW, et al. Migration patterns and breast cancer risk in Asian-American women. *J Natl Cancer Inst* 1993;85(22):1819–27.

6. Woodward M. *Epidemiology: Study Design and Data Analysis*, 3rd ed. Boca Raton, FL: Taylor & Francis; 2014.

7. Webb P, Bain C. *Essential Epidemiology*. Cambridge: Cambridge University Press; 2010.

8. Hill AB. The environment and disease: association or causation? *Proc R Soc Med* 1965;58:295–300.

9. International Agency for Research on Cancer. *International Agency for Research on Cancer (IARC) Monographs*. Lyon, France: International Agency for Research on Cancer; 2014.

10. Stewart BW, Wild CP, eds. *World Cancer Report 2014*. Lyon, France: International Agency for Research on Cancer, World Health Organization; 2014.

11. International Agency for Research on Cancer. Tobacco smoking. In *Personal Habits and Indoor Combustions*. IARC Monographs on the Evaluation of Carcinogenic Risks to Humans. Lyon, France: International Agency for Research on Cancer; 2012;100E:43–211.

12. International Agency for Research on Cancer. *Personal Habits and Indoor Combustions*. IARC Monographs on the Evaluation of Carcinogenic Risks to Humans. Lyon, France: International Agency for Research on Cancer; 2012;100E.

13. Secretan B, Straif K, Baan R, Grosse Y, El Ghissassi F, Bouvard V, et al. A review of human carcinogens – part E: tobacco, areca nut, alcohol, coal smoke, and salted fish. *Lancet Oncol* 2009;10(11):1033–4.

14. Warrell DAC, Cox TM, Firth JD. *Oxford Textbook of Medicine*, 5th ed. Oxford: Oxford University Press; 2010.

15. Detels R, Beaglehole R, Lansang MA, Gulliford M. *Oxford Textbook of Public Health*. Oxford: Oxford University Press; 2009.

16. Wipfli H, Samet JM. Global economic and health benefits of tobacco control: part 2. *Clin Pharmacol Ther* 2009;86(3):272–80.

17. Brinton LA. Reproductive and hormonal factors. In Stewart BW, Wild CP, eds., *World Cancer Report 2014*. Lyon, France: International Agency for Research on Cancer, World Health Organization; 2014, pp. 115–24.

18. Franco G. Bernardino Ramazzini and women workers' health in the second half of the XVIIth century. *J Public Health (Oxf)* 2012;34(2):305–8.

19. International Collaboration of Epidemiological Studies of Cervical C, Appleby P, Beral V, Berrington de Gonzalez A, Colin D, Franceschi S, et al. Carcinoma of the cervix and tobacco smoking: collaborative reanalysis of individual data on 13,541 women with carcinoma of the cervix and 23,017 women without carcinoma of the cervix from 23 epidemiological studies. *Int J Cancer* 2006;118(6):1481–95.

20. Humphrey PA. Cancers of the male reproductive organs. In Stewart BW, Wild CP, eds., *World Cancer Report 2014*. Lyon, France: International Agency for Research on Cancer, World Health Organization; 2014, pp. 453–65.

21. Rehm J, Shield K. Alcohol consumption. In Stewart BW, Wild CP, eds., *World Cancer Report 2014*. Lyon, France: International Agency for Research on Cancer, World Health Organization; 2014, pp. 96–105.

22. International Agency for Research on Cancer. *Alcohol Consumption and Ethyl Carbamate*. IARC Monographs on the Evaluation of Carcinogenic Risks to Humans. Lyon, France: International Agency for Research on Cancer; 2010, p. 96.

23. Baan R, Straif K, Grosse Y, Secretan B, El Ghissassi F, Bouvard V, Altieri A, Cogliano V. Carcinogenicity of alcoholic beverages. *Lancet Oncol* 2007;8(4):292–3.

24. Boffetta P, Hashibe M. Alcohol and cancer. *Lancet Oncol* 2006;7(2):149–56.

25. Poschl G, Seitz HK. Alcohol and cancer. *Alcohol Alcohol* 2004;39(3):155–65.

26. Arnold M, Pandeya N, Byrnes G, Renehan AG, Stevens GA, Ezzati M, et al. Global burden of cancer attributable to high body-mass index in 2012: a population-based study. *Lancet Oncol* 2014;16(1):36–46.

27. Byers T, Sedjo RL. Does intentional weight loss reduce cancer risk? *Diabetes Obes Metab* 2011;13(12):1063–72.

28. Willett W, Key T, Romieu I. Diet, obesity, and physical activity. In Stewart BW, Wild CP, eds., *World Cancer Report 2014*. Lyon, France: International Agency for Research on Cancer, World Health Organization; 2014, pp. 124–34.

29. Carneiro F. Stomach cancer. In Stewart BW, Wild CP, eds., *World Cancer Report 2014*. Lyon, France: International Agency for Research on Cancer, World Health Organization; 2014, pp. 383–92.

30. Parkin DM. Cancers attributable to dietary factors in the UK in 2010. IV. Salt. *Br J Cancer* 2011;105(Suppl 2):S31–3.

31. Gaziano JM, Sesso HD, Christen WG, Bubes V, Smith JP, MacFadyen J, et al. Multivitamins in the prevention of cancer in men: the Physicians' Health Study II randomized controlled trial. *JAMA* 2012;308(18):1871–80.

32. Gao X, LaValley MP, Tucker KL. Prospective studies of dairy product and calcium intakes and prostate cancer risk: a meta-analysis. *J Natl Cancer Inst* 2005;97(23):1768–77.

33. Siemiatycki J. Occupation. In Stewart BW, Wild CP, eds., *World Cancer Report 2014*. Lyon, France: International Agency for Research on Cancer, World Health Organization; 2014, pp. 134–43.

34. United Nations Scientific Committee on the Effects of Atomic Radiation. Effects of ionizing radiation. UNSCEAR 2006 Report to the General Assembly, with scientific annexes. New York, NY: United Nations; 2009.

35. Kesminiene A, Schüz J. Radiation: ionizing, ultraviolet, and electromagnetic. In Stewart BW, Wild CP, eds., *World Cancer Report 2014*. Lyon, France: International Agency for Research on Cancer, World Health Organization; 2014, pp. 143–51.

36. International Agency for Research on Cancer. Solar and ultraviolet radiation. In *Radiation: A Review of Human Carcinogens*. IARC Monographs on the Evaluation of Carcinogenic Risks to Humans. Lyon, France: International Agency for Research on Cancer; 2012;100D:35–102.

37. Cohen AJ. Pollution of air, water, and soil. In Stewart BW, Wild CP, eds., *World Cancer Report 2014*. Lyon, France: International Agency for Research on Cancer, World Health Organization; 2014, pp. 151–61.

38. World Health Organization. *Prevention*. Geneva: World Health Organization; 2007.

39. International Agency for Research on Cancer. *Biological Agents: A Review of Human Carcinogens*. IARC Monographs on the Evaluation of Carcinogenic Risks to Humans. Lyon, France: International Agency for Research on Cancer; 2012;100B:36–44.

40. de Martel C, Ferlay J, Franceschi S, Vignat J, Bray F, Forman D, et al. Global burden of cancers attributable to infections in 2008: a review and synthetic analysis. *Lancet Oncol* 2012;13(6):607–15.

41. Franceschi S, Herrero R. Infections. In Stewart BW, Wild CP, eds., *World Cancer Report 2014*. Lyon, France: International Agency for Research on Cancer, World Health Organization; 2014, pp. 105–15.

42. Nkondjock A, Ghadirian P. Epidemiology of breast cancer among BRCA mutation carriers: an overview. *Cancer Lett* 2004;205(1):1–8.

43. Parkin DM, Boyd L, Walker LC. 16. The fraction of cancer attributable to lifestyle and environmental factors in the UK in 2010. *Br J Cancer* 2011;105(Suppl 2):S77–81.

44. Ferlay J, Soerjomataram I, Dikshit R, Eser S, Mathers C, Rebelo M, Parkin DM, Forman D, Bray F. Cancer incidence and mortality worldwide: sources, methods and major patterns in GLOBOCAN 2012. *Int J Cancer* 2015;136(5):E359–86.

45. Cancer Research UK. Cancer incidence by age. London: Cancer Research UK; 2014. Available from http://www.cancerresearchuk.org/cancer-info/cancerstats/incidence/age/ (accessed 11 March 2015).

46. Peto R, Lopez AD, Pan H, Thun MJ. The full hazards of smoking and the benefits of stopping: cancer mortality and overall mortality. In Stewart BW, Wild CP, eds., *World Cancer Report 2014*. Lyon, France: International Agency for Research on Cancer, World Health Organization; 2014, pp. 839–51.

47. Cornfield J, Haenszel W, Hammond EC, Lilienfeld AM, Shimkin MB, Wynder EL. Smoking and lung cancer: recent evidence and a discussion of some questions. 1959. *Int J Epidemiol* 2009;38(5):1175–91.

2

Genetics and hereditary cancer syndromes, genetic polymorphisms and cancer

D GARETH EVANS

INTRODUCTION

In recent years there has been a burgeoning increase in the evidence for familial predisposition to cancer. This has gathered pace since the classic model of hereditary retinoblastoma was outlined in 1971 [1]. The supposition that some cancers were inherited has long been held by more than just a fringe community. The earliest report of cancer running in families dates back almost 200 years to a large cluster of breast cancer in the wife and family of a French physician named Broca, and clustering of gastric cancer in Napoleon's family [2]. The pioneering work of clinicians and researchers, including Henry Lynch and Mary-Claire King in the US in the 1960s to 1980s, provided anecdotal and some epidemiological evidence of the hereditary nature of a proportion of cancers (breast and colonic). However, the hereditary element was not proven until the advent of molecular biology, when mutations were identified in cancer-predisposing genes. It is, therefore, only in the last 25 years that molecular science has not only proven the strong hereditary nature of a small proportion of certain common cancers, but also demonstrated that polygenic inheritance of common genetic alterations (polymorphisms) accounts for a substantial further proportion.

MOLECULAR BASIS OF CANCER

That cancer is 'genetic' at the cellular level has been beyond dispute for some time. All tumours result from a combination of inactivating and promoting mutations/disruptions of two types of gene: tumour suppressor genes, which require inactivation to enable growth, and oncogenes, which require activation to promote cell division and proliferation. The great majority of these molecular events are acquired either through simple replication error (copying of DNA during cell division) or due to external DNA-damaging agents (radiation, chemicals and viruses) or by epigenetic factors such as ageing, which increase epigenetic gene silencing through methylation. Nevertheless, recent evidence has confirmed that predisposition to cancer involves a polygenic pattern with multiple common gene variations associated with small elevations in risk.

HEREDITARY CANCER

Occasionally, mutations in tumour suppressor genes can be inherited rather than acquired. Identifying the genes which cause hereditary tumour predisposition has given a major insight into many cancers. The role of cancer-predisposing genes in the aetiology of sporadic cancer has been the subject of a great deal of research, and much can still be learned from some of the more obscure cancer-prone syndromes. Broadly, tumour predisposition can be divided into rare genetic tumour-predisposing syndromes, where malignancy is a high-risk side effect, and a larger group which cannot be easily identified clinically from features in an individual, where there may be a strong family history of one or more common malignancies.

RETINOBLASTOMA

From epidemiological and genetic segregation work on retinoblastoma, a rare childhood malignancy of the eye, it became the model for much of our current knowledge of tumour suppressor genes. This often newborn or infancy eye malignancy was recognized as having a familial component as early as the nineteenth century. Approximately 50% of cases are due to inheritance of a mutation/deletion in one copy of the retinoblastoma gene (*RB*) (Table 2.1), and >90% of individuals who carry a mutation will develop retinoblastoma, usually bilaterally and often multifocally in the same retina. In 1971, Knudson proposed that the condition was caused by mutational events in both copies of the *RB* gene [1,3]. Those children that inherited a mutated copy required only one further mutational event in the other copy of *RB* and were far more likely to develop the malignancy, causing it to occur at a younger age and usually bilaterally. Sporadic cases required two mutations ('hits') in a retinal cell, as opposed to one in the familial situation (Figure 2.1), and thus bilateral tumours are incredibly unlikely to occur

and the unilateral tumours present later. This hypothesis, which has since been validated in a number of other conditions including type 2 neurofibromatosis [4] and *BRCA1* [5]-related breast and ovarian cancer, now bears the conceiver's name: the Knudson 'two-hit' hypothesis.

ROUTE TO DISCOVERING CANCER GENES

The discovery that bilateral retinoblastoma cases had constitutional deletions of chromosome 13 visible at the microscopic level concentrated research on that region [3]. One of the genes removed by the deletion in these cases, *esterase D*, then acted as a polymorphic genetic linkage marker for further studies. The *RB* gene, the first hereditary cancer gene, was finally localized and cloned using this gene linkage analysis in 1986 [6].

The same research approaches using chromosome and genetic linkage studies of individuals, their tumours and families have led to the discovery of nearly all the high-risk genes that cause cancer predisposition (Table 2.1). Indeed the majority of these genes were identified along with their

Table 2.1 Examples of autosomal dominant, recessive and X-linked syndromes predisposing to tumours and cancer, with their chromosomal location and protein product

Name of condition	Chromosomal location	Protein product/gene
Autosomal dominant		
Familial polyposis (FAP)	5q	APC
NF1	17q	Neurofibromin
NF2	22q	Merlin/Schwannomin
von Hippel–Lindau	3p	pVHL
MEN1	11q	Menin
MEN2	10q	RET
Tuberous sclerosis	9q	PTCH
	(TSC1) 11q	Hamartin
	(TSC2) 16q	Tuberin
Juvenile polyposis	18q and others	pBMPR1a, SMAD4
Peutz–Jeghers	19p and others	pSTK11/LKB1
Cowden	10q	PTEN
Tylosis	17q	Not found
Autosomal recessive		
Fanconi anaemia	14 loci	Many, including BRCA2
Bloom syndrome	15q	pBLM
Ataxia telangiectasia	11q	pATM
Xeroderma pigmentosum	7 types	2 types
Chediak–Higashi	1q	pLYST
Albinism	11q	OCA1, OCA2
Familial polyposis 2	1p	MUTYH1
Turcot syndrome	Several; see Lynch	PMS2, MLH1, MSH2, MSH6
X-Linked		
Bruton	Xq	BLk
Wiskott–Aldrich	Xp	CD43

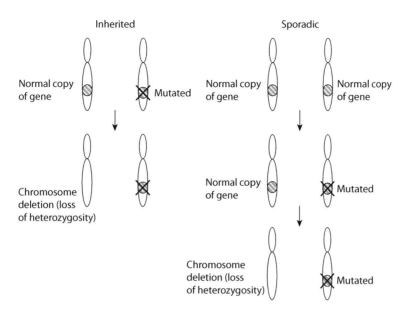

Figure 2.1 Knudson's two-hit hypothesis for retinoblastoma. The first hit, including the germline one, is usually a point mutation, with the second lost by large deletions often of the chromosome arm.

gene products (proteins) in a heady 6-year period between 1989 and 1995. The last 20 years has seen steady progress toward the understanding of how these genes function through their protein products and the development of the first line of gene-based therapies, such as trastuzumab, imatinib and a new group of synthetic lethal drugs, poly (ADP-ribose) polymerase (PARP) inhibitors to treat *BRCA1/2*-deficient cancers. However, much of the remaining inherited components have been unpicked in the last 4 years by genome-wide association studies (GWAS) to find the lower-risk genetic components [7,8].

CANCER-PREDISPOSING SYNDROMES

Cancer/tumour-predisposing syndromes are usually readily identifiable from a clinical phenotype (group of associated features) or by laboratory tests. The syndromes can be autosomal dominant, autosomal recessive or X-linked (Tables 2.1 and 2.2). It is the autosomal dominant disorders that have been of most interest as they are likely to represent the inheritance of a mutated copy of a tumour suppressor gene, which also predisposes the individual to common cancers. Although these conditions are generally uncommon, the tumour suppressor genes involved often play a fundamental role in the causation and initiation of sporadic cancers, which affect 35–40% of humans in the developed world in their lifetime. The identification of the genes causing genetic syndromes is still likely to lead to more bespoke treatments using gene-based therapies, as well as earlier identification, monitoring and, most ideally of all, prevention of common cancers.

FAMILIAL ADENOMATOUS POLYPOSIS

Familial adenomatous polyposis (FAP) is the paradigm condition by which translational researchers have

hoped to transpose knowledge of rare genetic disorders to a commonly occurring cancer. FAP is an autosomal dominant condition characterized by the development of hundreds to thousands of benign adenomatous polyps in the colorectum usually by 30 years of age [10]. If left without intervention this leads to the almost inevitable development of a colorectal cancer by 60 years of age. The condition may also be associated with osteomas, desmoid tumours and epidermal cysts, as well as an increased risk of other malignancies such as duodenal cancer, hepatoblastoma, glioma, medulloblastoma and thyroid cancer. The *APC* gene which causes autosomal dominant FAP was localized to chromosome 5q21–q22 by genetic linkage and cloned in 1991. FAP was one of the first conditions in which a clear genotype–phenotype correlation (connection between the genetic change in *APC* and the clinical picture) emerged. Patients with mutations in the 5′ exons 2–5 (early part of the gene reading frame) had a very mild clinical picture with late onset of polyps, whereas those with mutations from exon 9 to codon 1450 of exon 15 had a classical disease course with nearly all patients manifesting the typical congenital retinal pigmentation [11]. However, those with mutations beyond codon 1450 showed typical Gardner syndrome features (osteomas, cysts and desmoid disease) without congenital hypertrophy of the retinal pigment epithelium, but also had milder polyp disease [11]. The APC gene is fundamentally important in the initiation of the majority of 'sporadic' colorectal cancer, although the loss of both functioning copies of the gene is then acquired, rather than one inherited and one acquired, as seen in FAP. Use of genetic registers and genetic testing to target screening along with appropriately timed removal of the colon has led to an improvement in life expectancy in FAP of 15–30 years [12].

Table 2.2 Chromosomal location and implications of various dominant cancer syndromes

Disease	Location	Tumours/cancers	Probable earliest tumour	Lifetime risk without intervention	Start of screening	Life expectancy years [24]
FAP	5q	Adenomas, bowel cancer, thyroid cancer	First year? 4 years, 7 years	100%, 99%	10–16	63–70
NF1	17q	Neurofibroma, glioma, sarcoma, malignant peripheral nerve sheath tumour	First year, first year	100%, 12%	Birth	54–72
NF2	22q	Schwannomas, meningiomas, ependymoma	First year, first year, first year	100%, 60%, 10%	Birth	62–69
VHL	3p	Haemangioblastoma, renal carcinoma, phaeochromocytoma	1–2 years, 20 years, 10 years	90%, 70%	5 years, 15 years	49–53
MEN 1	11q	Parathyroid, insulinoma, gastrinoma	5 years	95%	5 years	Close to normal
MEN 2a	10q	Medullary thyroid cancer, parathyroid, phaeochromocytoma	3 years	80%	3–4 years	Reduced
MEN 2b	10q	As in MEN 2a, except parathyroid	1 year	100%	Birth	Reduced
Gorlin	9q	Basal cell carcinoma, medulloblastoma	5 years, 1 year	90%, 5%	Birth	73.4
Cowden	10q	Breast, thyroid	30 years, teenage	30%	35 years	Reduced in women
LFS	17p	Sarcoma (bone/soft tissue), adrenal, breast cancer, gliomas	First year	95%	First year	Severely reduced
BRCA1	17q	Breast/ovary/colon/prostate carcinoma	>16 years	80–90%	30 years	62 in women
BRCA2	13q	Breast/ovary/prostate carcinoma, male breast	>16 years	80–90%, 10%	30 years	68 in women
Lynch syndrome	2p, 3p, 2q, 7q	Colorectum, ovary, endometrium, ureter, gastric, pancreas	>16 years	80%	25 years	Reduced

OTHER AUTOSOMAL DOMINANT TUMOUR SYNDROMES

A number of other important dominantly inherited conditions are now well described both clinically and genetically. von Hippel–Lindau (VHL) predisposes to the development of retinal angiomas, haemangioblastomas of the cerebellum, renal cell carcinoma, phaeochromocytoma and renal, pancreatic and epididymal cysts [13,14]. Mutations in the VHL gene also play an important part in sporadic clear cell carcinoma of the kidney [15]. The neurofibromatoses consist of at least three separate disorders, NF1, NF2 and schwannomatosis, which give rise to an increased risk of mainly benign tumours of the nervous system and particularly the nerve sheath (schwanomas, neurofibromas). The main risk of malignancy occurs in NF1 where the predominant tumour, the neurofibroma, is associated with a 10–13% lifetime risk to each NF1-affected individual of developing malignant peripheral nerve sheath tumours

which have very poor survival [16]. NF2, the second type of neurofibromatosis, is largely associated with schwannomas and meningiomas of the neuro-axis, with most individuals being deafened by bilateral eighth nerve involvement [17].

Gorlin syndrome is characterized by the development of multiple jaw keratocysts and basal cell carcinomas as well as a 2–5% risk of childhood medulloblastoma [18]. Recently a second gene (*SUFU*) in addition to *PTCH* has been identified as a cause of Gorlin syndrome with a higher risk of medulloblastoma of around 25% [19]. Indeed *SUFU* is frequently involved in desmoplastic medulloblastoma. The multiple endocrine neoplasias are further conditions which predispose to benign tumours and at least one malignancy. In MEN1 the organs affected are the parathyroid glands, pituitary and pancreas and can lead to early death [20]. In MEN2 there is an association between medullary thyroid carcinoma and phaeochromocytoma [21]. MEN2 is unusual for the germline involvement of activating mutations in an oncogene (*RET*) which involves just one amino acid for the more severe infancy-onset MEN2b. Another example of inherited dominant involvement of an oncogene is with MET mutations that cause papillary renal carcinoma in Birt–Hogg–Dubé syndrome [22]. Additional important dominant conditions include Peutz–Jeghers [23] and juvenile polyposis, [24] both of which have a substantial risk of gastrointestinal tract malignancy. All of these cancer-predisposing syndromes have benefited from the identification of the causative gene and the targeted use of screening which in most of the conditions improves life expectancy [25]. This may mean intervention in childhood, particularly in MEN2 to remove the thyroid gland preventatively.

The rarer autosomal recessive and X-linked disorders are largely associated with immunodeficiency-related cancer risk or with loss of a DNA repair mechanism. The most notable from a surgical oncology perspective is the recessive form of Lynch syndrome caused by homozygous mutations in *PMS2*, *MSH2*, *MLH1* or *MSH6*, which gives an extremely high risk of childhood malignancy in addition to the typical Lynch syndrome cancers of the colorectum and endometrium. *PMS2*, which is least penetrant of the Lynch syndrome genes in its dominant form, is frequently involved at the recessive level and the resultant condition with multiple café au lait patches may be what was originally described as Turcot syndrome [26]. The second that also gives a high risk of colorectal cancer is MUTYH recessive polyposis. This should be investigated in families with multiple adenomatous polyps that do not follow a clear autosomal dominant inheritance and where APC testing is negative [27].

COMMON CANCER NON-'SYNDROMIC' CANCER PREDISPOSITION

There has been an enormous improvement in our understanding of the mechanisms of carcinogenesis in the last 25 years. Most cancers require a number of genetic mutations in a progenitor cell before an invasive tumour results. Virtually none will be caused solely by the loss of two copies of a single tumour suppressor gene as in retinoblastoma, and the number of driver mutations probably varies between 4 and 10 (many more are present on genome sequencing but most are bystanders). A combination of loss of function of tumour suppressor genes and activation of oncogenes is normally involved. The combination and order in which these mutations occur may alter the histological as well as invasive nature of the cancer, as seen with *BRCA1* mutations for breast and ovarian cancer [28,29]. There is clear epidemiological [30] and now genetic evidence that a minority of people who develop common cancers have inherited a dominantly inherited mutated gene, which puts them at high risk of malignancy, but this is usually not recognized as a syndrome apart from in the family history. Adenocarcinomas are more likely than carcinomas of squamous epithelium to have a strong hereditary component with 4–16% of all breast, ovarian and colon

cancer resulting from an inherited high-risk gene defect, although twin studies show that this figure rises to around 30% for any inherited component [31]. In addition to family history, cancers are more likely to be hereditary if they are early onset, bilateral, multifocal or are associated with other related primaries (such as breast with ovarian cancer or colorectal and endometrial). The germline inherited mutations in the *TP53* gene [32] (possibly the most important gene in cancer – often called the caretaker of the genome) in rare families with an often horrendous pattern of malignancy were the first major discovery in this area. Li–Fraumeni syndrome (LFS) links predisposition to sarcomas of the soft tissue, muscle and bone often in childhood with very early onset breast cancer, glioma, adrenal tumours and other tumours in children and adults. The risk of cancer approaches 100% for female mutation carriers by 50 years of age. While the condition is rare, affecting around 1 in 40,000 people, it is as common as *BRCA1* and *BRCA2* combined in very early onset apparently isolated breast cancer [33]. The breast cancers are predominantly HER2 overexpressed [34] and with a relatively high *de novo* mutation rate, women with HER2 positive invasive or high-grade comedo ductal carcinoma in situ under 30 years of age should be considered for *TP53* testing regardless of family history [33,35].

BREAST/OVARIAN CANCER

Breast cancer can occur as part of high-penetrance predisposition such as LFS, and also *BRCA1/2*, but may also be contributed to by mutations in other high-risk genes such as *PTEN*, *STK11* and *CDH1* and moderate risk genes such as *ATM*, *CHEK2*, *PALB2* and possibly *BRIP1*, the latter four giving lifetime risks of 20–40% (Table 2.3). Unsurprisingly, the greatest interest has focused on *BRCA1* and *BRCA2*, mutations which are carried by approximately 0.1% of the population each (this rises to 2.5% combined for three founder mutations in the Ashkenazi Jewish). This is because of the high lifetime risk of 40–85% of breast cancer with an associated 20–60% risk of ovarian cancer. Many women testing positive for mutations are now opting for risk-reducing surgery, with great publicity surrounding the actress Angelina Jolie's decision in 2013 [36]. Risk-reducing surgery can reduce risks of both cancers by more than 90%, with oophorectomy conferring protection against ovarian cancer and breast cancer [37–39]. Recently survival advantages have been published for those undergoing contralateral mastectomy after breast cancer [40] as well as for primary prevention [41]. The advent of more sensitive surveillance with MRI [42] with now a proven improvement in survival [43] and better treatments may reduce the use of risk-reducing mastectomy in the future. In the last few years much better risk prediction is possible, even within BRCA families, using information from mammographic density and multiple validated common single nucleotide polymorphisms (SNPs) [8,9,44]. There is also huge promise of improved outcomes from the use of PARP inhibitors in *BRCA1/2*-related tumours [45].

Table 2.3 Genes and SNPs predisposing to breast cancer

Gene	Other tumour susceptibility	Population frequency (%)	Proportion of breast cancer (%)	Proportion of HPHBC (%)	Proportion of familial breast cancer risk (%)	Lifetime risk in women (%), (RR)
BRCA1	Ovary/prostate	0.1	1.5	40	5–10	50–85
BRCA2	Ovary/prostate, pancreas	0.1	1.5	40	5–10	40–85
TP53 LFS	Sarcoma, glioma, adrenal	0.0025	0.02	2	0.1	80–90
PTEN Cowden's	Thyroid, colorectal	0.0005	0.004	0.3	0.02	25–50
CDH1	Gastric cancer	0.0005	0.004	0.3	0.02	30–60
CHEK2	Colorectal, prostate	0.5	0.5	0	2	18–20 (2.0)
ATM	HoZ (AR) lymphoma, leukaemia	0.5	0.5	0	2	20
STK11	Colorectal	0.001	0.001	0.6	0.04	40–60
BRIP1	HoZ-Fanconi (AR)	0.1	0.1	0	0.4	20 (2.0)
PALB2	HoZ-Fanconi (AR)	0.1	0.1	0	0.4	20–40 (2.0–4.0)
RAD51C	HoZ-Fanconi (AR)	0.001	0.1	0	0.2	15–20
77 SNPs [7–9]		5–46	0.5	0	20	11–13 (1.1–1.4)
Totals		100 for any	20	83	40	

Note: AR, autosomal recessive; HoZ, homozygous; HPHBC, highly penetrant hereditary breast cancer (e.g. >3 affected relatives).

PANEL GENE TESTING

Genetic testing for breast cancer predisposition until recently mainly involved testing BRCA1 and BRCA2 and occasionally targeted testing of TP53 [46]. However, since 2013 many commercial companies and health services have moved to testing panels of known cancer-predisposing genes, which may not even target the organs indicated from the family history [47,48], for example testing colorectal cancer genes in a breast cancer family. In a study of 198 women referred for BRCA1/2 testing, 57 (29%) harboured pathogenic mutations in BRCA1/2 [47]. A further 16 had what were classified as pathogenic mutations in the extended panel of 42 genes. However, the concept of what were 'actionable' mutations is debateable. The authors concluded that 15 women (11% of the non-BRCA1/2) had mutations that were actionable. However, four of these were MUTYH1 heterozygous mutations that do not even confer a twofold risk of colorectal cancer [49]. Many of the remainder were genes that still have an unknown breast cancer risk that almost certainly does not reach a high-risk definition (>40% lifetime risk) – NBN, BLM, SLX4, PRSS1 and ATM. Only three in fact met high-risk criteria, and two of these were for other cancers – CDKN2a (melanoma, pancreas) and MLH1 (colorectal, endometrial) – with only CDH1 meeting high-risk definition for breast cancer (Table 2.3). However, nearly all subjects carried a variant of 'uncertain significance' in at least one gene with an average of two per woman. Therefore in broader terms, only three women (2%) had a really useful result from the extended panel test with the problem of how to counsel nearly all of them on an uncertain result.

COLORECTAL CANCER

The other main organ in which high-risk dominant genes play an important role is the colorectum. Approximately 2–3% of colorectal cancer is due to inherited mutations in one of four DNA mismatch repair (MMR) genes (MLH1, MSH2, MSH6, PMS2) (Table 2.2) (a similar proportion to BRCA1/2 in breast cancer) that cause Lynch syndrome, previously known as hereditary non-polyposis colorectal cancer (HNPCC). MMR genes are important in the causation of about 13% of colorectal cancer that shows microsatellite instability. Inheriting a germline mutation confers about a 30–80% lifetime colorectal cancer risk without colonoscopy [50]. However, mutations also enhance risks of endometrial, ovarian, gastric and upper urinary tract cancers [51]. Identifying high-risk individuals can also save lives because bowel cancer can be prevented by regular colonoscopy.

OTHER COMMON CANCERS

High-risk predisposition to other cancers does occur but makes up less than 10% of a clinical genetics departments workload [52]. Endometrial cancer clearly has a strong hereditary component due to Lynch syndrome, and mutations in MLH1, MSH2 and MSH6 confer lifetime risks in excess of 40% [51]. Hereditary diffuse gastric cancer due to CDH1 mutations is rare but requires radical management with the recommendation for risk-reducing gastrectomy in mutation carriers due to the inefficacy of gastroscopy screening for early detection [53]. Hereditary melanoma due to CDKN2a, CDK4 or MITF mutations [54] is problematic because providing risk estimates to mutation carriers depends not only on the mutation but also on skin type, sun exposure and presence of moles, and in particular atypical moles that are not specifically linked to having the mutation. Although there is a strong inherited component to prostate cancer, no single gene clearly meets a high-risk category, although mutations in BRCA2 and HOXB13 [55] come very close and with screening in families with HOXB13 mutations [55] almost certainly does exceed a 40% lifetime risk.

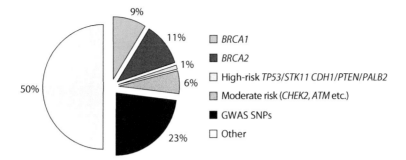

Figure 2.2 Proportion of the hereditary component of breast cancer identified.

GENETIC POLYMORPHISMS AND CANCER

The advent of GWAS has provided very strong evidence for the existence of polygenic risk for many common cancers. The first major breakthrough occurred with breast cancer in 2007 [7] with five loci being identified with validated increases in risk of 1.1- to 1.4-fold. Individually these SNPs are very common, usually with population frequencies of 5–49% for the minor allele. They also provide on an individual basis only a slight increase. However, evidence suggests that their effects are multiplicative even in the context of *BRCA1* and *BRCA2* [56]. By 2013, 77 validated SNPs had been published [57] and their use in combination potentially greatly improves risk stratification and prediction in the general population [58]. GWAS have been very successful also for colorectal cancer [59], prostate [60] and some other cancers, hastening more accurate risk prediction in these organs also. However, despite these major advances, only around 50% (Figure 2.2) of the hereditary component of the most well-elucidated cancer (breast) has so far been identified [57]. There is still much to do before family history of cancers can be discounted from any risk prediction process, and it still remains to be seen how family history and SNPs can be used together in risk prediction. As such SNPs may have the most to add in the population setting [61] and in very well-defined high-risk situations such as with *BRCA2* mutations in particular [40,56].

WHERE ARE THE REMAINING GENES?

While the lion's share of the high-risk predisposition to cancer has been elucidated, there remains a need to discover the remaining moderate risk and polygenic element. It is likely to be a few more years before 'generic' genetic tests for cancer which identify in excess of 70% of the familial component are developed. These are likely to test in excess of 200 genes and SNPs. In the meantime, there is still benefit to families from identifying the single high-risk genes. Indications on how to assess risks and who to refer for screening and genetic testing are available in more detailed texts [2,46,61].

CONCLUSION

The last 25 years has seen an enormous advance in understanding of cancer and its familial component. Genetic tests are now available for most high-risk conditions and generic tests may soon also be developed for all common cancers. Our increasing knowledge will also give rise to better targeting of surveillance and hopefully more gene-based treatments.

REFERENCES

1. Knudson AG. Mutation and cancer: statistical study of retinoblastoma. *Proc Natl Acad Sci USA* 1971;68:820–23.
2. Hodgson S, Foulkes WD, eds. *Inherited Susceptibility to Cancer*. Cambridge: Cambridge University Press, 1998.
3. Knudson AG, Meadows AT, Nichols WW, Hill R. Chromosomal deletion and retinoblastoma. *N Engl J Med* 1976;295:1120–23.
4. Woods R, Friedman JM, Evans DGR, Baser M, Joe H. Exploring the '2-hit hypothesis' in NF2: tests of 2-hit and 3-hit models of vestibular schwannoma development. *Genet Epidemiol* 2003;24:265–72.
5. Smith SA, Easton DF, Evans DGR, Ponder BAJ. Allele losses in the region 17q12-21 in familial ovarian cancer non-randomly involve the wild type chromosome. *Nat Genet* 1992;2:128–31.
6. Friend SH, Bernards R, Rogelj S, et al. A human DNA segment with properties of the gene that predisposes to retinoblastoma and osteosarcoma. *Nature* 1986;323:643–46.
7. Easton DF, Pharoah PDP, Dunning AM, et al. A genome-wide association study identifies multiple novel breast cancer susceptibility loci. *Nature* 2007;447(7148):1087–93.
8. Turnbull C, Ahmed S, Morrison J, et al. Genome-wide association study identifies five new breast cancer susceptibility loci. *Nat Genet* 2010;42(6):504–7.
9. Michailidou K, Hall P, Gonzalez-Neira A, et al. Large-scale genotyping identifies 41 new loci associated with breast cancer risk. *Nat Genet* 2013;45(4):353–61.
10. Evans DGR, Guy SP, Armstrong J, et al. Non penetrance and late appearance of polyps in families with familial adenomatous polyposis. *Gut* 1993;34:1389–93.

11. Davies DR, Armstrong JG, Thakker N, et al. Severe Gardner's syndrome in families with mutations restricted to a specific region of the APC gene. *Am J Hum Genet* 1995;57:1151–58.

12. Mallinson EK, Newton KF, Bowen J, et al. The impact of screening and genetic registration on mortality and colorectal cancer incidence in familial adenomatous polyposis. *Gut* 2010;59(10):1378–82.

13. Maher ER, Yates JR, Harries R, et al. Clinical features and natural history of von Hippel-Lindau disease. *Q J Med* 1990;77:1151–63.

14. Latif F, Tory K, Gnarra J, et al. Identification of the von Hippel-Lindau disease tumor suppressor gene. *Science* 1993;260:1317–20.

15. Martinez A, Fullwood P, Kondo K, et al. Role of chromosome 3p12-p21 tumour suppressor genes in clear cell renal cell carcinoma: analysis of VHL dependent and VHL independent pathways of tumorigenesis. *Mol Pathol* 2000;53(3):137–44.

16. Evans DGR, Baser ME, McGaughran J, et al. Malignant peripheral nerve sheath tumours in neurofibromatosis 1. *J Med Genet* 2002;39:311–14.

17. Evans DG. Neurofibromatosis type 2 (NF2): a clinical and molecular review. *Orphanet J Rare Dis* 2009;4:16.

18. Evans DGR, Farndon PA. Nevoid basal cell carcinoma syndrome. In *GeneReviews* at GeneTests: Medical Genetics Information Resource [database online]. University of Washington, Seattle, 1997–2014. Available at http://www.geneclinics.org.

19. Smith MJ, Beetz C, Williams SG, et al. Germline mutations in SUFU cause Gorlin syndrome-associated childhood medulloblastoma and redefine the risk associated with PTCH1 mutations. *J Clin Oncol* 2014;32(36):4155–61.

20. Ebeling T, Vierimaa O, Kytölä S, Leisti J, Salmela PI. Effect of multiple endocrine neoplasia type 1 (MEN1) gene mutations on premature mortality in familial MEN1 syndrome with founder mutations. *J Clin Endocrinol Metab* 2004;89(7):3392–96.

21. Machens A, Lorenz K, Sekulla C, et al. Molecular epidemiology of multiple endocrine neoplasia 2: implications for RET screening in the new millennium. *Eur J Endocrinol* 2013;168(3):307–14.

22. Spigelman AD, Murday V, Phillips RK. Cancer and the Peutz-Jeghers syndrome. *Gut* 1989;30(11):1588–90.

23. Howe JR, Roth A, Ringold JC, et al. Mutations in the SMAD4/DPC4 gene in juvenile polyposis. *Science* 1998;280(5366):1086–88.

24. Evans DG, Ingham SL. Reduced life expectancy seen in hereditary diseases which predispose to early-onset tumors. *Appl Clin Genet* 2013;6:53–61.

25. Schmidt L, Duh FM, Chen F, et al. Germline and somatic mutations in the tyrosine kinase domain of the MET proto-oncogene in papillary renal carcinomas. *Nat Genet* 1997;16(1):68–73.

26. De Rosa M, Fasano C, Panariello L, Scarano MI, Belli G, Iannelli A, Ciciliano F, Izzo P. Evidence for a recessive inheritance of Turcot's syndrome caused by compound heterozygous mutations within the PMS2 gene. *Oncogene* 2000;19(13):1719–23.

27. Sampson JR, Dolwani S, Jones S, et al. Autosomal recessive colorectal adenomatous polyposis due to inherited mutations of MYH. *Lancet* 2003;362(9377):39–41.

28. Lakhani SR, Reis-Filho JS, Fulford L, et al. Prediction of BRCA1 status in patients with breast cancer using estrogen receptor and basal phenotype. *Clin Cancer Res* 2005;11(14):5175–80.

29. Lakhani SR, Manek S, Penault-Llorca F, et al. Pathology of ovarian cancers in BRCA1 and BRCA2 carriers. *Clin Cancer Res* 2004;10(7):2473–81.

30. Claus EB, Risch N, Thompson D. Autosomal dominant inheritance of early onset breast cancer. *Cancer* 1994;73:643–51.

31. Peto J, Mack TM. High constant incidence in twins and other relatives of women with breast cancer. *Nat Genet* 2000;26:411–14.

32. Malkin D, Li FP, Strong LC, et al. Germline TP53 mutations in cancer families. *Science* 1990;250:1233–38.

33. Lalloo F, Varley J, Ellis D, et al. Family history is predictive of pathogenic mutations in BRCA1, BRCA2 and TP53 with high penetrance in a population based study of very early onset breast cancer. *Lancet* 2003;361:1101–2.

34. Wilson JR, Bateman AC, Hanson H, et al. A novel HER2-positive breast cancer phenotype arising from germline TP53 mutations. *J Med Genet* 2010;47(11):771–74.

35. Evans DG, Moran A, Hartley R, Dawson J, Bulman B, Knox F, Howell A, Lalloo F. Long term outcomes of breast cancer in women aged 30 years or younger, based on family history, pathology and BRCA1/BRCA2/TP53 status. *Br J Cancer* 2010:102(7):1091–98.

36. Evans DG, Barwell J, Eccles DM, et al. The Angelina Jolie effect: how high celebrity profile can have a major impact on provision of cancer related services. *Breast Cancer Res* 2014;16(5):442.

37. Hartmann LC, Schaid DJ, Woods JE, et al. Efficacy of bilateral prophylactic mastectomy in women with a family history of breast cancer. *N Engl J Med* 1999;340:77–84.

38. Rebbeck TR, Friebel T, Lynch HT, et al. Bilateral prophylactic mastectomy reduces breast cancer risk in BRCA1 and BRCA2 mutation carriers: the PROSE Study Group. *J Clin Oncol* 2004;22:1055–62.

39. Rebbeck TR, Lynch HT, Neuhausen SL, et al. Reduction in cancer risk after bilateral prophylactic oophorectomy in BRCA1 and BRCA2 mutation carriers. *N Engl J Med* 2002;346:1616–22.

40. Evans DG, Ingham SL, Baildam A, et al. Contralateral mastectomy improves survival in women with BRCA1/2-associated breast cancer. *Breast Cancer Res Treat* 2013;140(1):135–42.

41. Ingham SL, Sperrin M, Baildam A, et al. Risk-reducing surgery increases survival in BRCA1/2 mutation carriers unaffected at time of family referral. *Breast Cancer Res Treat* 2013; 142(3):611–18.

42. Leach MO, Boggis CR, Dixon AK, et al. Screening with magnetic resonance imaging and mammography of a UK population at high familial risk of breast cancer: a prospective multicentre cohort study (MARIBS). *Lancet* 2005;365:1769–78.

43. Evans DG, Kesavan N, Lim Y, et al. MRI breast screening in high-risk women: cancer detection and survival analysis. *Breast Cancer Res Treat* 2014;145(3):663–72.

44. Ingham SL, Warwick J, Byers H, et al. Is multiple SNP testing in BRCA2 and BRCA1 female carriers ready for use in clinical practice? Results from a large genetic centre in the UK. *Clin Genet* 2013;84(1):37–42.

45. Stebbing J, Ellis P, Tutt A. PARP inhibitors in BRCA1-/BRCA2-associated and triple-negative breast cancers. *Future Oncol* 2010;6(4):485–86.

46. McIntosh A, Shaw C, Evans G, et al. Clinical guidelines and evidence review for the classification and care of women at risk of familial breast cancer. London: National Collaborating Centre for Primary Care/University of Sheffield. NICE guideline CG014, 2004 (updated 2006 CG41, 2013 CG184). Available at http://www.nice.org.uk.

47. Kurian AW, Hare EE, Mills MA, et al. Clinical evaluation of a multiple-gene sequencing panel for hereditary cancer risk assessment. *J Clin Oncol* 2014;32(19):2001–9.

48. Hiraki S, Rinella ES, Schnabel F, et al. Cancer risk assessment using genetic panel testing: considerations for clinical application. *J Genet Couns* 2014;23(4):604–17.

49. Jones N, Vogt S, Nielsen M, et al. Increased colorectal cancer incidence in obligate carriers of heterozygous mutations in MUTYH. *Gastroenterology* 2009;137(2):489–94.

50. Barrow E, Aldhuaj W, Robinson L, et al. Colorectal cancer in HNPCC: cumulative lifetime incidence, survival and tumour distribution. A report of 121 families with proven mutations. *Clin Genet* 2008;74(3):233–42.

51. Barrow E, Robinson L, Aldhuaj W, et al. Extracolonic cancers in HNPCC: cumulative lifetime incidence and tumour distribution. A report of 121 families. *Clin Genet* 2009;75(2):141–49.

52. Wonderling D, Hopwood P, Cull A, et al. A descriptive study of UK cancer genetics services: an emerging clinical response to the new genetics. *Br J Cancer* 2001;85(2):166–70.

53. Fitzgerald RC, Hardwick R, Huntsman D, et al. Hereditary diffuse gastric cancer: updated consensus guidelines for clinical management and directions for future research. *J Med Genet* 2010;47(7):436–44.

54. Marzuka-Alcalá A, Gabree MJ, Tsao H. Melanoma susceptibility genes and risk assessment. *Methods Mol Biol* 2014;1102:381–93.

55. MacInnis RJ, Severi G, Baglietto L, et al. Population-based estimate of prostate cancer risk for carriers of the HOXB13 missense mutation G84E. *PLoS One* 2013;8(2):e54727.

56. Antoniou AC, Beesley J, McGuffog L, et al. Common breast cancer susceptibility alleles and the risk of breast cancer for BRCA1 and BRCA2 mutation carriers: implications for risk prediction. *Cancer Res* 2010;70(23):9742–54.

57. Brentnall AR, Evans DG, Cuzick J. Distribution of breast cancer risk from SNPs and classical risk factors in women of routine screening age in the UK. *Br J Cancer* 2014;110(3):827–28.

58. Eccles SA, Aboagye EO, Ali S, et al. Critical research gaps and translational priorities for the successful prevention and treatment of breast cancer. *Breast Cancer Res* 2013;15(5):R92.

59. Whiffin N, Hosking FJ, Farrington SM, et al. Identification of susceptibility loci for colorectal cancer in a genome-wide meta-analysis. *Hum Mol Genet* 2014;23(17):4729–37.

60. Eeles RA, Olama AA, Benlloch S, et al. Identification of 23 new prostate cancer susceptibility loci using the iCOGS custom genotyping array. *Nat Genet* 2013;45(4):385–91.

61. Lalloo F, Kerr B, Friedman J, Evans DGR, eds. *Risk Assessment and Management in Cancer Genetics*. Oxford: Oxford University Press, 2005.

3

Clinical trial design in surgical oncology

SERGE EVRARD AND PIPPA MCKELVIE-SEBILEAU

INTRODUCTION

Applying strict research methodology to clinical research in surgery is difficult, and many obstacles to trial design and execution are inherent to surgery [1]. The complexities of the disease and heterogeneity of surgical patients make them a more difficult group to study than non-surgical patients [2]. As a result, compared with other medical specialties, the quality of reporting in the surgical literature is low [3], and relevant research methodologies somewhere on the continuum between retrospective studies and randomized controlled trials (RCTs) are seriously underused. Surgical oncology, as for other local treatments, is no exception [4]. In this chapter, we will look at the specificities of clinical research in surgical oncology, with a particular focus on overcoming inherent barriers and improving the level of evidence-based research and reporting. The aim of this chapter is to convince young surgical oncologists that increasing the rate of prospective works is a major issue for their generation and, while the randomized trial is always beneficial, there are a lot of prospective studies of different natures which could dramatically enhance the quality of scientific knowledge in surgery.

WHY IS CONDUCTING CLINICAL TRIALS IN SURGERY DIFFERENT FROM OTHER MEDICAL DOMAINS?

The application of evidence-based care in surgery has improved over the past decade, but surgical treatments are still less likely to be investigated using full-scale and well-designed RCTs [1,5]. Various obstacles to RCTs and other forms of clinical research in surgery can be put forward.

First, difficulties in the standardization of the procedures and quality control may hinder reproducibility and external validity. Surgery comes from the Greek word *kheirourgía*, meaning manual activities. In contrast to drug trials where the intervention tested can be controlled down to the minutest dosage and timing detail, surgery is not a pill containing a precise quantity of specific molecules but a set of acts performed under the same denomination to treat a patient. Many studies outline the fact that one of the main prognostic factors regarding success of a surgical intervention is in fact the choice of the individual surgeon [6]. Achieving a surgical procedure is consequently something which cannot be standardized: it depends on the skill of the surgeon, decisions that will be made intraoperatively, as well as patient's characteristics like body mass index. Each surgical procedure is thus unique. Moreover, the definition and the execution of a procedure may vary between centres: the examples of the D1 and D2 lymphadenectomies in the Dutch trial is famous; a quality control review of the procedures by a Japanese expert surgeon revealed that some so-called D2 procedures were actually closer to those of a D1 procedure [7].

Achieving good quality control for a procedure for a surgical study is consequently a real challenge which greatly impacts the quality of the conclusions to be drawn. A famous example is the MacDonald trial [8] in gastric cancer where it was concluded that postoperative chemoradiotherapy after gastrectomy gave better results than gastrectomy alone. Actually the quality of the surgery was so poor (D0 and D1 lymphadenectomies) that postoperative chemoradiotherapy just had a catch-up role. Today, if a real radical gastrectomy is performed, no postoperative chemoradiotherapy is required.

A further barrier to clinical research in surgery is accrual difficulties, with one in five surgical RCTs discontinued early, mostly due to poor recruitment [9]. Accrual in surgical series is more difficult than for medical specialties. Surgeons' reputations are difficult to establish and can be challenged by randomization. Most of the time, surgical trials address specific questions: the more specific the question, the more restrictive the criteria for inclusion and the less patients are eligible to be recruited to the study. The purity of the issue addressed inversely affects the feasibility of the study. This can mean that clinical trials never get underway due to foreseen accrual difficulties, or the difficulties can be encountered during the study, with trials being stopped early, or in the case of a recent [10] intended RCT, more than 500 patients being downgraded to 'pilot' randomized trials with 100 patients. Another example is the conversion into a randomized phase II trial of the CLOCC trial (Chemotherapy + Local Ablation Versus Chemotherapy) which was initially designed as a phase III trial [11].

A further obstacle to randomization can be lack of clinical equipoise. Surgeons are known to be stubborn and are often convinced that what they do is the best for their patients when it is not the only manner to proceed. Travelling abroad will help the young surgeon to understand that various techniques and strategies can be used to treat the same patients with the same pathologies. Being aware of this is the beginning of surgical equipoise. However, the lack of equipoise may also come from the patient who comes with his or her own ideas about the best technique and who can refuse randomization. As such, prospective evaluation of emergent techniques should take place early in the process of clinical research before any popularization by the media [12].

Finally, funding issues often confound research objectives. Surgical endeavours in modern medicine are often not sufficiently recognized by funding agencies [2]. The proportion of public funding devoted to surgically oriented clinical research is very small compared to medical trials.

With study design in surgical intervention RCTs insufficiently described in more than 60% of published articles [13], efforts are required to improve the study designs used, as well as reporting methods.

PRAGMATIC APPROACH TO CLINICAL RESEARCH IN SURGICAL ONCOLOGY: RECONCILING THE LEVEL OF EVIDENCE AND FEASIBILITY

Various classification hierarchies of levels of evidence have been proposed, with the best evidence derived from the highest levels leading to enhanced care for patients and improved standards for surgeons and health care institutions. The Canadian Task Force on the Periodic Health Examination proposed a classification system from I to III in 1979 [14]. This level of evidence system was further developed and expanded upon by Sackett in 1989 for antithrombotic agents [15] (Table 3.1).

Both classifications agree that for therapeutic studies, only RCTs can provide level I evidence. However, some of the most important published surgical research is based on retrospective studies even in high-impact-factor journals [16–18], often because of the impossibility of randomizing patients between two very diverse treatment arms, although this is not always explicitly stated as the reason for not undertaking a RCT [17,19].

The IDEAL recommendations [12,20,21] for the assessment of surgery based on a five-stage description of surgical development are a good inventory of the difficulties of managing and organizing clinical research in surgery, and knowledge of these proposals is highly recommended. However, their scope remains fairly theoretical and the principles are difficult to apply within the time and funding constraints of actual surgical research. In the following

Table 3.1 Levels of evidence from the canadian task force on the periodic health examination and from Sackett

Level	Type of evidence
Canadian task force on the periodic health examination	
I	At least 1 RCT with proper randomization
II.1	Well-designed cohort or case-control study
II.2	Time series comparisons or dramatic results from uncontrolled studies
III	Expert opinions
Sackett levels of evidence	
I	Large RCTs with clear-cut results
II	Small RCTs with unclear results
III	Cohort and case-control studies
IV	Historical cohort or case-control studies
V	Case series, studies with no controls

Source: Adapted from Canadian Task Force on the Periodic Health Examination, *Can Med Assoc J* 1979;121(9):1193–254 and Sackett DL, *Chest* 1989;95(2 Suppl):2S–4S.

section, we propose a pragmatic critique of the various phases of clinical research in surgery, beginning with the inescapable phase III trial, before discussing alternative prospective designs.

Critique of randomized trials in surgery

Sometimes surgical innovations, initially reported mainly through case studies or small retrospective series, seem to be so modern and relevant that they are adopted into routine practice with loud acclamation, before finally being dethroned years later by a randomized trial, like for coronary artery stenting for stable coronary artery disease [22]. Surgical phase III trials are rare, representing only 8% of publications in 2006 [20]. Consequently, surgical journals place a lot of emphasis on encouraging surgeons to carry out and publish RCTs. While retrospective studies which are cheaper, faster and easier to carry out have a role in clinical research in surgery, RCTs are required, and clear and accurate reporting of RCT results is needed to provide evidence-based medicine. Despite being the gold standard, the RCT is not the only valid method to evaluate a new treatment. Some experimental studies comparing estimations of treatment effects by RCTs and non-randomized trials have not shown a definitive superiority of RCTs [23,24]. Schematically, RCTs have a major lack of generalizability as they require strict criteria of inclusion and exclusion. Indeed, as previously discussed, major accrual difficulties hinder surgical RCTs due to the rarity of patients meeting inclusion criteria. This highlights the issue of a lack of representativeness between RCT patients and those looking for real care in the real world. While RCTs are necessary, they should be preceded by other trial phases, in particular, to firmly establish criteria for sample size calculation and expected outcomes.

The Consolidated Standards of Reporting Trials (CONSORT) statement [25,26] was extended in 2008 to randomized trials of non-pharmacologic treatment (CONSORT NPT) [27], involving specificities such as the complexity of the intervention, expertise of the care provider and difficulties of blinding. Nagendran and colleagues [28] report worse adherence to the CONSORT NPT extension than to the original general CONSORT recommendations, possibly because there has been less time to adapt reporting practices and journal policy to the CONSORT NPT guidelines published in 2008, more than 10 years after the original CONSORT statement. They report limited awareness of the CONSORT NPT statement by authors, peer reviewers and editors. In a recent effort to increase adherence to these guidelines, the checklist was simplified to a 10-item reduced checklist [29].

The major risk of having few and poor-quality surgical RCTs is to produce counterfeit scientific money. An example is given by an article in the *Lancet* in 2002 [30] on a randomized trial on laparoscopy-assisted colectomy (LAC) versus open colectomy (OC) for treatment of non-metastatic colon cancer. The article concluded that LAC was more effective than OC for treatment of colon cancer in terms of morbidity, hospital stay, tumour recurrence and cancer-related survival. This trial was the first randomized work ever published on this topic; the place of LAC at this time was a pressing issue and the result was breaking news. All requirements of publishing in the *Lancet* were met except one, the quality of the methodology. Briefly, the paper was underpowered, multi-biased and it is not clear if the randomization design was written before or after patient accrual completion [31]. To prevent this issue, a trial should be considered to be prospective only if it is registered before starting the first inclusion. These results were never confirmed in further publication, and the two routes are nowadays considered to be equivalent [32]. It is easy to understand the danger of publishing such a so-called randomized trial not matching the CONSORT criteria. As randomized surgical trials are rare, they have a real prestige when undertaken and consequently, rigorous control of their quality is mandatory. That said, the reason why surgical RCTs often do not match CONSORT criteria is mainly because phase III frameworks are not designed for non-drug evaluation – a snake that bites its own tail. Indeed, all the reasons why clinical research is more difficult in surgery than in medicine are present and exacerbated in the phase III trial: lack of equipoise, difficulty in patient accrual, standardization and control of quality of the procedures, and finally the cost and the years required.

Moreover, as surgical randomized trials have difficulties in adhering to the CONSORT criteria, the risk is that, after several years of efforts, on publication, they will be criticized, considered biased and finally discarded. A good example of this 'trial bashing' can be observed in the ASTEC (efficacy of systematic pelvic lymphadenectomy in endometrial cancer) surgical trial investigating whether pelvic lymphadenectomy could improve survival of women with grade 1 endometrial cancer. Eighty-five centres in four countries and 1408 women participated. The results showed no evidence of benefit in terms of overall or recurrence-free survival. Six authors wrote letters to the editors to criticize the trial, outlining that the number of the retrieved lymph nodes was too small, the rate of low-risk patients was too high and peri-aortic lymph nodes were left in place. However, in the end, all authors concluded, more or less, that they will continue to undertake lymphadenectomies for such women. A similar controversy has ensued following the publication of the New EPOC trial in the *Journal of Clinical Oncology* [33].

In conclusion, there are two major potential drawbacks for surgical phase III trials: the first is the risk of a high level of investment of time and effort required in a study which several years later will be judged as having failed to demonstrate anything; the second one is the more serious risk of establishing a flawed hypothesis as the truth. Other alternative prospective designs are often more feasible, and compliance with statistical principles such as minimum sample size is more likely. They play a crucial role in clinical research in surgical oncology.

Critique and contribution of the alternative prospective trials applied to surgical oncology

PHASE 0

Phase 0 trials are also called exploratory investigational new drug studies or exploratory trials. The aim of these very early phase trials is to demonstrate biological efficacy of the molecule before the first phase I trial. They are generally used to help speed up and streamline the drug approval process by establishing very early on whether the drug or agent behaves in human subjects as was expected from preclinical studies. The principle is to give a small quantity of a new drug (1/100 of the effective dose) to a small group of patients (less than 10) over a short period (less than 7 days).

These studies are relatively difficult to organize as they have no individual benefit and require invasive biopsies. That is precisely why surgeons can play a major role in such trials. The idea is to take advantage of routine surgery to provide tumour tissue to assess drug response without the need for additional invasive biopsies. For example, early stage colon cancer just confirmed by a colonoscopy is treated by primary surgical removal usually after a short interval of 2–3 weeks during which a new pharmacological agent can be administered and its effect on the tumour thereby evaluated. A new preoperative colonoscopic biopsy may be required and can be refused by the patient, but the second specimen after a week of treatment will be the colectomy specimen. A phase 0 trial is consequently an excellent approach to link surgeons and biologists on a translational project. It is up to the surgeon to take the initiative of identifying suitable procedures (a standard surgery which can be organized without being disturbed by a short period of drug administration) and to enrol a biologist in the adventure of testing a new drug outside of an animal model for the first time.

PHASE I

Phase I trials designed to assess the safety of a new treatment in a small group of patients do not exist for surgical procedures. No framework exists for surgical innovation. For example, mandatory Conforme aux Exigences (CE) marking for a new surgical device can attest to the quality and safety of the device production and compliance with industry standards. It cannot, however, guarantee the legitimacy of indications for use and the role of use in humans. All of this has to be established after the device has been put on the market. For example, when the first generators of radiofrequencies for liver surgery appeared on the market at the end of the twentieth century, there were no recognized guidelines on how to use radiofrequency for this indication, for which lesions, which size, etc., and the first prospective evaluations were published around the same time in 2012 [34,35]. As such, health authorities need to establish a methodological framework for evaluating new surgical devices and techniques and their indications before widespread use, as for market approval of new drugs.

PHASE II

A phase II trial is carried out to establish the efficacy of a new treatment. The phase II framework is quite easily adaptable for surgery and is a largely untapped methodology in surgical trials. The principle is to define a priori a threshold for efficacy and non-efficacy. As short-term efficacy is focused on, the primary endpoint will favour the response rate rather than overall survival. If a response rate cannot be used, it can be replaced by progression-free survival. The number of patients to be included is calculated based on power calculations and is generally around 30–50, with the possibility of using several optimal designs and potentially reducing the required number of patients by introducing an intermediate level of analysis [36].

A phase II trial can be planned for one treatment alone or for two treatments. Two phase II trials can be run in parallel like for the Cascador study involving delayed coloanal anastomosis for medium and lower rectal cancer treatment (ID RCB no. 2010-A00299-30) or by randomization, like for the CLOCC trial [35]. In these two situations, comparisons between the two arms are not possible, but this type of trial enables one to assess the treatment effect in the same way in both groups at the same time. Randomized phase II trials are gaining more and more acceptance as they are cheaper and quicker to carry out than large phase III trials.

Imaging diagnostics is often a concern for surgeons. Phase II trials based on the model of an 'add-on' study are appropriate to evaluate such additional diagnostic measures in terms of modifications of the surgery. In the ULIIS study (Ultrasound Liver Intraoperative Imaging with SonoVue®, NCT01880554), the adjunct of a contrast agent to intraoperative ultrasound (IOUS) to track and treat colorectal liver metastases is being evaluated in comparison to IOUS alone, which is itself being compared to preoperative serial imaging. A rate of 15% was expected in the calculation when drawing the design.

PHASE IV

Phase IV trials are designed as post-marketing surveillance trials to monitor the risks, benefits and optimal use of a treatment once it has been approved for use. The previous phases (0–III) are assumed to have produced enough evidence to authorize the practice. The problem with respect to surgical practice is that preliminary phases are often skipped and phase IV studies become the first step of a regular methodological evaluation. As an example, colorectal liver metastases have been routinely resected all over the world for more than 30 years using one- or two-stage procedures, with or without portal vein obliteration and ablation, etc., without any prospective evaluation before 2012 when two phase II trials were published to evaluate the use of combined resection and ablation for advanced diseases [34,35].

When a practice has been accepted into clinical routines, and it is too late for a phase II or III trial, it is always possible to carry out a phase IV. There is indeed a lot to learn from outcome studies in surgical oncology. A recent strategic collaboration has been established between the European Society of Surgical Oncology (ESSO) and the European Organization for Research and Treatment of Cancer on outcome studies. The first of them is the CLIMB (Colorectal Liver Metastasis Database) study (NCT02218801) with a prospective multicentre database recording advanced cases of colorectal liver metastases which are initially unresectable and require chemoconversion or are operable up front (by combined resection and ablation). Morbidity and survival will be the endpoints, but a program to improve the quality of surgery is also scheduled. After the first hundred cases, some parameters will be chosen to become targets of a policy of improvement. Other projects are presently discussed for the future in colorectal liver metastases imaging such as the DREAM project (Diffusion-Weighted Magnetic Resonance Imaging Assessment of Liver Metastasis), in the breast or in oncogeriatrics.

CONCLUSIONS

There is no ideal design for optimal clinical research in surgery. Trade-offs between the exigency of a high level of scientific evidence and the dictatorship of feasibility are inevitable. Young generations of surgical oncologists must be convinced of the necessity to run a lot of trials or studies of different types depending on the issue addressed and providing that they have chosen a prospective design, accepting that in many cases randomization will not be possible. In parallel, journal editors and peer reviewers have a responsibility to endorse guidelines for the scientific quality of surgical research such as the CONSORT NPT statement or the IDEAL guidelines to increase the amount of evidence-based medicine in surgical oncology. Publication criteria should also be broadened to include other prospective research methodologies and to end the monopoly of the RCT in surgical oncology. If this condition is respected, major advancements in surgical knowledge can be expected in the future. The ESSO will accompany them.

REFERENCES

1. McCulloch P, Taylor I, Sasako M, Lovett B, Griffin D. Randomised trials in surgery: problems and possible solutions. *BMJ* 2002;324(7351):1448–51.
2. Weil RJ. The future of surgical research. *PLoS Med* 2004;1(1):e13.
3. Panesar SS, Thakrar R, Athanasiou T, Sheikh A. Comparison of reports of randomized controlled trials and systematic reviews in surgical journals: literature review. *J R Soc Med* 2006;99(9):470–2.
4. Menezes AS, Barnes A, Scheer AS, Martel G, Moloo H, Boushey RP, Sabri E, Auer RC. Clinical research in surgical oncology: an analysis of ClinicalTrials.gov. *Ann Surg Oncol* 2013;20(12):3725–31.
5. Farrokhyar F, Karanicolas PJ, Thoma A, Simunovic M, Bhandari M, Devereaux PJ, Anvari M, Adili A, Guyatt G. Randomized controlled trials of surgical interventions. *Ann Surg* 2010;251(3):409–16.
6. Martling A, Cedermark B, Johansson H, Rutqvist LE, Holm T. The surgeon as a prognostic factor after the introduction of total mesorectal excision in the treatment of rectal cancer. *Br J Surg* 2002;89(8):1008–13.
7. Bonenkamp JJ, Hermans J, Sasako M, van de Velde CJ, Welvaart K, Songun I, Meyer S, et al. Extended lymph-node dissection for gastric cancer. *N Engl J Med* 1999;340(12):908–14.
8. Macdonald JS, Smalley SR, Benedetti J, Hundahl SA, Estes NC, Stemmermann GN, Haller DG, et al. Chemoradiotherapy after surgery compared with surgery alone for adenocarcinoma of the stomach or gastroesophageal junction. *N Engl J Med* 2001;345(10):725–30.
9. Chapman SJ, Shelton B, Mahmood H, Fitzgerald JE, Harrison EM, Bhangu A. Discontinuation and non-publication of surgical randomised controlled trials: observational study. *BMJ* 2014;349:g6870.
10. Denost Q, Adam JP, Rullier A, Buscail E, Laurent C, Rullier E. Perineal transanal approach: a new standard for laparoscopic sphincter-saving resection in low rectal cancer, a randomized trial. *Ann Surg* 2014;260(6):993–9.
11. Ruers T, Punt CJ, van Coevorden F, Borel Rinkes I, Ledermann JA, Poston GJ, Bechstein W, Lentz M, Mauer M, Nordlinger B. Final results of the EORTC intergroup randomized study 40004 (CLOCC) evaluating the benefit of radiofrequency ablation (RFA) combined with chemotherapy for unresectable colorectal liver metastases (CRC LM). *J Clin Oncol* 2010;28(Suppl):712s(abs 10057).
12. McCulloch P, Altman DG, Campbell WB, Flum DR, Glasziou P, Marshall JC, Nicholl J, et al. No surgical innovation without evaluation: the IDEAL recommendations. *Lancet* 2009;374(9695):1105–12.
13. Jacquier I, Boutron I, Moher D, Roy C, Ravaud P. The reporting of randomized clinical trials using a surgical intervention is in need of immediate improvement: a systematic review. *Ann Surg* 2006;244(5):677–83.
14. The periodic health examination. Canadian Task Force on the Periodic Health Examination. *Can Med Assoc J* 1979;121(9):1193–254.
15. Sackett DL. Rules of evidence and clinical recommendations on the use of antithrombotic agents. *Chest* 1989;95(2 Suppl):2S–4S.
16. Adam R, Wicherts DA, de Haas RJ, Ciacio O, Levi F, Paule B, Ducreux M, Azoulay D, Bismuth H, Castaing D. Patients with initially unresectable colorectal liver metastases: is there a possibility of cure? *J Clin Oncol* 2009;27(11):1829–35.

17. Brouquet A, Abdalla EK, Kopetz S, Garrett CR, Overman MJ, Eng C, Andreou A, et al. High survival rate after two-stage resection of advanced colorectal liver metastases: response-based selection and complete resection define outcome. *J Clin Oncol* 2011;29(8):1083–90.

18. Elias D, Gilly F, Boutitie F, Quenet F, Bereder JM, Mansvelt B, Lorimier G, Dube P, Glehen O. Peritoneal colorectal carcinomatosis treated with surgery and perioperative intraperitoneal chemotherapy: retrospective analysis of 523 patients from a multicentric French study. *J Clin Oncol* 2010;28(1):63–8.

19. Curley SA. Radiofrequency ablation versus resection for resectable colorectal liver metastases: time for a randomized trial? *Ann Surg Oncol* 2008;15(1):11–3.

20. Barkun JS, Aronson JK, Feldman LS, Maddern GJ, Strasberg SM, Altman DG, Barkun JS, et al. Evaluation and stages of surgical innovations. *Lancet* 2009;374(9695):1089–96.

21. Ergina PL, Cook JA, Blazeby JM, Boutron I, Clavien PA, Reeves BC, Seiler CM, et al. Challenges in evaluating surgical innovation. *Lancet* 2009;374(9695):1097–104.

22. Boden WE, O'Rourke RA, Teo KK, Hartigan PM, Maron DJ, Kostuk WJ, Knudtson M, et al. Optimal medical therapy with or without PCI for stable coronary disease. *N Engl J Med* 2007;356(15):1503–16.

23. Benson K, Hartz AJ. A comparison of observational studies and randomized, controlled trials. *N Engl J Med* 2000;342(25):1878–86.

24. Concato J, Shah N, Horwitz RI. Randomized, controlled trials, observational studies, and the hierarchy of research designs. *N Engl J Med* 2000;342(25):1887–92.

25. Moher D, Hopewell S, Schulz KF, Montori V, Gotzsche PC, Devereaux PJ, Elbourne D, Egger M, Altman DG. CONSORT 2010 explanation and elaboration: updated guidelines for reporting parallel group randomised trials. *Int J Surg* 2012;10(1):28–55.

26. Moher D. CONSORT: an evolving tool to help improve the quality of reports of randomized controlled trials. Consolidated Standards of Reporting Trials. *JAMA* 1998;279(18):1489–91.

27. Boutron I, Moher D, Altman DG, Schulz KF, Ravaud P. Extending the CONSORT statement to randomized trials of nonpharmacologic treatment: explanation and elaboration. *Ann Intern Med* 2008;148(4):295–309.

28. Nagendran M, Harding D, Teo W, Camm C, Maruthappu M, McCulloch P, Hopewell S. Poor adherence of randomised trials in surgery to CONSORT guidelines for non-pharmacological treatments (NPT): a cross-sectional study. *BMJ Open* 2013;3(12):e003898.

29. Clavien PA, Lillemoe KD. A new policy to implement CONSORT guidelines for surgical randomized controlled trials. *Ann Surg* 2014;260(6):947–8.

30. Lacy AM, Garcia-Valdecasas JC, Delgado S, Castells A, Taura P, Pique JM, Visa J. Laparoscopy-assisted colectomy versus open colectomy for treatment of non-metastatic colon cancer: a randomised trial. *Lancet* 2002;359(9325):2224–9.

31. Evrard S, Mathoulin-Pelissier S, Kramar A. Open versus laparoscopy-assisted colectomy. *Lancet* 2003;361(9351):73–6.

32. Buunen M, Veldkamp R, Hop WC, Kuhry E, Jeekel J, Haglind E, Pahlman L, et al. Survival after laparoscopic surgery versus open surgery for colon cancer: long-term outcome of a randomised clinical trial. *Lancet Oncol* 2009;10(1):44–52.

33. Nordlinger B, Poston GJ, Goldberg RM. Should the results of the new EPOC trial change practice in the management of patients with resectable metastatic colorectal cancer confined to the liver? *J Clin Oncol* 2015 Jan 20;33(3):241–3.

34. Evrard S, Rivoire M, Arnaud J, Lermite E, Bellera C, Fonck M, Becouarn Y, Lalet C, Puildo M, Mathoulin-Pelissier S. Unresectable colorectal cancer liver metastases treated by intraoperative radiofrequency ablation with or without resection. *Br J Surg* 2012;99(4):558–65.

35. Ruers T, Punt C, Van CF, Pierie JP, Borel-Rinkes I, Ledermann JA, Poston G, et al. Radiofrequency ablation combined with systemic treatment versus systemic treatment alone in patients with non-resectable colorectal liver metastases: a randomized EORTC intergroup phase II study (EORTC 40004). *Ann Oncol* 2012;23(10):2619–26.

36. Simon R. Optimal two-stage designs for phase II clinical trials. *Control Clin Trials* 1989;10(1):1–10.

4

A critical overview of screening for cancer

KARSTEN JUHL JØRGENSEN

INTRODUCTION

Screening differs from the treatment of cancer in fundamental ways. While screening for some types of cancer clearly causes more good than harm, at a reasonable cost, screening can also harm healthy individuals, people that would not have been affected by the disease in the absence of screening. A balanced, evidence-based view is required, which is complex, as screening data are subject to a range of inherent biases which may make interpretation of benefits and harms difficult.

Screening differs from the treatment of symptomatic cancer in terms of the proportion of those subjected that can benefit. An effect on disease-specific mortality is only documented for four types of cancer screening (breast, colon, lung and cervical), but an effect on overall mortality is not shown for any type of cancer screening, despite hundreds of thousands of participants in the trials [1]. Even cancers that are perceived as common, such as breast and colon cancer, have a lifetime risk of causing death of 3% to 4%. A reduction of this risk of 10% to 25% thus affects very few, especially as a limited age range is invited.

Small effects place high demands on the quality of the evidence, as they are particularly susceptible to being erased or created by bias. Indeed, the harms of screening, such as radiation from computed tomography (CT),

perforations during colonoscopy, invasive diagnostic work-up of false positive findings and harms of overtreatment of cancer lesions that would not cause mortality or morbidity, will inevitably increase the risk of dying from other causes, which counters some of the benefit. Although the major benefit of screening, avoiding death from the cancer screened for, is immensely important, the harms can also be substantial, sometimes even lethal, and often affect many more individuals.

This causes an ethical dilemma. We have to weigh the benefit of avoiding a cancer death in one individual against harm inflicted by screening in completely different, healthy individuals who cannot benefit. It requires a value judgment to decide whether the benefits outweigh the harms and whether screening is justifiable. This dilemma is further complicated by an overarching, deontological principle: *primum non nocere* (above all, do no harm).

While science can inform value judgments by quantifying the benefits and harms, it cannot make these choices for us and there are no scientifically 'correct' answers. But screening for some types of cancer clearly causes more good than harm, at a reasonable cost, others have been abandoned, either because they did not offer the benefits hoped for or because the harms were found to outweigh them. Yet others are currently being debated as the balance between benefits and harms is delicate and divides opinion.

HOW CANCER SCREENING WORKS

There are two ways in which cancer screening may work: earlier detection of cancer (secondary prevention) and detection of the precursors of cancer (primary prevention). Sometimes, both mechanisms are at play. Cervical cancer screening is primary prevention, as it relies on removal of cellular changes that have not yet developed into cancer and it can therefore reduce both incidence and mortality. Breast screening is generally regarded as secondary prevention, as it aims to detect cancer earlier and cannot reduce incidence. Detection of ductal carcinoma *in situ* (DCIS) is by some regarded as primary prevention but has not resulted in a decline in rates of invasive breast disease, and so does not appear to be effective in this regard. The nomenclature here is somewhat contradictory and certainly confusing, because if one regards DCIS as a carcinoma, its detection through screening cannot also be primary prevention, as cancer is not prevented from occurring.

To be effective, earlier detection requires that screen detection can happen prior to metastases occurring. Some tumours metastasize when they are under the threshold for detection and the difference in size between screen-detected and clinically detected tumours is sometimes small. The value of earlier detection may therefore have been overstated, at least for some cancers. In addition, earlier detection often leads to the discovery of cancers that would never have progressed to become symptomatic or lethal (overdiagnosis). Secondary prevention therefore often leads to increased population incidence, as indeed it has in the case of breast cancer.

BIAS IN OBSERVATIONAL SCREENING STUDIES

Selection bias

It is tempting to compare disease-specific mortality in attendees versus non-attendees in screening, or in screen-detected versus clinically detected cancers. But the temptation should generally be resisted. Attendees and non-attendees are not immediately comparable, as attendees are predominantly the 'healthy, well-educated, affluent, physically fit, fruit and vegetable-eating non-smokers with long-lived parents' [2]. Attendees are therefore more likely to survive many kinds of disease, including cancer. This has been called the 'healthy screenee effect', a selection bias, similar to the healthy worker effect, and it is difficult to compensate reliably for, as its impact varies between settings and over time. Such studies are therefore expected to come out in favour of screening, even when screening has no benefit. The healthy screenee effect also means that screening is likely to increase social inequality in health, as attendees are those resourceful enough to worry about their future health.

Length bias

Screening selectively picks up cancers with a favourable prognosis because there is more time to detect a slow-growing cancer than a fast-growing one and studies that compare screen-detected with clinically detected cancers suffer from what is called length bias. These studies therefore also fail to compare like with like and predictably come out in favour of screening. Accurately correcting for length bias is impossible, especially when some of the screen-detected lesions are overdiagnosed cases that would never have caused symptoms or death, as such cases invariably have an excellent prognosis.

Lead time bias

A third bias also affects studies of screening effects: lead time bias. If screening successfully moves forward the time of diagnosis, patients will live longer with the diagnosis, regardless of whether they live to an older age. This bias means that the commonly used measure of effect in cancer treatment, survival time from diagnosis, becomes misleading and should not be used when assessing the efficacy of screening. Lead time bias is also important in studies that assess overdiagnosis. Screening is meant to increase incidence when it is introduced, as cancers that would have been detected at a later date are now detected earlier. In fact, if an incidence increase does not occur, screening has likely failed. But some of the incidence increase is caused by very slow-growing tumours that would never have caused problems, tumours that do not grow at all and sometimes tumours that regress [3]. Lead time estimates could in theory be used to calculate what proportion of the incidence increase that is due to the desired advancement of diagnosis and what proportion is due to overdiagnosis. The problem is that lead time is difficult to quantify and it has often been overestimated, which causes underestimates of overdiagnosis [4]. It may be further complicated by the fact that lead time may vary with the age cohort screened, as may be the case with breast cancer.

These biases are part of the reason that randomized trials are required prior to the implementation of cancer screening.

INFORMED CHOICE IN CANCER SCREENING

The information provided with an invitation to screening is often sparse. The benefits are exaggerated and harms either downplayed or not mentioned [5]. In addition, invitations often contain recommendations to attend, a pre-specified date of appointment, and invitations seem designed to make more people attend [5]. This practice may be based on good intentions, but it is paternalistic. After much criticism, the UK leaflet informing women about the benefits and harms of breast screening was revised in 2012. While the new leaflet was an improvement as it mentions overdiagnosis, it has important shortcomings and a pre-specified date of appointment is still included. This short-circuits the decision process, as it sends the message that breast screening is important, supported by a public authority, and that one is expected to attend. It also increases the risk that those who decline are left with a feeling of guilt, particularly if they are later diagnosed, which is an underappreciated harm of screening. Informed decisions in breast screening require that it is made explicitly clear that a genuine choice has to be made, that harms may outweigh benefits and that there are important, avoidable harms. These concerns are becoming more pressing in breast screening because, as we will see, it seems less attractive today than was initially hoped.

True informed choice is exceedingly hard to obtain. Providing thorough information on benefits and harms, quantified in absolute numbers so that they can be compared, is both necessary and an ethical prerequisite for screening, but requires time and resources and does not guarantee informed decisions. Most invitees will choose based on 'what they feel is right', rather than on facts and figures [6]. Providing the information does not free those who offer screening from responsibility.

CANCER SCREENING THAT MAY REDUCE BOTH INCIDENCE AND MORTALITY (PRIMARY PREVENTION)

Cervical cancer screening

Forty years ago, Archie Cochrane, after whom the Cochrane Collaboration is named, eloquently described the problems with cervical cancer screening [7]. He criticized that the programme began without evidence from randomized trials. The underlying hypothesis was simply assumed to be correct, and trials were considered 'unethical'. He described how mortality from cervical cancer was declining in many countries before screening and continued to decline largely unchanged after implementation. This makes it impossible to accurately quantify benefits and harms, both of which he believed existed. He also called into question whether the strategy of spending millions of pounds on a relatively rare though severe disease was an optimal one.

Cervical cancer screening was instrumental in prompting the WHO to commission the report in which Wilson and Jungner formulated 10 classic criteria for screening implementation, shown in Table 4.1. In 1968, they wrote: 'In theory, screening is an admirable method of combating disease … [but] in practice, there are snags. The central idea of early disease detection and treatment is essentially simple. However, the path to its successful achievement … is far from simple though sometimes it may appear deceptively easy' [8].

The situation in Denmark is similar to that in many other countries in the Western world. Screening began in the late 1960s, but mortality from cervical cancer had peaked 10 years earlier [9]. Incidence, however, increased

Table 4.1 Wilson and Jungner classic screening criteria

1. The condition sought should be an important health problem.
2. There should be an accepted treatment for patients with recognized disease.
3. Facilities for diagnosis and treatment should be available.
4. There should be a recognizable latent or early symptomatic stage.
5. There should be a suitable test or examination.
6. The test should be acceptable to the population.
7. The natural history of the condition, including development from latent to declared disease, should be adequately understood.
8. There should be an agreed policy on whom to treat as patients.
9. The cost of case-finding (including diagnosis and treatment of patients diagnosed) should be economically balanced in relation to possible expenditure on medical care as a whole.
10. Case-finding should be a continuing process and not a 'once and for all' project.

Source: From Wilson JMG, Jungner G, *Principles and Practice of Screening for Disease*, Geneva: World Health Organization, 1968, available from http://www.who.int/bulletin/volumes/86/4/07-050112BP.pdf

until the introduction of screening, culminating at 34 cases per 100,000 women, after which a sharp declined commenced [9]. It is tempting to attribute this decline to screening, but to reduce cancer incidence, screening must detect cervical intraepithelial neoplasia (CIN) and prevent its development into invasive cancer. With a 20-year latency period from infection to cancer [9], other factors than screening must have contributed as they did for mortality, and one cannot simply ascribe the reductions entirely to screening. Similar declines were also seen in stomach cancer (which is also of infectious origin but has no screening programme in the Western world), well before the advent of antibiotic therapy for ulcer disease. Separating the effect of screening from environmental factors and improved therapy is a common challenge in cancer screening.

Randomized trials in India have compared screening for cervical cancer with no screening and shown a benefit, though not as large as reductions observed in the population in general. Screening was offered to 224,929 women, while 138,624 served as controls [10]. Two-hundred fifty-four in the control arm and 327 in the intervention arm died from cervical cancer, a 21% reduction (95% confidence interval [CI] –23% to –7%; author's calculation) [10]. Transferring this result to other settings and screening methods is challenging, but the main problem was ethical concerns regarding whether it was acceptable for the US National Cancer Institute and the Bill and Melinda Gates Foundation to fund such trials, given that the intervention was known to reduce mortality [10,11].

Quantification of the benefit is important, because there are important harms, which are increasing with more sensitive tests, while vaccinations against human papilloma virus (HPV) may reduce the benefit over coming decades as the incidence of the disease falls. Many screened women will be recalled for further testing because results were inadequate, unclear or abnormalities were found. The vast majority will not have cancer, but recalls cause psychological stress. Based on an expected 60% mortality reduction with screening in the UK, it has been estimated that 1000 women should be screened for 35 years to avoid one death, requiring 7700 tests to be performed, resulting in 152 women with abnormal results at repeat testing, 53 biopsies confirming abnormalities, of which 17 would persist and lead to unnecessary cone excisions [12].

Overtreatment is inevitable as more than 80% of abnormalities would never develop into life-threatening disease [12]. Cone excisions negatively affect fertility and weaken the cervix, increasing the risk of premature delivery, and they may cause pain and sexual problems, as well as psychological harms [13].

Cervical cancer is a comparatively rare cause of death, with 75 fatalities among 5.6 million Danes in 2011, down from 344 in 1966 [9], and the costs and harms of initiatives to bring down mortality further must be considered. Liquid-based cytology has increased the referral and colposcopy rate [9], and while randomized trials that compared cytology-based screening with the addition of HPV testing have shown a reduction of 40% (95% CI –60% to –11%) in the incidence of invasive cervical cancer [14], HPV testing may increase overtreatment [15]. A 40% reduction in incidence seems impressive but translates into 25 fewer cases over 6.5 years in about half of the 176,464 included women [14] (author's calculation). The mortality reduction is unknown, but some avoided cancers would also have been treatable in the absence of HPV testing.

Invited age ranges and screening intervals vary and should be continuously re-evaluated; e.g. the recommendation from the US Preventive Services Task Force in 2012 extended screening intervals and raised the age at first screen to 21 years [13]. Perhaps the most pressing question is whether those vaccinated for HPV at a young age should be screened, and if so, at which interval and ages. However, a reduction in cervical cancer mortality with the vaccine has not been shown and will take 20–30 years to appear. Hopefully, the disease will become so rare that subjecting all women to the harms of screening, and society to the costs (£198 million per year in the UK [16]), will not be feasible. Establishing optimal screening intervals and age ranges is best done through randomized trials within established screening programmes.

Colorectal cancer screening

Colonoscopy and sigmoidoscopy screening is intended as primary prevention to find and remove polyps before they develop into cancer. Faecal occult blood testing (FOBT) is secondary prevention intended to find invasive cancers at an earlier stage. Polyps do not commonly bleed as cancers do and are therefore mostly incidental findings with FOBT, and reduced incidence is not expected.

While sigmoidoscopy screening and FOBT have not been tested directly against each other, they have been tested individually against no screening. Screening with sigmoidoscopy has been tested in five randomized trials (414,747 participants) and FOBT in four (329,614 participants) [17]. The reduction in disease-specific mortality with FOBT was 14% (95% CI –20% to –8%) and 28% (95% CI –35% to –21%) with sigmoidoscopy [17]. A Cochrane review indirectly compared the interventions in a network meta-analysis and the difference was slightly too small to be statistically significant, but results published since then have confirmed the difference [18]. Additionally, sigmoidoscopy reduced the incidence of cancer by 18% (95% CI –27% to –10%) while FOBT did not (–5%, 95% CI –12% to 2%) [17]. Again, the difference was not statistically significant, but updated results have confirmed it [18]. A further benefit with sigmoidoscopy is that only one test is needed, while FOBT requires 10–12 tests over 20–25 years. Sigmoidoscopy, however, is arguably even less appealing than stool sampling, which may affect uptake outside the setting of the randomized trials.

Many would likely prefer a test that reduces the risk of getting cancer, rather than 'only' reducing the risk of dying from it, especially when the risk of dying is further reduced as well. Regardless, FOBT is widely used in Europe. One possible explanation is that sigmoidoscopy screening was tested only after the decision to introduce FOBT in many countries. Since the trials, more sensitive FOBT tests have become available, but increased sensitivity may lead to a less favourable balance between the benefits and harms, as it may increase unnecessary testing more than it reduces disease-specific mortality [19].

Despite including several hundred thousand individuals, the trials of neither FOBT (relative risk 1.00, 95% CI 0.99–1.01) nor sigmoidoscopy screening (relative risk 0.98, 95% CI 0.95–1.01) influenced total mortality [17]. The effect of FOBT translates into 1 avoided death from colorectal cancer per 1000 subjects invited, while total mortality in the study period was 250 per 1000 [17]. Participation in most cancer screening will not measurably extend life for the average-risk person. In individuals with familial adenomatous polyposis (FAP) and hereditary non-polyposis colorectal cancer (HNPCC), where the underlying risk is much higher, it does.

As for cancer screening in general [20], harms were poorly documented in the trials and the psychological harms were particularly poorly investigated [17]. Overtreatment of polyps is likely less problematic than overdetection and overtreatment of invasive cancers, such as in breast and prostate cancer screening. But bleeding or death due to follow-up investigations with colonoscopy has implications for screening using this modality, common in North America. The US Preventive Services Task Force recommends screening with colonoscopy every 10 years between ages 50 and 75, although there are no randomized trials. The task force notes that serious harms occur in 2.8 per 1000 colonoscopies and that this risk is 10 times smaller with sigmoidoscopy [19]. An indirect comparison of observational studies of colonoscopy with randomized trials of sigmoidoscopy indicated that colonoscopy reduces mortality from proximal colorectal cancers, as well as from distal cancers [21], but observational studies have poor reliability in screening. Randomized trials that directly compare sigmoidoscopy with colonoscopy screening would be highly desirable.

CANCER SCREENING THAT MAY REDUCE MORTALITY BUT INCREASE INCIDENCE (SECONDARY PREVENTION)

Prostate cancer screening

Recommendations for prostate cancer screening with prostate-specific antigen (PSA) vary between countries and have changed considerably in recent years. The PSA test was intended to monitor growth and recurrence of prostate cancer, and its use for screening purposes was described by the discoverer, Richard J. Ablin, as a 'hugely expensive public health disaster', costing $3 billion per year in the United States [22].

Prostate cancer is the most common cancer in men. Autopsy studies indicate that if a man lives 100 years, he has a 100% risk of harbouring changes in his prostate that fulfil the pathological criteria for cancer [23]. Yet, the lifetime risk of being diagnosed is closely related to the use of PSA screening and is highest in the US, at about 16% [23], while the lifetime risk of dying from prostate cancer is about 3% [24]. Evidently, there is a large reservoir of cancer pathology that can be detected with screening, and incidence in the US and elsewhere has risen sharply with more testing and decreasing thresholds for PSA levels [23]. The test has caused massive overdiagnosis and overtreatment of lesions that would never have led to symptoms or death, which has diminished enthusiasm. Also, PSA can be elevated for a number of benign reasons, leading to false positive tests. Cancer must be excluded, often through biopsy, causing anxiety, pain and infections, apart from being genuinely unpleasant and having no benefit.

Two randomized trials were published in 2009 and summarized in a Cochrane review. One was performed in North America and showed no reduction in prostate cancer mortality (relative risk 1.13, 95% CI 0.75–1.70), but had contamination of the control group [25]. The second study was performed in Europe [26] and showed a 20% (relative risk 0.80%, 95% CI 0.65–0.98) reduction in prostate cancer mortality, but with widely varying results between contributing centres, from a large benefit in Sweden to no effect in Finland. For each man who avoided dying from prostate cancer, 47 men were diagnosed with a prostate cancer that would never have harmed them or come to attention without screening (overdiagnosis) [27]. Practically all of them received treatment, which include prostatectomy, radiotherapy and chemotherapy. This is painful and more than half become incontinent, impotent or suffer other sexual problems such as anorgasmia, with no benefit. Reduced mortality rates in the US with widespread screening could indicate some benefit, but improved therapy and increased disease awareness make interpretation difficult [23].

Screening for prostate cancer may be relevant in high-risk groups, such as men of African origin who have first-degree relatives with prostate cancer diagnosed at a young age. However, the test should only be offered after a thorough discussion of the uncertainties, benefits and harms, which should be disclosed in full, including that screening of high-risk men has not been tested in randomized trials. The PSA test is currently not justified for screening average-risk men at any age as standard practice.

Breast cancer screening

The debate around breast screening is heated and long-running. The benefits have been questioned and overdiagnosis has surfaced as a major concern. In 2009, the US Preventive Services Task Force recommended that the interval between screening rounds should be extended from 1 to 2 years and that women in their forties should no longer routinely be screened [28]. This is in line with European practice over decades, but the Task Force was met with fierce criticism in the US [29]. In the UK, sustained criticism and concerns about overdiagnosis led to the establishment of a panel of experts in various relevant topics who had not previously worked in the field of screening, in an attempt to avoid conflict of interest. Their review was published in 2012 and has been important in recognizing overdiagnosis as a serious harm. The authors estimated that screening causes three women to receive an unnecessary breast cancer diagnosis for every one woman who avoids a breast cancer death, but still considered the programme justified and recommended its continuation [30]. The estimated benefit was based on data from a Cochrane review [31], but unlike the Cochrane review, the authors of the Marmot report assumed that all trials that had contributed data were equally reliable [30]. While their estimated 20% reduction in disease-specific mortality is lower than that which formed the basis for the introduction of breast screening, it is still more optimistic than the estimate from the Cochrane review that 10 women are overdiagnosed for each woman who avoids dying from breast cancer [31].

Like all Cochrane reviews, the review on breast screening used standardized, empirically based quality criteria to assess the risk of bias in each trial (the Cochrane risk of bias tool) and found important differences, which was expected, as some trials showed large benefits and others none (Figure 4.1) [31]. When trials were assessed in sensitivity analyses, those with a low risk of bias showed little or no benefit, whereas trials with a high risk of bias showed large effects. The standardized approach to dealing with such a situation is clearly stated in the GRADE handbook; one should exclude the results of the trials at high risk of bias and consider only the results from the trials of low

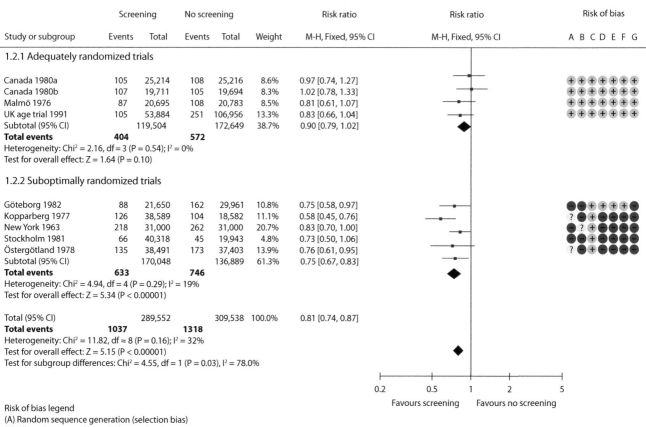

| Study or subgroup | Screening | | No screening | | | Risk ratio | Risk ratio | Risk of bias |
	Events	Total	Events	Total	Weight	M-H, Fixed, 95% CI	M-H, Fixed, 95% CI	A B C D E F G
1.2.1 Adequately randomized trials								
Canada 1980a	105	25,214	108	25,216	8.6%	0.97 [0.74, 1.27]		
Canada 1980b	107	19,711	105	19,694	8.3%	1.02 [0.78, 1.33]		
Malmö 1976	87	20,695	108	20,783	8.5%	0.81 [0.61, 1.07]		
UK age trial 1991	105	53,884	251	106,956	13.3%	0.83 [0.66, 1.04]		
Subtotal (95% CI)		119,504		172,649	38.7%	0.90 [0.79, 1.02]		
Total events	**404**		**572**					

Heterogeneity: Chi² = 2.16, df = 3 (P = 0.54); I² = 0%
Test for overall effect: Z = 1.64 (P = 0.10)

1.2.2 Suboptimally randomized trials								
Göteborg 1982	88	21,650	162	29,961	10.8%	0.75 [0.58, 0.97]		
Kopparberg 1977	126	38,589	104	18,582	11.1%	0.58 [0.45, 0.76]		
New York 1963	218	31,000	262	31,000	20.7%	0.83 [0.70, 1.00]		
Stockholm 1981	66	40,318	45	19,943	4.8%	0.73 [0.50, 1.06]		
Östergötland 1978	135	38,491	173	37,403	13.9%	0.76 [0.61, 0.95]		
Subtotal (95% CI)		170,048		136,889	61.3%	0.75 [0.67, 0.83]		
Total events	**633**		**746**					

Heterogeneity: Chi² = 4.94, df = 4 (P = 0.29); I² = 19%
Test for overall effect: Z = 5.34 (P < 0.00001)

Total (95% CI)		289,552		309,538	100.0%	0.81 [0.74, 0.87]		
Total events	**1037**		**1318**					

Heterogeneity: Chi² = 11.82, df = 8 (P = 0.16); I² = 32%
Test for overall effect: Z = 5.15 (P < 0.00001)
Test for subgroup differences: Chi² = 4.55, df = 1 (P = 0.03), I² = 78.0%

0.2   0.5   1   2   5
Favours screening   Favours no screening

Risk of bias legend
(A) Random sequence generation (selection bias)
(B) Allocation concealment (selection bias)
(C) Blinding of participants and personal (performance bias)
(D) Blinding of outcome assessment (detection bias)
(E) Incomplete outcome data (attrition bias)
(F) Selective reporting (reporting bias)
(G) Other bias

Figure 4.1 Forest plot and Cochrane Risk of Bias table for randomized trials of breast screening. (From Gøtzsche PC and Jørgensen KJ, *Cochrane Database Syst Rev*, 2013, 6, CD001877.)

risk of bias, as including studies of high risk of bias in the meta-analysis will lower the confidence in the estimated effect [32]. This is a cause for concern, and empirical evidence from ongoing breast screening programmes has added to this. For breast screening to be effective, it must reduce the rate of late stage cancers, but this seems not to be happening to any appreciable extent [33]. Observational studies with a 'control group' due to the staggered introduction of screening within countries [34–36], or comparisons of breast cancer mortality in similar countries that have introduced screening early or late [37], indicate that breast screening has contributed little to the substantial reductions in breast cancer mortality seen over the past decades. In Europe, the risk of dying from breast cancer has declined by about 50% in age groups below the screening age, while a 35% reduction in breast cancer–specific mortality was seen in the age group commonly invited for screening [38]. This means that factors other than screening, such as improved medical therapy, which has been more commonly used in younger age groups than older ones, can explain much of the observed reduction.

Screening has caused significant increases in the incidence of breast cancer wherever it has been introduced, which have not been compensated by later declines in incidence, despite decades with screening [39] (Figure 4.2). This is a hallmark of interventions that cause overdiagnosis. In addition to overtreatment with surgery, radiotherapy and chemotherapy, which can increase mortality from other causes, breast screening causes psychological harm in many women who experience false positive results. After 10 screening rounds, one-third of invited women will experience a false positive test [40].

Taking the quality of the individual trials into account and including information from observational studies, an expert panel under the Swiss Medical Board concluded in 2014 that breast screening was not justified as the harms outweighed the benefits, and that it should therefore not be introduced on a national basis [41]. Contrary to the UK, there is no national breast screening programme in Switzerland, where some cantons have organized screening and others not. Cantons with breast screening were recommended to end it [41].

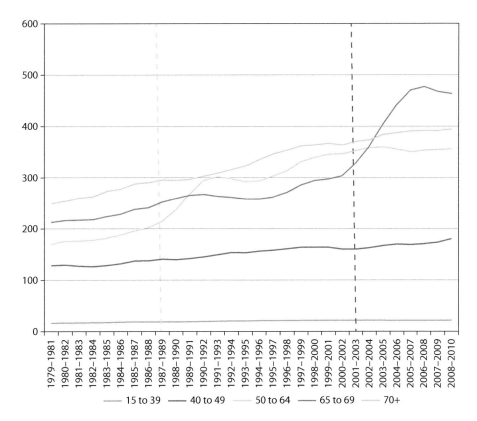

Figure 4.2 Incidence of invasive breast cancer and ductal carcinoma *in situ* combined in the UK. The vertical dotted lines indicate the introduction of breast screening in women aged 50 to 64 (green) and the extension to include women aged 65 to 70 (purple). (Data from Cancer Research UK: http://www.cancerresearchuk.org/health-professional/cancer-statistics/statistics-by-cancer-type/breast-cancer/incidence-invasive and http://www.cancerresearchuk.org/health-professional/cancer-statistics/statistics-by-cancer-type/breast-cancer/incidence-in-situ [accessed September 2015].)

Compared with the randomized trials 30 to 40 years ago, improved treatment has substantially reduced the absolute benefit of breast screening and the higher sensitivity of digital mammography, extending the age range to older women, and computer-assisted detection has increased the rate of overdiagnosis. Over the coming years, the acknowledgment of smaller benefits and greater harms than originally hoped for may change recommendations for breast screening, as it has in prostate cancer screening.

Lung cancer screening

Lung cancer has the highest mortality of almost any cancer and screening can be focused on a high-risk group: smokers. It therefore appears to be an obvious target disease for screening.

Despite this, screening for lung cancer using chest X-rays does more harm than good [42]. It did not reduce mortality from lung cancer but caused morbidity and mortality through diagnostic work-up of suspicious findings, many of which were harmless, and overdiagnosis of cancers that would not have caused morbidity and mortality. Smoking substantially increases morbidity and mortality from many other causes, which means that slow-growing cancers can be overdiagnosed, as attendees are more likely to

die prematurely. They are also more vulnerable to complications from surgery.

Based on four randomized trials, the US Preventive Services Task Force recommended annual screening for lung cancer with low-dose computed tomography (LDCT) [43]. The largest trial was the National Lung Screening Trial (NLST), which compared screening with LDCT to screening with chest X-rays in >50,000 people. It found a reduction in lung cancer mortality of 20% (95% CI −26.7% to −6.8%) after being stopped early at 6.5 years [43]. One of the main problems with this type of screening is the identification of incidental abnormalities which cause concern and may trigger further tests but result in no benefit. The ethical justification for the choice of comparator in the NLST trials can be questioned, especially as it makes a quantification of overdiagnosis impossible, but also as an intervention known not to be beneficial where used as a comparator. A Cochrane review recommended better quantification of harms and costs before introduction [42].

The costs are considerable and may be used more effectively on interventions with fewer harms. Smoking causes many more deaths from cardiovascular diseases, chronic obstructive pulmonary disease and other causes than lung cancer. Efforts to reduce tobacco use through increased prices are an effective means to obtain this.

CANCER SCREENING THAT DOES NOT REDUCE MORTALITY OR INCIDENCE

Ovarian cancer screening and screening for neuroblastoma in children illustrate the importance of doing randomized trials prior to the implementation of cancer screening, regardless of how appealing the theory and motivation to 'do something' may be. Screening for neuroblastoma was introduced in Japan prior to randomized trials. It is a solid abdominal tumour in children that can be detected with a urine test. Subsequently, two randomized trials showed no reduction in disease-specific mortality, but that twice as many children were diagnosed with cancer in the screened group [44,45]. The extra cancers would have spontaneously regressed, which is known to happen for this cancer. However, the ensuing overtreatment was harmful. Three of 149 diagnosed children in one of the studies died from complications to treatment, and screening caused substantial unnecessary worry. It is not known how many children in Japan were harmed by the programme.

A randomized trial was performed prior to introduction of ovarian cancer screening. This has likely avoided much harm and expense, at little or no cost in terms of avoided ovarian cancer deaths. The trial screened average-risk women with transvaginal ultrasound and the tumour marker CA-125 and showed a relative risk of ovarian cancer death of 1.18 (95% CI 0.82–1.71) [46]. After a median of 12.4 years following randomization, the trial was stopped as it had reached its 'boundary of futility'. There was no reduction in late stage tumours, but 3285 of the 34,253 women randomized to screening had a false positive result, for which 1080 had surgery and 15% of whom had at least one major complication, such as infection or cardiac or pulmonary complications. The UK Collaborative Trial of Ovarian Cancer Screening has randomized more than 200,000 women and results are expected in 2015 [46].

CONCLUSION

The value of earlier detection of cancer through screening is easily overestimated, but the desirable effect is small and the intuitive appeal is deceptive. Screening should not be undertaken without solid evidence that benefits outweigh harms, at a reasonable cost. It rarely saves resources, as those who avoid dying from the disease screened for will invariably die from another disease later on, the treatment of which also requires resources. The high cost of screening is not necessarily an argument against it, but even when benefits outweigh harms, screening should be compared to other interventions. Distributive justice and the harms that screening inflicts in healthy attendees should be at the forefront of considerations to spend resources most effectively, and on those who need them the most.

REFERENCES

1. Saquib N, Saquib J, Ioannidis J. Does screening for disease save lives in asymptomatic adults? Systematic review of meta-analyses and randomized trials. *Int J Epidemiol* 2015; doi: 10.1093/ije/dyu140.
2. Raffle AE, Gray M. *Screening: Evidence and Practise.* Oxford: Oxford University Press, 2007.
3. Zahl PH, Mæhlen J, Welch HG. The natural history of breast cancers detected by screening mammography. *Arch Intern Med* 2008;168:2311–6.
4. Gøtzsche PC, Mæhlen J, Jørgensen KJ, Zahl PH. Estimation of lead-time and overdiagnosis in breast cancer screening. *Br J Cancer* 2009;100;219.
5. Jørgensen KJ, Gøtzsche PC. Content of invitations for publicly funded screening mammography. *BMJ* 2006;332:538–41.
6. Loewenstein GF, Weber EU, Hsee CK, Welch N. Risk as feelings. *Psychol Bull* 2001;127(2):267–86.
7. Cochrane AL. *Effectiveness and Efficiency – Random Reflections on Health Services.* Chichester, UK: John Wiley & Sons, 2013.
8. Wilson JMG, Jungner G. *Principles and Practice of Screening for Disease.* Geneva: World Health Organization, 1968. Available from http://www.who.int/bulletin/volumes/86/4/07-050112BP.pdf (accessed 30 January 2015).
9. Lynge E, Rygaard C, Vazquez-Prada M, et al. Cervical cancer screening at crossroads. *Acta Pathol Microbiol Immunol Scand* 2014;122:667–73.
10. Suba EJ. US-funded measurements of cervical cancer death rates in India: scientific and ethical concerns. *Indian J Med Ethics* 2014;11(3):167–75.
11. Bagcchi S. Cervical cancer screening trials in India spark controversy. *BMJ* 2014;348:g3038.
12. Raffle AE, Alden B, Quinn M, et al. Outcomes of screening to prevent cancer: analysis of cumulative incidence of cervical abnormality and modeling of cases and deaths prevented. *BMJ* 2003;326:901–5.
13. National Cancer Institute. Pap and HPV testing. Available from http://www.cancer.gov/cancertopics/factsheet/detection/Pap-HPV-testing (accessed 30 January 2015).
14. Ronco G, Dillner J, Elfström KM, et al. Efficacy of HPV-based screening for prevention of invasive cervical cancer: follow-up of four European randomized controlled trials. *Lancet* 2014;383;524–32.
15. Malila N, Leinonen M, Kotaniemi-Talonen, et al. The HPV test has similar sensitivity but more overdiagnosis than the Pap test – a randomized health services study on cervical cancer screening in Finland. *Int J Cancer* 2013;132:2141–7.
16. Raffle AE. Challenges of implementing human papillomavirus (HPV) vaccination policy. *BMJ* 2007;335:375–7.

17. Holme Ø, Bretthauer M, Fretheim A, Odgaard-Jensen J, Hoff G. Flexible sigmoidoscopy versus faecal occult blood testing for colorectal cancer screening in asymptomatic individuals. *Cochrane Database Syst Rev* 2013;9:CD009259.

18. Holme Ø, Løberg M, Kalager M, et al. Effect of flexible sigmoidoscopy screening on colorectal cancer incidence and mortality: a randomized clinical trial. *JAMA* 2014;312:606–15.

19. Whitlock EP, Lin JS, Liles E, et al. *Final evidence summary: colorectal cancer: screening.* Rockville, MD: U.S. Preventive Services Task Force, 2008. Available from http://www.uspreventiveservices-taskforce.org/Page/SupportingDoc/colorectal-cancer-screening/final-evidence-summary4 (accessed 30 January 2015).

20. Heleno B, Thomsen MF, Rodrigues D, et al. Quantification of harms in cancer screening trials: literature review. *BMJ* 2013;347:f5334.

21. Brenner H, Stock C, Hoffmeister M. Effect of screening sigmoidoscopy and screening colonoscopy on colorectal cancer incidence and mortality: systematic review and meta-analysis of randomized controlled trials and observational studies. *BMJ* 2014;348:g2467.

22. Ablin RJ. The great prostate mistake. *New York Times*, 9 March 2010. Available from http://www.nytimes.com/2010/03/10/opinion/10Ablin.html?_r=0 (accessed 30 January 2015).

23. Hass GP, Delongchamps N, Brawley OW, et al. The worldwide epidemiology of prostate cancer: perspectives from autopsy studies. *Can J Urol* 2008;15:3866–71.

24. American Cancer Society. What are the key statistics about prostate cancer? Available from www.cancer.org/Cancer/ProstateCancer/DetailedGuide/prostate-cancer-keystatistics (accessed 30 January 2015).

25. Andriole GL, Grubb RL, Buys SS, et al. Mortality results from a randomized prostate-cancer screening trial. *N Engl J Med* 2009;360:1310–9.

26. Schröder FH, Hugosson J, Roobol MJ, et al. Screening and prostate-cancer mortality in a randomized European study. *N Engl J Med* 2009;360:1320–8.

27. Ilic D, Neuberger MM, Djulbegovic M, Dahm P. Screening for prostate cancer. *Cochrane Database Syst Rev* 2013;1:CD004720.

28. U.S. Preventive Services Task Force. Screening for breast cancer: U.S. Preventive Services Task Force recommendation statement. *Ann Intern Med* 2009;151:716–26.

29. Kopans DB. The recent US Preventive Services Task Force guidelines are not supported by the scientific evidence and should be rescinded. *J Am Coll Radiol* 2010;7:260–4.

30. Marmot M, Altman DG, Cameron DA, et al. The benefits and harms of breast cancer screening: an independent review. *Br J Cancer* 2013;108:2205–40.

31. Gøtzsche PC, Jørgensen KJ. Screening for breast cancer with mammography. *Cochrane Database Syst Rev* 2013;6:CD001877.

32. Shünemann H, Brozek J, Guyatt G, Oxman A, editors. GRADE handbook for grading quality of evidence and strength of recommendations. The GRADE Working Group, 2013. Available from www.guidelinedevelopment.org/handbook)

33. Autier P, Boniol M, Middleton R, et al. Advanced breast cancer incidence following population-based mammographic screening. *Ann Oncol* 2011;22:1726–35.

34. Jørgensen KJ, Zahl PH, Gøtzsche PC. Breast cancer mortality in organised mammography screening in Denmark. A comparative study. *BMJ* 2010;340:c1241.

35. Kalager M, Zelen M, Langmark F, Adami HO. Effect of screening mammography on breast-cancer mortality in Norway. *N Engl J Med* 2010;363:1203–10.

36. Olsen AH, Lynge E, Njor SH, et al. Breast cancer mortality in Norway after the introduction of mammography screening. *Int J Cancer* 2013;132:208–14.

37. Autier P, Boniol M, Gavin A, Vatten LJ. Breast cancer mortality in neighbouring European countries with different levels of screening but similar access to treatment: trend analysis of WHO mortality database. *BMJ* 2011;343:d4411.

38. Autier P, Boniol M, LaVecchia C, et al. Disparities in breast cancer mortality trends between 30 European countries: retrospective trend analysis of WHO mortality database. *BMJ* 2010;341:c3620.

39. Jørgensen KJ, Gøtzsche PC. Overdiagnosis in publicly organised mammography screening programmes: systematic review of incidence trends. *BMJ* 2009;339:b2587.

40. Elmore JG, Barton MB, Moceri VM, et al. Ten-year risk of false positive screening mammograms and clinical breast examinations. *N Engl J Med* 1998;338:1089–96.

41. Swiss Medical Board. Systemisches Mammographie – screening. Available from http://www.medical-board.ch/fileadmin/docs/public/mb/Fachberichte/2013-12-15_Bericht_Mammographie_Final_rev.pdf (accessed 30 January 2015).

42. Manser R, Lethaby A, Irving LB, Stone C, Byrnes G, Abramson MJ, Campbell D. Screening for lung cancer. *Cochrane Database Syst Rev* 2013;6:CD001991.

43. Humphrey LL, Deffebach M, Pappas M, et al. Screening for lung cancer with low-dose computed tomography: a systematic review to update the U.S. Preventive Services Task Force recommendation.

Evidence summary: lung cancer: screening. Rockville, MD: U.S. Preventive Services Task Force, 2014. Available from http://www.uspreventiveservicestaskforce.org/Page/SupportingDoc/lung-cancer-screening/evidence-summary4 (accessed 30 January 2015).

44. Woods WG, Gao RN, Shuster JJ, et al. Screening of infants and mortality due to neuroblastoma. *N Engl J Med* 2002;346:172–7.

45. Schilling FH, Spix C, Berthold F, et al. Neuroblastoma screening at one year of age. *N Engl J Med* 2002;346:1047–53.

46. Danforth KN, Im TN, Whitlock EP. Addendum to screening for ovarian cancer: evidence update for the US Preventive Services Task Force Reaffirmation Recommendation Statement. Ovarian cancer: screening. Rockville, MD: U.S. Preventive Services Task Force, 2014. Available from http://www.uspreventiveservicestaskforce.org/Page/SupportingDoc/ovarian-cancer-screening/addendum-to-screening-for-ovarian-cancer-evidence-update-for-the-us-preventive-services-task-force-reaffirmation-recommendation-statement (accessed 30 January 2015).

5

Principles of radiation therapy for surgeons

SASKIA RADEMAKERS, JOHAN BUSSINK AND PHILIP POORTMANS

INTRODUCTION

Radiation oncology is an important treatment modality in the multimodality management of cancer patients. About half of all oncological patients will be treated with radiation at some point during the course of their disease. Basic knowledge of radiation oncology can assist the oncologic surgeon in multidisciplinary decision making and patient referral. In this chapter an overview is given of the general principles, technical aspects, side effects and specific indications for clinical radiation therapy.

The aim of radiation therapy is to effectively treat the tumour-bearing area while at the same time minimizing the effect of radiation on the surrounding normal tissues. For this purpose, it is of paramount importance to identify exactly the region where a precise dose of radiation should be delivered. It is indeed the sensitivity of the normal tissues that limits the amount of radiation that can be delivered without excessive early or significant late toxicity. To limit treatment-related toxicity, apart from the proper identification of the target volume, radiation will be delivered in a course of several small fractions of the total dose over a predetermined period of time to obtain tumour control with a low risk of serious side effects.

We typically recognize three major groups of indications for radiation therapy in the management of cancer:

1. A course of *radical* or *curative* radiation therapy is planned where the probability of long-term survival after adequate local or locoregional therapy is high, and some normal tissue side effects of therapy, although undesirable, may be acceptable in this setting. The main advantage of primary non-surgical management of cancer is organ preservation with good functional or cosmetic outcome, with, in some cases, the scope for subsequent surgical salvage in the event of local disease recurrence.

   Radiation therapy as a single-modality treatment is effective for the cure of several types of cancer, for example early stage laryngeal cancer, skin cancer and prostate cancer [1–3]. In many cases a systemic modality (most often chemotherapy) is concomitantly administered to improve response rates and outcome, for example in head and neck, anal, rectal, oesophageal, lung and cervical cancer [4–6]. Chemoradiation has especially been demonstrated to improve locoregional control, for example in anal cancer [6]. In cervical cancer, it increases both local and systemic control [4], over radiation therapy alone. This might be explained by the radiosensitizing effect of chemotherapy resulting in increased locoregional control and subsequently less systemic progression, or could reflect the systemic cytotoxic effects of chemotherapy.

2. A course of *preoperative* or *postoperative* radiation therapy is delivered as an adjunct to the primary management modality to improve overall treatment efficacy. In this setting, radiation treatment is usually planned with a curative intention. In early breast cancer for instance, lumpectomy followed by postoperative radiation therapy is a valid alternative to mastectomy, with at least equivalent overall survival rates [7].

   Preoperative radiation therapy is used to downsize the primary tumour, thereby making some irresectable tumours resectable, and to reduce local disease recurrences, for example in rectal cancer [8]. In general, when radiation treatment is combined with surgery, a lower dose suffices compared to radiation as the sole treatment. In addition, in some cases, like in breast cancer, less extensive surgery can be performed when combined with radiation therapy.

3. *Palliative* radiation therapy is given for control of symptoms such as pain, cough or haemoptysis, for prevention of symptoms such as impending paralysis, or for temporary arrest of tumour growth. Palliative radiation therapy does not aim to improve survival. In contrast to radical or postoperative radiation therapy, where treatment schedules usually last a few weeks, palliative treatment schedules are of a short duration to minimize the burden for the patient. The treatment schedule is primarily dictated by the patient's life expectancy, the site (influencing the possible short-term side effects) and the volume of the tumour to be irradiated.

The optimal radiation therapy schedule in all three situations depends on the goal of the treatment, the tumour type, the expected acute and late normal tissue toxicity and the patient's condition.

GENERAL PRINCIPLES OF RADIATION THERAPY

Mechanism of action

The most commonly used type of ionizing radiation in a clinical setting is high-energy electromagnetic or photon radiation. A linear accelerator can produce photon beams with energies varying from 4 to 25 MV. Interaction of these photons with tissue leads to ionizations by liberating electrons. Subsequently, the released electrons can cause clusters of ionizations in the DNA, disrupting the structure of the DNA and leading to mitotic cell kill if the DNA double-strand breaks are not repaired adequately. The presence of oxygen enhances the effect of radiation by fixating the DNA damage, thereby preventing the DNA repair process (the oxygen effect) [9].

Following irradiation, a number of cells are likely to remain metabolically functional and may proliferate for several generations before they eventually die. Radiation is considered to have achieved its goal, if the capacity to produce a continuously expanding progeny (or colony formation; clonogenicity) of cancer cells is abolished.

The dose is prescribed in units of gray (1 Gy = the absorption of 1 J/kg of matter), which is the radiation dose absorbed by the tissue.

Factors influencing local tumour control

The most important biological factors influencing tumour and normal tissue response to fractionated radiation therapy are known as the 5R's: redistribution, reoxygenation, repair, repopulation and intrinsic cell radiosensitivity [10,11].

The radiosensitivity of cells varies throughout the different phases of the cell cycle, with cells in the S phase being the most resistant and cells in the late G2 and M phases the most sensitive. The progression of cells that survive radiation from a radioresistant phase of the cell cycle to a radiation-sensitive phase (*redistribution*) a few hours after irradiation enhances the response of tumours to radiation therapy. Similarly, the improvement in oxygenation (*reoxygenation*) of hypoxic cancer cells that survive radiation also increases tumour sensitivity to radiation therapy. Hypoxia is a well-known mechanism of radiation resistance, and hypoxic areas are present in many solid tumours [12]. The combination of hypoxia-modifying agents with radiation therapy has resulted in an enhancement of the therapeutic index of radiation therapy in certain tumours and is an area of considerable interest and research [13,14].

Cellular *repair* of radiation damage and repopulation are pivotal processes in the normal tissue as a response to radiation to prevent serious damage. In the tumour most of the DNA damage is repaired as well, although repair capacity is often altered, as for example in BRCA-mutated tumours, compared to normal cells.

Certain types of rapidly proliferating cancers also demonstrate a marked increase in growth rate (15–20 times faster) after the start of the radiation course. This 'accelerated *repopulation*' becomes apparent about 3–5 weeks (depending on the tissue) after the start of treatment [15,16]. Consequently, prolongation of a planned course of irradiation beyond a certain period may have a negative impact on local control of disease. For example, with squamous cell carcinoma of head and neck treated with primary radiation therapy, it has been estimated that an extra 0.6 Gy per day is required to counterbalance the effects of accelerated repopulation, when the overall treatment time exceeds 28 days [16]. The last R represents the inherent difference in *radiation sensitivity* between cells from different tumours, which makes some tumours more radioresponsive than others. For example, seminomas and lymphomas, which have a high intrinsic radiosensitivity, require smaller doses of radiation to achieve local tumour control or palliation [17–19]. Intrinsic radiosensitivity is most likely related to the extent to which cell types differ in their capacity to repair DNA damage.

Finally, tumour volume is an important factor determining local control. Several explanations can be found for this observation. First, a larger tumour volume contains more clonogenic stem cells, requiring a higher radiation dose. Second, hypoxia is often more pronounced in large tumours. Last, surrounding normal tissue will limit the dose of radiation that can be delivered safely with a large radiation volume.

Rationale of fractionation

A course of radiation therapy usually consists of multiple fractions per week over several weeks. The fractionation of a radiation treatment is important to minimize adverse effects and is based on the difference in shape of the radiation cell survival curve between normal tissue and malignant tumours. The radiation cell survival curve depicts the fraction of surviving cells as a function of the absorbed dose. The model that is widely used to describe the radiation cell survival curve *in vitro* is the linear-quadratic (LQ) model (20). Mathematically it is represented by the formula $S = \exp(-\alpha D - \beta D^2)$. The shape of the cell survival curve *in vitro* differs per cell line studied. *In vitro*, the α/β ratio is defined as the dose at which the linear and quadratic components of the curve are equal. For normal tissues and tumours the α/β value is calculated from adverse effects (normal tissues) or tumour control (tumours) reported in clinical trials. In general, tumours have a higher α/β value than normal tissue. The spinal cord for example has an α/β value of 2, and is therefore highly sensitive to changes in radiation therapy fraction size. In clinical practice this means for the spinal cord that when a lower dose per fraction is used, a higher total dose can be administered safely. Most tumours and acute radiation reactions have an α/β value >6 and are less sensitive to changes in fraction size and more sensitive to shortening of the overall treatment time. Exceptions to this general rule are melanoma and breast and prostate tumours.

This difference in fractionation sensitivity between tumour and normal tissue late effects explains the beneficial effect of fractionation. Figure 5.1 shows for normal tissue fibrosis ($\alpha/\beta = 2$ Gy) and tumour control ($\alpha/\beta = 10$) the equivalent dose in fractions of 2 Gy for different doses per fraction with equal total dose. A larger dose per fraction has a more pronounced effect on fibrosis (tissues with low α/β, steeper curve) than on tumour control probability (TCP) (tissues with high α/β, flatter curve) [21].

With the LQ model different fractionation regimens can be compared in terms of effectiveness and risk of late toxicity. In this respect it is important to realize that the consequences of changing the fractionation schedule differ per tissue.

Dose–response relationships

TCP curves are often used to relate the radiation dose with clinical outcome. TCP curves approximate a sigmoid

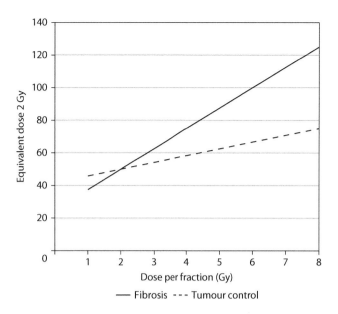

Figure 5.1 The equivalent dose in 2 Gy fractions for different doses per fraction, calculated with the linear-quadratic model for a total dose of 50 Gy. The dotted line represents tumour control with an α/β value of 10 Gy, and the solid line fibrosis with an α/β value of 2 Gy. A higher dose per fraction is detrimental for normal tissue complications.

shape (Figure 5.2), with a steep relationship between dose and TCP between 10% and 90% [22]. The shape and steepness of the TCP curve is affected by a number of factors, such as intrinsic radiosensitivity and heterogeneity in tumour cell kinetics [22,23]. The normal tissue complication probability (NTCP) curves are sigmoid shaped as well, depicting the relationship between radiation dose and probability of complications. To obtain a maximal therapeutic gain, the radiation therapy dose should result in maximal probability of tumour control combined with a minimal (or reasonably acceptable) likelihood of complications. In the ideal situation the TCP and NTCP curves are widely apart and tumour control can be achieved without complications. The separation between both curves is called the 'therapeutic window' [24].

A leftward shift of the TCP curve, resulting in a larger separation between the TCP and NTCP curves and a larger therapeutic gain, may result from factors such as smaller tumour burden or higher inherent tumour radiosensitivity. As illustrated in Figure 5.2, a worsening of the therapeutic index is seen with increase in tumour burden. In such situations, where the radiation dose needed to obtain tumour control is associated with a high probability of normal tissue toxicity, patients would be ideally managed with combination therapy, for example surgery followed by radiation therapy. In the situation of postoperative radiation therapy, when only subclinical disease is present, a lower radiation dose is required to eradicate the disease.

Time factor in radiation therapy

In radiation therapy treatment time is a crucial factor determining outcome. A prolongation of the overall treatment time is detrimental for tumour control rate (see also 'repopulation' in the 'Factors Influencing Local Tumour Control' section) [25] and shortening of the radiation course is applied to improve treatment results [26,27]. That is the reason that interruption of a radiation treatment should always be avoided. However, shortening of overall treatment time is associated with increased acute reactions and extreme acceleration is limited by acute toxicity [28].

Not only the duration of the radiation course is important, but also the total treatment time including surgery or chemotherapy should be kept as short as possible. In small cell lung cancer for example, overall survival is influenced by the time between start of chemotherapy and the end of radiation therapy [29]. The same principle applies to the time interval between surgery and radiation therapy, which should be kept as short as possible. Indirect evidence suggests that micrometastases grow at a faster rate than macroscopic disease [30]. Modelling studies based on clinical data have demonstrated that a delay in initiating postoperative treatment introduces a threshold in the dose–response curve of subclinical metastasis because existing subclinical cancer deposits continue to grow [30,31].

Clinical studies in squamous cell carcinoma of the head and neck have demonstrated that prolonging the interval between surgery and radiation therapy has an adverse effect on local control [32–34]. However, 1 day of interruption during postoperative radiation therapy has, most likely, a larger negative impact on TCP than 1 day of extension of the interval between surgery and radiation therapy [30,35]. These gaps in radiation therapy for subclinical disease may be detrimental from the first days of irradiation. Therefore, it is imperative that subsequent radiation therapy should be given as close as possible to the primary treatment and, even more important, that there is no prolongation of treatment, once it is initiated.

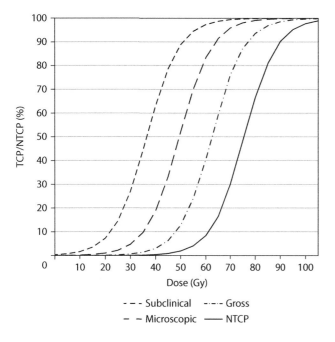

Figure 5.2 Theoretical curves showing the relationship between dose and tumour control probability in three situations: gross, microscopic and subclinical disease (dotted lines). The distance to the normal tissue complication rate curve (solid line) is called the therapeutic window.

RADIATION DELIVERY

External beam irradiation

External beam irradiation is the most applied technique of radiation delivery. Photon radiation produced by a linear accelerator is the most widespread type of external beam radiation therapy (EBRT). Photons can penetrate deeply into the patient and make all tumour locations accessible to irradiation. The higher the beam energy, the deeper is the penetration of the tissue. Each photon beam continues on its path beyond the tumour, so usually photon beams from different beam angles are directed to the target volume for more conformal treatment. This enables treatment of deeper-seated tumours with relative sparing of the skin and the surrounding normal tissue (Figure 5.3a). With modern techniques like intensity-modulated radiation therapy (IMRT), beam energies higher than 10 MV have no additional value and carry a few practical disadvantages in treatment planning and radiation shielding.

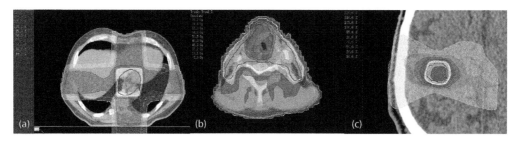

Figure 5.3 Examples of external beam radiation planning: (a) 3D-conformal radiation therapy, (b) intensity-modulated radiation therapy (IMRT) and (c) stereotactic radiation therapy. Colours represent the various isodose levels. The 95% isodose (yellow) encompasses the planning target volume (red line).

Superficial tumours can benefit from electron beam irradiation. An electron beam has a steeper fall-off in penetration depth than photon beam irradiation, relatively sparing the normal tissue behind the target volume. The depth of penetration can be controlled very well by the energy of the beam.

More recently proton irradiation, a form of particle therapy, has raised interest. The advantage of proton beam irradiation is the high dose peak (Bragg peak) at a certain depth with a steep dose fall-off behind the peak. The energy of the particle beam defines the depth of penetration, and hence the location of the maximum energy deposition. The normal tissue behind the target volume receives only a small percentage of the total dose, in theory enabling dose escalation while reducing side effects. The uncertainties regarding the exact localization of the steep dose peak in the patient make the planning and delivery of proton irradiation complex. Most applied methods in proton beam delivery are passive scattering and pencil beam scanning from one direction. Intensity-modulated proton therapy (IMPT) with multiple fields, which results in a superior dose distribution, is a complex technique that is not implemented in routine clinical practice yet. The uncertainties of dose deposition combined with the small day-to-day variations in setup in the patient are the main obstacles.

Well-established indications for proton treatment are skull base and paraspinal tumours, like chordoma and chondrosarcoma, paediatric neoplasms and uveal melanoma. Other applications, e.g. prostate, head and neck and lung, are under investigation. However, no clinical benefit over photon radiation treatment has been established yet, notwithstanding the considerably higher costs [36,37].

Brachytherapy

With brachytherapy a small radioactive source is placed into or close to the tumour, delivering a high radiation dose to the tumour with the possibility of sparing the surrounding normal tissue. In some superficially located tumours and a number of accessible tumours brachytherapy can have advantages. In the curative setting it is applied e.g. as a single-modality treatment in limited stage prostate cancer, involving the placement of radioactive iodine seeds into the prostate gland. The planned RT dose is emitted over several months with excellent results [38]. Another application in the curative setting is combination with EBRT in patients with cervical cancer. The applicator to position the radioactive source is placed into the uterus or vagina with the patient under sedation. Preferably MRI-based dose planning is performed, accounting for the location and sensitivity of the close-by organs at risk. The hollow guides of the applicator are then loaded for a short time with the radioactive source and the dose is administered in a few large dose fractions. In a palliative setting brachytherapy can be used to treat dysphagia in oesophageal cancer with subsequent good relief of symptoms [39].

Intra-operative radiation therapy

In selected cases intra-operative radiation therapy (IORT) is applied. Tumour sites can be exposed during an operation and radiation therapy can be delivered directly to the tumour bed. In recurrent rectal cancer [40] and in primary breast cancer [41] promising results are obtained with this technique. However, the dose delivered in a single fraction with IORT is rarely sufficient for definitive tumour control, and therefore IORT is usually combined with EBRT.

Treatment planning

Over the last 20 years the technical advances in radiation therapy planning have been huge, enabling more precise radiation delivery with fewer complications. In the past the target volume was assessed on an X-ray, while nowadays most radiation departments have a computed tomography (CT)–based planning system. On the planning CT both the target volume and the organs at risk can be visualized and delineated accurately to optimize dose delivery.

Irradiation beams can be chosen manually for a relatively simple planning, usually a limited number of beams from different directions (Figure 5.3a). A more complex planning can be calculated with several beams that are subdivided into multiple segments (IMRT) for a more homogeneous and conformal dose distribution (Figure 5.3b). With IMRT, a greater sparing of the organs at risk is possible, with fewer acute and late side effects [42,43]. A more sophisticated form of IMRT is volumetric arc therapy (VMAT). Radiation is delivered during the rotation of the machine, while varying the shape and intensity of the radiation beam, enabling irradiation from an infinite number of beam angles. The main advantage is a more conformal and homogeneous dose distribution and shorter treatment time [44].

Current developments

Stereotactic radiation therapy delivers a high dose of radiation to a small well-defined tumour volume, always with the aim to obtain definitive local tumour control often with curative intent. With this technique side effects are limited by minimizing the safety margins surrounding the tumour; i.e. side effects are not reduced by fractionation effects but by limiting the volume of normal tissue that is irradiated. If this treatment is given in a single fraction, it is often referred to as radiosurgery. Most often it will be given in a limited number of fractions, typically 1–8. A steep dose decline outside the treatment target can be achieved (Figure 5.3c). Position verification with a cone beam CT (CBCT) before each fraction is mandatory to safely deliver this type of radiation treatment. Clinical applications are expanding and comprise brain metastases, early stage lung cancer, liver tumours and bone metastases with high local control rates [45,46].

The main focus in the development of radiation treatment delivery is on image-guided radiation therapy (IGRT) and adaptive radiation therapy (ART). Frequent imaging during a course of image-guided radiation treatment enhances positioning accuracy and can reduce the margins required for setup uncertainties, consequently reducing the normal tissue dose. Imaging can be performed with two-dimensional kilo- or megavolt images or three-dimensional CBCT. A high dose close to delicate organs, like the optic nerve or brainstem, can be safely delivered, thanks to the use of CBCT.

Based on the imaging during treatment, the radiation plan can be adapted during the radiation course to account for changes in tumour mass or anatomy. Another possible approach is to make a collection of multiple radiation plans and choose each fraction of the optimal plan based on CBCT imaging.

The MRI-guided linear accelerator or cobalt machines that are currently being tested before clinical implementation theoretically have a great potential to combine IGRT with ART, increasing treatment accuracy, potentially reducing side effects and enabling increases in the therapeutic dose [47].

SIDE EFFECTS

The potential benefit of treatment has to be carefully balanced against radiation therapy–induced side effects in all situations. Radiation therapy–induced side effects can be broadly classified as early (acute) or late, based on the time frame of their manifestation. Early toxicities (Table 5.1) tend to arise during or shortly (days to weeks) after the start of radiation and can last from 6 weeks to 3 months after conclusion of the treatment. These acute reactions are usually due to direct damage to the parenchymal tissue cells that are sensitive to irradiation by depletion of stem cells that take care of repopulation and thereby recovery. Late toxicities can become apparent from 3 months after completion of radiation therapy (Table 5.1) and are attributed to damage to the microvasculature and mesenchymal cells. However, the exact aetiology is unknown and given the differences of the extent of toxicities observed between patients, inherent radiosensitivity of patients is likely to contribute to the development of late effects [48,49]. Long-term morbidity such as cardiovascular mortality [50] and the induction of secondary cancers [51] may occur as late as 10–20 years after completion of radiation therapy. It is therefore imperative to take into account all possible treatment-induced side effects that may have an overall impact on patient morbidity and mortality, prior to planning of radiation therapy. As the severity of side effects is dependent on the dose of radiation therapy and the volume of the organ that is irradiated (volume effect) [52], it is possible to limit the side effects by reducing the amount of normal tissue being irradiated using modern techniques. Advances in imaging and their

Table 5.1 Early and late side effects of radiotherapy

Organ	Early (acute) effects	Late effects
Skin	Erythema, pruritus, dry desquamation, moist desquamation, oedema	Fibrosis, atrophy, pigmentation, telangiectasia, alopecia, ulceration
Subcutaneous tissue	—	Fibrosis
Oral mucosa	Mucositis – pain	Fibrosis, atrophy, dryness
Bone/cartilage	—	Growth retardation, radionecrosis
Spinal cord	—	L'Hermitte syndrome, neurological symptoms
Salivary glands	Dryness, altered taste	Xerostomia
Oesophagus	Oesophagitis – dysphagia	Stricture, fistula
Kidney	—	Renal failure, hypertension
Lung	Cough, dyspnea	Radiation pneumonitis, fibrosis, diminished lung function
Liver	Radiation hepatitis – nausea, vomiting, raised hepatic transaminases	Diminished liver function
Stomach	Gastritis – indigestion, heartburn, excess wind	Bleeding
Small bowel	Enteritis – abdominal cramps, nausea, vomiting, diarrhea	Diarrhea, bleeding, fistula
Rectum	Proctitis – tenesmus, diarrhea	Tenesmus, bleeding
Bladder	Radiation cystitis – frequency, urgency, dysuria	Hemorrhagic cystitis, contracted bladder (capacity <100 cc)
Gonads	—	Sterility, genetic mutations
Systemic	Lethargy, anorexia	—
Hemapoietic	Anemia, leucopenia, thrombocytopenia	Myelofibrosis

integration in radiation therapy planning, and radiation delivery techniques, e.g. CT planning, integration of PET in planning, conformal radiation therapy, IMRT and IGRT, may allow full coverage of the target volume while appropriately reducing the volume of normal tissue that is irradiated during treatment [53–55], eventually minimizing the toxicities associated with radiation therapy. Treatment options of adverse late effects are limited. For late skin toxicity hyperbaric oxygen can be applied.

SPECIFIC APPLICATIONS

Although radiation therapy is a valuable treatment in many types of cancer, a few specific indications that illustrate the joint effort of surgeons and radiation oncologists are highlighted below. In these tumour types a combination of surgery and radiation therapy (and chemotherapy) is applied in the curative setting.

Breast cancer

Breast cancer is an excellent example of radiation therapy being used in the framework of an organ-sparing approach. In the 1980s breast-conserving therapy, combining surgery with postoperative whole breast radiation therapy, was introduced and is the standard of care for most patients with breast cancer nowadays. Radiation therapy successfully eliminates subclinical disease in the breast tissue surrounding the lumpectomy cavity. The results of mastectomy and breast-conserving therapy are similar with no difference in overall survival [56–58]. The addition of a higher radiation dose to the tumour bed even further reduces the risk of local recurrence [59]. Age is no contraindication for breast-conserving therapy; neither is a family history of breast cancer. A relative contraindication is the presence of a connective tissue disease like scleroderma or systemic lupus erythematosus (SLE). Numerous case reports suggest an increased risk of acute and late radiation toxicity in these patients. However, the results of several large retrospective series remain inconclusive and treatment decision should be made on an individual basis [60].

Although fibrosis is a frequent late toxicity of breast irradiation [61], good cosmetic outcome can be achieved in most patients with modern radiation therapy techniques by delivering a homogeneous dose distribution [62].

After mastectomy, tumour characteristics define the risk of local or regional recurrence and determine the need for postmastectomy radiation therapy [63]. The indications for locoregional radiation therapy, including any remaining regional lymph nodes, are based on the presence of axillary lymph nodes in the sentinel node or axillary lymph node dissection. Lymphoedema and limitation of shoulder movements are relevant late complications of axillary radiation therapy, although the rate of lymphoedema after radiation therapy is lower than the rate after axillary lymph node dissection [64].

Rectal cancer

Although surgery is the mainstay of treatment, preoperative radiation therapy has an established role in rectal cancer. Long-course preoperative chemoradiation is offered to patients with advanced local disease, as it increases the likelihood of achieving clinically relevant downsizing of the primary tumour and thereby the chance to obtain tumour-free resection margins and reduce the rate of local recurrences [65]. Postoperative radiation therapy has been proven to be less effective and associated with a higher complication rate [65] and no longer has a role in the treatment of rectal cancer.

The results of the Dutch TME trial and the MRC07 trial show a reduction in the relative risk of local recurrence in patients with resectable rectal cancer receiving short-course radiation therapy prior to total mesorectal excision [66,67]. The additive value of radiation therapy in low-risk patients can be questioned, as the absolute risk reduction in these patients is small [68]. The presence of lymph nodes on the preoperative MRI or the proximity of the tumour to the mesorectal fascia can be the factors to consider when deciding whether to offer preoperative radiation therapy to the patient [69]. These decisions should always be discussed in a multidisciplinary tumour board and the benefits and side effects, like anorectal and sexual dysfunction, have to be balanced. Short-course radiation therapy consisting of 25 Gy in five fractions can be applied to reduce the local recurrence rate in rectal cancer that requires no downstaging [8,67,70]. The total treatment time including radiation therapy and surgery should be restricted to 10 days to minimize the complication risk.

Symptoms like pain, bleeding or obstruction can be effectively palliated with short-course radiation therapy in patients with recurrent or metastatic disease.

Oesophageal cancer

Despite advances in multimodality treatment the outcome of oesophageal cancer remains poor.

In patients with resectable thoracic disease surgery is preceded by chemoradiaton (or chemotherapy alone) to the primary tumour and regional lymph nodes to improve overall survival [71,72]. In patients with irresectable disease chemoradiation without surgery can be administered with a cure rate of around 25% [73]. A higher radiation dose does not increase survival or locoregional control in one prematurely closed study [74], so whether a higher radiation dose is more effective remains unsure. For cancer arising in the cervical oesophagus radiation combined with chemotherapy is the preferred treatment over surgery alone, since survival appears to be the same, and major morbidity is avoided in most with chemoradiation [75].

Palliative radiation with EBRT, single-dose brachytherapy or a combination of both can be administered to diminish obstruction or bleeding of the primary tumour [39,76,77].

Dysphagia improves more rapidly after stent placement than after brachytherapy, but long-term relief of dysphagia is better after brachytherapy and stent placement has more complications [39].

Sarcoma

In the treatment of extremity soft-tissue sarcomas (STSs) radiation therapy has a role in improving local control in limb-sparing treatment, without improvement in overall survival [78,79]. Radiation therapy can effectively eradicate microscopic disease and achieve local control rates of 85–90% in high-grade extremity STS.

Radiation therapy can be applied pre- or postoperatively, depending on the tumour location, size of the tumour and institutional preference.

Surgical resections are more challenging in a previously irradiated field and a higher incidence of acute wound complications is seen with preoperative radiation therapy, particularly for lower-extremity lesions [80,81]. However, compared to postoperative radiation therapy, lower doses and smaller field sizes can be used with a reduced risk of irreversible late complications, like fibrosis, oedema and joint stiffness [82]. The use of IMRT seems beneficial with high local control rates and a dose reduction to the surrounding normal tissue compared to 3D-conformal radiation therapy [83,84]. Accurate delineation of the target volume can be achieved by matching with a diagnostic MRI, preferably made in the same position as used for radiation therapy.

CONCLUSION

Radiation therapy is and will remain for the foreseeable future an invaluable part of the multimodality approach in many types of cancer. The combination of surgery with a relatively low dose of radiation therapy can achieve high local control rates with acceptable morbidity. Higher radiation doses or a combination with radiosensitizing agents is needed in patients with macroscopic disease with a related higher risk of late radiation side effects. As individualization of cancer treatment is more frequent, a multidisciplinary approach is especially important, with input from specialists trained in oncology, radiologists and pathologists, so that the optimal management decision is made before embarking on treatment.

REFERENCES

1. Mendenhall, W. M., R. J. Amdur, C. G. Morris, and R. W. Hinerman. T1-T2N0 squamous cell carcinoma of the glottic larynx treated with radiation therapy. *J Clin Oncol* 19 (2001): 4029–4036.
2. van Hezewijk, M., C. L. Creutzberg, H. Putter, A. Chin, I. Schneider, M. Hoogeveen, R. Willemze, and C. A. Marijnen. Efficacy of a hypofractionated schedule in electron beam radiotherapy for epithelial skin cancer: analysis of 434 cases. *Radiother Oncol* 95 (2010): 245–249.
3. Grimm, P., I. Billiet, D. Bostwick, A. P. Dicker, S. Frank, J. Immerzeel, M. Keyes, et al. Comparative analysis of prostate-specific antigen free survival outcomes for patients with low, intermediate and high risk prostate cancer treatment by radical therapy. Results from the Prostate Cancer Results Study Group. *BJU Int* 109 (Suppl 1) (2012): 22–29.
4. Green, J., J. Kirwan, J. Tierney, C. Vale, P. Symonds, L. Fresco, C. Williams, and M. Collingwood. Concomitant chemotherapy and radiation therapy for cancer of the uterine cervix. *Cochrane Database Syst Rev* (2005): CD002225.
5. Forastiere, A. A., H. Goepfert, M. Maor, T. F. Pajak, R. Weber, W. Morrison, B. Glisson, et al. Concurrent chemotherapy and radiotherapy for organ preservation in advanced laryngeal cancer. *N Engl J Med* 349 (2003): 2091–2098.
6. Bartelink, H., F. Roelofsen, F. Eschwege, P. Rougier, J. F. Bosset, D. G. Gonzalez, D. Peiffert, M. van Glabbeke, and M. Pierart. Concomitant radiotherapy and chemotherapy is superior to radiotherapy alone in the treatment of locally advanced anal cancer: results of a phase III randomized trial of the European Organization for Research and Treatment of Cancer Radiotherapy and Gastrointestinal Cooperative Groups. *J Clin Oncol* 15 (1997): 2040–2049.
7. Early Breast Cancer Trialists' Collaborative Group, S. Darby, P. McGale, C. Correa, C. Taylor, R. Arriagada, M. Clarke, et al. Effect of radiotherapy after breast-conserving surgery on 10-year recurrence and 15-year breast cancer death: meta-analysis of individual patient data for 10,801 women in 17 randomised trials. *Lancet* 378 (2011): 1707–1716.
8. Kapiteijn, E., C. A. Marijnen, I. D. Nagtegaal, H. Putter, W. H. Steup, T. Wiggers, H. J. Rutten, et al. Preoperative radiotherapy combined with total mesorectal excision for resectable rectal cancer. *N Engl J Med* 345 (2001): 638–646.
9. Horsman, M., B. Wouters, M. Joiner, and J. Overgaard. The oxygen effect and fractionated radiotherapy. In *Basic Clinical Radiobiology*, 4th ed., edited by M. Joiner and A. van der Kogel, 207–209. London: Hodder Arnold, 2009.
10. Steel, G. G., T. J. McMillan, and J. H. Peacock. The 5Rs of radiobiology. *Int J Radiat Biol* 56 (1989): 1045–1048.
11. Withers, H. R. The four Rs of radiotherapy. In *Advances in Radiation Biology*, edited by J. T. Lett. New York: Academic Press, 1975.
12. Rademakers, S. E., P. N. Span, J. H. Kaanders, F. C. Sweep, A. J. van der Kogel, and J. Bussink. Molecular aspects of tumour hypoxia. *Mol Oncol* 2 (2008): 41–53.

13. Janssens, G. O., S. E. Rademakers, C. H. Terhaard, P. A. Doornaert, H. P. Bijl, P. van den Ende, A. Chin, et al. Accelerated radiotherapy with carbogen and nicotinamide for laryngeal cancer: results of a phase III randomized trial. *J Clin Oncol* 30 (2012): 1777–1783.

14. Overgaard, J., H. S. Hansen, M. Overgaard, L. Bastholt, A. Berthelsen, L. Specht, B. Lindelov, and K. Jorgensen. A randomized double-blind phase III study of nimorazole as a hypoxic radiosensitizer of primary radiotherapy in supraglottic larynx and pharynx carcinoma. Results of the Danish Head and Neck Cancer Study (DAHANCA) Protocol 5-85. *Radiother Oncol* 46 (1998): 135–146.

15. Roberts, S. A. and J. H. Hendry. Time factors in larynx tumor radiotherapy: lag times and intertumor heterogeneity in clinical datasets from four centers. *Int J Radiat Oncol Biol Phys* 45 (1999): 1247–1257.

16. Withers, H. R., J. M. Taylor, and B. Maciejewski. The hazard of accelerated tumor clonogen repopulation during radiotherapy. *Acta Oncol* 27 (1988): 131–146.

17. Fertil, B. and E. P. Malaise. Intrinsic radiosensitivity of human cell lines is correlated with radioresponsiveness of human tumors: analysis of 101 published survival curves. *Int J Radiat Oncol Biol Phys* 11 (1985): 1699–1707.

18. West, C. M. Invited review: intrinsic radiosensitivity as a predictor of patient response to radiotherapy. *Br J Radiol* 68 (1995): 827–837.

19. Haas, R. L., P. Poortmans, D. de Jong, B. M. Aleman, L. G. Dewit, M. Verheij, A. A. Hart, et al. High response rates and lasting remissions after low-dose involved field radiotherapy in indolent lymphomas. *J Clin Oncol* 21 (2003): 2474–2480.

20. Joiner, M. and S. Bentzen. Fractionation: the linear-quadratic approach. In *Basic Clinical Radiobiology*, 4th ed., edited by M. Joiner and A. van der Kogel, 102–109. London: Hodder Arnold, 2009.

21. Thames, H. D., Jr., H. R. Withers, L. J. Peters, and G. H. Fletcher. Changes in early and late radiation responses with altered dose fractionation: implications for dose-survival relationships. *Int J Radiat Oncol Biol Phys* 8 (1982): 219–226.

22. Zagars, G. K., T. E. Schultheiss, and L. J. Peters. Intertumor heterogeneity and radiation dose-control curves. *Radiother Oncol* 8 (1987): 353–361.

23. Suwinski, R., J. M. Taylor, and H. R. Withers. The effect of heterogeneity in tumor cell kinetics on radiation dose-response. An exploratory investigation of a plateau effect. *Radiother Oncol* 50 (1999): 57–66.

24. Bentzen, S. Dose-response relationships in radiotherapy. In *Basic Clinical Radiobiology*, 4th ed., edited by M. Joiner and A. van der Kogel, 63. London: Hodder Arnold, 2009.

25. Bese, N. S., J. Hendry, and B. Jeremic. Effects of prolongation of overall treatment time due to unplanned interruptions during radiotherapy of different tumor sites and practical methods for compensation. *Int J Radiat Oncol Biol Phys* 68 (2007): 654–661.

26. Overgaard, J., H. S. Hansen, L. Specht, M. Overgaard, C. Grau, E. Andersen, J. Bentzen, et al. Five compared with six fractions per week of conventional radiotherapy of squamous-cell carcinoma of head and neck: DAHANCA 6 and 7 randomised controlled trial. *Lancet* 362 (2003): 933–940.

27. Mauguen, A., C. Le Pechoux, M. I. Saunders, S. E. Schild, A. T. Turrisi, M. Baumann, W. T. Sause, et al. Hyperfractionated or accelerated radiotherapy in lung cancer: an individual patient data meta-analysis. *J Clin Oncol* 30 (2012): 2788–2797.

28. Kaanders, J. H., A. J. van der Kogel, and K. K. Ang. Altered fractionation: limited by mucosal reactions? *Radiother Oncol* 50 (1999): 247–260.

29. De Ruysscher, D., M. Pijls-Johannesma, S. M. Bentzen, A. Minken, R. Wanders, L. Lutgens, M. Hochstenbag, et al. Time between the first day of chemotherapy and the last day of chest radiation is the most important predictor of survival in limited-disease small-cell lung cancer. *J Clin Oncol* 24 (2006): 1057–1063.

30. Suwinski, R. and H. R. Withers. Time factor and treatment strategies in subclinical disease. *Int J Radiat Biol* 79 (2003): 495–502.

31. Withers, H. R. and R. Suwinski. Radiation dose response for subclinical metastases. *Semin Radiat Oncol* 8 (1998): 224–228.

32. Ang, K. K., A. Trotti, B. W. Brown, A. S. Garden, R. L. Foote, W. H. Morrison, F. B. Geara, D. W. Klotch, H. Goepfert, and L. J. Peters. Randomized trial addressing risk features and time factors of surgery plus radiotherapy in advanced head-and-neck cancer. *Int J Radiat Oncol Biol Phys* 51 (2001): 571–578.

33. Awwad, H. K., M. Lotayef, T. Shouman, A. C. Begg, G. Wilson, S. M. Bentzen, H. Abd El-Moneim, and S. Eissa. Accelerated hyperfractionation (AHF) compared to conventional fractionation (CF) in the postoperative radiotherapy of locally advanced head and neck cancer: influence of proliferation. *Br J Cancer* 86 (2002): 517–523.

34. Suwinski, R., A. Sowa, T. Rutkowski, J. Wydmanski, R. Tarnawski, and B. Maciejewski. Time factor in postoperative radiotherapy: a multivariate locoregional control analysis in 868 patients. *Int J Radiat Oncol Biol Phys* 56 (2003): 399–412.

35. Soyfer, V., R. Geva, M. Michelson, M. Inbar, E. Shacham-Shmueli, and B. W. Corn. The impact of overall radiotherapy treatment time and delay in initiation of radiotherapy on local control and distant metastases in gastric cancer. *Radiat Oncol* 9 (2014): 81.

36. Pearlstein, K. A. and R. C. Chen. Comparing dosimetric, morbidity, quality of life, and cancer control outcomes after 3D conformal, intensity-modulated, and proton radiation therapy for prostate cancer. *Semin Radiat Oncol* 23 (2013): 182–190.

37. Gray, P. J. and J. A. Efstathiou. Proton beam radiation therapy for prostate cancer – is the hype (and the cost) justified? *Curr Urol Rep* 14 (2013): 199–208.

38. Bowes, D. and J. Crook. A critical analysis of the long-term impact of brachytherapy for prostate cancer: a review of the recent literature. *Curr Opin Urol* 21 (2011): 219–224.

39. Homs, M. Y., E. W. Steyerberg, W. M. Eijkenboom, H. W. Tilanus, L. J. Stalpers, J. F. Bartelsman, J. J. van Lanschot, et al. Single-dose brachytherapy versus metal stent placement for the palliation of dysphagia from oesophageal cancer: multicentre randomised trial. *Lancet* 364 (2004): 1497–1504.

40. Hu, K. S. and L. B. Harrison. Results and complications of surgery combined with intra-operative radiation therapy for the treatment of locally advanced or recurrent cancers in the pelvis. *Semin Surg Oncol* 18 (2000): 269–278.

41. Barry, M. and V. Sacchini. Evaluating the role of intra-operative radiation therapy in the modern management of breast cancer. *Surg Oncol* 21 (2012): e159–e163.

42. Nutting, C. M., J. P. Morden, K. J. Harrington, T. G. Urbano, S. A. Bhide, C. Clark, E. A. Miles, et al. Parotid-sparing intensity modulated versus conventional radiotherapy in head and neck cancer (PARSPORT): a phase 3 multicentre randomised controlled trial. *Lancet Oncol* 12 (2011): 127–136.

43. Palma, D., E. Vollans, K. James, S. Nakano, V. Moiseenko, R. Shaffer, M. McKenzie, J. Morris, and K. Otto. Volumetric modulated arc therapy for delivery of prostate radiotherapy: comparison with intensity-modulated radiotherapy and three-dimensional conformal radiotherapy. *Int J Radiat Oncol Biol Phys* 72 (2008): 996–1001.

44. Teoh, M., C. H. Clark, K. Wood, S. Whitaker, and A. Nisbet. Volumetric modulated arc therapy: a review of current literature and clinical use in practice. *Br J Radiol* 84 (2011): 967–996.

45. Alexander, E., 3rd, T. M. Moriarty, R. B. Davis, P. Y. Wen, H. A. Fine, P. M. Black, H. M. Kooy, and J. S. Loeffler. Stereotactic radiosurgery for the definitive, noninvasive treatment of brain metastases. *J Natl Cancer Inst* 87 (1995): 34–40.

46. Timmerman, R., R. Paulus, J. Galvin, J. Michalski, W. Straube, J. Bradley, A. Fakiris, et al. Stereotactic body radiation therapy for inoperable early stage lung cancer. *JAMA* 303 (2010): 1070–1076.

47. Raaymakers, B. W., J. J. Lagendijk, J. Overweg, J. G. Kok, A. J. Raaijmakers, E. M. Kerkhof, R. W. van der Put, et al. Integrating a 1.5 T MRI scanner with a 6 MV accelerator: proof of concept. *Phys Med Biol* 54 (2009): N229–N237.

48. Rodningen, O. K., A. L. Borresen-Dale, J. Alsner, T. Hastie, and J. Overgaard. Radiation-induced gene expression in human subcutaneous fibroblasts is predictive of radiation-induced fibrosis. *Radiother Oncol* 86 (2008): 314–320.

49. West, C. M., S. E. Davidson, S. A. Elyan, R. Swindell, S. A. Roberts, C. J. Orton, C. A. Coyle, et al. The intrinsic radiosensitivity of normal and tumour cells. *Int J Radiat Biol* 73 (1998): 409–413.

50. Darby, S. C., D. J. Cutter, M. Boerma, L. S. Constine, L. F. Fajardo, K. Kodama, K. Mabuchi, et al. Radiation-related heart disease: current knowledge and future prospects. *Int J Radiat Oncol Biol Phys* 76 (2010): 656–665.

51. Deutsch, M., S. R. Land, M. Begovic, H. S. Wieand, N. Wolmark, and B. Fisher. The incidence of lung carcinoma after surgery for breast carcinoma with and without postoperative radiotherapy. Results of National Surgical Adjuvant Breast and Bowel Project (NSABP) clinical trials B-04 and B-06. *Cancer* 98 (2003): 1362–1368.

52. Dörr, W. and A. van der Kogel. The volume effect in radiotherapy. In *Basic Clinical Radiobiology*, 4th ed., edited by M. Joiner and A. van der Kogel, 192–195. London: Hodder Arnold, 2009.

53. Chen, L., R. A. Price, Jr., T. B. Nguyen, L. Wang, J. S. Li, L. Qin, M. Ding, E. Palacio, C. M. Ma, and A. Pollack. Dosimetric evaluation of MRI-based treatment planning for prostate cancer. *Phys Med Biol* 49 (2004): 5157–5170.

54. Grosu, A. L., M. Piert, W. A. Weber, B. Jeremic, M. Picchio, U. Schratzenstaller, F. B. Zimmermann, M. Schwaiger, and M. Molls. Positron emission tomography for radiation treatment planning. *Strahlenther Onkol* 181 (2005): 483–499.

55. Liu, H. H., X. Wang, L. Dong, Q. Wu, Z. Liao, C. W. Stevens, T. M. Guerrero, R. Komaki, J. D. Cox, and R. Mohan. Feasibility of sparing lung and other thoracic structures with intensity-modulated radiotherapy for non-small-cell lung cancer. *Int J Radiat Oncol Biol Phys* 58 (2004): 1268–1279.

56. Fisher, B., S. Anderson, J. Bryant, R. G. Margolese, M. Deutsch, E. R. Fisher, J. H. Jeong, and N. Wolmark. Twenty-year follow-up of a randomized trial comparing total mastectomy, lumpectomy, and lumpectomy plus irradiation for the treatment of invasive breast cancer. *N Engl J Med* 347 (2002): 1233–1241.

57. Veronesi, U., N. Cascinelli, L. Mariani, M. Greco, R. Saccozzi, A. Luini, M. Aguilar, and E. Marubini. Twenty-year follow-up of a randomized study

comparing breast-conserving surgery with radical mastectomy for early breast cancer. *N Engl J Med* 347 (2002): 1227–1232.

58. van Dongen, J. A., A. C. Voogd, I. S. Fentiman, C. Legrand, R. J. Sylvester, D. Tong, E. van der Schueren, P. A. Helle, K. van Zijl, and H. Bartelink. Long-term results of a randomized trial comparing breast-conserving therapy with mastectomy: European Organization for Research and Treatment of Cancer 10801 trial. *J Natl Cancer Inst* 92 (2000): 1143–1150.

59. Bartelink, H., P. Maingon, P. Poortmans, C. Weltens, A. Fourquet, J. Jager, D. Schinagl, et al. Whole-breast irradiation with or without a boost for patients treated with breast-conserving surgery for early breast cancer: 20-year follow-up of a randomised phase 3 trial. *Lancet Oncol* 16 (2015): 47–56.

60. Wo, J. and A. Taghian. Radiotherapy in setting of collagen vascular disease. *Int J Radiat Oncol Biol Phys* 69 (2007): 1347–1353.

61. Bartelink, H., J. C. Horiot, P. M. Poortmans, H. Struikmans, W. Van den Bogaert, A. Fourquet, J. J. Jager, et al. Impact of a higher radiation dose on local control and survival in breast-conserving therapy of early breast cancer: 10-year results of the randomized boost versus no boost EORTC 22881-10882 trial. *J Clin Oncol* 25 (2007): 3259–3265.

62. Donovan, E., N. Bleakley, E. Denholm, P. Evans, L. Gothard, J. Hanson, C. Peckitt, et al. Randomised trial of standard 2D radiotherapy (RT) versus intensity modulated radiotherapy (IMRT) in patients prescribed breast radiotherapy. *Radiother Oncol* 82 (2007): 254–264.

63. Early Breast Cancer Trialists' Collaborative Group, P. McGale, C. Taylor, C. Correa, D. Cutter, F. Duane, M. Ewertz, et al. Effect of radiotherapy after mastectomy and axillary surgery on 10-year recurrence and 20-year breast cancer mortality: meta-analysis of individual patient data for 8135 women in 22 randomised trials. *Lancet* 383 (2014): 2127–2135.

64. Donker, M., G. van Tienhoven, M. E. Straver, P. Meijnen, C. J. van de Velde, R. E. Mansel, L. Cataliotti, et al. Radiotherapy or surgery of the axilla after a positive sentinel node in breast cancer (EORTC 10981-22023 AMAROS): a randomised, multicentre, open-label, phase 3 non-inferiority trial. *Lancet Oncol* 15 (2014): 1303–1310.

65. Sauer, R., H. Becker, W. Hohenberger, C. Rodel, C. Wittekind, R. Fietkau, P. Martus, et al. Preoperative versus postoperative chemoradiotherapy for rectal cancer. *N Engl J Med* 351 (2004): 1731–1740.

66. Peeters, K. C., C. A. Marijnen, I. D. Nagtegaal, E. K. Kranenbarg, H. Putter, T. Wiggers, H. Rutten, et al. The TME trial after a median follow-up of 6 years: increased local control but no survival benefit in irradiated patients with resectable rectal carcinoma. *Ann Surg* 246 (2007): 693–701.

67. Sebag-Montefiore, D., R. J. Stephens, R. Steele, J. Monson, R. Grieve, S. Khanna, P. Quirke, et al. Preoperative radiotherapy versus selective postoperative chemoradiotherapy in patients with rectal cancer (MRC CR07 and NCIC-CTG C016): a multicentre, randomised trial. *Lancet* 373 (2009): 811–820.

68. Taylor, F. G., P. Quirke, R. J. Heald, B. Moran, L. Blomqvist, I. Swift, D. J. Sebag-Montefiore, P. Tekkis, G. Brown, and Mercury Study Group. Preoperative high-resolution magnetic resonance imaging can identify good prognosis stage I, II, and III rectal cancer best managed by surgery alone: a prospective, multicenter, European study. *Ann Surg* 253 (2011): 711–719.

69. Taylor, F. G., P. Quirke, R. J. Heald, B. J. Moran, L. Blomqvist, I. R. Swift, D. Sebag-Montefiore, P. Tekkis, G. Brown, and Group Magnetic Resonance Imaging in Rectal Cancer European Equivalence Study. Preoperative magnetic resonance imaging assessment of circumferential resection margin predicts disease-free survival and local recurrence: 5-year follow-up results of the MERCURY study. *J Clin Oncol* 32 (2014): 34–43.

70. Swedish Rectal Cancer Trial. Improved survival with preoperative radiotherapy in resectable rectal cancer. Swedish Rectal Cancer Trial. *N Engl J Med* 336 (1997): 980–987.

71. van Hagen, P., M. C. Hulshof, J. J. van Lanschot, E. W. Steyerberg, M. I. van Berge Henegouwen, B. P. Wijnhoven, D. J. Richel, et al. Preoperative chemoradiotherapy for esophageal or junctional cancer. *N Engl J Med* 366 (2012): 2074–2084.

72. Malthaner, R. A., S. Collin, and D. Fenlon. Preoperative chemotherapy for resectable thoracic esophageal cancer. *Cochrane Database Syst Rev* (2006): CD001556.

73. Cooper, J. S., M. D. Guo, A. Herskovic, J. S. Macdonald, J. A. Martenson, Jr., M. Al-Sarraf, R. Byhardt, et al. Chemoradiotherapy of locally advanced esophageal cancer: long-term follow-up of a prospective randomized trial (RTOG 85–01). Radiation Therapy Oncology Group. *JAMA* 281 (1999): 1623–1627.

74. Minsky, B. D., T. F. Pajak, R. J. Ginsberg, T. M. Pisansky, J. Martenson, R. Komaki, G. Okawara, S. A. Rosenthal, and D. P. Kelsen. INT 0123 (Radiation Therapy Oncology Group 94-05) phase III trial of combined-modality therapy for esophageal cancer: high-dose versus standard-dose radiation therapy. *J Clin Oncol* 20 (2002): 1167–1174.

75. Mendenhall, W. M., M. D. Sombeck, J. T. Parsons, M. E. Kasper, S. P. Stringer, and S. B. Vogel. Management of cervical esophageal carcinoma. *Semin Radiat Oncol* 4 (1994): 179–191.

76. Sreedharan, A., K. Harris, A. Crellin, D. Forman, and S. M. Everett. Interventions for dysphagia in oesophageal cancer. *Cochrane Database Syst Rev* (2009): CD005048.

77. Murray, L. J., O. S. Din, V. S. Kumar, L. M. Dixon, and J. C. Wadsley. Palliative radiotherapy in patients with esophageal carcinoma: a retrospective review. *Pract Radiat Oncol* 2 (2012): 257–264.

78. Yang, J. C., A. E. Chang, A. R. Baker, W. F. Sindelar, D. N. Danforth, S. L. Topalian, T. DeLaney, et al. Randomized prospective study of the benefit of adjuvant radiation therapy in the treatment of soft tissue sarcomas of the extremity. *J Clin Oncol* 16 (1998): 197–203.

79. Pisters, P. W., L. B. Harrison, D. H. Leung, J. M. Woodruff, E. S. Casper, and M. F. Brennan. Long-term results of a prospective randomized trial of adjuvant brachytherapy in soft tissue sarcoma. *J Clin Oncol* 14 (1996): 859–868.

80. O'Sullivan, B., A. M. Davis, R. Turcotte, R. Bell, C. Catton, P. Chabot, J. Wunder, et al. Preoperative versus postoperative radiotherapy in soft-tissue sarcoma of the limbs: a randomised trial. *Lancet* 359 (2002): 2235–2241.

81. Cannon, C. P., M. T. Ballo, G. K. Zagars, A. N. Mirza, P. P. Lin, V. O. Lewis, A. W. Yasko, R. S. Benjamin, and P. W. Pisters. Complications of combined modality treatment of primary lower extremity soft-tissue sarcomas. *Cancer* 107 (2006): 2455–2461.

82. Davis, A. M., B. O'Sullivan, R. Turcotte, R. Bell, C. Catton, P. Chabot, J. Wunder, et al. Late radiation morbidity following randomization to preoperative versus postoperative radiotherapy in extremity soft tissue sarcoma. *Radiother Oncol* 75 (2005): 48–53.

83. Alektiar, K. M., M. F. Brennan, J. H. Healey, and S. Singer. Impact of intensity-modulated radiation therapy on local control in primary soft-tissue sarcoma of the extremity. *J Clin Oncol* 26 (2008): 3440–3444.

84. Hong, L., K. M. Alektiar, M. Hunt, E. Venkatraman, and S. A. Leibel. Intensity-modulated radiotherapy for soft tissue sarcoma of the thigh. *Int J Radiat Oncol Biol Phys* 59 (2004): 752–759.

6

Intraoperative radiotherapy

WOJCIECH P POLKOWSKI AND DAVID A L MORGAN

PRINCIPLES OF IORT

Intraoperative radiotherapy (IORT) refers to the delivery of a large single fraction of radiation at the time of surgery to a surgically defined area, usually after resection of all, or most, macroscopic disease, with the aim of eradicating any residual microscopic foci of disease. Recent biological data suggest that such radiation may also impact upon disease recurrence through various, as yet ill-understood, effects on the tumour microenvironment. The use of IORT as a single dose of radiation also minimizes the treatment duration, which in itself may increase its effectiveness, as is also the case with the timing of its delivery, being given immediately after surgical resection, when the postulated effects on the tumour microenvironment are likely to be greatest. IORT is currently used in various techniques that show important differences in dose delivery: (1) high-dose-rate brachytherapy (HDR-IORT), (2) electron-beam radiation with dedicated fixed or mobile linear accelerators (intraoperative electron radiotherapy [IOERT]) and (3) orthovoltage (low-kilovolt X-ray beams) with dedicated mobile units (IO[X]RT). The mobile radiation therapy devices generate either megavoltage electrons (Mobetron and Novac-7/11) or kilovoltage photons (Intrabeam™ and Xoft) [1]. While megavoltage IOERT systems (cylindrical applicators) may be used either after removal of the tumour or for irradiation of unresectable (pancreatic) malignancies, kilovoltage systems with spherical applicators are mostly used directly on the tumour bed after excision. The use of different IORT techniques and devices varies with institutional preferences and target populations.

Advantages of IORT compared to EBRT

The surgically defined target for IORT is usually the tumour bed, with uninvolved and dose-limiting structures shielded or displaced from the immediate radiation field. IORT may be used when resection margins are narrow or involved by tumour and can be applied very specifically to an area at risk, under direct visual control, and with the ability to shield the surrounding structures from radiation.

IORT boost advantages in comparison to an external boost include, at least theoretically, smaller field sizes (because safety margins for daily positioning errors can be eliminated), the possibility to exclude organs at risk (like major nerves or skin) from the irradiation field and the reduction of overall treatment time.

In institutions that choose to have the availability of IORT as a component of treatment, a carefully constructed multidisciplinary team (MDT) needs to exist. This team should include a surgical oncologist, radiation oncologist, anaesthesiologist, operating nurse and radiation physicist. IORT demands close cooperation of radiation and surgical oncologists before and at the time surgery, thus creating an optimal MDT in one therapeutic session. This dramatically shortens time of hospitalization and therapy, compared to traditional fractionated external beam radiotherapy (EBRT). Additionally, the synergistic action of both local therapies, surgery and irradiation, increases the potential of local control, minimizes irradiation side effects by shielding of neighbouring and susceptible organs, and eliminates so-called geographical error.

The final goal of IORT is to enhance loco-regional tumour control. IORT can be safely used to increase the dose due to disease, because the tissues are properly moved away from the path of the radiation beam. IORT can also be used as a boost for EBRT by administration of a single high dose at the time of surgery.

Currently, IORT is mainly used to improve the therapeutic index. Many studies have suggested that the technique of IORT in patients with advanced or recurrent cancers may improve treatment results compared with conventional radiotherapy.

Disadvantages of IORT are prolongation of the surgical procedure and complex logistics. However, the usual irradiation time of the surgical field is 3–20 minutes, whereas simultaneous coordination of many specialists at one time of surgery is a matter of teamwork abilities. Therefore, these theoretical disadvantages should not pose major practical difficulties.

The best evidence of the advantages of IORT, as reflected by patient preferences regarding radiotherapy, comes from breast cancer treatment [2]. Time required for conventional EBRT is 3–6 weeks, whereas IORT adds about 30 minutes to breast-conserving surgery (BCS). This implies substantial gains in overall use of health service resources. Moreover, EBRT may damage ribs, intercostal nerves, heart or lungs and cause radiation-induced cancers, and IORT can achieve much lower doses to these organs, although late toxicity of IORT is currently unknown. A small increase in local recurrence rates, but no impairment of survival rates, has been seen following IORT, in certain populations [3].

EVIDENCE BEHIND THE USE OF IORT IN SURGICAL ONCOLOGY

For the last decade IORT has become an increasingly attractive method of local cancer treatment. It can be used for different cancer primaries, but most commonly it has been used for breast carcinoma, followed by (colo)rectal, prostate and pancreatic carcinomas and sarcomas [4]. For the treatment of early breast carcinoma, IORT alone may be used as an accelerated partial breast irradiation (APBI), or prior to EBRT of the whole breast or as a boost in order to increase a dose applied to the tumour bed.

Breast carcinoma

IORT ALONE RANDOMIZED CONTROLLED TRIALS: TARGIT-A AND ELIOT

In a proportion of patients with good prognostic factors, partial breast irradiation may be a risk-adapted strategy in radiotherapy following BCS. Recently updated results from an international, multicentre, randomized clinical trial (TARGIT-A) proved that for selected patients with a favourable prognosis, targeted IORT with low-energy photons (Figure 6.1) may be an acceptable alternative to conventional EBRT [5]. Although this form of IORT is presumed to be well tolerated, it may have deleterious effects on the early and late aesthetic outcomes. Application of the IORT by means of mobile linear accelerators makes the BCS even more demanding and complicated, especially in cases where expertise in oncoplastic techniques is required.

Two recently published randomized IORT trials for early stage breast cancer demonstrate acceptable recurrence rates for IORT, although worse than those achieved by whole breast irradiation (WBI) [3,5]. The ELIOT trial

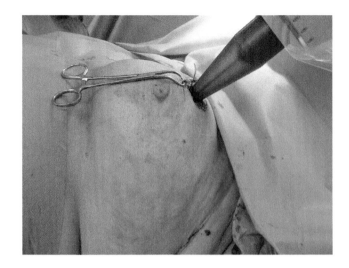

Figure 6.1 Intrabeam: the spherical applicator is temporarily sutured into the surgical cavity, to achieve a tight fit; the X-ray tube is introduced so that the X-ray source lies at the geometric centre of the sphere.

used electrons (IOERT), and the TARGIT-A trial used 50 kV X-rays (IOXRT). With a median follow-up of 5.8 years, the 5-year recurrence rates for ELIOT versus EBRT patients were 4.4% and 0.4%, respectively ($p = 0.0001$). A low-risk ELIOT group was identified with a 5-year recurrence rate of 1.5%. With a median follow-up of 29 months, the 5-year recurrence rates for the TARGIT-A versus EBRT patients were 3.3% and 1.3%, respectively ($p = 0.042$). Critical analysis of both trials has led to the conclusion that with 5.8 years of median follow-up, IOERT appears to have a subset of low-risk women for whom IOERT is acceptable. With 29 months of median follow-up the results of IORT with 50 kV devices are promising, but longer follow-up data are required. At the current time, single-fraction IOERT or IORT patients should be treated under strict institutional protocols [6,7]. However, there is evidence that early adoption of the TARGIT-A trial results would lead to minimal adverse impact, and substantially less resource use [8]. Although the follow-up in the TARGIT-A trial is immature and loco-regional recurrences occur after 5 years and even continue to rise beyond 10 years, the effects of all radiotherapy against local recurrences are predominantly concentrated within the first 5 years of follow-up. IORT of the tumour bed in combination with wide local excision applied in a risk-adapted manner seems appropriate local therapy for postmenopausal women (in particular women over the age of 70) with low-risk hormone receptor-positive tumours [9,10]. Individual patients' views should always be taken into account on this matter.

In 2009, the American Society for Radiation Oncology (ASTRO) and the Groupe Européen de Curiethérapie–European Society for Therapeutic Radiology and Oncology (GEC-ESTRO) separately formulated consensus definitions to classify patients into three risk groups toward the option of APBI outside a clinical trial, and both bodies produced similar categorizations [11,12]. Both these consensus documents defined three patient groups in terms of applicability of ABPI alone: (1) a *suitable* group, for whom ABPI outside of a clinical trial is acceptable; (2) a *cautionary* group, for whom caution and concern should be applied when considering ABPI outside of a clinical trial; and (3) an *unsuitable* group, for whom ABPI outside of a clinical trial is not generally considered warranted. Patients who choose treatment with IORT alone should be informed that WBI by means of EBRT is an established treatment with a much longer track record that has documented long-term effectiveness and safety. Concise characteristics of the three groups stated by the ASTRO/GEC-ESTRO statement are depicted in Table 6.1. It must be acknowledged that when these guidelines were written, they specifically excluded IORT from consideration among the types of APBI. It is a matter of contention whether the subsequent publication of two large randomized trials of IORT should necessitate expansion of the guidelines to include it: it is notable that retrospective analysis of the two trials has suggested that excellent results are obtained with IORT in patients who would be classified as 'suitable' by ASTRO and GEC-ESTRO.

The appropriateness of the division into the three groups was subsequently confirmed by secondary analysis of the ELIOT trial results, where ipsilateral in-breast recurrence, distant metastases and cause-specific survival, but not regional nodal failure, were significantly better in the suitable patients [13]. Outside the context of a clinical trial, and

before large-scale randomized clinical trial outcome data with mature follow-up, better characterization of aesthetic and late toxicity results become available, a very favourable subgroup of patients may be identified to have an acceptable recurrence rate after IORT alone, especially if adjuvant hormonal therapy is given [14].

BOOST = STANDARD

Boost irradiation with 16 Gy improves local control in breast cancer and is considered the standard of care in breast cancer treatment for younger patients [15]. Patients can benefit (lower rates of recurrences) from IORT when it is delivered as a boost, replacing the external boost at the end of EBRT [16]. The intraoperative boost at the time of surgery reduces the subsequent dose of EBRT, thus shortening the time required for the EBRT, albeit at the expense of time of BCS and operative field manipulation in the preserved breast.

The largest evidence for boost IORT preceding WBI originates from intraoperative electron treatments (Figure 6.2) with single doses around 10 Gy, providing outstandingly low local recurrence (LR) rates in any risk constellation also at long-term analyses. Compared to other boost methods, an intraoperative treatment has evident advantages [17].

Other sites

Whereas for breast cancer the use of IORT has mainly been as a way of reducing the burden of treatment (primarily

Table 6.1 Characteristics of the three patients groups stated by the ASTRO/GEC-ESTRO consensus for IORT alone outside of a clinical trial

	Suitable	Cautionary	Unsuitable
Patient factors			
Age (years)	>60	50–59	<50
BRCA 1/2	No	No	Yes
Pathological features			
T size	≤2 cm	2.1–3 cm	≥3 cm
T stage	T1	T0–T2	T3–T4
Margins	Negative	Close (≤2 mm)	Positive
Lympho-vascular invasion	No	Limited, focal	Extensive
ER	Positive	Negative	—
Multicentric	Unicentric	Unicentric	Present
Multifocal	Clinically unifocal	Clinically unifocal	Clinically multifocal
Histology of invasive carcinoma	Ductal	Lobular	—
Ductal carcinoma in situ (DCIS), extensive intraductal component (EIC)	No, no	Yes, yes (≤3 cm)	Yes, yes (>3 cm)
Lymph nodes			
N status	pNO[(i+,–)]	—	pN1, N2–3
Nodal surgery	Yes	Yes	No

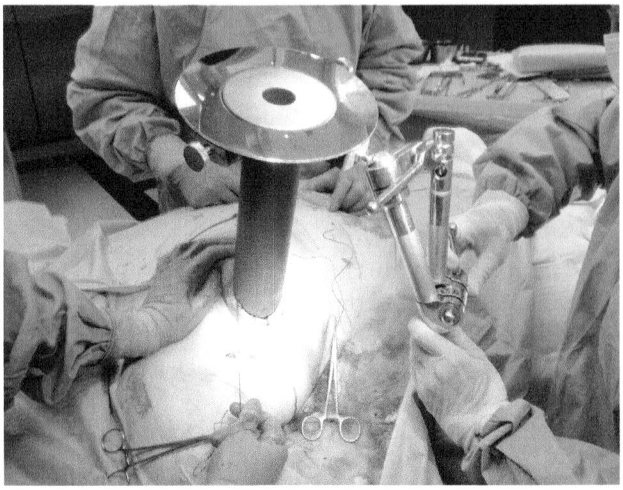

Figure 6.2 Electron-beam IORT: the tissues are onco-plastically rearranged to bring all excision margins into a 'block', against which an appropriately-sized electron applicator is placed, then attached to a small linac. (Courtesy of Dr Dawid Murawa from the Department of Surgical Oncology of the Greater Poland Cancer Centre in Poznań, Poland.)

for the patient, but also in health service resource usage), its use in other sites has very largely been in an attempt to achieve improved local control in circumstances where even radical surgery entails a high risk of failure. The perceived possible advantages of IORT in these circumstances have been alluded to earlier; the clinical situations in which these possibilities have been explored are numerous, but so far it remains impossible to ascertain whether the perceived potential of IORT can be translated into real clinical benefit in these circumstances. Outside the field of breast cancer, no randomized trials of IORT have been undertaken so high-level evidence, upon which decision making can be based, is lacking, even though thousands of patients have been so treated by now. Many large series have been published, as well as 'pooled' data and 'meta-analyses', but these cannot be accepted as high-level evidence in the absence of randomized comparison, particularly given the complexity of the patient population.

Series comprising more than a hundred patients have been published on recurrent colorectal cancer by Hahnloser et al. [18] and Haddock et al. [19], and on pancreatic cancer, both post-resection and unresectable, by Ogawa et al. [20,21], Morganti et al. [22], Nagai et al. [23] and Cai et al. [24]. Results are certainly encouraging, but again it must be said that their value is limited by the absence of a randomized comparator group.

CONCLUSION

Level 1 evidence on the use of IORT in surgical oncology has only been generated for breast cancer, so it cannot be considered to have been adequately evaluated for use at other sites, where it should still be regarded as a clinical option for use only under strict trial-based protocols. The low-level evidence that so far exists suggests that IORT performed after (or instead of) surgical resection is a safe and feasible procedure with a good therapeutic index that can improve treatment results by increasing local tumour control. Where IORT is used as an adjunct to surgical resection, it does not compensate for non-radical surgery in loco-regionally advanced cases, but may have real advantages over EBRT as surgical adjuvant treatment.

Even in breast cancer, the high-level evidence that does exist remains subject to differing interpretations: the view has been expressed by some authors that IORT is now a good ethical option for women with 'low-risk' breast cancer, for whom omission of radiotherapy altogether might be considered [25]. One exception might be boost delivery during BCS for early breast carcinoma, where a substantial body of evidence suggests its safe clinical practice, and a randomized clinical trial is currently testing this.

REFERENCES

1. Njeh CF, Saunders MW, Langton CM. Accelerated partial breast irradiation (APBI): a review of available techniques. *Radiation Oncology* 2010;5:90.
2. Alvarado MD, Conolly J, Park C, Sakata T, Mohan AJ, Harrison BL, et al. Patient preferences regarding intraoperative versus external beam radiotherapy following breast-conserving surgery. *Breast Cancer Research and Treatment* 2014;143(1):135–40.
3. Veronesi U, Orecchia R, Maisonneuve P, Viale G, Rotmensz N, Sangalli C, et al. Intraoperative radiotherapy versus external radiotherapy for early breast cancer (ELIOT): a randomised controlled equivalence trial. *Lancet Oncology* 2013;14(13):1269–77.
4. Krengli M, Calvo FA, Sedlmayer F, Sole CV, Fastner G, Alessandro M, et al. Clinical and technical characteristics of intraoperative radiotherapy. Analysis of the ISIORT-Europe database. *Strahlentherapie und Onkologie* 2013;189(9):729–37.
5. Vaidya JS, Wenz F, Bulsara M, Tobias JS, Joseph DJ, Keshtgar M, et al. Risk-adapted targeted intraoperative radiotherapy versus whole-breast radiotherapy for breast cancer: 5-year results for local control and overall survival from the TARGIT-A randomised trial. *Lancet* 2014;383(9917):603–13.
6. Silverstein MJ, Fastner G, Maluta S, Reitsamer R, Goer DA, Vicini F, et al. Intraoperative radiation therapy: a critical analysis of the ELIOT and TARGIT trials. Part 1 – ELIOT. *Annals of Surgical Oncology* 2014;21(12):3787–92.
7. Silverstein MJ, Fastner G, Maluta S, Reitsamer R, Goer DA, Vicini F, et al. Intraoperative radiation therapy: a critical analysis of the ELIOT and TARGIT trials. Part 2 – TARGIT. *Annals of Surgical Oncology* 2014;21(12):3793–9.

8. Esserman LJ, Alvarado MD, Howe RJ, Mohan AJ, Harrison B, Park C, et al. Application of a decision analytic framework for adoption of clinical trial results: are the data regarding TARGIT-A IORT ready for prime time? *Breast Cancer Research and Treatment* 2014;144(2):371–8.

9. Kaidar-Person O, Poortmans P, Klimberg S, Haviland J, Offersen B, Audisio R, et al. Haste makes waste: are the data regarding TARGIT-A IORT ready for prime time? *Breast Cancer Research and Treatment* 2014;147(1):221–2.

10. Esserman L, Hayes M, Alvarado M. Haste makes waste, but lack of urgency is opportunity lost. *Breast Cancer Research and Treatment* 2014;147(1):223–4.

11. Smith BD, Arthur DW, Buchholz TA, Haffty BG, Hahn CA, Hardenbergh PH, et al. Accelerated partial breast irradiation consensus statement from the American Society for Radiation Oncology (ASTRO). *International Journal of Radiation Oncology, Biology, Physics* 2009;74(4):987–1001.

12. Polgar C, Van Limbergen E, Potter R, Kovacs G, Polo A, Lyczek J, et al. Patient selection for accelerated partial-breast irradiation (APBI) after breast-conserving surgery: recommendations of the Groupe Europeen de Curietherapie–European Society for Therapeutic Radiology and Oncology (GEC-ESTRO) breast cancer working group based on clinical evidence (2009). *Radiotherapy and Oncology* 2010;94(3):264–73.

13. Leonardi MC, Maisonneuve P, Mastropasqua MG, Morra A, Lazzari R, Rotmensz N, et al. How do the ASTRO consensus statement guidelines for the application of accelerated partial breast irradiation fit intraoperative radiotherapy? A retrospective analysis of patients treated at the European Institute of Oncology. *International Journal of Radiation Oncology, Biology, Physics* 2012;83(3):806–13.

14. Kaidar-Person O, Yarnold J, Offersen BV, Poortmans P. Is current evidence about intraoperative partial breast irradiation sufficient for broad implementation in clinical practice? *European Journal of Surgical Oncology* 2014;40(7):791–3.

15. Poortmans PM, Collette L, Bartelink H, Struikmans H, Van den Bogaert WF, Fourquet A, et al. The addition of a boost dose on the primary tumour bed after lumpectomy in breast conserving treatment for breast cancer. A summary of the results of EORTC 22881-10882 'boost versus no boost' trial. *Cancer Radiotherapie* 2008;12(6–7):565–70.

16. Vaidya JS, Baum M, Tobias JS, Wenz F, Massarut S, Keshtgar M, et al. Long-term results of targeted intraoperative radiotherapy (Targit) boost during breast-conserving surgery. *International Journal of Radiation Oncology, Biology, Physics* 2011;81(4):1091–7.

17. Sedlmayer F, Reitsamer R, Fussl C, Ziegler I, Zehentmayr F, Deutschmann H, et al. Boost IORT in breast cancer: body of evidence. *International Journal of Breast Cancer* 2014;2014:472516.

18. Hahnloser D, Nelson H, Gunderson LL, Hassan I, Haddock MG, O'Connell MJ, et al. Curative potential of multimodality therapy for locally recurrent rectal cancer. *Annals of Surgery* 2003;237(4):502–8.

19. Haddock MG, Miller RC, Nelson H, Pemberton JH, Dozois EJ, Alberts SR, et al. Combined modality therapy including intraoperative electron irradiation for locally recurrent colorectal cancer. *International Journal of Radiation Oncology, Biology, Physics* 2011;79(1):143–50.

20. Ogawa K, Karasawa K, Ito Y, Ogawa Y, Jingu K, Onishi H, et al. Intraoperative radiotherapy for resected pancreatic cancer: a multi-institutional retrospective analysis of 210 patients. *International Journal of Radiation Oncology, Biology, Physics* 2010;77(3):734–42.

21. Ogawa K, Karasawa K, Ito Y, Ogawa Y, Jingu K, Onishi H, et al. Intraoperative radiotherapy for unresectable pancreatic cancer: a multi-institutional retrospective analysis of 144 patients. *International Journal of Radiation Oncology, Biology, Physics* 2011;80(1):111–8.

22. Morganti AG, Falconi M, van Stiphout RG, Mattiucci GC, Alfieri S, Calvo FA, et al. Multi-institutional pooled analysis on adjuvant chemoradiation in pancreatic cancer. *International Journal of Radiation Oncology, Biology, Physics* 2014;90(4):911–7.

23. Nagai S, Fujii T, Kodera Y, Kanda M, Sahin TT, Kanzaki A, et al. Prognostic implications of intraoperative radiotherapy for unresectable pancreatic cancer. *Pancreatology* 2011;11(1):68–75.

24. Cai S, Hong TS, Goldberg SI, Fernandez-del Castillo C, Thayer SP, Ferrone CR, et al. Updated long-term outcomes and prognostic factors for patients with unresectable locally advanced pancreatic cancer treated with intraoperative radiotherapy at the Massachusetts General Hospital, 1978 to 2010. *Cancer* 2013;119(23):4196–204.

25. Morgan DAL, Vaidya JS. In regard to Moran et al. and Smith et al. *International Journal of Radiation Oncology Biology Physics* 2014;90(4):967.

7

Principles of systemic therapy for surgeons

SUSANA ROSELLÓ, VALENTINA GAMBARDELLA, JUAN MIGUEL CEJALVO
AND ANDRÉS CERVANTES

INTRODUCTION

Most cancers are managed as part of a multidisciplinary team approach and it is essential that surgical oncologists are aware of the role played by non-surgical therapies in holistic cancer care. Knowledge of systemic therapies and radiotherapy techniques and how they may complement or even replace surgery is vital. In many cases, early stage tumors may be treated with a single modality of treatment, mainly surgery or radiotherapy, with curative results. However, sequential or concomitant multimodality treatments may enhance locoregional and systemic disease control. Multimodality strategies are constantly evolving as new drugs, new radiotherapy regimens and new surgical techniques are developed. Close collaboration with experts in each discipline is essential to keep abreast of the latest advances and every newly diagnosed cancer case must be reviewed by a properly constituted multidisciplinary team before any therapeutic decision is taken.

Systemic anticancer therapies have evolved rapidly over the last few decades with new, more effective chemotherapy drugs and regimens, and the advent of several new classes of agents forming molecularly targeted therapies comprising monoclonal antibodies, small molecular inhibitors, immunotherapy and cancer vaccines. Their mechanisms of action and side effect profiles differ significantly from classical chemotherapy agents. Targeted therapies allow individualized treatment according to the molecular characteristics of the tumor cells. This is increasingly being understood as tumor heterogeneity is better appreciated and new technologies to determine molecular subtypes (immunohistochemistry, gene arrays, FISH and DNA sequencing and array technology) move into the more affordable mainstream of clinical practice.

Selection of the best agent or multi-agent regimen must be individualized based not only on tumor immunophenotype but also on likely patient tolerance. It is well established in oncology to determine performance status (PS), according to the Eastern Cooperative Oncology Group (ECOG) system, and the impact of PS on tolerance of certain regimens is well characterized. Moreover tumor site histology, biological characteristics and stage at diagnosis are elements that need to be evaluated before planning each patient's individualized treatment schedule.

In this chapter we aim to define the different modalities of treatment ranging from preventive and curative to the management of incurable disease. There is a description of the most frequently used chemotherapy drugs with their characteristics and indications, with a special focus on new treatments such as monoclonal antibodies, small molecular therapies and immunotherapy.

MODALITIES OF SYSTEMIC THERAPY

Adjuvant chemotherapy is delivered after the known tumor is removed with surgery to treat patients with a high risk of recurrence. The goal of adjuvant treatment with curative intent is to prevent a possible cancer recurrence by eliminating microscopic residual tumor cells that may be present. Therapeutic endpoints in the adjuvant clinical setting are relapse-free and overall survival since there is no primary tumor response to measure. As an example, in the CONKO-001 phase III trial patients with complete resection of pancreatic cancer were randomly assigned either to adjuvant treatment with gemcitabine or to observation alone [1]. Patients randomized to adjuvant gemcitabine treatment had a prolonged overall survival compared with those randomized to observation alone (HR 0.76, $p = 0.01$). The trial showed a statistically significant absolute 10.3% improvement in the 5-year overall survival rate (20.7% vs. 10.4%) and a 4.5% improvement in the 10-year survival rate (12.2% vs. 7.7%), compared with observation alone.

Neoadjuvant or *primary chemotherapy* is given after a histologic diagnosis, but prior to the surgical procedure. The background of neoadjuvant therapy is the early exposure of disease to an effective treatment, avoiding the delay introduced by surgery and recovery from the operation. It allows *in vivo* assessment of the chemotherapy responsiveness of the primary tumor, and therefore of possible recurrent disease. Neoadjuvant chemotherapy enables direct and early observation of the response to treatment, which could lead to the offer of alternative effective salvage therapy in poor or non-responders. Moreover, the reduction of local disease extent may permit a less extensive surgical procedure (such as breast conservation rather than mastectomy for example) or, render initially inoperable disease operable. Other advantages are that preoperative treatment may also be better tolerated than postoperative treatment and pathologic complete response is an important prognostic factor in neoadjuvant chemotherapy trials. For example, in patients with resectable rectal cancer with high-risk factors defined by MRI, the recommended approach is preoperative short-course radiotherapy or long-course chemoradiotherapy (CRT) followed by total mesorectal excision surgery. Superiority of preoperative versus postoperative CRT has been demonstrated in several trials with lower local recurrence rates in the preoperatively irradiated group (7.1% vs. 10.1%, $p = 0.048$) [2]. Preoperative therapy is not only more efficient for rectal cancer patients, but also less toxic than postoperative treatment.

Chemotherapy given in initially unresectable metastatic disease with the purpose of achieving shrinkage of the tumor burden and facilitating a curative surgery is known as *conversion chemotherapy*. In selected cases of metastatic colorectal cancer (CRC) with initially unresectable disease, combination chemotherapy may favour a major response and a complete resection of the metastasis thereafter. This differs from the palliative treatment of extensive metastatic disease without options of curative surgery.

Palliative chemotherapy is given specifically to improve symptoms associated with incurable cancer. Despite improvements in treatment options, survival benefits tend to be modest. Chemotherapy may be helpful to provide some reduction in metastatic disease burden, relieving pain, cough, bleeding and other tumor-related symptoms.

In the adjuvant, neoadjuvant or metastatic setting, chemotherapy drugs may be used as single agents or in combination. Response rates achieved in the metastatic setting with single-agent therapy might be around 15–20% depending on cancer type, metastatic involvement and characteristics. Combination chemotherapy generally improves response rates with some increase in toxicity. In advanced disease, where the aim generally is not cure, it is very important to balance the possible advantage related to a specific drug and its toxic effects on overall quality of life and length of survival.

CHEMOTHERAPY

The history of chemotherapy for solid tumors began in 1940 when experiments with nitrogen mustard for the war effort were noted to inhibit white cell counts leading to their trial in the treatment of lymphomas and leukemias. Many pharmacologic agents have been developed since then to try to inhibit cancer cell's growth and metastatization. Chemotherapy drugs are traditionally classified into different groups according to either their principal mechanism of action or their biochemical properties (Table 7.1). Chemotherapy agents exert their effects by inhibiting proliferating cells, interfering with DNA, RNA or cell division, causing necrosis or hyperactivation of the apoptotic pathway.

Alkylating agents

The first drugs used in oncology were the alkylating agents, such as cyclophosphamide, ifosfamide, procarbazine, temozolomide, dacarbazine and streptozotocin. These drugs are able to induce cell death through the production of DNA strand breaks. The alkylation process results in the formation of covalent bonds between two nucleophilic molecules causing interstrand or intrastrand cross-links on different DNA bases between a carbon atom and the nitrogen, oxygen or sulfur of another compound. This process induces reactions of substitution of nucleic bases, DNA alterations and finally DNA damage and subsequent cell death [3].

Platinum derivatives

The platinum compounds, widely used in clinical oncology, bind DNA with covalent adducts, causing irreversible alteration and subsequent cell death. Three different drugs belong to this class: cisplatin, carboplatin and oxaliplatin. Their use as single agents or in combination is very diffuse in clinical oncology, for instance in both non–small and small cell lung cancer, mesothelioma, ovarian cancer, CRC, pancreatic cancer, bladder cancer and germinal carcinoma. Comparative trials have revealed a substantial equivalent activity of these compounds, but despite such data, each one has a specific clinical indication. Moreover despite the similar mechanisms of action each one of them is characterized by peculiar pharmacokinetic activity and different

Table 7.1 Most frequently used chemotherapy agents

Family	Drug	Indications	Toxicity
Alkylating agents	Cyclophosphamide	Breast, Hodgkin's lymphoma (HL), non-Hodgkin's lymphoma (NHL), leukemia, ovarian, sarcoma, neuroblastoma, Wilm's tumor, multiple myeloma	Gastrointestinal (GI): Nausea and vomiting Hematologic toxicity Urologic: Hemorrhagic cystitis Dermatologic: Alopecia, skin hyperpigmentation Cardiac: With high-dose therapy Other: Syndrome of inappropriate antidiuretic hormone (SIADH) secretion, lung fibrosis, amenorrhea/testicular atrophy, liver toxicity
	Ifosfamide	Sarcomas, ovarian, testicular, NHL, lung, breast, cervix, bladder	GI: Nausea and vomiting, liver toxicity Hematologic toxicity Urologic: Hemorrhagic cystitis, renal failure Dermatologic: Alopecia Other: Encephalopathy
	Dacarbazine	Melanoma, HL, sarcomas	GI: Nausea, vomiting, liver toxicity Hematologic toxicity Flu-like syndrome Skin: Photosensitivity, alopecia Neurologic: Neuropathy, ataxia, lethargy, seizures Other: Carcinogenesis, teratogenesis
	Temozolomide	Brain tumors, melanoma	GI: Nausea, vomiting, liver toxicity Hematologic toxicity Other: Rash, constipation, headache, asthenia, photosensitivity
Platinum agents	Cisplatin	Lung, ovarian, bladder, testicular, germinal carcinoma, head and neck, cervix, esophageal, gastric	GI: Nausea, vomiting, anorexia, diarrhea, liver toxicity Hematologic toxicity Renal: Nephrotoxicity, electrolytic abnormalities Neurologic: Peripheral sensory neuropathy, seizures, encephalopathy, ototoxicity Hypersensitivity reactions Other: Alopecia, myalgia, fertility reduction, vascular events, SIADH secretion

(Continued)

Table 7.1 *(Continued)* Most frequently used chemotherapy agents

Family	Drug	Indications	Toxicity
	Carboplatin	Ovarian, NSCLC, esophageal, head and neck, bladder, endometrial	GI: Nausea, vomiting, liver toxicity Hematologic toxicity Renal: Electrolytic abnormalities Neurologic: Peripheral neuropathy, ototoxicity Hypersensitivity reactions
	Oxaliplatin	Colorectal, gastric, pancreatic	GI: Nausea, vomiting, diarrhea Hematologic toxicity Neurologic: Peripheral sensory neuropathy, laryngopharyngeal dysesthesia Hypersensitivity reactions Other: Renal toxicity, ototoxicity
Antimetabolites	Methotrexate	Leukemia, breast, carcinomatous meningitis, head and neck, bladder, NHL, gestational trophoblastic cancer, osteosarcoma	GI: Mucositis, nausea, vomiting, liver toxicity Hematologic toxicity Renal: Acute renal failure Lung: Pneumonitis Neurologic: Aphasia, behavioral abnormalities, acute chemical arachnoiditis after intrathecal administration Skin: Rash, photosensitivity, radiation recall Other: Osteoporosis, anaphylaxis
	Pemetrexed	NSCLC, mesothelioma	GI: Nausea, vomiting, mucositis, diarrhea, liver toxicity Hematologic toxicity Skin: Hand–foot syndrome
	5-Fluorouracil	Breast, colorectal, esophageal, gastric, pancreatic, anal carcinoma, head and neck	GI: Nausea, vomiting, mucositis, diarrhea Hematologic toxicity Skin: Hand–foot syndrome, photosensitivity Neurologic: Headache, somnolence, ataxia Cardiac: Chest pain, ECG changes, cardiac enzyme elevation Other: Conjunctivitis

(Continued)

Table 7.1 *(Continued)* Most frequently used chemotherapy agents

Family	Drug		Indications	Toxicity
	Capecitabine		Breast, colorectal, gastric	GI: Nausea, vomiting, diarrhea, mucositis, liver toxicity Hematologic toxicity Skin: Hand–foot syndrome Cardiac: Chest pain, ECG changes, cardiac enzyme elevation Other: Neurotoxicity, ophthalmologic disorders
	Gemcitabine		NSCLC, pancreatic, bladder, breast, ovarian, sarcoma	GI: Nausea, vomiting, diarrhea, mucositis, liver toxicity Hematologic toxicity Flu-like syndrome Skin: Maculopapular skin rash Lung: Pneumonitis Renal: Proteinuria, hematuria, hemolytic-uremic syndrome Infusional reaction
Topoisomerase I inhibitors	Irinotecan		Colorectal (CRC), NSCLC, gastric, pancreatic, ovarian	GI: Early-form diarrhea (cholinergic syndrome), late-onset diarrhea, nausea, vomiting, liver toxicity Hematologic toxicity Other: Alopecia, asthenia
	Topotecan		Squamous cell lung cancer (SCLC), cervix, ovarian	Hematologic toxicity GI: Nausea, vomiting, diarrhea, liver toxicity Other: Headache, arthralgias, myalgias, hematuria, alopecia
Topoisomerase II inhibitors	Etoposide		SCLC, germinal cancer, HL, NHL, Kaposi's sarcoma	Hematologic toxicity GI: Nausea, vomiting, anorexia, diarrhea, mucositis Skin: Alopecia, skin hyperpigmentation, radiation recall Hypersensitivity reaction with chills, fever, bronchospasm
	Anthracyclines	Doxorubicin	Breast cancer, sarcomas, HL, NHL, gastric, ovarian, liver, thyroid, leukemia	GI: Nausea, vomiting, diarrhea, mucositis Hematologic toxicity Acute cardiotoxicity: Arrhythmias, ECG changes Chronic cardiotoxicity: Dilated cardiomyopathy, dose dependent Skin: Alopecia, hyperpigmentation nails, radiation recall

(Continued)

Table 7.1 *(Continued)* Most frequently used chemotherapy agents

Family	Drug	Indications	Toxicity
	Epirubicin	Breast, gastric	GI: Nausea, vomiting, diarrhea, mucositis Cardiotoxicity: Same as doxorubicin but less severe Hematologic toxicity Skin: Alopecia, hyperpigmentation, radiation recall
	Liposomal doxorubicin (Myocet)	Breast	Hematologic toxicity GI: Nausea, vomiting, diarrhea, mucositis Cardiotoxicity: Same as doxorubicin but less severe
	Liposomal doxorubicin (Doxil, Caelyx)	Sarcomas, ovarian, breast, multiple myeloma, liver	Hematologic toxicity GI: Nausea, vomiting, diarrhea, mucositis Cardiotoxicity: Same as doxorubicin but less severe Skin: Hand–foot syndrome, alopecia, hyperpigmentation Infusion reactions
Vinka alkaloids	Vinorelbine	NSCLC, breast, ovarian, HL	GI: Nausea, vomiting, stomatitis, constipation, diarrhea, liver toxicity Hematologic toxicity Neurotoxicity Other: Hypersensitivity reactions, SIADH secretion
	Vinflunine	Urothelial tract carcinoma	Hematologic toxicity GI: Constipation, nausea, vomiting Cardiotoxicity: QT prolongation, ischemic cardiac events Other: Encephalopathy, SIADH secretion
Taxanes	Paclitaxel	Breast, ovarian, NSCLC, esophageal, prostate, AIDS-related Kaposi's sarcoma	GI: Nausea, vomiting, diarrhea, mucositis, liver toxicity Hematologic toxicity Neurologic: Peripheral sensory neuropathy Hypersensitivity reaction: Dyspnea, rash, hypotension Cardiac: Bradycardia, arrhythmias Skin: Alopecia, onycholysis

(Continued)

Table 7.1 *(Continued)* Most frequently used chemotherapy agents

Family	Drug	Indications	Toxicity
	Docetaxel	Breast, ovarian, NSCLC, prostate, gastric, head and neck, bladder, sarcomas	Hematologic toxicity GI: Mucositis, diarrhea, liver toxicity Hypersensitivity reactions Fluid retention syndrome Skin: Alopecia, maculopapular rash, discoloration nails Neurologic: Peripheral sensory neuropathy
	Nab-paclitaxel	Pancreatic, breast	Hematologic toxicity GI: Nausea, vomiting, diarrhea, liver toxicity Neurologic: Peripheral sensory neuropathy Skin: Alopecia, photosensitivity Other: Arthralgia, myalgia, sore mouth
	Cabazitaxel	Prostate	Hematologic toxicity GI: Diarrhea, nausea, vomiting, constipation Hypersensitivity reactions
Miscellaneous	Bleomycin	NHL, HL, germ cell tumors, skin, cervix, vulva, sclerosing agent for malignant pleural effusion	GI: Nausea, vomiting, mucositis Lung: Interstitial pneumonia Skin: Erythema, hyperpigmentation, alopecia Hypersensitivity reaction with fever, chills
	Mitomycin C	Anal carcinoma, gastric, pancreatic	GI: Nausea, vomiting, mucositis Hematologic toxicity Other: Hemolytic-uremic syndrome, interstitial pneumonitis, hepatic veno-occlusive disease
	Eribulin	Breast	Hematologic toxicity Skin: Alopecia Neurologic: Peripheral neuropathy GI: Nausea, vomiting, diarrhea, constipation Other: Arthralgia, myalgia, asthenia

toxicity profiles. Generally these drugs are used as part of combination regimens, but they represent a cornerstone of medical oncology even as single agents or in combination with radiotherapy [4].

Antimetabolites

Another strategy adopted in oncology is trying to induce cell death using drugs that substitute normal metabolites. Antifolates, purine and pyrimidine analogues act like false metabolites blocking normal cellular function. Folate metabolism is essential for cellular activity, and alterations to this system are responsible for causing cell death. Antifolate agents include methotrexate and pemetrexed. Pemetrexed has demonstrated great activity in lung adenocarcinoma. This cancer has a low expression of thymidylate synthase, the main target of pemetrexed. Because of these biological features, the use of pemetrexed in combination with cisplatin is able to prolong overall and progression-free survival in advanced lung adenocarcinoma [5,6].

Both purine and pyrimidine analogues, such as 5-fluorouracil (5FU), gemcitabine and capecitabine, are useful drugs in daily clinical practice in oncology. Fluoropyrimidines are the cornerstone of most treatments in GI tumors. 5FU as a single agent or 5FU-based combinations represent a very helpful tool in the neoadjuvant, adjuvant or metastatic setting and may even be useful as a radiosensitizing drug. Most of the antimetabolites act during the S phase of the cell cycle when proliferation is prominent, but they can also act in phase G1, G2 or M [7].

Topoisomerase inhibitors

Another strategy to induce cell death is by inhibiting cellular DNA replication by damaging topoisomerase I or II. DNA topoisomerases are enzymes that regulate the topological state of DNA during all cell processes such as replication, transcription, recombination and chromatin remodelling.

Topoisomerase I is a ubiquitous nuclear enzyme which catalyzes the reaction of superhelical DNA generating a transient single-strand break in double-stranded DNA. Its function is to preserve the three-dimensional conformation of DNA by removing torsional stress generated during replication and transcription. Inhibition of topoisomerase I activities is lethal and leads to cell death. The topoisomerase II enzyme mediates the ATP-dependent induction of nicks in the double-stranded DNA, allowing relaxation of superhelical DNA during replication and transcription. These agents interfere with enzyme functions by stabilizing a reaction intermediate in which DNA strands are cut and covalently linked to tyrosine residues of the protein forming a cleavable complex. Topoisomerase I inhibitors include irinotecan and topotecan. Irinotecan is widely used in gastrointestinal malignancies as a single agent or in combination. The association with 5FU improves notably overall and progression-free survival in metastatic CRC. Recently its activity has been underlined in gastric cancer.

Topoisomerase II inhibitors include etoposide and anthracyclines. Anthracyclines such as doxorubicin and epirubicin, and products like pegylated liposomal doxorubicin are commonly used in oncology and their activity is related to their capacity to induce many biological reactions, but mainly topoisomerase II inhibition, DNA intercalation, helicase inhibition and production of reactive oxygen species damaging DNA and membranes. They represent one of the cornerstones of breast cancer treatment, but also have activity in ovarian cancer and sarcomas [8].

Anti-tubulin agents

Another potential mechanism to attack cancer cells is by damaging the microtubules which regulate mitosis. Microtubules are polymeric filaments composed of alpha-tubulin and beta-tubulin heterodimers. Microtubules have crucial roles in cell division and growth. Two different mechanisms of action are used by microtubules targeting agents: First, by binding tubulin they prevent the formation of the microtubule, which is important during mitosis. This is the mechanism of action of the vinka alkaloids such as vincristine, vinblastine, vinorelbine and vinflunine. The second mechanism by which chemotherapy agents may attach microtubules is that of the taxane group (paclitaxel, docetaxel, cabazitaxel, nab-paclitaxel), which prevents the disassembly of microtubules, so inhibiting normal function. Both taxanes and vinka alkaloids are used in many tumors as single agents or in combination. Notably vinflunine represents the only active drug usable as a second line in patients with metastatic bladder carcinoma. Taxanes are indispensable drugs in clinical practice with significant antitumor activity in ovarian, lung, breast, gastroesophageal and pancreatic malignancies [9].

SYSTEMIC HORMONAL THERAPIES

In hormone-sensitive cancers, such as breast or prostate cancer, inhibition of the hormonal stimulus is an essential therapeutic strategy. In breast cancer, the expression of oestrogen and progesterone receptors characterizes a particular subtype of cancer known as luminal type, which is very sensitive to hormonal therapies. High oestrogen receptor expression is also usually associated with reduced chemotherapy sensitivity. Many antioestrogen drugs have been developed and they are widely used in the metastatic, adjuvant and neoadjuvant settings. One of the oldest and most widely used is tamoxifen, a selective oestrogen receptor modulator (SERM), which binds to the oestrogen receptor and either antagonizes its effects on breast tissue or acts as an agonist at other sites such as bone and endometrium. It binds to the ER on the nuclear membrane and inhibits intranuclear transduction. Tamoxifen is indicated in adjuvant and metastatic settings. In the adjuvant setting treatment is usually reserved for premenopausal women. Another antioestrogens currently used in clinical practice include fulvestrant, a pure oestrogen receptor antagonist able to competitively bind the oestrogen receptor with high affinity inducing its downregulation. This drug is indicated for metastatic hormone receptor positive breast cancer where it is able to prolong both progression-free survival and overall survival [10,11]. In all settings the drug is relatively safe and well tolerated with the main side effect being hot flashes, but it is also associated with a slightly increased risk of venous thromboembolism and endometrial cancer [12].

In postmenopausal women ovarian-derived oestrogen levels are very low and the peripheral process of aromatization whereby adrenal androgens are converted to oestrogens becomes the most relevant source of endogenous production. In women with hormone-dependent tumors developing postmenopausally, aromatase inhibitors have a greater efficacy and enhanced side effect profile than tamoxifen [13]. These agents might be divided according to the biochemical structure into steroidal and non-steroidal and into reversible and irreversible. Classically they can be used in the adjuvant, neoadjuvant or metastatic setting.

Unlike tamoxifen which has a bone density protective effect, aromatase inhibitors may cause osteoporosis, which should be monitored for [14].

Recently these drugs have been used in combination with other target agents such as everolimus, an mTOR inhibitor, in order to overcome hormone resistance [15]. Sometimes in specific situations complete hormonal blockade is needed. Luteinizing hormone-releasing hormone (LHRH) analogues are able, after an initial stimulation of gonadotropin release (sometimes known as a flare), to fully inhibit gonadotropin formation, thanks to receptor downregulation. This results in a decreased level of oestrogen, progesterone and testosterone. These agents, which are given by monthly injection, may be used in the treatment of both oestrogen-sensitive breast cancer and androgen-sensitive prostate cancer. Examples include goserelin and leuprolide.

In androgen-sensitive prostate cancer a leading role in treatment is effected by antiandrogens. Examples include flutamide and bicalutamide. These are competitive antagonists of the androgen receptor inhibiting androgen binding and preventing translocation of the androgen receptor complex. Antiandrogens do not inhibit pituitary LH secretion. They can be divided into steroidal and non-steroidal and into reversible and non-reversible subtypes [16].

TARGETED AGENTS AND TAILORED MEDICINE

The concept of cancer treatment during recent years has dramatically changed. Oncologic treatment has transitioned from the use of non-specific cytotoxic drugs to the era of targeted agents such as antibodies or small tyrosine kinase inhibitors, which are playing an increasingly important role in a growing number of tumor types (Figure 7.1, Table 7.2). Various molecules implicated in cancer development and metastasis have been identified and studied as possible pharmacological targets.

Anti-HER agents

Perhaps the most widely known pathway targeted by molecularly targeted therapies is the ERBB family of proteins which are recognized as key drivers in carcinogenesis. Since the beginning of the 1980s, research has been confirming the ERBB network as a potential target for anticancer drugs. The transmembrane members of the epidermal growth factor family, potent mediators of cell growth and survival, are made up of four tyrosine kinase receptors: epidermal growth factor receptor (EGFR) or HER1, HER2, HER3 and HER4. After binding of extracellular ligands, these receptors activate an important signalling cascade promoted by the activation of their tyrosine kinase domain. Activation of the pathway is mediated by dimerization that may occur between two different receptors of the same family or the same receptor. The most important downstream pathways activated are Ras–Raf–MEK–ERK and PI3K–Akt–mTOR. Gain of function in

EGFR (receptor overexpression) can be observed in many epithelial tumors and many neoplasms are directly dependent on its activation [17,18].

EGFR plays a crucial role in the carcinogenesis of CRC, and it is a fascinating target in metastatic CRC patients. In many randomized clinical trials, the use of anti-EGFR monoclonal antibodies both as single agents and in combination with chemotherapy has shown a clear benefit in overall survival and progression-free survival in RAS wild-type colon cancer patients. Initially the immunohistochemical expression of EGFR was thought to be a relevant predictive biomarker. Further analysis, however, led to the conclusion that anti-EGFR antibodies were active only in KRAS wild-type tumors (with no mutations on codons 12 and 13 of exon 2). Recently, it has been shown that other RAS mutations (codon 61 of exon 3 and codons 117 and 146 of exon 4 of KRAS and exons 2, 3 and 4 of NRAS) need to be tested. Exon 2 KRAS mutations occur in 40% of CRC cases, and the other KRAS and NRAS mutations in 10–15% of patients. The activity of the anti-EGFR antibodies is confined to RAS wild-type tumors. Two different monoclonal antibodies have been developed and are now approved for use in the clinical metastatic setting: cetuximab and panitumumab. Cetuximab is a chimeric IgG1 monoclonal antibody able to induce an important antibody-dependent cell-mediated cytotoxicity reaction. Panitumumab is a fully humanized IgG2 monoclonal antibody. Both these drugs may be used in RAS wild-type metastatic CRC patients. Outcomes are enhanced still further if they are combined with oxaliplatin and irinotecan. Cetuximab is also approved in locally advanced head and neck tumors achieving, when combined with radiotherapy, higher response rates, prolonged disease-free survival (DFS) and overall survival compared with radiotherapy alone [19,20].

Genetic alterations of the EGFR have been identified in non–small cell lung cancer (NSCLC), where in patients with deletions in exons 19 and 21 of EGFR, there is tumor dependency on EGFR activation. The incidence of EGFR mutations in the Caucasian population is about 10% and is higher in never-smokers, adenocarcinoma subtype, in women and also in East Asian patients. Activating epidermal growth factor receptor mutations is predictive for response to the EGFR tyrosine kinase inhibitors gefitinib and erlotinib, improving response rate, progression-free survival and quality of life when compared with chemotherapy as first-line therapy. Gefitinib and erlotinib are both reversible small tyrosine kinase inhibitors able to block this signalling pathway by binding to the ATP site. Another drug able to interact with tyrosine kinase is afatinib [21–23].

Another important ERBB family receptor is HER2. Particular subtypes of breast and gastric cancer overexpress HER2 and in its alteration could be considered 'driver'. In early breast cancer, one of the most important prognostic and predictive factors is the overexpression of HER2, allowing for selection of patients for anti-HER2 directed treatments. Targeting HER2 represents a fundamental part of treatment both in adjuvant HER2 positive breast cancer

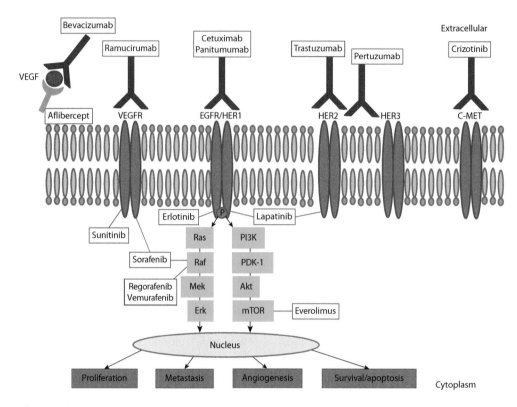

Figure 7.1 Signalling pathways.

patients and in HER2 positive metastatic breast cancer patients. Trastuzumab, an IgG1 humanized monoclonal antibody, binds the extracellular receptor inhibiting the proliferation of HER2-dependent cancer cells. When given in combination with chemotherapy, as widely demonstrated in randomized clinical trials, trastuzumab reduces the risk of relapse in the adjuvant setting and enhances survival in metastatic patients; this translates into 10% absolute improvement in 3-year DFS and a 3% increase in 3-year overall survival [24]. Another anti-HER2 directed drug is lapatinib. This is a dual EGFR/HER2 tyrosine kinase inhibitor that can be used in trastuzumab-resistant HER2 positive breast cancer in association with chemotherapy and after the failure of first-line anti-HER2 treatment with trastuzumab. This drug is able to inhibit the HER2 signalling pathway even with the truncated version of the HER2 receptor (p95HER2), which is overexpressed in 25% of patients with HER2-dependent breast cancer. It can be used even after a first failure treatment with trastuzumab [25]. In patients who have trastuzumab-resistant, metastatic breast cancer, a new drug consisting of trastuzumab bound to the chemotherapy agent emtansine, TDM1, has been recently developed. The chemotherapy agent is effectively targeted to the HER2 receptor overexpressing cancer cells. In randomized clinical trials this agent has demonstrated the capacity to reverse trastuzumab resistance [26]. Metastatic gastric cancer patients may also benefit from testing for HER2 expression. In HER2 amplified gastric cancer (10–15% of cases), a phase III trial demonstrated clinically and statistically significant improvements in response rate, progression-free

survival and overall survival with the addition of trastuzumab to a cisplatin–fluoropyrimidine chemotherapy combination regimen (median OS 13.8 vs. 11.1 months, HR 0.74, 95% CI 0.60–0.91, $p = 0.0048$). This regimen now represents the standard of care for these patients [27].

In recent years another important drug that blocks the dimerization of HER2 has been developed. Pertuzumab is now available in metastatic breast cancer and when combined with both trastuzumab and chemotherapy is able to notably prolong survival [28].

BRAF inhibitors

The downstream pathway of the EGFR may be hyperactivated in the presence of mutations of the RAS or BRAF genes. While there are presently no inhibitors of RAS, BRAF mutations are able to be targeted. Approximately 6–8% of CRC tumors carry a mutated BRAF gene. RAS mutations and BRAF mutations are usually mutually exclusive. The BRAF mutation is a strong negative prognostic biomarker: indeed, patients with a BRAF mutant metastatic CRC have a very poor prognosis. Drugs able to act against BRAF V600, such as vemurafenib or dabrafenib, have shown great activity in metastatic melanoma. Trials are now underway in BRAF mutated CRC patients [29].

Antiangiogenic agents

The regulation of angiogenesis is a complex process and the result of a balance of stimulating peptides (vascular

Table 7.2 Most frequently used targeted therapies

Anti-EGFR	Cetuximab, panitumumab	Colorectal, head and neck	Skin: Maculopapular rash, paronychia Hypersensitivity reactions GI: Nausea, vomiting, diarrhea Hematologic toxicity Other: Hypomagnesemia
	Gefitinib, erlotinib, afatinib	NSCLC	GI: Nausea, diarrhea, anorexia, mucositis Skin: Rash, dry skin, paronychia Other: Asthenia, conjunctivitis, interstitial pneumonia
Anti-HER2	Trastuzumab	Breast, gastric	Cardiotoxicity: Decrease in left ventricular ejection fraction Hypersensitivity reactions
Anti-HER1–HER2	Lapatinib	Breast	GI: Diarrhea, constipation Skin: Rash
Anti-HER2–HER3	Pertuzumab	Breast	Hematologic toxicity GI: Diarrhea, constipation Skin: Rash Other: Asthenia, taste change
BCR-ABL	Imatinib	GISTs, leukemia	GI: Nausea, vomiting, diarrhea, constipation Hematologic toxicity Skin: Rash, changes in hair colour Other: Hemorrhage (GI, brain)
Antiangiogenic	Bevacizumab, aflibercept, ramucirumab	NSCLC, CRC	Hematologic toxicity Vascular: Increased blood pressure, deep venous thrombosis Cardiac: Thromboembolic heart failure Other: Asthenia, proteinuria
Antiangiogenic TKIs	Sunitinib, sorafenib, regorafenib, axitinib, pazopanib	Renal cancer, HCC, CRC, GISTs, sarcomas	GI: Diarrhea, mucositis Vascular: Increased blood pressure, hemorrhage, epistaxis Arterial/venous thromboembolic event Other: Fistula, hand–foot syndrome

endothelial growth factor [VEGF], fibroblast growth factor [FGF], interleukins 4 and 8 [IL-4, IL-8] and others) and endogenous inhibitory factors. Three vascular endothelial growth factor receptors are known: VEGFR 1, 2 and 3. Their activation, in particular VEGF mediated, triggers a sequence of downstream events (involving even RAS–RAF and PI3K pathways), resulting in endothelial proliferation, enhanced cancer cell survival and migration with the formation of new blood vessels. Other pathways implicated in the neo-angiogenesis process include different integrins and proteases [30]. Attacking neo-angiogenesis, that is the development of new blood vessels, is one of the most interesting challenges in cancer treatment and several anti-angiogenic agents are currently in clinical use. Two classes of drug are available: monoclonal antibodies against vascular growth factors and tyrosine kinase inhibitors against angiogenesis-implicated receptors. Unfortunately, despite the wide use of these agents in oncology, there are no markers to predict response. The first drug developed to try to block angiogenesis and thereby inhibit cancer growth was bevacizumab. This is a recombinant IgG1 monoclonal antibody able to bind VEGFA inhibiting the interaction with the endothelial VEGF receptors 1 and 2 (VEGFR 1 and 2). Bevacizumab is widely used in oncology, in particular in metastatic colorectal cancer, NSCLC, ovarian cancer and breast cancer patients, leading to an improvement in progression-free survival and overall survival. Other anti-angiogenic drugs have been recently approved for cancer treatment [31,32]. Aflibercept is a recombinant fusion protein containing VEGF-binding portions from the extracellular domains of human VEGFR 1 and 2, fused to the Fc portion of human immunoglobulin G1. This drug blocks the activity of VEGFA, VEGFB and placental growth factor (PDGF) by acting as a high-affinity ligand trap to prevent these ligands from binding to their endogenous receptors. Actually aflibercept is indicated in second-line metastatic CRC patients where a randomized clinical trial has demonstrated an improvement of both progression-free survival and overall survival [33]. Another antiangiogenic agent is ramucirumab, a human IgG1 monoclonal antibody VEGFR 2 antagonist, which prevents ligand binding and receptor-mediated pathway activation in endothelial cells. This drug has been recently developed and its activity has been confirmed in metastatic gastric, colorectal and NSCLC patients, revealing a benefit in terms of overall survival and progression-free survival [34]. Multi-tyrosine kinase inhibitors of angiogenic pathways currently in use are sorafenib, sunitinib, axitinib, pazopanib and regorafenib. Sorafenib is used in unresectable hepatocellular carcinoma. Sunitinib, pazopanib and axitinib are indicated in clear renal cell carcinoma. Pazopanib is also indicated in sarcomas, while regorafenib is now indicated in metastatic CRC and gastrointestinal stromal tumors (GISTs) [35–40].

mTOR inhibitors

The PI3K–AKT–mTOR signalling pathway regulates many processes in neoplastic cells. Upstream of this pathway and hence feeding into it are the HER, PDGFR and IGFR pathways, which influence many different types of cancer. It is a principal regulator of many processes of neoplastic and non-neoplastic cells, including proliferation, survival, growth and motility. Evidence of dysregulation of the PI3K pathway has been described in many tumors, especially in breast cancer, renal cell carcinoma and neuroendocrine tumors, and many drugs are now under development or testing as part of phase II or III clinical trials. One of the most important targetable molecules is mTOR: the mTOR inhibitor everolimus inhibits mTORC1 and is an active drug in metastatic renal carcinoma and neuroendocrine tumors and now is used in association with aromatase inhibitors

in metastatic luminal-type breast cancer in order to reverse secondary hormone resistance. The evidence of an active role in cancer development and progression of the pathway leads to the use of inhibitors in different kinds of cancers [41,42].

ALK inhibitors

Another important oncogenic driver in NSCLC patients is the presence of the EML4-ALK fusion gene, resulting from an inversion in chromosome 2. It is encountered more frequently in never-smokers, the adenocarcinoma subtype and in younger patients, representing probably about 5% of all lung adenocarcinomas. ALK activity can be efficiently targeted by the TKI crizotinib, an oral small-molecule tyrosine kinase inhibitor targeting ALK (anaplastic lymphoma receptor tyrosine kinase), MET and ROS1 tyrosine kinases. Many clinical trials have demonstrated clinical superiority compared to chemotherapy in overall survival, progression-free survival and quality of life in well-selected patients. Second-generation ALK inhibitors are now in use in order to reverse crizotinib resistance [43].

IMMUNOTHERAPY

One of the most investigated fields in oncology is the linkage between immune surveillance and the development of cancer based on the hypothesis that the immune system can suppress the development or progression of spontaneous malignancies. The idea that some cancer cells could evade this protective system has led to the development of new drugs stimulating the immune response to recognize and kill tumor cells. Strategies to stimulate effector immune cells include vaccination with tumor antigens, treatment with cytokines such as IL-2 or interferon-α, enhancement of antigen presentation by stimulation of Toll-like receptor 7, 8 or 9, administration of dendritic cells or the use of a CD40-targeted agonistic antibody. Further stimulatory strategies include the possibility to stimulate T cell activity by using antibodies targeting the tumor necrosis factor receptor, members 4-1BB, OX40 or glucocorticoid-induced tumor necrosis factor receptor (TNFR)–related protein. Actually in oncology many drugs are in development and many association regimens are in study.

One of the most important drugs already used in clinical practice is ipilimumab, an antagonistic CTLA4-targeted antibody that acts to overcome the T cell inhibitory pathways elicited by CTLA4. This agent is currently used in melanoma and has shown activity in prostate cancer patients [44].

During recent years, great attention has been given to the possibility to adopt therapeutic vaccines for cancer treatment. Despite many unsuccessful trials, recently in hormone-resistant prostate cancer patients, sipuleucel-T, an autologous active cellular immunotherapy, has shown efficacy in reducing mortality and prolonging overall survival among men with metastatic castration-resistant prostate cancer. No effect on the time to disease progression was observed [45].

Another relevant class of agents is the immune checkpoint inhibitors, also known as anti-PDL-1/PD-1 drugs, such as pembrolizumab, nivolumab or atezolizumab. They have a significant role in the treatment of solid tumors such as melanoma, renal cell carcinoma, squamous lung or head and neck cancers and colorectal tumor with microsatellite instability (MSI). According to data taken from preclinical studies, combinatorial approaches between different immunotherapy agents, targeted agents or chemotherapy may be optimal but further clinical trials are awaited. Recent work in cancer genomics, in particular the sequencing of breast and colon carcinomas, showed that there were almost 100 missense mutations per tumor that could lead to the creation of neo-antigens with the potential to be recognized by the immune system. This could explain the high antitumor activity observed when advanced CRC patients with high levels of MSI are treated with pembrolizumab [46]. Currently, there is a lack of predictive diagnostic biomarkers to rationally choose combinations of immunotherapy for individual patients or cancer types [47].

SUMMARY

As can be seen above systemic anticancer therapies are progressing rapidly and are a vital component of many multimodal cancer treatment regimens in the adjuvant, neoadjuvant and metastatic setting. New agents are being continually developed in response to our increasing knowledge about the molecular heterogeneity and characteristics of cancer. It is likely that increasingly tailored approaches will continue to improve outcomes for individual cancer patients.

However, this progress is very costly. Exploratory and development research and subsequent clinical trials to bring such agents to clinical approval is a hugely expensive and time-consuming process leaving drug companies little time to recoup costs before patent protection expires. In many countries the costs of these agents are very high and drug regulatory authorities urgently need to look at ways of rationalizing this process to make these agents affordable.

REFERENCES

1. Oettle H, Neuhaus P, Hochhaus A, et al. Adjuvant chemotherapy with gemcitabine and long-term outcomes among patients with resected pancreatic cancer. The CONKO-001 Randomized Trial. *JAMA* 2013;310(14):1473–1481.

2. Sauer R, Liersch T, Merkel S, et al. Preoperative versus postoperative chemoradiotherapy for locally advanced rectal cancer: results of the German CAO/ARO/AIO-94 randomized phase III trial after a median follow-up of 11 years. *J Clin Oncol* 2012;30:1926–1933.

3. Helleday T, Petermann E, Lundin C, et al. DNA repair pathways as targets for cancer therapy. *Nat Rev Cancer* 2008;8:193–204.

4. Kelland L. The resurgence of platinum-based cancer chemotherapy. *Nat Rev Cancer* 2007;7:573–584.

5. Gonen N, Assaraf YG. Antifolates in cancer therapy: structure, activity and mechanisms of drug resistance. *Drug Resist Update* 2012;15(4):183–210.

6. Scagliotti GV, Parikh P, von Pawel J, et al. Phase III study comparing cisplatin plus gemcitabine with cisplatin plus pemetrexed in chemotherapy-naive patients with advanced-stage non–small-cell lung cancer. *J Clin Oncol* 2008;26(21):3543–3551.

7. Longley D, Harkin DP, Johnston PJ. 5-Fluorouracil: mechanisms of action and clinical strategies. *Nat Rev Cancer* 2003;3:330–338.

8. Pommier Y. Topoisomerase I inhibitors: camptothecins and beyond. *Nat Rev Cancer* 2006;6:789–802.

9. Jackson JR, Patrick DR, Dar MM, et al. Targeted antimitotic therapies: can we improve on tubulin agents? *Nat Rev Cancer* 2007;7:107–117.

10. Goldhirsch A, Wood WC, Coates AS. Strategies for subtypes – dealing with the diversity of breast cancer: highlights of the St Gallen International Expert Consensus on the Primary Therapy of Early Breast Cancer. *Ann Oncol* 2011;22(8):1736–1747.

11. Robertson JFR, Llombart-Cussac A, Rolski J. Activity of fulvestrant 500 mg versus anastrozole 1 mg as first-line treatment for advanced breast cancer: results from the FIRST study. *J Clin Oncol* 2009;27(27):4530–4535.

12. Chen JY, Kuo SJ, Liaw YP, et al. Endometrial cancer incidence in breast cancer patients correlating with age and duration of tamoxifen use: a population based study. *J Cancer* 2014;5(2):151–155.

13. Howell A, Cuzick J, Baum M, et al. Results of the ATAC (Arimidex, Tamoxifen, Alone or in Combination) trial after completion of 5 years' adjuvant treatment for breast cancer. *Lancet* 2005;365(9453):60–62.

14. Eastell R. Aromatase inhibitors and bone. *J Steroid Biochem Mol Biol* 2007;106(1–5):157–161.

15. Baselga J, Campone M, Piccart M. Everolimus in postmenopausal hormone-receptor positive advanced breast cancer. *N Engl J Med* 2012;366:520–529.

16. Sharifi N, Gulley JL, Dahut WL, et al. Androgen deprivation therapy for prostate cancer. *JAMA* 2005;294(2):238–244.

17. Yarden Y, Sliwkowski MX. Untangling the ErbB signalling network. *Nat Rev Mol Cell Biol* 2001;2(2):127–137.

18. Ciardiello F, Tortora G. EGFR antagonists in cancer treatment. *N Engl J Med* 2008;358:1160–1174.

19. Van Cutsem A, Cervantes B, Nordlinger B, et al. Metastatic colorectal cancer ESMO clinical practice guidelines. *Ann Oncol* 2014;25(Suppl. 3):iii1–iii9.

20. Vermorken JB, Mesia R, Rivera F. Platinum-based chemotherapy plus cetuximab in head and neck cancer. *N Engl J Med* 2008;359:1116–1127.

21. Mok T, Wu YL, Thongprasert S. Gefitinib or carboplatin–paclitaxel in pulmonary adenocarcinoma. *N Engl J Med* 2009;361:947–957.

22. Rosell R, Carcereny E, Gervais R, et al. Erlotinib versus standard chemotherapy as first-line treatment for European patients with advanced EGFR mutation-positive non-small-cell lung cancer (EURTAC): a multicentre, open-label, randomised phase 3 trial. *Lancet* 2012;13(3):239–246.

23. Sequist LV, Chih-Hsin Yang J, Yamamoto N. Phase III study of afatinib or cisplatin plus pemetrexed in patients with metastatic lung adenocarcinoma with EGFR mutations. *J Clin Oncol* 2013;31(27):3327–3334.

24. Cardoso F, Costa A, Norton L, et al. Advanced breast cancer: ESO-ESMO consensus guideline. *Ann Oncol* 2014;25(10):1871–1888.

25. Geyer CE, Forster J, Lindquist D. Lapatinib plus capecitabine for HER2-positive advanced breast cancer. *N Engl J Med* 2006;355:2733–2743.

26. Krop JE, Kim SB, González-Martín A, et al. Trastuzumab emtansine versus treatment of physician's choice for pretreated HER2-positive advanced breast cancer (TH3RESA): a randomised, open-label, phase 3 trial. *Lancet Oncol* 2014;15:689–699.

27. Bang YJ, Van Cutsem E, Feyereislova A. Trastuzumab in combination with chemotherapy versus chemotherapy alone for treatment of HER2-positive advanced gastric or gastro-oesophageal junction cancer (ToGA): a phase 3, open-label, randomised controlled trial. *Lancet* 2010;376(9742):687–697.

28. Baselga J, Cortez J, Kim SB, et al. Pertuzumab plus trastuzumab plus docetaxel for metastatic breast cancer. *N Engl J Med* 2012;366(2):109–119.

29. Chapman PB, Hauschild A, Robert C. Improved survival with vemurafenib in melanoma with BRAF V600E mutation. *N Engl J Med* 2011;364:2507–2516.

30. Ellis LM, Hicklin DJ. VEGF-targeted therapy: mechanisms of anti-tumour activity. *Nat Rev Cancer* 2008;8:579–591.

31. Sandler A, Gray R, Perry MC. Paclitaxel–carboplatin alone or with bevacizumab for non–small-cell lung cancer. *N Engl J Med* 2006;355:2542–2550.

32. Burger R, Brady MF, Bookman MA. Incorporation of bevacizumab in the primary treatment of ovarian cancer. *N Engl J Med* 2011;365:2473–2483.

33. Van Cutsem E, Tabernero J, Lakomy R, et al. Addition of aflibercept to fluorouracil, leucovorin, and irinotecan improves survival in a phase III randomized trial in patients with metastatic colorectal cancer previously treated with an oxaliplatin-based regimen. *J Clin Oncol* 2012;30(28):3499–3506.

34. Fuchs CS, Tomasek J, Yong CJ, et al. Ramucirumab monotherapy for previously treated advanced gastric or gastro-oesophageal junction adenocarcinoma (REGARD): an international, randomised, multicentre, placebo-controlled, phase 3 trial. *Lancet* 2014;383:31–39.

35. Motzer RJ, Hutson TE, Tomczak P. Sunitinib versus interferon alfa in metastatic renal-cell carcinoma. *N Engl J Med* 2007;356:115–124.

36. Motzer RJ, Hutson YE, Cella D. Pazopanib versus sunitinib in metastatic renal-cell carcinoma. *N Engl J Med* 2013; 369:722–731.

37. Llovet JM, Ricci S, Mazzaferro V. Sorafenib in advanced hepatocellular carcinoma. *N Engl J Med* 2008;359:378–390.

38. Motzer RJ, Escudier B, Tomczak P. Axitinib versus sorafenib as second-line treatment for advanced renal cell carcinoma: overall survival analysis and updated results from a randomised phase 3 trial. *Lancet Oncol* 2013;14(6):552–562.

39. Grothey A, Van Cutsem E, Sobrero A. Regorafenib monotherapy for previously treated metastatic colorectal cancer (CORRECT): an international, multicentre, randomised, placebo-controlled, phase 3 trial. *Lancet* 2013;381(9863):303–312.

40. Demetri GD, Reichardt P, Kang YK. Efficacy and safety of regorafenib for advanced gastrointestinal stromal tumours after failure of imatinib and sunitinib (GRID): an international, multicentre, randomised, placebo-controlled, phase 3 trial. *Lancet* 2013;381(9863):295–302.

41. Yao JC, Shah MH, Ito T. Everolimus for advanced pancreatic neuroendocrine tumors. *N Engl J Med* 2011;364:514–523.

42. Motzer RJ, Escudier B, Oudard S. Efficacy of everolimus in advanced renal cell carcinoma: a double-blind, randomised, placebo-controlled phase III trial. *Lancet* 2008;372(9637):449–456.

43. Shaw AT, Kim DW, Nakagawa K. Crizotinib versus chemotherapy in advanced ALK-positive lung cancer. *N Engl J Med* 2013;368:2385–2394.

44. Hodi FS, O'Day SJ, McDermott DF. Improved survival with ipilimumab in patients with metastatic melanoma. *N Engl J Med* 2010;363: 711–723.

45. Kantoff PW, Higano CS, Shore ND. Sipuleucel-T immunotherapy for castration-resistant prostate cancer. *N Engl J Med* 2010;363(5):411–422.

46. Le DT, Uram JN, Bartlett BR, et al. PD1 blockade in tumors with mismatch repair deficiency. *N Engl J Med* 2015; 372:2509–2520.

47. Sharma P, Wagner K, Wolchok JD, et al. Novel cancer immunotherapy agents with survival benefit: recent successes and next steps. *Nat Rev Cancer* 2011;11:805–812.

8

Quality assurance in surgical oncology

MICHEL W J M WOUTERS

INTRODUCTION

In the last decades cancer care has developed rapidly. The ever-expanding technological advances, together with the widespread adoption of multidisciplinary cancer care, have led to more complex treatment processes. Simultaneously, in most Western countries the number of cancer patients is rising and will continue to do so, with concurrently a rise in the number of elderly patients, leading to a greater risk of treatment-related morbidity and mortality.

These developments force us to constantly evaluate the way cancer care is provided. Processes of care, including diagnostic procedures, multidisciplinary decision making, minimally invasive, combined modality and targeted treatments, are becoming more and more complex, demanding specific knowledge, expertise and infrastructure in the institutions that provide such care. In this complex environment, to ensure that every patient gets the optimal care available, there is a need to define the standard of care and the acceptable level of variation.

At the same time, surgical oncologists are more and more aware of the need for constant evaluation of the processes and outcomes of care they provide, not only for external accountability to payers, policy makers and the public, but especially to use this information to evaluate and improve care for their patients, continuously.

VARIATION IN QUALITY OF CARE

Ever since the publication of the Harvard Medical Practice Study [1] and the Institute of Medicine's report *To Err Is Human* [2], attention has focused on quality and safety in health care. A plethora of articles have reported on variation in patient safety and quality of care delivered by different types of hospitals [3–5]. In particular, reported differences in patient outcomes between low- and high-volume providers in high-risk cancer procedures, like pancreaticoduodenectomies and esophagectomies, have attracted the attention of the medical profession as well as the public [6,7]. The first reports on this issue were published at the end of the twentieth century. Initially there was solid criticism on the methodological quality of these volume–outcome studies: the majority were based on administrative instead of clinical data, lacking important information on differences in hospitals' case mix and limited to postoperative mortality as the sole determinant of outcome. During the last decade more and more studies on the volume–outcome relationship for high-risk cancer procedures have been added to the literature, including extensive case mix adjustments and using several outcome parameters, like morbidity, mortality, long-term survival and quality of life. Next to high procedural volume, other attributes of hospitals, like their teaching status or specialized setting (e.g. cancer centres), have been linked to superior outcomes in complex cancer procedures [3,8,9]. This suggests substantial opportunities for improving outcomes through the selective referral of cancer patients to centres with high procedural volumes of these high-risk operations [10]. On the other hand, doubts remain about actual improvement in outcome after concentrating high-risk cancer operations in centres selected exclusively for their procedural volume [11,12]. The differences found in volume studies between high- and low-volume providers might only be true for groups of hospitals on average, without adequate discrimination in quality of care between individual hospitals, for example to select future referral centres for complex surgical procedures like esophagectomies and pancreatectomies.

GUIDELINES

Traditionally, data on differences in quality of care between providers have been scarce. In most Western countries quality of cancer care is advanced by the development of evidence-based clinical guidelines. These provide oncologists with a series of recommendations on clinical care, supported by the best available evidence in the literature, though, until recently, there was hardly any information on the adherence to these guidelines in daily clinical practice and the variation between providers. Guidelines are based on results of clinical trials in which inclusion and exclusion criteria ensure homogeneous patient groups. Elderly patients and patients with multiple comorbidities can be underrepresented in these trials, which hampers the adoption of guideline recommendations in the 'real world'. Several studies have evaluated guideline adherence, which revealed substantial unexplained variation between providers [13]. Reducing variation in guideline adherence, but more importantly, investigating the reasons behind this variation and identifying care processes that lead to better outcomes (outcomes research), is an opportunity to improve cancer care on a population basis [14].

QUALITY ASSURANCE

Quality assurance has been defined as the complete set of systematic actions that are required to achieve a treatment result that meets a certain standard [15]. Generally, in surgical oncology evidence-based guidelines fall short of ensuring that every cancer patient gets optimal care. Next to the fact that guidelines are not applicable to certain subgroups of patients, there are hardly any (evidence-based) recommendations that go further than which procedure has to be performed. Standardization of surgical techniques and active quality control are tools to implement quality assurance in cancer surgery. For example, quality assurance has been an essential part of the Dutch Total Mesorectal Excision (TME) trial [16,17] that investigated the efficacy of preoperative short-term radiotherapy in rectal cancer patients treated with TME surgery. It was considered crucial that the study was quality controlled,

for the performance of the surgical TME technique as well as for the radiation fields and pathological examination. Therefore all surgeons participating in the study were trained, with instruction videos and workshops, and the first five operations performed were supervised by a trainer. Completeness of the mesorectal excision and circumferential resection margin (CRM) involvement were reported routinely and proved to be a strong instrument for predicting recurrent disease [15].

Among others, the Dutch trial showed that quality control is feasible within the framework of a randomized clinical trial, though many have experienced that the introduction of standardization and quality control in daily clinical practice is much more challenging. On the other hand, quality assurance gives an opportunity to optimize care processes for every cancer patient and improve the outcomes considerably. Recently, Van Leersum and colleagues reported the results of the Dutch Surgical Colorectal Audit (DSCA) which was initiated in 2009 [18], 10 years after the end of the Dutch TME trial. Their study showed that in 2009 a CRM was reported in only 48% of rectal cancer resections in the Netherlands. After the DSCA started feeding back these results to the surgical teams, pathology reporting improved markedly within 3 years of auditing, with 93% of CRMs reported in 2013. In the same time period, CRM positivity fell from 14% in 2009 to 4.9% in 2013.

MEASURING QUALITY

Several studies emphasized the importance of measuring and feeding back quality information to care providers. According to the definition of the Institute of Medicine, quality of care is a multidimensional concept, encompassing safety, effectiveness, timeliness, efficiency and patient centredness. The way quality is measured depends largely on the availability of reliable data. Only recently, large and detailed multicentre clinical databases have become available, mainly from northwestern Europe, the United States and Canada [19–21]. In general, simple and readily available clinical outcomes have been used to evaluate the quality of surgical care. To reveal real differences in quality of care, measurements of variation between providers have to be adjusted for case mix and chance variation. Subsequently, to understand variation, it is important to consider relationships between structure, process of care and clinical outcomes, as was described by Donabedian [22].

Structure

Structural variables describe the setting in which care is provided, which can be attributes of the hospital (infrastructure, volume), multidisciplinary teams or individual physicians. These structural variables, for instance procedural volume, availability of a plastic surgeon, high-level ICU or on-site radiotherapy department, can be related to patient outcomes, especially by the influence they have on the process of care. Hospital volume is a structural measure that has been related to outcome of surgical procedures in an overwhelming number of studies [23]. However, the extent of this relationship varies widely by type of procedure and by country or region. As mentioned above, the relationship between hospital volume and outcome has proven to be true on average; however, as a quality measure it may fall short in identifying high leverage processes of care in hospitals with excellent outcomes. Focusing on 'procedural volume' has limited ability to move the medical field forward in better understanding the complex clinical processes that lead to success or failure [14].

Process of care

Process components of care refer to the interactions between the provider (i.e. physician) and the patient, for example the delivery of adequate staging investigations to detect distant metastases in patients considered for curative surgery. To use process measures to evaluate quality levels in surgical oncology, it has to be determined which care processes lead to the better outcomes. The development of evidence-based guidelines has provided standards for diagnostic and treatment policies used by clinicians [24]. Measuring the implementation of these standards in routine patient care could give insight into the quality provided by an institution. Regretfully, the empirical evidence of relationships between measurable process variables and outcome is limited [23], though recent studies show that hospitals in which guideline adherence is high also have better outcomes [25].

Clinical outcome

The ultimate outcome in (surgical) oncology is survival, in which the 'quality of survival' also has to be taken into account. The surgical cancer patient is at risk of poor outcomes twice in their cancer journey. First, treatment-related morbidity can affect a patient's quality of life and can even lead to mortality. In addition, surgical complications can lead to omission of adjuvant therapies, lowering a patient's chances for long-term survival [26]. Second, inadequate patient selection, staging and therapy can lead to 'unnecessary' recurrences, though they can also effect functional outcomes, cosmesis and health-related quality of life.

Direct outcome measurements are preferable in the evaluation of treatment quality, because they have face validity for both physicians and patients.

There are several limitations to direct outcome measurement. First, all relevant case mix factors should be available to make reliable outcome comparisons between institutions [27,28]. Second, an early outcome parameter should be available to allow control and evaluation of the quality of the care process. For many tumours, like breast, colorectal and prostate cancer, the endpoint 'recurrence-free survival' is far too temporally delayed to permit continuous evaluation and improvement of care processes. Proxy outcome measures, directly related to the long-term outcome, like the CRM in rectal cancer surgery, can be used to solve this problem. Third, when evaluating differences in outcome between institutions, the reliability of comparisons is largely dependent on sample sizes. For low-volume cancer procedures the number of cases per hospital (denominator) and the number of complications (nominator) can be too small to evaluate quality of care within a reasonable period of time [29]. Finally, in quality assessment various outcome parameters can interact. For example, complication rates after colorectal surgery can be reduced substantially by omitting a primary anastomosis and performing a colostomy in the majority of patients. Likewise, local recurrence rates of patients with advanced rectal cancer can be improved with neo-adjuvant chemoradiation, though radiation may lead to more perineal wound complications. Such improvements in outcome on one parameter (anastomotic leakage and local recurrence rates) at the expense of another (colostomy and wound complication rate) ask for a more comprehensive approach in outcome assessment.

QUALITY INDICATORS

Quality indicators give an indication of the quality of the patient care delivered and can be used for quality assurance. Quality indicators can also be categorized as structure, process or outcome indicators. All must be relevant to the important aspects of cancer care and comply with high-quality standards. Therefore, there must be adequate scientific evidence that the recommendations from which they are derived are related to the various dimensions of quality: clinical effectiveness, safety, timeliness, patient centredness and efficiency (validity). For example, perioperative blood loss can be a valid quality indicator for hepatic resections, though it may be hardly relevant for breast cancer surgery.

In addition, quality indicators should measure the quality in a correct and consistent way (reliability) and be able to detect changes in the care process (responsiveness) [30]. The false-negative rate in sentinel node procedures for melanoma was 4.8% in the final report of the MSLT I trial [31]. As a quality indicator, the false-negative rate may hardly be responsive to further improvements of the biopsy technique, for example by image-guided surgery, though the same quality indicator can be very useful to monitor the performance of surgeons (in training) in a melanoma centre.

QUALITY IMPROVEMENT

Acknowledging the differences in (infra)structure, care processes and patient outcome between physicians, institutions, regions and countries, efforts to reduce undesired variation could lead to real benefits for cancer patients worldwide. Traditionally, improvement of quality of surgical care is the domain of professional organizations, like the British Association of Surgical Oncologists (BASO) in the United Kingdom and the Society for Surgical Oncology (SSO) in the United States. Until recently, quality improvement efforts were based on the transfer of knowledge and skills through surgical oncology education and training, the development of evidence-based guidelines and the organization of scientific meetings.

Despite these initiatives, actual information on variation in quality of care in routine practice is generally lacking. The implementation process following development of evidence-based guidelines is seldom monitored and reasons for non-adherence are largely unknown. The gradual introduction of studies comparing outcomes between providers has changed this situation and has given rise to more and more research groups evaluating hospital variation in quality of care. Nowadays, three relatively new instruments contribute to quality improvement in surgical oncology.

Selective referral

The potential benefits of selective referral of patients to hospitals with higher procedural volumes and dedicated infrastructures have been speculated upon by many authors [11]. In response to an Institute of Medicine report on building a safer health care system [2], in 2000, several large employers in the United States formed the Leapfrog Group. The objective of Leapfrog is to improve the quality and safety of medical care by steering surgical patients to hospitals likely to have the best results. For example, since 2003 Leapfrog has a volume standard for esophagectomy of 13 procedures per institution per year. On average, Leapfrog hospitals have lower risk-adjusted mortality rates, though between hospitals meeting the Leapfrog standard there is still important variation in outcomes, including a fivefold variation in mortality [32]. Apparently, procedural volume as a proxy for quality of care can fall short in identifying hospitals providing 'excellent' cancer care. Simunovic et al. published the results of centralization of pancreatic surgery in two provinces in Canada, Ontario and Quebec [33]. In a 10-year period, pancreatic surgery was concentrated in high-volume hospitals in both provinces to the same extent. However, only in Ontario did this result in actual improvements in outcomes of pancreatic surgery patients. The difference was that in Ontario centralization was accompanied by an audit of results, which were fed back to participating surgeons.

Quality control

Alternative approaches to selective referral include strategies that aim to improve quality of care in *all* hospitals treating a certain group of cancer patients. Such an approach seems most appropriate for high-volume cancer surgery performed in significant volumes by almost all hospitals, like breast and colorectal cancer surgery. Quality assurance is such a strategy and focuses on the implementation and monitoring of a complete set of systematic actions that are required to achieve a certain standard of care. Since variability in care processes and surgical techniques can lead to irreproducible results, quality control is used in clinical trials, in which the quality of surgery is essential for the

outcome [34]. Adequate quality control in daily practice is more challenging, though it could make use of a set of quality indicators covering the essential aspects of diagnostic procedures and treatments performed by surgical oncologists.

Surgical audit

An instrument that combines the relative merits of monitoring guideline adherence, quality assurance, outcome measurement and selective referral is surgical audit. Medical (or surgical) audit as a quality improvement tool was first defined by Ernest Amory Codman, a surgeon at the Harvard University Hospital, in 1912: 'the systematic critical analysis of the quality of medical care, including the procedures used for diagnosis, treatment and resulting outcome for the patient, carried out by those personally engaged in the activity concerned' [35]. In surgical oncology, audits can be carried out on different levels, on the level of individual surgeons or on a hospital, regional or (inter) national level. The basic essential of surgical auditing is the audit cycle that involves the definition of quality standards, collecting data to measure current practice, setting benchmarks and implementing improvements. This concept of auditing is closely related to quality assurance and provides continuous feedback on a set of quality standards and outcomes to the participating surgeons.

Several nationwide clinical audit programs have been developed in the United States and northwestern Europe in the last two decades [36,37]. In Norway local recurrence rates dropped from 28% to 7% as a result of a national audit program for rectal cancer surgery. In the United States the National Surgical Quality Improvement Program (NSQIP) that began more than 20 years ago in the Veterans Affairs hospitals reported marked reductions in morbidity (45%) and mortality (27%) after surgery in the participating hospitals [36]. This was accomplished by a peer-controlled program of continuous and timely feedback of case mix–adjusted outcomes of surgical care. More recently, similar results have been shown after adoption of the NSQIP program by the private sector [38].

The reason for clinical auditing being a powerful instrument for quality improvement is found in the combination and integration of several quality improvement tools. First, the peer-controlled development of data sets covering a set of quality standards based on evidence-based guidelines explicates which aspects of the care process are believed to be essential for optimization of clinical outcomes. Through data collection, as well as the reporting process, these sets of standards are spread within the surgical community (knowledge transfer). The continuous data collection, often executed or supervised by the clinicians themselves, gives constant attention to these quality aspects. In addition, clinicians are provided with rigorous feedback of their outcomes relative to those of their peers (benchmarking).

That feedback itself can be very effective in improving outcomes was shown in the DSCA, which was initiated in the Netherlands in 2009. This nationwide peer-reviewed, quality-controlled, outcome-based and case mix–adjusted clinical audit program feeds back benchmarked information on the quality of colorectal cancer treatment to the participating surgeons. All hospitals participate and case ascertainment is very high (>96%) [18]. An extensive set of process and outcome indicators is reported and fed back to the surgical teams through a secure web-based environment (*My*DSCA), which is updated on a weekly basis. In the first 4 years of the audit guideline adherence improved significantly, with a substantial reduction of variation between hospitals. More importantly, a remarkable drop in morbidity and mortality after colorectal resections was shown, with a 30% drop in the risk for postoperative mortality after colon resections, from 4.5% in 2009 to 3.2% in 2012.

OUTCOMES RESEARCH

Next to its direct influence on quality of care, one of the most important side effects of the development of nationwide data collection systems is the detailed clinical 'real world' information that is retrieved by these surgical audits. Apart from quality assurance and the initiation of local improvement initiatives, reliable databases with essential information on (differences in) care processes and outcome may move the whole medical field forward. Recognizing groups of patients at risk for adverse outcome, revealing the underlying mechanisms and identifying processes of care with better outcomes are the central issues in outcomes research. The ultimate goal is to transfer best practices found in centres with excellent results to all hospitals treating these patients. For example, Ghaferi and colleagues reported recently on hospital differences in mortality after esophagectomy, gastrectomy and pancreatectomy [39]. They found that complication rates did not differ significantly between hospitals. Instead, differences seemed to be associated with the ability of hospitals to effectively rescue patients once complications occurred (failure to rescue). The adequate way surgical teams in hospitals with low mortality rates react on symptoms or signs of complications may be of benefit for all patients having this kind of surgery. Moreover, many clinical questions stay unanswered because certain (sub)groups of patients are not included in randomized controlled trials addressing these questions. Some trials are simply not feasible. Large population-based databases provide the opportunity to investigate these questions for the benefit of patient care.

INTERNATIONAL BENCHMARKING

Considerable variation exists in cancer management and outcome between Western countries. Differences in treatment patterns between these countries provide the opportunity to learn from each other. International data collection, analysis and benchmarking can reveal 'best practices' in

cancer management, in addition to the available evidence. Several international initiatives to combine data from different countries have been taken. In surgical oncology the European Registry of Cancer Care (EURECCA) started in 2007 as an initiative of the European Society for Surgical Oncology (ESSO) to improve the quality of cancer care by data registration, feedback, improvement initiatives and sharing of knowledge between surgical oncologists from different countries in Europe [40]. EURECCA started with organizing consensus conferences for colon and rectal cancer in 2012, to synchronize data collection in regional or national surgical audits throughout Europe [41]. Today there are seven tumour site groups, covering colorectal, gastro-esophageal, hepato-pancreatico-biliary, breast, prostate and melanoma. These international expert groups meet twice a year to promote, monitor and synchronize data collection in Europe and discuss the clinical questions to be addressed.

TRANSPARENCY

It is generally believed that transparency in hospital-specific quality information is a catalyst for quality improvement. Additional to the benefits of clinical auditing, public reporting of a hospital's outcomes could stimulate improvement initiatives in under- as well as high-performing hospitals. Moreover, transparency could steer patients to the hospitals with better outcomes for certain kinds of cancer procedures, giving these the opportunity to specialize in treating such a group of patients. Nonetheless, in many Western countries there is hardly any provider-specific outcome information available to the public [42]. In addition, apart from the detailed clinical information that is being collected in national audit programs, there is still a lack of patient reported experiences and outcomes in cancer care. Routine collection of functional outcomes and health-related quality of life provides tremendous opportunities to re-evaluate cancer treatments and further improve patient outcomes in surgical oncology.

REFERENCES

1. Brennan, T.A., et al. Incidence of adverse events and negligence in hospitalized patients: results of the Harvard Medical Practice Study I. 1991. *Qual Saf Health Care* 2004;13(2):145–51; discussion 151–2.
2. Institute of Medicine. *To Err Is Human: Building a Safer Health System.* Washington, DC: Institute of Medicine Committee on Quality of Health Care in America, 1999.
3. Birkmeyer, J.D., et al. Hospital volume and surgical mortality in the United States. *N Engl J Med* 2002;346(15):1128–37.
4. Lemmens, V.E., et al. Mixed adherence to clinical practice guidelines for colorectal cancer in the southern Netherlands in 2002. *Eur J Surg Oncol* 2006;32(2):168–73.

5. Li, W.W., et al. The influence of provider characteristics on resection rates and survival in patients with localized non-small cell lung cancer. *Lung Cancer* 2008;60(3):441–51.

6. Wouters, M.W., et al. The volume-outcome relation in the surgical treatment of esophageal cancer: a systematic review and meta-analysis. *Cancer* 2012;118(7):1754–63.

7. Gooiker, G.A., et al. Systematic review and meta-analysis of the volume-outcome relationship in pancreatic surgery. *Br J Surg* 2011;98(4):485–94.

8. Birkmeyer, N.J., et al. Do cancer centers designated by the National Cancer Institute have better surgical outcomes? *Cancer* 2005;103(3):435–41.

9. Chowdhury, M.M., H. Dagash, and A. Pierro. A systematic review of the impact of volume of surgery and specialization on patient outcome. *Br J Surg* 2007;94(2):145–61.

10. Birkmeyer, J.D., E.V. Finlayson, and C.M. Birkmeyer. Volume standards for high-risk surgical procedures: potential benefits of the Leapfrog initiative. *Surgery* 2001;130(3):415–22.

11. Birkmeyer, J.D. and J.B. Dimick. Potential benefits of the new Leapfrog standards: effect of process and outcomes measures. *Surgery* 2004;135(6):569–75.

12. Wouters, M.W., et al. Volume- or outcome-based referral to improve quality of care for esophageal cancer surgery in the Netherlands. *J Surg Oncol* 2009;99(8):481–7.

13. Wouters, M.W., M.L. Jansen-Landheer, and C.J. van de Velde. The Quality of Cancer Care initiative in the Netherlands. *Eur J Surg Oncol* 2010;36(Suppl. 1):S3–S13.

14. Wouters, M. Outcome-based referral to improve quality of care in upper GI surgery. *J Surg Oncol* 2008;98(5):307–8.

15. Peeters, K.C. and C.J. van de Velde. Surgical quality assurance in breast, gastric and rectal cancer. *J Surg Oncol* 2003;84(3):107–12.

16. Kapiteijn, E., et al. Preoperative radiotherapy combined with total mesorectal excision for resectable rectal cancer. *N Engl J Med* 2001;345(9):638–46.

17. Peeters, K.C., et al. The TME trial after a median follow-up of 6 years: increased local control but no survival benefit in irradiated patients with resectable rectal carcinoma. *Ann Surg* 2007;246(5):693–701.

18. Van Leersum, N.J., et al. The Dutch surgical colorectal audit. *Eur J Surg Oncol* 2013;39(10):1063–70.

19. Khuri, S.F., et al. The Department of Veterans Affairs' NSQIP: the first national, validated, outcome-based, risk-adjusted, and peer-controlled program for the measurement and enhancement of the quality of surgical care. National VA Surgical Quality Improvement Program. *Ann Surg* 1998;228(4):491–507.

20. Pahlman, L., et al. The Swedish rectal cancer registry. *Br J Surg* 2007;94(10):1285–92.

21. Wibe, A., et al. Nationwide quality assurance of rectal cancer treatment. *Colorectal Dis* 2006;8(3):224–9.

22. Donabedian, A. Evaluating the quality of medical care. *Milbank Mem Fund Q* 1966;44 (3 Suppl.):166–206.

23. Courrech Staal, E.F., et al. Quality-of-care indicators for oesophageal cancer surgery: a review. *Eur J Surg Oncol* 2010;36(11):1035–43.

24. Eddy, D.M. Clinical policies and the quality of clinical practice. *N Engl J Med* 1982;307(6):343–7.

25. Kolfschoten, N.E., et al. Combining process indicators to evaluate quality of care for surgical patients with colorectal cancer: are scores consistent with short-term outcome? *BMJ Qual Saf* 2012;21(6):481–9.

26. Hendren, S., et al. Surgical complications are associated with omission of chemotherapy for stage III colorectal cancer. *Dis Colon Rectum* 2010;53(12):1587–93.

27. Wouters, M.W., et al. High-volume versus low-volume for esophageal resections for cancer: the essential role of case-mix adjustments based on clinical data. *Ann Surg Oncol* 2008;15(1):80–7.

28. Kolfschoten, N.E., et al. Variation in case-mix between hospitals treating colorectal cancer patients in the Netherlands. *Eur J Surg Oncol* 2011;37(11):956–63.

29. Dimick, J.B., H.G. Welch, and J.D. Birkmeyer. Surgical mortality as an indicator of hospital quality: the problem with small sample size. *JAMA* 2004;292(7):847–51.

30. Wollersheim, H., et al. Clinical indicators: development and applications. *Neth J Med* 2007;65(1):15–22.

31. Morton, D.L., et al. Final trial report of sentinel-node biopsy versus nodal observation in melanoma. *N Engl J Med* 2014;370(7):599–609.

32. Varghese, T.K., Jr., et al. Variation in esophagectomy outcomes in hospitals meeting Leapfrog volume outcome standards. *Ann Thorac Surg* 2011;91(4):1003–9; discussion 1009–10.

33. Simunovic, M., et al. Assessing the volume-outcome hypothesis and region-level quality improvement interventions: pancreas cancer surgery in two Canadian provinces. *Ann Surg Oncol* 2010;17(10):2537–44.

34. Peeters, K.C. and C.J. van de Velde. Quality assurance of surgery in gastric and rectal cancer. *Crit Rev Oncol Hematol* 2004;51(2):105–19.

35. Neuhauser D. Ernest Amory Codman MD. *Quality & Safety in Health Care* 2002;11(1):104–105.

36. Khuri, S.F., J. Daley, and W.G. Henderson. The comparative assessment and improvement of quality of surgical care in the Department of Veterans Affairs. *Arch Surg* 2002;137(1):20–7.

37. van Gijn, W., et al. Nationwide outcome registrations to improve quality of care in rectal surgery. An initiative of the European Society of Surgical Oncology. *J Surg Oncol* 2009;99(8):491–6.

38. Khuri, S.F., et al. Successful implementation of the Department of Veterans Affairs' National Surgical Quality Improvement Program in the private sector: the Patient Safety in Surgery Study. *Ann Surg* 2008;248(2):329–36.

39. Ghaferi, A.A., J.D. Birkmeyer, and J.B. Dimick. Hospital volume and failure to rescue with high-risk surgery. *Med Care* 2011;49(12):1076–81.

40. Breugom, A.J., et al. Quality assurance in the treatment of colorectal cancer: the EURECCA initiative. *Ann Oncol* 2014;25(8):1485–92.

41. van de Velde, C.J., et al. EURECCA colorectal: multidisciplinary management: European consensus conference colon and rectum. *Eur J Cancer* 2014;50(1):1e1–34.

42. Kuenen, J.W., R. Mohr, S. Larsson, and W. van Leeuwen. Zorg voor Waarde. Amsterdam: Boston Consulting Group, 2011.

9

Palliative care in surgical oncology

IAIN LAWRIE AND MARI LLOYD-WILLIAMS

Suffering has four components: physical, psychological, social and spiritual. When defined this way, palliative care is applicable across the spectrum of cancer care and not merely at the end of life [1].

INTRODUCTION

To many, the specialties of surgery and palliative medicine must appear worlds apart. Surgery is often viewed as a heroic, life-saving and essentially physical domain, of the Cartesian school of thought where body is independent of mind, and where results are assessed in terms of death, disability or cure [2], death being regarded as failure, the least acceptable outcome [3]. Palliative care is seen by some as a less dynamic branch of medicine, where patients and families are metaphorically shielded from the nastier aspects of their disease, and where intervention and practical management are viewed secondary to comfort and emotional support for the duration of the illness, often until death. Neither of these impressions is warranted.

In this chapter, we present an overview of palliative care in surgical oncology. The nature and origins of both palliative care and palliative surgery are discussed before the application of palliative care principles to a number of specific clinical problems. The place of palliative care in oncology, examples of good practice and potential barriers to an effective palliative care approach are then considered. Finally, we look toward the continued integration and future development of this approach in the field of surgical oncology.

BACKGROUND

Care of patients with malignant disease, of the dying and, in different forms, hospice care has been practiced since the very beginnings of medicine [4]. The technological advances of the twentieth century focused medical attention on pathology and cure, often accompanied by a denigration of treatment aimed at symptomatic relief. However, as the limitations of modern medicine were acknowledged, a common element of palliative care emerged in the form of an holistic approach to patient care. This 'whole person' approach places emphasis not only on the physical aspects of diagnosis and treatment of disease, but also on comfort, freedom from distress and support of the individual and the family [5].

Palliative care developed new prominence in 1967, with the opening of St Christopher's Hospice, England, as the first research and teaching hospice and a centre for provision of both patient and family care in the hospice itself, in the community and, for families, into bereavement. This was followed in the 1970s by diverse developments of the modern hospice movement across Europe and the US. Palliative care as a distinct medical specialty is a relatively recent development of the mid-1980s, and since then has developed rapidly throughout the world with local, national and international organizations founded to share good practice, provide education and collaborate in research.

Several definitions of palliative care have been proposed and, in many respects, it can take different forms depending on the context in which it is practiced. The World Health Organization (WHO) defines palliative care as 'the active total care of patients whose disease is not responsive to curative treatment' [6]. This includes the control of pain and other distressing symptoms and of psychological, social and spiritual problems. It affirms life and regards death as a normal process, its goal being to achieve the best quality of life for patients and families.

Surgery has its roots in palliation of both symptoms and disease and, until the twentieth century, the vast majority of medical and surgical procedures were palliative in nature. Procedures for palliation of symptoms of bowel obstruction, for drainage of abscesses and for removal of tumours were common. The management of patients with burns is probably the most developed example of palliative care in surgery [7], where the primary aims are relief of pain and quality of life. The now commonplace procedure of coronary artery bypass grafting was initially developed to relieve the pain of angina before its place as a life-prolonging technique was evident [7]. Palliative surgery today still accounts for a significant proportion of both cancer and general surgery practice [8,9].

It is clear, therefore, that both the historical basis of surgery and its present-day practice are intimately connected to many of the basic tenets of palliative care. The relief of suffering has long been the primary intention of surgeons and has helped develop medical practice in the prolongation of life for patients with both early and advanced disease.

Surgical palliative care encapsulates far more than malignant disease. Many illnesses, both acute and chronic, require palliation. However, practice relating to cancer is the main focus of attention of this chapter.

SELECTED COMPONENTS OF PALLIATIVE CARE

Numerous physical and non-physical symptoms can cause distress and suffering for the patient with advanced disease. However, satisfactory symptom control can usually be accomplished when symptoms are both looked for and recognized, with 'a direct organized approach' to care [10].

Pain

Pain is common in patients with cancer, occurring in up to 75% of patients [11], and effective pain management is crucial. Pain is an 'unpleasant sensory and emotional experience' [12] and is what the experiencing person says it is [13]. The most important component of management is a thorough and accurate assessment of a patient's pains. Many different components contribute to pain and a multimodal approach to pain relief may be necessary (Figure 9.1). A number of tools for assessment of pain are available [15–17].

There is no such thing as the perfect analgesic, and patients may require different classes, strengths, forms and dosages of analgesic during the course of their illness. The basis of effective pain relief remains the analgesic ladder [18], originally designed for the management of cancer pain but equally applicable to other situations (Figure 9.2). Attention to both background pain and incident or 'breakthrough' pain is important. There is little point in a patient being comfortable at rest but being prevented from activity due to pain.

Analgesics can be split into three classes: non-opioids, opioids and adjuvants (Table 9.1). The analgesic ladder advocates a step-wise titration of analgesia to the needs of the individual patient, with both non-opioid and adjuvant analgesics being retained at each step. Non-opioids are the starting point toward effective pain relief and may be

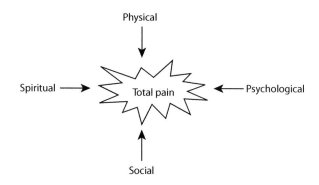

Figure 9.1 The concept of total pain. (Adapted from Twycross R, *Introducing Palliative Care*, 3rd ed., Oxford: Radcliffe Medical Press, 1997: 66.)

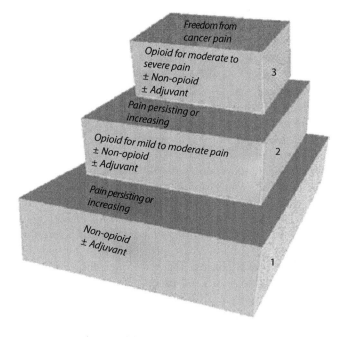

Figure 9.2 The World Health Organization analgesic ladder. (Reproduced from World Health Organization, *WHO Guidelines: Cancer Pain Relief*, 2nd ed., Geneva: World Health Organization, 1996. With permission.)

supplemented by adjuvant analgesics according to the type and probable cause of pain. Opioid analgesics include those for mild to moderate pain (step 2 opioids) and others for moderate to severe pain (step 3 opioids). Step 2 analgesics display a 'ceiling' effect for analgesia [14] and, with increasing severity of pain, it may be necessary to progress to a stronger opioid (step 3). When using strong opioids with which they are unfamiliar, clinicians should liaise with palliative care or pain specialist colleagues.

Apprehension regarding the use of opioids, displayed by both patients and professionals, can be a barrier to effective pain relief. These fears are largely unfounded. Neither addiction nor tolerance occurs when opioids are used to manage pain [19]. Respiratory depression can occur when large doses of opioids are given for acute pain or in error, and sedation is usually a short-lived feature of early opioid use or dose increase.

Nausea and vomiting

Nausea and vomiting are distressing symptoms present in up to 70% of patients with advanced cancer [20–22] and four causes (gastric stasis, intestinal obstruction, drugs and chemicals) account for the majority of cases [14–23]. Identification of possible causes is imperative and should guide management. Reversible causes, such as uncontrolled pain, medication side effects, constipation and hypercalcemia, should be corrected where possible. Non-physical causes, such as anxiety, should always be considered.

Antiemetic drugs act on specific receptors, thus emphasizing the importance of accurate assessment of possible etiologies. Where gastric stasis or functional bowel obstruction is suspected, a prokinetic antiemetic (e.g. metoclopramide) would be an appropriate first-line choice. Acting principally on the chemoreceptor trigger zone in the area postrema, haloperidol is effective for chemical causes of nausea and vomiting, whether biochemical or drug induced. An antispasmodic and antisecretory antiemetic (e.g. hyoscine butylbromide) is useful where colic is present, or where a reduction in gastrointestinal secretions is appropriate. Finally, for organic bowel obstruction, motion-induced symptoms and raised intracranial pressure cyclizine, which acts on the vomiting centre, is appropriate. An 'antiemetic ladder' has been proposed (Figure 9.3) [5].

Antiemetics should be prescribed regularly as well as 'as needed' and the route of administration should be considered. If oral absorption is likely to be affected by persistent vomiting, a continuous subcutaneous infusion (CSCI) is most appropriate. Unless the identified cause is self-limiting, it is advisable to continue antiemetic treatment.

Should first-line antiemetic treatment be ineffective, trial of a broad-spectrum drug such as levomepromazine is sensible. Other drugs which can be used in the management of

Table 9.1 Analgesics classified according to the World Health Organization ladder

Step 1	Step 2	Step 3	Adjuvants
Paracetamol	Co-codamol	Morphine	Corticosteroids
Non-steroidal anti-inflammatory drugs	Dihydrocodeine	Oxycodone	Antidepressants
	Tramadol	Hydromorphone	Antiepileptics
		Methadone	Antispasmodics
		Buprenorphine	Muscle relaxants
		Fentanyl	

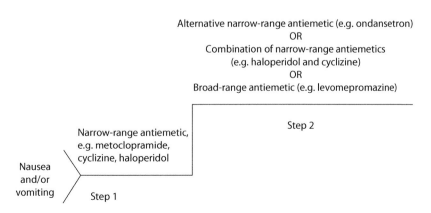

Figure 9.3 Proposed antiemetic ladder. (Adapted from Watson M, et al., eds., *Oxford Handbook of Palliative Care*, Oxford: Oxford University Press, 2005.)

nausea and vomiting include corticosteroids as an adjuvant in bowel obstruction, $5HT_3$ receptor antagonists such as granisetron or tropisetron in bowel obstruction or in patients who have had chemotherapy or abdominal radiotherapy, and octreotide, a somatostatin analog, for reduction of secretions where hyoscine butylbromide has been ineffective.

Bowel obstruction

Malignant bowel obstruction, most frequently seen in bowel and pelvic carcinoma, occurs in 3–15% of advanced cancers [24]. It can occur anywhere in the gastrointestinal tract and may be the result of the cancer itself, drug induced (e.g. opioids, antimuscarinics), related to constipation or previous treatment (e.g. surgery, radiation), or an unrelated benign condition [25]. Obstruction can cause considerable distress to the patient and is often accompanied by nausea, vomiting and abdominal pain and distension.

Surgery for obstruction is often indicated where a procedure is technically feasible, it carries clear benefits and the patient is sufficiently fit, but is often not possible, especially in cases of diffuse intra-abdominal disease, rapidly recurring ascites or where there has been previous radiotherapy or extensive surgery. That said, 40–70% of patients will have relief of their obstruction following surgery, although perioperative mortality can be high [26].

Medical management of bowel obstruction rarely includes the use of a nasogastric tube or intravenous fluids [14,27]. Drugs are usually administered by CSCI in order to be effective and pain is controlled using an appropriate opioid. Gut motility can be improved using a prokinetic drug such as metoclopramide, possibly with dexamethasone to reduce bowel edema. However, if colic is a feature, prokinetic medications and stimulant laxatives should be avoided and hyoscine butylbromide should be used instead. Where constipation is thought to be a feature, a stool-softening laxative may be used. Finally, management of associated nausea, which can be troublesome, can be effected by means of either metoclopramide (no colic) or drugs such as haloperidol and cyclizine. Vomiting, often a feature of obstruction, may be improved by the measures already mentioned. However, if hyoscine butylbromide is inadequate, octreotide may be indicated to reduce the volume of such vomits. As with all CSCIs, drug compatibility should be checked prior to administration.

Dyspnea

Dyspnea, seen in 40–80% of palliative care patients [28], is a source of considerable functional limitation and distress. The pathophysiological mechanisms of breathlessness are complex and remain unclear, and fatigue, muscle weakness, anxiety, pleural effusion, direct tumour effects and distortion of mechanoreceptors can all contribute [5].

After correction of reversible causes, management of dyspnea can be difficult. Non-pharmacological strategies and interventions include pulmonary rehabilitation and activity-related education, positioning, use of oxygen and non-invasive positive pressure ventilation. Pharmacological intervention relies mainly on the use of opioids, benzodiazepines and, possibly, buspirone. Opioids reduce the ventilatory response to raised carbon dioxide or reduced oxygen levels [25,29], reduce anxiety and the sensation of breathlessness and may act peripherally on local lung receptors [30]. Opioid-naïve patients should be commenced on small doses of oral morphine regularly and the dose titrated according to response. If patients already taking opioids find benefit from additional doses, their regular opioid can be titrated. Benzodiazepines such as diazepam, lorazepam and midazolam have been used and, although often empirically effective, evidence is lacking.

Communication

It is vital at all stages of a terminal illness to communicate well with patients and their relatives. What is said and what the patient may hear or understand may be very different, leading to misunderstanding and, not infrequently, bitterness and resentment against the bearer of the bad news [31].

While many patients may have an inkling that all is not well, the desire to hear good news can prevent information from being heard and assimilated. Giving bad news in whatever setting is never easy – nor should it be – but certain steps can help a diagnosis or prognosis to be communicated in an understandable way. Showing empathy and concern (e.g. saying, 'I realize this is very difficult for you') can do much to avoid the feelings of abandonment which many patients feel when they are told that a diagnosis is terminal. Often, relatives will try to protect the patient and ask for them not to be told bad news. For the professional, where does loyalty lie? Ultimately, their main responsibility is to the patient. Collusion can pull families apart at a time when they most need to be close to each other. Offering to speak to patients with their relatives present can be helpful. Information needs to be given honestly, but always with the assurance that symptoms can be palliated – 'there is nothing more that can be done to help you' is both cruel and untrue and should never be said. In addition to communicating with patients and relatives, it is also important to communicate what has been told to patients and management decisions, both within the hospital team and to primary care colleagues, to ensure that patients receive a consistent message.

Anorexia and cachexia

Cachexia (muscle wasting and marked weight loss) is common in patients with advanced malignant disease and may be due to any combination of direct tumour effect, nausea, cytokine action, medication, psychological factors and unresolved pain [27]. Both anorexia and cachexia can lead to extreme fatigue and weakness, and are associated with reduced survival in many illnesses.

Management is complex and multidisciplinary. While artificial nutrition, for example via enteral tube feeding, is possible, it is not always beneficial or appropriate in patients with advanced cancer. However, the legal and ethical debate regarding artificial nutrition and hydration in advanced disease is beyond the scope of this book. That aside, attention must be paid to concerns regarding body image, skin care to prevent decubitus ulcers, dental review if appropriate and occupational therapy involvement for help with activities of daily living.

Specific medical treatment, using megestrol acetate, steroids or thalidomide, may be of some use, but no medical management has proven effectiveness. Advice regarding nutrition and trial of commercial dietary supplements are often appropriate. However, when faced with advanced, often terminal disease, emphasis should remain on patient choice, and 'adequate' nutrition should not be an unshakable goal at the expense of this and of patient quality of life.

Psychosocial problems

Patients may experience a number of different emotions when treatment is no longer curative. Distress is normal and is not on its own pathological, and it is difficult to distinguish appropriate sadness at the end of life from treatable depressive illness. Up to 32% of patients develop a significant mood disorder in advanced cancer [32]. Certain types of cancer, such as pancreatic cancer, are associated with an increased incidence of depression. Depression is frequently missed and may present as anger, profound sadness or irritability. Depression should always be suspected in a patient for whom the control of physical symptoms (e.g. pain) is difficult [33] and also in patients who appear more unwell than their disease stage suggests. Patients are often reluctant to mention depression, so it is important that mood is assessed as frequently as pain or any other symptom. A simple question such as 'how are you feeling in your mood?' can allow patients the opportunity to share their symptoms. Screening tools are also available and the Edinburgh Depression Scale is one of the most sensitive in the palliative care population [34]. Depression should be treated with an appropriate antidepressant and psychosocial support from members of the treating team. Appropriate antidepressants include citalopram, mirtazapine and venlafaxine. A small dose of steroids (e.g. dexamethasone 4–6 mg once daily) can help increase mood quickly and improve general well-being while waiting for an antidepressant to work.

End-of-life care

At some point in most patients' final illness, it becomes apparent that they are in a phase of terminal deterioration and that no further traditional active intervention is either appropriate or beneficial. This, however, does not mean that no further active intervention is necessary. Palliative care strives to challenge the attitude that 'there is nothing more we can do'[3,14] and serves to prevent patients' possible feelings of abandonment by professionals involved in their care [14,35,36].

A good death is one which is appropriate for the individual patient and the challenge is to provide care tailored to the patient, while fostering independence, autonomy and control. Factors which are considered important at the end of life are shown in Table 9.2. Good communication is essential, as is control of symptoms which may distress the patient, while also discontinuing any medication, observation or intervention which does not fulfil this aim.

Quality of life in the last few days and hours of life largely depends on the care the patient has previously received. Careful thought and planning can achieve this and is within the capabilities of all health professionals.

Bereavement

When a patient dies, the grief felt may take many forms. In the first few hours, there may be numbness, denial or even relief that suffering is over, or anger at the patient for dying. Relatives appreciate support given at the time of death. Information regarding death certification and the practicalities of registering the death is helpful, as can be asking whether they wish to see the chaplain or other members of the team who may have been particularly involved in the patient's care. Good communication with the primary care team is essential as they will be the key support for the family in the community. It is also important to acknowledge that the team may well also feel a sense of bereavement if they have cared for the patient over a long period of time. Allowing team members time to share any thoughts or feelings after a death can be helpful in allowing staff also to move on. Some deaths will impact more than others on the team and the provision of support from chaplaincy or occupational health can be helpful in such situations.

Table 9.2 Important factors at the end of life

Dignity of patient and caregivers

Respect for the patient's wishes

Effective and timely communication with patient and caregivers

Management of pain and other symptoms

Attention to psychological, social and spiritual concerns

Continuity of care

Access to specialist palliative care services where appropriate

Effective interprofessional communication

Provision of appropriate treatments and discontinuation of those inappropriate at the end of life

DISCUSSION

Palliation has long been part of the surgeon's remit and, as a result of advances in oncology and the changing demographics of death [37], this role has expanded. Several definitions of palliative surgery have been proposed [36,38,39] and, while this can cause confusion, many acknowledge the importance of alleviation of symptoms and improvement in quality of life [40]. Palliative care need not be synonymous with end-of-life care, however [9]. Major components of the palliative care approach are symptom control and psychological support, both of which are applicable in most clinical situations.

Significant advances have been made in the integration of skills from both disciplines. The various British royal surgical colleges, the American College of Surgeons, the American Thoracic Society, the Society of Critical Care Medicine and others have agreed that palliative care will increasingly influence the care of patients [3]. The Promoting Excellence in End-of-Life Care national program [41] in the US and the prominence of both palliative care and end-of-life care in the new syllabus of the Intercollegiate Surgical Curriculum Project [42] in the UK are excellent examples of such integration.

However, potential barriers to an effective palliative care approach in surgical oncology exist. The lack of a universally accepted definition of surgical palliative care has been mentioned. This may influence clinicians' perception, as lack of clarity, coupled with surgeons' conceptualization of success and failure in terms of death, disability and cure [3,7,43], could prevent cultural change. The background of the surgeon has been described as leading to lack of awareness of non-physical suffering [36] and of 'heroic optimism' [43], which may, in turn, prevent attention to palliative care principles in favour of attempts at cure. Indeed, until recently there has been a lack of formal education in palliative and end-of-life care in surgical training [9,37,44,45] and little in the literature [9,36,39,46,47].

Problems related to communication can impact negatively on the relationship between surgeon and patients with malignant disease. Lack of common language in discussing disease and management can be troublesome. Uncertainty regarding prognosis can pose significant challenges and the surgeon may find it difficult to be candid with the patient regarding their illness for fear of removing hope [9,36]. This may be a reflection of discomfort with emotional challenges associated with managing advanced illness, but may be more the result of difficulty in acknowledging death as 'a natural end-point of the normal process of dying' [39], where the emphasis of care addresses patient needs rather than prognosis.

THE FUTURE

It is clear that palliative care principles have been acknowledged by surgeons and are being integrated into basic and postgraduate training and practice, and that both disciplines could 'benefit by coming together … [to] … reclaim the lost ground of the surgeon–patient relationship' [39]. The prevailing bias toward separating care into a curative and then a palliative phase ('cure, then comfort') is not acceptable. Provision of palliative care alongside comprehensive, possibly curative care should be available to every patient at an early stage [48]. This would represent a shift toward patient-centred care [1] (Figure 9.4).

The integration of a palliative care approach into general hospital practice has demonstrated improved terminal care [49,50]. Such practice centres on outcomes that are meaningful to the patient and thus may be a focus for further research. Some work into quality of life in surgical oncology has been undertaken [2,51], a relatively new focus in palliative surgery [52]. This increased interest in quality of life should be welcomed and developed further, and may help surgeons to identify appropriate procedures for patients with advanced disease [2] and reflect goals important to patients themselves [9].

In palliative surgery there is a lack of evidence-based benefit and risk in many instances [40]. There can be a reluctance to involve palliative care patients in research, perhaps due to ethical concern or fear of creating false hope of cure. Such concern is largely unnecessary. Patients are often keen to be involved in clinical trials, if not for their own benefit, then for the 'common good' and researchers should not avoid them through any such fears or thoughts that the trial would be weakened [1].

CONCLUSION

It is encouraging to reflect on the origins of palliation in surgical oncology and recent developments toward further integration of the specialties. Important lessons have been

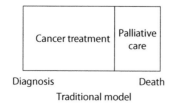

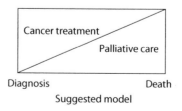

Figure 9.4 Traditional and suggested place of palliative care in cancer management. (Adapted from Twycross R, *Introducing Palliative Care*, 3rd ed., Oxford: Radcliffe Medical Press, 1997: 66.)

learned through the realization that quality of life, rather than patient prognosis or survival, is an appropriate focus for professional involvement in patients with advanced disease. A palliative care approach to patient care is within the capabilities of all professionals involved in patient care and can only serve to improve such care to the benefit of patients, families and professionals themselves.

The closer to the bedside, the better [7].

REFERENCES

1. Meyers FJ, Linder J. Simultaneous care: disease treatment and palliative care throughout illness. *J Clin Oncol* 2003; 21: 1412–5.
2. Langenhoff BS, Krabbe PFM, Wobbes T, et al. Quality of life as an outcome measure in surgical oncology. *Br J Surg* 2001; 88: 643–52.
3. Mosenthal AC, Lee KF, Huffman J. Palliative care in the surgical intensive care unit. *J Am Coll Surg* 2002; 194: 75–83.
4. Saunders C. Introduction – history and challenge. In Saunders C, Sykes N, eds., *The Management of Terminal Malignant Disease*, 3rd ed. London: Edward Arnold, 1993: 1–14.
5. Watson M, Lucas C, Hoy A, Back I, eds. *Oxford Handbook of Palliative Care*. Oxford: Oxford University Press, 2005.
6. World Health Organization. Cancer pain relief and palliative care. Technical Report Series 804. Geneva: World Health Organization, 1990.
7. Dunn GP, Milch RA. Introduction and historical background of palliative care: where does the surgeon fit in? *J Am Coll Surg* 2001; 193: 325–8.
8. Krouse RS, Nelson RA, Farrell BR, et al. Surgical palliation at a cancer center: incidence and outcomes. *Arch Surg* 2001; 136: 773–8.
9. McCahill LE, Krouse RS, Chu Z, et al. Decision making in palliative surgery. *J Am Coll Surg* 2002; 195: 411–22.
10. Byock I. Completing the continuum of cancer care: integrating life-prolongation and palliation. *CA Cancer J Clin* 2000; 50: 123–32.
11. Bonica JJ. Cancer pain: current status and future needs. In Bonica JJ, ed., *The Management of Pain*, 2nd ed. Philadelphia, PA: Lea & Febiger, 1990: 400–45.
12. International Association for the Study of Pain (IASP), Subcommittee on Taxonomy. Descriptions of chronic pain syndromes and definitions of pain terms. *Pain* 1986; S3: 1–226.
13. McCaffery M. *Nursing Management of the Patient in Pain*. Philadelphia, PA: JB Lippincott, 1972.
14. Twycross R. *Introducing Palliative Care*, 3rd ed. Oxford: Radcliffe Medical Press, 1997: 66.
15. Melzack R. The McGill pain questionnaire. In Melzack R, ed., *Pain Measurement and Assessment*. New York: Raven Press, 1983: 41–48.
16. Jensen MP, Karoly P, Braver S. The measurement of clinical pain intensity: a comparison of six methods. *Pain* 1986; 27: 117–26.
17. Bennett MI. The LANSS pain scale – the Leeds assessment of neuropathic symptoms and signs. *Pain* 2001; 92: 147–57.
18. World Health Organization. *WHO Guidelines: Cancer Pain Relief*, 2nd ed. Geneva: World Health Organization, 1996.
19. Bennett M, Forbes K, Faull C. The principles of pain management. In Faull C, Carter Y, Daniels L, eds., *Handbook of Palliative Care*, 2nd ed. Oxford: Blackwell Publishing, 2005: 116–49.
20. Grond S, Zech D, Diefenbach C, et al. Prevalence and pattern of symptoms in patients with cancer pain: a prospective evaluation of 1635 cancer patients referred to a pain clinic. *J Pain Symptom Manage* 1994; 9: 372–82.
21. Dunlop GM. A study of the relative frequency and importance of gastrointestinal symptoms, and weakness in patients with far advanced cancer. *Palliat Med* 1989; 4: 37–43.
22. Meuser T, Pietruck C, Radbruch L, et al. Symptoms during cancer pain treatment following WHO-guidelines: a longitudinal follow-up study of symptom prevalence, severity and etiology. *Pain* 2001; 93: 247–57.
23. Lichter I. Results of antiemetic management in terminal illness. *J Palliat Care* 1993; 9: 19–21.
24. Ripamonti C, Mercadante S. Pathophysiology and management of malignant bowel obstruction. In Doyle D, Hanks G, Cherny N, et al., eds., *Oxford Textbook of Palliative Medicine*, 3rd ed. Oxford: Oxford University Press, 2004: 496–507.
25. Twycross R, Wilcock R. *Symptom Management in Advanced Cancer*, 3rd ed. Abingdon, UK: Radcliffe Medical Press, 2001: 111–5.
26. Dunn GP, Milch RA, Mosenthal AC, et al. Palliative care by the surgeon: how to do it. *J Am Coll Surg* 2002; 194: 509–37.
27. Chilton A, Faull C. The management of gastrointestinal symptoms and advanced liver disease. In Faull C, Carter Y, Daniels L, eds., *Handbook of Palliative Care*, 2nd ed. Oxford: Blackwell Publishing, 2005: 150–84.
28. Bruera E. The frequency and correlates of dyspnoea in patients with advanced cancer. *J Pain Symptom Manage* 2000; 19: 357–62.
29. Wade R, Booth S, Wilcock A. The management of respiratory symptoms. In Faull C, Carter Y, Daniels L, eds., *Handbook of Palliative Care*, 2nd ed. Oxford: Blackwell Publishing, 2005: 185–207.
30. Zebraski SE, Kochenash SM, Raffa RB. Lung opioid receptors: pharmacology and possible target for nebulized morphine in dyspnea. *Life Sci* 2000; 66: 2221–31.
31. Heaven C, Maguire P. Communication issues. In Lloyd-Williams M, ed., *Psychosocial Issues in Palliative Care*. Oxford: Oxford University Press, 2003: 13–34.

32. Hotopf M, Chidgey J, Addington-Hall J, Lan Ly K. Depression in advanced disease: a systematic review. Part 1: prevalence and case finding. *Palliat Med* 2002; 16: 81–97.

33. Lloyd-Williams M, Dennis M, Taylor F. A prospective study to determine the association between physical symptoms and depression in patients with advanced cancer. *Palliat Med* 2004; 18: 558–63.

34. Lloyd-Williams M, Friedman T, Rudd N. The criterion validation of the EDS for the assessment of depression in patients with advanced metastatic disease. *J Pain Symptom Manage* 2000; 20: 259–65.

35. Dunphy JE. Annual discourse on caring for the patient with cancer. *N Engl J Med* 1976; 295: 313–9.

36. Dunn GP. Restoring palliative care as a surgical tradition. *Bull Am Coll Surg* 2004; 89: 23–9.

37. Easson AM, Crosby JA, Librach SL. Discussion of death and dying in surgical textbooks. *Am J Surg* 2001; 182: 34–9.

38. McCahill LE, Krouse R, Chu D, et al. Indications and use of palliative surgery – results of Society of Surgical Oncology survey. *Ann Surg Oncol* 2002; 9: 104–112.

39. Palliative Care Workgroup. Office of promoting excellence in end-of-life care: surgeons' palliative care workgroup report from the field. *J Am Coll Surg* 2003; 197: 661–86.

40. Hofmann B, Hâheim LL, Søreide JA. Ethics of palliative surgery in patients with cancer. *Br J Surg* 2005; 92: 802–9.

41. Bryock I, Twohig JS. Expanding the realm of the possible. *J Palliat Med* 2003; 6: 331–3.

42. Intercollegiate Surgical Curriculum Project. http://www.ISCP.ac.uk/2006.

43. Buchman TG, Cassell J, Ray SE, et al. Who should manage the dying patient? Rescue, shame, and the surgical ICU dilemma. *J Am Coll Surg* 2002; 194: 665–73.

44. Goldberg R, Guandanoli E, LaFarge S. A survey of housestaff attitudes towards terminal care education. *J Cancer Educ* 1987; 2: 163.

45. Rappaport W, Prevel C, Witzke D, et al. Education about death and dying during surgical residency. *Am J Surg* 1991; 161: 690–2.

46. Carron AT, Lynn J, Keaney P. End-of-life care in medical textbooks. *Ann Intern Med* 1999; 130: 82–6.

47. Rabow MW, Hardie GE, Fair JM, et al. End-of-life care content in 50 textbooks from multiple specialties. *JAMA* 2000; 283: 771–8.

48. Fisher JA, Parker MC. Joint surgical/palliative care ward round in a district general hospital. *Palliat Med* 1999; 13: 249–50.

49. Manfredi P, Morrison S, Morris J, et al. Palliative care consultations: how do they impact the care of hospital patients? *J Pain Symptom Manage* 2002; 24: 91–6.

50. Virik K, Glare P. Profile and evaluation of a palliative medicine consultation service within a tertiary teaching hospital in Sydney, Australia. *J Pain Symptom Manage* 2002; 23: 17–25.

51. McCahill LE, Smith DD, Borneman T, et al. A prospective evaluation of palliative outcomes for surgery of advanced malignancies. *Ann Surg Oncol* 2003; 10: 654–63.

52. Lee KF, Purcell GP, Hinshaw DB, et al. Clinical palliative care for surgeons: part 1. *J Am Coll Surg* 2004; 198: 303–19.

10

Communication and psychological needs of the cancer surgery patient

CLARE BYRNE AND GRAEME J POSTON

BACKGROUND

When confronted by cancer, patients may experience a sense of loss of control, fear and even anger. The principal concern with the psychological aspects of cancer is to alleviate the emotional distress which affects patients. There is a current trend to view psychological care within the context of 'supportive care' in a multidisciplinary team approach [1]. Supportive care refers to a culture of care that has evolved from the palliative care ethos and focuses on generic cancer teams assisting the patient and their carers to cope with cancer and its treatments at all stages of the cancer journey. It helps the patient to maximize the benefits of treatment and to live as well as possible with the effects of the disease.

The key principles underpinning supportive care are [1]:

- A focus on quality of life
- A whole person approach
- Care to include the patient and those who matter to them
- Respect for patient autonomy and choice
- An emphasis on open and sensitive communication

Communication that assists patients and their carers to express emotions and concerns can reduce fears and anxiety, and promote working together in the cancer experience. An individualized approach to information can empower patients to be involved in decision making and exercise choice, resulting in a greater sense of control and self-esteem.

HISTORICAL PERSPECTIVE

Communication with, and the psychological response by, patients to their cancer was barely investigated before the 1950s, when it was commonplace not to disclose a cancer diagnosis. Outcomes tended to be restricted to survival time and recurrence-free survival. Cancer surgeons traditionally obtained consent for surgery without discussing the definite diagnosis, or likelihood of a diagnosis, of cancer, and following surgery, cancer was not revealed as the diagnosis because it was considered as something that it was best for the patient not to know. At this time there was also a commonly believed assumption that because anxiety and depression were natural, inevitable reactions to cancer, psychological treatment was not feasible. Set against this model of care, systematic enquiry that included the patient perspective on how patients felt about their cancer, and their quality of life, was simply not accessible.

Decades before this, many radical surgical procedures for the treatment of cancer had been developed and utilized, surgery being the main treatment approach for cancer. Much of the seminal work had been undertaken at the Memorial Hospital in New York. At this same unit, some of the first studies into the psychological aspects of cancer surgery were undertaken by Sutherland (a psychiatrist), who examined psychological adaptation to mastectomy and colostomy [2,3]. However, Sutherland and others [4] struggled to have these psychological studies accepted as necessary, let alone scientific, as psychology was not viewed as an important aspect of cancer patient management.

It was during the 1960s that a more enlightened view of the ethical issues surrounding disclosure of a cancer diagnosis to patients started to be acknowledged. Alongside this, the importance of the relationship between the psychological effects of cancer and cancer treatments such as surgery also began to develop and measurement of outcomes in cancer care began to include the psychological issues of quality of life of individuals affected by cancer.

In the US, papers were presented by cancer surgeons at academic meetings [5] and published in recognized journals [6], resulting in an increased recognition of the psychological needs in the management of the patient with cancer. Practical guidance was provided [6], which is still very pertinent today and included how to:

- Establish rapport with the patient in the preoperative period
- Allay the patient's fears
- Inform the patient that incurable cancer was found at surgery
- Establish close communication with the patient whose cancer was found to be incurable at surgery

Across the Atlantic, developments in the hospice movement in the UK saw a shift from relying only on the measurement of clinical outcomes to the measurement of factors that were likely to be of direct concern to patients, such as cancer and depression or discussion about preferred place to die [7]. In cancer surgery, a number of studies arose through psychiatric and psychological academic links with oncology units [8]. Some of this early work involved those affected by breast cancer, both in the acute phase around diagnosis and during treatment [8,9] and at the stage of recurrence, development of metastases or dissemination [10]. Therapeutic interventions for the psychological management of cancer patients were also developed in those having breast cancer surgery [11], and for those who presented with advanced breast disease [12].

COMMUNICATION SKILLS IN CANCER

The ability to communicate with patients is a core requirement for all health care professionals. Much of the research in this field has been undertaken in cancer care and disability [13–15]. Having the skills to elicit patient concerns, and to appropriately respond to them, to individualize patient information and to involve patients in decision preferences about their care calls upon a range of both interpersonal and communication skills [16,17].

Studies have shown repeatedly that many health care professionals do not have such skills [16–19], and it is the lack of these skills which seems to be the main reason why communication breaks down. It has been identified that these skills are not innate in most health care professionals, and need to be developed to a level of competence and confidence through research-based communication skills training [19,20].

INFORMATION AND CANCER

The information given to cancer patients about their diagnosis, treatment options and concerns about the future can have a profound impact on their psychological well-being [21]. Increasing evidence in cancer studies points to a need for an individualized approach to information giving [15,22], as too much or too little (in areas such as treatment options or prognosis) can contribute to psychological distress. The challenge seems to lie in assessing what information individual patients require, rather than using routine ways of supplying information, which ignores the individual's needs or preferences [15].

Of concern in patients faced with surgery as an option for treatment of their cancer, while informed consent necessitates full information to patients, it does not currently require an interpretation or expression of comprehension of that information. Lack of access to not only an adequate level of information, but also interpretation and application of accepted treatment guidelines (including potential risks and even uncertain benefits), appears to be a crucial issue in the provision of information and patient autonomy [23]. It is also suggested that supportive, individualized information strategies may have positive consequences for accruing patients to clinical trials [24].

DECISION MAKING AND CANCER

The concept of user involvement in the development, monitoring and delivery of cancer treatment has been accompanied by a reduction in the paternalistic approach to patients, where patient opinion and decisions about treatment are valued as an essential component, and where consideration of the whole person, including their carers, is incorporated into a more holistic and supportive approach to care. Patients' attitudes, their coping resources and their ability and willingness to be involved in decisions about their management may be influenced by previous experience of disclosure and information received [25,26]. Furthermore, how patients feel about how they have been included and involved in decision making can result in dissatisfaction and non-compliance [27], and may contribute to an adverse outcome [28].

Decision making is not just a one-way process of the health care professional telling the patient what will be. In today's environment, the 'expert patient' [28] is better informed than their predecessor and many will expect to be involved in the decision process that determines their treatment. In many cancers, combination therapy utilizing surgery, chemotherapy, radiotherapy and biotherapy may be the norm. Different ways of describing the outcomes of treatment can have a dramatic impact on patient treatment decisions [29]. This has implications for not only what is said, but also how it is said and by whom, and contributes to the complexity faced by health care professionals in supporting patients through information giving and decision making [23].

Translating scientific data from clinical trials into layman's language contributes to the dilemma for health care professionals. Patient involvement in decision making seems to be influenced by [25]:

- Conflicting expectations between doctor and patient about the most appropriate treatment
- Unexpected information
- Issues related to treatment costs and benefits
- Lack of clear treatment recommendations from the oncologist

Marked differences in decision-making role preferences, but similarities in information needs, have been identified [26]. In breast cancer patients only 52% chose a passive role in decision making compared to 78% of colorectal cancer patients and 80% of colorectal patients and 61% of breast cancer patients recalled the doctor making treatment decisions. The main concerns for information in both patient cohorts were in relation to:

- Cure
- Spread of disease
- Treatment options

A later study [30] confirmed that while patients wanted information and to feel included in the consultation, they did not necessarily want to be involved in decisions about their care.

PSYCHOLOGICAL DISTRESS AND CANCER

Anxiety

Most patients will be apprehensive about their cancer, and some may experience stronger psychological responses including feelings of anxiety, resentment, anger and even panic attacks [31]. Anxiety in the patient with cancer may be induced by the patient perceiving threats to survival and well-being, as well as their uncertainty about the future [31]. Applying this to the patient faced with cancer surgery, anxiety may be compounded by fear of death from surgery or

anaesthetic, as well as fear of pain and mutilation. Integral to this major significant area influencing the level of anxiety is the stage of cancer [31]. While patients with early stage cancer can often have a long life expectancy and anticipation of curative surgery, patients diagnosed with advanced cancer or those with a recurrence or metastatic spread have to face the emotional consequences of imminent death. This emotional burden usually causes intense emotional reactions, including clinical states of anxiety.

Depression

Depression in the patient with cancer, like anxiety, is one of the most difficult psychological problems to identify [32], and some suggest it may be underestimated [33]. As a simple cut-off point it is said to be significant when the sadness response (e.g. depressed mood, insomnia, fatigue, feelings of worthlessness, diminished ability to think) to a disclosure of a cancer diagnosis or poor prognosis lasts more than 2 weeks [34]. A useful concept when considering whether a patient is depressed is that the patient who blames the illness for how they are feeling is probably experiencing sadness, whereas the patient who blames themselves for their illness and how they are feeling may well be depressed [32]. The surgeon and the whole health care team should be receptive to any signs of depression in the patient.

The concern is that if health care professionals assess depression as a normal feature of cancer, there is a risk that depressed cancer patients may go undiagnosed and untreated [35]. It has been suggested that there is some reluctance among many health care professionals to initiate and explore psychological issues with their patients, as they are concerned that this will exacerbate patients' distress [35]. Another reason suggested is that health professionals feel powerless to influence the situation and so do not intervene [35]. However, other studies [17,18,20] indicate that the main reason why they do not pursue these sensitive issues with patients is the lack of communication and interpersonal skills of health care professionals to draw out and explore patients' concerns and so fail to identify and meet their information needs and decision-making preferences.

PSYCHOLOGICAL NEEDS OF THE CANCER SURGERY PATIENT

The psychological needs of the patient having cancer surgery are similar to those of any patient having surgery. They include:

- An ability to understand the need for surgery and the procedure proposed
- Having the resources to deal with the physical and mental discomfort involved to achieve the intention of improved health and survival

Surgery plays a crucial role in the curative treatment of cancer, so the stigma of cancer and its threat to survival can add to the psychological demands on an individual and their family or carers. Developing rapport with the patient, acknowledging the existence of stress factors, and supplying empathetic support and information from the point of disclosure of diagnosis, and especially during the preoperative period, can have an impact on how patients cope with their cancer and their postoperative recovery and rehabilitation, including their psychological well-being.

The majority of patients affected by cancer will undergo some sort of surgical procedure, as surgical oncology is not just the removal of a tumor but can include diagnosis and staging of cancer, by, for example, biopsy at staging laparoscopy, prevention, reconstruction, palliation and supportive surgery.

The impact of cancer surgery, and where the procedure sits within the context of the individual's cancer journey, coping resources and responses must be considered. The meaning a patient attaches to the surgical procedure will vary according to both their previous experience and the aims of the surgery. This may also be influenced by the explorative or definitive nature of the surgery, whether the tumor is resectable, and any functional consequences including loss or deficit. The meaning an individual attaches to a biopsy taken for diagnostic purposes at staging laparoscopy, a curative liver resection, or palliative surgery to relieve gastric outflow obstruction in cholangiocarcinoma will be different for each individual.

PSYCHOLOGICAL ADAPTATION

Medical variables

Medical variables that may influence psychological adaptation to cancer surgery include:

- Site, stage and potential for curability either with surgery alone or as part of a multimodal approach to treatment
- Functional deficit as a consequence of surgery
- Rehabilitation available including reconstruction
- The surgeon and other health care professionals' acknowledgment of and management of the patient's psychological needs

Patient variables

Patient variables that may influence psychological adaptation to cancer surgery include:

- Meaning attached to the cancer diagnosis (or potential diagnosis)
- The risks and benefits the patient perceives of the surgical procedure, including the anaesthetic
- The functional consequences
- The individual patient's psychological response and ability to cope with both the stress of surgery and the cancer diagnosis

- History of psychiatric disorder, particularly depression
- Response to surgeon and relationship established

PREOPERATIVE CARE

How the patient presents for possible surgery for cancer and how they are adapting and coping with their cancer diagnosis may well be influenced by how they have been managed during their cancer journey. Patients who have experienced a protracted diagnosis associated with doubt about their symptoms, poor disclosure of diagnosis and delay in receiving an appointment to meet with the cancer specialist may be more psychologically maladjusted to their cancer diagnosis than someone whose experience has been well managed with prompt referral from their general practitioner through a speedy process of investigations (accompanied by information and support from health care professionals along the way), and timely recall to discuss diagnosis and ongoing management options.

As such, it is important at the time of meeting with the patient for the first time for the surgeon to assess the patient's experience and understanding of why they are there, to check their understanding of their diagnosis, to elicit any concerns and to identify and clarify any misconceptions they may have about their cancer. It is only then that the surgeon can start to explore surgical treatment options with the patient. Encouraging the inclusion of a family member or friend to be present acts as resource to the patient for support and also acknowledges the carer's important role in the patient's life as well as their potential involvement in care and rehabilitation after discharge.

While preoperative information to the patient could almost be seen as a checklist, how that information is divulged in response to an individual assessment of the patient's information needs and concerns should be accompanied by a collaborative and proactive approach with the patient, as it may be that the patient when asked if they have any questions or concerns will respond, 'But I don't know what I need to know'. Again, inclusion of the carer should be encouraged. Providing the patient with a preclinic list of questions may help them prepare questions to ask, and endorse that it is okay to ask questions. An example of such a list is given in Table 10.1.

Questions that acknowledge that the patient may have concerns, such as 'how are you feeling about this surgery?' encourage them to explore fears, and to voice any related anxieties they may have about probable pain, discomfort or any physical changes. If surgery involves loss of a limb, formation of a stoma or the sexual organs, such open-ended questions allow the patient to explore concerns they may have about sexual function and body image.

Important issues to explore with the patient include:

- The purpose of surgery – is it prophylactic, diagnostic, staging, curative or palliative?
- The benefits of the surgery proposed.

Table 10.1 List of questions to be given to patients prior to attendance at clinic to help them prepare their own questions

Attending hospital and undergoing tests can be quite an anxious time for you. While we try very hard to give you all the information you require to understand and decide about the most appropriate treatments available to you, you and your family may have questions to ask. However, these may only occur to you after you have met with the consultant. *So, why not write them down?*

Other patients with cancer have found it useful to ask some of the following questions:

- What are the results of my tests?
- Where exactly is the tumor and how big is it?
- Is it malignant or non-malignant?
- Has the tumor spread to any other areas?
- What treatments are available to me?
- Do I need surgery or do I need chemotherapy?
- Would I benefit from a combination of treatments?
- Why is this particular treatment recommended for me?
- Can I be cured?
- What will happen if I don't have treatment?
- What are the chances of the tumor returning or spreading?
- Is this a unit specializing in my type of tumor?
- Who will be treating me?
- Has the doctor received specialist training for treating my type of tumor?
- What will the treatment entail, e.g. time in hospital, side effects, the risks involved, the number of treatments I will need?
- Once I have had my treatment how will I be followed up?
- Is there anyone I can talk to who has had my type of treatment?

- The risks of surgery for the individual (complications, peri- or postoperative death) taking into account other comorbidity.
- What kind of surgery will be performed and what preoperative preparation is required (e.g. bowel prep, fasting). Proposed incision, postoperative drains, infusions and pain control.
- Admission to a high-dependency area if necessary.
- Treatment options if inoperable disease is found at time of surgery.
- Proposed admission date, preoperative screening, anticipated recovery time and potential discharge plan.
- Control of postoperative pain, including pain assessment, methods of pain control (e.g. epidural, patient-controlled analgesia), and managing pain and discomfort postdischarge.

- Anticipated rehabilitation postdischarge.
- Location of carer on day of surgery, and contact telephone number. Access to carer accommodation during patient stay.

Having access to a contact number of a member of the multidisciplinary team such as a clinical nurse specialist or nurse practitioner who ideally has been present at the consultation and is available to discuss any related concerns or queries can be useful to both the patient and their carer, but also acts as a support to the surgeon, knowing that any concerns will be acknowledged, and when possible addressed, prior to the patient's admission. Following discussion at the outpatient appointment, patients and their carers may find it helpful to write down information, and a summary sheet can be provided with the following headings:

- Your diagnosis
- The need for any further investigations
- Treatment options discussed
- The next stage of treatment
- The questions and answers we have explored together

ENHANCING PHYSICAL WELL-BEING AND PSYCHOLOGICAL DISTRESS

The cancer patient awaiting surgery may be affected by a number of symptoms associated with their cancer, including side effects of tumor mass, tumor obstruction, tumor toxicity and side effects of chemotherapy or radiotherapy. Assessing and alleviating physical symptoms such as pain, nausea, vomiting, diarrhea, fatigue or anorexia can contribute to both the patient's physical and mental recovery. Proactive preoperative treatment and management of these side effects are more likely to equip the patient to deal better with the trauma of surgery and the challenges of recovery. Immediate postoperative needs of all surgical patients including cancer patients are primarily physical and the usual postoperative care protocols should be adhered to.

PREPARING THE PATIENT FOR UNEXPECTED FINDINGS AT TIME OF SURGERY

An important area of information to discuss with patients preoperatively is the issue of finding inoperable disease at the time of surgery. Acknowledging that this can happen (despite improvements in radiological imaging and access to staging laparoscopy) and exploring strategies for alternative management of the patient's cancer are important areas to cover, preferably in the company of their family or carer. Preparing the patient in such a way sows the seeds for dealing with the 'open and close' situation more positively and maintains hope by reminding the patient that although surgery has not been possible, and that their cancer may therefore be incurable, there are other treatment options that will be considered to manage their cancer.

POSTOPERATIVE PSYCHOLOGICAL NEEDS

When the patient is rousing from anaesthetic it has to be anticipated that they will start to ask questions such as 'Was it cancer?', 'Is it all gone?' and 'Has it spread anywhere else?' Answering questions at this stage should be avoided until the patient has recovered from the anaesthetic and the surgeon is able to explain the findings at surgery and the procedure performed, or not, to the patient accompanied preferably by their relative or carer.

It is of further historical interest to note that in relation to discussing incurable disease found at surgery it has been suggested that:

> If the doctor-patient relationship is one which each feels free to communicate with the other, telling the patient that he is incurable, although never easy, is less painful. Here, again, if we listen to the patient he will let us know when he can be told and how much he can tolerate hearing.
>
> Once the essentials of truth are explained in the proper manner, the way becomes clear for the next phase … hope … the words 'incurable' and 'hopeless' are not synonymous. To tell a patient that his condition is hopeless is both cruel and technically incorrect. Incurability is a state of mind, a giving up – a situation that must be avoided at all cost. A patient can tolerate knowing he is incurable; he cannot tolerate hopelessness [6].

For the patient who has inoperable disease found at surgery, the surgeon and the multidisciplinary team should anticipate and encourage discussion with the patient and carer in the postoperative period about the implications of inoperable disease, and support the adjustment to the fact that inoperable in most cancers also means incurable. Again, the clinical nurse specialist or nurse practitioner who knows the patient is best placed to support the individual and their carers and to meet their information needs. Setting up an early appointment with the medical oncologist to discuss palliative treatment options can be beneficial, prior to or soon after discharge.

PSYCHOLOGICAL ISSUES

Psychological issues to be explored in the context of the aims of surgery include:

- Prophylactic
- Diagnostic
- Definitive
- Reconstructive
- Palliative
- Supportive surgery

Prophylactic surgery and psychological needs

Prophylactic surgery is usually considered in those individuals who have a family history of a certain type of cancer such as breast, ovarian or colorectal cancer, and in whom an underlying condition or a genetic predisposition may put them at higher risk of developing the disease [36]. The psychological challenges to an individual faced with the decision to undergo surgery to remove currently benign tissue or organs to prevent the development of cancer may be compounded by the knowledge that they have a genetic defect that can be passed on with or without surgery. While surgery at this time might prevent the disease developing, there are also consequences to quality of life following surgical removal of body parts resulting in, for example, altered body image, sexual function and how an individual feels about their self-image and confidence. Benefits may not always be as great as the individual had anticipated [37]. However, this also has to be weighed against the alternative of intensive screening which may cause both reassurance with good results and at times distress in both the time leading up to the screening and when results are not favourable [38].

For women with breast cancer it is necessary to acknowledge their social situation. Often, these women come from families where grandmothers, mothers, aunts and cousins have been diagnosed, treated and died from breast cancer. As such, they live within an environment of uncertainty and fear of not only the occurrence of breast cancer but also the effectiveness of treatments such as mastectomy, chemotherapy and radiotherapy. Ultimately, they live with the fear of living with cancer and the uncertainty of survival, and this along with concerns about their husband or partner and children may influence their decision to undergo prophylactic mastectomy.

Supporting individuals faced with the prospect of prophylactic surgery is crucial. Accurate information about the benefits of surgery according to evidence available as well as the risks of surgery, and reconstructive surgery as an option, must be explored. Time and timing are important. The decision should not be rushed. It is suggested that eliciting patient's concerns about their decision in the context of their role and responsibilities within their family and society, their age, occupation, culture, and religion and their own subjective assessment of the risk of developing cancer, as well as their previous experiences with illness, death and the medical system, is important to consider [39].

While prophylactic surgery might relieve an individual of the fear of developing cancer, the effects of the operation may take some adjustment, and this aspect must be acknowledged and discussed with the individual both prior to and as part of a rehabilitation following surgery to prepare them for both the physical discomfort of surgery and their altered body image. After surgery, ongoing psychological support is essential, as this is the time when they may be concerned about how they now appear to their husband or wife, whether they are as attractive with a stoma or having had a mastectomy. As such, the impact on their sexuality can be severely affected, in the way of not only sexual function, but also their self-image and self-confidence.

Psychological issues related to loss in, for example, young women that surgery will result in their inability to breast-feed in the future, set against the thought that they may never have developed cancer anyway, are issues that must be acknowledged during the process of preparing the patient for prophylactic surgery.

Diagnostic surgery and psychological needs

When malignancy is suspected, the accuracy of information gained during the diagnostic process is crucial in order that the most effective treatment decisions can be made. While diagnostic imaging such as computed tomography (CT) or magnetic resonance (MR) scan and biochemistry and tumor markers can often confirm diagnosis, where there is uncertainty, a surgical procedure may be required. The major role for surgery at this stage is to acquire a sample of tissue for histological diagnosis, and techniques include fine-needle aspiration, excisional biopsy, endoscopic biopsy, bone marrow biopsy, examination under anaesthetic and biopsy at staging laparoscopy.

While many of these procedures may seem simple and routine to health care professionals, for the individual patient affected by the uncertainty of their presenting symptoms, the time leading up to and including diagnosis can be associated with great anxiety and fear. While they may seek an answer, the fear of what the results may show and the impact the diagnosis may have on their life as well as on those close to them, their role in their family or their job compounds this anxiety. The coordination and management of the diagnostic phase is important as it can greatly affect the adjustment to and coping with a diagnosis of cancer. Waiting for an appointment, waiting for a scan and waiting for results can increase anxiety and fear associated with uncertainty and loss of control, as well as fear that if it is cancer it will be growing and getting worse. Part of this coordination should include access to a key member of the cancer multidisciplinary team, such as a clinical nurse specialist who can acknowledge any concerns, provide both support and information about how investigations are proceeding and act as a resource and coordinator during this crucial aspect of the patient's journey. This is particularly important as many diagnostic procedures take place in an outpatient or day case setting where the time available to assess patients' concerns and meet their psychological needs may be limited. Another aspect of time and timing is delay in coming to definitive surgery which can affect the quality of life in newly diagnosed cancer patients [40].

Definitive surgery and psychological reaction

The aim of definitive surgery is to remove the cancerous tumor as well as a safe margin of normal tissue surrounding it [41].

In many patients with solid tumors, where the disease is confined to the anatomical site of origin, and the tumor is small (e.g. Dukes A cancer of the colon), this may be excised through a local resection, and will be the optimal chance of cure. However, it also carries with it anxiety in the patient that surgery has a successful outcome.

When discussing treatment options with the patient, it is important to know the stage of the cancer in order to know whether surgery might effect a cure, or whether combination treatment including surgery and adjuvant treatment such as chemotherapy might be necessary. Sometimes it is only after the tumor is excised and examined by the histopathologist that this essential staging information can be secured and the chances of cure or need for further treatment decided.

Where the tumor is large and there is a suspicion or evidence of metastatic spread, a more radical resection is usually necessary. This involves not only resection of the tumor but also resection of local and regional tissue, the lymphatics and a margin of tumor-free tissue, in an attempt to prevent further metastatic spread and local recurrence.

Psychological reactions to cancer surgery can be related to the site of surgery and the extent of functional loss [42,43]. Adverse emotional reactions correlate with the psychological significance of the loss, especially with the face, breast, genitals or colon [42,43]. Site-specific problems also arise when surgery results in a major loss of a particular function. Examples of this include loss of normal bowel function with the formation of a colostomy, and the loss of normal speech when laryngectomy is performed [43,44].

Surgery as part of a multimodal approach to cancer treatment

When cancer is first detected, about 50% of all patients will have metastatic disease, with a probable high incidence of undiagnosed, occult metastases. Surgery, therefore, is often used as a localized treatment and as part of a multimodal approach to increase chance of cure and to prolong disease-free survival.

The use of multimodal therapies does have consequences that need to be considered if surgery is part of the treatment plan. The timing of chemotherapy or radiotherapy before or after surgery can affect how the body copes with surgery, for example risk of chest infection or wound infection where neutropenia is a side effect of chemotherapy, and delayed wound healing where radiotherapy has caused fibrosis and damage to lymphatic and vascular channels. The patient needs to be aware of these considerations, such as allowing the body to recover following chemotherapy and prior to surgery, as they may associate delay of surgery with a less favourable outcome, rather than it being a considered decision within their treatment plan.

As well as curative intent, surgery with other treatment modalities may also be performed to debulk a tumor in for example ovarian cancer or in metastatic neuroendocrine cancer. However, debulking is usually only of benefit when it is used in conjunction with other treatments, such as chemotherapy, to control the residual disease left behind. Reduction of tumor mass can improve the outcome of radiotherapy or chemotherapy.

Traditionally, the presence of metastatic disease in the liver or the lungs has precluded the chance of cure. However, in such cancers as colorectal cancer, there is increasing evidence to show that surgical resection of liver metastases can play a part in cure [45] and as part of a multimodal, palliative oncological approach.

Furthermore, disease-free survival is also improving in those colorectal cancer patients who later develop lung metastases and undergo pulmonary resection [45]. However, treatment of metastatic disease very much depends on the primary cancer, and this is an important information issue for patients, and needs to be actively addressed by health care professionals, to ensure that patients understand why surgical treatment options might, or might not, be available to them. For example, surgery is not a treatment option for liver metastases in the presence of pancreas cancer or breast cancer, but may be considered in a primary ocular melanoma or for lung metastases in soft tissue sarcoma.

Reconstructive surgery and psychological needs

Radical cancer surgery can often result in marked physical deformity or loss of function. This physical loss also carries with it the risk of major psychological distress and social isolation. Approaches to reconstructive surgery to improve anatomical defects, function and cosmetic appearance have developed in an attempt to restore an individual to as normal a life as possible following cancer surgery. Examples of reconstructive surgery include breast reconstruction, skin grafting, head and neck surgery, and artificial joints in sarcoma patients.

Reconstructive surgery must be considered as part of the treatment plan when considering surgery as an option, as in many cases, for example breast surgery, reconstruction may be carried out at the time of the initial operation. Health care professionals need to consider that not only are patients often grappling with their diagnosis of cancer and radical surgery such as mastectomy, but also a further psychological challenge for patients is the decision whether to have reconstructive surgery at this time or later [42]. Options for reconstruction should be discussed clearly with the patient and having support of the presence of a spouse or family member may help. While breast reconstruction is often considered to be in the individual's best interest and can minimize some of the negative consequences of breast cancer [42], it can be undertaken at a later date if the individual would prefer or cannot decide.

In head and neck cancer surgery, reconstruction is not an option as it is a necessary part of the surgery to excise the tumor. Overall, head and neck surgery is viewed as more complex than other regions as it carries challenges to the surgeon in both essential and social functions as well as the individual's appearance.

Studies have shown that as well as coping with a cancer diagnosis, patients who have had head and neck cancer surgery view themselves as different from how they were, physically, emotionally and in their self-identity, and this can result in a negative outcome in their relationship with others and their sexuality [43]. Techniques in head and neck surgery are improving all the time in an attempt to reduce physical disfigurement and loss of function, and to optimize cosmetic appearance. However, a major difficulty in this cancer type is finding the balance between surgical excision and reconstruction, with the challenge and prospect of early local recurrence in relation to physical and psychological morbidity and quality of life [44]. It has to be considered that the loss of ability to eat and talk, or to be physically disfigured is a high price to pay if prognosis is limited [41].

While a diagnosis of cancer has associated physiological, psychological and social challenges, the decision or the ability to have reconstructive surgery can affect an individual's lifestyle and sense of self [42]. Reconstruction can facilitate self-esteem, promote return to a normal lifestyle and help the individual to cope with their diagnosis and treatment. When exploring diagnosis and treatment options, health care professionals need to provide a supportive environment where options and information about consequences of surgical treatment can be discussed and concerns acknowledged. Where appropriate, careful emotional and physical planning and information about reconstruction must be included so that the individual can come to an informed decision. It has to be stressed [39] that while reconstructive surgery will result in 'a breast' or 'a tongue', it will not be the same as the real thing, in that a reconstructed breast will not feel or move in the same way or have the same sensual feeling. Likewise the replacement of a tongue with a platform of tissue (a latissimus dorsi myocutaneous flap) may help to restore some of the ability to swallow and maintain intelligible speech, but it will not be the same. As such, a balance needs to be made between optimism and realism, and between quality of life and length of life.

Individuals having reconstructive surgery and their spouse or carers will also need support with adjusting to their new self and their new identity. While uncertainties will still exist about the outcome of treatment, and future prognosis, reconstructive surgery may play a vital role in allowing the individual to face that uncertain future [41]. New approaches to psychological support that include the patient's partner in a psychosocial model of support have demonstrated some success in breast cancer [46]. Findings of a randomized controlled trial indicate that such an intervention increases quality of life, reduces uncertainty and improves family communication. Patients and their family members gained benefit from help focusing on the here and now, as well as strategies for supporting one another.

Palliative surgery and psychological needs

When cure is no longer an option, surgery can be effective for relieving symptoms that develop in the advanced stages of cancer. Examples of palliative surgery include:

- Treatment of a fungating breast wound
- Relief of bowel obstruction in ovarian cancer
- Debulking of a tumor to control discharge, the formation of fistulae or hemorrhage
- Prevention of hemorrhage when a tumor is pressing on a vital blood vessel
- Prophylactic or therapeutic pinning of metastases in long bones
- Spinal surgery to prevent or stabilize spinal cord compression
- Debulking of tumor to control infiltration of nerves which cause neuropathic pain
- Insertion of intraepidural or intrathecal catheters for spinal opioids or neuro-lytic blocks for pain in such cancers as pancreas or gallbladder cancer

The aim of palliative surgery is to relieve suffering and minimize the symptoms of the disease, so that if the quality of life will not be improved, or if there is an unnecessary risk of morbidity or mortality, then palliative surgery should not be considered. Individuals and their spouse or carers need to be informed of the aims of palliative surgery, so that they can be realistic in their expectations of the surgery and make an informed decision. Some individuals may refuse palliative surgery, preferring to spend what time they have left without submitting themselves to a hospital stay or the risks of surgery, while others may welcome the surgical intervention and see it as a treatment that may prolong their life. Again, individuals should be supported in their decision, as the signs and symptoms that require palliative surgery are invariably those of progressive disease, and as such realistic expectations of surgery should be reiterated, and the patient supported to understand these. Palliative surgery needs to be considered on an individual basis and the decision based on each individual's symptoms and their current quality of life against how surgery might improve that quality.

Supportive surgery and psychological needs

Supportive surgery for the individual with cancer may include any of the following:

- Providing venous and arterial access for the administration of cytotoxic drugs
- Providing venous and arterial access for the administration of nutritional support
- The ablation of functioning ovaries in women less than 50 years old with early breast cancer

The use of an indwelling catheter such as a Hickman line has been shown to have made a marked improvement to not only the safety of administering cytotoxic drugs, but also the quality of life of the individual with cancer [47], though the altered body image seems to be underresearched, and this should be assessed with the individual when considering use of an indwelling catheter. The reason why the line is proposed needs careful discussion with the individual and their spouse or carer. Whether the line is going to be used with the intention of a curative procedure, such as bone marrow transplant, or is to be used for palliative intervention such as palliative chemotherapy when the goal is to prolong life but not cure should be discussed. Furthermore, the individual and their spouse or carer need to be taught about all aspects of care, function and maintenance of the line, to ensure that they understand the implications and are prepared and supported to care for it safely.

Cancer surgery and carers

Increasing evidence demonstrates the need to involve family members or carers at all stages of the patient's cancer journey [48] with consequences for their psychological health if excluded [48,49]. There is a trend toward shorter hospital stay, and once fit for discharge following cancer treatment including surgery, most individuals continue their rehabilitation at home being cared for by a spouse or carer. The emergence of 'informal carers', usually a family member or close friend, who provide unpaid assistance for their dependent relatives living in the community is becoming more specifically recognized on the health and social care policy agenda [50]. However, there are still significant gaps in our understanding of family care with concern about the fact that caring relationships are rarely seen as reciprocal and tend to be interpreted as unrewarding and damaging, with an emphasis on the physical burden of caring [50].

Carers and psychological distress

Studies looking at the experiences of carers have helped to inform the factors which predict psychological distress in carers in cancer and palliative care [48,51,52]. The emphasis on information need is prevalent in many of these cancer studies, with carers indicating that they would have welcomed more information and support at an earlier stage [48], someone to talk to [52], and that their information needs are different than those of patients and should be assessed on an individual basis [51]. Understanding details related to the illness seemed to help carers cope with the situation [51], and fear of not knowing what to do or expect greatly increased carers' stress, as did poor coordination of care [52]. Overall carers would have appreciated more educational input from health care professionals.

The attitude of health care professionals who view the carer 'not as a person in their own right, but merely as an appendage to the patient' or even 'a co-worker' may contribute to increased levels of psychological distress [53].

While carers are apparently recognized in policy, there are still uncertainties as to whether carers are providers or users of services, or whether they should be acknowledged as experts in their own right [50].

SUMMARY

While the communication and psychological needs associated with cancer surgery reflect those of an individual undergoing any type of surgery, the added impact of a cancer diagnosis, its uncertainty and threat to life make increased demands on coping resources for psychological well-being. The meaning of surgery to the patient with cancer is important and will vary for each individual. In order for health care professionals to give the care that is necessary, effective communication skills and an understanding of the range of psychological responses to cancer and cancer surgery are essential. It would appear that preparation for surgery through preoperative discussion, acknowledgment of uncertainties, information exchange and support in decision making can make a difference, and can influence the postoperative course and adjustment. Inclusion of spouse or carer at all stages, with appropriate information and involvement, can enhance both the patient's and the carer's psychological well-being and may result in a more favourable outcome of the cancer surgery experience.

REFERENCES

1. Jeffrey D. What do we mean by psychosocial care in palliative care? In Lloyd-Williams M, ed., *Psychosocial Issues in Palliative Care.* Oxford: Oxford University Press, 2003: 1–5.
2. Sutherland AM, Orbach CE. Psychological impact of cancer and cancer surgery: II. Depressive reactions associated with surgery for cancer. *Cancer* 1953; 6: 958–62.
3. Bard M, Sutherland AM. Psychological impact of cancer and its treatment: IV. Adaptation to radical mastectomy. *Cancer* 1955; 8: 652–72.
4. Renneker R, Cutler M. Psychological problems of adjustment to breast cancer. *JAMA* 1952; 148: 833–8.
5. Pack GT. Counselling the cancer patient: surgeon's counsel. In *The Physician and the Total Care of the Cancer Patient: A Symposium Presented at the 1961 Scientific Session of the American Cancer Society.* New York: American Cancer Society, 1962: 56–61.
6. Stehlin JS, Beach KH. Psychological aspects of cancer therapy. *JAMA* 1966; 197: 140–4.
7. Hinton J. The physical and mental distress of the dying. *QJ Med* 1963; 32: 1–21.
8. Maguire GP, Lee EG, Bevington DJ, et al. Psychiatric problems in the first year after mastectomy. *Br Med J* 1978; 1: 963.
9. Greer S, Morris T. Psychological attributes of women who develop breast cancer; a controlled study. *J Psychosom Res* 1975; 19: 147–53.
10. Schmale AH. Psychological reactions to recurrences, metastases, or disseminated cancer. *Int J Radiat Oncol Biol Phys* 1976; 1: 515–20.
11. Maguire GP, Tait A, Brooke M, et al. Effect of counselling on the psychiatric morbidity associated with mastectomy. *Br Med J* 1980; 281: 1454–6.
12. Hopwood P, Howell A, Maguire P. Psychiatric morbidity in patients with advanced cancer of the breast: prevalence measured by two self-rating questionnaires. *Br J Cancer* 1991; 64: 349–52.
13. Taylor KM. Telling bad news: physicians and the disclosure of undesirable information. *Sociol Health Illn* 1988; 10: 109–32.
14. Fallowfield LJ. No news is not good news. *Psychooncology* 1995; 4: 197–202.
15. Maguire P. Breaking bad news. *Eur J Surg Oncol* 1998; 24: 188–91.
16. Maguire P, Faulkner A, Booth K, et al. Helping cancer patients disclose their concerns. *Eur J Cancer* 1996; 32A: 78–81.
17. Heaven CM, Maguire P. Training hospice nurses to elicit patient concerns. *J Adv Nurs* 1996; 23: 280–6.
18. Booth K, Maguire P, Butterworth T, et al. Perceived professional support and the use of blocking behaviours by hospice nurses. *J Adv Nurs* 1996; 24: 522–7.
19. Fallowfield L, Jenkins V, Farewell V, et al. Efficacy of a cancer research UK communication skills training model for oncologists: a randomised controlled trial. *Lancet* 2002; 359: 650–6.
20. Wilkinson S, Roberts A, Aldridge J. Nurse-patient communication in palliative care; an evaluation of a communication skills programme. *Palliat Med* 1998; 12: 13–22.
21. Butow PN, Kazemi JN, Beeney NJ, et al. When the diagnosis is cancer: patient communication experiences and preferences. *Cancer* 1996; 77: 2630–7.
22. Fallowfield LJ, Hall A, Maguire P, et al. Psychological outcomes of different treatment policies in women with early breast cancer outside a clinical trial. *Br Med J* 1990; 301: 575–80.
23. Poston GJ, Byrne CH. Decision making for patients with colorectal cancer liver metastases. *Ann Surg Oncol* 2006; 13: 10–1.
24. Wright JR, Whelan TJ, Schiff S, et al. Why cancer patients enter randomised clinical trials: exploring the factors that influence their decision. *J Clin Oncol* 2004; 22: 12–8.
25. Sanders T, Skevington S. Participation as an expression of patient uncertainty: an exploration of bowel cancer consultations. *Psychooncology* 2004; 13: 675–88.
26. Beaver K, Bogg J, Luker KA. Decision making role preferences and information needs: a comparison of colorectal and breast cancer. *Health Expect* 1999; 2: 266–76.

27. Dowsett SM, Saul JL, Butow PN, et al. Communication style in the cancer consultation: preferences for a patient-centred approach. *Psychooncology* 2000; 9: 147–56.

28. Coulter A. Paternalism or partnership? Patients have grown-up and there's no going back. *Br Med J* 1999; 319: 719–20.

29. Martin RCG, Studts JL, McGuffin SA, et al. Method of presenting oncology treatment outcomes influences patient treatment decision making in metastatic colorectal cancer. *Ann Surg Oncol* 2006; 13: 86–95.

30. Beaver K, Jones D, Susnerwala S, et al. Exploring decision making preferences of people with colorectal cancer. *Health Expect* 2005; 8: 103–13.

31. Maguire P. Psychosocial interventions to reduce affective disorders in cancer patients: research priorities. *Psychooncology* 1995; 4: 113–9.

32. Lloyd-Williams M. Screening for depression in palliative care. In Lloyd-Williams M, ed., *Psychosocial Issues in Palliative Care*. Oxford: Oxford University Press, 2003: 105–18.

33. Ibbotson T, Maguire P, Selby P, et al. Screening for anxiety and depression in cancer patients. *Eur J Cancer* 1994; 30A: 37–40.

34. Barraclough J. *Cancer and Emotion: Practical Guide to Psychooncology*. Chichester: Wiley, 1994.

35. Block S. Assessing and managing depression in the terminally ill patient. *Ann Intern Med* 2000; 132: 209–18.

36. Rosenberg SA. Principles of cancer management: surgical oncology. In De Vita VT, Hellman S, Rosenberg SA, eds., *Cancer: Principles and Practice of Oncology*, 5th ed. Philadelphia: Lippincott-Raven, 1997: 1, 295–306.

37. Grann VR, Panageas KS, Whang W, et al. Decision analysis of prophylactic mastectomy and oophorectomy in BRCA1-positive or BRAC2-positive patients. *J Clin Oncol* 1998; 16: 979–85.

38. Fentiman IS. Prophylactic mastectomy: deliverance or delusion? *Br Med J* 1998; 317: 1402–3.

39. Downing J. Surgery. In Corner J, Bailey C, eds., *Cancer Nursing: Care in Context*. London: Blackwell Science, 2001: 156–78.

40. Visser MR, van Lanschot JJ, van der Velden J, et al. Quality of life in newly diagnosed cancer patients waiting for surgery is seriously impaired. *J Surg Oncol* 2006; 93: 571–7.

41. Davidson T, Sacks N. Principles of surgical oncology. In Horwich A, ed., *Oncology: A Multidisciplinary Textbook*. London: Chapman & Hall, 1995: 101–15.

42. Neill KM, Armstrong N, Burnett CB. Choosing reconstruction after mastectomy: a qualitative analysis. *Oncol Nurs Forum* 1998; 25: 743–50.

43. Gamba A, Romano M, Grosso IM, et al. Psychosocial adjustment of patients surgically treated for head and neck cancer. *Head Neck* 1992; 14: 218–23.

44. Rhys-Evans F. Tumours of the head and neck. In Saunders C, ed., *Nursing the Patient with Cancer*. London: Prentice Hall, 1996: 178–201.

45. Poston GJ. Surgical strategies for colorectal liver metastases. *Surg Oncol* 2004; 13: 125–36.

46. Northouse L. Factors affecting couples adjustment to recurrent breast cancer. *Res Nurs Health* 1995; 18: 515–24.

47. Alexander H. Vascular access and specialised techniques of drugs delivery. In De Vita VT, Hellman S, Rosenberg SA, eds., *Cancer: Principles and Practice of Oncology*, 5th ed. Philadelphia: Lippincott-Raven, 1997: 1, 725–34.

48. Payne S, Smith P, Dean S. Identifying the concerns of informal carers in palliative care. *Palliative Med* 1999; 13: 37–44.

49. Davis BD, Cowley SA, Ryland RK. The effects of terminal illness on patients and their carers. *J Adv Nurs* 1996; 23: 512–20.

50. Nolan M, Grant G, Keady J. The Carers Act: realising the potential. *Br J Community Health Nurs* 1996; 1: 317–22.

51. Rose KE. A qualitative analysis of the information needs of informal carers of terminally ill cancer patients. *J Clin Nurs* 1999; 8: 81–91.

52. Beaver K, Luker KA, Woods S. Primary care services received during terminal illness. *Int J Palliative Nurs* 2000; 6: 220–7.

53. Twigg J. Models of carers: how do social care agencies conceptualise their relationship with informal carers? *J Soc Policy* 1989; 18: 53–66.

11

Nutrition in cancer and cancer surgery

SERGIO SANDRUCCI, LAURA ESPOSITO AND MARCO BRAGA

INTRODUCTION

Malnutrition is observed in about 40% of cancer patients. The Academy of Nutrition and Dietetics and the American Society for Parenteral and Enteral Nutrition guidelines consensus statement identified malnutrition as an 'acute, subacute or chronic state of nutrition, in which a combination of varying degrees of overnutrition or undernutrition with or without inflammatory activity has led to a change in body composition and diminished function' [1]. It is characterized by weight loss, hypoalbuminemia, decreased skeletal muscle mass and reduced fat storage; it has been shown to increase morbidity (including a higher rate of toxicities during chemotherapy and radiotherapy), hospital length of stay (LOS) and treatment costs; decrease performance status and quality of life (QoL) [2]; and finally, has a negative impact on survival [3].

More than half of all patients with cancer have cancer-related surgery. Malnutrition prior to surgery may prolong recovery owing to poor wound healing or infectious complications [4]. Patients with certain cancers, such as cancers of the head, neck, stomach and bowel, may be malnourished at diagnosis; therefore, nutrition intervention is often warranted for these individuals prior to surgery. Nutrition-related side effects may also occur as a result of surgery. Surgical resections or excision may result in adverse effects on gastrointestinal (GI) function, depending on the tumour site and the extent of the surgery.

For early stage cancer patients, nutritional support in the form of either enteral or parenteral feeding, as appropriate based on the functionality of the GI tract, may help patients in a preoperative setting, or when aggressive, potentially beneficial cancer treatment may result in greater evidence of caloric depletion [5]. However, for many cancer patients, particularly those with advanced disease, caloric supplementation can be of limited value because of metabolic upset induced by the disease.

Understanding the consequences of malnutrition and of the physiopathology of weight loss mechanisms in the oncologic patient is mandatory to set up adequate treatments to prevent surgical complications in malnourished subjects.

MALNUTRITION IN THE PREOPERATIVE CANCER PATIENT

The impact of malnutrition on operative morbidity and mortality is well described in cancer patients [6–9], and the extent of weight loss at the time of cancer diagnosis is prognostic for survival. More than 10% loss of usual body weight appears to be especially problematic, as is a rate of weight loss of greater than 2.75% per month [10,11]. Malnutrition is also a significant factor that affects the QoL in cancer patients [12].

Undernutrition and negative energy balance have substantial effects on energy stores and organ function. Systemic inflammation induced by cancer is associated with a greater need for glucose as substrate, leading to breakdown of lean body mass; muscle is converted via gluconeogenesis to glucose for use by inflammatory tissue and cells of the immune system [13]. The consequence is a rapid loss of muscle mass and decrease of muscle function. An increase in fatty acid turnover occurs, with decreased production of ketone bodies, insulin resistance and fat accumulation in various organs.

A loss of more than 20% of body protein has a negative effect on respiratory muscle structure and function (maximal voluntary ventilation and respiratory muscle strength). Moreover, a loss of intestinal absorptive surface area is frequently observed during malnutrition. The attendant diarrhoea due to malabsorption exacerbates malnutrition, and intestinal barrier function can be impaired by bacterial overgrowth and inflammation.

Almost all immune functions, especially cell-mediated immunity, are negatively affected by undernutrition [14]. This is due particularly to impaired function of T-lymphocytes, complement activity, phagocytosis, chemotaxis and intracellular destruction of bacteria. When starvation is accompanied by systemic inflammation (e.g., trauma, sepsis), immune function is further depressed, which is associated with accelerated loss of muscle mass.

Body composition measurement is a method to assess nutritional status, and various techniques based on atomic, molecular, organ or tissue composition are available. However, from the clinical and nutritional point of view, it is relevant only to measure fat tissue and fat-free mass – a two-compartment model. For more sophisticated measurements, a four-compartment model can be used: fat tissue, bone mass, extracellular water and the cellular compartment (Table 11.1) [15]. Regular measurement of body weight and calculating changes in body mass index (BMI) are also clinically relevant and useful (Table 11.2).

Asking patients about weight loss continues to be the simplest, best validated method for assessing nutritional status in cancer patients. In a multicentre trial on cancer

Table 11.1 Body compartments and methods of measurement

Two-Compartment Model

Compartment
- Fat tissue and fat-free mass
  - Subcutaneous skinfold measurements
  - Underwater weighing
  - Dual-energy X-ray absorptiometry (DEXA)
  - Magnetic resonance imaging (MRI) or computed tomography (CT) scan
  - Bioimpedance analysis (BIA)

Four-Compartment Model

Compartment
- Fat tissue
  - Subcutaneous skinfold measurements
  - Underwater weighing
  - DEXA
  - MRI or CT scan
  - BIA
- Extracellular water
  - Bromide space – dilution method
  - BIA
- Body cell mass
  - Total body nitrogen – nitrogen neutron activation
  - Total body water minus extracellular water
- Bone mass
  - DEXA

Table 11.2 BMI and its interpretation

BMI	Interpretation
<18.5	Severe undernutrition
<20	Mild undernutrition
20–25	Normal range
25–30	Overweight
30–35	Obesity
35–40	Severe obesity
>40	Morbid obesity

Note: BMI = body weight (kg)/body height (m)^2.

patients, univariate and multivariate analyses showed that patient-reported weight loss of >5% of premorbid weight predicted a shortened survival. These data provide solid evidence that a patient-reported history of weight loss remains an extremely powerful tool for assessing malnutrition [16].

To calculate daily energy requirements, daily energy expenditure should be assessed. Resting energy expenditure (REE), the energy needed to preserve basic vital functions, can be measured by indirect calorimetry. However, in clinical practice, REE is more frequently estimated by equations, including the Harris–Benedict formula. An easy and practical approach to estimate REE consists of multiplying body weight and the daily energy requirements of body weight. This ranges from 20 to 35 kcal/kg body weight (BW) (Table 11.3) [15].

Patients diagnosed with cancer experience changes in energy expenditure which are more varied and do not occur with all tumour types [17].

REE can range from 60% to 150% of expected energy expenditure. Additionally, some patients with elevated energy requirements are able to gain weight, although this weight gain tends to consist of increases in body fat while the person continues to lose lean body mass.

Weight-loss and weight-stable patients with cancer had similar REEs when adjusted for fat-free mass but were different in terms of the acute-phase response (APR). The APR is believed to be one of many factors that contribute to elevations in the REE in patients with cancer, which in turn could promote weight loss. In addition, the commonly used Harris–Benedict equation (HBE) was in poor agreement with measured REE in both groups and, therefore, was not suitable for REE prediction in a clinical setting.

Some investigators examining dietary intake, REE and weight loss in adults primarily with GI tumours, and considering the relationship between these factors and survival rates, reported that 48.5% of patients were hypermetabolic, 50% were normometabolic and 1.4% were hypometabolic. Because dietary intake did not differ between normometabolic and hypermetabolic patients, and because neither tumour type nor gender was related to energy and protein intake, weight loss could not be solely accounted for by diminished intake. So, a failure in feedback regulation between dietary intake in relation to energy expenditure may add to the weight loss experienced by many cancer patients, and the wide variability

Table 11.3 Estimating energy requirements for cancer patients[a]

Harris–Benedict Formula

Men BMR = 66.473 + (13.7516 × weight in kg) + (5.0033 × height in cm) – (6.7550 × age in years)

Women BMR = 655.0955 + (9.5634 × weight in kg) + (1.8496 × height in cm) – (4.6756 × age in years)

- Normometabolic patients: 25–30 kcal/kg/day
  - Hypermetabolic or weight gain desired: 30–35 kcal/kg/day
- Obese patients: 21–25 kcal/kg/day (when weight maintenance is the goal; energy needs may be increased when nutritional status is deteriorating)

Source: Harris JA, Benedict FG, Proc Natl Acad Sci 1918;4(12): 370–3.
Note: BMR, basal metabolic rate.
[a] More than 35 kcal/kg/day may be required to maintain or promote weight gain in some situations.

in energy expenditure reported thereby contributes to the challenge of accurately predicting energy requirements in this patient population.

Nutritional screening and nutritional assessment should be a mandatory and regular part of the medical care of cancer patients, given the increased risk of disease- and therapy-related undernutrition [18].

Nutritional screening needs to be simple, rapid and easily performed on admission. This procedure serves as a baseline and dictates appropriate nutritional intervention. Several screening tools exist based on actual body weight, recent weight loss and recent food intake: the Subjective Global Assessment (SGA), the Patient-Generated Subjective Global Assessment (PG-SGA) (a modification of SGA for oncological patients), the Nutritional Risk Screening (NRS), the Malnutrition Universal Screening Tool (MUST), the Malnutrition Screening Tool (MST), and the Mini Nutritional Assessment (MNA) (Table 11.4) [19–21].

Nutritional assessment is a more detailed evaluation of nutritional status, clinically indicated in oncological patients because of their higher risk for malnutrition. This is more detailed, and possibly more effective, to guide provision of nutritional support. Nutritional assessment can be divided into:

- Measurement of nutrient balance (nutrition intake and output)
- Measurement of body composition (BMI, anthropometry, bioimpedance analysis [BIA])
- Measurement of inflammatory activity (C-reactive protein, leukocyte count)
- Measurement of function (muscle function [dynamometry], respiratory function, immune function)

For all methods of nutritional assessment, measurements must be repeated at various time intervals according to clinical status and needs, because it is the directional change that guides therapy. Each test has its unique

Table 11.4 Nutritional screening tools

Subjective Global Assessment (SGA)
- Patient's history (weight loss, change in dietary intake, GI symptoms, functional capacity)
- Physical examination (muscles, subcutaneous fat, edema, ascites)
- Clinician's overall subjective judgment
  - Good nutritional status – A
  - Moderate malnutrition – B
  - Severe malnutrition – C

Patient-Generated Subjective Global Assessment (PG-SGA)
- Patient portion:
  - Weight loss in past month, past 6 months
  - Current oral intake compared to baseline
  - Current physical activity compared to baseline
- Clinician component:
  - Disease and related metabolic demands
  - Cancer, wound, age >65, AIDS, pulmonary/cardiac cachexia
  - Metabolic demands
  - Fevers, sepsis, steroids
  - Physical exam and assessment

Nutritional Risk Screening (NRS)
- BMI <20.5
- Body weight loss during last 3 months
- Low dietary intake during last week
- Disease severity

Patients with a total score of ≥ 3 are classified as nutritionally at risk [19]

Malnutrition Universal Screening Tool (MUST)
- BMI score
- Unplanned weight loss during last 3–6 months
- Acute disease effect score/no nutritional intake for 5 days [20]

Malnutrition Screening Tool (MST)
Two questions related to:
- Recent unintentional weight loss
- Low food intake because of decreased appetite

This tool provides a score between 0 and 5, with a score ≥2 indicating a risk of undernutrition [21]

Mini Nutritional Assessment (MNA)
Similar to the MUST with additional questions on neuropsychological functional status, physical mobility and food intake. Scoring works in the opposite direction to the MUST with a lower score indicating a higher risk of malnutrition

advantages and limitations. However, their interpretation must take into consideration the underlying disease, the ongoing therapy and the overall clinical picture.

METABOLIC EFFECTS OF CANCER

Weight loss in cancer patients and its devastating consequences may be present in as many as 80% of patients with advanced malignancies [10,11].

Cachexia is a multifactorial syndrome, characterized by weight loss (at least 5% or weight loss greater than 2% in individuals already showing depletion according to value of body mass index [<20 kg/m^2]), muscle and adipose tissue wasting (sarcopenia) and inflammation [22]. The complex syndrome of cancer cachexia (CCS) is a pathological state where loss of muscle or muscle and fat occurs manifested in the cardinal feature of emaciation, weakness affecting functional status, an impaired immune system and metabolic dysfunction. CCS is characterized by increased cycling (synthesis and catabolism) of a variety of metabolic intermediaries, including amino acids, fatty acids and carbohydrates.

Cancer cachexia is identified as an independent predictor of shorter survival and increased risk of treatment failure and toxicity. It reduces the QoL and accounts for more than 20% of all cancer-related deaths [23,24]. In contrast to starvation, CCS results in the loss of both adipose and skeletal muscle mass, while visceral muscle mass is preserved and hepatic mass increases. Weight loss associated with CCS generally cannot be stopped or reversed with increases in nutrient intake alone. Appetite stimulants are only minimally effective for treatment of CCS.

Lymphoma, leukemia, breast cancer and soft-tissue sarcoma have some of the lowest frequencies of weight loss, while more aggressive lymphomas, colon, prostate and lung cancers are associated with an approximately 50% incidence of weight loss. The highest incidence and severity is seen in pancreatic and gastric cancer, wherein approximately 85% of patients experience cachexia. The extent of undernutrition parallels the type of neoplasm, with more severe malnutrition observed with upper GI and pancreatic cancers, and less severe malnutrition with lymphomas, breast cancers and sarcomas [10] (Table 11.5).

Although there is no universally accepted model that adequately explains the etiology of CCS in all patients, CCS is caused in part by pro-inflammatory cytokines such as tumour necrosis factor (TNF), interferon-γ and interleukins-1 and -6. Tumour-produced substances such as proteolysis-inducing factor, lipid-mobilizing factor and mitochondria-uncoupling proteins 1, 2 and 3 also affect nutrient metabolism.

TNF-α is believed to play a central role in the body's response to a variety of immunologic challenges [25]. In the presence of injury, infection and inflammation, TNF is important to local host defences. Unfortunately, its systemic effects may be deleterious. The administration of TNF leads to metabolic changes that are associated

Table 11.5 Malnutrition and cancer

General cancer population	60–63%
Acute non-lymphocytic leukemia	39%
Breast	9–36%
Bronchial carcinoma	66%
Colon	54%
Colorectal	60%
Diffuse lymphoma	55%
Esophagus	79%
Gastric	83%
Head and neck	72%
Larynx	40%
Lung (all types)	50%
Neuroblastoma	56%
Non-Hodgkin's lymphoma	31–48%
Oral cavity	41–63%
Pancreas	83%
Prostate	56%
Rectum	40%
Sarcoma	39%

with cachexia, such as lipolysis, muscle catabolism and increased glucose turnover and utilization. TNF enhances lipolysis through activation of hormone sensitive lipase (HSL). It also decreases lipogenesis by inhibiting production of lipoprotein lipase.

Interferon-γ possesses biological activities that overlap those of TNF. Its effects on fat and protein metabolism are similar in that it potentiates lipolysis, inhibits lipoprotein lipase and decreases protein synthesis [26].

Interleukin-1 and IL-6 are the cytokines shown to play important roles in cancer cachexia. Interleukin-1 seems to act centrally to induce anorexia by causing early satiety and increases proteolysis peripherally [26,27] However, the major contribution of IL-1 to the development of cancer cachexia may reside in its ability to enhance the production and release of IL-6 [28]. Interleukin-6 can be detected in the serum of tumour-bearing animals, where it functions to increase hepatic gluconeogenesis and proteolysis [29,30]. In animal models, IL-6 has been shown to induce a more severe wasting than TNF.

In addition to cytokines, several hormones and neuropeptides have recently been identified as having important functions relating to cancer cachexia. Leptin is an adipocyte-derived hormone that regulates adipose tissue mass. It reduces appetite, increases REE and regulates insulin levels [31]. Leptin affects appetite and energy expenditure via hypothalamic neuropeptides. Specifically, a loss in body fat reduces leptin levels and thereby decreases REE. Conversely, food intake resulting in a gain of body fat will prompt an increase in REE. This process is mediated by increased activity of ghrelin and neuropeptide Y (NPY) and decreased production of corticotropin-releasing factor (CRF) and melanocortin [32].

NUTRITIONAL SUPPORT IN SURGICAL PATIENTS WITH CANCER

It is well established that poor nutritional status is associated with poor postoperative outcomes in cancer patients [4]. Weight loss of 10% has been often quoted as a cut-off point, but unless associated with hypoalbuminemia or other organ dysfunction, this magnitude of weight loss does not appear to increase postoperative complications [33]. For weight loss alone to influence the postoperative prognosis, a higher percentage is required, probably 15% or more.

Besides the degree of weight loss, it is important to consider the BMI at baseline; some works have effectively demonstrated a statistically significant difference in length of hospital stay across BMI categories, and they have shown a trend to increased complications in patients with a lower BMI, although not statistically significant [34]. Other studies have demonstrated that BMI independently can predict survival, while weight change is not an independent predictor [35].

It must be noted that many of the parameters used to define nutritional status are also acute-phase reactants or markers of severity of disease. It is evident that severity of disease is also associated with poor outcomes. Therefore, although nutritional status is undoubtedly important, it is not surprising that nutrition-directed interventions are only modestly effective. The magnitude of the contribution of nutrition-based therapies to cancer outcomes is likely modest in comparison to disease-directed therapies.

Nutrition-directed therapies should not be expected to benefit well-nourished patients. In fact, there are clear data that some nutrition-directed therapies such as the routine use of parenteral nutrition in well-nourished patients are actually harmful [36]. A prerequisite for the use of nutritional therapy in surgery patients must therefore be the presence of malnutrition. Based on a validated assessment of preoperative nutrition status, a practical approach can be developed to optimize outcomes.

Traditional nutrition assessment parameters such as serum albumin, total lymphocyte count, skin test reactivity (as markers of immunocompetence), anthropometric changes (triceps skinfold test) and body composition may be confounded by the severity of the underlying cancer [37]. For example, hypoalbuminemia is associated with poor healing, sepsis and increased surgical mortality and morbidity [36].

However, APR proteins in the perioperative setting can confound the use of traditional nutrition indicators such as serum albumin and prealbumin. There is some evidence that neither serum albumin nor weight loss alone is a specific predictor of perioperative complications; however, they may be useful in the context of multivariable models [38].

Several nutrition assessment formulas have been developed to predict morbidity and mortality in surgical patients [39]. However, cancer patients are unique in their physiology: no single parameter is a definitive,

all-encompassing factor that comprehensively captures the nutritional state of a cancer patient. That being said, the ideal screening tool for such a task needs to offer ease of use, reliability, validity, sensitivity and cost-effectiveness [40]. One of the most widely used screening tools is the PG-SGA (Table 11.4) [41]. Longitudinal use of the PG-SGA can help determine the response to the nutritional care plan and guide modifications as appropriate [42].

Evidence-based guidelines for the use of nutrition support (enteral and parenteral) have been developed by multiple organizations, including the American Society for Parenteral and Enteral Nutrition (ASPEN) and the European Society for Parenteral and Enteral Nutrition (ESPEN) [43]. Table 11.6 summarizes the ASPEN guidelines.

The oral route for nutritional care is optimal because it is generally very safe and cost-effective. Preferably via

Table 11.6 Nutrition support guideline recommendations during adult anticancer treatment (ASPEN Clinical Guidelines)

1. Patients with cancer are nutritionally at risk and should undergo nutrition screening to identify those who require formal nutrition assessment with development of a nutrition care plan.
2. Nutrition support therapy should not be used routinely in patients undergoing major cancer operations.
3. Perioperative nutrition support therapy may be beneficial in moderately or severely malnourished patients if administered for 7–14 days preoperatively, but the potential benefits of nutrition support must be weighed against the potential risks of the nutrition support therapy itself and of delaying the operation.
4. Nutrition support therapy should not be used routinely as an adjunct to chemotherapy.
5. Nutrition support therapy should not be used routinely in patients undergoing head and neck, abdominal or pelvic irradiation.
6. Nutrition support therapy is appropriate in patients receiving active anticancer treatment who are malnourished and who are anticipated to be unable to ingest or absorb adequate nutrients for a prolonged period of time (7–14 days).
7. The palliative use of nutrition support therapy in terminally ill cancer patients is rarely indicated.
8. Omega-3 fatty acid supplementation may help stabilize weight in cancer patients on oral diets experiencing progressive, unintentional weight loss.
9. Patients should not use therapeutic diets to treat cancer.
10. Immune-enhancing enteral formulas containing mixtures of arginine, nucleic acids and essential fatty acids may be beneficial in malnourished patients undergoing major cancer operations.

education and supplementation in the form of protein powders and supplements, patients can optimize their caloric intake to be nutritionally robust. If there are anatomic or physiologic factors that prohibit oral intake, access to the GI tract may be obtained via a gastrostomy or a jejunostomy feeding tube. The enteral route for nutritional support is generally preferred over parenteral nutrition because it is more cost-effective and is associated with fewer infection-related complications [43]. If enteral nutritional support is not feasible (e.g., bowel obstruction, malabsorption secondary to short gut syndrome and enterocutaneous fistulae), then the parenteral route is an option.

Preoperative nutritional support

Preoperative nutritional support has been hypothesized to benefit patients undergoing cancer surgery by mitigating the consequences of suboptimal nutrition on postoperative morbidity and mortality. The routine (routine referring to administration regardless of the patient's nutrition status) use of preoperative parenteral nutrition is not appropriate [36,42]. Patients with mild malnutrition do not benefit from TPN and actually have more infectious complications. In contrast, in severely malnourished patients who receive TPN, the rate of non-infectious complications and 'healing' complications (e.g., wound dehiscence, anastomotic leak, fistula formation) is significantly lower. So, the use of preoperative TPN should be limited to patients who are severely malnourished unless there are other specific indications. There is growing evidence that traumatic and surgical insult is associated with a period of relative immune suppression, which may expose patients to subsequent risk of infection. Despite significant changes in elective surgical care and newer antimicrobial agents, postoperative infectious complications remain common, adding to length of hospital stay, healthcare costs and potential excess mortality.

Recently, the main focus of clinical nutrition has moved from the issue of simply covering energy and nitrogen requirements (nutritional support) to the new concept of supplementing selected nutritional substrates because of their specific pharmacological effects (nutritional therapy). Immunonutrition is probably one of the best examples of the application of nutritional therapy in the clinical scenario [44]. The main purpose is to modulate the postoperative metabolic response by giving perioperative nutritional formulas supplemented with specific nutrients such as arginine, glutamine, omega-3 fatty acids, nucleotides and others. The main target of these new diets is not solely to provide energy and nitrogen, but to modulate inflammatory, post-injury response and to counteract postoperative immune impairment which may per se increase patient susceptibility to infectious complications.

Glutamine constitutes more than half of the body's amino acid pool [45]. Although considered to be a non-essential amino acid, catabolism-inducing states like surgery, sepsis and trauma can lead to a spike in its consumption, outstripping the body's production. For this reason, glutamine should be viewed as a 'conditionally essential' amino acid [46]. One of glutamine's major functions is to shuttle nitrogen between organs and serve as fuel for rapidly proliferating cells such as enterocytes, lymphocytes and fibroblasts [47]. Glutamine is also central to multiple processes in intermediary metabolism such as the synthesis of purines and pyrimidines, modification of proteins and lipids to allow for signal transduction and secretion, and neutralization of oxidative stress associated with rapid metabolism and other causes [48].

Arginine, like glutamine, is a non-essential amino acid that becomes conditionally essential during catabolic states [49]. In cancer patients, arginine improves nitrogen balance and boosts host immune function. Arginine deficiency after surgical stress was reported more than 30 years ago, although the mechanisms behind this have remained unknown for years. When given alone, arginine reduced the incidence of wound complications and hospital LOS, and improved both disease-free and overall survival in head and neck cancer patients [50,51].

Synthetic polyribonucleotides stimulate immune function, possibly via modulation of intracellular regulatory enzymes [49]. Nucleic acids seem to modulate both the cell-mediated and humoral immune systems through an increased production of interferon.

Essential polyunsaturated fatty acids (PUFAs) of either the omega-6 (n-6) series derived from linoleic acid or the omega-3 (n-3) series derived from linolenic acid can alter the expression of membrane-bound receptors. They are also central to the synthesis of intermediate compounds, such as prostaglandins, leucotrienes and hydroxyacids. Omega-3 PUFAs increase the production of eicosanoids that improve immune response, while attenuating inflammatory response [52].

In the last few years, four meta-analyses have been published on the clinical impact of perioperative immunonutrition [53–56]. In all the included randomized clinical trials (RCTs) control groups received an isoenergetic, isonitrogenous standard enteral formula. Postoperative mortality was similar in the immunonutrition and control groups. The most important finding was that immunonutrition significantly reduced the overall morbidity rate, particularly postoperative infectious complications. Moreover, immunonutrition shortened length of hospital stay, probably as a direct consequence of a lower postoperative complication rate. The best results have been obtained when arginine and omega-3 fatty acids were given together. It could be speculated that they may act synergistically to modulate both immune and inflammatory postoperative responses and consequently to improve short-term postoperative outcomes. Moreover, beneficial effects on clinical outcome have been found in both malnourished and well-nourished patients and in both GI and non-GI surgery. An early postoperative increase of myeloid-derived cells expressing arginase 1 which deplete arginine has been recently reported [55]. Coupled with a poor arginine intake this can lead to an arginine deficiency state and consequently to a suppression of T-lymphocyte function. We can speculate that arginine supplementation can overcome this deficiency and omega-3 fatty acids can blunt upregulation of myeloid-derived cells and decrease arginase 1 expression. Further studies are required to better elucidate other possible interactions between arginine, omega-3 fatty acids and nucleotides. Moreover, dose–response studies should better clarify which is the optimal dose of each substrate to maximize benefits in surgical patients.

Perioperative nutrition support

As in most clinical settings, judgment for the use of perioperative nutrition is paramount. The 2009 ASPEN clinical guidelines for nutritional support therapy during adult anticancer treatment state that perioperative nutrition support therapy may be beneficial in moderately or severely malnourished patients if administered for 7–14 days preoperatively. However, they state that the potential benefits of nutrition support must be weighed against the potential risks of the nutrition support therapy itself delaying the operation [43]. Their review of the data indicates that the majority of parenteral versus standard oral intake studies find no differences in morbidity or mortality with the use of parenteral nutrition versus a standard oral diet [12,36,42,43,57–60]. Additionally, little difference has been found in morbidity and mortality in studies comparing enteral to parenteral nutrition. Enteral nutrition is favoured because it is thought to be more cost-effective and facilitate glycaemic management. Based on the review of the available studies, it appears that most studies report no difference in morbidity or mortality in enteral nutrition versus standard oral intake in patients with malignancy. This has been studied in both the preoperative and postoperative setting [37,58,61,62].

SPECIAL CONSIDERATIONS ACCORDING TO TUMOUR TYPE

There is a relation between weight loss and tumour type: malnutrition appears more common in GI, head and neck and lung tumour than in other types of cancer, and it is associated with a poor prognosis [63].

Conversely, patients with favourable subtypes of non-Hodgkin's lymphomas, breast cancer, acute non-lymphocytic leukemia and sarcoma have the lowest prevalence of weight loss (31–41%).

GI cancer patients are considered at high risk for malnutrition, and the prevalence of preoperative malnutrition among them has been reported as nearly 10–20%. Incidence rates of weight loss or malnutrition range from 79% to 100% for esophageal cancer, from 44% to 87% for gastric cancer and from 40% to 72% for head and neck cancer.

Head and neck cancer may cause dysphagia and odynophagia; more than 50% of patients with advanced head and neck cancer have a markedly impaired nutrition and significant involuntary weight loss at the time of diagnosis.

Furthermore, these patients may have underlying chronic malnutrition at presentation due to alcohol or tobacco abuse and unhealthy dietary habits [64].

Sometimes primary mediastinal tumours, such as lymphoma, as well as metastatic tumours, such as lung tumours, may cause dysphagia due to esophageal involvement. Esophageal cancer typically causes progressive dysphagia, odynophagia and regurgitation, and about 50–80% of these patients present with malnutrition at diagnosis.

Common presenting symptoms of gastric cancer include loss of appetite, early satiety and abdominal discomfort. In the colorectal cancer population specifically, rates of malnutrition have been documented to be between 20% and 56% [65]. The presenting symptoms of pancreatic cancer can include pain, loss of appetite, steatorrhoea or dyspepsia and the prevalence of malnutrition ranges from 50% to 88% depending on the type of assessment utilized [66].

ENHANCED RECOVERY AFTER SURGERY

The purpose of the enhanced recovery after surgery (ERAS) pathway is to reduce postoperative stress and improve clinical practice by incorporating evidence-based medicine into patient management [67]. To fully implement an ERAS pathway, a multidisciplinary team involving at least surgeons, an anaesthesiologist and nurses is necessary. Optimal pain control, prevention of fluid overload and aggressive postoperative rehabilitation, including the early recovery of oral feeding and mobilization, should improve short-term outcomes after surgery [68]. Several items have been incorporated into the ERAS pathway (Figure 11.1). All recommendations for specific items are strongly supported by high-level published evidence.

There is a strong level of evidence against the routine use of NG/NJ decompression following GI surgery. Surgical morbidity was not significantly influenced by decompression [69–71]. The most recent of the meta-analyses and the Cochrane review concluded that patients without routine decompression experienced significantly less pulmonary complications, earlier time to flatus, earlier time to oral dietary intake and a shorter hospital stay.

A nil-by-mouth regimen for several days postoperatively has traditionally been enforced for patients who undergo GI surgery [72]. A large Norwegian multicentre trial randomized major upper GI and HPB surgery patients to food at will from postoperative day 1 [73]. Of 447 patients included, 77 were subject to total gastrectomy and a significant reduction in the number of intra-abdominal abscesses was demonstrated for those allowed food at will in this subgroup. Importantly, no trial has reported any adverse outcome from any attempt at introducing patient-controlled or early scheduled food for patients undergoing GI surgery. One may assume that total calorie intake is low for the first days and that some patients will need additional sip feeds or artificial tube or catheter feeding. A recent educational review on nutritional care for patients undergoing esophagus and

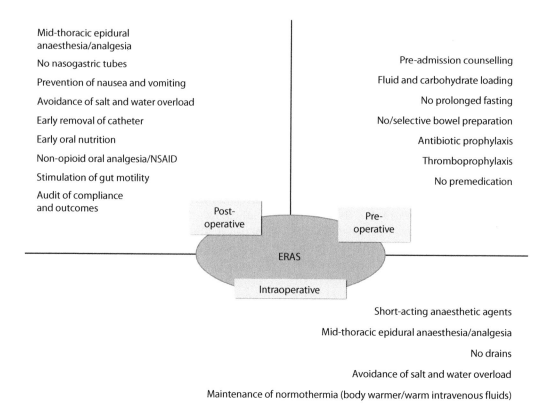

Mid-thoracic epidural
anaesthesia/analgesia

No nasogastric tubes

Prevention of nausea and vomiting

Avoidance of salt and water overload

Early removal of catheter

Early oral nutrition

Non-opioid oral analgesia/NSAID

Stimulation of gut motility

Audit of compliance
and outcomes

Post-operative

Pre-admission counselling

Fluid and carbohydrate loading

No prolonged fasting

No/selective bowel preparation

Antibiotic prophylaxis

Thromboprophylaxis

No premedication

Pre-operative

ERAS

Intraoperative

Short-acting anaesthetic agents

Mid-thoracic epidural anaesthesia/analgesia

No drains

Avoidance of salt and water overload

Maintenance of normothermia (body warmer/warm intravenous fluids)

Figure 11.1 ERAS pathway.

gastric surgery recommends nutritional support postoperatively in patients who have not reached 60% of desired intake by the first week following surgery [74]. Nutritional support should preferably be by high-energy oral sip feeds. Enteral tube feeding is indicated where oral intake is not possible and parenteral nutrition only when the gut is not working or is inaccessible. While robust data are lacking, it appears wise and safe to provide more intensive nutritional support both pre- and postoperatively to severely malnutritioned patients. Mechanical bowel preparation (MBP) may cause dehydration and fluid and electrolyte imbalance, especially in the elderly [75]. Meta-analyses of trials performed on patients undergoing colonic surgery have not shown MBP to be beneficial [76,77].

Reduced postoperative pain has not been demonstrated following pre-emptive use of analgesics [78], but medications for chronic pain should be continued perioperatively. Pre-induction anxiolytic medication might increase sedation postoperatively on postoperative day 1 [79,80], and the benefits of this are uncertain. However, short-acting drugs to alleviate anxiety may be helpful during insertion of an epidural catheter in some patients. Also, a carbohydrate-rich drink has been shown to attenuate anxiety [81].

Continuous epidural analgesia (EDA) with or without opioids provides significantly less postoperative pain than parenteral opioids after open abdominal surgery. A Cochrane review demonstrated that EDA is better than patient-controlled intravenous opioid analgesia in relieving pain 72 h after open abdominal surgery [82] and epidural

administration of local anaesthetic leads to lower occurrence of ileus after laparotomy than systemic or epidural opioids. EDA is also associated with fewer complications as well as an improvement in pulmonary function, decreased risk of postoperative pneumonia, better arterial oxygenation after abdominal or thoracic surgery [83] and reduced insulin resistance [84].

A comparative non-randomized study has indicated that an ERAS protocol with early mobilization, metoclopramide and removal of nasogastric tube on day 1 or day 2 reduced the rate of postoperative nausea and vomiting (PONV) after pancreaticoduodenectomy [85]. Until further evidence becomes available for gastric cancer surgery, the suggestions for patients undergoing colorectal surgery [86] should be applicable: Patients with two risk factors (non-smokers, females, a history of motion sickness or PONV, postoperative administration of opioids) [87] should be given prophylaxis with dexamethasone upon induction or a serotonin receptor antagonist at the end of surgery [88]. High-risk individuals (three risk factors) should receive general anaesthesia with propofol and remifentanil and no volatile anaesthetics and dexamethasone 4–8 mg at the commencement of surgery, with the addition of a serotonin receptor antagonist or droperidol, or 25–50 mg metoclopramide 30–60 min before the end of surgery [89]. Ondansetron can be used for prophylaxis and treatment.

Numerous meta-analyses and RCTs [90–93] have shown that preventing hypothermia during major abdominal surgery reduces the occurrence of wound infections, cardiac complications, bleeding and transfusion requirements, as well as the duration of post-anaesthetic recovery. Prolonging systemic warming in the perioperative period (2 h before and after surgery) confers further benefits.

Both overload of salt and water and hypovolemia in the perioperative period increase postoperative complication rates [94–96], suggesting that near-zero fluid balance should be achieved perioperatively. Deciding the correct amount required is complicated by the use of epidurals as it causes vasodilatation and hypovolemia with hypotension, often diagnosed and treated as fluid depletion. This may result in the administration of large volumes of fluid instead of a vasopressor. Thus, to avoid unnecessary fluid overload, vasopressors should be considered for intra- and postoperative management of epidural-induced hypotension. Delayed resumption of gut function combined with surgical trauma leads to a lengthened recovery period in patients undergoing major GI surgery. Extended bed rest is associated with several unwanted effects [97]. Literature is wanting on this matter, but the present authors support the use of written day-to-day instructions for patients with detailed targets postoperatively. This improves autonomy and cooperation with patients. Day-to-day progress can be documented with simple monitoring devices.

Enhanced recovery protocols for perioperative care have proven valuable in reducing complications after surgery, improving overall outcomes and shortening LOS, thus also saving resources. Updated and evidence-based guidelines are now available for colonic and rectal resections and pancreaticoduodenecomies [98–100]. In a recent meta-analysis including 16 RCTs, the ERAS pathway does not increase postoperative mortality and anastomotic leak rates after elective colorectal surgery [101]. This clearly confirms that the early recovery of oral feeding after surgery has no detrimental effect on anastomotic healing. A common idea in the surgical community is that the ERAS pathway reduces LOS, while increasing the hospital readmission rate. Data from the RCTs confirm that the ERAS pathway significantly shortens LOS, while readmission rates remain similar to those of the control group. The ERAS pathway significantly reduced overall postoperative morbidity, particularly non-surgical complications. Not surprisingly, respiratory and cardiovascular complication rates were very low in the ERAS group because of beneficial effects of fluid restriction, avoidance of long-acting opioids and earlier mobilization. Evidence of the significant reduction of non-surgical complications is consistent with the beneficial effects of the ERAS pathway in the elderly, and in patients with severe comorbidities [102].

CONCLUSION

Nutritional state is adversely affected in cancer patients which may have a significant impact on surgical and cancer-related outcomes. Measures to enhance nutritional status in those with malnutrition in the pre-, peri- and postoperative period may be beneficial and new evidence-based guidelines are now available to guide best practice. Enhanced recovery programmes which incorporate nutritional strategies are increasingly recognized as beneficial in reducing outdated surgical dogma and improving outcomes.

REFERENCES

1. White JV, Guenter P, Jensen G, Malone A, Schofield M, Academy Malnutrition Work Group, A.S.P.E.N. Malnutrition Task Force, A.S.P.E.N. Board of Directors. Consensus statement: Academy of Nutrition and Dietetics and American Society for Parenteral and Enteral Nutrition: characteristics recommended for the identification and documentation of adult malnutrition (Undernutrition). *JPEN J Parenter Enteral Nutr* 2012;36:275–83.
2. Senesse P, Assenat E, Schneider S, Chargari C. Nutritional support during oncologic treatment of patients with gastrointestinal cancer: who could benefit? *Cancer Treat Rev* 2008;34(6):568–75.
3. Jemal A, Siegel R, Wand E, Hao Y, Thun MJ. Cancer statistics 2009. *Cancer J Clin* 2009;59(4):225–49.
4. Maureen B, Huhmann DA. Nutrition support in surgical oncology. *Nutr Clin Pract* 2009;24:520–6.
5. Weimann A, Braga M, Harsanyi L, Laviano A, Ljungqvist O, Soeters P, et al. Vestweber ESPEN guidelines on enteral nutrition: surgery including organ transplantation. *Clin Nutr* 2006;25:224–44.
6. August D, Huhmann M. Nutritional care of cancer patients. In Norton J, Barie P, Bollinger R, Chang A, Lowry S, Mulvihill S, et al., eds., *Surgery: Basic Science and Clinical Evidence*, 2nd ed. New York, NY: Springer, 2008, pp. 2123–49.
7. Puccio M, Nathanson L. The cancer cachexia syndrome. *Semin Oncol* 1997;24(3):277–87.
8. Studley H. Percentage of weight loss. *JAMA* 1936;106:458–60.
9. Mullen JT, Davenport DL, Hutter MM, Hosokawa PW, Henderson WG, Khuri SF, et al. Impact of body mass index on perioperative outcomes in patients undergoing major intra-abdominal cancer surgery. *Ann Surg Oncol* 2008;15(8):2164–72.
10. Dewys WD, Begg C, Lavin PT, Band PR, Bennett JM, Bertino JR, et al. Prognostic effect of weight loss prior to chemotherapy in cancer patients. Eastern Cooperative Oncology Group. *Am J Med* 1980;69(4):491–7.
11. Tan BH, Fearon KC. Cachexia: prevalence and impact in medicine. *Curr Opin Clin Nutr Metab Care* 2008;11(4):400–7.
12. Lis CG, Gupta D, Lammersfeld CA, Markman M, Vashi PG. Role of nutritional status in predicting quality of life outcomes in cancer – a systematic review of the epidemiological literature. *Nutr J* 2012;11:27.

13. Andreoli A, De Lorenzo A, Cadeddu F, Iacopino L, Grande M. New trends in nutritional status assessment of cancer patients. *Eur Rev Med Pharmacol Sci* 2011;15:469–80.

14. Van Cutsem E, Arends J. The causes and consequences of cancer-associated malnutrition. *Eur J Oncol Nurs* 2005;9(Suppl. 2):S51–63.

15. Laviano A, Sobotka L, Meguid MM. Basic concepts of nutrition. In Van Halteren H, Jatoi A, eds., *ESMO Handbook of Nutrition and Cancer.* Lugano, Switzerland: ESMO Press, 2011, pp. 3–18.

16. Martin L, Watanabe S, Fainsinger R, Lau F, Ghosh S, Quan H, et al. Prognostic factors in patients with advanced cancer: use of the Patient-Generated Subjective Global Assessment in survival prediction. *J Clin Oncol* 2010;28(28):4376–83.

17. Soeters PB, ReijvenPL, van Bokhorst-de van der Scheuren MA. A rational approach to nutritional assessment. *Clin Nutr* 2008;27:706–16.

18. Charmey P, Cranganu A. Nutrition screening and assessment in oncology. In Maran M, Roberts S, eds., *Clinical Nutrition in Oncology Patients.* Burlington, MA: Jones & Bartlett Learning, 2010, pp. 21–44.

19. Kondrup J, Rasmussen HH, Hamberg O, Stanga Z. Ad Hoc ESPEN Working Group. Nutritional risk screening (NRS 2002): a new method based on an analysis of controlled clinical trials. *Clin Nutr.* 2003;22(3):321–36.

20. Stratton RJ, Hackston A, Longmore D, Dixon R, Price S, Stroud M, King C, Elia M. Malnutrition in hospital outpatients and inpatients: prevalence, concurrent validity and ease of use of the 'malnutrition universal screening tool' ('MUST') for adults. *Br J Nutr.* 2004;92(5):799–808.

21. Ferguson ML, Bauer J, Gallagher B, Capra S, Christie DR, Mason BR. Validation of a malnutrition screening tool for patients receiving radiotherapy. *Australas Radiol.* 1999;43(3):325–7.

22. Fearon K, Strasser F, Anker SD, Bosaeus I, Bruera E, Fainsinger RL, et al. Definition and classification of cancer cachexia: an international consensus. *Lancet Oncol* 2011;12(5):489–95.

23. Kumar NB, Kazi A, Smith T, Crocker T, Yu D, Reich RR. Cancer cachexia: traditional therapies and novel molecular mechanism-based approaches to treatment. *Curr Treat Options Oncol* 2010;11(3–4):107–7.

24. Mercadante S, Valle A, Porzio G, Aielli F. Prognostic factors of survival in patients with advanced cancer admitted to home care. *J Pain Symptom Manage* 2013;45:56–62.

25. Garcia-Martinez C, Costelli P, Lopez-Soriano FJ, Argiles JM. Is TNF really involved in cachexia? *Cancer Invest* 1997;15(1):47–54.

26. Toomey D, Redmond HP, Bouchier-Hayes D. Mechanisms mediating cancer cachexia. *Cancer* 1995;76(12):2418–26.

27. Ramos EJ, Suzuki S, Marks D, Inui A, Asakawa A, Meguid MM. Cancer anorexia-cachexia syndrome: cytokines and neuropeptides. *Curr Opin Clin Nutr Metab Care* 2004;7(4):427–34.

28. Fischer E, Marano MA, Barber AE, Hudson A, Lee K, Rock CS, et al. Comparison between effects of interleukin-1 alpha administration and sublethal endotoxemia in primates. *Am J Physiol* 1991;261(2 Pt. 2):R442–52.

29. Gelin J, Moldawer LL, deMan P, Svanborg-Eden C, Lowry SF, et al. Appearance of hybridoma growth factor/interleukin-6 in the serum of mice bearing a methylcholanthrene-induced sarcoma. *Biochem Biophys Res Commun* 1988;157(2):575–9.

30. Argiles JM, Lopez-Soriano FJ. The role of cytokines in cancer cachexia. *Med Res Rev* 1999;19(3): 223–48.

31. Smiechowska J, Utech A, Taffet G, Hayes T, Marcelli M, Garcia JM. Adipokines in patients with cancer anorexia and cachexia. *J Invest Med* 2010;58(3):554–9.

32. Suzuki H, Asakawa A, Amitani H, Nakamura N, Inui A. Cancer cachexia – pathophysiology and management. *J Gastroenterol* 2013;48(5):574–94.

33. Windsor JA, Hill GL. Weight loss with physiologic impairment: a basic indicator of surgical risk. *Ann Surg* 1988;207(3):290–6.

34. Beaton J, Carey S, Solomon MJ, Tan KK, Young J. Preoperative body mass index, 30-day postoperative morbidity, length of stay and quality of life in patients undergoing pelvic exenteration surgery for recurrent and locally-advanced rectal cancer. *Ann Coloproctol* 2014;30(2):83–7.

35. Karnell LH, Sperry SM, Anderson CM, Pagedar NA. Influence of body composition on survival in patients with head and neck cancer. *Head Neck* 2014; doi: 10.1002/hed.23983.

36. The Veterans Affairs Total Parenteral Nutrition Cooperative Study Group. Perioperative total parenteral nutrition in surgical patients. *N Engl J Med* 1991;325(8):525–32.

37. Huhmann MB, August DA. Perioperative nutrition support in cancer patients. *Nutr Clin Pract* 2012;27(5):586–92.

38. Jensen GL. Inflammation as the key interface of the medical and nutrition universes: a provocative examination of the future of clinical nutrition and medicine. *JPEN J Parenter Enteral Nutr* 2006;30(5):453–63.

39. Hirsch S, de Obaldia N, Petermann M, Covacevic S, Burmeister R, Llorens P, et al. Nutritional status of surgical patients and the relationship of nutrition to postoperative outcome. *J Am Coll Nutr* 1992; 11(1):21–4.

40. ASPEN Board of Directors and the Clinical Guidelines Task Force. Guidelines for the use of parenteral and enteral nutrition in adult and pediatric patients. *JPEN J Parenter Enteral Nutr* 2002;26(1 Suppl.):1SA–138SA.

41. Bauer J, Capra S, Ferguson M. Use of the scored Patient-Generated Subjective Global Assessment (PG-SGA) as a nutrition assessment tool in patients with cancer. *Eur J Clin Nutr* 2002;56(8):779–85.

42. Ferguson M. Patient-Generated Subjective Global Assessment. *Oncology* 2003;17(2 Suppl. 2):13–4.

43. August DA, Huhmann MB, American Society for Parenteral and Enteral Nutrition Board of Directors. A.S.P.E.N. clinical guidelines: nutrition support therapy during adult anticancer treatment and in hematopoietic cell transplantation. *JPEN J Parenter Enteral Nutr* 2009;33(5):472–500.

44. Braga M. Perioperative immunonutrition and gut function. *Curr Opin Clin Nutr Metab Care* 2012;15(5):485–8.

45. Wang Y, Jiang ZM, Nolan MT, Jiang H, Han HR, Yu K, et al. The impact of glutamine dipeptide supplemented parenteral nutrition on outcomes of surgical patients: a meta-analysis of randomized clinical trials. *JPEN J Parenter Enteral Nutr* 2010;34(5):521–9.

46. Coster J, McCauley R, Hall J. Glutamine: metabolism and application in nutrition support. *Asia Pac J Clin Nutr* 2004;13(1):25–31.

47. Savarese DM, Savy G, Vahdat L, Wischmeyer PE, Corey B. Prevention of chemotherapy and radiation toxicity with glutamine. *Cancer Treat Rev* 2003; 29(6):501–13.

48. DeBerardinis RJ, Cheng T. Q's next: the diverse functions of glutamine in metabolism, cell biology and cancer. *Oncogene* 2010;29(3):313–24.

49. Heys SD, Gough DB, Khan L, Eremin O. Nutritional pharmacology and malignant disease: a therapeutic modality in patients with cancer. *Br J Surg* 1996;83(5):608–19.

50. De Luis DA, Izaola O, Cuellar L, Terroba MC, Martin T, Aller R. High dose of arginine enhanced enteral nutrition in postsurgical head and neck cancer patients. A randomized clinical trial. *Eur Rev Med Pharmacol Sci* 2009;13(4):279–83.

51. Buijs N, van Bokhorst-de van der Schueren MA, Langius JA, Leemans CR, Kuik DJ, Vermeulen MA, et al. Perioperative arginine-supplemented nutrition in malnourished patients with head and neck cancer improves long-term survival. *Am J Clin Nutr* 2010;92(5):1151–63.

52. van der Meij BS, van Bokhorst-de van der Schueren MA, Langius JA, Brouwer IA, van Leeuwen PA. n-3 PUFAs in cancer, surgery, and critical care: a systematic review on clinical effects, incorporation, and washout of oral or enteral compared with parenteral supplementation. *Am J Clin Nutr* 2011;94(5):1248–56.

53. Cerantola Y, Hubner M, Grass F, Demartines N, Schafer M. Immunonutrition in gastrointestinal surgery. *Br J Surg* 2011;98:37–48.

54. Marik PE, Zaloga GP. Immunonutrition in high-risk surgical patients: a systematic review and analysis of the literature. *JPEN J Parenter Enteral Nutr* 2010;34:378–86.

55. Drover JW, Dhaliwal R, Weitzel L, Wischmeyer PE, Ochoa JB, Heyland DK. Perioperative use of arginine-supplemented diets: a systematic review of the evidence. *J Am Coll Surg* 2011;212:385–99.

56. Marimuthu K, Varadhan KK, Ljungqvist O, Lobo DN. A meta-analysis of the effect of combinations of immune modulating nutrients on outcome in patients undergoing major open gastrointestinal surgery. *Ann Surg* 2012;255:1060–68.

57. Meijerink WJ, von Meyenfeldt MF, Roufl art MM, Soeters PB. Efficacy of perioperative nutritional support. *Lancet* 1992;340(8812):187–8.

58. Foschi D, Cavagna G, Callioni F, Morandi E, Rovati V. Hyperalimentation of jaundiced patients on percutaneous transhepatic biliary drainage. *Br J Surg* 1986;73(9):716–9.

59. August DA, Kushner RF. The 1995 A.S.P.E.N. standards for nutrition support: hospitalized patients. *Nutr Clin Pract* 1995;10(6):206–7.

60. Foschi D, Toti GL, Del Soldato P, Ferrante F, Galeone M, Rovati V. Adaptive cytoprotection: an endoscopic study in man. *Am J Gastroenterol* 1986;81(11):1035–7.

61. Heslin MJ, Latkany L, Leung D, Brooks AD, Hochwald SN, Pisters PW, et al. A prospective, randomized trial of early enteral feeding after resection of upper gastrointestinal malignancy. *Ann Surg* 1997;226(4):567–77.

62. Enomoto TM, Larson D, Martindale RG. Patients requiring perioperative nutritional support. *Med Clin N Am* 2013;97:1181–200.

63. Arends J, Bodoky G, Bozzetti F, Fearon K, Muscaritoli M. ESPEN guidelines on enteral nutrition: non surgical oncology. *Clin Nutr* 2006;25:245–59.

64. Chasen MR, Bhargava R. A descriptive review of the factors contributing to nutritional compromise in patients with head and neck cancer. *Support Care Cancer* 2009;17(11):1345–51.

65. Read JA, Choy ST, Beale PJ, Clarke SJ. Evaluation of nutritional and inflammatory status of advanced colorectal cancer patients and its correlation with survival. *Nutr Cancer* 2006;55:78–85.

66. La Torre M, Ziparo V, Nigri G, Cavallini M, Balducci G, Ramacciato G. Malnutrition and pancreatic surgery: prevalence and outcomes. *J Surg Oncol* 2013; 107(7):702–8.

67. Fearon KC, Ljungqvist O, Von Meyenfeldt M, Revhaug A, Dejong CH, Lassen K, et al. Enhanced recovery after surgery: a consensus review of clinical care for patients undergoing colonic resection. *Clin Nutr* 2005;24(3):466–77.

68. Veenhof AAFA, Vlug MS, Van Der Pas MHGM, Sietses C, van der Peet DL, de Lange-de Klerk ES, et al. Surgical stress response and postoperative immune function after laparoscopy or open surgery with fast track or standard perioperative care: a randomized trial. *Ann Surg* 2012;255:216–21.

69. Chen K, Mou YP, Xu XW, Xie K, Zhou W. [Necessity of routine nasogastric decompression after gastrectomy for gastric cancer: a meta-analysis]. *Zhonghua Yi Xue Za Zhi* 2012;92(26):1841–4.

70. Yang Z, Zheng Q, Wang Z. Meta-analysis of the need for nasogastric or nasojejunal decompression after gastrectomy for gastric cancer. *Br J Surg* 2008;95(7):809–16.

71. Nelson R, Edwards S, Tse B. Prophylactic nasogastric decompression after abdominal surgery. *Cochrane Database Syst Rev* 2007;(3):CD004929.

72. Lassen K, Dejong CH, Ljungqvist O, Fearon K, Andersen J, Hannemann P, et al. Nutritional support and oral intake after gastric resection in five northern European countries. *Dig Surg* 2005;22(5):346–52.

73. Lassen K, Kjaeve J, Fetveit T, Trano G, Sigurdsson HK, Horn A, et al. Allowing normal food at will after major upper gastrointestinal surgery does not increase morbidity: a randomized multicenter trial. *Ann Surg* 2008;247(5):721–9.

74. Mariette C, De Botton ML, Piessen G. Surgery in esophageal and gastric cancer patients: what is the role for nutrition support in your daily practice? *Ann Surg Oncol* 2012;19(7):2128–34.

75. Holte K, Nielsen KG, Madsen JL, Kehlet H. Physiologic effects of bowel preparation. *Dis Colon Rectum* 2004;47(8):1397–402.

76. Guenaga KF, Matos D, Castro AA, Atallah AN, Wille-Jorgensen P. Mechanical bowel preparation for elective colorectal surgery. *Cochrane Database Syst Rev* 2005;(1):CD001544.

77. Cao F, Li J, Li F. Mechanical bowel preparation for elective colorectal surgery: updated systematic review and meta-analysis. *Int J Colorectal Dis* 2012;27(6):803–10.

78. Moiniche S, Kehlet H, Dahl JB. A qualitative and quantitative systematic review of preemptive analgesia for postoperative pain relief: the role of timing of analgesia. *Anesthesiology* 2002;96(3):725–41.

79. Caumo W, Hidalgo MP, Schmidt AP, Iwamoto CW, Adamatti LC, Bergmann J, et al. Effect of pre-operative anxiolysis on postoperative pain response in patients undergoing total abdominal hysterectomy. *Anaesthesia* 2002;57(8):740–6.

80. Walker KJ, Smith AF. Premedication for anxiety in adult day surgery. *Cochrane Database Syst Rev* 2009;(4):CD002192.

81. Hausel J, Nygren J, Lagerkranser M, Hellstrom PM, Hammarqvist F, Almstrom C, et al. A carbohydrate-rich drink reduces preoperative discomfort in elective surgery patients. *Anest Analg* 2001;93(5):1344–50.

82. Werawatganon T, Charuluxanun S. Patient controlled intravenous opioid analgesia versus continuous epidural analgesia for pain after intra-abdominal surgery. *Cochrane Database Syst Rev* 2005;(1):CD004088.

83. Popping DM, Elia N, Marret E, Remy C, Tramer MR. Protective effects of epidural analgesia on pulmonary complications after abdominal and thoracic surgery: a meta-analysis. *Arch Surg* 2008;143(10):990–9.

84. Uchida I, Asoh T, Shirasaka C, Tsuji H. Effect of epidural analgesia on postoperative insulin resistance as evaluated by insulin clamp technique. *Br J Surg* 1988; 75(6):557–62.

85. Balzano G, Zerbi A, Braga M, Rocchetti S, Beneduce AA, Di Carlo, V. Fast-track recovery programme after pancreatico-duodenectomy reduces delayed gastric emptying. *Br J Surg* 2008; 95(11):1387–93.

86. Lassen K, Soop M, Nygren J, Cox PB, Hendry PO, Spies C, et al. Consensus review of optimal perioperative care in colorectal surgery: Enhanced Recovery After Surgery (ERAS) Group recommendations. *Arch Surg* 2009;144(10):961–9.

87. Rusch D, Eberhart L, Biedler A, Dethling J, Apfel CC. Prospective application of a simplified risk score to prevent postoperative nausea and vomiting. *Can J Anaesth* 2005;52(5):478–84.

88. Carlisle JB, Stevenson CA. Drugs for preventing postoperative nausea and vomiting. *Cochrane Database Syst Rev* 2006;(3):CD004125.

89. Wallenborn J, Gelbrich G, Bulst D, Behrends K, Wallenborn H, Rohrbach A, et al. Prevention of postoperative nausea and vomiting by metoclopramide combined with dexamethasone: randomised double blind multicentre trial. *BMJ* 2006;333(7563):324.

90. Scott EM, Buckland R. A systematic review of intraoperative warming to prevent postoperative complications. *AORN J* 2006;83(5):1090–113.

91. Nesher N, Zisman E, Wolf T, Sharony R, Bolotin G, David M, et al. Strict thermoregulation attenuates myocardial injury during coronary artery bypass graft surgery as reflected by reduced levels of cardiac-specific troponin I. *Anesth Analg* 2003;96(2):328–35.

92. Rajagopalan S, Mascha E, Na J, Sessler DI. The effects of mild perioperative hypothermia on blood loss and transfusion requirement. *Anesthesiology* 2008;108(1):71–7.

93. Wong PF, Kumar S, Bohra A, Whetter D, Leaper DJ. Randomized clinical trial of perioperative systemic warming in major elective abdominal surgery. *Br J Surg* 2007;94(4):421–6.

94. Brandstrup B, Tonnesen H, Beier-Holgersen R, Hjortso E, Ording H, Lindorff-Larsen K, et al. Effects of intravenous fluid restriction on postoperative complications: comparison of two

perioperative fluid regimens: a randomized assessor-blinded multicenter trial. *Ann Surg* 2003; 238(5):641–8.

95. Chowdhury AH, Lobo DN. Fluids and gastrointestinal function. *Curr Opin Clin Nutr Metab Care* 2011;14(5):469–76.

96. Lobo DN. Fluid overload and surgical outcome: another piece in the jigsaw. *Ann Surg* 2009;249(2):186–8.

97. Kehlet H, Wilmore DW. Multimodal strategies to improve surgical outcome. *Am J Surg* 2002;183(6):630–41.

98. Gustafsson UO, Scott MJ, Schwenk W, Demartines N, Roulin D, Francis N, et al. Guidelines for perioperative care in elective colonic surgery: Enhanced Recovery After Surgery (ERAS) Society recommendations. *World J Surg* 2013;37(2):259–84.

99. Lassen K, Coolsen MM, Slim K, Carli F, de Aguilar-Nascimento JE, Schafer M, et al. Guidelines for perioperative care for pancreaticoduodenectomy: Enhanced Recovery After Surgery (ERAS) Society recommendations. *World J Surg* 2013;37(2):240–58.

100. Nygren J, Thacker J, Carli F, Fearon KC, Norderval S, Lobo DN, et al. Guidelines for perioperative care in elective rectal/pelvic surgery: Enhanced Recovery After Surgery (ERAS) Society recommendations. *World J Surg* 2013;37(2):285–305.

101. Greco M, Capretti G, Beretta L, Gemma M, Pecorelli N, Braga M. Enhanced recovery program in colorectal surgery: a meta-analysis of randomized controlled trials. *World J Surg* 2014;38:1531–41.

102. Pawa N, Cathcart PL, Arulampalam TH, et al. Enhanced recovery program following colorectal resection in the elderly patient. *World J Surg* 2012;36(2):415–23.

12

Image-guided surgery

LEONORA S F BOOGERD, HENRICUS J M HANDGRAAF, MARTIN C BOONSTRA,
ALEXANDER L VAHRMEIJER AND CORNELIS J H VAN DE VELDE

INTRODUCTION

The diagnostic accuracy of preoperative imaging modalities, such as MRI and CT scan, has improved considerably over the last decades, but their ability to detect small-sized tumours remains suboptimal [1]. In addition, translation of these images to the surgical theatre is often challenging as they do often not depict the actual situation in the patient's body. Image-guided surgery (IGS), using near-infrared (NIR) fluorescence, is a promising intraoperative imaging modality that can assist surgeons to identify tumour tissue, lymph nodes and vital structures [2]. This relatively novel imaging modality gives real-time feedback during surgical procedures by revealing the location of the targeted tissue. Hence, it may improve patient outcomes, for example, by reducing the number of positive resection margins or by decreasing the risk of iatrogenic damage to vital structures. This chapter provides an overview of the technique, applications and future perspectives of NIR fluorescence IGS.

NEAR-INFRARED FLUORESCENCE IMAGING

Technique

NIR fluorescence IGS uses specific molecules, so-called fluorophores, that can emit light after excitation [3]. Fluorophores emitting light in the NIR wavelength spectrum (700–900 nm) are of particular interest, because autofluorescence and light absorbance of normal tissue structures, such as blood or fatty tissue, are low in these wavelength spectra [4]. Consequently, relatively deep tissue penetration can be achieved enabling

visualization of structures up to a depth of 10 mm [5,6]. Furthermore, this light is invisible to the human eye and therefore does not alter the surgical field. The requirements for NIR fluorescence imaging are, besides fluorophores, an imaging system consisting of a light source that is able to excite fluorophores combined with a camera that can detect the emitted fluorescence (Figure 12.1).

Since the introduction of IGS in 1998, various commercially available NIR fluorescent imaging systems have been developed, either for open, laparoscopic or robotic surgery [7]. Imaging systems all have to deal with specific challenges to optimize their utility, such as enabling sufficient fluorescence excitation, low-attenuation optics for NIR light and enough sensitivity to detect low concentrations of NIR fluorophores [5]. A high fluence rate of the excitation light would be optimal to achieve deep tissue penetration. However, the safety of the technique is partly dependent on illumination levels: high levels can burn tissue and photobleach contrast agents [8]. Therefore, fluence rates are currently restricted to the range of 10–25 mW/cm².

Along with NIR fluorescence images, most imaging systems are also capable of showing normal white light images [7]. Some imaging systems have the ability to display a real-time overlay of the fluorescence and normal light image, which enhances anatomical orientation of the origin of the fluorescent signal. At present there is significant variation between the different NIR imaging systems in terms of the wavelength of the excitation light, internal optics, usability and costs. No established fluorescence imaging standard is available resulting in difficulties comparing the performance of imaging devices in an objective manner [9]. At this moment, the only two NIR fluorescent

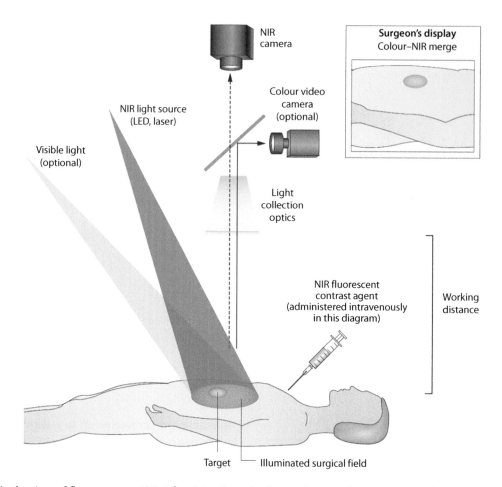

Figure 12.1 Mechanism of fluorescence IGS. After injection of a fluorophore, either intravenously, peritumourally or topically, its localization can be visualized by NIR fluorescence imaging. During surgery, the NIR light source can be positioned above the surgical field with a distance of approximately 20–30 cm, or can be encased within a fibre optic scope for minimally invasive and robotic surgery. Some NIR fluorescence imaging systems can simultaneously display colour, NIR fluorescence and overlay images in real time during surgery and thereby enhance anatomical orientation. (Reprinted from Vahrmeijer AL, et al., *Nat Rev Clin Oncol* 2013;10(9):507–18. With permission from Macmillan Publishers Ltd.: *Nature Medicine*. Copyright © 2013.)

contrast agents approved for clinical use by the US Food and Drug Administration (FDA) and European Medicine Agency (EMA) are methylene blue (MB) and indocyanine green (ICG).

CLINICAL INDICATIONS

Sentinel lymph node mapping

The sentinel lymph node (SLN) mapping procedure can be improved by using NIR fluorescence IGS [2]. Currently, SLN mapping is performed by a peritumoural injection of a radiotracer or blue dye. The radioactive tracer is injected several hours or the day before surgery, and subsequently the SLNs can be mapped preoperatively using either single-photon emission computed tomography (SPECT)/CT or lymphoscintigraphy. During surgery, the radioactive signal can be traced using a handheld gamma probe. Blue dye is injected peritumourally in the operating room, prior to the first incision, providing visual guidance to the surgeon.

However, not all SLNs stain blue. For example, in only 69% of vulvar cancer patients could blue SLNs be identified [10]. Nonetheless, the combined approach results in high SLN detection rates and low numbers of false negative lymph nodes and is currently the standard of care in melanoma, breast and vulvar cancer patients [11–13]. However, due to the high costs of using radioactivity, poor availability in some countries, the risk of radiation exposure, discoloration of the surgical field and long-lasting tattooing of the skin by using blue dye, there is still a need for improvement.

ICG is used as the preferred NIR fluorescent dye for SLN mapping. For decades, ICG has been approved for use to determine cardiac output, hepatic function and ophthalmic perfusion [14]. At first, application of ICG as a lymphatic tracer was based on its intrinsic green colour, resulting in relatively low contrast and consequently low SLN detection rates [15,16]. However, its fluorescent characteristics have resulted in superior SLN detection rates compared to blue dye alone [17]. After peritumoural injection of a low dose of ICG (1.6 ml of 500 μM), the lymphatic drainage can be traced in real time using a NIR imaging system. Lymphatic vessels and lymph nodes can sometimes even be identified percutaneously, which facilitates the procedure and may decrease incisional length and postoperative morbidity [18]. The use of ICG as NIR fluorescent tracer has been studied in SLN procedures in head and neck, breast, skin, gastrointestinal, urological and gynaecological cancer patients (Figure 12.2a) [10,19–23]. ICG emits light with a wavelength of 820 nm, is cleared almost exclusively by the liver and has a half-life time in blood of 150–180 s [24]. Allergic reactions after administration are rare and have been documented in less than 1:10,000 patients, but only in doses above 0.5 mg/kg [14]. The doses used in NIR fluorescence imaging are lower: between 0.1 and 0.5 mg/kg [25]. Although use of NIR fluorescence light results in deeper tissue penetration (up to 10 mm) than use of a conventional blue dye (1 mm), the relatively superficial tissue penetration still remains a problem for SLN detection in obese patients.

Furthermore, injection of ICG alone as a lymphatic tracer has been shown to result in fluorescent staining of second-tier nodes. Therefore, ICG has been non-covalently absorbed to albumin nanocolloid, hypothesizing that an increased hydrodynamic diameter would possibly lead to less staining of higher-tier nodes and a better retention in the SLN [2,26]. In Europe, an albumin-based tracer is most commonly used, since ICG already shows high affinity for albumin, while in the US a sulphur-based colloid is commonly used [27]. A hybrid tracer, combining ICG and 99m technetium nanocolloid (ICG:99mTc), has been studied in several feasibility trials for SLN mapping [28]. Although those studies were intended as feasibility studies, ICG outperformed blue dye as a tracer. Moreover, one combined preoperative injection of ICG:99mTc resulted in similar sensitivity rates. Intraoperative injections of blue dye may be omitted in the near future [29]. However, a recent study suggested that omitting a radiotracer might become reliable with use of NIR imaging and blue

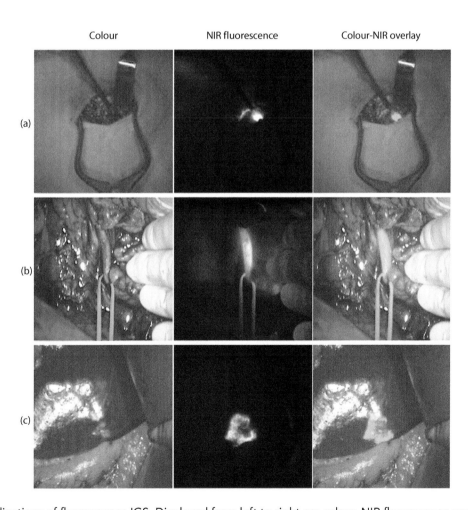

Figure 12.2 Applications of fluorescence IGS. Displayed from left to right are colour, NIR fluorescence and colour-NIR overlay images. (a) Example of sentinel lymph node detection in a patient with breast cancer after periareolar injection of 1.6 ml of 0.5 mM indocyanine green. A lymphatic vessel leading to the SLN is clearly visible. The surgical field is not altered by staining of any dye. (b) Example of ureter visualization after intravenous administration of 1 mg/kg methylene blue. (c) Example of colorectal liver metastasis identification after preoperative injection (24 h before surgery) of 10 mg of indocyanine green. A fluorescent rim pattern surrounding the colorectal liver metastasis clearly marks the border of the tumour.

dye. In 714 early breast cancer patients a detection rate of 99.6% of SLNs was achieved by using ICG together with blue dye and a low rate of axillary lymph node recurrence was noted (0.4%) [30].

Identification of vital structures

Morbidity after surgery depends partly on the extent of damage to vital structures, such as nerves, ureters and bile ducts. Although improvements in surgical techniques, for example, the introduction of laparoscopic and robotic surgery, have decreased morbidity rates, iatrogenic damage is sometimes inevitable. One step closer to preservation of vital structures is highlighting these structures using NIR fluorescence imaging. Currently, nerves are identified during surgery by inspection, potentially in combination with electromyographic (EMG) monitoring. However, nerve damage is still frequently observed, resulting in pain, numbness, weakness or paralysis. Preclinical studies have already shown accurate identification of nerves as small as 50 μm using the specific peptide NP41, but none of these agents have been clinically approved and evaluated yet [31,32].

Bile duct imaging can be achieved by an intravenously injected low dose of ICG (2.5–20 mg) prior to surgery [33]. Since ICG is almost exclusively cleared by the liver into the bile, it can be used to explore the biliary anatomy with NIR imaging. Injecting ICG directly prior to or during surgery results in highly fluorescent liver tissue, concealing the bile ducts. However, after 4–8 h the liver tissue gradually darkens, leaving only the bile ducts fluorescent [34]. Improved anatomical orientation may decrease complication rates, for example, in patients with an aberrant biliary anatomy or severe adhesions or those undergoing major liver surgery.

Another delicate structure that is sensitive to damage is the ureter. In a clinical feasibility study, the ureter was successfully visualized with MB as a NIR fluorophore (Figure 12.2b) [35]. MB is fluorescent at 700 nm and is partly cleared by the kidneys. Similarly to ICG, MB was first used for its intrinsic blue color [36]. However, due to the high doses required for direct visualization (7.5 mg/kg), it can result in serious adverse events, such as toxic metabolic encephalopathy [37]. In strongly diluted concentrations, MB reveals its fluorescent properties [38]. Intravenous injection of doses of 0.5–1.0 mg/kg MB resulted in good visualization of the ureters, and no serious adverse events are reported at these low dose levels [35]. However, as MB is a suboptimal fluorophore, improvement can be expected when novel 800 nm fluorophores, such as ZW800-I, become available for clinical use. The quantum yield, i.e. brightness of the fluorescent signal, of ZW800-I is four times higher and ZW800-I is cleared exclusively by the kidneys, potentially resulting in a much brighter signal in the ureters [39].

Perfusion angiography

Sufficient blood supply is of vital importance in the creation of intestinal anastomosis. Although complications, such as stricture or leakage, have multifactorial causes, any means of minimizing or avoiding them is desirable [40]. A reliable, relatively easy and low-risk method to assess the vascularization of an anastomosis is NIR fluorescence angiography. Several studies have shown the feasibility of NIR fluorescence angiography during intestinal surgery by using low doses of ICG [41,42] Intravenous injection of 0.5 mg/kg ICG led to real-time feedback about the perfusion of the organ of interest. A retrospective study compared 332 colorectal cancer patients who underwent surgery and intraoperative laser fluorescence angiography with 306 matched controlled colorectal cancer patients [43]. In the first group, only 7 (3.5%) surgical revisions due to anastomotic leakages were performed compared to 15 (7.5%) in the control group. Furthermore, use of fluorescence led in 16% of patients to a change of the initially planned point of transection of the bowel by revealing insufficient perfusion. Objective criteria for insufficient blood flow are yet to be determined, for example because quantification of the fluorescence signal is not directly correlated to actual perfusion. Nonetheless, in the hands of an experienced surgeon, NIR fluorescence angiography may contribute to reduced anastomotic complication rates. To further assess the added value of NIR fluorescence angiography for perfusion of bowel anastomoses, more extensive studies are needed.

Fluorescence angiography has also been proven to be helpful in reconstructive cancer surgery [44]. By intraoperative identification of vascular perfusion of free or pedicled flaps, optimally perfused flaps can be ensured and venous outflow can be monitored [45].

Tumour identification

Intraoperative tumour imaging has already been shown to be feasible using the nonspecific fluorescent dyes ICG and MB. Liver metastases and hepatocellular carcinoma (HCC) can be identified due to the inherent properties of ICG. Metastases are identifiable by a fluorescent rim, caused by stasis of ICG in compressed liver parenchyma. Healthy hepatocytes clear ICG from the blood within approximately 24 h. Compression by tumour tissue causes obstructed bile canaliculi. In addition, compression and inflammation lead to an increased presence of immature hepatocytes, in which ICG tends to accumulate. As a result, superficially located liver metastases, even as small as 1 mm, can be identified by a characteristic fluorescent rim pattern surrounding the metastases (Figure 12.2c). van der Vorst and colleagues showed that NIR fluorescence imaging, 24 or 48 h after intravenous injection of either 10 or 20 mg ICG, detected additional superficial lesions that were otherwise undetectable [46] in 12.5% of patients (5 out of 40) with colorectal liver metastases.

In pancreatic cancer patients, additional metastases were identified in 8 out of 49 patients (16%) [47]. In patients with uveal melanoma with liver metastases, laparoscopic fluorescence imaging identified multiple additional liver lesions in two out of three patients [48]. NIH imaging is especially valuable in the detection of small, superficially located liver metastases, since intraoperative ultrasound (IOUS) is only able to detect more deeply located metastases (>6 mm) [49]. In addition, the resolution of CT is too low to accurately detect lesions smaller than 10 mm [50]. Due to the limited penetration capacity of NIR fluorescence imaging to only 10 mm, IOUS and CT are still the imaging modalities of choice for deeper lying lesions. Ishizawa and colleagues were the first to demonstrate NIR fluorescence detection of HCC after a preoperative injection of ICG, resulting in a clear fluorescence signal throughout the tumour [51].

Currently, three types of fluorescence can be classified in HCC patients: uniform, partial and rim. The type of fluorescence is associated with tumour pathology. Well- or moderately differentiated HCCs show mostly uniform fluorescence, whereas poorly differentiated HCCs show partial or rim-type fluorescence [52]. In addition to NIR detection of liver metastases and HCCs, tumour imaging after an intravenous injection of ICG has been attempted in pancreatic cancer patients hypothesizing that accumulation of the NIR fluorophore in tumorous lesions would occur based on the *enhanced permeation and retention* (EPR) principle [53]. Due to a combination of newly formed, porous blood vessels and poorly developed lymphatic vessels in tumour tissue, large molecules such as ICG are retained in the tumour [54]. The EPR effect mainly depends on the physical characteristics of the injected macromolecules and therefore leads to nonspecific targeting [55].

Although in breast cancer patients the EPR effect has been shown to result in adequate tumour detection, neither pancreatic cancer lesions nor metastatic ovarian cancer lesions could be identified after systemic injection of ICG. A possible explanation for this failure might be the difference in tumour biology [53,56,57].

MB was originally used to visualize enlarged parathyroid adenomas and neuroendocrine tumours; administration of a high dose of MB (up to 7.5 mg/kg) resulted in macroscopically visible blue staining of the tumour [36,37]. After dilution, using its fluorescent characteristics, NIR detection of various types of (neuro)endocrine tumours by administration of 1 mg/kg MB appeared feasible [58,59]. However, the exact mechanism of tracer uptake in these tumours remains unclear. A recent study showed visualization of hyperparathyroid adenomas after a single injection of 0.5 mg/kg, and MB has also been successfully used for tumour identification in breast cancer patients [58,60].

Since the first report of intraoperative use of fluorescein for the detection of brain tumours in 1948, fluorescence imaging has been applied in neurosurgical procedures [61]. Oral administration 3 h before surgery of 5-aminolevulinic acid (5-ALA), a precursor of the haemoglobin synthesis pathway, leads to accumulation of fluorescing protoporphyrin IX (PpIX) in malignant tumour tissue [62,63]. By using a specifically modified neurosurgical microscope, PpIX can be identified by excitation with violet-blue light. In a large phase III multicentre randomized controlled trial

(RCT) in 2006, Stummer and colleagues demonstrated the benefit of fluorescence-guided resection of malignant gliomas using 5-ALA compared to conventional white light resection. Compared to conventional surgery, use of 5-ALA resulted in a higher number of complete tumour resections (65% vs. 36%) and significantly prolonged 6-month progression-free survival (41% vs. 21%) [61]. Application of 5-ALA is currently approved for resection of high-grade malignant gliomas.

Although broadly applied in clinical trials, neither 5-ALA, ICG nor MB is a tumour-specific fluorophore. Identification of novel targets, based on the various hallmarks of cancer, has paved the way for development of tumour-specific fluorophores [64]. To accomplish tumour-specific targeting, a tumour-specific ligand, such as an antibody or nanobody, has to be conjugated to a (NIR) fluorescent dye. Both ICG and MB cannot easily be conjugated due to their chemical properties, but novel conjugable NIR fluorophores include IRDye 800CW (LI-COR Biosciences, Lincoln, Nebraska) and ZW800-I (Curadel Surgical Innovations, Wayland, Massachusetts). They share favourable characteristics such as emission at a wavelength range of 800 nm, small size and low toxicity, but only IRDye 800CW is currently available for clinical use [2].

A milestone in tumour-targeted NIR fluorescence imaging was the first in-human trial with folate–fluorescein isothiocyanate (FITC) for visualization of metastatic ovarian cancer [65]. The folate receptor is known to be upregulated in ovarian cancer and targeting of this receptor with folate-FITC, i.e. folate conjugated to a 500 nm fluorophore, resulted in otherwise undetected tumour lesions. Clinical trials using antibody-based targeting ligands conjugated to IRDye 800CW, such as bevacizumab and cetuximab, targeting, respectively, the vascular endothelial growth factor-A (VEGF-A) and the epidermal growth factor receptor (EGRF), are currently under trial in breast, colon and head and neck cancer patients.

FUTURE PERSPECTIVES

NIR fluorescence imaging has proven its feasibility in many clinical indications. However, before this technique can progress to routine patient care, large RCTs have to confirm its utility and efficacy. Imaging systems are still relatively expensive and specific training is required to use them. Furthermore, fluorophores should be optimized, for example to increase penetration capacity or to improve retention in targeted tissue.

A new era in IGS has recently begun with the description of the first clinical study using a tumour-targeted probe [65]. In addition, a large number of preclinical studies are currently underway to identify novel targets and molecules for tumour-specific IGS. Targets can be antibodies, but other ligands such as fragments of antibodies, nanobodies, small peptides or much larger nanoparticles are also undergoing evaluation for clinical translation [66]. One example of a small peptide is cyclic arginine–glycine–aspartic acid (cRGD) targeting specific integrins, such as αvβ3, which are involved in angiogenesis. The peptide itself has already been clinically tested in several positron emission tomography (PET) and SPECT studies [67,68]. Conjugated to an 800 nm fluorophore, this probe showed tumour-specific targeting in several mouse models. Translation of these types of probes to the clinic is to be expected in the near future.

Along with developments of tumour-targeted probes, optimization of imaging systems should follow simultaneously, including improvements in sensitivity, efficacy, ergonomics and options such as multispectral imaging [69]. In addition to all these developments, cost efficiency remains a key factor that should be addressed before IGS can be widely implemented in the clinic setting [9].

CONCLUSION

IGS has only recently been introduced into the field of surgery, but its feasibility has been confirmed for a wide range of clinical indications, such as intraoperative identification of SLNs, vital structures, vascular perfusion and tumour tissue identification. In the near future, large clinical trials should focus on patient outcomes and cost efficiency. However, the real advantages of fluorescence IGS are to be expected from tumour-targeted probes. This will potentially result in highly specific detection of malignant cells during oncological surgery, an increase in the rate of radical tumour resections and a decrease in the morbidity and mortality of such surgery. However, there are still some challenges that have to be overcome before IGS can become standard of care.

REFERENCES

1. Frangioni JV. New technologies for human cancer imaging. *J Clin Oncol* 2008;26(24):4012–21.
2. Vahrmeijer AL, Hutteman M, van der Vorst JR, et al. Image-guided cancer surgery using near-infrared fluorescence. *Nat Rev Clin Oncol* 2013;10(9):507–18.
3. Vahrmeijer AL, Frangioni JV. Seeing the invisible during surgery. *Br J Surg* 2011;98(6):749–50.
4. Frangioni JV. In vivo near-infrared fluorescence imaging. *Curr Opin Chem Biol* 2003;7(5):626–34.
5. Keereweer S, van Driel PB, Snoeks TJ, et al. Optical image-guided cancer surgery: challenges and limitations. *Clin Cancer Res* 2013;19(14):3745–54.
6. Chance B. Near-infrared images using continuous, phase-modulated, and pulsed light with quantitation of blood and blood oxygenation. *Ann N Y Acad Sci* 1998;838:29–45.
7. Zhu B, Sevick-Muraca EM. A review of performance of near-infrared fluorescence imaging devices used in clinical studies. *Br J Radiol* 2015;88(1045):20140547.
8. Gioux S, Choi HS, Frangioni JV. Image-guided surgery using invisible near-infrared light: fundamentals of clinical translation. *Mol Imaging* 2010;9(5):237–55.
9. Snoeks TJ, van Driel PB, Keereweer S, et al. Towards a successful clinical implementation of fluorescence-guided surgery. *Mol Imaging Biol* 2014;16(2):147–51.
10. Handgraaf HJM, Verbeek FP, Tummers QR, et al. Real-time near-infrared fluorescence guided surgery in gynecologic oncology: a review of the current state of the art. *Gynecol Oncol* 2014;135(3):606–13.
11. Morton DL, Thompson JF, Cochran AJ, et al. Sentinel-node biopsy or nodal observation in melanoma. *N Engl J Med* 2006;355(13):1307–17.
12. Giuliano AE, Kirgan DM, Guenther JM, et al. Lymphatic mapping and sentinel lymphadenectomy for breast cancer. *Ann Surg* 1994;220(3):391–8.
13. van der Zee AG, Oonk MH, de Hullu JA, et al. Sentinel node dissection is safe in the treatment of early-stage vulvar cancer. *J Clin Oncol* 2008;26(6):884–9.
14. Schaafsma BE, Mieog JS, Hutteman M, et al. The clinical use of indocyanine green as a near-infrared fluorescent contrast agent for image-guided oncologic surgery. *J Surg Oncol* 2011;104(3):323–32.
15. Motomura K, Inaji H, Komoike Y, et al. Combination technique is superior to dye alone in identification of the sentinel node in breast cancer patients. *J Surg Oncol* 2001;76(2):95–9.
16. Motomura K, Inaji H, Komoike Y, et al. Sentinel node biopsy in breast cancer patients with clinically negative lymph-nodes. *Breast Cancer* 1999;6(3):259–62.
17. van der Vorst JR, Schaafsma BE, Verbeek FP, et al. Randomized comparison of near-infrared fluorescence imaging using indocyanine green and 99(m) technetium with or without patent blue for the sentinel lymph node procedure in breast cancer patients. *Ann Surg Oncol* 2012;19(13):4104–11.
18. Hutteman M, van der Vorst JR, Gaarenstroom KN, et al. Optimization of near-infrared fluorescent sentinel lymph node mapping for vulvar cancer. *Am J Obstet Gynecol* 2012;206(1):89–5.
19. van der Vorst JR, Schaafsma BE, Verbeek FP, et al. Near-infrared fluorescence sentinel lymph node mapping of the oral cavity in head and neck cancer patients. *Oral Oncol* 2013;49(1):15–9.
20. Tong M, Guo W, Gao W. Use of fluorescence imaging in combination with patent blue dye versus patent blue dye alone in sentinel lymph node biopsy in breast cancer. *J Breast Cancer* 2014;17(3):250–5.
21. Cloyd JM, Wapnir IL, Read BM, et al. Indocyanine green and fluorescence lymphangiography for sentinel lymph node identification in cutaneous melanoma. *J Surg Oncol* 2014;110(7):888–92.
22. Can MF, Yagci G, Cetiner S. Systematic review of studies investigating sentinel node navigation surgery and lymphatic mapping for gastric cancer. *J Laparoendosc Adv Surg Tech A* 2013;23(8):651–62.

23. Schaafsma BE, Verbeek FP, Elzevier HW, et al. Optimization of sentinel lymph node mapping in bladder cancer using near-infrared fluorescence imaging. *J Surg Oncol* 2014;110(7):845–50.

24. Shimizu S, Kamiike W, Hatanaka N, et al. New method for measuring ICG Rmax with a clearance meter. *World J Surg* 1995;19(1):113–8.

25. Boni L, David G, Mangano A, et al. Clinical applications of indocyanine green (ICG) enhanced fluorescence in laparoscopic surgery. *Surg Endosc* 2014;29(7):2046–55.

26. Buckle T, van Leeuwen AC, Chin PT, et al. A self-assembled multimodal complex for combined pre- and intraoperative imaging of the sentinel lymph node. *Nanotechnology* 2010;21(35):355101.

27. Morton DL, Bostick PJ. Will the true sentinel node please stand? *Ann Surg Oncol* 1999;6(1):12–4.

28. Brouwer OR, Buckle T, Vermeeren L, et al. Comparing the hybrid fluorescent-radioactive tracer indocyanine green-99mTc-nanocolloid with 99mTc-nanocolloid for sentinel node identification: a validation study using lymphoscintigraphy and SPECT/CT. *J Nucl Med* 2012;53(7):1034–40.

29. Brouwer OR, van den Berg NS, Matheron HM, et al. A hybrid radioactive and fluorescent tracer for sentinel node biopsy in penile carcinoma as a potential replacement for blue dye. *Eur Urol* 2014;65(3):600–9.

30. Inoue T, Nishi T, Nakano Y, et al. Axillary lymph node recurrence after sentinel lymph node biopsy performed using a combination of indocyanine green fluorescence and the blue dye method in early breast cancer. *Breast Cancer* 2014; doi: 10.1007/s12282-014-0573-8.

31. Whitney MA, Crisp JL, Nguyen LT, et al. Fluorescent peptides highlight peripheral nerves during surgery in mice. *Nat Biotechnol* 2011;29(4):352–6.

32. Park MH, Hyun H, Ashitate Y, et al. Prototype nerve-specific near-infrared fluorophores. *Theranostics* 2014;4(8):823–33.

33. Schols RM, Connell NJ, Stassen LP. Near-infrared fluorescence imaging for real-time intraoperative anatomical guidance in minimally invasive surgery: a systematic review of the literature. *World J Surg* 2015;39(5):1069–79.

34. Verbeek FP, Schaafsma BE, Tummers QR, et al. Optimization of near-infrared fluorescence cholangiography for open and laparoscopic surgery. *Surg Endosc* 2014;28(4):1076–82.

35. Verbeek FP, van der Vorst JR, Schaafsma BE, et al. Intraoperative near infrared fluorescence guided identification of the ureters using low dose methylene blue: a first in human experience. *J Urol* 2013;190(2):574–9.

36. Dudley NE. Methylene blue for rapid identification of the parathyroids. *Br Med J* 1971;3(5776):680–1.

37. Keaveny TV, Tawes R, Belzer FO. A new method for intra-operative identification of insulinomas. *Br J Surg* 1971;58(3):233–4.

38. Winer JH, Choi HS, Gibbs-Strauss SL, et al. Intraoperative localization of insulinoma and normal pancreas using invisible near-infrared fluorescent light. *Ann Surg Oncol* 2010;17(4):1094–100.

39. Choi HS, Gibbs SL, Lee JH, et al. Targeted zwitterionic near-infrared fluorophores for improved optical imaging. *Nat Biotechnol* 2013;31(2):148–53.

40. Girard E, Messager M, Sauvanet A, et al. Anastomotic leakage after gastrointestinal surgery: diagnosis and management. *J Visc Surg* 2014;151(6):441–50.

41. Ris F, Hompes R, Cunningham C, et al. Near-infrared (NIR) perfusion angiography in minimally invasive colorectal surgery. *Surg Endosc* 2014;28(7):2221–6.

42. Diana M, Noll E, Diemunsch P, et al. Enhanced-reality video fluorescence: a real-time assessment of intestinal viability. *Ann Surg* 2014;259(4):700–7.

43. Kudszus S, Roesel C, Schachtrupp A, et al. Intraoperative laser fluorescence angiography in colorectal surgery: a noninvasive analysis to reduce the rate of anastomotic leakage. *Langenbecks Arch Surg* 2010;395(8):1025–30.

44. Lee BT, Hutteman M, Gioux S, et al. The FLARE intraoperative near-infrared fluorescence imaging system: a first-in-human clinical trial in perforator flap breast reconstruction. *Plast Reconstr Surg* 2010;126(5):1472–81.

45. Newman MI, Samson MC, Tamburrino JF, et al. Intraoperative laser-assisted indocyanine green angiography for the evaluation of mastectomy flaps in immediate breast reconstruction. *J Reconstr Microsurg* 2010;26(7):487–92.

46. van der Vorst JR, Schaafsma BE, Hutteman M, et al. Near-infrared fluorescence-guided resection of colorectal liver metastases. *Cancer* 2013;119(18):3411–8.

47. Yokoyama N, Otani T, Hashidate H, et al. Real-time detection of hepatic micrometastases from pancreatic cancer by intraoperative fluorescence imaging: preliminary results of a prospective study. *Cancer* 2012;118(11):2813–9.

48. Tummers QR, Verbeek FP, Prevoo HA, et al. First experience on laparoscopic near-infrared fluorescence imaging of hepatic uveal melanoma metastases using indocyanine green. *Surg Innov* 2015;22(1):20–25.

49. Nomura K, Kadoya M, Ueda K, et al. Detection of hepatic metastases from colorectal carcinoma: comparison of histopathologic features of anatomically resected liver with results of preoperative imaging. *J Clin Gastroenterol* 2007;41(8):789–95.

50. Niekel MC, Bipat S, Stoker J. Diagnostic imaging of colorectal liver metastases with CT, MR imaging, FDG PET, and/or FDG PET/CT: a meta-analysis of prospective studies including patients who have not previously undergone treatment. *Radiology* 2010;257(3):674–84.

51. Ishizawa T, Fukushima N, Shibahara J, et al. Real-time identification of liver cancers by using indocyanine green fluorescent imaging. *Cancer* 2009;115(11):2491–504.

52. Ishizawa T, Masuda K, Urano Y, et al. Mechanistic background and clinical applications of indocyanine green fluorescence imaging of hepatocellular carcinoma. *Ann Surg Oncol* 2014;21(2):440–8.

53. Hutteman M, van der Vorst JR, Mieog JS, et al. Near-infrared fluorescence imaging in patients undergoing pancreaticoduodenectomy. *Eur Surg Res* 2011;47(2):90–7.

54. Matsumura Y, Maeda H. A new concept for macromolecular therapeutics in cancer chemotherapy: mechanism of tumoritropic accumulation of proteins and the antitumor agent smancs. *Cancer Res* 1986;46(12 Pt. 1):6387–92.

55. Maeda H, Wu J, Sawa T, et al. Tumor vascular permeability and the EPR effect in macromolecular therapeutics: a review. *J Control Release* 2000;65(1–2):271–84.

56. Hagen A, Grosenick D, Macdonald R, et al. Late-fluorescence mammography assesses tumor capillary permeability and differentiates malignant from benign lesions. *Opt Express* 2009;17(19):17016–33.

57. Tummers QR, Hoogstins CE, Peters AA, et al. The value of intraoperative near-infrared fluorescence imaging based on enhanced permeability and retention of indocyanine green: feasibility and false-positives in ovarian cancer. Submitted for publication.

58. van der Vorst JR, Schaafsma BE, Verbeek FP, et al. Intraoperative near-infrared fluorescence imaging of parathyroid adenomas with use of low-dose methylene blue. *Head Neck* 2014;36(6):853–8.

59. van der Vorst JR, Vahrmeijer AL, Hutteman M, et al. Near-infrared fluorescence imaging of a solitary fibrous tumor of the pancreas using methylene blue. *World J Gastrointest Surg* 2012;4(7):180–4.

60. Tummers QR, Verbeek FP, Schaafsma BE, et al. Real-time intraoperative detection of breast cancer using near-infrared fluorescence imaging and methylene blue. *Eur J Surg Oncol* 2014;40(7):850–8.

61. Moore GE, Peyton WT. The clinical use of fluorescein in neurosurgery; the localization of brain tumors. *J Neurosurg* 1948;5(4):392–8.

62. Stummer W, Pichlmeier U, Meinel T, et al. Fluorescence-guided surgery with 5-aminolevulinic acid for resection of malignant glioma: a randomised controlled multicentre phase III trial. *Lancet Oncol* 2006;7(5):392–401.

63. Stummer W, Stocker S, Novotny A, et al. In vitro and in vivo porphyrin accumulation by C6 glioma cells after exposure to 5-aminolevulinic acid. *J Photochem Photobiol B* 1998;45(2–3):160–9.

64. Keereweer S, Van Driel PB, Robinson DJ, et al. Shifting focus in optical image-guided cancer therapy. *Mol Imaging Biol* 2014;16(1):1–9.

65. van Dam GM, Themelis G, Crane LM, et al. Intraoperative tumor-specific fluorescence imaging in ovarian cancer by folate receptor-alpha targeting: first in-human results. *Nat Med* 2011;17(10):1315–9.

66. Warram JM, de Boer E, Sorace AG, et al. Antibody-based imaging strategies for cancer. *Cancer Metastasis Rev* 2014;33(2–3):809–22.

67. Beer AJ, Kessler H, Wester HJ, et al. PET imaging of integrin alphaVbeta3 expression. *Theranostics* 2011;1:48–57.

68. Verbeek FP, van der Vorst JR, Tummers QR, et al. Near-infrared fluorescence imaging of both colorectal cancer and ureters using a low-dose integrin targeted probe. *Ann Surg Oncol* 2014;21(Suppl. 4):S528–37.

69. Themelis G, Yoo JS, Ntziachristos V. Multispectral imaging using multiple-bandpass filters. *Opt Lett* 2008;33(9):1023–5.

13

The role of interventional radiology in the management of cancer patients

SHAHZAD ILYAS, TARUN SABHARWAL AND ANDY ADAM

INTRODUCTION

Intervention radiology (IR) is a specialty that has revolutionized patient care. It has had an impact on the diagnosis and treatment of patients in all medical and surgical specialties. Using evolving, innovative and often complex techniques, under image guidance, patient care can be delivered in an efficient and effective manner. The emergence of this specialty has been made possible by enormous technological advances over the past several decades in relation to catheter and instrument design, imaging systems and radiological expertise.

Many invasive surgical procedures have been replaced or enhanced by IR procedures, resulting in reduced morbidity, mortality and hospital stay for patients. *Interventional oncology* is a branch of IR which uses interventional techniques in the diagnosis, treatment or palliation of patients with cancer. It is vital that interventional oncology is practiced within a multidisciplinary setting, in order to assess how best IR services can enhance patient management, throughout the care pathway [1].

Interventional procedures undertaken in the management of cancer patients can be divided into three main groups, depending on their primary intent: diagnostic procedures, supportive and palliative procedures, and disease-modifying and therapeutic procedures (Tables 13.1 and 13.2).

ROLE OF INTERVENTIONAL RADIOLOGY IN THE DIAGNOSIS OF CANCER

The gold standard for definitive diagnosis of many tumours is histological confirmation, following which non-invasive imaging allows accurate assessment and staging of the malignancy. These steps are vital in order to appropriately treat the cancer.

Image guidance allows direct visualization of the lesion, allowing the safe passage of a needle into the diseased tissue, thereby improving efficacy and minimizing the risk of damaging adjacent structures [2]. Most organ systems and regions of the body can be biopsied using image guidance, resulting in a minimally invasive procedure with a high level of accuracy and low complication rate [2]. Cross-sectional imaging allows accurate biopsy planning, by identifying lesion location as well as surrounding structures that should be avoided during the procedure. In cases where lesions are present in more than one organ, percutaneous biopsy can be used to concurrently confirm histological diagnosis, allowing accurate staging of the cancer. Another increasingly important role of percutaneous biopsy is to obtain microbiological diagnosis of lesions suspicious for opportunistic infections in oncology patients with febrile neutropenia [3].

In cases where surgical biopsy remains the preferred diagnostic approach, image guidance can be of preoperative

Table 13.1 Supportive and palliative interventional procedures

Procedure	Examples of indications
Drainage	Malignant obstruction of renal and biliary tract, pleural effusion and ascites
Stenting	Malignant strictures: Bile duct, gastrointestinal, tracheobronchial, ureteric, SVC or IVC obstruction
Feeding	Tunnelled lines, PICC lines, radiological inserted gastrostomy (RIG)
Palliative embolization	Hormone-producing metastases, primary hepatocellular carcinoma, skeletal metastases, neo-adjuvant portal vein embolization
Filter	IVC
Vertebroplasty	Vertebral metastasis, multiple myeloma and osteoporosis

Table 13.2 Disease-modifying and therapeutic procedures

Procedure	Examples of indications
Ablation • Cryoablation • Microwave ablation • Radiofrequency ablation	Renal, liver, lung and bone tumours
Intra-arterial procedures • Embolization • Chemoembolization (TACE) • Selective internal radiation therapy	Hepatocellular carcinoma, liver metastasis

assistance by localizing the tumour, thereby preventing extensive surgical access in order to identify the lesion.

The modality used for guidance during percutaneous biopsies depends on the location of the lesion and the level of operator experience. Lesions, which are either superficial or located within a solid organ such as the liver or kidney, can be biopsied using ultrasound guidance. This has the benefit of real-time imaging allowing accurate and safe manipulation of the biopsy needle into the target lesion, while avoiding exposure to ionizing radiation during the procedure [3]. CT guidance offers the benefit of enhanced anatomical delineation, allowing more precise needle localization within the target lesion and avoidance of surrounding structures such as bowel loops, which may not be clearly visualized on ultrasound. CT guidance is particularly useful in biopsying retroperitoneal, pelvic and thoracic lesions as these are generally difficult to identify on ultrasound. They can be performed using static images or CT fluoroscopy, which provides near-real-time imaging allowing accurate monitoring of the biopsy needle trajectory. The main disadvantage of using CT guidance is the associated radiation dose to the patient, which is dependent on the total scan time, patient's body mass and scan parameters such as peak tube kilovoltage and milliamperage. Fluoroscopic images are generally acquired at a lower milliamperage than standard static CT images, resulting in lower radiation to the patient; however, the radiation dose to the performing clinical is increased.

SUPPORTIVE/PALLIATIVE PROCEDURES

Malignancy can result in several complications following dysfunction of organs and systemic systems, the majority of which can be treated by minimally invasive interventional procedures. Hence interventional oncology can play a significant role in the palliative and supportive management of cancer patients with unresectable tumours, by relieving symptoms without the need for a general anaesthetic and prolonged hospital stay. The majority of procedures are performed under local anaesthesia with mild sedation if required and can have a significant impact on the patient's quality of life.

Drainage procedures and stenting

RENAL TRACT

Malignant obstruction of the urinary tract can be due to retroperitoneal adenopathy, extrinsic tumour compression or direct tumour invasion. Management requires decompression of the urinary collecting system by means of a percutaneous nephrostomy. Obstruction can be unilateral or bilateral and induced by a wide range of malignancies, but most commonly those of gastrointestinal, urological or gynaecological origin. Percutaneous nephrostomies can also be used to redirect urinary flow in cases of recto-vesical or recto-vaginal fistulas caused by pelvic malignancies or in cases of haemorrhagic cystitis secondary to chemotherapy.

Diversion of the urine allows the lower urinary system to become 'dry' and hence tissues to heal. Providing direct access to the urinary system not only drains the urine but also allows access for further uro-radiological intervention such as antegrade ureteric stenting. Indications for percutaneous nephrostomy in an emergency setting are urinary tract sepsis, rapidly deteriorating renal function, hyperkalaemia and metabolic acidosis.

The pelvicalyceal system is initially punctured under ultrasound guidance using a fine-gauge needle. Contrast medium is subsequently injected through the needle under fluoroscopic guidance, in order to delineate the anatomy and identify the level of obstruction. Samples are often sent for microbiological and cytological analysis. The actual nephrostomy drain has a pigtail configuration at its distal end, with multiple side holes, which are positioned within the renal pelvis. The proximal end is attached to an external drainage bag; however, if long-term drainage is required, then an antegrade stent can be placed, following manipulation of a guidewire and catheter beyond the obstruction, allowing the patient to be 'bag free'. Contrast studies may demonstrate complete obstruction of the ureters; however, hydrophilic guidewires can often be advanced through the obstruction by finding the narrow luminal channel. Percutaneous dilation of the ureteric stricture is often required in these cases prior to advancing the larger-calibre ureteric stent.

BILIARY TRACT

Patients with irresectable malignant biliary strictures commonly present with yellow discolouration and pruritus secondary to obstructive jaundice. These symptoms can be relieved by insertion of a biliary stent, therefore restoring drainage of bile. The majority of these patients have an underlying pancreatic neoplasm, which extrinsically compresses the distal bile duct and can be treated via endoscopic retrograde stent placement. In patients with more proximal or central obstruction of the common bile duct or when endoscopic retrograde cholangiopancreatography (ERCP) fails to relieve the obstruction, a percutaneous transhepatic approach can be taken in order to access the biliary system for stent placement.

Fluoroscopic or now more commonly ultrasound guidance is used to gain percutaneous access into the peripheral hepatic ducts, followed by injection of contrast medium (percutaneous transhepatic cholangiography [PTC]) in order to delineate the anatomy of the biliary tree identifying the location of the obstruction. Static bile within a dilated biliary system can become infected, and hence these patients often present with severe sepsis. Extensive manipulation and stent placement in such cases can result in a sudden systemic influx of organisms, resulting in septic shock. Therefore a staged approach is often recommended with initial placement of either an external or internal drain, in order to allow decompression of the biliary system, followed by insertion of a stent at a later date after the sepsis has settled. Prior to initiating percutaneous biliary procedures, all patients should be administered appropriate prophylactic

intravenous antibiotics to minimize septic complications. Other complications apart from sepsis, associated with percutaneous biliary drainage, include haemorrhage and localized inflammatory and infective processes such as abscess formation, cholecystitis, peritonitis or pancreatitis. Metal stents have a 6-month patency rate of approximately 50% and hence are almost exclusively used in patients with terminal cancer [4]. Occluded metal stents cannot be removed, but placing another stent coaxially within the first can restore its patency.

PLEURAL EFFUSIONS

Malignant pleural effusions can be a significant cause of morbidity in oncology patients, commonly presenting with cough, shortness of breath and chest pain [5]. Drainage of pleural effusions is most commonly undertaken under ultrasound or CT guidance. A diagnostic thoracocentesis may initially be performed in certain cases to aid primary diagnosis or staging of malignancy, by undergoing cytology evaluation [6]. Therapeutic thoracocentesis may provide temporary symptomatic relief; however the fluid often re-accumulates in malignant disease and therefore requires a more permanent solution. Initially this may involve inserting a chest drain (tube thoracostomy), using a Seldinger technique. The actual drainage tubes can vary in diameter, with small-calibre drains used in cases with simple serious collections and larger-calibre drains reserved for more viscous collections. More definitive treatment requires pleurodesis [7]. In order for this to be successful the effusions have to be adequately drained, which also prevents accumulation of the therapeutic agents within the pleural space. A sclerosing agent (doxycycline, bleomycin or talc) is then injected through the tube thoracotomy.

In cases where sclerotherapy is contraindicated, cannot be tolerated or has failed, a permanent tunnelled pleural catheter can be inserted, known as the Denver Biomedical PleurX® catheter (Denver Biomaterials, Inc., Golden, Colorado). This is essentially a small-bore chest tube that is designed to remain in place for prolonged periods, allowing intermittent drainage of the pleural space through a one-way valve.

ASCITES

Patients with intraperitoneal spread of tumour accumulate large-volume intractable ascites that require frequent paracentesis in order to relieve discomfort. Patients often experience symptoms of abdominal pressure resulting in shortness of breath, nausea and limited mobility. These patients have a poor prognosis, with management of symptoms focusing on palliation rather than definitive treatment. Paracentesis is the most common method of treatment and the most effective at relieving symptoms. Some patients require weekly or even daily paracentesis, which can have a greater risk of complications due to multiple passes of a needle into the abdomen. Implanted peritoneal catheters can be placed in these patients, such as the PleurX catheter (Denver Biomaterials), which is a 15.5 F silicone catheter with multiple side holes and is inserted percutaneously. These are the same catheters used for the long-term drainage of malignant pleural effusions. They are tunnelled for a short distance under the skin of the abdominal wall to minimize the risk of infection, with the distal end ideally positioned within the posterior pelvis in order to maximize drainage. Patients can be instructed on how to perform drainages at home, therefore reducing the frequency of hospital visits.

Gastrointestinal tract

OESOPHAGUS

Oesophageal stents are important tools for palliative treatment of inoperable oesophageal malignancies. A range of self-expanding stents can be deployed across the narrowed region, in order to relieve dysphagia and hence improve quality of life. Placement of the stent can be performed under fluoroscopic or endoscopic guidance and is associated with minimal morbidity and mortality. Self-expanding stents can be covered, partially covered or uncovered. Covered stents have the advantage of preventing tumour ingrowth in addition to the fact that they can be removed; however, they have a significantly higher risk of stent migration than uncovered stents. A stent should ideally bridge the stricture and extend 2–4 cm beyond each end. Hence a stricture located proximally or distally can be difficult to stent [8]. Severely stenosed or even occluded oesophageal lumens can be crossed using small-calibre catheters and wires, which reduce the risk of perforation, followed by accurate positioning and deployment of the stent under fluoroscopic guidance. Stent placement across the gastro-oesophageal junction can lead to aspiration secondary to reflux disease. Studies have demonstrated that using stents with an anti-reflux mechanism across this region can result in a significant reduction in gastro-oesophageal reflux.

Complications following oesophageal stenting can be classified into early or delayed [9]. Early complications occur either immediately or within 2–4 weeks post-procedure, while late complications occur 2–4 weeks after deployment [10]. Among both early and late complications, the most common complication is stent migration, occurring in 7–75% of cases (Table 13.3) [11].

Table 13.3 Early and late complications, following oesophageal stenting [12]

Early complications	Late complications
Bleeding	Stent occlusion
Fever	Stent migration
Chest pain	Tumour ingrowth
Perforation	Oesophageal fistulas
Stent migration	Re-occurrence of stenosis
Globus sensation	
Gastro-oesophageal reflux disease	

Source: Baron TH, *New England Journal of Medicine*, vol. 344, pp. 1681–1687, 2001.

Covered metallic stents can be used in the management of oesophageal fistulas, secondary to malignant disease, which unlike benign fistulas do not tend to heal spontaneously. If untreated, patients can suffer from malnutrition and thoracic sepsis [13]. Covered stents immediately seal the fistula, allowing the patients to resume a normal diet within 24 h.

GASTRODUODENAL AND COLORECTAL

Self-expanding stents play an important role in the palliative treatment of inoperable gastroduodenal and acute colonic obstruction. This group of patients tend to be frail, suffering from dehydration and electrolyte imbalance, making them poor surgical candidates. The use of self-expanding stents provides a minimally invasive approach to relieving the obstruction and improving the quality of life of these patients, who would otherwise have to undergo a possible morbid surgical procedure or may have limited treatment options because of multiple comorbidities.

TRACHEOBRONCHIAL

Patients with malignant airway obstruction can suffer from considerable respiratory distress. Self-expanding stents can provide palliative support for non-operable lesions; however, this is ideally done as a combined procedure between a bronchoscopist and an interventional radiologist, under general anaesthesia. The stricture is visualized on bronchoscopy and often the extent of the stricture is marked with radio-opaque markers. Prior to deploying a self-expanding stent under fluoroscopic guidance, the stricture may be dilated in order to allow the non-traumatic advancement of the stent through the narrow lumen. Patients may experience significant symptomatic improvement, with re-expansion of the collapsed lung.

VENOUS OBSTRUCTION AND THROMBOEMBOLIC DISEASE

Mediastinal tumours or large primary and secondary central lung lesions can result in extrinsic compression of the superior vena cava (SVC), which can be partial or complete and in extreme cases can also result in tumour invasion. Occlusion of venous drainage from the head, neck and upper limbs can result in extensive swelling of these areas and is frequently further complicated by venous thrombosis.

Venocavography is performed via a percutaneous transfemoral approach, in order to identify the exact location and length of stenosis. If extensive thrombus is present within the cava, then selective intravenous thrombolysis may be required. The cava is initially dilated, prior to insertion of a self-expandable stent, which restores flow immediately, often resulting in rapid relief of symptoms. Malignant obstruction of the inferior vena cava (IVC) is managed in a similar fashion.

Malignancy is an established risk factor for venous thromboembolism. Percutaneous insertion of an IVC filter can trap thrombus, originating in the deep veins of the lower limb, preventing the occurrence of potentially life-threatening pulmonary emboli (PE).

An IVC filter is indicated in patients with lower-limb venous thrombosis in whom anticoagulation is contraindicated, who have a bleeding disorder or who develop recurrent PE despite adequate anticoagulation therapy [14].

Acute occlusive lower-limb venous disease, if not treated adequately, can result in chronic venous disease and post-thrombotic syndrome (PTS). This can have a negative impact on the patient's health and quality of life. There are several endovascular techniques that can be used to manage acute venous thrombus, including catheter-directed thrombolysis and mechanical thrombectomy devices. Catheter-directed thrombolysis involves the targeted infusion of high-dose thrombolytic agents through multi-side-hole infusion catheters directly into the thrombus, resulting in a lower risk of haemorrhage and higher patency rate than systematic thrombolysis. In symptomatic patients with chronically occluded pelvic veins flow can be re-established following venous angioplasty and stenting.

Feeding

PERCUTANEOUS GASTROSTOMY AND GASTROJEJUNOSTOMY

Patients with upper gastrointestinal obstruction secondary to head, neck or oesophageal malignancy may not be able to tolerate oral intake in advanced stages of the disease, therefore requiring nutritional support often by gastrostomy or gastrojejunostomy [15]. This avoids the need for nasogastric and intravenous lines, which can be physically uncomfortable for patients and result in psychological distress. If ascites is present, then paracentesis prior to tube insertion is essential in order to prevent leakage and the risk of peritonitis. Gastrojejunostomies are preferred over gastrostomies in cases where there is gastric outlet obstruction or gastro-oesophageal reflux.

Percutaneous image-guided placement of feeding tubes directly into the stomach has a higher technical success rate and reduced associated morbidity than endoscopic or surgical placement [16]. Endoscopy may also not be technically possible in such patients with severe luminal stenosis. The most common complications associated with enteric feeding tubes include infection and tube dislodgement. If the tube has been in place for more than 2 weeks, then the track becomes established and can be re-cannulated, without the need for re-puncturing the stomach.

CENTRAL VENOUS ACCESS

Medium- and long-term vascular access is essential in most cancer patients with terminal disease, in order to administer medication, chemotherapy and parenteral nutrition, as well as allow regular blood sampling without the repeated need for venipuncture. Under a combination of ultrasound and fluoroscopic guidance, a variety of long-term venous lines (e.g. tunnelled central catheters, peripherally inserted central catheters [PICCs] and venous ports) can be positioned with the tips at the cavo-atrial junction or right atrium. The procedure is performed following administration of local anaesthesia, under strict aseptic conditions. Procedural complications are typically related to injury of surrounding structures or catheter malposition, which are significantly lower using fluoroscopic guidance than blind techniques guided by anatomical landmarks. Long-term complications include line occlusion, thrombosis and line-related infection, rates of which are unaffected by the insertion technique. The risk of developing thrombosis is higher in cancer patients than in the general population and is further increased by placement of a central venous line within the vein. Unfortunately venous thromboembolic prophylaxis has not been shown to reduce the incidence of thrombosis in patients with central venous access [17]. Most patients, once diagnosed with venous thrombosis, are treated with anticoagulation therapy, with the duration depending on the extent of the thrombus and response to initial therapy [17].

Palliative embolization

Minimally invasive image-guided occlusion of arteries or veins through selectively placed catheters can be used either to stop bleeding, as an adjunct to surgery, or more commonly as a method of palliation to alleviate symptoms such as pain. The injection of embolic agents is usually performed via a percutaneous puncture, following administration of local anaesthesia and intravenous sedation. It provides an attractive alternative to surgery, which has the added risk of a general anaesthesia. In certain cases it may be the only therapeutic option available. There are a wide variety of embolic agents available, which can broadly be allocated into one of three categories (Table 13.4). The type of agent used depends on the type and site of lesion being embolized and the desired outcome.

Embolization can provide significant symptomatic relief in patients with large bulky tumours. Selective arterial catheterization of the feeding artery, followed by bland embolization with particles, can result in disruption of the afferent blood supply, which induces hypoxia and inhibits tumour growth. Over time ischaemia causes the tumour to reduce in size, leading to a reduction in mass effect. A variety of tumours throughout the body can be treated in this manner, providing palliative relief for end-stage cancer patients.

Table 13.4 Embolic agents used in the management of oncology patients

Liquid	N-butyl cyanoacrylate (glue), lipiodol, alcohol
Mechanical	Detachable balloons, coils, plug
Particulate	Gelfoam, polyvinyl alcohol (PVA), acrylic gelatin microspheres

Arterial embolization can also be beneficial in the management of hormone-secreting neoplasms (e.g. metastatic neuroendocrine tumours), which are non-operable. Depriving the tumour of blood reduces the production of hormones, which can result in a significant clinical improvement within hours of the procedure.

Portal vein embolization (PVE) is also used to augment the size of a future liver remnant, prior to partial liver resection [18] secondary to a hepatic tumour. The liver is a unique organ, as it has the capacity to regenerate, if part of it is removed. Embolization of the portal vein branches, supplying segments of the liver to be resected, diverts blood flow into the future remnant liver. This has a dual effect in that first the affected part of the liver shrinks, which is subsequently resected, and second the remaining normal liver compensates by growing in size. This reduces the risk of patients suffering from liver failure, due to lack of remaining liver tissue. PVE is commonly performed at least 4 weeks prior to surgery in order to allow the liver sufficient time to regenerate. The procedure itself involves percutaneous portal vein puncture, under ultrasound guidance. A portal venogram is performed in order to delineate the various branches of the portal vein, followed by selective cannulation of the main branches supplying the segments to be resected. Embolization is performed with coils, plugs, particles, glue or more commonly a combination of these materials.

Embolization also plays a key role in the therapeutic management of cancer, which is discussed in more detail later in this chapter.

Vertebroplasty and kyphoplasty

Vertebroplasty and kyphoplasty are techniques used to treat painful vertebral compression fractures, which can occur due to either osteoporosis or malignancy. Malignant causes of vertebral compression fractures include multiple myeloma, lymphoma, bone metastasis and aggressive haemangiomas. The procedure is indicated in patients with debilitating pain due to vertebral compression fractures, which cannot be controlled using conventional analgesia and therapy, such as bed rest and the use a supportive brace.

The procedure is performed under conscious sedation or a general anaesthesia and involves percutaneous access into the vertebral body, using fluoroscopic or CT guidance. A large-bore needle is positioned within the vertebral body, via a transpedicular route for the lumbar spine or an intercostovertebral route for the thoracic spine [13]. Vertebroplasty involves the injection of polymethyl methacrylate (bone cement) into the partially collapsed vertebral body, mixed with contrast medium. The cement mixture is deliberately kept viscous in order to prevent leakage into adjacent structures. Kyphoplasty involves the placement and inflation of balloons into the vertebral body to create a cavity before injecting the cement. This not only results in alleviation of pain but also restores vertebral body height, reducing the focally exaggerated kyphosis within the spine and preventing further fractures of adjacent vertebral bodies due to abnormal load bearing.

DISEASE-MODIFYING AND THERAPEUTIC PROCEDURES

Over the past few decades interventional oncology has significantly evolved to offer a wide variety of minimally invasive treatment options for cancer patients. The role of interventional oncology is no longer restricted to performing palliative or salvage procedures in patients who have terminal cancer and have exhausted all other medical and surgical options. Image-guided procedures now form an integral part of the cancer treatment pathway at an early stage, at times being performed as the primary treatment option, but more commonly in combination with conventional therapy.

Disease-modifying or therapeutic procedures offered in interventional oncology can be divided into those which involve percutaneous ablation and those which are performed via an intra-arterial approach resulting in the selective treatment of lesions.

Ablation

Ablation results in the local destruction of the tumour and is generally reserved for patients with localized metastatic disease, recurrent malignancy in areas of previous radiation therapy and primary neoplasms in patients who are poor surgical candidates. Ablation techniques are not considered curative but can result in survival rates equal to those of surgery in most cases. In addition, ablation has the advantage over surgery of having reduced morbidity and mortality, with the ability to perform procedures as an outpatient at a lower cost. Ultrasound, CT or MRI guidance is used to percutaneously position the probes accurately within the lesions.

Percutaneous techniques of tumour ablation can be categorized into heating (radiofrequency ablation [RFA], microwave therapy and high-intensity focused ultrasound) and freezing (cryoablation). All these techniques result in cell death by coagulative necrosis. Locally developed post-ablation imaging protocols using CT or MRI should be employed to monitor post-procedural changes within the tissue and to detect any residual or recurrent disease.

CRYOABLATION

Cryoablation has been used in multiple organs including kidneys, liver, lungs, prostate and even musculoskeletal lesions. Multiple probes are often used to increase the field of treatment. It causes cell death through the application of subfreezing temperatures, which are achieved with the use of argon gas under high pressure [19]. The subfreezing temperatures are transmitted through the cryoprobe to the tissues being ablated. Cell death occurs due to a combination of diminished blood flow, dehydration of cells and formation of ice crystals resulting in apoptosis. Ice formation and microvascular thrombosis also induce tissue ischaemia, which reduces bleeding [20]. The temperature at the probe, located in the centre of the lesion, is around –130°C, with temperatures increasing to 0°C at the edge of the lesion.

RADIOFREQUENCY ABLATION

RFA is the most widely used ablation technique and involves the use of electromagnetic energy in the radiofrequency range, which causes ionic agitation resulting in frictional heat and eventual cell death. RFA can be used to treat several types of tumours including hepatocellular and metastatic liver lesions, in addition to renal, adrenal, lung and musculoskeletal tumours.

Most RFA procedures are performed following conscious sedation. At least two grounding pads are placed on the patient, equidistant from the target lesion. Once the probes are adequately positioned within the tumour they are connected in a closed-loop circuit to a monopolar or bipolar energy source [21]. The tissues around the tip of the electrode are heated beyond temperatures of 50°C resulting in thermal damage of tissues and cell death. The size and shape of the necrosed lesion depend on the gauge of the probe, duration of therapy, length of the exposed tip and temperature achieved at the tip. Cell death occurs between the temperatures of 50°C and 100°C, beyond which the tissues become charred. Cooling the probes with saline during ablation can prevent charring of the tissues and hence reduces the impedance of the tissues adjacent to the probe.

The procedure is generally well tolerated and serious complications, consisting of intraperitoneal haemorrhage or abscess formation, are rare.

MICROWAVE ABLATION

Microwave ablation uses electromagnetic energy at a frequency of 900 MHz, which causes agitation of water molecules within the targeted tissues resulting in fictional heat and cell death via coagulation necrosis. There is no current transmitted through the patient and hence grounding pads are not needed.

Studies comparing RFA and microwave ablation have shown comparable therapeutic results and complication rates [22,23], particularly in the treatment of hepatocellular carcinoma. However, certain studies have demonstrated that RFA results in a higher survival rate and a lower recurrence rate [24].

Intra-arterial procedures

Catheter-directed embolization could be used as a primary mode of treatment in cases of inoperable primary tumours, while it can also increase survival times in metastatic disease. Similar to ablation, a wide spectrum of tumours can be treated including renal, lung, adrenal and most commonly liver.

Prior to the procedure it is vital to perform either contrast-enhanced CT or MRI, in order to delineate the arterial supply to the lesion and aid transcatheter embolization. In order to avoid non-targeted embolization it is vital to be as selective as possible when trying to cannulate the feeding vessel to the tumour, prior to embolization.

The liver tolerates the procedure because of its dual blood supply from the hepatic and portal veins. The portal vein provides the majority of nutrients to the normal liver, while hepatic tumours derive their blood supply from the hepatic artery. It is therefore essential to check if the portal vein is patent prior to embolization, in order to avoid hepatic necrosis.

EMBOLIZATION

Bland mechanical embolization can be achieved using coils and plugs, but most commonly either polyvinyl alcohol (PVA) particles or acrylic microspheres are used. In the majority of lesions, the absence of arterial enhancement of a previously hypervascular lesion, when re-imaged 4–6 weeks following the procedure, indicates a favourable outcome. Aggressive hypervascular tumours tend to recruit new arterial channels and therefore the procedure may need to be repeated several times in order to control tumour growth.

TRANSARTERIAL CHEMOEMBOLIZATION

Transarterial chemoembolization (TACE) is a modification of the above embolization technique, which is used to treat hepatic tumours. Following selective catheterization of the artery supplying the hepatic lesion, a combination of chemotherapy drugs and embolic agents is directly injected into the artery. Hepatic tumours rely on the hepatic artery, as opposed to the portal vein, for the majority of their blood supply. The embolic agent causes ischaemia of the tumour cells and also reduces the flow rate within the tumour vasculature, therefore increasing contact time between the cytotoxic agent and malignant cells.

The advantage of TACE compared to systemic chemotherapy is that it provides targeted delivery of the chemotherapy agent, at the site of the lesion, therefore providing a higher local and lower systemic concentration. The procedure may need to be repeated several times until the entire tumour bed is devascularized [25].

More recently there has been development of non-resorbable drug-eluting beads, which can incorporate the chemotherapeutic drug. The drug is retained at the site of disease for a longer period of time, therefore improving its pharmacokinetic profile and reducing systemic effects. Beads loaded with doxorubicin have shown promising results when treating non-operable hepatocellular cancer, with lower peak plasma concentration at 5 min than for patients receiving conventional TACE [26].

SELECTIVE INTERNAL RADIATION THERAPY

Radioembolization is a form of brachytherapy used in the focused treatment of malignant liver lesions [27]. Beta-emitting radioactive particles are delivered directly into the tumour following selective catheter placement. The most commonly used radioisotope is yttrium 90 (^{90}Y), which is incorporated in resin or glass microspheres measuring 20–40 µm. Beta radiation has a very low penetration and hence only results in local necrosis of tissue [28].

The procedure is commonly performed in two stages. Stage 1 involves performing a mesenteric angiogram in order to identify any arterial variants. The right gastric and gastroduodenal arteries are embolized in order to avoid non-targeted spread of the beads, following which the main hepatic artery is cannulated and a small concentration of ^{99m}Tc-MAA is administered. The patient is then transferred for a nuclear medicine lung scan in order to identify any arteriovenous shunting through the liver to the pulmonary circulation, which can result in radiation pneumonitis. The second stage is undertaken if there is no shunting to the lungs. The hepatic artery is cannulated with a microcatheter, followed by slow injection of the beads under fluoroscopic guidance. A microcatheter is used in order to limit the flow rate of ^{90}Y and therefore reduce the chance of reflux. The procedure is generally well tolerated; however, patients may experience mild nausea, fatigue and abdominal discomfort.

Selective internal radiation therapy has demonstrated favourable results when treating unresectable hepatocellular carcinoma [28,29]. It has also been reported to achieve a meaningful response and disease stabilization in patients with advanced metastatic liver disease and may be extremely useful in dealing with chemorefractory colorectal cancer [30].

CONCLUSION

Over the past few decades interventional oncology has significantly evolved to meet the challenges of managing complex cancer patients. It plays an integral role in the multidisciplinary management of these patients, offering both palliative and therapeutic image-guided minimally invasive procedures. It has played a key role in improving the quality of life and life expectancy of cancer patients, in addition to reducing the burden on nursing care.

REFERENCES

1. Chow DS and Itagaki MW. Interventional oncology research in the United States: slowing growth, limited focus, and a low level of funding. *Radiology*, vol. 257, no. 2, pp. 410–417, 2010.

2. Gupta S, Wallace MJ, Cardella JF, Kundu S, Miller DL, and Rose SC. Quality improvement guidelines for percutaneous needle biopsy. *Journal of Vascular and Interventional Radiology*, vol. 21, no. 7, pp. 969–975, 2010.

3. Arellano RS, Maher M, Gervais DA, Hahn PF, and Mueller PR. The difficult biopsy: let's make it easier. *Current Problems in Diagnostic Radiology*, vol. 32, no. 5, pp. 218–226, 2003.

4. Rossi P, Bezzi M, Rossi M, et al. Metallic stents in malignant biliary obstruction: results of a multicenter European study of 240 patients. *Journal of Vascular and Interventional Radiology*, vol. 5, no. 2, pp. 279–285, 1994.

5. Uzbeck MH, Almeida FA, Sarkiss MG, et al. Management of malignant pleural effusions. *Advances in Therapy*, vol. 27, no. 6, pp. 334–347, 2010.

6. Lombardi G, Zustovich F, Nicoletto MO, Donach M, Artioli G, and Pastorelli D. Diagnosis and treatment of malignant pleural effusion: a systematic literature review and new approaches. *American Journal of Clinical Oncology*, vol. 33, no. 4, pp. 420–423, 2010.

7. Shaw P and Agarwal R. Pleurodesis for malignant pleural effusions. *Cochrane Database of Systematic Reviews*, no. 1, article ID CD002916, 2004.

8. Hindy P, Hong J, Lam-Tsai Y, and Gress F. A comprehensive review of esophageal stents. *Gastroenterology and Hepatology (N Y)*, vol. 8, no. 8, pp. 526–534, 2012.

9. Martinez JC, Puc MM, and Quiros RM. Esophageal stenting in the setting of malignancy. *ISRN Gastroenterology*, vol. 2011, article ID 719575, 2011.

10. Hindy P, Hong J, Lam-Tsai Y, and Gress F. A comprehensive review of esophageal stents. *Gastroenterology and Hepatology (N Y)*, vol. 8, no. 8, pp. 526–534, 2012.

11. Sharma P, Kozarek R, and Practice Parameters Committee of American College of Gastroenterology. Role of esophageal stents in benign and malignant diseases. *American Journal of Gastroenterology*, vol. 105, pp. 258–273, 2010.

12. Baron TH. Expandable metal stents for the treatment of cancerous obstruction of the gastrointestinal tract. *New England Journal of Medicine*, vol. 344, pp. 1681–1687, 2001.

13. Sabharwal T, Fotiadis N, and Adam A. The role of interventional radiology in the palliative care of patients with cancer. In Hanks G, Cherny N, Christakis NA, et al., eds., *Oxford Textbook of Palliative Medicine*, 4th ed. Oxford: Oxford University Press.

14. Grassi CJ, Swan TL, Cardella JF, et al. Quality improvement guidelines for percutaneous permanent inferior vena cava filter placement for the prevention of pulmonary embolism. *Journal of Vascular and Interventional Radiology*, vol. 14, no. 9, part 2, pp. S271–S275, 2003.

15. Chan SC, Ko SF, Ng SH, et al. Fluoroscopically guided percutaneous gastrostomy with modified gastropexy and a large-bore balloon-retained catheter in patients with head and neck tumors. *Acta Radiologica*, vol. 45, no. 2, pp. 130–135, 2004.

16. Wollman B, D'Agostino HB, Walus-Wigle JR, Easter DW, and Beale A. Radiologic, endoscopic, and surgical gastrostomy: an institutional evaluation and meta-analysis of the literature. *Radiology*, vol. 197, no. 3, pp. 699–704, 1995.

17. Baskin JL, Pui CH, Reiss U, et al. Management of occlusion and thrombosis associated with long-term indwelling central venous catheters. *Lancet*, vol. 374, no. 9684, pp. 159–169, 2009.

18. Smith KA and Kim HS. Interventional radiology and image-guided medicine: interventional oncology. *Seminars in Oncology*, vol. 38, no. 1, pp. 151–162, 2011.

19. Beland M, Mueller PR, and Gervais DA. Thermal ablation in interventional oncology. *Seminars in Roentgenology*, vol. 42, no. 3, pp. 175–190, 2007.

20. O'Neill SB, O'Connor OJ, Ryan MF, and Maher MM. Interventional radiology and the care of the oncology patient. *Radiology Research and Practice*, vol. 2011, article ID 160867, 2011.

21. Gillams AR. Image guided tumour ablation. *Cancer Imaging*, vol. 5, pp. 103–109, 2005.

22. Shibata T, Iimuro Y, Yamamoto Y, et al. Small hepatocellular carcinoma: comparison of radio-frequency ablation and percutaneous microwave coagulation therapy. *Radiology*, vol. 223, pp. 331–337, 2002.

23. Boutros C, Somasundar P, Garrean S, Saied A, and Espat NJ. Microwave coagulation therapy for hepatic tumors: review of the literature and critical analysis. *Surgical Oncology*, vol. 19, no. 1, pp. e22–e32, 2010.

24. Ohmoto K, Yoshioka N, Tomiyama Y, et al. Comparison of therapeutic effects between radio-frequency ablation and percutaneous microwave coagulation therapy for small hepatocellular carcinomas. *Journal of Gastroenterology and Hepatology*, vol. 24, no. 2, pp. 223–227, 2009.

25. O'Connor OJ, Buckley JM, and Maher MM. Interventional radiology in oncology. *Cancer Treatment and Research*, vol. 143, pp. 493–511, 2008.

26. Varela M, Real MI, Burrel M, et al. Chemoembolization of hepatocellular carcinoma with drug eluting beads: efficacy and doxorubicin pharmacokinetics. *Journal of Hepatology*, vol. 46, pp. 474–481, 2007.

27. Ahmadzadehfar H, Biersack HJ, and Ezziddin S. Radioembolization of liver tumors with yttrium-90 microspheres. *Seminars in Nuclear Medicine*, vol. 40, no. 2, pp. 105–121, 2010.

28. Deleporte A, Flamen P, and Hendlisz A. State of the art: radiolabeled microspheres treatment for liver malignancies. *Expert Opinion on Pharmacotherapy*, vol. 11, no. 4, pp. 579– 586, 2010.

29. Geschwind JF, Salem R, Carr BI, et al. Yttrium-90 microspheres for the treatment of hepatocellular carcinoma. *Gastroenterology*, vol. 127, pp. S194–S205, 2004.

30. Cosimelli M, Golfieri R, Cagol PP, et al. Multi-centre phase II clinical trial of yttrium-90 resin microspheres alone in unresectable, chemotherapy refractory colorectal liver metastases. *British Journal of Cancer*, vol. 103, no. 3, pp. 324–331, 2010.

14

Minimal access and robotic surgery

DOMENICO D'UGO, ALBERTO BIONDI AND MARIA CARMEN LIROSI

INTRODUCTION

A combined therapeutic approach and personalized cancer care by a multidisciplinary oncology team [1] result in the greatest advantages for patients; as regards local disease control, innovations in technology produce their best results only through constant application of updated knowledge and techniques in all medical specialties that are involved in the loco-regional treatment of cancer. Fellowship-trained surgeons with a high-volume practice are more likely to be focused on a particular disease process or group of operations, resulting in increased technical expertise and greater knowledge of the disease [2–4]. It is therefore crucial that surgeons are correctly trained in the specific oncologic principles of surgical oncology as well as in modern minimally invasive technologies.

The most important question for laparoscopic surgery in surgical oncology is whether similar short-term and long-term outcomes for cancer are achievable compared with conventional open surgery. Oncologic outcomes and principles remain the foundation of any procedure to cure malignancies, so any laparoscopic procedure should follow the same standard of care as open surgery, especially margins of resection and lymphadenectomy [5]. With this in mind, it is also established that laparoscopic surgery has many advantages over open surgery, if the operation is performed competently: there is a significant reduction in postoperative pain and analgesic need, and gastrointestinal function returns to normality more rapidly. There is also less scarring and fewer wound complications (wound infections, dehiscence, incisional hernias). The postoperative length of stay is also an important factor in favour of the laparoscopic approach. Moreover, there is a well-recognized role of laparoscopy in decreasing the pro-inflammatory and immunologic response to surgery that could be related to an improved immediate or even long-term oncologic result [6–8]. There is also a decrease in postoperative adhesion formation and re-laparoscopy is available if complications are suspected.

HISTORY OF LAPAROSCOPY

Hippocrates was the first to describe insertion of instruments through various orifices in order to visualize internal anatomy and pathology, but the modern endoscopic and laparoscopic era dates to the early nineteenth century, when Philipp Bozzini described a 'Lichtleiter' cystoscope (1805) [9]. Kelling of Dresden reported a truly laparoscopic procedure in dogs in 1902 [10,11], and Jacobaeus of Stockholm claimed the first human laparoscopies and thoracoscopies in 1910 [12]. Veress, a Hungarian, devised his spring-loaded needle in 1938 to collapse the lung in patients with tuberculosis [3].

Harold Hopkins, in the 1950s, invented the Rod Lens [14]: this made the laparoscope more rigid and robust, giving a brighter image, less liable to distortion. It was originally marketed by Karl Storz, constituting the basis of most modern laparoscopes.

The German gynaecologist Semm performed an 'incidental' appendicectomy in 1982 (removal of a normal appendix during a diagnostic procedure) and was duly castigated, heavily by the German Surgical Society [15]. The first human laparoscopic cholecystectomy was described by Muhe in 1985 and popularized after 1987 by Mouret [16,17].

Semm developed the basic laparoscopic instrumentation (hook scissor, endoloop applicator, devices to prevent loss of intraperitoneal insufflated CO_2, clip applicators, atraumatic forceps); in 1975 he designed a suture loop (the Roeder loop) to

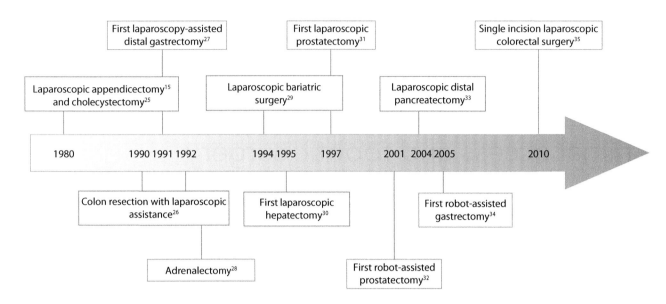

Figure 14.1 Timeline: key events in the history of mini-invasive surgery.

allow adequate haemostasis and perfected intra- and extra-corporeal knot-tying techniques [18–21]. Berci in Los Angeles pioneered the use of laparoscopy for the management of diagnostic dilemmas, especially in emergency and oncologic cases [22–24]. Once initiated, laparoscopic surgery advanced with great rapidity for neoplastic diseases [15,25–35] (Figure 14.1).

APPLICATIONS, INDICATIONS AND EVIDENCE FOR EFFICACY

In the past, concerns about port-site metastasis in laparoscopic surgery for cancer have been raised, but they have never been subsequently confirmed [36,37].

In a review by Zmora and colleagues, the port-site recurrence rate in their laparoscopic experience in colorectal cancers was 0.62%, similar to the rate reported for open resections [38]. In addition, in a review from the MD Anderson Cancer Center, there was no increase in port-site recurrences in patients undergoing laparoscopy compared with laparotomy for gastrointestinal cancers [39].

Zanghì and colleagues in their meta-analysis on 13 randomized controlled studies reported no statistically significant differences in wound, port-site recurrence and peritoneal seeding between laparoscopic colorectal surgery and conventional open surgery [40]. Studies also report a low incidence of port-site recurrences after staging laparoscopy (0–2%), which is similar to that after open explorations for cancer patients [41].

Diagnostic and staging laparoscopy

Laparoscopy may assist in the more accurate staging of digestive cancers, enabling direct inspection of intra-abdominal organs, obtaining biopsies and peritoneal fluid for cytology, together with the possible use of a laparoscopic ultrasound probe. Preoperative staging laparoscopy avoids unnecessary laparotomies, being the most useful tool for

ruling out occult peritoneal metastases; it shortens the time to initiation of neoadjuvant chemotherapy in gastrointestinal/intra-abdominal cancers, with the benefits of more precise staging. It can be performed just before the planned surgery or as a separate diagnostic procedure for many different abdominal neoplasms.

HEPATOCELLULAR CARCINOMA

Identification of patients who have unresectable hepatocellular carcinoma by staging laparoscopy possibly combined with laparoscopic ultrasound may spare patients from non-therapeutic laparotomy and alter treatment plans, decreasing morbidity, hospital stay and costs and allowing an early start to adjuvant therapy (levels 2 and 3 evidence) [42,43].

The most common findings that preclude resection are bilobar intrahepatic metastases, cirrhosis combined with inadequate functional hepatic reserve, peritoneal or lymph node metastases, vascular involvement and invasion of adjacent organs. Known unresectable hepatic diseases such as major vessel or organ invasion would be a contraindication for staging laparoscopy. Laparoscopic ultrasound can detect 9.5% more tumours (most <1 cm) than CT alone (level 2 evidence) [44]. Staging laparoscopy correctly identifies 63% to 67% of patients with unresectable disease (levels 2 and 3 evidence) [44].

Diagnostic laparoscopy combined with laparoscopic ultrasound spares approximately one in five patients a non-therapeutic laparotomy (levels 2 and 3 evidence) [44,45].

BILIARY TRACT TUMOURS

Intrahepatic cholangiocarcinoma is commonly found to be unresectable due to the presence of intrahepatic or peritoneal metastases. Staging laparoscopy is indicated for stage T2 or T3 hilar cholangiocarcinoma without evidence of overt unresectable or metastatic disease on imaging [46].

Staging laparoscopy can identify previously unsuspected peritoneal or superficial liver metastases (level 3 evidence) [47], detecting unresectable disease with a sensitivity of 60% (level 2 evidence) [48]. Due to the few published studies on the use of staging laparoscopy for patients with biliary tract cancer patients, no level 1 evidence exists [49].

HEPATIC METASTASES

Due to the improved quality of imaging, the indications for diagnostic laparoscopy for hepatic metastases have decreased over the years. Staging laparoscopy with laparoscopic ultrasound is indicated in resectable liver metastases and is helpful in finding unexpected extrahepatic metastases or additional hepatic metastases and can identify more accurately the size, number and location of all lesions (level 2 evidence) [50–53].

As described by Jarnagin and colleagues, patients that may benefit from staging laparoscopy are those who have more than two poor-outcome factors as described by the clinical risk score (lymph node–positive colon cancer, disease-free interval shorter than 12 months, more than one hepatic tumour, CEA greater than 200 ng/ml within 1 month of surgery, size of largest hepatic tumour greater than 5 cm) [51]. A highly selected group of patients with non-colorectal, non-neuroendocrine metastases also come to hepatic resection. In this subset of patients, given the unclear benefit of resection and the relatively high yield, diagnostic laparoscopy is recommended before hepatectomy, being indicated to identify systemic or unresectable disease, thus avoiding an unnecessary laparotomy [54].

PANCREATIC CANCER

Despite better-quality preoperative imaging, many patients with pancreatic cancer still have unresectable disease at laparotomy. Compared to open exploration, staging laparoscopy reduces surgical morbidity and shortens recovery time with no delay to administration of adjuvant therapy or palliation [55–61].

Staging laparoscopy has been shown to identify undiagnosed intra-abdominal disease with a median sensitivity of 94% (93–100%), a specificity of 88% (80–100%) and an accuracy of 89% (87–89%) [62,63]. In such cases, laparoscopic ultrasound can be used to evaluate the deep hepatic parenchyma, vascular invasion (portal vein, mesenteric vessels, celiac trunk, hepatic artery), the entire pancreas and even periportal and para-aortic lymph nodes [63–65].

Some studies suggest that tumours larger than 3 cm are more likely to be associated with a higher incidence of positive peritoneal cytology and occult metastatic disease (level 3 evidence) [66], and this would justify the added time and cost of laparoscopy. On the other hand, CA 19-9 levels of less than 150 UI/ml have been associated with a lower likelihood of metastatic disease and consequently a lower yield on staging laparoscopy (level 3 evidence) [67].

GASTRIC CANCER

In most current treatment algorithms, staging laparoscopy is mainly indicated for patients with T3/T4 gastric cancer without evidence of distant metastases. Patients with M1 disease are referred for systemic chemotherapy and palliative resection in case of obstruction, haemorrhage or perforation, while patients with early stage gastric cancer (T1/T2) should proceed directly to surgical resection without staging laparoscopy.

The minimally invasive detection of occult metastases after a conventional work-up based on computed tomography or ultrasound avoided unnecessary laparotomy for up to one-third of patients with newly diagnosed gastric cancers [68,69]. In these cases, staging laparoscopy reduced operative and hospitalization time and perioperative morbidity and, in addition, laparoscopy had a fundamental role in selecting patients for neoadjuvant therapies [70].

The accuracy of laparoscopy was superior to that of the other imaging techniques (CT and ultrasound) in detecting peritoneal, hepatic and nodal metastases (levels 2 and 3 evidence), and its accuracy is reported to be from 89% to 100% in different series [71–73].

Ascites may be aspirated and sent for cytology, as may peritoneal fluid washings obtained from both upper quadrants and the pelvis. In patients with localized disease the rate of positive peritoneal cytology is generally low [76]; on the other hand, a cytologic positivity strongly correlates with the extent of disease (level 3 evidence) [74–77].

Laparoscopic ultrasound may also be used to detect intraparenchymal liver metastases, local extension of gastric cancer into adjacent organs (pancreas, splenic vessels), or para-aortic and coeliac lymphadenopathy [70]; nevertheless the use of laparoscopic ultrasound as a staging modality for gastric cancer is still unproven.

ESOPHAGEAL CANCER

The added value of precise staging is the differentiation of patients with early stage tumours who are candidates for immediate curative resection from those with locally advanced, resectable cancers who may benefit from neoadjuvant therapy. Staging laparoscopy should be therefore applied in patients with esophageal cancer without evidence of bulky nodes at preoperative staging, while it is contraindicated for patients with known metastatic disease [78–80].

Laparoscopy, with or without laparoscopic ultrasound, shows a high sensitivity in finding radiologically occult metastasis (peritoneal metastases 71%, nodal metastases 78%, liver metastases 86%, level 2 evidence) with a reported accuracy of 75–80% (level 3 evidence) [79–81]. Despite these reports, in the literature, no level 1 evidence exists regarding staging laparoscopy in esophageal cancer, and the few studies that have been performed have taken place in highly specialized centres and may not be fully generalizable.

LYMPHOMA

Staging laparoscopy in patients with Hodgkin's lymphoma may be useful to determine the stage and location of the disease and define appropriate treatment or prognosis, although in most cases such staging is now adequately achieved by CT scanning and core biopsy [82,83].

Staging laparoscopy in non-Hodgkin's lymphoma may spare patients the morbidity of a laparotomy and provide tissue to confirm the diagnosis when core needle biopsy is non-diagnostic [84], although again this is much less frequently needed in modern practice. Intraoperative ultrasound may be applied to parenchymal organs in addition to abdominal nodal masses [85,86].

Apart from pure staging purposes, laparoscopy can also be used for patients who need splenectomy as part of their treatment, with less postoperative pain, faster recovery and earlier definitive treatment.

Laparoscopic gastrointestinal cancer surgery: Levels of evidence

Many palliative procedures, such as gastrointestinal bypass, gastrostomy and jejunostomy, colostomy, are easily carried out with minimally invasive surgery [87], with benefits which are claimed to be greater for unresectable cancer patients, even if no evidence has been published on this particular indication.

As regards primary tumour resections with the intent of cure (R0), laparoscopic surgery has gained the widest diffusion into standard clinical practice in the management of colorectal malignancy. Many authors agree that minimally invasive surgery is now the gold standard in this field. Recent multicentre trials (COST trial, COLOR trial, CLASSIC trial, ALCCAS trial) [88–92] have confirmed the oncological safety of laparoscopic colorectal resection with equivalent long-term oncologic outcomes compared to open surgery and clear proof of 'non-inferiority'.

Koh and colleagues [93] and Liang and colleagues [94] have confirmed the safety and superiority of laparoscopic gastric resection for gastric gastrointestinal stromal tumours compared to open surgery. Retrospective studies have also demonstrated that despite the longer operating time, laparoscopic-assisted distal gastrectomy has lower complication rates and similar total number of retrieved lymph nodes as the open distal gastrectomy group [95,96].

Hwang and colleagues [97] and Song and colleagues [98] reported similar 5-year overall survival rates comparing laparoscopically assisted distal gastrectomy and open distal gastrectomy.

Kim and colleagues, in a multicentre study, confirmed that the overall survival rate after case matching (by body mass index, operative technique, extent of lymphadenectomy, operator and cancer stage) did not show any significant differences between open gastrectomy and laparoscopic gastrectomy for all stages of cancer [99].

Recently very promising results have also been reported for laparoscopic surgery for esophageal cancer [100–102], pancreatic cancer [103–105] and left-sided liver resection [106,107], but only in selected centres.

In contrast, total gastrectomy, pancreatico-duodenectomy and major hepatic resections should be considered as pioneering procedures, reserved for expert laparoscopic cancer surgeons (Table 14.1) [108].

Details of surgical techniques will be largely described in the organ-based chapters of this book; in all cases, besides the perfect knowledge of all surgical steps, advanced laparoscopic techniques for malignant disease should be initiated and carried out only in selected centres with surgical experience in both laparoscopy and cancer surgery. Moreover, the author believes that every new laparoscopic program in surgical oncology should be tutored, monitored and validated by short-term surgical morbidity and longer-term oncological outcomes.

SURGICAL TRAINING

The surgical education landscape is changing due to the rapid development of health care technologies and this fact, combined with the 'digital native' generation of learners who are now entering surgical training programs, is challenging traditional apprenticeship programs. Gone are the days of 'see one, do one, teach one': modern-day

Table 14.1 Indications to laparoscopic surgery for cancer

	Laparoscopic surgery	Open surgery	Level of evidence
Colon	Standard	Accepted	1
Rectum	Becoming standard	Standard	2
Esophagus	Accepted	Standard	2
Distal stomach	Accepted	Standard	2
Proximal stomach	Being standard	Standard	3
Minor liver resection	Being standard	Standard	3
Pancreas body–tail	Being standard	Standard	3
Pancreas head	Pioneeristic	Standard	4
Major liver resection	Pioneeristic	Standard	4
Small bowel	Being standard	Standard	5
Gallbladder	Pioneeristic	Standard	5
Biliary tree	Pioneeristic	Standard	5

surgery needs the implementation of new models of training. Until the year 2000, a huge group of surgeons required laparoscopic training when a few teachers were available and most were being trained through variable industry-funded courses. L Swanstrom and N Soper, co-chairmen in 1997 of the SAGES Continuing Education Committee, were among the first to share the idea of teaching the basic skills of laparoscopy through standardizing a threefold program: didactics, clinical judgment and manual skills – called Fundamentals in Laparoscopic Surgery (FLS). The impact on general surgery has been impressive: In 2008, the American Board of Surgery mandated that all residents seeking board certification pass the FLS exam. In 2012, in a public statement, SAGES and the American Cancer Society (ACS) recommended that all general surgeons who perform laparoscopy be certified through the FLS program. The concept of measurable outcomes has permeated the way that laparoscopic surgery is taught today; with the birth of many national preceptorship programs throughout the world, the verification of surgical training has become a new model for other traditional programs.

In this context, the use of a technology-based educational assessment, such as simulation, has a fundamental role: simulated patient management eliminates risk to real patients and offers experience of a wide range of scenarios in a more efficient manner. Trainees may learn procedures through interactive video tutorials and synthetic models in order to practice tasks in 'box trainers' (Figure 14.2) and learn entire procedures [109–111].

The success of this form of training is now evident from the large number of laparoscopic courses available worldwide, but the acquisition of basic skills for proficiency in laparoscopic surgery is not to be interpreted as a licence to perform unsupervised laparoscopic procedures: direct patient care and operating privileges could be contingent on passing multimodal standardized modules in clinical management, surgical skills and procedure simulations, and a brand new 'science' is emerging behind the validation of simulations for health care, at the intersection between clinical, educational, and technical and engineering.

One of the major problems with box training is the trainer time, since an expert is necessary for evaluation and feedback. In contrast, in 'virtual reality training' (Figure 14.3), a computer evaluates every movement of the trainee and provides feedback after completion of the task (e.g. reports the number of movements, reports the distance moved by each hand, traces the path of movements). Using these simulators, trainees can practice standardized laparoscopic tasks repeatedly, with instant objective feedback of performance. Virtual reality training is one of the many methods used in laparoscopic surgical training and is currently aimed at improving cognitive, psychomotor and technical skills, of both surgical residents during their studies and experienced surgeons for maintaining their overall skill; the latter could perform a 'warm-up' exercise before the real operation.

The scope of this technology should be coupled with validated training programs incorporating inbuilt measures of performance before progressing to real procedures [112].

Such systems allow repeated practice of standardized tasks and provide unbiased and objective measurements of laparoscopic performance. However, their widespread application in surgical training programs has not been generally accepted, because evidence that simulator training improves surgical skills in the operating room is lacking.

Many papers have demonstrated that the trained group perform operations significantly faster than those who have not been trained [113].

Grantcharov and colleagues, in a randomized clinical trial, examined the impact of virtual reality surgical simulation on the improvement of psychomotor skills relevant to the performance of laparoscopic cholecystectomy, demonstrating that surgeons who received virtual reality training performed laparoscopic cholecystectomy significantly faster than the control group and showed significantly greater improvement in error rates and in economy of movement scores [114].

Surgical societies and regulatory bodies, such as the Society of American Gastrointestinal and Endoscopic Surgeons (SAGES) and the European Association of Endoscopic Surgeons (EAES), stipulated minimum requirements for those performing laparoscopic surgery, with an emphasis on training both in and outside the operating theatre [115,116].

Virtual simulation should be incorporated into current training programs to develop validated curricula for basic, intermediate and advanced-level laparoscopic training. The correct frequency of training and whether tutors need to be present at all times should be determined. Competency levels should be defined using a national approach, enabling

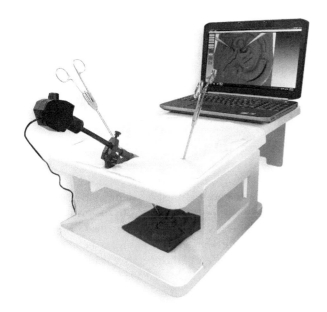

Figure 14.2 Box trainer.

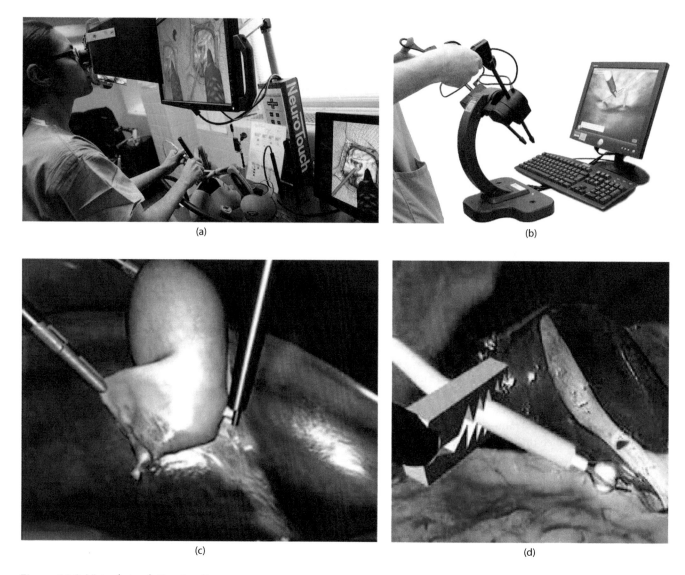

Figure 14.3 Virtual simulation (a–d).

standardization of training programs; in the meanwhile it has been suggested that surgical telementoring may be a solution to enhance and improve surgical education [117].

Telementoring permits an expert surgeon, who remains in his or her own hospital, to instruct a non-expert on how to perform a new laparoscopic technique [117] using oral instructions or tele-demonstration, a visually assisted mentoring system (Figure 14.4) [118].

To become technically proficient at laparoscopic colorectal resections may require a much longer training period than simpler procedures such as cholecystectomy [119,120]. Numerous studies have reported on the length of the learning curve using different training methods and end points over the past 20 years, resulting in a suggested number of cases of between 11 and 110 [121,122].

Junior surgeons might initially attend an intensive basic laparoscopic skills program, followed by intermediate and advanced skills training [123,124]. Telementoring can contribute to reducing the length of the learning curve in complex laparoscopic surgeries.

Surgical simulation, telementoring and telepresence surgery (guidance given to the surgeon by another surgeon who is not in the operating room) are unique benefits of 'robotic technology' [125–128].

ROBOTIC SURGERY

Since the 1980s, surgical robots (remotely controlled devices aiding the positioning and manipulation of surgical instruments) have been developed with the primary goal of helping in technically demanding procedures while the surgeon is in a comfortable position sitting at a console, with a three-dimensional view of the operative field, full control of camera and instruments, absence of a fulcrum effect, elimination of hand tremor and 7 versus 4 degrees of freedom of movement.

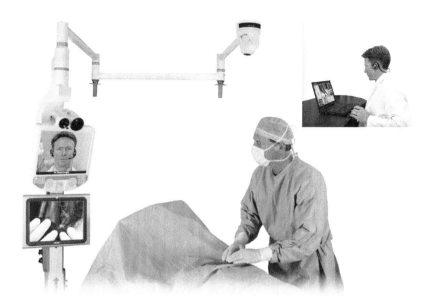

Figure 14.4 Telementoring.

The use of robotic technology in minimally invasive surgery was first described in 1985. Following FDA approval in 2000 and after the promising results of the nerve sparing prostatectomy, robotics has been widely adopted in urology, gynaecology and later in general surgery. To date the da Vinci® system (Intuitive Surgical, Sunnyvale, California) is the sole commercially available robotic platform and has undergone several evolutions from the first model introduced in 1999. Currently about 3000 da Vinci systems of different generations are working on a global scale; the number of robot-assisted procedures that are performed worldwide has tripled from 80,000 in 2007 to 205,000 in 2009 [129].

One of the big theoretical advantages of the robotic platform in surgery is the shorter learning curve compared with conventional laparoscopy, but even if robotic training programs have become part of many surgical residency programs, an official credentialing in robotic surgery has not yet been established [130].

There certainly are some disadvantages of robotic-assisted surgery, including the absence of tactile feedback, instrument collisions and the need to reposition the instruments in wide surgical fields; many emphasize the high costs, time-consuming procedures and lack of clinical evidence in the absence of standard requirements for robot-assisted laparoscopy training.

Although the most common use for robotics was to treat urologic oncologic conditions (i.e. prostate cancer), it has also been adopted for gynaecologic, thoracic, and head and neck surgeries. In general surgery, robotic-assisted surgery is used for resections for colon and rectal cancers, pancreatectomy for pancreatic cancer, adrenalectomy for adrenal lesions, hepatectomy for liver lesions and gastrectomy for gastric cancer.

For several procedures, there is evidence that robotics offers short-term benefits such as shorter lengths of stay and lower intraoperative blood loss, with safety profiles and oncologic outcomes comparable to those of open and conventional laparoscopic approaches. However, data on long-term oncologic and functional outcomes are generally lacking.

Robotic-assisted laparoscopic radical prostatectomy (RALP) for prostate cancer is by far the most commonly performed robotic operation [131]. In a large comparative meta-analysis RALP was associated with lower estimated blood loss than open and laparoscopic approaches and fewer blood transfusions than open approaches, and length of stay was shorter than those for open and laparoscopic approaches. RALP had lower incidences of readmissions, reoperations, nerve injury, rectal injury and fistulae, deep vein thromboses and sepsis than laparoscopic surgery. Compared with open radical prostatectomy, RALP had fewer readmissions, ureteral injuries, deep vein thromboses, hematomas, lymphoceles, anastomotic leaks and wound infections. However, bowel injuries were more frequent with RALP versus open radical prostatectomy. In addition, the likelihood of reoperation, vessel, nerve, bladder and rectal injuries, as well as ileus, was comparable for robotic versus open approaches [132].

In summary, RALP oncological outcomes appear to be at least equivalent to other approaches, but with additional costs.

Recent studies comparing robotic and laparoscopic partial nephrectomies demonstrated reduced complications, shorter ischemia time, lower blood loss, shorter postoperative stay and a lower conversion rate to open surgery in favour of robotics [133].

The median costs between different approaches were not significantly different so that robotic partial nephrectomy seems safe and cost-effective particularly for complex tumours [134].

Robot-assisted radical cystectomy for the treatment of bladder cancer is still under investigation and although promising, all the available studies were conducted in high-volume centres [135]. To date, the largest series comparing 104 open versus 83 robot-assisted cystectomies showed fewer 30-day complications in the robotic group [136].

Since the Food and Drug Administration approval for myomectomy and hysterectomy in 2005, robotics has been applied increasingly in gynaecologic oncology, mainly for radical hysterectomy for cervical cancer and staging surgery with lymphadenectomy in endometrial cancer. Most of the publications on robotic surgery are still retrospective or descriptive. Literature reviews demonstrate the feasibility and favourable short-term surgical outcomes of a robotic approach for gynaecologic surgery [137,138].

In the last 5 years a number of case series of robotic lung resection have been published [139]. However, all available studies are retrospective and non-comparative with potential patient and tumour selection biases. The robotic approach confers advantages over open surgery similar to Video-Assisted Thoracoscopic Surgery (VATS) and is safe with outcomes comparable to VATS. However, existing data do not demonstrate superiority over VATS, and comparative effectiveness studies are needed to explore short-term outcomes such as pain and respiratory function and to assess cost differences [140].

Many experienced laparoscopic surgeons have reported that compared with laparoscopic gastrectomy, robotic gastrectomy is safe and effective [141]. The current indications for robotic surgery are similar to laparoscopic surgery and are based on the recommendation of the Japanese Gastric Cancer Association guidelines [142].

Results of a meta-analysis revealed that compared with laparoscopic surgery, use of robotic surgery for gastric cancer significantly decreases intraoperative blood loss and results in comparable morbidity and mortality. However, the operative time of robotic gastrectomy was significantly longer than those of open and laparoscopic surgery [143].

In Korea, a multicentre prospective observational study (Multi-Institutional Study on the Assessment of Robotic Surgery for Gastric Cancer, NCT01309256) that is comparing robotic and laparoscopic surgery for gastric cancer is currently ongoing. This study will investigate cost-effectiveness, patient quality of life, learning curve of the surgeon and feasibility. The results of this study will contribute data that address questions about clinical indications and efficacy of robotic surgery in the field of gastric cancer treatment. It must be stressed that costs in robotic gastrectomy are undoubtedly higher than in open and laparoscopic gastrectomy and a detailed analysis of this aspect is still lacking, especially where a self-pay health care system is in force.

The use of robotic systems for performing minimally invasive colectomy was first reported in 2002 by Weber et al [144].

The results from recent meta-analysis of case series or comparative non-randomized studies combining both rectal resections and abdominal colectomies concluded that conversion rates and perioperative morbidity were similar for the colectomy group, and considerably lower for robotic anterior resection of the rectum, with an adequate lymph node harvest [145].

Similar to other laparoscopic complex procedures, robotics in colorectal minimally invasive surgery has been introduced to overcome limitations of laparoscopic instruments. These limitations are particularly relevant during rectal dissection within the pelvis as they result in difficult retraction, crowding and clashing of instruments. In this field the robotic platform is able to eliminate tremor of the surgeons' hand and improve imaging controlled by the surgeon rather than the assistant, and wrist movement of robotic instruments allows for more precise dissection of tissue planes. This is why most of the published literature on robotic colorectal resection is focused on rectal resection. Meta-analysis of the available non-randomized studies comparing robotic and laparoscopic rectal resection suggests a lower conversion rate to open surgery for robotic procedures, with similar operative times and other short-term outcomes [146].

Moreover some authors had reported reduced rates of circumferential resection margin involvement and autonomic nerve dysfunction in patients undergoing robotic total mesorectal excision [147,148].

Also in colorectal robotic surgery, the main obstacle is definitely thought to be the high cost. In all cost-analyzed studies, every author reported higher costs than in laparoscopic or open surgeries [149].

Further data from the international, multicentre, randomized ROLARR trial comparing robotic-assisted versus standard laparoscopic surgery for rectal cancer in terms of both short-term perioperative and longer-term outcomes are awaited in the near future [150].

Robotics in liver surgery have so far been limited; nevertheless, from the limited number of cases reported in the literature, robotic surgery for major liver resection appears to be a feasible procedure for primary and metastatic disease. Robotic hepatectomy appears to be safe when performed by experienced surgeons and offers results similar to those of laparoscopic and open approaches. However, these results coming from small series performed by experienced surgeons are not generalizable [151].

Robotic surgery has recently been applied to pancreatectomy by various hybrid techniques (i.e. laparoscopic resection and robotic reconstruction). No clear benefit or advantage over laparoscopy has been established with the application of robotics in pancreatic surgery [152].

Health care cost issues

The rapid diffusion of robotics is currently driven by a non-evidence-based enthusiasm for the technology. Hospitals, which compete with one another to attract surgeons and patients, decide by themselves to purchase robots even without an evident economic benefit, since it is well known that one major disadvantage of robotic surgery is the high cost. Robotic surgical systems have high fixed costs, with prices ranging from $1 million to $2.5 million for each unit. The systems also require costly maintenance (around $110,000 annually) and require the use of additional disposable instruments and more operating time. Estimates of the net per-procedure cost of robot assistance vary with assumptions about the frequency with which a robot will be used. Health care cost analysis estimates that in 2007, on average, the additional variable cost of using a robot-assisted procedure was about $1600. Including the cost of the robot itself, the additional costs rose to about $3200 [153].

Of particular interest is the case of prostate cancer: while non-surgical treatment options do exist with similar long-term outcomes, a US survey showed an increase of more than 60% in the number of prostatectomies between 2005 and 2008 despite a decrease in the incidence of prostate cancer. The short-term benefits associated with robotic prostatectomy may encourage patients to opt for surgery rather than non-surgical treatment. These data suggest that robotic surgery may have contributed to divert prostate cancer patients from non-surgical to surgical treatments, increasing both the cost per surgical procedure and the overall number of cases treated surgically.

To date, the available evidence fails to show that the long-term outcomes of robot-assisted surgery are superior to those of laparoscopic procedures, which are generally associated with only modest additional cost, short-term benefits, more rapid recovery and similar outcomes in terms of survival and cure rates [154].

Shorter lengths of stay have resulted in decreased overall hospital charges and lower 'social costs' have also been demonstrated from many laparoscopic procedures in surgical oncology, with the exception of robotics.

In the future cost-effectiveness studies may play a critical role in this process. Well-designed, large-scale, multicentre trials and comparative evaluations are needed to determine which patients benefit from open surgical approaches and which from laparoscopic and robot-assisted approaches. Government, hospitals, insurance providers, surgeons and patients could use this information to make a responsible choice about the adoption and use of these new technologies.

REFERENCES

1. Balch CM, Bland KI, Brennan MF, Cameron JL, Chabner BA, Copeland EM 3rd, Hoskins WJ, et al. What is a surgical oncologist? *Ann Surg Oncol* 1994;1:2–4.

2. Wong SL, Revels SL, Yin H, Stewart AK, McVeigh A, Banerjee M, Birkmeyer JD. Variation in hospital mortality rates with inpatient cancer surgery. *Ann Surg 2014*; 261(4):632–36.

3. Reames BN, Ghaferi AA, Birkmeyer JD, Dimick JB. Hospital volume and operative mortality in the modern era. *Ann Surg* 2014;260:244–51.

4. Bilimoria KY, Phillips JD, Rock CE, Hayman A, Prystowsky JB, Bentrem DJ. Effect of surgeon training, specialization, and experience on outcomes for cancer surgery: a systematic review of the literature. *Ann Surg Oncol* 2009; 16:1799–808.

5. Sharma B, Baxter N, Grantcharov T. Outcomes after laparoscopic techniques in major gastrointestinal surgery. *Curr Opin Crit Care* 2010;16:371–6.

6. Goldfarb M, Brower S, Schwaitzberg SD. Minimally invasive surgery and cancer: controversies part 1. *Surg Endosc* 2010;24:304–34.

7. Gitzelmann CA, Mendoza-Sagaon M, Talamini MA. Cell-mediated immune response is better preserved by laparoscopy than laparotomy. *Surgery* 2000;127:65–71.

8. Mendoza-Sagaon M, Gitzelmann CA, Herreman-Suquet K, Pegoli W Jr, Talamini MA, Paidas CN. Immune response: effects of operative stress in a pediatric model. *J Pediatr Surg* 1998;33:388–93.

9. Bozzini PH. Lichtleiter, eine Erfindung zur Anschauung innerer Theile und Krankheiten nebst der Abbildung. *J Practis Arzneyk Wunderarzneyk* 1806;24:107–24.

10. Kelling G. Ueber Oesophagoskopie, Gastroskopie und Kölioskopie. *Munch Med Wochenschr* 1902;1:21–24.

11. Lau WY, Leow CK, Li AK. History of endoscopic and laparoscopic surgery. *World J Surg* 1997;21:444–53.

12. Jacobaeus HC. Ueber die Möglichkeit die Zystoskopie bei Untersuchungen seröser Höhlungen anzuwenden. *Munch Med Wochenschr* 1910;57:2090–92.

13. Verres J. Neues instrument zur ausfuhrung von brust-punktmonen und pneumothorax behandlung. *Dtsch Med Wochenschr* 1938;64:1480.

14. Hopkins HH. On the diffraction theory of optical images. *Proc R Soc Lond* 1953;A217:408.

15. Semm K. History. In *Operative Gynecologic Endoscopy*, JS Sanfilippo, RL. Levine, eds. New York: Springer-Verlag, 1989.

16. Muhe E. Die erste Cholecystectomie durch das Laparoskop. *Langenbecks Arch Chir* 1986;369:804.

17. Muhe E. Laparoscopic cholecystectomy – late results. *Langenbecks Arch Chir.* 1991;Suppl.:416–423.

18. Semm K. Das Pneumoperitoneum mit CO_2. In *Endoslopie – Methoden, Ergebnisse*, L Demling, R Ottenjann, eds. Munich: Banaschewski, 1967, p. 167.

19. Semm K. Tissue-puncher and loop-ligation: new aids for surgical therapeutic pelviscopy (laparoscopy): endoscopic intra-abdominal surgery. *Endoscopy* 1978;10:119.

20. Semm K. Advances in pelviscopic surgery (appendectomy). *Curr Probl Obstet Gynecol* 1982;5(10):1.

21. Semm K. *Endoscopic intraabdominal surgery.* Kiel, Germany: Christian-Albrechts-Universitat, 1984.

22. Berci G, Davids J. Endoscopy and television. *BMJ* 1962;1:1610.
23. Berci G, Schulman AG, Morgenstern L, Paz-Partlow M, Cuschier A, Wood RA. Television choledochoscopy. *Surg Gynecol Obstet* 1985;160:176.
24. Berci G, Brooks PG, Paz-Partlow M. TV laparoscopy – a new dimension in visualization and documentation of pelvic pathology. *J Reprod Med* 1986;31:585.
25. Litynski GS. *Highlights in the history of laparoscopy.* Frankfurt, Germany: Barbara Bernert Verlag, 1996, pp. 165–168.
26. Jacobs M, Verdeja JC, Goldstein HS. Minimally invasive colon resection (laparoscopic resection). *Surg Laparosc Endosc* 1991;1:144–50.
27. Kitano S, Iso Y, Moriyama M, Sugimachi K. Laparoscopy assisted Billroth I gastrectomy. *Surg Laparosc Endosc* 1994;4:146–8.
28. Gagner M, Lacroix A, Bolté E. Laparoscopic adrenalectomy in Cushing's syndrome and pheochromocytoma. *N Engl J Med* 1992;327:1033.
29. Wittgrove AC, Clark GW, Tremblay LJ. Laparoscopic gastric bypass, Roux-en-Y: preliminary report of five cases. *Obes Surg* 1994;4:353–7.
30. Hashizume M, Takenaka K, Yanaga K, Ohta M, Kajiyama K, Shirabe K, Itasaka H, Nishizaki T, Sugimachi K. Laparoscopic hepatic resection for hepatocellular carcinoma. *Surg Endosc* 1995;9:1289–91.
31. Schuessler WW, Schulam PG, Clayman RV, Kavoussi LR. Laparoscopic radical prostatectomy: initial short-term experience. *Urology* 1997;50:854–7.
32. Abbou CC, Hoznek A, Salomon L, Olsson LE, Lobontiu A, Saint F, Cicco A, Antiphon P, Chopin D. Laparoscopic radical prostatectomy with a remote controlled robot. *J Urol* 2001;165:1964–6.
33. Gagner M, Pomp A, Herrera MF. Early experience with laparoscopic resections of islet cell tumors. *Surgery* 1996;120(6):1051–4.
34. Song J, Oh SJ, Kang WH, Hyung WJ, Choi SH, Noh SH. Robot-assisted gastrectomy with lymph node dissection for gastric cancer: lessons learned from an initial 100 consecutive procedures. *Ann Surg* 2009;249:927–32.
35. Boni L, Dionigi G, Cassinotti E, Di Giuseppe M, Diurni M, Rausei S, Cantore F, Dionigi R. Single incision laparoscopic right colectomy. *Surg Endosc* 2010;24:3233–6.
36. Kuhry E, Schwenk WF, Gaupset R, Romild U, Bonjer HJ. Long-term results of laparoscopic colorectal cancer resection. *Cochrane Database Syst Rev* 2008;2:CD003432.
37. Nussbaum DP, Speicher PJ, Ganapathi AM, Englum BR, Keenan JE, Mantyh CR, Migaly J. Laparoscopic versus open low anterior resection for rectal cancer: results from the national cancer data base. *J Gastrointest Surg* 2015;19:124–32.
38. Zmora O, Weiss EG. Trocar site recurrence in laparoscopic surgery for colorectal cancer. Myth or real concern? *Surg Oncol Clin N Am* 2001;10:625–38.
39. Pearlstone DB, Feig BW, Mansfield PF. Port site recurrences after laparoscopy for malignant disease. *Semin Surg Oncol* 1999;16:307–12.
40. Zanghì A, Cavallaro A, Piccolo G, Fisichella R, Di Vita M, Spartà D, Zanghì G, Berretta S, Palermo F, Cappellani A. Dissemination metastasis after laparoscopic colorectal surgery versus conventional open surgery for colorectal cancer: a meta-analysis. *Eur Rev Med Pharmacol Sci* 2013;17:1174–84.
41. Velanovich V. The effects of staging laparoscopy on trocar site and peritoneal recurrence of pancreatic cancer. *Surg Endosc* 2004;18:310–313.
42. Jarnagin WR, Bodniewicz J, Dougherty E, Conlon K, Blumgart LH, Fong Y. A prospective analysis of staging laparoscopy in patients with primary and secondary hepatobiliary malignancies. *J Gastrointest Surg* 2000;4:34–43.
43. Lo CM, Lai EC, Liu CL, Fan ST, Wong J. Laparoscopy and laparoscopic ultrasonography avoid exploratory laparotomy in patients with hepatocellular carcinoma. *Ann Surg* 1198;227:527–32.
44. Foroutani A, Garland AM, Berber E, String A, Engle K, Ryan TL, Pearl JM, Siperstein AE. Laparoscopic ultrasound vs. triphasic computed tomography for detecting liver tumors. *Arch Surg* 2000;135:933–8.
45. Kim HJ, D'Angelica M, Hiotis SP, Shoup M, Weber SM. Laparoscopic staging for liver, biliary, pancreas, and gastric cancer. *Curr Probl Surg* 2007;44:228–69.
46. Weber SM, DeMatteo RP, Fong Y, Blumgart LH, Jarnagin WR. Staging laparoscopy in patients with extrahepatic biliary carcinoma. *Ann Surg* 2002;235:392–9.
47. van Delden OM, de Wit LT, Nieveen van Dijkum EJM, Smits NJ, Gouma DJ, Reeders JW. Value of laparoscopic ultrasonography in staging of proximal bile duct tumors. *J Ultrasound Med* 1997 16:7–12.
48. Tilleman EH, de Castro SM, Busch OR, Bemelman WA, van Gulik TM, Obertop H, Gouma DJ. Diagnostic laparoscopy and laparoscopic ultrasound for staging of patients with malignant proximal bile duct obstruction. *J Gastroint Surg* 2002;6:426–43.
49. Chang L, Stefanidis D, Richardson WS, Earle DB, Fanelli RD. The role of staging laparoscopy for intraabdominal cancers: an evidence-based review. *Surg Endosc* 2009;23:231–41.
50. Thaler K, Kanneganti S, Khajanchee Y, Wilson C, Swanstrom L, Hansen P. The evolving role of staging laparoscopy in the treatment of colorectal hepatic metastasis. *Arch Surg* 2005;140:727–34.

51. Jarnagin WR, Conlon K, Bodniewicz J, Dougherty E, Dematteo RP, Blumgart LH, Fong Y. A clinical scoring system predicts the yield of diagnostic laparoscopy in patients with potentially resectable hepatic colorectal metastases. *Cancer* 2001;91:1121–8.

52. Goletti O, Celon G, Galatioto C, Viaggi B, Lippolis PV, Pieri L, Cavina E. Is laparoscopic sonography a reliable and sensitive procedure for staging colorectal cancer? *Surg Endosc* 1198;12:1236–41.

53. Rahusen FD, Cuesta MA, Borgstein PJ, Bleichrodt RP, Barkhof F, Doesburg T, Meijer S. Selection of patients for resection of colorectal metastases to the liver using diagnostic laparoscopy and laparoscopic ultrasonography. *Ann Surg* 1999;230:31–37.

54. D'Angelica M, Jarnagin W, DeMatteo R, Conlon K, Blumgart LH, Fong Y. Staging laparoscopy for potentially resectable noncolorectal, nonneuroendocrine liver metastases. *Ann Surg Oncol* 2002;9:204–9.

55. Pietrabissa A, Caramella D, Di Candio G, Carobbi A, Boggi U, Rossi G, Mosca F. Laparoscopy and laparoscopic ultrasonography for staging pancreatic cancer: critical appraisal. *World J Surg* 1999;23:998–1002.

56. Awad SS, Colletti L, Mulholland M, Knol J, Rothman ED, Scheiman J, Eckhauser FE. Multimodality staging optimizes resectability in patients with pancreatic and ampullary cancer. *Am Surg* 1197;63:634–8.

57. Conlon KC, Dougherty E, Klimstra DS, Coit DG, Turnbull AD, Brennan MF. The value of minimal access surgery in the staging of patients with potentially resectable peripancreatic malignancy. *Ann Surg* 1996;223:134–40.

58. Pisters PW, Lee JE, Vauthey JN, Charnsangavej C, Evans DB. Laparoscopy in the staging of pancreatic cancer. *Br J Surg* 2001;88:325–37.

59. Nieveen van Dijkum EJ, Romijn MG, Terwee CB, de Wit LT, van der Meulen JH, Lameris HS, Rauws EA, Obertop H, van Eyck CH, Bossuyt PM, Gouma DJ. Laparoscopic staging and subsequent palliation in patients with peripancreatic carcinoma. *Ann Surg* 2003;237:66–73.

60. Liu RC, Traverso LW. Diagnostic laparoscopy improves staging of pancreatic cancer deemed locally unresectable by computed tomography. *Surg Endosc* 2005;19:638–42.

61. Stefanidis D, Grove KD, Schwesinger WH, Thomas CR Jr. The current role of staging laparoscopy for adenocarcinoma of the pancreas: a review. *Ann Oncol* 2006;17:189–99.

62. Gloor B, Todd KE, Reber HA. Diagnostic workup of patients with suspected pancreatic carcinoma: the University of California–Los Angeles approach. *Cancer* 1997;79:1780–6.

63. Jimenez RE, Warshaw AL, Rattner DW, Willett CG, McGrath D, Fernandez-del Castillo C. Impact of laparoscopic staging in the treatment of pancreatic cancer. *Arch Surg* 2000;135:409–14.

64. Luque-de Leon E, Tsiotos GG, Balsiger B, Barnwell J, Burgart LJ, Sarr MG. Staging laparoscopy for pancreatic cancer should be used to select the best means of palliation and not only to maximize the resectability rate. *J Gastrointest Surg* 1999;3:111–7.

65. Schachter PP, Avni Y, Shimonov M, Gvirtz G, Rosen A, Czerniak A. The impact of laparoscopy and laparoscopic ultrasonography on the management of pancreatic cancer. *Arch Surg* 2000;135:1303–7.

66. Morganti AG, Brizi MG, Macchia G, Sallustio G, Costamagna G, Alfieri S, Mattiucci GC, et al. The prognostic effect of clinical staging in pancreatic adenocarcinoma. *Ann Surg Oncol* 2005;12:145–51.

67. Connor S, Bosonnet L, Alexakis N, Raraty M, Ghaneh P, Sutton R, Neoptolemos JP. Serum CA19–9 measurement increases the effectiveness of staging laparoscopy in patients with suspected pancreatic malignancy. *Dig Surg* 2005;22:80–5.

68. Burke EC, Karpeh MS, Conlon KC, Brennan MF. Laparoscopy in the management of gastric adenocarcinoma. *Ann Surg* 1997;225:262–7.

69. Lehnert T, Rudek B, Kienle P, Buhl K, Herfarth C. Impact of diagnostic laparoscopy on the management of gastric cancer: prospective study of 120 consecutive patients with primary gastric adenocarcinoma. *Br J Surg* 2002;89:471–5.

70. Goh PM, So JB. Role of laparoscopy in the management of stomach cancer. *Semin Surg Oncol* 1999;16:321–6.

71. Stell DA, Carter CR, Stewart I, Anderson JR. Prospective comparison of laparoscopy, ultrasonography and computed tomography in the staging of gastric cancer. *Br J Surg* 1996;83:1260–2.

72. D'Ugo DM, Pende V, Persiani R, Rausei S, Picciocchi A. Laparoscopic staging of gastric cancer: an overview. *J Am Coll Surg* 2003;196:965–74.

73. Burke EC, Karpeh MS, Conlon KC, Brennan MF. Laparoscopy in the management of gastric adenocarcinoma. *Ann Surg* 1997;225:262–7.

74. Conlon KC. Staging laparoscopy for gastric cancer. *Ann Ital Chir* 2001;72:33–7

75. Ribeiro U Jr, Safatle-Ribeiro AV, Zilberstein B, Ucerino D, Yagi OK, Bresciani CC, Jacob CE, Iryia K, Gama-Rodrigues J. Does the intraoperative peritoneal lavage cytology add prognostic information in patients with potentially curative gastric resection? *J Gastrointest Surg* 2006;10:170–6.

76. Bentrem D, Wilton A, Mazumdar M, Brennan M, Coit D. The value of peritoneal cytology as a preoperative predictor in patients with gastric carcinoma undergoing a curative resection. *Ann Surg Oncol* 2005;12:347–53.

77. de Manzoni G, Verlato G, Di Leo A, Tomezzoli A, Pedrazzani C, Pasini F, Piubello Q, Cordiano C. Peritoneal cytology does not increase the prognostic information provided by TNM in gastric cancer. *World J Surg* 2006;30:579–84.

78. Krasna MJ, Reed CE, Nedzwiecki D, Hollis DR, Luketich JD, DeCamp MM, Mayer RJ, Sugarbaker DJ. CALGB 9380: a prospective trial of the feasibility of thoracoscopy/laparoscopy in staging esophageal cancer. *Ann Thorac Surg* 2001;71:1073–9.

79. Heath EI, Kaufman HS, Talamini MA, Wu TT, Wheeler J, Heitmiller RF, Kleinberg L, Yang SC, Olukayode K, Forastiere AA. The role of laparoscopy in preoperative staging of esophageal cancer. *Surg Endosc* 2000;14:495–9.

80. Bonavina L, Incarvone R, Lattuada E, Segalin A, Cesana B, Peracchia A. Preoperative laparoscopy in management of patients with carcinoma of the esophagus and of the esophagogastric junction. *J Surg Oncol* 1997;65:171–4.

81. Romijn MG, van Overhagen H, Spillenaar Bilgen EJ, Ijzermans JN, Tilanus HW, Lameris JS. Laparoscopy and laparoscopic ultrasonography in the staging of oesophageal and cardial carcinoma. *Br J Surg* 1998;85:1010–2.

82. Asoglu O, Porter L, Donohue JH, Cha SS. Laparoscopy for the definitive diagnosis of intraabdominal lymphoma. *Mayo Clin Proc* 2005;80:625–31.

83. Baccarani U, Carroll BJ, Hiatt JR, Donini A, Terrosu G, Decker R, Chandra M, Bresadola F, Phillips EH. Comparison of laparoscopic and open staging in Hodgkin's disease. *Arch Surg* 1998;133:517–22.

84. Silecchia G, Raparelli L, Perrotta N, Fantini A, Fabiano P, Monarca B, Basso N. Accuracy of laparoscopy in the diagnosis and staging of lymphoproliferative diseases. *World J Surg* 2003;27:653–8.

85. Casaccia M, Torelli P, Cavaliere D, Panaro F, Nardi I, Rossi E, Spriano M, Bacigalupo A, Gentile R, Valente U. Laparoscopic lymph node biopsy in intra-abdominal lymphoma: high diagnostic accuracy achieved with a minimally invasive procedure. *Surg Laparosc Endosc Percutan Tech* 2007;17:175–8.

86. Zanghì G, Arena M, Di Stefano G, Benfatto G, Basile F. The role of laparoscopy and intraoperative ultrasound in the diagnosis and staging of lymphomas. *G Chir* 2012;33:71–3.

87. Torab FC, Bokobza B, Branicki F. Laparoscopy in gastrointestinal malignancies. *Ann N Y Acad Sci* 2008;1138:155–61.

88. Clinical Outcomes of Surgical Therapy Study Group. A comparison of laparoscopically assisted and open colectomy for colon cancer. *N Engl J Med* 2004;350:2050–9.

89. Veldkamp R, Kuhry E, Hop WC, Jeekel J, Kazemier G, Bonjer HJ, Haglind E, Påhlman L, Cuesta MA, Msika S. Laparoscopic surgery versus open surgery for colon cancer: short-term outcomes of a randomised trial. *Lancet Oncol* 2005;6:477–84.

90. Guillou PJ, Quirke P, Thorpe H, Walker J, Jayne DG, Smith AM, Heath RM, Brown JM. Short-term endpoints of conventional versus laparoscopic-assisted surgery in patients with colorectal cancer (MRC CLASICC trial): multicentre, randomised controlled trial. *Lancet* 2005;365:1718–26.

91. Lacy AM, García-Valdecasas JC, Delgado S, Castells A, Taurá P, Piqué JM, Visa J. Laparoscopy-assisted colectomy versus open colectomy for treatment of non-metastatic colon cancer: a randomised trial. *Lancet* 2002;359:2224–9.

92. Hewett PJ, Allardyce RA, Bagshaw PF, Frampton CM, Frizelle FA, Rieger NA, Smith JS, Solomon MJ, Stephens JH, Stevenson AR. Short-term outcomes of the Australasian randomized clinical study comparing laparoscopic and conventional open surgical treatments for colon cancer: the ALCCaS trial. *Ann Surg* 2008;248:728–38.

93. Koh YX, Chok AY, Zheng HL, Tan CS, Chow PK, Wong WK, Goh BK. A systematic review and meta-analysis comparing laparoscopic versus open gastric resections for gastrointestinal stromal tumors of the stomach. *Ann Surg Oncol* 2013;20:3549–60.

94. Liang JW, Zheng ZC, Zhang JJ, Zhang T, Zhao Y, Yang W, Liu YQ. Laparoscopic versus open gastric resections for gastric gastrointestinal stromal tumors: a meta-analysis. *Surg Laparosc Endosc Percutan Tech* 2013;23:378–87.

95. Lee SE, Kim YW, Lee JH, Ryu KW, Cho SJ, Lee JY, Kim CG, et al. Developing an institutional protocol guideline for laparoscopy-assisted distal gastrectomy. *Ann Surg Oncol* 2009;16:2231–6.

96. Kim HH, Hyung WJ, Cho GS, Kim MC, Han SU, Kim W, Ryu SW, Lee HJ, Song KY. Morbidity and mortality of laparoscopic gastrectomy versus open gastrectomy for gastric cancer: an interim report – a phase III multicenter, prospective, randomized Trial (KLASS Trial). *Ann Surg* 2010;251:417–20.

97. Hwang SH, Park Do J, Jee YS, Kim MC, Kim HH, Lee HJ, Yang HK, Lee KU. Actual 3-year survival after laparoscopy-assisted gastrectomy for gastric cancer. *Arch Surg* 2009;144:559–64.

98. Song J, Lee HJ, Cho GS, Han SU, Kim MC, Ryu SW, Kim W, Song KY, Kim HH, Hyung WJ, Korean Laparoscopic Gastrointestinal Surgery Study (KLASS) Group. Recurrence following laparoscopy-assisted gastrectomy for gastric cancer: a multicenter retrospective analysis of 1,417 patients. *Ann Surg Oncol* 2010;17:1777–86.

99. Kim HH, Han SU, Kim MC, Hyung WJ, Kim W, Lee HJ, Ryu SW, Cho GS, Song KY, Ryu SY. Long-term results of laparoscopic gastrectomy for gastric cancer: a large-scale case-control and case-matched Korean multicenter study. *J Clin Oncol* 2014;7:627–33.

100. Briez N, Piessen G, Bonnetain F, Brigand C, Carrere N, Collet D, Doddoli C, Flamein R, Mabrut JY, Meunier B. Open versus laparoscopically-assisted oesophagectomy for cancer: a multicentre randomised controlled phase III trial – the MIRO trial. *BMC Cancer* 2011;11:310.

101. Maas KW, Biere SS, Scheepers JJ, Gisbertz SS, Turrado Rodriguez VT, van der Peet DL, Cuesta MA. Minimally invasive intrathoracic anastomosis after Ivor Lewis esophagectomy for cancer: a review of transoral or transthoracic use of staplers. *Surg Endosc* 2012;26:1795–802.

102. Schumer E, Perry K, Melvin WS. Minimally invasive esophagectomy for esophageal cancer: evolution and review. *Surg Laparosc Endosc Percutan Tech* 2012;22:383–6.

103. Kendrick ML, Cusati D. Total laparoscopic pancreaticoduodenectomy: feasibility and outcome in an early experience. *Arch Surg* 2010;145:19–23.

104. Corcione F, Pirozzi F, Cuccurullo D, Piccolboni D, Caracino V, Galante F, Cusano D, Sciuto A. Laparoscopic pancreaticoduodenectomy: experience of 22 cases. *Surg Endosc* 2013;27:2131–6.

105. Ammori BJ, Ayiomamitis GD. Laparoscopic pancreaticoduodenectomy and distal pancreatectomy: a UK experience and a systematic review of the literature. *Surg Endosc* 2011;25:2084–99.

106. Vibert E, Perniceni T, Levard H, Denet C, Shahri NK, Gayet B. Laparoscopic liver resection. *Br J Surg* 2006;93:67–72.

107. Dagher I, Belli G, Fantini C, Laurent A, Tayar C, Lainas P, Tranchart H, Franco D, Cherqui D. Laparoscopic hepatectomy for hepatocellular carcinoma: a European experience. *J Am Coll Surg* 2010;211:16–23.

108. Bencini L, Bernini M, Farsi M. Laparoscopic approach to gastrointestinal malignancies: toward the future with caution. *World J Gastroenterol* 2014;20:1777–89.

109. Derossis AM, Fried GM, Abrahamowicz M, Sigman HH, Barkun JS, Meakins JL. Development of a model for training and evaluation of laparoscopic skills. *Am J Surg* 1998;175:482–7.

110. Majeed AW, Reed MW, Johnson AG. Simulated laparoscopic cholecystectomy. *Ann R Coll Surg Engl* 1992;74:70–1.

111. Mughal M. A cheap laparoscopic surgery trainer. *Ann R Coll Surg Engl* 1992;74:256–7.

112. Gallagher AG, Satava RM. Virtual reality as a metric for the assessment of laparoscopic psychomotor skills. Learning curves and reliability measures. *Surg Endosc* 2002;16:1746–52.

113. Seymour NE, Gallagher AG, Roman SA, O'Brien MK, Bansal VK, Andersen DK, Satava RM. Virtual reality training improves operating room performance: results of a randomized, double-blinded study. *Ann Surg* 2002;236:458–63.

114. Grantcharov TP, Kristiansen VB, Bendix J, Bardram L, Rosenberg J, Funch-Jensen P. Randomized clinical trial of virtual reality simulation for laparoscopic skills training. *Br J Surg* 2004;91:146–50.

115. European Association of Endoscopic Surgeons. Training and assessment of competence. *Surg Endosc* 1994;8:721–2.

116. Society of American Gastrointestinal Endoscopic Surgeons. Granting of privileges for laparoscopic general surgery. *Am J Surg* 1991;161:324–5.

117. Bogen EM, Augestad KM, Patel HR, Lindsetmo RO. Telementoring in education of laparoscopic surgeons: an emerging technology. *World J Gastrointest Endosc* 2014;6:148–55.

118. Santomauro M, Reina GA, Stroup SP, L'Esperance JO. Telementoring in robotic surgery. *Curr Opin Urol* 2013;23:141–5.

119. Schlachta CM, Mamazza J, Seshadri PA, Cadeddu M, Gregoire R, Poulin EC. Defining a learning curve for laparoscopic colorectal resections. *Dis Colon Rectum* 2001;44:217–22.

120. Tekkis PP, Senagore AJ, Delaney CP, Fazio VW. Evaluation of the learning curve in laparoscopic colorectal surgery: comparison of right-sided and left-sided resections. *Ann Surg* 2005;242:83–91.

121. Miskovic D, Ni M, Wyles SM, Tekkis P, Hanna GB. Learning curve and case selection in laparoscopic colorectal surgery: systematic review and international multicenter analysis of 4852 cases. *Dis Colon Rectum* 2012;55:1300–10.

122. Dinçler S, Koller MT, Steurer J, Bachmann LM, Christen D, Buchmann P. Multidimensional analysis of learning curves in laparoscopic sigmoid resection: eight-year results. *Dis Colon Rectum* 2003;46:1371–78.

123. Shenvi SC. First-place essay – revolution: surgical training: time for a revolution. *Bull Am Coll Surg* 2014;99:17–9.

124. Brunt LM. Celebrating a decade of innovation in surgical education. *Bull Am Coll Surg* 2014;99:10–5.

125. Sanchez BR, Mohr CJ, Morton JM, Safadi BY, Alami RS, Curet MJ. Comparison of totally robotic laparoscopic Roux-en-Y gastric bypass and traditional laparoscopic Roux-en-Y gastric bypass. *Surg Obes Relat Dis* 2005;1:549–54.

126. Lim PC, Kang E, Park do H. Learning curve and surgical outcome for robotic-assisted hysterectomy with lymphadenectomy: case-matched controlled comparison with laparoscopy and laparotomy for treatment of endometrial cancer. *J Minim Invasive Gynecol* 2010;17:739–48.

127. Smith JA Jr, Herrell SD. Robotic-assisted laparoscopic prostatectomy: do minimally invasive approaches offer significant advantages? *J Clin Oncol* 2005;23:8170–5.

128. Menon M, Tewari A, Baize B, Guillonneau B, Vallancien G. Prospective comparison of radical retropubic prostatectomy and robot-assisted anatomic prostatectomy: the Vattikuti Urology Institute experience. *Urology* 2002;60:864–8.

129. Barbash GI, Glied SA. New technology and health care costs – the case of robot-assisted surgery. *N Engl J Med* 2010;363:701–4.

130. Herron DM, Marohn M, SAGES-MIRA Robotic Surgery Consensus Group. A consensus document on robotic surgery. *Surg Endosc* 2008;22:313–25.

131. Trinh QD, Sammon J, Sun M, Ravi P, Ghani KR, Bianchi M, Jeong W, et al. Perioperative outcomes of robot-assisted radical prostatectomy compared with open radical prostatectomy: results from the nationwide inpatient sample. *Eur Urol* 2012;61:679–85.

132. Tewari A, Sooriakumaran P, Bloch DA, Seshadri-Kreaden U, Hebert AE, Wiklund P. Positive surgical margin and perioperative complication rates of primary surgical treatments for prostate cancer: a systematic review and meta-analysis comparing retropubic, laparoscopic, and robotic prostatectomy. *Eur Urol* 2012;62:1–15.

133. Cha EK, Lee DJ, Del Pizzo JJ. Current status of robotic partial nephrectomy (RPN). *BJU Int* 2011;108:935–41.

134. Yu HY, Hevelone ND, Lipsitz SR, Kowalczyk KJ, Hu JC. Use, costs and comparative effectiveness of robotic assisted, laparoscopic and open urological surgery. *J Urol* 2012;187:1392–8.

135. Orvieto MA, DeCastro GJ, Trinh QD, Jeldres C, Katz MH, Patel VR, Zorn KC. Oncological and functional outcomes after robot-assisted radical cystectomy: critical review of current status. *Urology* 2011;78:977–84.

136. Ng CK, Kauffman EC, Lee MM, Otto BJ, Portnoff A, Ehrlich JR, Schwartz MJ, Wang GJ, Scherr DS. A comparison of postoperative complications in open versus robotic cystectomy. *Eur Urol* 2010;57:274–81.

137. Reza M, Maeso S, Blasco JA, Andradas E. Meta-analysis of observational studies on the safety and effectiveness of robotic gynaecological surgery. *Br J Surg* 2010;97:1772–83.

138. Yim GW, Kim YT. Robotic surgery in gynecologic cancer. *Curr Opin Obstet Gynecol* 2012;24:14–23.

139. Louie BE. Robotic lobectomy for non-small cell lung cancer. *Indian J Surg Oncol* 2013;4:125–31.

140. Yu HY, Friedlander DF, Patel S, Hu JC. The current status of robotic oncologic surgery. *CA Cancer J Clin* 2013;63:45–56.

141. Woo Y, Hyung WJ, Pak KH, Inaba K, Obama K, Choi SH, Noh SH. Robotic gastrectomy as an oncologically sound alternative to laparoscopic resections for the treatment of early-stage gastric cancers. *Arch Surg* 2011;146:1086–92.

142. Japanese Gastric Cancer Association. Japanese gastric cancer treatment guidelines 2010 (ver. 3). *Gastric Cancer* 2011;14:113–23.

143. Xiong B, Ma L, Zhang C. Robotic versus laparoscopic gastrectomy for gastric cancer: a meta-analysis of short outcomes. *Surg Oncol* 2012;21:274–80.

144. Weber PA, Merola S, Wasielewski A, Ballantyne GH. Telerobotic-assisted laparoscopic right and sigmoid colectomies for benign disease. *Dis Colon Rectum* 2002;45:1689–94.

145. Antoniou SA, Antoniou GA, Koch OO, Pointner R, Granderath FA. Robot-assisted laparoscopic surgery of the colon and rectum. *Surg Endosc* 2012;26:1–11.

146. Papanikolaou IG. Robotic surgery for colorectal cancer: systematic review of the literature. *Surg Laparosc Endosc Percutan Tech* 2014;24:478–83.

147. Baik SH, Ko YT, Kang CM, Lee WJ, Kim NK, Sohn SK, Chi HS, Cho CH. Robotic tumor-specific mesorectal excision of rectal cancer: short-term outcome of a pilot randomized trial. *Surg Endosc* 2008;22:1601–8.

148. Pigazzi A, Ellenhorn JD, Ballantyne GH, Paz IB. Robotic-assisted laparoscopic low anterior resection with total mesorectal excision for rectal cancer. *Surg Endosc* 2006;20:1521–1525.

149. Kim CW, Kim CH, Baik SH. Outcomes of robotic-assisted colorectal surgery compared with laparoscopic and open surgery: a systematic review. *J Gastrointest Surg* 2014;18:816–30.

150. Collinson FJ, Jayne DG, Pigazzi A, Tsang C, Barrie JM, Edlin R, Garbett C, Guillou P, Holloway I, Howard H. An international, multicentre, prospective, randomised, controlled, unblinded, parallel-group trial of robotic-assisted versus standard laparoscopic surgery for the curative treatment of rectal cancer. *Int J Colorectal Dis* 2012;27:233–41.

151. Leung U, Fong Y. Robotic liver surgery. *Hepatobiliary Surg Nutr* 2014;3:288–94.

152. Liang S, Hameed U, Jayaraman S. Laparoscopic pancreatectomy: indications and outcomes. *World J Gastroenterol* 2014;20:14246–54.

153. Barbash GI, Glied SA. New technology and health care costs – the case of robot-assisted surgery. *N Engl J Med* 2010;363:701–4.

154. Lee L, Li C, Landry T, Latimer E, Carli F, Fried GM, Feldman LS. A systematic review of economic evaluations of enhanced recovery pathways for colorectal surgery. *Ann Surg* 2014;259:670–6.

15

Surgery for older cancer patients

PONNANDAI S SOMASUNDAR, LYNDA WYLD AND RICCARDO A AUDISIO

INTRODUCTION

Cancer is a disease of the elderly: this is true for the majority of cancer types. The average life expectancy of the western population has increased significantly in the last 40 years and is predicted to rise further such that most babies born in the western world since 2000 will live to see their 100th birthday [1]. In the EU, life expectancy from birth is expected to increase further from 76.7 years in 2010 to 84.6 in males and from 82.5 to 89.1 in females. The population in the US of those older than 65 has been projected by the US censor bureau to be about 90 million by 2050. In the EU, similar projections have been made with the European Commission projecting the percentage of those older than 65 to rise from the present level of 17% to 30% of the EU's predicted total population of 517 million by 2060 (data from the European Commission). As a consequence of this increase in the age demographic of Western populations, the incidence of most common cancers will increase, as will the need for surgical therapies in these older cancer patients.

Older age is associated with a number of both physiological and pathological changes which may impact on treatment tolerance and life expectancy: nutritional imbalances, polypharmacy, psychosocial issues, the number and severity of comorbidities, cognitive impairment and impaired functional reserve in all organ systems resulting in frailty. Appropriate management of these patients depends on identifying and quantifying these changes for each individual followed by complex treatment planning specifically tailored to their needs via a true multidisciplinary approach.

The majority of solid organ malignancies like GI cancers, lung cancer, head and neck cancers and sarcoma are optimally treated by surgical excision. However, as the patients' age increases surgical complication rates, mortality, length of stay and intensive care unit admissions increase [2] and affect the oncological outcomes. Surgery and general anaesthesia may impair, either temporarily or permanently, the functional status of the individual. For example, recovery following abdominal surgery, when evaluated using a measure of functional exercise capacity, showed two-thirds of people had not re-attained baseline levels 9 weeks after surgery [3,4].

Older patients often present with cancer at a later stage than younger patients or present as an emergency. This reflects reduced symptom awareness and the lack of routine screening in this age group. Emergency presentation with cancer is commonly associated with increased morbidity and mortality and is one of the reasons for inferior outcomes in this age group.

The other major contributing factor to inferior cancer outcomes in this age group is non-standard treatment. There is a global lack of trial data relating to cancer therapies in those older than 70, and hence evidence-based guidelines are lacking. Treatment plans are often modified because of concerns about treatment tolerance and surgery is often omitted despite evidence that in many cancer types it improves survival in this age group [5–7].

Older cancer patients have been disadvantaged as a consequence of inappropriate treatment which is clearly demonstrated by a lack of improvement in cancer-related survival rates.

Good-quality research is needed, ideally from randomized controlled trials (RCTs), but where this is difficult, from good-quality prospective cohort studies, and in all cases accurate, detailed assessment of fitness and frailty will enable comparison between treatment modalities.

ASSESSING OLDER PATIENTS

Geriatric patients are unique, with multiple complex medical problems, impaired physiological and functional reserves, geriatric syndromes (such as dementia, falls, malnutrition, sensory impairments) and restrictions in personal and social resources, which result in a decreased ability to recover fully from stressors such as surgery [8].

The elderly frail patient who undergoes surgery is more likely to experience postoperative complications (e.g. delirium, pneumonia and urinary tract infection), prolonged hospital stays, discharge to nursing homes or long-term care facilities, amplified financial burdens and higher mortality rates than fit patients [9].

Patients undergoing surgery are usually evaluated by the surgeon with a physical examination, some routine laboratory tests and sometimes a preoperative cardiological opinion. Expert input from a geriatrician is rarely requested [10] The American Society of Anesthesiologists physical status classification (ASA class) is the anesthesiology tool utilized worldwide: ASA class is not sensitive enough to identify patients who are at risk of developing postoperative complications [11,12]. These geriatric surgical patients have unique impairments that need further assessment beyond the conventional preoperative evaluation [13]. The Comprehensive Geriatric Assessment (CGA) is used by geriatricians in their evaluations, a multidisciplinary approach for the evaluation of the elderly population that often reveals information missed by routine history or physical examination alone. Its advantages include prolongation of life, prevention of geriatric syndromes (postoperative delirium for example), the prevention of institutionalization and improvements in postoperative subjective well-being [14]. CGA is a systematic approach to assessing physical functioning, comorbidity, polypharmacy, nutrition, cognition and emotional status in elderly patients. The solid evidence supporting this approach has been shown by RCTs proving that a geriatric intervention guided by a CGA has positive effects on health, functional status and mortality [15,16]. Despite this CGA is still not routinely used in the assessment of elderly oncology patients. Nevertheless, a sizeable number of review articles promote the introduction of CGA as a routine assessment in elderly patients with cancer. In addition some observational studies suggest that the evaluated domains have predictive value in elderly cancer patients receiving chemotherapy or undergoing surgery [17].

There are several validation studies currently ongoing to validate CGA-based approaches in older cancer patients. The CGA was studied by Kristjansson and colleagues on elective colorectal cancer patients. They did a prospective observational cohort study which confirmed that a CGA-based stratification predicted complications in elderly patients undergoing elective colorectal cancer surgery. Patients who were frail had a significantly higher morbidity than patients in the fit and intermediate groups. In addition, the rate of postoperative complications was not related to increasing age, ASA classification or tumour stage [12]. Sun Wook Kim and colleagues performed a study which included patients undergoing intermediate-risk or high-risk elective operations in whom CGA was performed on a prospective basis. The most significant findings of this study were that in the postoperative setting 1-year all-cause mortality rate, length of hospital stay and likelihood of discharge to a nursing facility could be predicted from particular components of the CGA in older surgical patients. A predictive model based on the CGA showed unfavourable outcomes with better accuracy than the conventional ASA classification. A higher score is correlated with a greater mortality risk [18].

In a regular surgical oncology practice CGA is difficult to adopt as the assessments are time-consuming and there is no particular model to help the physician improve the outcomes. The morbidity or mortality prediction is good, but unless appropriate interventions are instituted the outcomes may not improve. The trend of declining 30-day morbidity and mortality in the face of an increasing incidence of cancer among older patients, with multiple comorbidities, and complex treatment schedules underscores the important and significant advances in surgical and aesthetic techniques in recent years. Several organizations are now focusing on cancer survivorship and community reintegration after cancer treatment.

Research is needed to tackle the development and application of interventions that will prevent or reduce negative outcomes of cancer and its treatment. A handful of studies have looked into CGA-guided interventions. Two randomized studies addressed the effect of a CGA in the outpatient setting of older cancer patients who had undergone surgery. McCorkle and colleagues [19] performed a study where geriatric nurse practitioners conducted a CGA in the patients' home for cancer patients treated surgically. In a month-long period both patients and their caregivers received three home visits and five phone calls for comprehensive clinical assessments, monitoring and teaching, including skill training. There was a survival advantage, with a 2-year survival rate of 67% in the group with intervention compared with 40% in the control group.

Goodwin and colleagues [20] assessed the effect of nurse-based care management in the treatment of older women with breast cancer. They identified that patients in the CGA-directed intervention group were significantly more likely to return to normal function within 2 months after completion of surgery compared with controls. It has been identified that CGA-guided interventions have a positive impact on health outcomes, including a reduction in the risk of falls, prevention of disability progression, unplanned hospitalization and nursing home admission, providing appropriate evidence supporting the use of a multidimensional approach in older patients [21].

CGA is time-consuming and its use may be better restricted to a subgroup of older patients identified as vulnerable by the use of simple screening tools such as the Groningen Frailty Index or the Vulnerable Elders Survey [17]. It has been found that disability is associated with increased rates of adverse outcomes [22], preventable hospitalization and utilization of health care resources [23].

Interventions should be designed to prevent disability to potentially generate large health care savings, and in addition they also must lead to important reductions in the physical, emotional, social and financial problems attributable to disability to the individual patient [24–26].

Attempts made to improve outcomes such as functional decline without having any prior injury are very limited. A prospective study by Gill and colleagues involving 188 frail older patients studied the effect of home-based physical therapy. The intervention focused on improving underlying impairments, including muscle strength, balance, ability to transfer from one position to another and mobility. Use of the intervention was associated with less functional decline over a subsequent 12-month period [27]. This so-called 'pre-habilitation,' or exercise before surgery, may be useful in frail elderly patients who are undergoing cancer surgery. The essential requirements for pre-habilitation are not yet fully defined. A 4-week period of pre-habilitation for muscle strength has been shown to improve recovery after a total knee arthroplasty among patients 50 to 60 years of age [28], but the evidence is limited for oncologic surgery.

Malnourishment is well known to be associated with adverse postoperative outcomes such as abdominal abscess, chest infection, wound infection, urinary tract infection, bacteremia/septicemia, wound dehiscence, anastomotic leak, renal dysfunction and hepatic failure. The percentage of patients experiencing major complications increases as nutritional status deteriorates and is more than doubled even in the presence of mild nutritional impairment [29]. Nutritional deficits, either global or specific, are more common in older patients, and their assessment is a routine component of the CGA. Correction of these preoperatively may confer benefit in older patients.

DISEASE SITE-SPECIFIC SURGICAL RESECTION CONSIDERATIONS IN OLDER PATIENTS

Chronological age is still considered to be an indication for refusal of treatment by many surgeons and physicians: biological age is a much more appropriate but less easily definable parameter. A survey of a large group of primary care providers in France showed that chronological age of the patient was strongly associated with the decision not to refer patients with advanced cancer (not defined) to oncologic specialties (odds ratio 0.55; 95% confidence interval [CI] 0.35–0.86; $p = 0.009$) [30]. Similar findings were also seen in a survey of 1408 French medical and radiation oncologists to whom breast cancer patients were referred, where significant differences in treatment plans were observed depending on patient age alone [31].

In solid cancers, surgical resection when feasible is one of the most successful modalities of therapy. The age of the patient as a factor helping to decide on surgery is becoming less important for adequate and appropriate surgery. The belief of this surgical philosophy is different in different parts of the world, as it is not uncommon for surgeons to routinely perform cancer resections on patients with multiple comorbidities and increased frailty. The Eindhoven Cancer Registry study found an acceptance rate of 95% for surgical resection in non-metastatic colorectal cancer patients who were elderly. This study involved 8000 patients aged 50 to 80 years with colon, rectal and other cancers [32]. A study comparing colorectal cancer resection outcomes among 32,621 Veterans Administration patients in the US between temporal cohorts of 1987 to 1993 and 1994 to 2000 found that significantly more patients aged 80 or more received surgical resection in the latter time period [33]. Nascimbeni and colleagues looked at the temporal trends in patients undergoing colorectal cancer resections and compared outcomes between 1975 to 1984 and 1995 to 2004. They found that patients aged 75 years or more increased from 19% to 29% and those aged 85 years or more doubled from 3% to 6% [34].

Inadequate treatment in older cancer patients is associated with poor survival [34]. Rates of surgery in elderly cancer patients have increased in recent years which may be a factor in the improvements in outcomes seen in this age group. One study of the treatment and survival of older (>75 years of age) cancer patients in the Danish National Cancer Registry identified that the proportion of patients who were denied treatment or received only palliative therapy decreased by 35% from 19.8% in the period 1977 to 1982 to 13.1% in the period 1995 to 1999. This study also found that the proportion receiving 'curative' therapy increased from 36% to 49.2% during these same time intervals [35].

However, major cancer surgery may not be appropriate for everyone in this age group and, after full assessment, it is sometimes necessary to elect less radical options than major visceral resections. This is critically relevant for those patients undergoing major thoracic and abdominal resections as they have the greatest operative risks [36]. As with most solid malignancies lung cancer is primarily a disease of the elderly. Greater than 65% of lung cancer patients are older than 65 [37]. In these patients the standard of care for any age with resectable lung cancer has been anatomic lung lobectomy: the relative risks and efficacy of lesser resections (i.e. segmentectomy) are being evaluated in clinical trials [38]. In one of the large randomized trials lobectomy was associated with a mortality of 1.4% and no increased risk was found to be associated with advanced age [39]. Unfortunately this and several smaller studies have not characterized the elderly in adequate detail. There are several alternative therapies for lung cancer which may be used in those too frail for major surgery, such as ablation or radiotherapy. The criteria used for identifying such patients are not clearly defined [40,41].

Greater than half of all colon cancer patients are diagnosed when older than 65 years, and about 70% are diagnosed at early stages, when surgical resection is the cornerstone of treatment [42]. In colonic carcinoma curative resection is well tolerated in the elderly, and age alone should not be an indication for less aggressive therapy. The postoperative mortality and morbidity in the elderly are influenced by the presence of comorbidities [43]. Hence careful patient selection for surgical procedures is important, because frail elderly patients are at higher risk for complications than their counterparts who are not frail [11]. At present laparoscopic surgery seems to be associated with improved short-term outcomes in selected series of elderly colorectal patients. In a systematic review [44] of comparative outcomes of elderly and non-elderly patients with rectal cancer, postoperative morbidity was as high as 40% in elderly patients, not significantly higher than in younger patients. In those patients who survived the first year after surgery, they showed similar outcomes as their younger counterparts [45].

There has recently been an improvement in the outcomes for older patients undergoing liver resections for primary and secondary cancer due to improvements in anaesthesia, postoperative management and surgical techniques [46]. However, morbidity and mortality remain high compared with other types of surgery. There have been several retrospective studies which have shown that liver resection can be performed safely in elderly, but their length of hospital stay and their discharge to rehabilitation facilities are higher than those of their younger counterparts [47]. For example, in one series of 856 patients undergoing major hepatectomy [48] age was independently associated with surgical mortality (odds ratio 1.039; 95% CI 1.021–0.058; $p = 0.0029$). Another large series evaluated 7764 patients who underwent liver resection for colorectal liver metastases [49]. In comparison with patients younger than age 70, those older than 70 had increased 60-day mortality (3.8% vs. 1.6%; $p < 0.001$) and increased complication rates (32.3% vs. 28.7%; $p < 0.001$). It is clear that hepatectomy can be performed safely on some patients in this age group with careful selection of patients for fitness and preoperative optimization.

When feasible, pancreatic resection is the mainstay of treatment for pancreatic cancer. Multiple large population-based studies in the pancreatic literature suggest worse short-term outcomes in older, compared to younger patients [50,51]. In one large series of elderly patients undergoing major pancreatic or hepatobiliary operations when analyzed, chronological age was not a significant risk factor, although the consensus is that physiologic age is an essential consideration [52–54]. When the contribution of chronologic age was isolated statistically using logistic regression modelling with pseudo r^2 analysis in one of the world's largest series of pancreaticoduodenectomy, age alone was found to contribute less than 1% to morbidity and mortality, whereas chronic obstructive pulmonary disease and coronary artery disease had a nearly fourfold and fivefold increased impact, respectively [52]. Hence liver and pancreas resections can be performed safely, although older patients are at higher risk for perioperative mortality, which reinforces the need for better assessment tools and perioperative interventions.

POSTOPERATIVE CARE

Management of the elderly postoperative patient is different from that of younger patients. The older cancer population is at increased risk of complications including malnutrition, delirium, urinary incontinence, pressure ulcers, depression, falls, infection, functional decline, adverse drug effects and death [55]. In hospitalized older adults one-third of them develop delirium during hospitalization. Education of patients and the families of the elderly about postoperative delirium to prepare them for this is important. Screening of individuals for geriatric syndromes such as delirium and to implement interventions that have been shown to prevent delirium, accidental falls and acute functional decline in the hospital is also important [56]. The 4AT tool has recently been reported as a useful and quick instrument to identify delirium and cognitive impairment in the postoperative period [57].

OUTCOMES

It is important to understand that outcomes studied in elderly patients should not be restricted to short-term outcomes and survival [36,58]. Improvements in anaesthetic techniques, surgical techniques and technologies have made short-term mortality very rare even among the elderly. A more detailed analysis of postoperative outcomes in older colorectal cancer patients suggests that most studies primarily evaluate 30-day morbidity and mortality [17,59]. Few studies have looked at results of long-term, patient-centred outcomes defined as postoperative functional and physical status, psychological and cognitive status, quality of life, disposition (i.e. long-term care placement vs. community integration) and longitudinal symptoms resulting from cancer therapy [60,61]. Patients who are elderly undergoing surgery have different issues that need to be addressed: there is certainly more to life after surgery than just survival. These patients have a relatively shorter lifespan than younger patients and hence preserving functional independence is key to maintaining an acceptable quality of life [62], with a substantial group experiencing protracted disability at 6 months after major abdominal operations and several components of physical and mental functioning never returning to preoperative levels. These long-term and functional outcomes are still insufficiently studied and there are limited data available to inform both doctors' and patients' expectations for these outcomes.

AGE RELATED VARIANCE IN TUMOR BIOLOGY AND STAGE

Undoubtedly tumour biology and biological behaviour may differ between young and older patients. An excellent example is the changing pattern of oestrogen (ER) and HER-2 receptor expression in older women where the percentage ER positivity is roughly equal to the age of the patient. This has obvious implications for treatment and prognosis. Grade is also lower in breast cancer in older women. Somewhat counter to this, however, is that breast cancers are larger and more likely to be advanced in older women, but this relates to the lack of screening in this age group and reduced breast symptom awareness, not to disease biology.

Colon cancer is another example. The Surveillance, Epidemiology, and End Results (SEER) database revealed fewer cases of lymph node involvement in older patients with colon adenocarcinoma: when adequately staged (≥12 lymph nodes harvested) lymph node involvement decreased significantly as the patients got older: 33% in those <70 years old compared with 27% in those aged 70 to 79 years and 23% in patients ≥80 years old. Patients were divided into several groups, 20–49, 50–64, 65–74, 75–84 and ≥85 years: the relative risks of node positivity were 1, 0.95, 0.85, 0.80 and 0.74, respectively. This study also showed that patients who had ≥12 lymph nodes harvested had a better prognosis and that the number of lymph nodes harvested also decreased as age increased [63,64]. As the patients get older and the cancer treatment is directed toward the elderly cancer biology should also be a factor to better treat these individuals.

CONCLUSIONS

The treatment of the elderly with cancer is a challenge. We learn to define older patients by their chronological age as it is easier to define than their biological age. Surgical and medical oncologists must move away from age-based practice toward global health-based practice to ensure that all patients receive appropriate and adequate cancer treatment. The physiological status of the individual patient should be formally assessed using a comprehensive CGA. Treatment modalities should be appropriately instituted within a multidisciplinary team ideally with input from a geriatrician in complex cases. Appropriate interventions in the perioperative period, including pre-habilitation should help to improve outcomes. More research is needed to achieve a better understanding of tumour biology so that appropriately individualized treatment can be offered. Outcome measures such as functional decline and disability monitoring should be adopted in the future as survival alone may not appropriately tell the story of the elderly undergoing cancer treatment.

REFERENCES

1. Christensen K, Doblhammer G, Rau R, Vaupel JW. Ageing populations: the challenges ahead. *The Lancent* 2009;374(9696):1196–1208.
2. Al-Refaie WB, Parsons HM, Habermann EB, Kwaan M, Spencer MP, Henderson WG, Rothenberger DA. Operative outcomes beyond 30-day mortality: colorectal cancer surgery in oldest old. *Ann Surg* 2011;253:947–952.
3. Carli F, Mayo N, Klubien K, et al. Epidural analgesia enhances functional exercise capacity and health-related QOL after colonic surgery: randomized trial. *Anesthesiology* 2002;97:540–549.
4. Christensen T, Kehlet H. Postoperative fatigue. *World J Surg* 1993;17:220–225.
5. Hurria A, Leung D, Trainor K, et al. Factors influencing treatment patterns of breast cancer patients age 75 and older. *Crit Rev Oncol Hematol* 2003;46:121–126.
6. Audisio RA, Bozzetti F, Gennari R. The surgical management of elderly cancer patients: recommendations of the SIOG surgical task force. *Eur J Cancer* 2004;40:926–938.
7. Zbar AP, Gravitz A, Audisio RA. Principles of surgical oncology in the elderly. *Clin Geriatr Med* 2012;28:51–71.
8. Fried LP, Tangen CM, Walston J. Frailty in older adults: evidence for a phenotype. *J Gerontol A Biol Sci Med Sci* 2001;56:M146–M156.
9. Saxton A, Velanovich V. Preoperative frailty and QOL as predictors of postoperative complications. *Ann Surg* 2011;253(6):1223–1229.
10. Audisio RA, Osman N, Audisio NM, et al. How do we manage breast cancer in elderly patients? A survey among physicians of British Association of Surgical Oncologists (BASO). *Crit Rev Oncol Hematol* 2004;52(2):135–141.
11. de Cassia Braga Ribeiro K, Kowalski LP. APACHE II, POSSUM, and ASA scores and the risk of perioperative complications in patients with oral or oropharyngeal cancer. *Arch Otolaryngol Head Neck Surg* 2003;129(7):739–745.
12. Kristjansson SR, Nesbakken A, Jordhoy MS, et al. Comprehensive geriatric assessment can predict complications in elderly patient after elective surgery for colorectal cancer: a prospective observation cohort study. *Crit Rev Oncol Hematol* 2010;76(3):208–217.
13. Robinson TN, Eiseman B Wallace JL, et al. Redefining geriatric preoperative assessment using frailty, disability and co-morbidity. *Ann Surg* 2009;250:449–455.
14. Cohen MR, Naeim A. Assessing the older cancer patient. In Huria A, Balducci L, eds., *Geriatric Oncology, Treatment, Assessment and Management.* New York, NY: Springer, 2009.
15. Stuck AT, Siu Al, Wieland GD, et al. CGA: a meta-analysis of controlled trials. *Lancet* 1993;342:1032–1036.
16. Ferucci L, Guralnik JM, Cavazzini C, et al. The frailty syndrome: a critical issue in geriatric oncology. *Crit Rev Oncol Hematol* 2003;46:127–137.
17. Audisio RA, Pope D, Ramesh HS, et al. Shall we operate? Preoperative assessment in elderly cancer patients (PACE) can help. A SIOG surgical task force prospective study. *Crit Rev Oncol Hematol* 2008;65:156–163.
18. Kim SW, Han HS, Jung HW, et al. Multidimensional frailty score for the prediction of postoperative mortality risk. *JAMA Surg* 2014;149(7):633–640.
19. McCorkle R, Strumpfr NE, Nuahmah IF, et al. A specialized home care intervention improves survival among older post-surgical cancer patients. *J Am Geriatr Soc* 2000;48:1707–1713.

20. Goodwin JS, Satish S, Anderson ET, et al. Effect of nurse case management on the treatment of older women with breast cancer. *J Am Geriatr Soc* 2003;51:1252–1259.

21. Cohen HJ, Feussner JR, Lavori P. A controlled trial of inpatient and outpatient geriatric evaluation and management. *N Engl J Med* 2002;346:905–912.

22. Manton KG. A longitudinal study of functional change and mortality in the United States. *J Gerontol* 1988;43:153–161.

23. Guralnik JM, Alecxih L, Branch LG, et al. Medical and long-term care costs when older persons become more dependent. *Am J Public Health* 2002;92:1244–1245.

24. Coughlin TA, Mcbride TD, Peozek M, et al. Home care for the disabled elderly: predictors and expected costs. *Health Serv Res* 1992;27:453–479.

25. Kennie DC, Reid J, Richardson IR, et al. Effectiveness of geriatric rehabilitative care after fractures of proximal femur in elderly women: a randomized controlled trial. *BMJ* 1988;297:1083–1086.

26. Tinetti ME, Baker DI, Gottschalk M, et al. Systematic home-based physical and functional therapy for older persons after hip fracture. *Arch Phys Med Rehabil* 1997;78:1237–1247.

27. Gill TM, Baker DI, Gottschalk M, et al. A program to prevent functional decline in physically frail, elderly persons who live at home. *N Engl J Med* 2002;347:1068–1074.

28. Jaggers JR, Simpson CD, Frost KL, et al. Prehabilitation before knee arthroplasty increases postsurgical function: a case study. *J Strength Cond Res* 2007;21:632–634.

29. Huisman M, Audisio R, Ugolini G, et al. Increased risk of major postoperative complications in oncogeriatric surgical patients with an impaired nutritional status. The preop study. *J Geriatr Oncol* 2013;4(Suppl. 1):S19–S20.

30. Delva F, Marien E, Fonck M, et al. Factors influencing general practitioners in the referral of elderly cancer patients. *BMC Cancer* 2011;5.

31. Protière C, Viens P, Rousseau F, Moatti JP. Prescribers' attitudes toward elderly breast cancer patients. Discrimination or empathy? *Crit Rev Oncol Hematol* 2010;75(2):138–150.

32. Janssen-Heijnen ML, Houterman S, Lemmens VE, et al. Prognostic impact of increasing age and co-morbidity in cancer patients: a population-based approach. *Crit Rev Oncol Hematol* 2005;55:231–240.

33. Davila JA, Rabeneck L, Berger DH, et al. Postoperative 30-day mortality following surgical resection for colorectal cancer in veterans: changes in the right direction. *Dig Dis Sci* 2005;50:1722–1728.

34. Nascimbeni R, Di Fabio F, Di Betta E, et al. The changing impact of age on colorectal cancer surgery. A trend analysis. *Colorectal Dis* 2009;11:13–18.

35. Iversen LH, Pedersen L, Riis A, et al. Age and colorectal cancer with focus on the elderly: trends in relative survival and initial treatment from a Danish population-based study. *Dis Colon Rectum* 2005;48:1755–1763.

36. Al Refale WB, Parson HM, Henderson WG, et al. Major cancer surgery in the elderly: results from the American College of Surgeons National Surgical Quality Improvement Program. *Ann Surg* 2010;251:311–318.

37. Jaklitsch M, Billmeier S. Preoperative evaluation and risk assessment for elderly thoracic surgery patients. *Thorac Surg Clin* 2009;19:301–312.

38. Schuchert MJ, Pettiford BL, Luketich JD, et al. Parenchymal-sparing resections: why, when, and how. *Thorac Surg Clin* 2008;18:93–105.

39. Allen MS, Darling GE, Pechet TT, et al. Morbidity and mortality of major pulmonary resections in patients with early-stage lung cancer: initial results of the randomized, prospective ACOSOG Z0030 trial. *Ann Thorac Surg* 2006;81:1013–1019.

40. Wu CY, Chen JS, Lin YS, et al. Feasibility and safety of nonintubated thoracoscopic lobectomy for geriatric lung cancer patients. *Ann Thorac Surg* 2013;95:405–411.

41. Mun M, Kohno T. Video-assisted thoracic surgery for clinical stage I lung cancer in octogenarians. *Ann Thorac Surg* 2008;85:406–411.

42. National Cancer Institute, Surveillance, Epidemiology, and End Results (SEER) Program. SEER stat fact sheets: colon and rectum cancer. 2008. http://seer.cancer.gov/statfacts/html/colorect.html.

43. Hermans E, van Schaik PM, Prins HA, et al. Outcome of colonic surgery in elderly patients with colon cancer. *J Oncol* 2010;2010:865–908.

44. Manceau G, Karoui M, Werner A, et al. Comparative outcomes of rectal cancer surgery between elderly and non-elderly patients: a systematic review. *Lancet Oncol* 2012;13:e525–e536.

45. Dekker JW, van den Broek CB, Bastiaannet E, et al. Importance of the first postoperative year in the prognosis of elderly colorectal cancer patients. *Ann Surg Oncol* 2011;18:1533–1539.

46. Jarnagin WR, Gonen M, Fong Y, et al. Improvement in perioperative outcome after hepatic resection: analysis of 1,803 consecutive cases over the past decade. *Ann Surg* 2002;236:397–406.

47. Cho SW, Steel J, Tsung A, et al. Safety of liver resection in the elderly: how important is age? *Ann Surg Oncol* 2011;18(4):1088–1095.

48. Reddy SK, Barbas AS, Turley RS, et al. Major liver resection in elderly patients: a multi-institutional analysis. *J Am Coll Surg* 2011;212:787–795.

49. Adam R, Frilling A, Elias D, et al. Liver resection of colorectal metastases in elderly patients. *Br J Surg* 2010;97:366–376.

50. Riall TS, Reddy DM, Nealon WH, Goodwin JS. The effect of age on short-term outcomes after pancreatic resection: a population-based study. *Ann Surg* 2008;248(3):459–465.

51. Finlayson E, Fan Z, Birkmeyer JD. Outcomes in octogenarians undergoing high-risk cancer operation: a national study. *J Am Coll Surg* 2007;205(6):729–734.

52. Makary MA, Winter JM, Cameron JL, et al. Pancreaticoduodenectomy in the very elderly. *J Gastrointest Surg* 2006;10(3):347–356.

53. Petrowsky H, Clavien PA. Should we deny surgery for malignant hepato-pancreatico-biliary tumors to elderly patients? *World J Surg* 2005;29(9):1093–1100.

54. di Sebastiano P, Festa L, Buchler MW, di Mola FF. Surgical aspects in management of hepato-pancreaticobiliary tumours in the elderly. *Best Pract Res Clin Gastroenterol* 2009;23(6):919–923.

55. Creditor MC. Hazards of hospitalization of the elderly. *Ann Intern Med* 1993;118:219–223.

56. Inouye SK. Delirium in older persons. *N Engl J Med* 2006;354:1157–1165.

57. 4AT-Rapid Assessment Test for Delirium. Available at http://www.the4at.com.

58. Massrweh NN, Legner VJ, Simons RG, et al. Impact of advancing age on abdominal surgical outcomes. *Arch Surg* 2009;144:1108–1114.

59. Kingston RD, Jeacock J, Walsh S, et al. The outcome of surgery for colorectal cancer in the elderly: a 12-year review from the Trafford Database. *Eur J Surg Oncol* 1995;21:514–516.

60. Ulander K, Jeppsson B, Grahn G. Quality of life and independence in activities of daily living preoperatively and at follow-up in patients with colorectal cancer. *Support Care Cancer* 1997;5:402–409.

61. Temple PC, Travis B, Sachs L, et al. Functioning and well-being of patients before and after elective surgical procedures. *J Am Coll Surg* 1995;181:17–25

62. Lawrence VA, Hazuda HP, Cornell JE, et al. Functional independence after major abdominal surgery in the elderly. *J Am Coll Surg* 2004;199:762–772.

63. Owonikoko TK, Ragin CC, Belani CP, et al. Lung cancer in elderly patients: an analysis of the surveillance, epidemiology, and end results database. *J Clin Oncol* 2007;25:5570–5577.

64. Khan H, Olszewshki AJ, Somasundar P. Lymph node involvement in colon cancer patients decreases with age; a population based analysis. *Eur J Surg Oncol* 2014;40(11):1474–1480.

16

Cancer of unknown primary

NICHOLAS PAVLIDIS

INCIDENCE AND AETIOLOGY

Cancer of unknown primary (CUP) is characterized as a clinical disorder where patients present with histologically confirmed metastatic cancer for which standard diagnostic investigations failed to identify the primary site [1]. Median age at presentation is 65 years and is more common in men. It accounts for 3–5% of all human cancers with an overall incidence per 100,000 population per year of 7–12 cases in the US, 4–6 in Switzerland and 18–19 in Australia. It is considered to be the seventh or eighth most frequent malignant tumour.

CUP's aetiology and biology are poorly understood. Several investigators support the hypothesis that CUP represents a distinct biological and clinical entity which carries a unique molecular signature that differentiates it from typical metastatic cancers of known primaries [2].

PRESENTATION

CUP is mostly associated with a short history of symptoms and signs, with an aggressive clinical course, and often presents with a unique natural history of unpredictable metastatic spread from that of a known primary cancer [1]. CUP is classified into favourable and unfavourable groups where several clinicopathological subsets according to age, sex, histopathology, clinical presentation and metastatic sites are included. Patients with unfavourable CUPs represent 80% of all CUPs [3].

Histopathologically, CUP is divided into adenocarcinomas of well or moderate differentiation (60%), undifferentiated or poorly differentiated adenocarcinomas (30%), squamous cell carcinomas (5%) and undifferentiated neoplasms (5%) [1,3].

CLINICOPATHOLOGICAL SUBSETS

Since 2003, CUP has been distinguished into two separated groups, the favourable and the unfavourable groups. Favourable subsets are those patients who respond to local or systemic treatments and enjoy a longer survival [3]. Table 16.1 illustrates the various CUP clinicopathological subsets.

1. *Women with adenocarcinoma involving axillary nodes.* The primary site is most often hidden in the breast and the presentation is similar to stage II breast cancer (N_2 or N_3 disease). The most common histology is ductal adenocarcinoma, with 40% having positive oestrogen receptors. Mean age is 52 years [4].
2. *Women with papillary adenocarcinoma of peritoneal cavity or primary peritoneal carcinoma.* Similar clinical presentation with advanced ovarian cancer. Median age 60 years. Histopathological diagnosis should always be serous or papillary adenocarcinoma with a frequently raised serum CA 125 marker. In comparison with primary ovarian cancer patients, primary peritoneal carcinoma affects older women, has bulkier disease and overexpresses HER-2 oncogene and Ki-67, probably carrying a somehow worse prognosis [5].
3. *Squamous cell carcinoma involving cervical nodes.* It mainly affects men of approximately 60 years old and constitutes 5% of all head and neck cancers. They present with a painless unilateral mass, usually of level II lymph nodes. Diagnosis and investigation for the primary site include fine-needle aspiration (specificity 95%), panendoscopy, CT scan (sensitivity 22%), MRI (sensitivity 36%) and PET scan (sensitivity up to 60%) [6].

Table 16.1 Clinicopathological subsets of CUP patients

Favourable subsets

1. Women with adenocarcinoma involving axillary lymph nodes
2. Women with papillary adenocarcinoma of peritoneal cavity
3. Squamous cell carcinoma involving cervical lymph nodes
4. Poorly differentiated neuroendocrine carcinomas; Merkel cell carcinoma of unknown primary (localized disease)
5. Adenocarcinoma with a colon profile (CK20$^+$, CK7$^-$, CDX2$^+$)
6. Men with blastic bone metastases and elevated PSA (adenocarcinoma)
7. Isolated inguinal adenopathy (squamous carcinoma)
8. Patients with a single, small, potentially respectable tumour

Unfavourable subsets

1. Adenocarcinoma metastatic to the liver or other organs
2. Poorly differentiated carcinoma with or without midline distribution
3. Non-papillary malignant ascites (adenocarcinoma)
4. Multiple cerebral metastases (adeno or squamous Ca)
5. Multiple lung/pleural metastases (adenocarcinoma)
6. Multiple metastatic bone disease (adenocarcinoma)
7. Squamous cell carcinoma of the abdominal cavity

Table 16.2 Required work-up for detecting the primary site

Pathology work-up

- Histopathology
- Specific immunohistochemical staining

Work-up for all CUP patients

- Full blood count
- Biochemistry
- Urinalysis
- Testing for occult blood in stools
- Chest radiography
- CT scan of thorax, abdomen and pelvis

Work-up for selected CUP subsets

- Mammography (for all women)
- Breast MRI
- Testicular ultrasonography
- PET or CT scan
- Endoscopy
- Tumour markers (AFP, β-HCG, PSA, CA 125, CA 15-3)

Immunohistochemistry is of paramount importance since it differentiates between (1) the type of cancer (carcinoma, sarcoma, melanoma, lymphoma), (2) the type of carcinoma (adenocarcinoma, germ-cell tumour, hepatocellular, renal, thyroid, neuroendocrine or squamous cell carcinoma) and (3) the primary site of an adenocarcinoma (lung, breast, ovarian, colon, pancreas, biliary tract or prostate) (Tables 16.2 and 16.3). Cytokeratins are also extensively used, especially CK7 and CK20 for detecting the primary site (Table 16.4) [11].

- *Molecular diagnosis.* Gene profiling microarray assays on cDNA or mRNAs platforms have an accuracy rate of 90–95% in detecting the primary site. Whether this innovative diagnostic technology will lead to specific treatment with better patient outcomes remains uncertain, although several prospective randomized trials are still ongoing [12–15].
- *Imaging technology.* CT scans provide a diagnostic accuracy of 55% mainly in pancreatic, colorectal and lung cancer, while MRI can detect primary breast cancer in 70% of cases [1]. Fluoro-deoxyglucose (FDG) PET accuracy ranges between 25% and 45% and is more sensitive in detecting hidden head and neck cancers or lung cancer [16,17]. Also, ^{68}Gα-DOTA-NOC receptor PET/CT is helpful in identifying neuroendocrine tumours or their metastatic sites [18].
- *Endoscopy.* In general they have low accuracy rates and low sensitivity or specificity. The only cases in which endoscopy could become useful are those patients who present clinically with relevant symptoms or signs, as well as in patients with specific immunohistopathological findings [1,3].

4. *Poorly differentiated neuroendocrine carcinoma.* The majority of patients present with poorly differentiated neuroendocrine tumours, while a minority present with well-differentiated low-grade histology. Metastatic sites most frequently affected include retroperitoneal, mediastinal or peripheral nodes and less frequently involve the liver and bones [7].
5. *Adenocarcinoma with a colon profile (CK20$^+$, CK7$^-$, CDX2$^+$).* This recently described CUP subset is more common in women. Clinical presentation includes the involvement of abdominal nodes (51%), peritoneal surfaces (50%), liver (30%) and ascites (27%) [8,9].
6. *Unfavourable subsets of metastatic visceral or skeletal CUP.* These are the most frequent CUP subsets and account for almost 80% of all CUP patients. They carry a poor prognosis with short survival. Histologically, around 60% are moderate to poorly differentiated adenocarcinomas, and the remainder are undifferentiated tumours. Liver is the most commonly affected organ (40–50%), followed by lymph nodes (35%), lungs (31%), bones (28%) and the brain (15%) [1,3,10].

Investigation of the primary site

- *Immunohistopathology.* Immunohistopathology is one of the most important diagnostic aids.

Table 16.3 Immunohistochemistry staining for investigating CUP cases

	Diagnosis
Step 1	
AE1 or AE3 pan-cytokeratin	Carcinoma
Common leukocyte antigen	Lymphoma
S100, HMB-45	Melanoma
S100, vimentin	Sarcoma
Step 2	
CK7 or CK20, PSA	Adenocarcinoma
PLAP, OCT4, AFP, human chorionic gonadotropin	Germ-cell tumour
Hepatocyte paraffin 1, canalicular pCEA, CD10 or CD13	Hepatocellular carcinoma
RCC, CD10	Renal cell carcinoma
TTF1, thyroglobulin	Thyroid carcinoma
Chromogranin, synaptophysin, PGP9.5, CD56	Neuroendocrine carcinoma
CK5 or CK6, p63	Squamous cell carcinoma
Step 3	
PSA, PAP	Prostate
TTF1	Lung
GCDFP-15, mammaglobin, ER	Breast
CDX2, CK20	Colon
CDX2 (intestinal epithelium), CK20, CK7	Pancreas or biliary
ER, CA 125, mesothelin, WT1	Ovary

Table 16.4 Cytokeratins staining used in CUP

	Cytokeratins
Colon	CK7$^-$/CK20$^+$
Stomach	CK7$^-$/CK20$^+$, CK7$^+$/CK20$^+$
Biliary	CK7$^+$/CK20$^-$, CK7$^+$/CK20$^+$
Pancreas	CK7$^+$/CK20$^-$, CK7$^+$/CK20$^+$
Lung	CK7$^+$/CK20$^-$
Ovarian, non-mucinous	CK7$^+$/CK20$^-$
Ovarian, mucinous	CK7$^-$/CK20$^+$, CK7$^+$/CK20$^+$
Breast	CK7$^+$/CK20$^-$
Urothelial	CK7$^+$/CK20$^+$
Endometrium	CK7$^+$/CK20$^-$
Prostate	CK7$^-$/CK20$^-$
Renal	CK7$^-$/CK20$^-$
Liver	CK7$^-$/CK20$^-$

- *Serum tumour markers.* Almost 70% of CUP patients express elevated epithelial serum tumour markers (CEA, CA 125, CA 15-3, CA 19-9) in a non-specific manner, lacking any diagnostic, prognostic or predictive value. However, in certain clinicopathological subsets it might be diagnostically helpful, i.e. prostate-specific antigen (PSA) in men with osteoblastic bone metastases, CA 125 in women with primary serous papillary peritoneal adenocarcinoma or CA 15-3 in females with axillary adenocarcinoma [19].

Treatment

Treatment depends on the specific clinicopathological subset. It includes surgical procedures, local radiotherapy or systemic chemotherapy (Table 16.5).

WOMEN WITH ADENOCARCINOMA INVOLVING AXILLARY NODES

These cases should be managed as stage II breast cancer with complete axillary dissection, ipsilateral breast radiotherapy followed by adjuvant chemotherapy or hormone therapy depending on the biomarkers. Patients who do not receive local treatment are associated with high locoregional relapse rates (40–55%). Survival is longer in patients who received primary breast radiotherapy, as well as in patients with adjuvant systemic treatment. A 72% mean 5-year survival has been reported [1,4,20,21].

WOMEN WITH SEROUS PAPILLARY ADENOCARCINOMA OF PERITONEAL CAVITY

This CUP subset should be treated similarly to stage III and IV ovarian cancer. Surgical cytoreduction, followed by platinum and paclitaxel chemotherapy, is recommended. Response rates of 80% have been reported, with 30–40% complete responders and a median survival of 36 months. Some reports have demonstrated poorer survival of patients with primary peritoneal carcinoma when compared to primary ovarian cancer (due to reasons stated in the Clinicopathological Subsets section) [1,5,22].

SQUAMOUS CELL CARCINOMA INVOLVING CERVICAL NODES

Patients with N_1 or N_{2a} disease without extracapsular extension could be treated with surgery alone, including excisional biopsy, radical or modified radical neck dissection or bilateral tonsillectomy. Locoregional control is around 80–90%, and 5-year overall survival up to 65%. Postoperative radiotherapy is indicated following excisional or incisional biopsy, extracapsular extension, stage N_{2b} or higher, nodes fixed to adjacent structures or in patients with low performance status and comorbidities. The irradiation fields include the involved nodal stations (65–70 Gy), the uninvolved sites (50 Gy) and the mucosal sites (50–60 Gy) [1,6]. Chemoradiation could be indicated in N_2 or N_3 cases with cisplatin-based chemotherapy. However, chemoradiation could be associated with significant grade 3 toxicities [23].

Table 16.5 Recommended treatment for CUP patients

CUP subset	Recommended therapy	Survival
Women with adenocarcinoma involving axillary nodes	Axillary nodal dissection mastectomy or breast irradiation following by chemo-hormonotherapy according to risk factors	Mean 5 years: 72%
Women with papillary adenocarcinoma of peritoneal cavity	Optimal surgical debulking and platinum-based chemotherapy	Mean: 36 months
Squamous cell carcinoma involving cervical nodes	Neck dissection or irradiation of bilateral neck and mucosa (±chemotherapy)	Mean 5 years: 60–65%
Poorly differentiated neuroendocrine carcinoma	Platinum–etoposide combination chemotherapy	Median: 15.5 months 2-year survival: 33–50% Long-term survivors: 10–15%
Adenocarcinoma with a colon cancer profile	Colorectal combination chemotherapy regimens	Median: 20–36 months
Men with bone metastases and elevated serum PSA	LHRH agonists or anti-androgens	—
Patients with limited disease (isolated inguinal nodal metastases or a single metastatic lesion)	Local surgical excision with or without local irradiation	—
Unfavourable subsets	Platinum-based empirical chemotherapy	Median: 9–12 months

POORLY DIFFERENTIATED NEUROENDOCRINE CARCINOMAS

This group of patients should be treated with platinum-based or platinum–taxane combination chemotherapy. Response rates are up to 55%, with 20% complete responders having been reported, overall survival of 15 months and almost 10–15% long-term survivors [1,7].

Recently, a 2-year survival benefit has been reported in patients with unknown primary stage III$_B$ Merkel cell carcinoma, which compares well to patients with known primary NET (76.9% vs. 36.4%) [24].

ADENOCARCINOMA WITH A COLON PROFILE (CK20$^+$, CK7$^-$, CDX2$^+$)

This subset of patients should be treated as advanced colorectal cancer. The overall response rate is 50%, with 15% complete and 35% partial responses, and a median survival of 21–37 months [1,8,9].

OTHER FAVOURABLE SUBSETS

Male patients with metastatic bone metastases and elevated serum PSA should be managed as advanced prostate cancer [1]. Patients with isolated inguinal nodal metastases or a single metastatic lesion should undergo local dissection, with or without local radiotherapy [11].

TREATMENT OF UNFAVOURABLE SUBSETS

Unfortunately, this group of CUP patients represents 80% of cases. They are usually treated with empirical chemotherapy, mostly with platinum or taxane combinations. Response rates are around 20% and median survival is 6 months. A recent meta-analysis has shown that no type of chemotherapy has demonstrated any survival benefit in these subsets [25–27]. Specific targeted treatment in CUP patients following gene profiling microarray tests has not yet been proven. Since there are no prospective randomized studies available, we have to wait until some already ongoing trials start to report.

REFERENCES

1. Pavlidis N, Pentheroudakis G. Cancer of unknown primary site. *Lancet* 2012;379:1428–35.
2. Kamposioras K, Pentheroudakis G, Pavlidis N. Exploring the biology of cancer of unknown primary: breakthroughs and drawbacks. *Eur J Clin Invest* 2013;43(5):491–500.
3. Pavlidis N, Briasoulis E, Hainsworth J, Greco FA. Diagnostic and therapeutic management of cancer of an unknown primary. *Eur J Cancer* 2003;39:1990–2005.
4. Pentheroudakis G, Lazaridis G, Pavlidis N. Axillary nodal metastases from carcinoma of unknown primary (CUPAX): a systemic review of published evidence. *Breast Cancer Res Treat* 2010;119:1–11.
5. Pentheroudakis G, Pavlidis N. Serous papillary peritoneal carcinoma: unknown primary tumor, ovarian cancer counterpart or a distinct entity? A systemic review. *Crit Rev Oncol Hematol* 2010;75:27–42.

6. Pavlidis N, Pentheroudakis G, Plataniotis G. Cervical lymph node metastases of squamous cell carcinoma from an unknown primary site: a favourable prognosis subset of patients with CUP. *Clin Transl Oncol* 2009;11:340–8.

7. Stoyianni A, Pentheroudakis G, Pavlidis N. Neuroendocrine carcinoma of unknown primary: a systematic review of the literature and comparative study with other neuroendocrine tumours. *Cancer Treat Rev* 2011;37:358–65.

8. Hainsworth JD, Schnabel CA, Erlander MG, et al. A retrospective study of treatment outcomes in patients with carcinoma of unknown primary site and a colorectal cancer molecular profile. *Clin Colorectal Cancer* 2012;11(2):112–8.

9. Varadhachary GR, Karanth S, Qiao W, et al. Carcinoma of unknown primary with gastrointestinal profile: immunohistochemistry and survival data for this favorable subset. *Int J Clin Oncol* 2014;19(3):479–84.

10. Lazaridis G, Pentheroudakis G, Fountzilas G, Pavlidis N. Liver metastases from cancer of unknown primary (CUPL): a retrospective analysis of presentation, management and prognosis in 49 patients and systematic review of the literature. *Cancer Treat Rev* 2008;34:693–700.

11. Oien KA. Pathologic evaluation of unknown primary cancer. *Semin Oncol* 2009;36:8–37.

12. Monzon F, Koen TJ. Diagnosis of metastatic neoplasms: molecular approaches for identification of tissue of origin. *Arch Pathol Lab Med* 2010;134:216–24.

13. Bridgewater J, van Laar R, Floore A, Van TVL. Gene expression profiling may improve diagnosis in patients with carcinoma of unknown primary. *Br J Cancer* 2008;98:1425–30.

14. Greco FA, Spigel DR, Yardley DA, et al. Molecular profiling in unknown primary cancer: accuracy of tissue of origin prediction. *Oncologist* 2010;15:500–6.

15. Pentheroudakis G, Spector Y, Krikelis D, et al. Global microRNA profiling in favorable prognosis subgroups of cancer of unknown primary (CUP) demonstrates no significant expression differences with metastases of matched known primary tumors. *Clin Exp Metastasis* 2013;30(4):431–9.

16. Seve P, Billotey C, Broussolle C, et al. The role of 2-deoxy-2[F-18]fluoro-D-glucose positron emission tomography in disseminated carcinoma of unknown primary site. *Cancer* 2007;109:292–99.

17. Keller F, Psychogios G, Linke R, et al. Carcinoma of unknown primary in the head and neck: comparison between positron emission tomography (PET) and PET/CT. *Head Neck* 2011;33:1569–75.

18. Prasad V, Ambrosini V, Hommann M, et al. Detection of unknown primary neuroendocrine tumours (CUP-NET) using (68) Gα-DOTA-NOC receptor PET/CT. *Eur J Nucl Med Mol Imaging* 2010;37:67–77.

19. Pentheroudakis G, Pavlidis N. Serum tumor markers. In Wick MR, ed., *Metastatic Carcinomas of Unknown Origin*. New York, NY: Demos Medical Publishing, 2008: 165–75.

20. Masinghe SP, Faluyi OO, Kerr GR, Kunkler IH. Breast radiotherapy for occult breast cancer with axillary nodal metastases – does it reduce the local recurrence and increase overall survival? *Clin Oncol (R Coll Radiol)* 2011;23(2):95–100.

21. Barton SR, Smith IE, Kirby AM, et al. The role of ipsilateral breast radiotherapy in management of occult primary breast cancer presenting as axillary lymphadenopathy. *Eur J Cancer* 2011;47(14):2099–106.

22. Chao KC, Chen YJ, Juang CM, et al. Prognosis for advanced-stage peritoneal serous papillary carcinoma and serous ovarian cancer in Taiwan. *Taiwan J Obstet Gynecol* 2013;52(1):81–4.

23. Fakhrian K, Thamm R, Knapp S, et al. Radio(chemo) therapy in the management of squamous cell carcinoma of cervical lymph nodes from an unknown primary site. A retrospective analysis. *Strahlenther Onkol* 2012;188(1):56–61.

24. Tarantola JI, Vallow LA, Halyard MY, et al. Unknown primary Merkel cell carcinoma: 23 new cases and a review. *J Am Acad Dermatol* 2013;68(3):433–40.

25. Golfinopoulos V, Pentheroudakis G, Salanti G, et al. Comparative survival with diverse chemotherapy regimens for cancer of unknown primary site: multiple-treatments meta-analysis. *Cancer Treat Rev* 2009;35:570–3.

26. Greco AF, Pavlidis N. Treatment for patients with unknown primary carcinoma and unfavorable prognostic factors. *Semin Oncol* 2009;36:65–74.

27. Petrakis D, Pentheroudakis G, Voulgaris E, Pavlidis N. Prognostication in cancer of unknown primary (CUP): development of a prognostic algorithm in 311 cases and review of the literature. *Cancer Treat Rev* 2013;39(7):701–8.

Disease site specific surgical oncology

17

Oral cancer

AKASH AGARWAL, ARUN CHATURVEDI AND SANJEEV MISRA

INTRODUCTION

Oral cancer is one of the most common head and neck malignancies. It accounts for a large number of cancers in the Indian subcontinent, where tobacco chewing is very common. The age-standardized rates in India are as high as 9.6 per 100,000 males and 6.3 per 100,000 females [1], the highest in the world.

The oral cavity includes the following subsites: lips, buccal mucosa, oral (anterior two-thirds) tongue, hard palate, alveolar ridges (upper and lower gingival), floor of mouth (FOM) and retromolar trigone (RMT).

ETIOLOGY

Head and neck cancers are predominantly related to lifestyle factors such as consumption of tobacco, alcohol and areca nut. Tobacco is the main cause implicated in the etiopathogenesis of oral cancers. It produces nitrosamines which cause destruction of the xenobiotic mechanism by free radical generation. Tobacco can be consumed either by smoking as in cigarettes or in a smokeless form along with areca nut in quids. Alcohol is also a potent carcinogen in the development of oral cancers. There is a synergistic effect of tobacco and alcohol in causing oral cancer.

Human papilloma virus (HPV) is also known to cause oral and oropharyngeal cancers. Eating fresh fruits and vegetables has a preventive effect.

The mucosa of the upper aerodigestive tract is globally exposed to the effects of carcinogens, leading to multiple synchronous and metachronous tumours (field carcinogenesis).

PATHOLOGY

Most oral cancers are primary squamous cell cancers. Grossly, the lesions are generally ulcerative, proliferative or ulceroproliferative. The disease spreads locally by invading adjacent structures – muscle, bone or skin. The predominant route of spread of oral squamous cell cancers is through the regional lymph nodes. The lymphatics of the oral cavity drain into the neck nodes, levels I–III (Table 17.1). Skip metastasis to levels IV and V is unusual. The exception to this is the tongue, where skip metastasis to level V can occur in as many as 15% of cases [2]. Lesions approaching or crossing the midline may also drain to the contralateral neck nodes. Distant metastasis is uncommon and occurs with advanced locoregional or recurrent disease. Lungs, bones and liver are the most frequent metastatic sites.

Lymphatic spread of oral cancer is dependent on a number of factors. Larger tumours (T stage), thicker, more deeply invasive tumours, high-grade tumours and those with lymphovascular invasion have higher propensity to metastasize to the regional lymph nodes [3,4].

Table 17.1 Neck nodal levels

Neck nodal level	Boundaries
IA (submental triangle)	Anterior belly of digastrics (bilateral) and arch of mandible
IB (submandibular triangle)	Anterior and posterior belly of digastrics and body of mandible
II	Skull base to level of hyoid, midline to posterior border of SCM
III	Level of hyoid to lower border of cricoid, midline to posterior border of SCM
IV	Lower border of cricoids to clavicle, midline to posterior border of SCM
V (posterior triangle)	Posterior border of SCM to anterior border of trapezius, clavicle inferiorly
VI	Hyoid to suprasternal notch, bilaterally carotid arteries
VII	Inferior to suprasternal notch, superior mediastinum

POTENTIALLY MALIGNANT DISORDERS

Abnormalities previously classified as precancerous lesions (localized) and conditions (generalized) have now been termed 'potentially malignant disorders', which conveys the fact that not all disorders described under this term may transform into cancer [5]. The common disorders are leukoplakia and erythroplakia (precancerous lesions), oral submucous fibrosis (SMF), lichen planus and discoid lupus erythematosus (precancerous conditions).

SCREENING

The presence of a preinvasive stage and the ease of visualization of the oral cavity make it potentially amenable to screening. A large randomized controlled trial (RCT) from India has shown screening to reduce oral cancer–related mortality by 12% in the overall population and 24% in tobacco and alcohol users after 15 years follow-up [6]. Clearly this strategy is only appropriate in high disease burden countries and so would be unlikely to be cost-effective in most European countries unless targeted at high-risk population subgroups.

CHEMOPREVENTION

Head and neck cancers were the first tumours which were targeted for chemoprevention. However, despite three RCTs, none have shown to decrease the risk of second primary cancers by treating patients with either retinoids or β-carotene [7].

CLINICAL FEATURES

Patients commonly present with an oral ulcer or growth (Figures 17.1 through 17.4). Occasionally patients may present with subtle complaints of ill-fitting dentures or

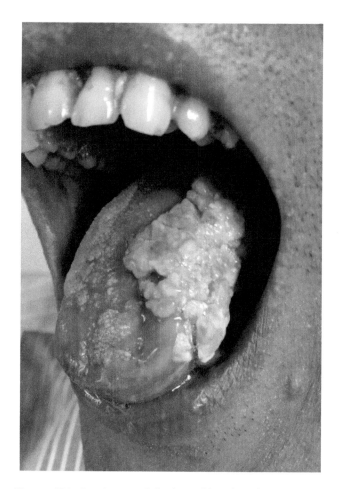

Figure 17.1 Carcinoma of the lateral border of the tongue.

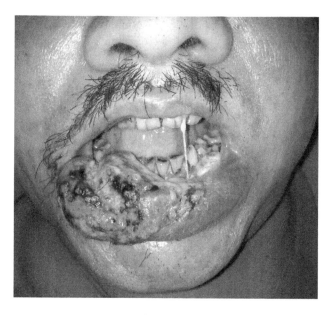

Figure 17.2 Carcinoma of the lower lip.

a non-healing tooth extraction site. Pain is a late feature and is generally localized to the ear. Inability to protrude the tongue (ankyloglossia) and trismus are indicators of advanced disease. However, care should be taken to exclude SMF as a cause of trismus, especially in Indian

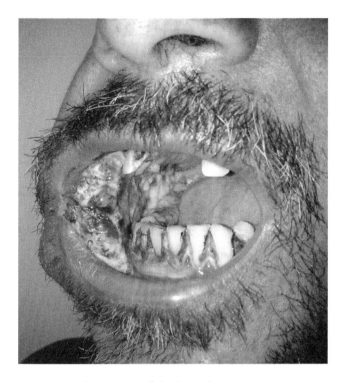

Figure 17.3 Carcinoma of the buccal mucosa.

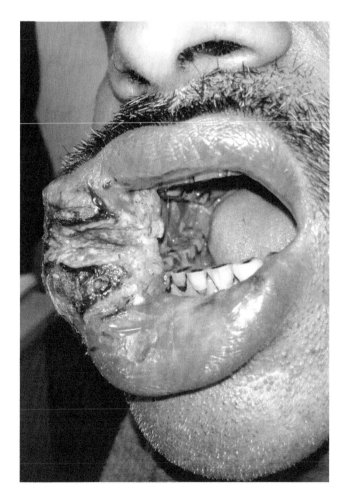

Figure 17.4 Carcinoma of the buccal mucosa and commissure.

subcontinent patients. Some patients may present with cervical lymphadenopathy as the only symptom.

DIAGNOSTIC WORK-UP

Imaging

The need for and modality of imaging are dictated both by disease subsite and the extent of disease. Small lesions confined to the lip or buccal mucosa or the anterior part of the tongue may not necessarily require any imaging. On the other hand, lesions in the gingi-vobuccal sulcus, alveolus or RMT and larger lesions of the tongue will require further imaging in the form of contrast-enhanced computerized tomography (CECT) or magnetic resonance imaging (MRI), as in the case of the tongue. Orthopantomogram (OPG) X-ray can be used to document bony invasion; however, it is not as sensitive as a CT scan with 3D bone reconstruction (Figure 17.5).

Neck nodes can be evaluated by high-resolution ultrasonography of the neck, or alternatively by CECT. In patients who are planning to undergo a CECT for the primary, the scan can be extended to include the neck also.

The chest is evaluated by plain X-ray; any suspicious lesion can be further characterized by CECT. In the absence of clinical or radiological suspicion, a CECT of the thorax is not routinely recommended.

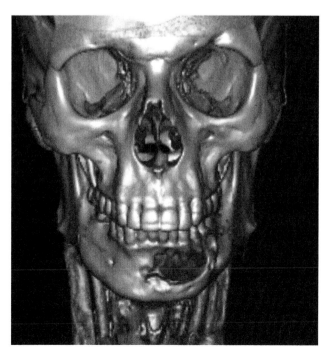

Figure 17.5 Mandibular destruction seen in CT 3D reconstruction.

Biopsy

An incisional biopsy of the lesion can be performed in the outpatient clinic under local anaesthesia. However, care should be taken to avoid taking non-representative necrotic tissue from the centre of large lesions. Examination under anaesthesia is important as it allows proper assessment of the extent of disease especially in patients with painful lesions and those with trismus and posteriorly based tongue lesions. In some centres, pan-endoscopy is recommended as part of initial evaluation, to exclude the presence of a second primary lesion in the upper aerodigestive tract.

STAGING

The currently followed staging method is the UICC-AJCC TNM staging system (Table 17.2) [8].

MANAGEMENT

The management of oral cancer depends on the stage of the disease. Early lesions can be treated by a single modality – either surgery or radiotherapy. Surgery has the advantage of early recovery and the ability to perform repeated surgeries in case of recurrence or development of a new primary. However, surgery may leave the patient with significant functional or cosmetic defects. Radiotherapy has the advantage of being non-invasive, but its repeated use is limited by cumulative dose toxicity. The choice of treatment modality will depend on the site of disease and presence of SMF. Advanced disease will frequently require multimodality treatment – surgery followed by adjuvant radiotherapy or chemoradiotherapy or chemoradiation alone, or chemoradiation followed by salvage surgery. Patients with advanced disease may suffer from malnutrition. Nutritional support is important prior to starting treatment.

Surgical management

The basic principle of surgery for oral cancers is wide resection of the lesion with a 1 cm circumferential margin of normal healthy tissue (Figure 17.6). This can result in full-thickness loss of skin or excision of an adjacent subsite. To gain access for posterior lesions, a lip split can be combined with a cheek flap or with a paramedian mandibulotomy and lateral swing.

Principles of mandibulectomy

An intact mandible is essential for facial cosmesis, speech and proper occlusion of the teeth for mastication. Efforts are made to preserve the mandible, whenever possible, without compromising the surgical margins. Patients with minimal erosion of the superior part of the mandible and those with small-volume paramandibular disease are best treated by a marginal mandiblectomy. In this, the superior tooth bearing part of the mandible is resected en bloc with the

Table 17.2 TNM staging of oral cancers with stage grouping

TX	Primary tumour cannot be assessed.
T0	No evidence of primary tumour.
Tis	Carcinoma in situ.
T1	Tumour ≤2 cm in greatest dimension.
T2	Tumour >2 cm but ≤4 cm in greatest dimension.
T3	Tumour >4 cm in greatest dimension.
T4a	Moderately advanced local disease
	(Lip) Tumour invades through cortical bone, inferior alveolar nerve, floor of mouth or skin of face, that is, chin or nose.
	(Oral cavity) Tumour invades adjacent structures only (e.g., through cortical bone [mandible or maxilla] into deep [extrinsic] muscle of tongue [genioglossus, hyoglossus, palatoglossus, and styloglossus], maxillary sinus or skin of face).
T4b	Very advanced local disease.
	Tumour invades masticator space, pterygoid plates or skull base and/or encases internal carotid artery.
NX	Regional lymph nodes cannot be assessed.
N0	No regional lymph node metastasis.
N1	Metastasis in a single ipsilateral lymph node, ≤3 cm in greatest dimension.
N2a	Metastasis in single ipsilateral lymph node, >3 cm but ≤6 cm in greatest dimension.
N2b	Metastases in multiple ipsilateral lymph nodes, none >6 cm in greatest dimension.
N2c	Metastases in bilateral or contralateral lymph nodes, none >6 cm in greatest dimension.
N3	Metastasis in a lymph node, >6 cm in greatest dimension.
M0	No distant metastasis.
M1	Distant metastasis.

Stage	T	N	M
0	Tis	N0	M0
I	T1	N0	M0
II	T2	N0	M0
III	T3	N0	M0
	T1	N1	M0
	T2	N1	M0
	T3	N1	M0
IVA	T4a	N0	M0
	T4a	N1	M0
	T1	N2	M0
	T2	N2	M0
	T3	N2	M0
	T4a	N2	M0
IVB	Any T	N3	M0
	T4b	Any N	M0
IVC	Any T	Any N	M1

Source: With kind permission from Springer Science+Business Media: *AJCC Cancer Staging Atlas*, 2012, pp. 41–53, Compton, et al.

primary tumour leaving a minimum 1 cm vertical height of the intact mandible. Marginal mandiblectomy is contraindicated in cases with gross clinical and radiological involvement of mandible, large-volume paramandibular disease, in edentulous patients and where the residual mandibular segment height is <1 cm.

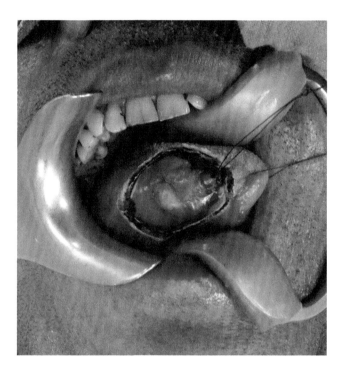

Figure 17.6 Wide excision of carcinoma tongue.

Table 17.3 Conditions with >20% chances of lymph node metastases

Tongue lesions: T1 >4 mm thickness, T2 or beyond, any thickness
Floor of mouth lesions: T1 >1.5 mm thickness, T2 or beyond, any thickness
Buccal mucosa and other subsites: T3 and beyond
Presence of lymphovascular involvement

Management of neck nodes

In patients with clinically negative nodes, the indications for nodal dissection are based on the risk of occult nodal metastases. In patients with >20% risk of nodal metastases (Table 17.3) an elective nodal dissection (END) is indicated. An END is also indicated in patients with a short neck (whose evaluation is difficult), those unreliable for follow-up and those where the neck is entered to excise the primary lesion. The preferred surgery is a supraomohyoid neck dissection (SOND), which is the removal of the level I–III lymph nodes and an extended supraomohyoid neck dissection (removal of levels I–IV) for lesions of the tongue. In node negative neck low-risk patients (<20% risk of cervical lymph node metastases), periodic evaluation is necessary to recognize nodal recurrence early.

A recently reported RCT by D'Çruz et al. has shown a significant benefit, in terms of both disease-free and overall survival, of END over therapeutic node dissection (TND) in early stage clinically node negative oral squamous cell cancer. END at the time of primary surgery compared to watchful waiting followed by TND in relapsing patients shows an absolute overall survival benefit of 12.5 percentage points and a disease-free survival benefit of 23.6 percentage points [9].

In patients with positive nodes on preoperative evaluation, a comprehensive nodal dissection is indicated (Table 17.4). A radical neck dissection is rarely performed except for extensive nodal disease. A modified neck dissection, with preservation of the spinal accessory nerve, internal jugular vein (IJV) or sternocleidomastoid (SCM) muscle, is preferred because of better functional and cosmetic outcomes.

Reconstruction

The need for and type of reconstruction depends on the extent of surgical resection and the resultant defect. The goal is to provide a complete and early functional restoration, which enables the patient to ingest food and vocalize and to provide a good cosmetic result. Defects can either be closed primarily or be reconstructed by skin grafts, local flaps (nasolabial, palatal) or regional flaps (pectoralis major myocutaneous flap, deltopectoral flap). However, the

Table 17.4 Types of neck dissections

Type	Lymph node levels removed	Structures removed in addition to lymph nodes		
		SCM	IJV	SAN
Radical neck dissection (RND)	I–V	Yes	Yes	Yes
Modified neck dissection (MND) type I	I–V	Yes	Yes	No
Modified neck dissection (MND) type II	I–V	Yes	No	No
Modified neck dissection (MND) type III	I–V	No	No	No
Supraomohyoid neck dissection	I–III	No	No	No
Extended supraomohyoid neck dissection	I–IV	No	No	No

emphasis today is on achieving high-quality reconstruction using microvascular free flaps. These flaps can be either fasciocutaneous (free radial artery flap, anterolateral thigh free flap) or osseocutaneous (free fibular flap), which are reliable substitutes providing function and cosmesis.

Radiotherapy

Patients at risk for locoregional recurrence are given adjuvant radiation, either alone or combined with chemotherapy as chemoradiation. The criteria for the need for adjuvant radiotherapy are the presence of large-volume primary disease (T3/4), a large nodal burden (N2/3) with extracapsular involvement, high-grade tumours, perineural invasion, close margins or involvement of level IV or V lymph nodes.

In patients with a high risk of recurrence (positive surgical margins, extracapsular invasion), radiotherapy combined with chemotherapy has the benefit of better locoregional control [10], though with increased toxicity. This is based on the combined analysis of two large RCTs which showed a benefit of chemoradiation compared with radiotherapy alone [11,12]. Commonly used doses are in the range of 60–66 Gy at 2 Gy per fraction given 5 days a week.

Definitive chemoradiation is given in patients who are not candidates for curative surgical resection (T4b lesions). Cisplatin is given along with 70 Gy radiation in 35 fractions.

Preoperative radiotherapy is generally not recommended because of difficulty with subsequent surgery. However, it may be given in a select group of patients who have fixed neck nodes and those who will have an extensive surgery or reconstructive procedure which might delay administration of postoperative radiation.

Chemotherapy

Chemotherapy alone is not curative in oral cancers. However, it can be given in combination with other treatment modalities – radiotherapy and surgery – either as adjuvant or neoadjuvant therapy, or alone in the palliative settings. Meta-analysis of chemotherapy in head and neck cancer (MACH-NC) was first published in 2000 and subsequently updated in 2009 [13]. This update showed a benefit of addition of chemotherapy to the locoregional treatment.

A subsite analysis of this meta-analysis has shown a 5.1% absolute 5-year overall survival benefit of adding chemotherapy to oral cancer treatment plans. However, when analyzed with respect to the timing of the chemotherapy, it failed to show significant benefit in the adjuvant and neoadjuvant setting (hazard ratio [HR], [95% confidence interval], 0.83 [0.69, 1.01] and 0.94 [0.84, 1.06]), with benefit derived only in concurrent use with radiotherapy (HR [95% confidence interval] 0.81 [0.73, 0.90]) [14].

Neoadjuvant chemotherapy (NACT) is used in oral cancers with the aim of organ preservation (mandible) and downstaging of disease. There is only limited evidence that it has achieved either of these goals [15]. A recent study from India has shown a survival benefit in oral cancer

patients who were responders to neoadjuvant chemotherapy (NACT), and could undergo definitive surgery [16].

Palliative chemotherapy has been shown to improve survival in patients with metastatic disease, not suitable for curative treatment. Commonly used agents are taxanes, platinum agents, methotrexate and 5-fluorouracil (5FU), either alone or in combination.

Targeted therapy

Anti-epidermal growth factor receptor (EGFR) agents have been used as potential targets in treating oral cancers. Erbitux in First-Line Treatment of Recurrent or Metastatic Head and Neck Cancer (EXTREME) was a phase III trial which compared outcomes in patients with metastatic or recurrent head and neck cancers who were randomized to receive either cisplatin +5FU alone or in combination with cetuximab, an anti-EGFR monoclonal antibody. The patients receiving cetuximab had significantly better overall survival with an acceptable side effect profile when compared with patients in the other arm [17].

MANAGEMENT OF RECURRENT LESIONS

The management of recurrent cancer depends on the extent and site of recurrence. All patients with recurrence should be restaged to see all potential sites of metastasis.

For patients with disease localized to the primary site or to the neck nodes, surgical resection, if possible, should be done. Surgical resection provides the best outcomes, with long-term survival providing higher disease-specific and overall survival than patients who did not undergo surgery [18]. For patients with unresectable disease, palliative treatment is recommended.

REHABILITATION

Rehabilitation is an important aspect for patients undergoing treatment for oral cancers. The most common problems encountered are xerostomia, loss of sphincter mechanism of the oral commissure, difficulty in swallowing and mastication and speech difficulties.

Xerostomia is generally a sequel of radiation therapy and is treated with saliva substitutes and patient education to drink liquids prior to eating solid food and is useful in preventing aspiration. Radiation also leads to fibrosis of the oral cavity. Exercises to maintain mouth opening and tongue mobility are important. In patients who develop a palatal defect, the placement of a prosthesis is helpful in preventing nasal regurgitation of food and restoring quality of speech.

FOLLOW-UP

Patients who have been treated for oral cancer should be followed up at regular intervals to look for any signs of recurrence. Initially, for the first year, the patients should be seen every 3 months and imaging conducted whenever required. Subsequently, patients can be followed up at longer intervals.

OROPHARYNX

The boundaries of oropharynx are from the level of the hard palate superiorly to the hyoid inferiorly, from the anterior tonsillar pillars anteriorly to the posterior pharyngeal wall posteriorly. It includes the posterior third of the tongue, the tonsils and the walls of the pharynx.

There is evidence of the role of HPV in the pathogenesis of oropharyngeal cancers, and there is evidence of a better prognosis associated with these HPV positive patients [19]. The primary treatment for oropharyngeal cancers is chemoradiation, as surgical procedures can lead to more functional disabilities. However, surgery is useful in addressing small and recurrent lesions which leave patients with less functional compromise.

REFERENCES

1. Forman D, Bray F, Brewster DH, Gombe Mbalawa C, Kohler B, Piñeros M, et al. Cancer incidence in five continents, vol. X [electronic version]. Lyon: International Agency for Research on Cancer, 2013. http://ci5.iarc.fr (accessed 2 July 2015).
2. Byers RM, Weber RS, Andrews T, McGill D, Kare R, Wolf P. Frequency and therapeutic implications of "skip metastases" in the neck from squamous carcinoma of the oral tongue. *Head Neck* 1997;19(1):14–9.
3. Pentenero M, Gandolfo S, Carrozzo M. Importance of tumor thickness and depth of invasion in nodal involvement and prognosis of oral squamous cell carcinoma: a review of the literature. *Head Neck* 2005;27(12):1080–91.
4. Goerkem M, Braun J, Stoeckli SJ. Evaluation of clinical and histomorphological parameters as potential predictors of occult metastases in sentinel lymph nodes of early squamous cell carcinoma of the oral cavity. *Ann Surg Oncol* 2010; 17(2):527–35.
5. Warnakulasuriya S, Johnson NW, van der Waal I. Nomenclature and classification of potentially malignant disorders of the oral mucosa. *J Oral Pathol Med* 2007;36(10):575–80.
6. Sankaranarayanan R, Ramadas K, Thara S, Muwonge R, Thomas G, Anju G, et al. Long term effect of visual screening on oral cancer incidence and mortality in a randomized trial in Kerala, India. *Oral Oncol* 2013;49(4):314–21.
7. Mendenhall WM, Werning JW, Pfister DG. Treatment of head and neck cancer. In DeVita VT Jr, Lawrence TS, Rosenberg SA, eds., *Cancer: Principles and Practice of Oncology*. 9th ed. Philadelphia: Lippincott Williams & Wilkins, 2011, pp. 729–80.

8. Compton CC, Byrd DR, Garcia-Aguilar J, Kurtzman SH, Olawaiye A, Washington MK (eds.). Lip and oral cavity. *AJCC Cancer Staging Atlas*. New York: Springer, 2012, pp. 41–53.
9. D'Çruz AK, Vaish R, Kapre N, Dandekar M, Gupta S, Hawaldar R, et al. Elective versus therapeutic neck dissection in node-negative oral cancer. *N Engl J Med* 2015;373(6):521–9.
10. Bernier J, Cooper JS, Pajak TF, van Glabbeke M, Bourhis J, Forastiere A, et al. Defining risk levels in locally advanced head and neck cancers: a comparative analysis of concurrent postoperative radiation plus chemotherapy trials of the EORTC (#22931) and RTOG (#9501). *Head Neck* 2005;27(10):843–50.
11. Bernier J, Domenge C, Ozsahin M, Matuszewska K, Lefèbvre JL, Greiner RH, et al. Postoperative irradiation with or without concomitant chemotherapy for locally advanced head and neck cancer. *N Engl J Med* 2004;350(19):1945–52.
12. Cooper JS, Pajak TF, Forastiere AA, Jacobs J, Campbell BH, Saxman SB, et al. Postoperative concurrent radiotherapy and chemotherapy for high-risk squamous-cell carcinoma of the head and neck. *N Engl J Med* 2004;350(19):1937–44.
13. Pignon JP, le Maître A, Maillard E, Bourhis J, MACH-NC Collaborative Group. Meta-analysis of chemotherapy in head and neck cancer (MACH-NC): an update on 93 randomised trials and 17,346 patients. *Radiother Oncol* 2009;92(1):4–14.
14. Blanchard P, Baujat B, Holostenco V, Bourredjem A, Baey C, Bourhis J, et al. Meta-analysis of chemotherapy in head and neck cancer (MACH-NC): a comprehensive analysis by tumour site. *Radiother Oncol* 2011;100(1):33–40.
15. Licitra L, Grandi C, Guzzo M, Mariani L, Lo Vullo S, Valvo F, et al. Primary chemotherapy in resectable oral cavity squamous cell cancer: a randomized controlled trial. *J Clin Oncol* 2003;21(2):327–33.
16. Patil VM, Prabhash K, Noronha V, Joshi A, Muddu V, Dhumal S, et al. Neoadjuvant chemotherapy followed by surgery in very locally advanced technically unresectable oral cavity cancers. *Oral Oncol* 2014;50(10):1000–4.
17. Vermorken JB, Mesia R, Rivera F, Remenar E, Kawecki A, Rottey S, et al. Platinum-based chemotherapy plus cetuximab in head and neck cancer. *N Engl J Med* 2008;259(11):1116–27.
18. Liao CT, Chang JT, Wang HM, Ng SH, Hsueh C, Lee LY, et al. Salvage therapy in relapsed squamous cell carcinoma of the oral cavity: how and when? *Cancer* 2008;112(1):94–103.
19. Ang KK, Harris J, Wheeler R, Weber R, Rosenthal DI, Nguyen-Tân PF, et al. Human papillomavirus and survival of patients with oropharyngeal cancer. *N Engl J Med* 2010;363(1):24–35.

18

Salivary gland tumors

ARUN CHATURVEDI, AKASH AGARWAL AND SANJEEV MISRA

INTRODUCTION

Salivary gland neoplasms are uncommon tumors with diverse pathology, biological behaviour, clinical course and management. An understanding of the diversity and the natural history of various histopathological tumor types is fundamental to sound clinical management. Annual incidence rates for malignant salivary gland tumors (SGTs) range from <0.05 to 2.3 per 100,000 in males and up to 1.7 per 100,000 in females [1], and they constitute 3–4% of head and neck cancers [2].

ANATOMY

Salivary tissue is distributed in the paired major salivary glands and smaller aggregates of minor salivary glands. The paired major salivary glands include the parotid, submandibular and sublingual glands. The minor salivary glands are distributed as hundreds of aggregates of salivary tissue in the mucosa of the upper aerodigestive tract (oral cavity, palate, uvula, peritonsillar area, pharynx, larynx and paranasal sinuses) [2].

ETIOLOGY

The etiology of SGTs is largely unknown. Occupational exposures shown to be associated with SGTs are rubber manufacturing, asbestos mining, hairdressing salons and wood and nickel industry [3,4]. Association of irradiation,

immunosuppression, Epstein–Barr virus and HIV infection with SGTs has been shown [5–7]. A past history of Hodgkin's lymphoma, medulloblastoma, UV radiation exposure or basal cell cancer of the skin has also been associated with salivary gland malignancy [8–12].

PATHOLOGY

SGTs have diverse histopathology and represent perhaps the most heterogeneous group of tumors from any tissue [13]. The WHO [14] and Armed Forces Institute of Pathology (AFIP) classifications [12], based on recognizable morphological patterns, are complex. Some of these tumors are known to be benign, while others have varied biological behaviour and aggressiveness which are reflected by the grade of the tumor. The grade of the tumor is an important prognostic factor. However, treatment outcome may relate more to clinical stage and grade must be considered in context to the tumor's stage.

Pleomorphic adenomas are the most common benign SGT and constitute 65% of parotid and half of all SGTs. Mucoepidermoid carcinoma is the most common malignant SGT (10% of all and 35% of malignant SGTs) [15,16]. The most common site is the parotid gland [2,16,17].

The majority (80%) of SGTs occur in the parotid glands and are benign. Malignant tumors constitute 15–32% of parotid, 41–45% of submandibular and 70–90% of sublingual SGTs [5,15].

Childhood salivary gland tumors

These are rarer than in adults. Most of the SGTs in children are benign tumors and tumor-like conditions. In a series on those less than 14 years old, 22.5% had a salivary gland carcinoma (epithelial–myoepithelial, salivary duct and mucoepidermoid). Metastasis (4%) and lymphomas (1.5%) were reported in a minority of patients [18].

PROGNOSTIC FACTORS

Several prognostic factors have been described for SGTs – site, histopathology, grade, T stage, presence of nodal disease, facial nerve involvement, fixation to deeper structures and skin, and distant metastasis [19,20]. The clinical stage of the tumor, particularly the T stage, may be the most important prognostic factor. It may be even more important than the histopathological grade [21,22]. The '4 cm rule' may be used as a prognostic guide. Tumors less than 4 cm will do well regardless of grade and histopathological type [15]. Prognostic factors similar to major SGTs have also been described for minor SGTs and are used for deciding the optimal treatment strategy [23].

CLINICAL FEATURES

The majority (80%) of SGTs arise from the parotid gland and present as a painless, localized swelling. SGTs present as swellings or lumps developing over a variable period of time at the site of major salivary glands (Figure 18.1). Tumors which are benign or low grade have a long history of a painless, slowly progressive swelling. High-grade aggressive malignant tumors usually have a shorter, rapidly progressive course with subsequent development of clinical features of facial nerve involvement and lymphatic spread of disease. The risk of malignancy in pleomorphic adenoma is 1.5% up to 5 years and 9.5% after 15 years [24]. There is a 7.1% risk of cancer with recurrent benign mixed tumors.

Advanced disease may present with trismus and skin ulceration (Figure 18.2). Deep lobe parotid tumors are uncommon (10%) and present as an oropharyngeal swelling or medialization of tonsil.

Rarely patients may present with metastatic disease. Patients with malignant SGT may develop metastatic disease over a long period. Over a period of 10 years metastatic disease may occur in about 30–40% patients, the most common sites being lungs (80%) and bones (15%) [25,26].

Minor SGTs may present at various sites in the upper aerodigestive tract as a submucosal swelling. Symptoms depend on the particular site of disease. A higher proportion of patients (50% of palate tumors) have a malignancy than major salivary glands [15].

DIAGNOSTIC WORK-UP

Tissue diagnosis

Fine Needle Aspiration Cytology (FNAC) is an inexpensive and reliable method to diagnose SGTs and has a high sensitivity (above 80% in large series) and specificity (87–99%) [27]. Tumor seeding is negligible and FNAC is simple and safe. Accuracy can be improved by combining it with Ultrasonography (USG) guidance [25].

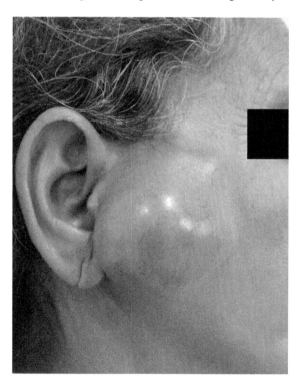

Figure 18.1 Tumor of the parotid gland.

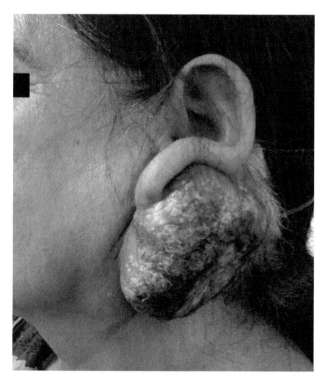

Figure 18.2 Advanced parotid tumor with skin ulceration.

Core needle biopsy may be needed when FNAC is inconclusive and can be safely done for parotid and submandibular neoplasms. Open biopsy is not recommended. Frozen section assessment of histopathology is not reliable and has limited application.

Imaging

Ultrasound imaging, though operator dependent, can provide useful initial information [25] about the site and nature of the primary disease and also the presence and extent of cervical lymphadenopathy.

Contrast-enhanced computed tomography (CECT) is valuable in diagnosing deep lobe tumors and defining the extent of locoregional disease in large tumors.

Magnetic resonance imaging (MRI) is the preferred imaging modality [28] and has the added advantage of better anatomical detail including relation to the facial nerve. MRI can also distinguish between tumor and obstructed secretions.

The role of FDG-PET in SGTs is still investigational.

Staging

The AJCC-UICC TNM classification [29] is used for staging salivary gland cancers (Table 18.1). Minor salivary gland cancers are staged according to their anatomic site.

MANAGEMENT

Surgery

PAROTID GLAND

Superficial parotidectomy is the standard treatment for benign parotid tumors. Conservative total parotidectomy may be needed in close to 10% patients who have deep lobe involvement. The facial nerve is especially at risk in recurrent lesions with dense scarring.

Surgery is the mainstay for treatment of malignant SGTs. Good initial treatment is crucial to long-term survival. This involves adequate surgical resection with clear margins. Surgical treatment may be a superficial, total, deep lobe, radical or extended parotidectomy. For the vast majority of tumors in the superficial lobe of parotid a superficial parotidectomy with clear resection margins is an appropriate surgical treatment (Figure 18.3). Deep lobe tumors require either a total parotidectomy or a deep lobe resection only, if possible.

Unless clinically involved, effort is made to preserve the facial nerve in all cases (Figure 18.4). Only when the nerve is inseparably encased in tumor tissue would a nerve resection be justified. The patient must be prepared for possible facial nerve sacrifice. Immediate nerve grafting using the greater auricular nerve may be done in this situation. Alternatively, interpositional sural nerve graft, hypoglossal–facial nerve transfer or free muscle flap with or without cross-face sural nerve graft can be done. Other regional

Table 18.1 AJCC T stage of salivary gland tumors[a]

Tx	Primary tumor cannot be assessed
T0	No evidence of primary tumor
Tis	Carcinoma in situ
T1	Tumor = 2 cm in greatest dimension without extraparenchymal extension (clinical or macroscopic evidence of invasion of the soft tissues, not microscopic evidence)
T2	Tumor >2 cm but not more than 4 cm in greatest dimension without extraparenchymal extension
T3	Tumor >4 cm and/or tumor has extraparenchymal extension
T4a	Tumor invades the skin, mandible, ear canal and/or facial nerve
T4b	Tumor invades skull base and/or pterygoid plates and/or encases carotid artery

Stage	T	N	M
0	Tis	N0	M0
I	T1	N0	M0
II	T2	N0	M0
III	T3	N0	M0
	T1	N1	M0
	T2	N1	M0
	T3	N1	M0
IVA	T4a	N0	M0
	T4a	N1	M0
	T1	N2	M0
	T2	N2	M0
	T3	N2	M0
	T4a	N2	M0
IVB	T any	N3	M0
	T4b	n any	M0
IVC	T any	N any	M1

Source: With kind permission from Springer Science+Business Media: *AJCC Cancer Staging Atlas*, 2012, pp. 41–53, Compton, et al.

[a] N and M categories are same as other head and neck sites.

muscle transpositions and static facial support techniques are also available [30]. Eyelid gold implants may be done to prevent corneal damage.

NECK

Neck node metastases are more common in the submandibular gland (40%) than the parotid gland (25%) [25]. Elective neck node dissection is not recommended for malignant parotid tumors. In high-grade tumors an intraoperative frozen section assessment of level 2 nodes may be used to indicate the need for a formal comprehensive radical neck dissection [31]. Occult metastasis rates are higher in patients with high-grade, advanced T stage tumors with extracapsular extension and facial paralysis [32].

Where lymph nodes are clinically involved, a therapeutic comprehensive neck dissection is indicated.

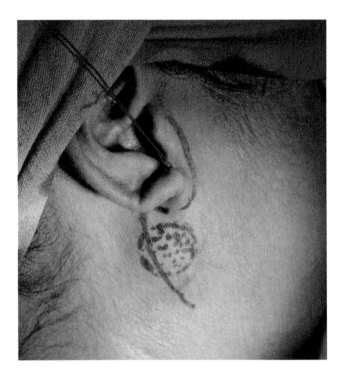

Figure 18.3 Skin incision for parotidectomy.

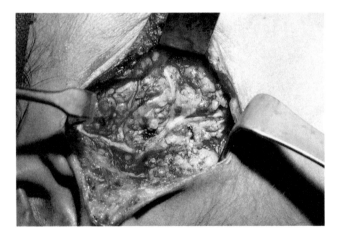

Figure 18.4 Branches of facial nerve exposed after superficial parotidectomy.

SUBMANDIBULAR GLAND

Submandibular tumors require a margin-free excision of the submandibular gland. For malignant tumors a formal level 1 or a supraomohyoid neck dissection is done. In patients with locally advanced disease additional resection of adherent or involved structures, e.g. lingual or hypoglossal nerve, muscles or mandibular margin, may be needed. Metastatic nodal disease would require a comprehensive neck dissection.

MINOR SALIVARY GLAND

Minor SGTs require a wide-margin (5 mm or more) resection similar to that done for squamous cell cancer.

Radiotherapy

Though historically considered radioresistant, radiotherapy plays an important role in the adjuvant postoperative setting and as the definitive treatment for unresectable SGTs.

Adjuvant radiotherapy is indicated for the management of SGTs which are high grade, recurrent or have close or positive resection margins. Additionally, tumors which are advanced T stage (invading adjacent structures), have nodal involvement, and perineural and angiolymphatic invasion may also benefit from adjuvant postoperative radiotherapy [25,31]. Doses ranging from 60 to 66 Gy have been used.

Definitive radiotherapy is indicated for unresectable malignant SGTs. Fast neutron beam radiotherapy is recommended in this situation [33]. The limited availability and toxicity of neutron beam radiation prevent it from being standard treatment [34]. Accelerated hyperfractionated photon beam radiation therapy has also provided good locoregional control [35].

The role of adjuvant chemoradiotherapy (CT-RT) is not well established. Few studies have shown better overall survival using adjuvant CT-RT in high-risk patients and also in the definitive setting [36–39].

Chemotherapy

This is used for palliating symptomatic patients with metastatic disease. Due to rarity and heterogeneity of these tumors, there is lack of phase III clinical trials evaluating the role of chemotherapy. The recommendations are based on large case series and few phase II trials. Numerous chemotherapeutic agents have been used, either alone or in combination, but none with very encouraging results [40]. Cisplatin, mitoxantrone, cyclophosphamide, 5-fluorouracil (5FU), gemcitabine, vinorelbine, paclitaxel and docetaxel have been used as single-agent chemotherapy. A combination of platinum and taxanes, cyclophosphamide, doxorubicin and cisplatin and several other combinations have been reported [40].

Targeted therapies

Due to the increased understanding of molecular aberration in SGTs, the use of targeted agents has been examined [40]. The most common agents include the tyrosine kinase inhibitors, monoclonal antibodies and proteosome inhibitors. Trastuzumab and lapatinib are the most promising among these. However, the use of these agents is still limited to clinical trials.

Advances in molecular pathogenesis have elucidated the key role of fusion oncogenes in SGTs. This has opened the way to developing novel targeted agents [25].

RECURRENT DISEASE

Treatment outcomes and prognosis in recurrent malignant SGTs are poor. Treatment depends on the tumor histopathology, site and extent of recurrence, previous treatment and individual factors.

Surgical resection, if possible, followed by radiation therapy or reirradiation can be used depending on the nature and extent of recurrence. Radiotherapy (preferably fast neutron beam) or palliative chemotherapy may be needed if this is not feasible. Metastatic lung disease, if solitary, can be resected [26]. Skeletal metastasis can be managed by surgery, radiation, chemotherapy or biphosphonates as indicated. Salivary gland metastasis may have an indolent course with prolonged survival despite the advanced nature of the disease.

FOLLOW-UP

Most (70%) recurrences occur within the first 3 years [26]. Follow-up at 3–6 months is recommended in the initial 3 years. After 3 years, follow-up can be done every 6 months and once a year after 5 years. Since late relapse can occur, yearly follow-up may be continued for up to 20 years.

CONCLUSIONS

SGTs are relatively uncommon. However, they pose a challenge to the surgeon by their histological diversity, unpredictable behaviour and tendency for long-term recurrences.

REFERENCES

1. Forman D, Bray F, Brewster DH, Gombe Mbalawa C, Kohler B, Piñeros M, et al. Cancer incidence in five continents, vol. X [electronic version]. Lyon: International Agency for Research on Cancer, 2013. http://ci5.iarc.fr (accessed 2 July 2015).
2. Mendenhall WM, Werning JW, Pfister DG. Treatment of head and neck cancer. In DeVita VT Jr, Lawrence TS, Rosenberg SA, eds., *Cancer: Principles and Practice of Oncology*, 9th ed. Philadelphia: Lippincott Williams & Wilkins, 2011, pp. 729–80.
3. Swanson GM, Burns PB. Cancers of the salivary gland: workplace risks among women and men. *Ann Epidemiol* 1997;7(6):369–74.
4. Horn-Ross PL, Ljung BM, Morrow M. Environmental factors and the risk of salivary gland cancer. *Epidemiology* 1997;8(4):414–9.
5. Eveson JW, Cawson RA. Tumours of the minor (oropharyngeal) salivary glands: a demographic study of 336 cases. *J Oral Pathol Med* 1985;14(6):500–9.
6. Bell RB, Dierks EJ, Homer L, Potter BE. Management and outcome of patients with malignant salivary gland tumors. *J Oral Maxillofac Surg* 2005;63(7):917–28.
7. Serraino D, Boschini A, Carrieri P, Pradier C, Dorrucci M, Dal Maso L, et al. Cancer risk among men with, or at risk of, HIV infection in southern Europe. *AIDS.* 2000;14(5):553–9.
8. Dong C, Hemminki K. Second primary neoplasms among 53 159 haematolymphoproliferative malignancy patients in Sweden, 1958–1996: a search for common mechanisms. *Br J Cancer* 2001;85(7):997–1005.
9. Goldstein AM, Yuen J, Tucker MA. Second cancers after medulloblastoma: population-based results from the United States and Sweden. *Cancer Causes Control* 1997;8(6):865–71.
10. Milán T, Pukkala E, Verkasalo PK, Kaprio J, Jansén CT, Koskenvuo M, et al. Subsequent primary cancers after basal-cell carcinoma: a nationwide study in Finland from 1953 to 1995. *Int J Cancer* 2000;87(2):283–8.
11. Spitz MR, Tilley BC, Batsakis JG, Gibeau JM, Newell GR. Risk factors for major salivary gland carcinoma. A case-comparison study. *Cancer* 1984;54(9):1854–9.
12. Ellis GL, Auclair PL. *Tumors of the Salivary Glands, Atlas of Tumor Pathology: Third Series.* Washington, DC: Armed Forces Institute of Pathology, 1996.
13. Brandwein MS, Ferlito A, Bradley PJ, Hille JJ, Rinaldo A. Diagnosis and classification of salivary neoplasms: pathologic challenges and relevance to clinical outcomes. *Acta Otolaryngol* 2002;122(7):758–64.
14. Barnes L, Eveson JW, Reichart P, Sidransky D, eds. *Pathology and Genetics of Head and Neck Tumours*, 3rd ed. Lyon: International Agency for Research on Cancer, 2005.
15. Speight PM, Barrett AW. Salivary gland tumours. *Oral Dis* 2002;8(5):229–40.
16. Guzzo M, Andreola S, Sirizzotti G, Cantu G. Mucoepidermoid carcinoma of the salivary glands: clinicopathologic review of 108 patients treated at the National Cancer Institute of Milan. *Ann Surg Oncol* 2002;9(7):688–95.
17. Goode RK, Auclair PL, Ellis GL. Mucoepidermoid carcinoma of the major salivary glands: clinical and histopathologic analysis of 234 cases with evaluation of grading criteria. *Cancer* 1998;82(7):1217–24.
18. Muenscher A, Diegel T, Jaehne M, Ussmüller J, Koops S, Sanchez-Hanke M. Benign and malignant salivary gland diseases in children A retrospective study of 549 cases from the Salivary Gland Registry, Hamburg. *Auris Nasus Larynx* 2009;36(3):326–31.
19. Terhaard CH, Lubsen H, Van der Tweel I, Hilgers FJ, Eijkenboom WM, Marres HA, et al. Salivary gland carcinoma: independent prognostic factors for locoregional control, distant metastases, and overall survival: results of the Dutch Head and Neck Oncology Cooperative Group. *Head Neck* 2004;26(8):681–92.
20. Vander Poorten VL, Balm AJ, Hilgers FJ, Tan IB, Loftus-Coll BM, Keus RB, et al. The development of a prognostic score for patients with parotid carcinoma. *Cancer* 1999;85(9):2057–67.

21. Vander Poorten VL, Balm AJ, Hilgers FJ, Tan IB, Loftus-Coll BM, Keus RB, et al. Prognostic factors for long term results of the treatment of patients with malignant submandibular gland tumors. *Cancer* 1999;85(10):2255–64.

22. Spiro RH. Factors affecting survival in salivary gland cancers. In: McGurk M, Renehan AG, (eds.). Controversies in the Management of Salivary Gland Disease. Oxford, UK: Oxford University Press, 2001, pp.143–50.

23. Vander Poorten VL, Balm AJ, Hilgers FJ, Tan IB, Keus RB, Hart AA. Stage as major long term outcome predictor in minor salivary gland carcinoma. *Cancer* 2000;89(6):1195–204.

24. Phillips PP, Olsen KD. Recurrent pleomorphic adenoma of the parotid gland: report of 126 cases and a review of the literature. *Ann Otol Rhinol Laryngol* 1995;104(2):100–4.

25. Carlson J, Licitra L, Locati L, Raben D, Persson F, Stenman G. Salivary gland cancer: an update on present and emerging therapies. *Am Soc Clin Oncol Educ Book* 2013:257–63.

26. Thiagarajan S, Nair VS, Joshi P, Chaturvedi P. A review of salivary gland neoplasms and its management. *Online J Otolaryngol* 2014;4(3):41–60.

27. Tyagi R, Dey P. Diagnostic problems of salivary gland tumors. *Diagn Cytopathol* 2015;43(6):495–509.

28. Shah GV. MR imaging of salivary glands. *Magn Reson Imaging Clin N Am* 2002;10(4):631–62.

29. Compton CC, Byrd DR, Garcia-Aguilar J, Kurtzman SH, Olawaiye A, Washington MK. Major salivary glands. In Compton CC, Byrd DR, Garcia-Aguilar J, Kurtzman SH, Olawaiye A, Washington MK, eds., *AJCC Cancer Staging Atlas*. New York, NY: Springer, 2012, pp. 105–12.

30. Anderson RG. Facial nerve disorders and surgery. *Selected Readings Plastic Surg* 2006;10(14):1–41.

31. Andry G, Hamoir M, Locati LD, Licitra L, Langendijk JA. Management of salivary gland tumors. *Expert Rev Anticancer Ther* 2012;12(9):1161–8.

32. Armstrong JG, Harrison LB, Thaler HT, Friedlander-Klar H, Fass DE, Zelefsky MJ, et al. The indications for elective treatment of the neck in cancer of the major salivary glands. *Cancer* 1992;69(3):615–9.

33. Laramore GE, Krall JM, Griffin TW, Duncan W, Richter MP, Saroja KR, et al. Neutron versus photon irradiation for unresectable salivary gland tumors: final report of an RTOG-MRC randomized clinical trial. Radiation Therapy Oncology Group. Medical Research Council. *Int J Radiat Oncol Biol Phys* 1993;27(2):235–40.

34. Terhaard CH, Lubsen H, Rasch CR, Levendag PC, Kaanders HH, Tjho-Heslinga RE, et al. The role of radiotherapy in the treatment of malignant salivary gland tumors. *Int J Radiat Oncol Biol Phys* 2005;61(1):103–11.

35. Wang CC, Goodman M. Photon irradiation of unresectable carcinomas of salivary glands. *Int J Radiat Oncol Biol Phys* 1991;21(3):569–76.

36. Pederson AW, Salama JK, Haraf DJ, Witt ME, Stenson KM, Portugal L, et al. Adjuvant chemoradiotherapy for locoregionally advanced and high-risk salivary gland malignancies. *Head Neck Oncol* 2011;3:31.

37. Rosenberg L, Weissler M, Hayes DN, Shockley W, Zanation A, Rosenman J, et al. Concurrent chemoradiotherapy for locoregionally advanced salivary gland malignances. *Head Neck* 2012;34(6):872–6.

38. Schoenfeld JD, Sher DJ, Norris CM Jr, Haddad RI, Posner MR, Balboni TA, et al. Salivary gland tumors treated with adjuvant intensity-modulated radiotherapy with or without concurrent chemotherapy. *Int J Radiat Oncol Biol Phys* 2012;82(1):308–14.

39. Tanvetyanon T, Qin D, Padhya T, McCaffrey J, Zhu W, Boulware D, et al. Outcomes of postoperative concurrent chemoradiotherapy for locally advanced major salivary gland carcinoma. *Arch Otolaryngol Head Neck Surg* 2009;135(7):687–92.

40. Lagha A, Chraiet N, Ayadi M, Krimi S, Allani B, Rifi H, et al. Systemic therapy in the management of metastatic or advanced salivary gland cancers. *Head Neck Oncol* 2012;4:19.

19

Paranasal sinus cancers

SAMEER GUPTA, AKASH AGARWAL AND SANJEEV MISRA

INTRODUCTION

Paranasal sinus malignancies are rare, constituting approximately 3% of all head and neck malignancies [1]. Significant advances in the diagnosis and management of paranasal sinus malignancies have led to accurate delineation of tumor extent and safe excision of tumors, even involving the cranial base, with cosmetically acceptable outcomes. Microvascular free tissue transfer has made it possible to reconstruct these large defects effectively. Three-dimensional conformal radiation therapy (RT) and intensity-modulated radiation therapy (IMRT) allow optimal radiation dosimetry to the tumor while sparing normal surrounding tissue.

ANATOMY

The maxillary sinus (also called the *antrum of Highmore*), the largest of the paranasal sinuses, is pyramidal in shape. The ethmoid air cells consist of numerous thin-walled cavities situated in the ethmoid labyrinth and bounded by the frontal, maxillary, sphenoid and palatine bones on both sides. They are arranged in three groups – anterior, middle and posterior. The frontal sinuses are located above the superciliary arches. The sphenoid sinus begins at the most posterior and superior portion of the nasal cavity. The optic nerve and internal carotid artery are closely related to the superolateral wall of the sphenoid sinus.

Infratemporal fossa

It is located below and medial to the zygomatic arch bounded anteriorly by posterior surface of maxilla; superiorly by greater wing of sphenoid and squamous temporal bone; medially by lateral pterygoid plate and laterally by the ramus of mandible.

Lymphatic drainage

The lymphatic drainage of the paranasal sinuses goes primarily to the retropharyngeal and lateral pharyngeal nodes at the base of the skull, and subsequently to the upper jugular lymph nodes. Regional lymph node involvement at initial presentation is reported in approximately 10% of patients, but the overall reported risk of nodal involvement is close to 30% and is most commonly seen with maxillary sinus cancer [2]. The development of regional metastases is a poor prognostic indicator.

ETIOLOGY

Factors associated with an increased risk include occupational exposures including leather, textile, wood dust and formaldehyde. Air pollution, tobacco smoke, viral infection (human papilloma virus [HPV]) and metals such as nickel have also been associated with an increased risk [3].

PATHOLOGY

The most common epithelial neoplasm arising in the paranasal sinuses is squamous cell carcinoma followed by adenocarcinoma [4]. The majority of these tumors (88%) arise in the maxillary sinus followed by the ethmoid sinus (7%), with cancers of the sphenoid and frontal sinuses being uncommon (5%). Most patients (85%) present with T3 or T4 cancers [4].

CLINICAL FEATURES

Early disease is often asymptomatic or mimics common benign conditions such as chronic sinusitis, allergy or nasal polyposis. Common presenting symptoms include nasal obstruction, nasal discharge (mucoid or bloody), anosmia and headache. Failure of these symptoms to respond to appropriate medical therapy should alert the physician to the possibility of malignancy. Invasion of adjoining structures is an obvious but late manifestation of the disease and may present as soft tissue swelling of the face, non-healing ulcer in the palate, proptosis, epiphora, blurred vision, diplopia or middle ear effusion. Associated neck masses may represent metastasis in cervical lymph nodes.

DIAGNOSTIC WORK-UP

Imaging

Contrast-enhanced computerized tomography (CECT) in coronal and axial planes is the initial study of choice. Contrast enhancement improves tumor definition from adjacent soft tissues, while bone windows delineate the bony architecture [5]. Coronal images delineate involvement of the orbital floor and skull base, particularly the cribriform plate (Figures 19.1 and 19.2). Axial images demonstrate tumor extension through the posterior wall of the maxillary sinus into the pterygopalatine and infratemporal fossae.

MRI is preferred for better delineation of soft tissue extent, identification of perineural and intracranial extension and also to distinguish between retained secretions and tumor tissue. MRI is also helpful for postoperative monitoring and can be of particular importance in detecting recurrence [6].

Prosthetic or dental work-up

Evaluation by a maxillofacial prosthodontist is required to obtain a preoperative dental impression for creation of a postoperative prosthesis.

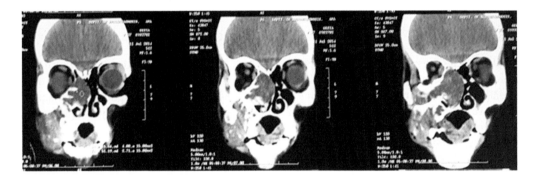

Figure 19.1 Serial coronal CT demonstrating superior, medial, lateral and inferior extension of maxillary sinus carcinoma.

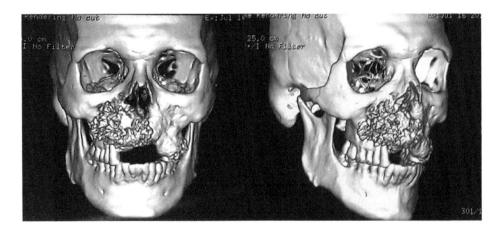

Figure 19.2 3D CT reconstruction of carcinoma of the maxilla involving the anterior bony wall.

Biopsy

Tumors confined to the maxillary sinus can be accessed endoscopically by creation of a wide antrostomy near the region of the natural ostium. Alternatively, biopsy can be done by the Caldwell–Luc approach. Tumors of the ethmoid sinus can be approached endoscopically or by an external ethmoidectomy approach via a Lynch incision. Frontal sinus tumors are rare and trephination through the floor of the sinus is used for biopsy of the lesions. The sphenoid sinus is easily approached endoscopically in the vast majority of cases.

STAGING

Ohngren (1933) divided the antrum into anteroinferior and superoposterior sections by an imaginary line drawn from the angle of the mandible to the medial canthus of the eye (Ohngren's line) [7]. Cancers located above the line (suprastructure) have a worse prognosis, as these tumors are in proximity to major vascular, neural and intracranial structures, and margin negative resection is difficult to achieve.

The American Joint Committee on Cancer (AJCC) staging system is widely used for classifying paranasal sinus (PNS) malignancies [8]. The N and M categories for PNS cancers are similar to those for oral cavity carcinoma (Table 19.1).

TREATMENT

Surgery

Surgical resection alone or in combination with adjuvant therapy remains the mainstay of treatment for cancers of the PNS. Surgery is indicated where a margin negative resection (R0) of the tumor can be attained with acceptable morbidity. The development of new craniofacial approaches has extended the indications for surgery to include patients with skull base and even limited intracranial extension. Microvascular free flap reconstruction and prosthetic rehabilitation have reduced morbidity following extensive resection.

The various surgical approaches used for PNS cancers are lateral rhinotomy, transoral, the Weber–Fergusson approach, midfacial degloving and the combined craniofacial approach.

Medial maxillectomy is indicated for tumors involving the lateral wall of the nasal cavity or medial wall of the maxillary antrum. A lateral rhinotomy or the Weber–Fergusson incision is most commonly employed.

Subtotal maxillectomy is done for tumors of the hard palate, gum and maxillary antrum involving the infrastructure of maxilla. A modified Weber–Ferguson incision is commonly used for adequate exposure and facilitating appropriate monobloc resection. The anterior wall of the maxilla is divided just below the infraorbital foramen (Figure 19.3).

Table 19.1 T stage of paranasal sinus tumors with stage grouping

TX	Primary tumor cannot be assessed.
T0	No evidence of primary tumor.
Tis	Carcinoma in situ.

Maxillary sinus

T1	Tumor limited to maxillary sinus mucosa with no erosion or destruction of bone.
T2	Tumor causing bone erosion or destruction including extension into the hard palate and/or middle nasal meatus, except extension to posterior wall of maxillary sinus and pterygoid plates.
T3	Tumor invades any of the following: bone of the posterior wall of maxillary sinus, subcutaneous tissues, floor or medial wall of orbit, pterygoid fossa or ethmoid sinuses.
T4a	Moderately advanced local disease. Tumor invades anterior orbital contents, skin of cheek, pterygoid plates, infratemporal fossa, cribriform plate, or sphenoid or frontal sinuses.
T4b	Very advanced local disease. Tumor invades any of the following: orbital apex, dura, brain, middle cranial fossa, cranial nerves other than maxillary division of trigeminal nerve (V_2), nasopharynx, or clivus.

Nasal cavity and ethmoid sinus

T1	Tumor restricted to any one subsite, with or without bony invasion.
T2	Tumor invading two subsites in a single region or extending to involve an adjacent region within the nasoethmoidal complex, with or without bony invasion.
T3	Tumor extends to invade the medial wall or floor of the orbit, maxillary sinus, palate, or cribriform plate.
T4a	Moderately advanced local disease. Tumor invades any of the following: anterior orbital contents, skin of nose or cheek, minimal extension to anterior cranial fossa, pterygoid plates, or sphenoid or frontal sinuses.
T4b	Very advanced local disease. Tumor invades any of the following: orbital apex, dura, brain, middle cranial fossa, cranial nerves other than (V_2), nasopharynx or clivus.

(Continued)

Table 19.1 *(Continued)* T stage of paranasal sinus tumors with stage grouping

Stage	T	N	M
0	Tis	N0	M0
I	T1	N0	M0
II	T2	N0	M0
III	T3	N0	M0
	T1	N1	M0
	T2	N1	M0
	T3	N1	M0
IVA	T4a	N0	M0
	T4a	N1	M0
	T1	N2	M0
	T2	N2	M0
	T3	N2	M0
	T4a	N2	M0
IVB	T any	N3	M0
	T4b	N any	M0
IVC	T any	N any	M1

Source: With kind permission from Springer Science+Business Media: *AJCC Cancer Staging Atlas*, 2012, pp. 41–53, Compton, et al.

Total maxillectomy is indicated for tumors filling the maxillary antrum. A modified Weber–Fergusson incision is employed. Osteotomies are performed as shown in Figure 19.4. The surgical defect is covered using split-thickness skin graft followed by a preformed surgical prosthesis or alternatively by a microvascular free flap.

Anterior craniofacial resection

Combined intracranial and extracranial approaches allow en bloc extirpation of paranasal tumors that abut or penetrate the skull base. A bicoronal incision is made along with an appropriate facial incision depending on the site and extent of tumor. The placement of osteotomies and the extent of resection are dictated by the extent of tumor. Watertight reconstruction of the skull base is usually achieved by a vascularized pericranial flap to prevent CSF leak and meningitis.

Management of the neck

The incidence of palpable cervical metastases range from 3% to 16%, with most series reporting an average incidence of 10% [9]. In patients with a clinically

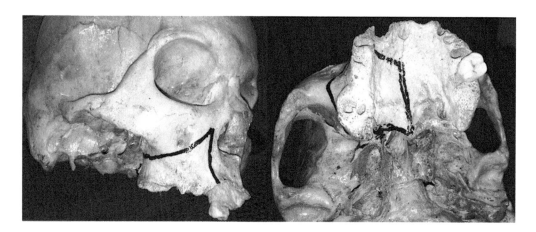

Figure 19.3 Osteotomy markings in subtotal maxillectomy.

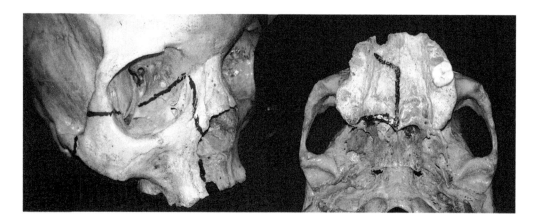

Figure 19.4 Osteotomy markings in total maxillectomy.

node negative neck, elective neck irradiation effectively reduces the relapse rate in the neck. For patients with clinical evidence of nodal metastases, combined modality of treatment with neck dissection and post operative adjuvant radiotherapy with or without chemotherapy offers the best chance of disease control.

Radiotherapy

RT is used in paranasal sinus cancer either as an adjuvant to surgery or in the palliative setting. It is also used in combination with chemotherapy for definitive treatment. Adjuvant RT is indicated in early lesions (T1, T2) with positive resection margins, perineural spread, adenoid cystic histology and all T3 and T4a lesions [10]. The usual dose of RT in the adjuvant setting is 60–74 Gy [11]. Three-dimensional CRT and IMRT significantly reduce the radiation doses to the brain and ipsilateral parotid gland compared with conventional treatment [12,13].

Chemotherapy

Chemotherapy may be given as induction therapy or as part of a chemoradiation protocol in the adjuvant or palliative setting. Concurrent chemoradiation seems to enhance local control and disease-specific survival in patients with advanced PNS malignancies [14]. Excellent long-term local control, overall survival and disease-free survival may be achieved in patients with locoregionally advanced PNS cancers treated with induction chemotherapy (consisting of three cycles of cisplatin and 5-fluorouracil [5 FU]) followed by surgery and postoperative concurrent chemoradiotherapy [15]. These results have been shown to be superior to those treated with surgery and RT alone.

Principles of reconstruction and rehabilitation

Oronasal separation is required to achieve effective speech and deglutition. This is done by a prosthetic obturator or tissue flaps. To minimize the risk of CSF leak, meningitis and pneumocephalus, cranionasal separation is essential. Options for repairing large dural defects include temporalis fascia, pericranium or fascia lata grafts. Bony defects of the anterior skull base can be repaired using vascularized or non-vascularized bone grafts and bone cement [16]. Loss of three maxillary supports – nasomaxillary, zygomaticomaxillary and pterygomaxillary – results in superio-posterior deviation of the alar base of the nose, inferior displacement of the orbit and flattening of the malar eminence and posterior–superior deviation of the upper lip, respectively. Skeletal reconstruction options include autogenous calvarial bone grafts, demineralized bone grafts or alloplastic implants like titanium mesh and bone cement accompanied by adequate soft tissue coverage. Prosthetic dentures are the easiest method of dental restoration. Early initiation of jaw opening exercises using stacked wooden tongue blades or TheraBite is important in preventing or minimizing postoperative trismus.

OUTCOMES AND PROGNOSIS

Aggressive multimodality treatment offers good local control and acceptable survival rates ranging from 65% to 75% [17]. Factors influencing prognosis and outcome for patients include tumor stage, site, histology, extent of resection, surgical margins, adjuvant therapy and performance status [18].

REFERENCES

1. Hanna E, Vural E, Teo C, Farris P, Breau R, Suen JY. Sinonasal tumors: the Arkansas experience. *Skull Base Surg* 1998;8:15.
2. Porceddu S, Martin J, Shanker G, Weih L, Russell C, Rischin D, et al. Paranasal sinus tumors: Peter MacCallum Cancer Institute experience. *Head Neck* 2004;26(4):322–30.
3. Sunderman FW Jr. Nasal toxicity, carcinogenicity, and olfactory uptake of metals. *Ann Clin Lab Sci* 2001;31(1):3–24.
4. Waldron JN, O'Sullivan B, Gullane P, Witterick IJ, Liu FF, Payne D, et al. Carcinoma of the maxillary antrum: a retrospective analysis of 110 cases. *Radiother Oncol* 2000;57(2):167–73.
5. Sievers KW, Greess H, Baum U, Dobritz M, Lenz M. Paranasal sinuses and nasopharynx CT and MRI. *Eur J Radiol* 2000;33(3):185–202.
6. Lloyd G, Lund VJ, Howard D, Savy L. Optimum imaging for sinonasal malignancy. *J Laryngol Otol* 2000;114(7):557–62.
7. Ohngren LG. Malignant tumors of the maxillo-ethmoidal region. *Acta Otolaryngol* 1933;19:476.
8. Compton CC, Byrd DR, Garcia-Aguilar J, Kurtzman SH, Olawaiye A, Washington MK. Nasal cavity and paranasal sinuses. In Compton CC, Byrd DR, Garcia-Aguilar J, Kurtzman SH, Olawaiye A, Washington MK, eds., *AJCC Cancer Staging Atlas*. New York: Springer, 2012, pp. 91–104.
9. Le QT, Fu KK, Kaplan MJ, Terris DJ, Fee WE, Goffinet DR. Lymph node metastasis in maxillary sinus carcinoma. *Int J Radiat Oncol Biol Phys* 2000;46(3):541–9.
10. Hoppe BS, Stegman LD, Zelefsky MJ, Rosenzweig KE, Wolden SL, Patel SG, et al. Treatment of nasal cavity and paranasal sinus cancer with modern radiotherapy techniques in the postoperative setting – the MSKCC experience. *Int J Radiat Oncol Biol Phys* 2007;67(3): 691–702.
11. Tufano RP, Mokadam NA, Montone KT, Weinstein GS, Chalian AA, Wolf PF, et al. Malignant tumors of the nose and paranasal sinuses: hospital of the University of Pennsylvania experience 1990–1997. *Am J Rhinol* 1999;13(2):117–23.

12. Grégoire V, De Neve W, Eisbruch A, Lee N, Van den Weyngaert D, Van Gestel D. Intensity-modulated radiation therapy for head and neck carcinoma. *Oncologist* 2007;12(5):555–64.

13. Ogawa K, Toita T, Kakinohana Y, Adachi G, Kojya S, Itokazu T, et al. Postoperative radiotherapy for squamous cell carcinoma of the maxillary sinus: analysis of local control and late complications. *Oncol Rep* 2001;8(2):315–9.

14. Rischin D, Porceddu S, Peters L, Martin J, Corry J, Weih L. Promising results with chemoradiation in patients with sinonasal undifferentiated carcinoma. *Head Neck* 2004;26(5):435–41.

15. Lee MM, Vokes EE, Rosen A, Witt ME, Weichselbaum RR, Haraf DJ. Multimodality therapy in advanced paranasal sinus carcinoma: superior long-term results. *Cancer J Sci Am* 1999;5(4):219–23.

16. Hasegawa M, Torii S, Fukuta K, Saito K. Reconstruction of the anterior cranial base with the galeal frontalis myofascial flap and the vascularized outer table calvarial bone graft. *Neurosurgery* 1995;36(4):725–9.

17. Dulguerov P, Jacobsen MS, Allal AS, Lehmann W, Calcaterra T. Nasal and paranasal sinus carcinoma: are we making progress? A series of 220 patients and a systematic review. *Cancer* 2001;92(12):3012–29.

18. Dulguerov P, Allal AS. Nasal and paranasal sinus carcinoma: how can we continue to make progress? *Curr Opin Otolaryngol Head Neck Surg* 2006;14(2):67–72.

20

Skull base tumours

AMIT GOYAL, SAMEER GUPTA AND SANJEEV MISRA

INTRODUCTION

The skull base is a conventionally difficult to access region, sitting on the juncture of many important anatomical regions. Anatomically, the skull base is divided into three subdivisions: anterior, middle and posterior skull base, which can be further subdivided into median and lateral areas (Figure 20.1). Management of skull base tumours is governed by involvement of bony boundaries and the neurovascular structures traversing through its various compartments.

Skull base tumours have their origin from one of the three anatomical areas: intracranially from basal neurovascular structures and meninges, arising *de novo* from the skull base region and arising extracranially involving the skull base and cranial base, from below.

PATHOLOGY

Skull base tumours are relatively rare. The most common benign tumours are meningiomas and vestibular schwannomas (Table 20.1). Among malignant tumours, chondrosarcomas and chordomas are more common [1]. Chondrosarcomas originate from primitive mesenchymal cells or from the embryonic rest of the cartilaginous matrix of the cranium. The incidence of primary intracranial chondrosarcomas is estimated to be <0.16% of all intracranial tumours and 6% of all skull base lesions [2]. The majority of these tumours are slow growing and rarely metastasize [3]. Skull base chordomas arise from the remnants of the primitive notochord at the spheno-occipital synchondrosis [1]. They are generally slow-growing, radioresistant tumours that are locally aggressive and invasive [4].

Though the most common sellar region tumour is a pituitary adenoma, various malignancies may also involve this region, e.g. granular cell tumours, chordoma, nasopharyngeal carcinoma, spindle cell oncocytoma of the adenohypophysis, medulloepithelioma, pituitary carcinoma or metastatic tumours.

Carcinoma of the temporal bone represents 1 in 5000 to 20,000 oncologic cases [5,6], with an incidence of between 1 and 6 cases per million population per year [7,8]. These tumours have been associated with chronic suppurative otitis media (chronic inflammation leading to squamous metaplasia), exposure to chemicals and previous radiotherapy exposure [9]. Human papilloma virus (HPV) has also been implicated as an etiological factor. These tumours have an aggressive nature and spread along preformed vascular and neural pathways, invading adjacent structures. Nodal metastases are uncommon in early disease, but may occur in 10–20% cases of advanced disease [10,11].

CLINICAL FEATURES

The clinical features depend on the stage, site of pathology and rate of growth (Table 20.2). Symptoms are produced mainly by involvement of adjacent neurovascular structures.

DIAGNOSIS

CT scan and MRI are indispensable tools in the diagnosis and management of skull base lesions and are used to visualize the intricate relationship of these lesions with important structures, i.e. the orbit, cavernous sinus, internal carotid artery (ICA) and cranial nerves. They allow the surgeon

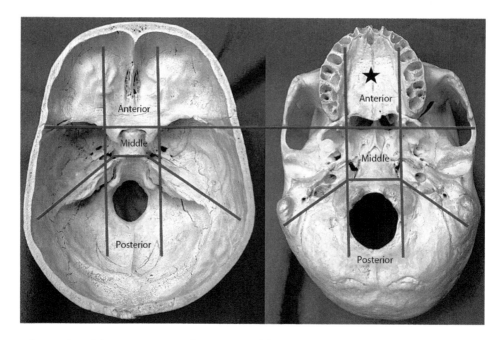

Figure 20.1 Approximate pictorial representation of anterior, middle and posterior subdivisions of skull base divided into median and lateral compartments. (*The maxilla and palatine bones are covering the caudal aspect of the anterior skull base.)

Table 20.1 Malignancies involving the skull base region

1. Tumours of mesenchymal origin
   a. Chondrosarcoma
   b. Chordoma
   c. Esthesioneuroblastoma
   d. Primitive neuroectodermal tumour
2. Tumours of cranial and paraspinal nerves
   a. Malignant peripheral nerve sheath tumour (MPNST)
3. Germ cell tumours
   a. Germinoma
   b. Teratoma with malignant transformation
   c. Yolk sac tumour
   d. Embryonal cell carcinoma
   e. Choriocarcinoma
4. Tumours of cutaneous/epithelial origin
   a. Squamous cell carcinoma
   b. Melanoma
   c. Endolymphatic sac tumour
5. Tumours of glandular origin
   a. Ceruminous gland carcinoma
   b. Adenoid cystic carcinoma
   c. Endolymphatic sac tumour
6. Vascular tumours
   a. Haemangiopericytoma
7. Haematopoietic tumours
   a. Leukemia
   b. Lymphoma
   c. Plasmacytoma
8. Primary central nervous system lymphoma
9. Metastatic tumours
10. Tumours of temporal bone

to plan and customize the optimal surgical approach for a given lesion (Figure 20.2). Digital subtraction angiography is useful in assessing the vascularity of these lesions preoperatively and embolizing feeding vessels, wherever possible. The balloon occlusion test of the ICA can be performed in the same sitting to assess the contralateral blood flow for feasibility of ICA ligation or occlusion.

TREATMENT

Landmark events which have revolutionized the management strategies and improved surgical outcomes for skull base malignancies are the introduction of the operating microscope, microvascular surgery and pedicled or free flaps for reconstruction, stereotactic radiosurgery, targeted organ-sparing high-beam radiotherapy techniques, new chemotherapeutic agents, the advent of rigid fibre-optic endoscopes including 3D stereo endoscopes, image-guided navigation and most notably, dedicated skull base teams.

Surgery

Historically, anterior skull base lesions were managed by open and often combined approaches (Table 20.3). In 1941, Dandy attempted removal of facial tumours by the transcranial route. Later in 1954, Klopp used combined transfacial and transcranial routes, thus beginning the era of formal craniofacial resections (CFRs), resulting in significantly improved outcomes of surgery for anterior skull base tumours [12]. The basic surgical challenge in CFR is to reach deeply situated tumours, via extensive facial skeleton mobilization or brain retraction, with minimum

Table 20.2 Symptomatology in skull base malignancies

Skull base region	Structure involved	Clinical presentation
Anterior skull base		
Central and lateral	Olfactory nerve	Hyposmia, anosmia
	Frontal lobe	Personality change
	Increased intracranial pressure	Headache, vomiting, ocular palsies, papilloedema
	Orbit and optic nerve	Proptosis, extraocular movement paralysis, blindness, diplopia
	Nasal cavity	Nasal obstruction, discharge, epistaxis
Middle skull base		
Central	Pituitary gland	Pituitary hypo/hypersecretion along with compression features like headache and vision loss, field defects
	Hypothalamus	Hormonal changes, diabetes insipidus
	Increased intracranial pressure	Headache, vomiting, ocular palsies, papilloedema
	Sphenoid sinus	Vision loss and field defects (due to involvement of optic nerve and chiasma), headache
Paracentral (cavernous)	Optic nerve at apex	Visual disturbances, diplopia or even blindness
	Cranial nerves 3–6	Facial hypo/anaesthesia, restricted eye movement
Lateral	Trigeminal divisions	Paraesthesias, facial pain
	Lateral orbit	Visual disturbances, gaze restriction, proptosis, diplopia
	Infratemporal fossa	Facial pain and swelling
	Eustachian tube	Hearing loss, ear ache
	Temporal bone	Hearing loss, facial palsy, tinnitus, dizziness, ear discharge/bleeding, ear ache
Posterior skull base		
Upper central (petroclival–clival)	Cranial nerves 3–10	Facial hypo/anaesthesia, lateral gaze restriction, hearing loss, tinnitus, gait instability, gaze restriction, loss of taste, facial deviation/palsy, voice change
	Cerebellum	Features of cerebellar compression and hydrocephalus
Lower central (foramen magnum)	Cranial nerves 9 and 10	Swallowing difficulties, change in voice
	Cranial nerves 11 and 12	Tongue deviation
	Sensorimotor long tracts	Weakness, stereoagnosis, cape shape anaesthesia in neck, dysesthesia and atrophy of hand
Upper lateral (CP angle)	Cranial nerves 7 and 8	Tinnitus, hearing loss, facial weakness/palsy
	Cranial nerves 5 and 6	Facial parasthesia, lateral gaze restriction
	Cranial nerves 9 and 10	Swallowing difficulties, change in voice
Lower lateral (jugular foramen)	Cranial nerves 9–12	Swallowing difficulties, change in voice, deviation of tongue

surgical morbidity. Visualization and navigation around deeper corners are also restricted. The main complications are related to tumour recurrence, reconstruction of defects and CSF leaks.

Rigid endoscopy through natural air passages (nose and sinuses) to approach skull base tumours offers excellent visualization. The use of angled scopes and both nostrils in the 'two surgeons four hands technique', allows simultaneous use of more instruments and increased space for navigation (Figure 20.3). Use of high-speed drills and powered shaver systems by endoscopic endonasal approaches (EEAs) has enabled surgeons to reach beyond defined bony anatomical compartments and remove deep-seated tumours. The resultant bony and dural defects are smaller in comparison to CFR, resulting in a decreased incidence of postoperative complications. Another advantage is enhanced visualization of the origin of the tumour even in seemingly extensive tumours.

Initially EEAs were considered against the oncological principle of 'en bloc resection' due to piecemeal removal of tumours. Recent experience has shown that the primary aim of achieving a negative tumour resection margin is eminently possible with EEAs. There is no large randomized study comparing the outcomes of open and endoscopic

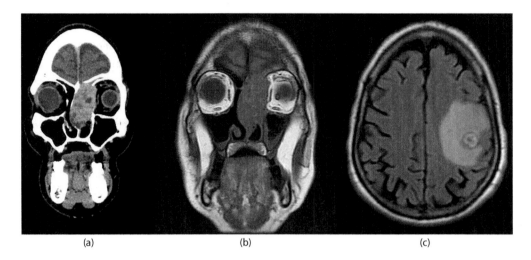

(a) (b) (c)

Figure 20.2 **(a)** CT PNS showing erosion of cribriform plate by tumour with intracranial extension. **(b)** MRI PNS of the same patient confirming dural invasion with involvement of frontal lobe by the tumour. **(c)** MRI brain showing brain metastasis in same patient.

Table 20.3 Surgical approaches for skull base malignancies

Anterior skull base

1. Sagittal (median) plane endonasal endoscopic approaches
   Transfrontal, transcribriform, transplanum, transsellar, transclival, transodontoid
2. Coronal (paramedian) endonasal endoscopic approaches
   Transorbital, transsphenoidal (medial), transpterygoid± nasoantral window/medial maxillectomy, premaxillary
3. Transfacial approaches
   Midfacial degloving, maxillary swing technique, transpalatal, Lefort I osteotomy
   Combined transfacial and transcranial craniofacial resection

Lateral skull base

1. Transtemporal
   Translabyrinthine, transcochlear, retrolabyrinthine
2. Infratemporal
   Fisch types A–C, transparotid, extended rhytidectomy, facial biflap procedure, lateral facial and lateral temporal sphenoid approaches, subtemporal preauricular approaches
3. Intracranial
   Temporal craniotomy, middle cranial fossa approach, subtemporal craniectomy, retrosigmoid approach

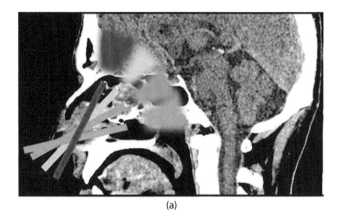

(a)

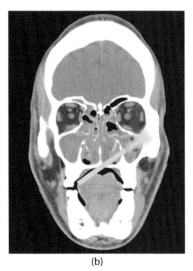

(b)

Figure 20.3 Endoscopic endonasal approaches (EEAs). **(a)** Sagittal approaches giving access to anterior, middle and posterior cranial fossae (red, transfrontal and transcribriform; yellow, transplanum; blue, transsellar; green, transclival and transodontoid). **(b)** Coronal approaches (endoscopic removal of medial and posterolateral walls of maxilla gives access to pterygopalatine and infratemporal fossa and through them to middle cranial fossa).

approaches, but available literature clearly demonstrates similar oncological results with both approaches [13–16]. EEAs may be best suited for approaching skull base tumours in pediatric patients, where extensive mobilization of the facial skeleton in CFR may have negative effects on future facial growth.

The patient selection for endoscopic techniques is based on the nature of the pathology (location, diagnosis and vascularity), patient characteristics (age and medical comorbidities), surgeon attributes (training, experience and expertise) and available institutional resources (adjunctive services, intensive care unit and operating room equipment).

Direct involvement of the orbit (necessitating exenteration), skin or anterior table of the frontal sinus is the main contraindication for EEAs. Cranial nerves and ICA on both sides define the limits of the surgical field for EEAs. Any tumour crossing them may need a combined approach.

Use of the microscope has revolutionized the management of lateral skull base tumours. Infratemporal approaches by Fisch, later modified by Gardner, Schramm and Sekhar, are used to address tumours from the nasopharynx to the infratemporal region and the petrous apex up to the sigmoid sinus with excellent results and acceptable morbidity [12].

Carcinoma of the external auditory canal (EAC) and middle ear should be treated primarily by a lateral or subtotal temporal bone resection combined with a parotidectomy and neck dissection. Local resection of the EAC alone is not sufficient, even in T1 tumours [17]. Disease extent, positive margins, dural involvement, facial nerve paralysis, cranial nerve involvement and moderate to severe pain on presentation have been associated with inferior outcomes [18]. The available reconstruction options are given in Table 20.4.

Radiotherapy

Due to the proximity of critical structures such as the brain stem, cranial nerves, optic chiasm and optic pathways, which are prone to irreversible damage by radiation, radiation therapy for skull base tumours is challenging. Radiobiologically, these structures behave as serial organs and even a small point of high-dose therapeutic radiation can produce serious toxicities. The lower tolerated dose to these vital neural structures reduces the window of therapeutic ratio available and compromises the total tumouricidal dose which can be delivered and thus the outcomes. Skull base is a site where high-precision and novel radiation therapy technology such as stereotactic radiation therapy, proton therapy and particle therapy has been tried with promising preliminary results.

Meningiomas (WHO grades I to III) have shown better survival rates with adjuvant radiation therapy than surgery alone. Several studies using high-precision fractionated stereotactic radiotherapy (FSRT) or stereotactic

Table 20.4 Reconstruction options during skull base surgery for malignancies

Grafts	• Skin
	• Fascia
	• Fat or dermis fat
	• Allografts – dura, dermis, bone
Local flaps	• Forehead and scalp flaps – Cutaneous
	• Galeal-pericranial – fascial
	• Temporal system – muscle, fascial, osseus
	• Hadad–Bassagasteguy flap – septonasal mucosal flap[a]
	• Lateral nasal wall mucosal flap
	• Inferior turbinate mucosal flap
Regional flaps	• Pectoralis major – myocutaneous
	• Latissimus dorsi – myocutaneous
	• Inferior trapezius – myocutaneous
Free flaps	• Radial forearm – fasciocutaneous
	• Rectus abdominis – myofasciocutaneous
	• Subscapular – osseo/myofasciocutaneous
	• Latissimus dorsi – myocutaneous
	• Gastro-omental – fascial/mucosal
Alloplast implants	• Titanium plate
	• Hydroxyapatite cement
	• Porous polyethylene
	• Resorbable plate

[a] With the fast-growing trend of endoscopic skull base surgeries, nasoseptal flaps (especially the Hadad flap) have revolutionized the reconstruction of anterior and middle skull base defects and reduced the incidence of postoperative CSF leaks significantly.

radiosurgery (SRS) have produced 5-year control rates of 86–100% [19,20]. Adjuvant radiotherapy has not shown improved outcomes in chordomas and chondrosarcomas [21], but particle therapy has yielded an overall survival of 86% at 3 years in small groups of patients [22], although longer follow-up is needed. Rhabdomyosarcoma is quite sensitive to both chemotherapy and radiation therapy. Multimodal therapy gives excellent 5-year survival rates of 97% in the absence of risk factors and up to 71% in stage III tumours [23].

Chemotherapy

Multimodality treatment using combinations of surgery, radiotherapy and chemotherapy is shown to improve outcomes in most skull base malignancies like sarcomas, epithelial tumours and esthesioneuroblastoma. The feasibility of hyperosmolar mannitol was assessed as a liquid tumour embolizing agent *in vitro* and found to be toxic to endothelial cells and meningioma cells showing potential for future clinical use [24].

Despite the availability of numerous treatment options, it is always prudent to follow a team approach with informed decisions, taken after carefully assessing the risk-to-benefit ratio of each offered modality, on an individualized basis.

REFERENCES

1. Almefty K, Pravdenkova S, Colli BO, Al-Mefty O, Gokden M. Chordoma and chondrosarcoma: similar, but quite different, skull base tumors. *Cancer* 2007;110(11):2457–67.

2. Maslehaty H, Petridis AK, Kinzel A, Binay Y, Scholz M. Chondrosarcoma of the petrous bone: a challenging clinical entity. *Head Neck Oncol* 2013;5(2):13.

3. Gelderblom H, Hogendoorn PC, Dijkstra SD, van Rijswijk CS, Krol AD, Taminiau AH, et al. The clinical approach towards chondrosarcoma. *Oncologist* 2008;13(3):320–9.

4. Walcott BP, Nahed BV, Mohyeldin A, Coumans JV, Kahle KT, Ferreira MJ. Chordoma: current concepts, management, and future directions. *Lancet Oncol* 2012;13(2):e69–76.

5. Barrs DM. Temporal bone carcinoma. *Otolaryngol Clin North Am* 2001;34(6):1197–218.

6. Manolidis S, Pappas D Jr, Von Doersten P, Jackson CG, Glasscock ME 3rd. Temporal bone and lateral skull base malignancy: experience and results with 81 patients. *Am J Otol* 1998;19(6 Suppl.):S1–15.

7. Isipradit P, Wadwongtham W, Aeumjaturapat S, Aramwatanapong P. Carcinoma of the external auditory canal. *J Med Assoc Thai* 2005;88(1):114–7.

8. Kuhel WI, Hume CR, Selesnick SH. Cancer of the external auditory canal and temporal bone. *Otolaryngol Clin North Am* 1996;29(5):827–52.

9. Lim LH, Goh YH, Chan YM, Chong VF, Low WK. Malignancy of the temporal bone and external auditory canal. *Otolaryngol Head Neck Surg* 2000;122(6):882–6.

10. Moffat DA, Wagstaff SA, Hardy DG. The outcome of radical surgery and postoperative radiotherapy for squamous carcinoma of the temporal bone. *Laryngoscope* 2005;115(2):341–7.

11. Moody SA, Hirsch BE, Myers EN. Squamous cell carcinoma of the external auditory canal: an evaluation of a staging system. *Am J Otol* 2000;21(4):582–8.

12. Donald PJ. History of skull base surgery. *Skull Base Surg* 1991;1(1):1–3.

13. Eloy JA, Vivero RJ, Hoang K, Civantos FJ, Weed DT, Morcos JJ, et al. Comparison of transnasal endoscopic and open craniofacial resection for malignant tumors of the anterior skull base. *Laryngoscope* 2009;119(5):834–40.

14. Nicolai P, Battaglia P, Bignami M, Bolzoni Villaret A, Delù G, Khrais T, et al. Endoscopic surgery for malignant tumors of the sinonasal tract and adjacent skull base: a 10-year experience. *Am J Rhinol* 2008;22(3):308–16.

15. Hanna E, DeMonte F, Ibrahim S, Roberts D, Levine N, Kupferman M. Endoscopic resection of sinonasal cancers with and without craniotomy: oncologic results. *Arch Otolaryngol Head Neck Surg* 2009;135(12):1219–24.

16. Nicolai P, Castelnuovo P, Bolzoni Villaret A. Endoscopic resection of sinonasal malignancies. *Curr Oncol Rep* 2011;13(2):138–44.

17. Kollert M, Draf W, Minovi A, Hofmann E, Bockmühl U. Carcinoma of the external auditory canal and middle ear: therapeutic strategy and follow up. *Laryngorhinootologie* 2004;83(12):818–23.

18. Testa JR, Fukuda Y, Kowalski LP. Prognostic factors in carcinoma of the external auditory canal. *Arch Otolaryngol Head Neck Surg* 1997;123(7):720–4.

19. Condra KS, Buatti JM, Mendenhall WM, Friedman WA, Marcus RB Jr, Rhoton AL. Benign meningiomas: primary treatment selection affects survival. *Int J Radiat Oncol Biol Phys* 1997;39(2):427–36.

20. Minniti G, Amichetti M, Enrici RM. Radiotherapy and radiosurgery for benign skull base meningiomas. *Radiat Oncol* 2009;14(4):42.

21. Bohman LE, Koch M, Bailey RL, Alonso-Basanta M, Lee JY. Skull base chordoma and chondrosarcoma: influence of clinical and demographic factors on prognosis: a SEER analysis. *World Neurosurg* 2014;82(5):806–14.

22. Kim PJ, Kobayashi W, Chen YL, Hornicek FC, Ebb DH, Choy E, et al. Radiotherapy in the management of mesenchymal chondrosarcomas. *Int J Radiat Oncol Biol Phys* 2010;78(3 Suppl.):S613.

23. Wharam MD Jr. Rhabdomyosarcoma of parameningeal sites. *Semin Radiat Oncol* 1997;7(3):212–6.

24. Feng L, Kienitz BA, Matsumoto C, Bruce J, Sisti M, Duong H, et al. Feasibility of using hyperosmolar mannitol as a liquid tumor embolization agent. *AJNR Am J Neuroradiol* 2005;26(6):1405–12.

21

Cancer of larynx and hypopharynx

DHAIRYASHEEL SAVANT, TANVEER ABDUL MAJEED, PUNEET PAREEK, AMIT GOYAL
AND AKASH AGARWAL

INTRODUCTION

Carcinoma larynx accounts for approximately 2% of all cancers and 25% of all head and neck malignancies [1]. Hypopharyngeal cancer is uncommon; approximately 3900 new cases are diagnosed in the United States each year [2]. Larynx includes three subsites, namely supraglottis, glottis and subglottis. Hypopharynx includes posterior pharyngeal wall (PPW), pyriform sinus (PFS) and postcricoid area.

ETIOLOGY

Smoking and alcohol are the most common etiological factors and both have synergistic effect. Tobacco is responsible for the projected increase in the incidence in developing countries [3]. Other possible factors are human papilloma virus–related laryngeal papillomas, Plummer–Vinson syndrome and occupational exposure to welding fumes, chromium, nickel and asbestos.

PATHOLOGY

The majority of the laryngeal and hypopharyngeal cancers are squamous cell carcinomas (SCCs). Pyriform fossa cancers arising from the medial wall are known as marginal zone cancers and form the most common subsite. Carcinoma in situ is common on vocal cords.

CLINICAL FEATURES

Symptoms depend on location and size of the primary subsite involved. Common features are change in voice and difficulty, pain or cough during swallowing. Other presentations may include pain in throat or ear, cough, blood mixed with sputum, neck swelling and difficulty breathing.

DIAGNOSTIC WORK-UP

Endoscopy

Rigid or flexible fibre-optic laryngoscopy is useful in the diagnosis and documentation of laryngeal lesions (Figure 21.1). It can be combined with biopsy in the same sitting for patients with adequate airway. Patients with compromised airway or submucosal tumors are evaluated and biopsied under anaesthesia. Endoscopy can be combined with narrow-band imaging and autofluorescence, especially in evaluating potentially malignant disorders.

Imaging

Tumors of larynx and hypopharynx are best evaluated by direct visualization. However, the submucosal extent and any suspicious involvement of adjacent cartilage, muscles

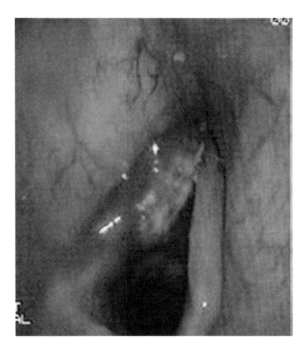

Figure 21.1 Ulceroproliferative growth (squamous cell carcinoma) involving left vocal cord.

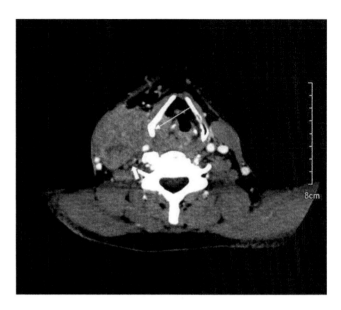

Figure 21.3 Axial contrast-enhanced CT section showing mass involving the right paralaryngeal space and right thyroid lamina (arrow), with mass effect upon the great vessels of the neck. The right internal jugular vein (IJV) is compressed and displaced posteriorly (thick arrow) with a large necrotic node anterior to it.

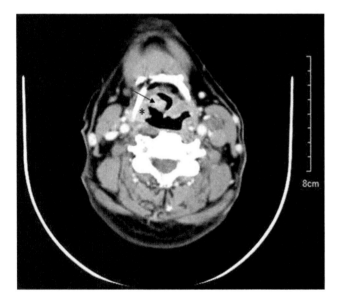

Figure 21.2 Axial contrast-enhanced CT section showing irregular soft tissue thickening in the supraglottic larynx (arrow) extending across the midline and effacing the right pyriform sinus (asterisk).

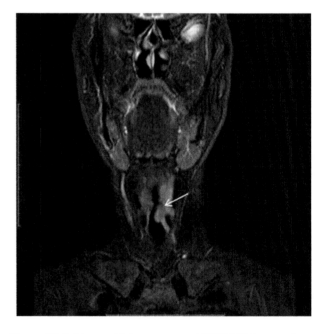

Figure 21.4 Coronal fat-suppressed T2W MR image showing mass (arrow) involving the left vocal cord with supra- and infraglottic extensions.

or soft tissue are best done with appropriate imaging [4] (Figures 21.2 through 21.4). Contrast-enhanced magnetic resonance imaging (MRI) is superior to computerized tomography (CT). Cross-sectional imaging is also done as a part of modern intensity-modulated radiation therapy to create appropriate volumes for treatment planning. The FDG PET scan has a limited role because of poor spatial resolution and specificity. However, because of high

negative predictive value, it may be recommended before aggressive treatment for a recurrence [5].

Staging

The currently followed staging method is the UICC/AJCC TNM staging system (Table 21.1) [6,7]. The N and M categories are similar to those of oral cancers.

Table 21.1 T stage of subsites of larynx and hypopharynx with stage grouping

Supraglottis

TX	Primary tumor cannot be assessed.
T0	No evidence of primary tumor.
Tis	Carcinoma *in situ*.
T1	Tumor limited to one subsite of supraglottis with normal vocal cord mobility.
T2	Tumor invades mucosa of more than one adjacent subsite of supraglottis or glottis or region outside the supraglottis (e.g., mucosa of base of tongue, vallecula, and medial wall of pyriform sinus) without fixation of the larynx.
T3	Tumor limited to larynx with vocal cord fixation and/or invades any of the following: postcricoid area, pre-epiglottic space, paraglottic space and/or inner cortex of thyroid cartilage.
T4a	Moderately advanced local disease. Tumor invades through the thyroid cartilage and/or invades tissues beyond the larynx (e.g., trachea, soft tissues of neck including deep extrinsic muscle of the tongue, strap muscles, thyroid or esophagus).
T4b	Very advanced local disease. Tumor invades prevertebral space, encases carotid artery or invades mediastinal structures.

Subglottis

TX	Primary tumor cannot be assessed.
T0	No evidence of primary tumor.
Tis	Carcinoma *in situ*.
T1	Tumor limited to the subglottis.
T2	Tumor extends to vocal cord(s) with normal or impaired mobility.
T3	Tumor limited to larynx with vocal cord fixation.
T4a	Moderately advanced local disease. Tumor invades cricoid or thyroid cartilage and/or invades tissues beyond the larynx (e.g., trachea, soft tissues of neck including deep extrinsic muscles of the tongue, strap muscles, thyroid, or esophagus).
T4b	Very advanced local disease. Tumor invades prevertebral space, encases carotid artery or invades mediastinal structures.

Glottis

TX	Primary tumor cannot be assessed.
T0	No evidence of primary tumor.
Tis	Carcinoma *in situ*.
T1	Tumor limited to the vocal cord(s) (may involve anterior or posterior commissure) with normal mobility.
T1a	Tumor limited to one vocal cord.
T1b	Tumor involves both vocal cords.
T2	Tumor extends to supraglottis and/or subglottis and/or with impaired vocal cord mobility.
T3	Tumor limited to the larynx with vocal cord fixation and/or invasion of paraglottic space and/or inner cortex of the thyroid cartilage.
T4a	Moderately advanced local disease. Tumor invades through the outer cortex of the thyroid cartilage and/or invades tissues beyond the larynx (e.g., trachea, soft tissues of neck including deep extrinsic muscle of the tongue, strap muscles, thyroid or esophagus).
T4b	Very advanced local disease. Tumor invades prevertebral space, encases carotid artery or invades mediastinal structures.

Hypopharynx

TX	Primary tumor cannot be assessed.
Tl	Tumor limited to one subsite of hypopharynx and 2 cm or less in greatest dimension.
T2	Tumor invades more than one subsite of hypopharynx or an adjacent site, or measures more than 2 cm but not more than 4 cm in greatest diameter without fixation of the hemilarynx.
T3	Tumor more than 4 cm in greatest dimension or with fixation of the hemilarynx or extension to esophagus.

(Continued)

Table 21.1 *(Continued)* T stage of subsites of larynx and hypopharynx with stage grouping

Hypopharynx

T4a   Tumor invades thyroid/cricoid cartilage, hyoid bone, thyroid gland or central compartment soft tissue.

T4b   Tumor invades the prevertebral fascia, encases the carotid artery or involves mediastinal structures.

Stage grouping

Stage	T	N	M
0	Tis	N0	M0
I	T1	N0	M0
II	T1	N1	M0
	T2	N0	M0
	T2	N1	M0
III	T1	N2	M0
	T2	N2	M0

Source: With kind permission from Springer Science+Business Media: *AJCC Cancer Staging Atlas,* 2012, pp. 41–53, Compton, et al.

MANAGEMENT

Surgical management

In the last few decades, emphasis has been given to the function and organ preservation techniques of management for these cancers. In early laryngeal cancers, both surgery and irradiation are equally effective, though speech and voice outcomes are better in patients treated with irradiation. Early glottic cancers perform better in 5-year survival rates than supraglottic cancers [8].

Early laryngeal cancers can be treated with function-preserving surgical approaches like vertical partial laryngectomy or horizontal supraglottic laryngectomy. The surgical paradigm is now shifting toward minimally invasive surgery. Minimally invasive surgical options available are transoral CO_2 laser microsurgery and transoral robotic surgery (TORS).

Superficially infiltrative squamous cancers of the supraglottis, glottis and hypopharynx are best suited for transoral CO_2 laser resection. These are cases where the vocal cords are freely mobile, without gross invasion of the pre-epiglottic or paraglottic space and absence of laryngeal widening or pharyngeal bulge. Trans-regional superficial cancers may also be addressed by transoral laser resection, and so can a few T3 lesions in experienced hands. Bulky and anterior commissure lesions are better managed with open approaches [9].

TORS has several advantages over open approaches in selected cases of supraglottic laryngectomy. These include avoidance of the external incision, preservation of uninvolved structures, shorter hospitalization and improved postoperative function with reduced need for gastric and tracheostomy tube placement. In comparison to transoral laser microsurgery, TORS has the advantage of en bloc resection with negative margins due to better maneuverability and improved vision in the supraglottic region [10]. Both of the above techniques have shown a lower incidence of pharyngo-cutaneous fistula. The presence of neck nodes is not a contraindication, as neck dissection may be done concurrently or a few days later [9].

Advanced laryngeal cancers are treated by total laryngectomy. Organ preservation techniques by chemoradiation have been popularized in recent times. However, long-term studies have shown inferior survival rates following organ preservation. The functional outcomes in terms of speech and swallowing may also be at times inferior, defeating the very purpose of organ preservation [11,12].

Early laryngeal cancers with N0 neck may be managed with close observation since the incidence of occult node positivity is low, especially for glottic cancers [13]. The presence of positive nodes adversely affects survival and should be managed by comprehensive neck dissection.

Radiation and chemoradiation

For early laryngeal and hypopharyngeal tumors, radiation therapy is preferred, as it can achieve local control rates approaching 90%. A recent Cochrane systematic review showed that equipoise remains between radiotherapy and endolaryngeal surgery as both treatment modalities offer laryngeal preservation with similar survival rates [14]. Locally advanced tumors can be treated with chemoradiation. Concomitant chemoradiation produces better survival than induction chemotherapy and radiotherapy or radiotherapy alone with significantly better laryngeal preservation [15]. Failures after radiation therapy can be effectively salvaged by surgery [16,17]. A 66 to 70 Gy equivalent dose is sufficient to achieve high control rates. Even with early superficial involvement of cartilage organ preservation can be achieved. With larger-volume disease or involvement of cartilage and soft tissues of the neck, surgery becomes a preferred primary modality with adjuvant radiation therapy.

Adjuvant radiation therapy to a dose of 60 Gy in conventional fractionation can increase the local control rates in patients treated with surgery as the primary modality of treatment [18]. Patients presenting with advanced stage and poor performance status may require a short course of palliative radiation to reduce suffering from fungating nodes, bleeding and pain. Tracheostomy may become necessary for airway obstruction.

Chemotherapy and targeted therapy

Concurrent chemoradiation produces superior overall survival and local control than neoadjuvant or adjuvant chemotherapy. In the Meta-Analysis of Chemotherapy in Head and Neck Cancer (MACH-NC), 63 randomized trials were included and there were more than 5000 patients with laryngeal and hypopharyngeal cancer. Concomitant chemoradiation increased the 5-year absolute survival benefit by approximately 5% [19]. The addition of neoadjuvant chemotherapy to concurrent chemoradiation does not have any benefit over chemoradiation [20].

The addition of targeted therapy in the form of cetuximab to definitive radiation has shown better survival than radiotherapy alone [21]. Palliative chemotherapy for recurrent or metastatic tumors of the larynx or hypopharynx does not produce significant benefits. Drugs such as cisplatin, bleomycin, mitomycin, taxanes and methotrexate have limited progression-free survival ranging from weeks to a few months. The addition of cetuximab to cisplatin has achieved better survival in this group [22]. Patients with advanced tumors and poor performance status should be given palliative and supportive care.

MANAGEMENT OF RECURRENT LESIONS

Small recurrent lesions amenable to surgery should be resected. While 60% of T3 glottic cancers recurring after radiation therapy alone are salvageable by cordectomy, partial laryngectomy or total laryngectomy, only up to 50% of those recurring after surgery alone can be salvaged by radiation therapy [23]. Recurrence after partial laryngopharyngectomy can be treated with total laryngopharyngectomy. Post-radiation recurrent neck disease can be addressed by salvage neck dissection. Chemoradiation therapy can be offered to patients who had not received it earlier. For patients with unresectable disease, palliative treatment is recommended.

FOLLOW-UP

Patients should be evaluated every 3 to 4 months for the initial 2 years and less frequently thereafter. Most of the recurrences occur within 2 years of treatment. Imaging should be done if required. Patients treated with radiation therapy should be evaluated for hypothyroidism and should receive regular dental care and prophylaxis.

REHABILITATION FOLLOWING SURGERY FOR LARYNGEAL CANCER

Important functional concerns after laryngectomy are loss of smell, changes in swallowing and respiration patterns and most notably loss of speech. Various options for development of laryngeal speech are available: nonsurgical (esophageal speech and electrolarynx) and surgical (neo-glottic reconstruction, trachea–esophageal shunts and tracheoesophageal puncture [TEP]). Among surgical options, TEP is popular with good results and low complication rates. TEP can be primary (at the time of laryngectomy) or secondary (a few days after laryngectomy). Various indwelling and non-indwelling voice prostheses can be used along with TEP, e.g., Blom–Singer prosthesis (duck bill prosthesis), Panje button, Groningen button and Provox prosthesis.

With training and motivation, useful and reasonably comprehensible speech may be expected in post-laryngectomy patients with TEP and voice prosthesis. Anosmia due to loss of airflow in the nasal passage may be managed by nasal airflow-inducing maneuver (NAIM), 'the polite yawning' technique, as described by Hilgers [24].

Loss of upper airway resistance shifts the 'equal pressure point' to the periphery in the pulmonary tract leading to excessive sputum production and coughing. It also leads to loss of warming, humidifying and filtering action of the upper airway. All of these may be effectively managed by a heat and moisture exchanger (HME).

REFERENCES

1. Varghese BT, Babu S, Desai KP, Bava AS, George P, Iype EM, et al. Prospective study of outcomes of surgically treated larynx and hypopharyngeal cancers. *Indian J Cancer* 2014;51(2):104–8.
2. Kuo P, Chen MM, Decker RH, Yarbrough WG, Judson BL. Hypopharyngeal cancer incidence, treatment, and survival: temporal trends in the United States. *Laryngoscope* 2014;124(9):2064–9.
3. Dikshit R, Gupta PC, Ramasundarahettige C, Gajalakshmi V, Aleksandrowicz L, Badwe R, et al. Million Death Study Collaborators. Cancer mortality in India: a nationally representative survey. *Lancet* 2012;379(9828):1807–16.
4. Connor S. Laryngeal cancer: how does the radiologist help? *Cancer Imaging* 2007;28(7):93–103.
5. Yoo J, Henderson S, Walker-Dilks C. Evidence-based guideline recommendations on the use of positron emission tomography imaging in head and neck cancer. *Clin Oncol (R Coll Radiol)* 2013;25(4):e33–66.
6. Compton CC, Byrd DR, Garcia-Aguilar J, Kurtzman SH, Olawaiye A, Washington MK. Larynx. In Compton CC, Byrd DR, Garcia-Aguilar J, Kurtzman SH, Olawaiye A, Washington MK, eds., *AJCC Cancer Staging Atlas.* New York: Springer, 2012, pp. 79–90.

7. Compton CC, Byrd DR, Garcia-Aguilar J, Kurtzman SH, Olawaiye A, Washington MK. Pharynx. In Compton CC, Byrd DR, Garcia-Aguilar J, Kurtzman SH, Olawaiye A, Washington MK, eds., *AJCC Cancer Staging Atlas*. New York: Springer, 2012, pp. 55–77.

8. Jones AS, Fish B, Fenton JE, Husband DJ. The treatment of early laryngeal cancers (T1-T2 N0): surgery or irradiation? *Head Neck* 2004;26(2):127–35.

9. Pradhan S, Mehta M, Hakeem A, Tubachi J, Kannan R. Transoral resection of laryngeal and hypopharyngeal cancers. *Indian J Surg Oncol* 2010;1(2):207–11.

10. Ozer E, Alvarez B, Kakarala K, Durmus K, Teknos TN, Carrau RL. Clinical outcomes of transoral robotic supraglottic laryngectomy. *Head Neck* 2013;35(8):1158–61.

11. Gourin CG, Conger BT, Sheils WC, Bilodeau PA, Coleman TA, Porubsky ES. The effect of treatment on survival in patients with advanced laryngeal carcinoma. *Laryngoscope* 2009;119(7):1312–7.

12. Karatzanis AD, Psychogios G, Waldfahrer F, Kapsreiter M, Zenk J, Velegrakis GA, et al. Management of locally advanced laryngeal cancer. *J Otolaryngol Head Neck Surg* 2014;43:4.

13. Layland MK, Sessions DG, Lenox J. The influence of lymph node metastasis in the treatment of squamous cell carcinoma of the oral cavity, oropharynx, larynx, and hypopharynx: N0 versus N+. *Laryngoscope* 2005;115(4):629–39.

14. Warner L, Chudasama J, Kelly CG, Loughran S, McKenzie K, Wight R, et al. Radiotherapy versus open surgery versus endolaryngeal surgery (with or without laser) for early laryngeal squamous cell cancer. *Cochrane Database Syst Rev* 2014;12:CD002027.

15. Forastiere AA, Goepfert H, Maor M, Pajak TF, Weber R, Morrison W, et al. Concurrent chemotherapy and radiotherapy for organ preservation in advanced laryngeal cancer. *N Engl J Med* 2003;349(22):2091–8.

16. Nakamura K, Shioyama Y, Kawashima M, Saito Y, Nakamura N, Nakata K, et al. Multi-institutional analysis of early squamous cell carcinoma of the hypopharynx treated with radical radiotherapy. *Int J Radiat Oncol Biol Phys* 2006;65(4):1045–50.

17. Hinerman RW, Mendenhall WM, Amdur RJ, Stringer SP, Villaret DB, Robbins KT. Carcinoma of the supraglottic larynx: treatment results with radiotherapy alone or with planned neck dissection. *Head Neck* 2002;24(5):456–67.

18. Rosenthal DI, Mohamed AS, Weber RS, Garden AS, Sevak PR, Kies MS, et al. Long-term outcomes after surgical or nonsurgical initial therapy for patients with T4 squamous cell carcinoma of the larynx: a 3-decade survey. *Cancer* 2015;121(10):1608–19.

19. Blanchard P, Baujat B, Holostenco V, Bourredjem A, Baey C, Bourhis J, et al. Meta-analysis of chemotherapy in head and neck cancer (MACH-NC): a comprehensive analysis by tumour site. *Radiother Oncol* 2011;100(1):33–40.

20. Haddad R, O'Neill A, Rabinowits G, Tishler R, Khuri F, Adkins D, et al. Induction chemotherapy followed by concurrent chemoradiotherapy (sequential chemoradiotherapy) versus concurrent chemoradiotherapy alone in locally advanced head and neck cancer PARADIGM: a randomised phase 3 trial. *Lancet Oncol* 2013;14(3):257–64.

21. Bonner JA, Harari PM, Giralt J, Azarnia N, Shin DM, Cohen RB, et al. Radiotherapy plus cetuximab for squamous-cell carcinoma of the head and neck. *N Engl J Med* 2006;354(6):567–78.

22. Vermorken JB, Mesia R, Rivera F, Remenar E, Kawecki A, Rottey S, et al. Platinum-based chemotherapy plus cetuximab in head and neck cancer. *N Engl J Med* 2008;259(11):1116–27.

23. Mendenhall WM, Parsons JT, Stringer SP, Cassisi NJ, Million RR. Stage T3 squamous cell carcinoma of the glottic larynx: a comparison of laryngectomy and irradiation. *Int J Radiat Oncol Biol Phys* 1992;23(4):725–32.

24. Hilgers FJ, van Dam FS, Keyzers S, Koster MN, van As CJ, Muller MJ. Rehabilitation of olfaction after laryngectomy by means of a nasal airflow-inducing maneuver: the "polite yawning" technique. *Arch Otolaryngol Head Neck Surg* 2000;126(6):726–32.

22

Breast cancer

MARJUT LEIDENIUS, LYNDA WYLD, ISABEL T RUBIO, TIBOR KOVACS, TUOMO MERETOJA,
JOHANNA MATTSON, PHILIP POORTMANS, PÄIVI HEIKKILÄ AND DAVID EVANS

BREAST CANCER INCIDENCE, AETIOLOGY AND RISK FACTORS

Breast cancer is the most common cancer in women worldwide and also the leading cause of cancer deaths. It accounts for approximately 25% of all new cancer diagnoses and 15% of all cancer deaths in females. The incidence of breast cancer is higher in developed countries than in developing countries, with the age-standardized incidence rate estimated at 74 per 100,000 in developed areas and 31 per 100,000 in less developed areas of the world [1]. The global incidence of breast cancer is increasing. An estimated cumulative probability of breast cancer incidence in individual women aged 15–79 years was 5.5% globally in 2010 [2].

Several well-established risk factors for breast cancer have been identified, mainly in large epidemiological studies. These may vary somewhat according to breast cancer subtypes.

General risk factors include increasing age, previous high-dose radiation to the chest area and a previous history of breast cancer. Alcohol consumption increases the risk of breast cancer linearly even with moderate consumption.

Hormonal factors play a major role in the aetiology of breast cancer and many known risk factors are hormone related. These include young age at menarche and high age at menopause, nulliparity, older age at first birth, no lactation, high mammographic breast density, recent use of hormonal contraceptives, long-term use of hormonal replacement therapy and obesity. Bilateral oophorectomy reduces the risk of breast cancer, and the earlier in life the oophorectomy is performed, the greater the risk reduction. Higher postmenopausal bone density is associated with increased risk of breast cancer, probably due to higher endogenous or exogenous oestrogen levels.

A strong family history of breast cancer substantially increases the risk of developing breast cancer. Having a mother or sister diagnosed with breast cancer increases a woman's risk of breast cancer two- to threefold. The majority of women with a familial tendency have only a moderately increased risk due to genetic changes called single nucleotide polymorphisms (SNPs), which may act singly or in combination with other SNPs and other risk factors, and these women cannot presently be offered gene testing to fully characterize their risk. However, a small percentage have dominantly inherited a potent genetic mutation, such as BRCA1 or BRCA2. These and other high-risk gene mutations are discussed in more detail below.

Finally, the spectrum of benign breast diseases includes high-risk lesions, which refer to any histological finding in the breast associated with a subsequently increased risk of breast cancer. Proliferative disease with atypia is associated with a fourfold or higher risk of subsequent breast cancer; these findings include atypical ductal hyperplasia (ADH), atypical lobular hyperplasia (ALH) and lobular carcinoma in situ (LCIS). Proliferative disease without atypia confers an approximately twofold increase in breast cancer risk. These findings include papilloma, radial scar, columnar hyperplasia, usual ductal hyperplasia and sclerosing adenosis [3].

GENETICS AND BREAST CANCER RISK MANAGEMENT

A progressively increasing percentage of all diagnosed breast cancer cases are thought to develop due to inherited susceptibility of either potent single genes or SNPs. A rapidly expanding number of breast cancer susceptibility genes have now been identified. The first to be identified were BRCA1 and BRCA2 which were discovered in 1994 and 1995, respectively [4,5]. Germ line mutations of these genes are autosomal dominant disorders accounting for approximately 25–30% of all hereditary breast cancers. These mutations have been estimated to confer a cumulative lifetime breast cancer risk of as high as 80% for both BRCA1 and BRCA2, and an ovarian cancer risk of approximately 40% for BRCA1 and 20% for BRCA2. BRCA2 is also associated with pancreatic cancer as well as male breast cancer and prostate cancer at young age [6,7].

Other high-penetrant dominantly inherited gene mutations associated with breast cancer risk include mutations in TP53, PTEN, CDH1 and STK11 genes (Table 22.1). These mutations account for approximately 5% of all hereditary breast cancer cases. Germ line mutations in the TP53 gene may cause a clinically and genetically heterogeneous Li–Fraumeni syndrome that predisposes to various malignancies including sarcomas, brain tumours, leukemia, adrenocortical tumours, lung tumours and a lifetime cumulative breast cancer risk of approximately 56–90% [8]. Identifiable PTEN mutations are found in 80% of patients with Cowden syndrome, which is associated with a lifetime breast cancer risk of 25–50% [9]. Hereditary diffuse gastric cancer syndrome is associated with a CDH1 gene mutation and confers a high risk of diffuse gastric cancer and an estimated lifetime lobular breast cancer risk of up to 50% [10]. Peutz–Jeghers syndrome is caused by mutations in the STK11 gene, manifesting as hamartomatous polyposis and a predisposition to malignant tumours of

Table 22.1 Highly penetrant breast cancer gene mutations

Syndrome	Gene	Cancers	Lifetime risk of breast cancer for females (%)
Breast–ovarian	BRCA1	Female breast, ovarian	40–80
Breast–ovarian	BRCA2	Female and male breast, ovarian, prostate, pancreatic	20–80
Li–Fraumeni	TP53	Breast, sarcoma, leukemia, brain, adrenocortical, lung	56–90
Cowden's	PTEN	Breast, thyroid, endometrial	25–50
Peutz–Jeghers	STK11	Breast, ovarian, pancreatic, uterine, testicular, colon	32–54
Hereditary diffuse gastric cancer	CDH1	Early onset diffuse gastric cancer, lobular breast cancer	60

Source: Modified from Apostolou P and Fostira F, *Biomed Res Int*, 2013;747318:2013.

the gastrointestinal tract, ovary, uterine and cervix and also breast cancer, with a lifetime breast cancer risk of up to 50% [11].

A number of identified moderate- to low-risk breast cancer susceptibility genes include ATM, BRIP1, CHEK2, NBS1, RAD50, RAD51B-D, PALB2 and XRCC2 which together account for approximately 5% of all hereditary breast cancers (Table 22.2). Additionally, more than 60 moderate-risk susceptibility genes have been identified accounting for 14% of all hereditary breast cancers. Thus, approximately half of the hereditary breast cancer cases are caused by still unidentified hereditary mechanisms [11].

There is also increasing awareness of the role of SNPs in conveying increased breast cancer risk. This is an area of extensive research at the present time with large international consortia gathering evidence from massive cohorts of women [12]. Interpretation of the risks associated with these polymorphisms is complex as there may be as many as 1000 of significance and they may have a multiplicative effect on risk [13,14].

There are several management strategies for women at high risk of developing breast cancer either due to an extensive family history or due to a known genetic mutation. The majority of evidence regarding risk-reducing strategies is based on BRCA1 and BRCA2 carriers. Risk-reducing measures range from surveillance to chemoprevention and risk-reducing surgery to both breasts and ovaries.

Surveillance of high-risk women is currently based on annual MRI screening in addition to traditional mammograms. Intensive MRI and mammogram screening has been shown to improve survival when compared with no intensive screening [15]. As expertise about the impact of complex inherited genetic profile is combined with more ready availability of next-generation sequencing, it may be possible to target screening more appropriately to women at high risk [16]. Chemoprevention by selective oestrogen receptor modulators (SERMs) in premenopausal women reduces breast cancer risk in the high-risk women by approximately one-third. Chemoprevention is associated with considerable adverse effects which need to be taken into account as they may affect patient's adherence to the treatment, and the risks of endometrial cancer and thromboembolic disease must be discussed with the patient [17,18]. There is now good evidence that up to 5 years of aromatase inhibitor therapy (exemestane or anastrozole) in postmenopausal high-risk women is also associated with an even greater breast cancer risk reduction than prophylactic SERMs (Figure 22.1) [19,20].

Risk-reducing bilateral mastectomy reduces the risk of consequent breast cancer to less than 10%, and Ingham and colleagues (2013)[21] have recently found that bilateral risk-reducing mastectomy in gene carriers does confer a survival advantage if performed before the woman

Table 22.2 Moderate-risk breast cancer genes

Gene	Cancers	Lifetime risk of breast cancer %
ATM	Breast, ovarian	20–50
CHEK2	Breast, colorectal, ovarian, bladder	25–37
PALB2	Breast, pancreatic, ovarian, male breast	20–40
RAD51C	Breast, ovarian	Variable
BRIP1	Breast, ovarian	Variable
ABRAXAS	Breast	Variable

Source: Modified from Apostolou P and Fostira F, *Biomed Res Int*, 2013;747318:2013.

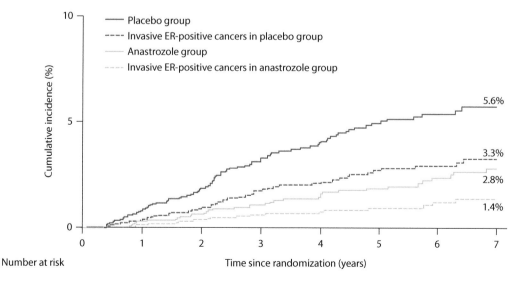

Figure 22.1 Kaplan–Meier chart showing the cumulative incidence of breast cancer (ER positive only or all types) in women taking 5 years of prophylactic anastrozole or placebo. (Data reprinted from Cuzick J, et al., *Lancet*, 381: 1827–34, 2013. With permission from Elsevier.)

develops cancer. Removal of a healthy contralateral breast in a gene carrier who has developed cancer in the breast is somewhat more contentious, but there is emerging evidence that this not only prevents further cancers and improves quality of life by reducing cancer anxiety but also has a significant impact on survival in selected cases [22]. In most cases risk-reducing mastectomy is combined with reconstructive surgery to minimize aesthetic and psychosocial impacts.

Bilateral salpingo-oophorectomy effectively reduces the risk of ovarian cancer by 99% but also that of breast cancer by approximately 50% in BRCA mutation carriers if performed premenopausally [23].

These management strategies need to be discussed in detail with the patient as they may potentially have significant effects on psychosocial and sexual well-being.

PREMALIGNANT AND HIGH-RISK LESIONS

The advent of ever more sensitive breast imaging and core biopsies has increased the identification of a number of benign breast pathologies that are considered premalignant or that are markers of elevated risk of developing breast cancer. These biopsy findings can broadly be divided into three categories: non-proliferative changes, proliferation without atypia and atypical proliferation, accounting for approximately 65%, 30% and 5% of all diagnosed benign breast lesions, respectively.

The non-proliferative changes are associated with a low relative cancer risk (RR) of 1.2 to 1.4. These include simple cysts, fibrosis, fibroadenoma, columnar cell change, apocrine metaplasia and mild ductal hyperplasia. Proliferative diseases confer a higher RR of 1.7 to 2.1 and include usual ductal hyperplasia, sclerosing adenosis, columnar hyperplasia, papilloma and radial scar. Atypical proliferative diseases are associated with an estimated fourfold or higher breast cancer risk and these findings include ADH, ALH and LCIS. Biopsy findings that are associated with uncertain but probably increased relative breast cancer risk include flat epithelial atypia (FEA), apocrine atypia, secretory atypia and mucocele-like tumour with atypia. Atypical hyperplasia may also manifest in papillomas, radial scars and other lesions, increasing their RR. Management strategies of biopsy findings depend on the relative cancer risk and should always include analysis of the radiologic–pathologic concordance of the findings. Possible management strategies include surgical excision, surveillance and preventive interventions [3].

The rationale for surgical excision of a high-risk lesion is based not so much on the radical removal of the entire lesion but rather on the potential sampling error by the core biopsy and the possibility of an adjacent carcinoma. Upgrade rates of up to 30%, from benign to malignant diagnosis between core biopsy and surgical excision specimen, have been reported. The risk of upgrade increases with core biopsy finding showing atypia, the biopsy being performed with smaller-gauge needles and with larger

lesions on imaging [24,25]. Vacuum-assisted biopsy provides a wider sample and is increasingly recognized as an alternative to surgical excision for some of these lesions.

There is a general consensus that a surgical excision should be considered in patients with discordance between radiological and pathological findings, in symptomatic patients and in patients with high-risk lesions. These high-risk lesions include ADH, papillary lesions with atypia, radial scar with atypia and the pleomorphic variant of LCIS. There is less evidence on the management of common type LCIS (classical LCIS), ALH, FEA and other atypical lesions. Many researchers tend to lean toward surgical excision due to little evidence on surveillance alone [3,24] although recent data suggest that in carefully selected cases, surveillance with short-term follow-up may be appropriate [25,26]. Vacuum-assisted large-volume biopsy may be used in certain circumstances to widely sample or excise some lesions.

Evidence suggests that ADH, ALH and LCIS, but possibly also all other atypical biopsy findings, represent non-obligate precursors to cancer. Yet, they are also associated with an increased risk of both ipsilateral and contralateral breast cancer (CBC), representing an increased constitutional lifetime breast cancer risk. Therefore, patients with atypical biopsy findings should also be offered surveillance. Generally, the surveillance constitutes annual mammograms [3,24].

Finally, there is a growing body of evidence showing a substantial breast cancer risk reduction by SERMs or aromatase inhibitors in women with high-risk lesions (ADH, ALH and LCIS). Chemoprevention is, however, associated with considerable adverse effects which may affect patient compliance [17].

BREAST CANCER PATHOLOGY, PROGNOSTIC AND PREDICTIVE FACTORS

Breast cancer is a highly heterogeneous disease with diverse morphology, differing response to systemic therapies and variable clinical outcomes. Breast cancer can be divided into numerous subtypes according to histological morphologies, as well as biological and molecular characteristics. A number of traditional pathological determinants, as well as the more recent molecular characteristics, have an impact on an individual patient's prognosis and may predict the possible benefit of systemic therapies.

Pathology

The histopathological work-up of the surgical breast specimen includes meticulous evaluation of tumour resection margins together with evaluation of tumour morphology and differentiation. Immunohistochemistry is routinely used to evaluate several tumour biology-related variables.

In situ carcinoma is differentiated from invasive carcinoma by microscopic evaluation and can be facilitated by immunohistochemical staining of the myoepithelium in problematic cases.

The histopathological classification of breast cancer is based on the WHO classification of tumours that is adopted worldwide. The most common histological type is invasive carcinoma of no special type, previously known as invasive ductal carcinoma, not otherwise specified (75% of all breast cancers). Invasive lobular carcinoma is the second largest group representing 10–15% of all breast cancers. The mere histopathological tumour type has little prognostic or predictive value, as it groups together tumours with very different biological and clinical profiles. Some of the more infrequent breast cancer types do have prognostic implications, as they are associated with excellent prognosis. These include pure tubular, cribriform, secretory, invasive papillary, low-grade mucinous, adenoid cystic and low-grade adenosquamous carcinomas [27,28].

Prognostic and predictive factors

Prognostic factors predict the natural history of a patient's breast cancer unrelated to systemic therapy, whereas predictive factors predict the response to a specific treatment. Prognostic factors include tumour size, lymph node stage and extent of distant tumour spread, all of which constitute the American Joint Committee on Cancer tumour, node and metastasis (TNM) staging system (see Table 22.5) [29].

Histological tumour grade, usually described using the modified Bloom and Richardson system into grade 1, 2 or 3 based on tubule formation, nuclear pleomorphism and mitotic count, is widely recognized to have prognostic significance. Lymphovascular invasion in breast cancer is known to predict axillary metastases, recurrence and long-term survival [30].

IMMUNOHISTOCHEMICALLY DETERMINED FACTORS

A number of biological prognostic and predictive factors in breast cancer are determined from the tumour by immunohistochemistry as routine clinical practice. The hormone receptor status of breast cancer has been used since the 1970s as a predictive factor for endocrine treatment responsiveness and as a prognostic marker for early recurrence. Currently, both oestrogen receptor (ER) and progesterone receptor (PgR) status should be routinely assessed by standardized immunohistochemistry techniques. The ER and PgR status is commonly considered positive with 1% or more tumour cells staining positive on immunohistochemistry, although also the actual percentage of receptor positive tumour cells should be reported [28,31]. Approximately 70% of all breast cancers are ER positive, but the rate varies with age being very roughly equivalent to the age of a patient (e.g. 40% of breast cancers in 40-year-olds, 90% in 90-year-olds).

Human epidermal growth factor receptor type 2 (HER-2) gene amplification occurs in approximately 14–20% of primary breast cancers and the majority of these cases are oestrogen receptor negative. HER-2 gene amplification is a predictor of decreased survival and also of poor response to traditional chemotherapy. However, HER-2 protein overexpression provides a target for anti-HER-2 directed therapy (e.g. trastuzumab, pertuzumab, trastuzumab–emtansine/TDM1) which has been shown to benefit the outcome for these patients significantly. The assessment of HER-2 status is commonly performed as a combination of preliminary immunohistochemistry and in equivocal cases validation by *in situ* hybridization [28,31,32].

Tumour proliferation in breast cancer has been established as one of the most important prognostic factors. Traditionally the proliferative activity of breast cancer has been evaluated by the mitotic count, which is also part of the standard histological grading system. Molecular techniques for assessing the tumour proliferation include immunohistochemical staining of proliferation-related antigens, most commonly Ki-67 which identifies the percentage of cells in cycle versus those which are quiescent. Ki-67 is a useful addition in predicting the response to chemotherapy in hormone receptor positive and HER-2 negative patients. However, universal adoption of Ki-67 into routine clinical practice has been hindered by the lack of standardization of the assay and its interpretation [31,33].

MOLECULAR SUBTYPES AND SURROGATE IMMUNOHISTOCHEMISTRY

The molecular basis of breast cancer heterogeneity has been further elaborated during the last decade by gene expression profiling, performed by DNA microarray or RT-PCR techniques. On the basis of the gene expression signatures, a number of molecular subtypes, mapping to the ER, PgR, HER-2 and Ki-67 status of the breast cancer, have been identified [34]. On the basis of this molecular subtype classification, several commercially available assays have been developed, which predict patient outcome or response to systemic therapies on the basis of the tumour's gene signature profile [31]. The molecular subtypes can be approximated by surrogate immunohistochemistry assessing the hormone receptor status, HER-2 status and Ki-67, in combination (Table 22.3). However, the molecular genotypes and immunophenotypes do not completely overlap, with occasional discrepancies [33].

Risk prediction models

A number of risk prediction models have been developed with the common objective of identifying patients whom might or might not benefit from adjuvant chemotherapy. The commercial gene profiling assays aim at just this and have been incorporated into clinical practice in many centres. The most widely studied and validated assays are Oncotype DX and MammaPrint, both of which predict recurrence-free survival. Oncotype DX includes 21 genes,

Table 22.3 Surrogate definitions of major molecular subtypes of breast cancer

	Oestrogen (ER) and progesterone (PgR) receptor expression	HER-2 receptor expression	Proliferative marker Ki-67 expression	Multigene assay recurrence score (if available)
Luminal A	ER positive PgR positive	Negative	Low	Low
Luminal B (HER-2 negative)	ER positive PgR negative	Negative	High	High
Luminal B (HER-2 positive)	ER positive PgR any	Positive	Any	Not applicable
HER-2 enriched	Negative	Positive	Any	Not applicable
Triple negative	Negative	Negative	Any	Not applicable

Source: Modified from Goldhirsch A, et al., Ann Oncol, 2013;24:2206–23.

while MammaPrint includes 70 genes [35,36]. The role and clinical importance of these commercial gene profiling assays will be further elaborated by ongoing randomized trials TAILORx and MINDACT [37,38]. TAILORx has just published some of its results which validate the use of Oncotype DX in the identification of very low recurrence risk patients in whom chemotherapy may be safely avoided [39].

Perhaps the most adopted and validated risk prediction models are the Adjuvant! OnLine and the Nottingham Prognostic Index (NPI), which are based on classical prognostic factors and not gene profiling. Adjuvant! OnLine aims to predict overall survival, recurrence-free survival and systemic treatment benefit, while the NPI predicts recurrence-free survival [35,36]. Adjuvant! OnLine has some limitations in that it does not allow HER-2 receptor status or Ki-67 to be factored in, whereas more recently an online prognostic tool, PREDICT, has been developed which does, based on UK data (http://www.predict.nhs.uk/predict.html) [40,41].

BREAST SCREENING

There is a large amount of data in favor of breast cancer screening, dating back several decades. These studies estimate that the mortality from breast cancer can be reduced by up to 30% in screened populations [42]. Screen-detected breast cancers are usually smaller, lower grade and less frequently associated with lymph node involvement when compared with clinically detected breast cancers, resulting in better survival rates. Even in comparable stages, screen-detected breast cancers appear to have a better outcome than non-screen-detected cancers [43–46].

Despite this, screening has remained a controversial subject [47,48]. A recent comprehensive independent review in the UK concluded that screening is effective at saving lives, with an estimated mortality reduction of around 20% [49]. There is, however, a cost in terms of 'overdiagnosis'. This reflects the fact that for every life saved from a potentially fatal breast cancer, several women will have had unnecessary biopsy for benign lesions, plus a number will have had treatment for a non-life-threatening breast cancer. Wide-ranging rates of overdiagnosis have been reported; however, those studies that accounted for cancer incidence during screening and for lead time have estimated overdiagnosis at only 1% to 10% [50–53].

Implementation and quality assurance in breast screening across Europe

Population breast screening programmes have been established in many European countries for several decades, but the implementation of these programmes varies between countries.

There have only been two randomized controlled trials (RCTs) comparing breast screening intervals, both comparing annual versus 3-yearly mammography [54,55]. Neither showed conclusive evidence in favor of the shorter screening interval. The EU recommends screening the 50–69 age group at an interval of 2 years.* Most EU countries use a screening interval of 2 years, with the UK and Malta being the exception, using a 3-year interval.

There is evidence that screening in the 40–50 age group reduces mortality by around 17% [56], but this has not been shown to be statistically significant [57]. Because the incidence of breast cancer and the effectiveness of mammography are lower among women in their forties than among women 50 years of age or older, mammography screening results in less absolute benefit and greater absolute risk for women 40–49 years of age than for women 50 years of age or older.

In order to maximize the effectiveness of breast screening, comprehensive European quality assurance guidelines

---

* Perry NM. Multi-disciplinary aspects of quality assurance in the diagnosis of breast disease. 2006. (This is a revised version of the original EUSOMA position paper published in 2001 [European Journal of Cancer 2001;37:159–172].) Available from http://www.eusoma.org/Engx/Guidelines/Other/OtherQA_D.aspx?cont=QA_D

Table 22.4 Key surgical quality measures for screen-detected breast cancers in the UK NHS Breast Screening Quality Assurance Programme

Measure	Minimum standard
Waiting time for biopsy results	Less than 1 week in 90% of cases
Surgeon case load per year	10 screened cancers
Rate of non-operative diagnosis	More than 90% invasive cancers diagnosed on percutaneous biopsy
Rates of benign diagnostic open biopsy	Less than 15 per 10,000 women in the prevalent screen
Specimen weight of benign open biopsy	More than 90% less than 20 g
Surgical localization rates of impalpable lesions	More than 98% correctly identified

have been produced, which set out organizational, clinical and professional standards for screening programmes. They also set minimum and recommended targets for a large number of quality measures such as recall rate, cancer detection rate and benign biopsy rate. A small selection of these targets are indicated in Table 22.4 based on the UK Screening Quality Assurance Programme.* Implementation of these guidelines, together with a locally organized QA structure, helps to ensure that screening programmes maintain adequate cancer detection rates, while minimizing the effects of overdiagnosis.

DIAGNOSIS AND STAGING IN BREAST CANCER

Diagnosis

Diagnosis of breast cancer is based on the concept of triple assessment. This approach applies in the context of the symptomatic patient and in the assessment of screen-detected abnormalities. Triple assessment consists of:

1. Clinical examination
2. Appropriate imaging
3. Tissue sampling

The imaging modalities typically used as first-line investigations are mammography and ultrasound (US). These are proven, readily available methods which can provide a high degree of diagnostic accuracy in most cases. MRI is more often used as a second-line

investigation, in cases where mammography and US prove non-diagnostic or equivocal.

MAMMOGRAPHY AND TOMOSYNTHESIS

Screen-film mammography (Figure 22.2) has been largely superseded by full-field digital mammography (FFDM) over the past 10 years. FFDM offers increased contrast resolution and dynamic range, together with the ability to manipulate and optimize the image [58,59]. FFDM has been shown to increase the accuracy of mammography in the under 50 age group and in those with densely glandular breast tissue [60].

A more recent development of digital mammography is digital breast tomosynthesis (DBT). This technology utilizes a mammography unit with a rotating X-ray tube, which moves through an arc while taking several X-ray exposures. These exposures are then reconstructed into many thin parallel slices. This technology helps to alleviate the difficulties with overlying structures and dense glandular tissue, making cancers more clearly visualized [61]. Several trials are currently underway assessing the feasibility of using DBT in the screening population. Initial results have shown a relative increase in cancer detection rates of between 32% and 51%, when using FFDM plus DBT compared with FFDM alone [62,63].

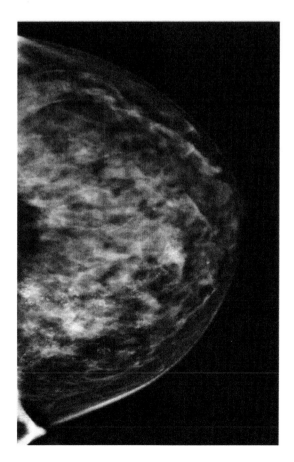

Figure 22.2 Screen-film mammogram showing a large invasive cancer with typical density and spiculation.

---

* See https://www.gov.uk/government/uploads/system/uploads/attachment_data/file/465694/nhsbsp20.pdf

ULTRASOUND

Ultrasound (US) has a long history in breast imaging, being in use for more than 40 years. It is readily available, well tolerated and does not involve ionizing radiation. Modern high-frequency ultrasound machines are able to demonstrate masses less than 5 mm in size, and accurately differentiate between solid and cystic lesions. In some cases, microcalcifications may also be visualized, allowing US-guided sampling.

There is no evidence that stand-alone screening with US reduces breast cancer mortality, but there are some data showing increased sensitivity when used together with mammography, compared with mammography alone, in higher-risk groups [64]. It is used routinely as the first-line imaging investigation of symptomatic lumps in the under-40 age group. It is also used in the assessment of screen-detected abnormalities, for axillary lymph node staging and in real-time guidance for interventional procedures.

MRI

Breast MRI has for many years been used as a problem-solving tool, in cases where there was diagnostic uncertainty or discordant imaging or pathology findings, and for evaluation of breast implant integrity. More recently, it has also been used to screen women in higher-risk groups. Sensitivity of MRI for cancer detection in these patients is almost double (77% vs. 40%) compared with mammography [65].

MRI has also been shown to be the most accurate method of determining response to primary chemotherapy, and in staging, more accurately measures tumour size in lobular carcinoma where it also has value in detecting multifocal or multicentric disease (Figure 22.3) [66–70].

BREAST BIOPSY

A tissue diagnosis of a breast lesion can be obtained by a number of methods, the most common of which are fine-needle aspiration (FNA), core biopsy (CB) and vacuum-assisted core biopsy (VACB). All of these sampling techniques are best performed using imaging guidance, which can be ultrasound, X-ray stereotaxis or MRI.

FNA is a simple, minimally invasive test that gives immediate cytological information. It is less accurate than core biopsy, with sensitivity reported between 35% and 95% and specificity between 46% and 100% [71]. Neither is it able to differentiate between *in situ* and invasive malignancy. However, it remains useful in evaluating axillary lymph nodes for metastasis, particularly where the proximity of the axillary artery and vein may make core biopsy difficult [72].

Automated core biopsy, generally using a 14 G needle, is widely regarded as the preferred method for obtaining a diagnosis in the majority of cases. The accuracy of CB is significantly higher than that of FNA, particularly for non-palpable or small lesions [73–75]. It is possible to distinguish between invasive and *in situ* disease, determine tumour subtype and perform immunohistochemistry on core samples. It has limitations, however, with lower accuracy in diagnosis of atypical lesions and lesions related to screen-detected calcification.

VACB utilizes a larger-gauge needle, typically between 11 and 7 G, and most VACB systems are able to obtain multiple tissue samples without repeated removal of the biopsy needle. Therefore VACB has the ability to quickly obtain a significantly larger volume of tissue than 14 G CB. A single 11 G VACB core is approximately six times larger than a 14 G core (100 mg vs. 17 mg) (Figure 22.4) [76].

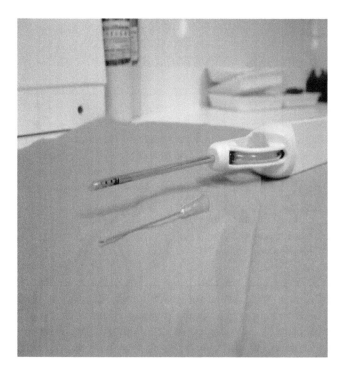

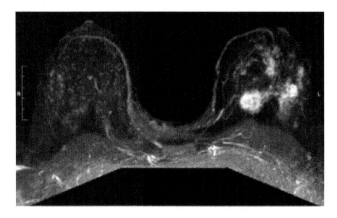

Figure 22.3 MRI of both breasts showing enhancement of a multifocal cancer in the post-gadolinium contrast phase.

Figure 22.4 Photograph showing the comparative size of a VACB needle and a standard 14 G needle.

Surgical upgrade rates, from atypia to ductal carcinoma in situ (DCIS) and from DCIS to invasive disease, are decreased by more than 50% where VACB is used in preference to CB [77].

VACB can also be used as a therapeutic procedure, enabling benign lesions such as fibroadenomas and papillary lesions, without atypia, to be removed without the need for a surgical excision. Radial scars without atypia may also be safely left without surgical excision following adequate sampling with a VACB [78].

Staging

There are two main hypotheses that explain breast cancer dissemination: it is either a heterogeneous disease that may remain localized throughout its course and spread over time through lymphatics (the Halstedian theory) [79] or it is a systemic disease when first diagnosed (the Fisher theory) [80,81]. The American Joint Committee on Cancer (AJCC) has designated staging by size of the tumour (T), regional lymph node involvement (N) and metastasis (M) (TNM) to define breast cancer (Table 22.5) [82]. The AJCC staging system groups patients with respect to prognosis and has been regularly updated to include prognostic indicators and new technologies (sentinel lymph node, molecular tests, size of axillary metastasis, number of axillary nodes metastasis, etc.). In the future, a major challenge will be that the TNM classification will incorporate the advances in cancer biology that predict cancer outcome and response to treatment better than just the anatomical-based staging [83,84]. Treatment decision making in breast cancer should be based on several factors that include patient and tumour characteristics and clinical staging. Generally, the recommended work-up and staging of invasive breast cancer includes history and physical exam, laboratory test (CBC count, liver function test, diagnostic mammography, breast ultrasound if needed, axillary ultrasound for determination of clinical nodal status) and pathology report (tumour grade, hormone receptors, HER-2 status). Use of MRI is optional as there is no consensus on whether the detection of additional foci improves patient outcomes. EUSOMA has issued a consensus on the indications and recommendations on the use of MRI in breast cancer [85].

Additional imaging in order to diagnose distant metastases is performed depending on the tumour and nodal stage, according to national or local guidelines as well as according to the most common sites of breast cancer distant metastases (bone, liver, lungs). In some institutes, this staging imaging consists of chest X-ray, abdominal ultrasound and bone scan; CT scan is performed only in patients with suspicious findings in chest X-ray or abdominal ultrasound. In other institutions, CT scan is performed, instead of chest X-ray and abdominal ultrasound.

In addition, staging imaging is indicated in patients with symptoms or laboratory test results suspicious for distant metastases. These include abdominal ultrasound, chest X-ray or CT scan, bone scan or brain MRI, according to the

Table 22.5 Simplified version of the UICC/AJCC TNM staging system for breast cancer

TNM stage	Definition
Primary cancer	
Tx	Primary not assessed
T0	No evidence of a primary cancer (e.g. in cases with metastases with an occult primary)
Tis	Subgroup as either DCIS, LCIS or Paget's disease
T1	Primary less than 2 cm (subgroup as mic: less than 1 mm of microinvasion; [a] 1–5 mm, [b] 5–10 mm and [c] 10–20 mm)
T2	20–50 mm primary
T3	More than 50 mm primary
T4	Locally advanced tumour of any size as a result of the presence of (a) chest wall invasion; (b) skin invasion, peau d'orange, ulceration or nodules; (c) both a and b; or (d) inflammatory cancer
Nodes	
Nx	Nodes not assessed
N0	No nodal disease (includes isolated tumour cells <0.2 mm on IHC (i+/−) or RT-PCR analysis (Mol+/−)
N1	Mobile ipsilateral nodal disease (includes micrometastases N1mi if 0.2–2 mm)
N2	Either (a) matted or fixed ipsilateral nodes or (b) ipsilateral internal mammary nodes only
N3	Either (a) infraclavicular, (b) internal mammary *and* axillary or (c) supraclavicular
Metastases	
Mx	Metastases not assessed
M0	No distant metastases
M1	Distant metastases present

Source: Edge SB, et al., eds., in *AJCC Cancer Staging Manual*, 7th ed., New York: Springer, 2010, pp. 347–76.

symptoms and signs in the clinical examination or laboratory test results.

PET/CT with F18-fluoro-2-deoxy-D-glucose (FDG) has gained widespread clinical applications in oncology, and the information provided reflects the metabolic activity of the tumour. Therefore false negative results are more common in slowly proliferating grade I tumours, while nonmalignant conditions, such as inflammation, may lead to false positive findings. FDG PET/CT is not indicated or recommended in the routine staging of early breast cancer, although it may show distant metastases not detected with other imaging methods. The role of FDG PET/CT in evaluating locoregional nodal status for initial staging of breast cancer has not yet been defined in clinical practice and different studies have reported sensitivity that ranges from 30% to 60% and specificity from 95% to 100% [86].

Most of the guidelines do not recommend the use of CA-15.3, CA-27.29 and CEA for screening, diagnosis or staging of breast cancer, not even for surveillance after primary treatment [87].

SURGERY OF THE BREAST IN EARLY PRIMARY BREAST CANCER

Breast conservation

ONCOPLASTIC BREAST CONSERVATION

Breast conservation surgery became the treatment of choice for early breast cancer in the past decades. Studies conducted have confirmed that breast conservation (BC) with adjuvant radiotherapy to the residual breast tissue gives similar disease control and survival rates as simple mastectomy [88,89].

The two major long-term goals that have to be achieved by BC are:

1. Complete surgical excision of the tumour (local control with low local recurrence [LR] rates)
2. Acceptable aesthetic outcome with good symmetry achieved [90]

Indications for breast conservation are early breast cancer without skin or fascia involvement, tumour size not exceeding 30–40% of the original breast volume, unifocal lesions or multifocal lesions situated in the same quadrant, in general tumours that can be removed from the breast with microscopically clear surgical resection margins and acceptable cosmetic outcome with regard to the shape, contour and size of the remaining breast.

An extended indication of BC is for tumours downsized by neoadjuvant chemotherapy or systemic endocrine treatment where incomplete or complete pathological response is achieved [91,92]

Contraindications for BC are:

1. Any contraindications for adjuvant radiotherapy (previous radiotherapy including mantle radiotherapy for Hodgkin's disease)
2. Extensive skin or chest wall involvement, tumours larger than 40% of the original breast volume
3. When BC would lead to a significant breast deformity and poor aesthetic outcome
4. Extensive malignant microcalcifications or inflammatory carcinoma
5. Multifocal (two or more foci in same quadrant) or multicentric (different quadrants) cancers represent a relative contraindication

With the introduction of oncoplastic surgery (OPLS) (meaning plastic surgical techniques used for breast cancer surgery with the goal of improving aesthetic outcomes without compromising oncological results), larger tumours can be excised with oncological safety and the contraindications for breast conservation have significantly reduced.

In case of multifocal or multicentric disease, OPLS can make BC technically possible, but patients have to be carefully counselled regarding the risk of incomplete surgical excision and the higher likelihood of re-excision and increased risk of locoregional recurrence [93,94].

BC with adjuvant radiotherapy gives equivalent survivals with total mastectomy, demonstrated by long-term follow-up results in several randomized trials [88,89,95,96]. Clear surgical resection margins are needed to reduce the risk of locoregional recurrence [97], but there is a lack of agreement on what clear resection margin means, leading to a discussion about 'bigger is not better' [98]. Definitions of clear margins range from 'no ink on the tumour surface' to 10 mm or more. Accordingly, the rate of surgical margin re-excision varies significantly between centres. The need for further surgery causes major distress to patients and often interferes with aesthetic outcomes of BC and raises treatment costs.

The 2014 SSO-ASTRO Consensus Guideline based on the meta-analysis of margin width and ipsilateral breast recurrence from a systematic review of 33 studies including 28,162 patients recommends 'the use of no ink on tumour as the standard for an adequate margin in invasive cancer in the era of multidisciplinary therapy, this being associated with low LR rates and has the potential to decrease re-excision rates, improve cosmetic outcomes and decrease healthcare costs' [99].

Due to early diagnosis (screening) and downsizing with neoadjuvant chemotherapy or hormonal treatment, potentially BC can be performed in 70–80% of breast cancers. Unfortunately there are breast units where the mastectomy rates are still around 50%. Causes mainly are related to limited access to adjuvant radiotherapy, patient choice (to minimize the risk of locoregional recurrence) or surgeon judgment (to achieve better local control, avoid breast deformity) and lack of training in oncoplastic techniques.

Factors influencing the aesthetic outcomes in BC and responsible for poor cosmesis are small-sized breasts, ptotic breast shape, large tumour size, tumour location (central, upper-inner, lower-inner quadrants), multifocal or when more than 20% of the breast volume has to be resected [100–102].

Oncoplastic breast conservation surgery allows the breast surgeon to extend the indications for BC without compromising oncological principles and aesthetic outcomes; extensive resections of more than 20% of the breast volume are possible without significant deformity and could reduce the rate of re-excisions for close margins [103]. OPLS became 'fashionable' in the last decade and some surgeons may feel that not doing a more complex oncoplastic resection is not in line with current treatment guidelines. This could lead to overtreatment and exposing patients to unnecessary procedures with increased complication rates. In general terms complex oncoplastic procedures should be offered to patients with large lesions, small breasts or both, where traditional BC (simple lumpectomy) seems impossible or will lead to major breast deformity.

General principles of OPLS are as follows:

1. Use OPLS for definitive cancer surgery only and not for diagnostic excisional biopsy.
2. Evaluate disease extent in detail (MRI if unclear with traditional imaging).
3. Document with pre- and postoperative medical photography.
4. Use multiple bracketed wire or seed localization for extensive lesions (4 cm).
5. Use intraoperative US (IOUS) or ROLL, radioactive seed (RSL) or wire localization for non-palpable lesions.
6. Use radiopaque markers for the cavity (to mark tumour location for adjuvant radiotherapy planning).
7. Orient surgical specimen for margin assessment.

The oncoplastic decision-making process (what procedure to offer the patient, intended benefits, outcomes, likeliness of achieving clear margins) is based on the OPLS technique classification proposed by Clough et al [104,105]. The selection criteria for the techniques include the planned excision volume, breast volume, tumour location and glandular density (BIRADS 1–4).

As a general principle, large tumours of 3–4 cm diameter, where the excised volume is more than 20% of the breast volume, in patients with small cup size breasts and in patients opting for breast conservation following downsizing with neoadjuvant treatment, level 2 oncoplastic techniques have a major role in obtaining clear margins with acceptable aesthetic outcomes.

Level 1 oncoplastic techniques are applied when there is a less than 20% volume loss and they consist of:

1. Extensive undermining in the skin-sparing mastectomy plane to facilitate both tumour resection and glandular redistribution once the tumour has been removed.
2. Nipple–areola complex (NAC) undermining and centralization.
3. Full-thickness glandular excision down to the pectoralis fascia.
4. Dual-plane glandular mobilization (pectoralis fascia level).
5. The glandular defect is closed with tissue re-approximation.

Level 2 oncoplastic techniques (see Figure 22.5) are performed in patients with a more than 20% breast volume loss and they are called therapeutic mammoplasties (TMPLs). These are volume redistribution techniques meant to optimize the breast shape and volume following tumour resection. Usually a smaller breast is created by glandular remodelling, there is a need for contralateral symmetrization and the procedure can improve the breast aesthetics without compromising the oncological resection.

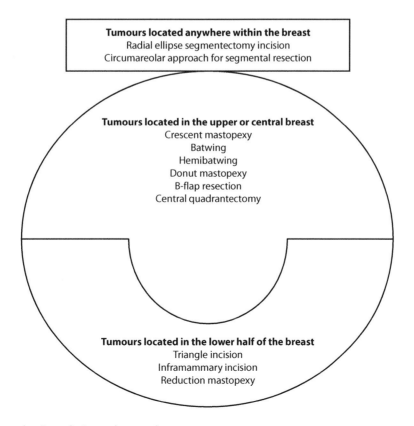

Figure 22.5 Level 2 oncoplastic techniques by quadrant.

TMPLs may be classified according to tumour location [106]:

1. *Upper-central breast tumours.* Crescent mastopexy (Figure 22.6), batwing (Figure 22.7) or hemibatwing, donut mastopexy, B-flap resection (Grisotti type) (Figure 22.8), inferior pedicle reduction mastopexy (wise pattern which may be used with a variety of nipple pedicles depending on the location of the tumour and the degree of ptosis (Figure 22.9)
2. *Lower quadrant tumours.* Inframammary incision, superior pedicle reduction mastopexy, inferior pedicle reduction mastopexy (Figure 22.9)
3. *Anywhere in the breast.* Circumareolar approach for segmental resection (Figure 22.10)
4. *Outer quadrant tumours.* Lateral mammoplasty with NAC medialization

Central quadrant techniques can help in avoiding a square shape to the breast or a flattened breast and may permit preservation of the NAC even in tumours situated close to it. It can help achieve a complete oncological resection with clear surgical resection margins (Figures 22.6 and 22.7).

The crescent TMPL works like a mastopexy, leading to an elevation of the NAC and mild correction of ptosis, allowing the excision of a crescent-shaped dermo-glandular tissue block, in tumours without nipple–areola involvement, situated above the NAC between the 10 and 1 o'clock position. The skin overlying the tumour is removed [106].

The batwing TMPL is indicated in tumours without nipple involvement, in the upper central breast, permits a breast ptosis correction and elevates the lower half of the breast and nipple–areola. When marking, the nipple–areola should always remain on the breast meridian in order to avoid displacement. The glandular advancement flaps are created at the pectoralis fascia level to allow tension-free closure. Contralateral symmetrization is usually needed.

Due to extensive tissue mobilization, oncoplastic procedures have a higher complication rate than traditional wide local excisions, and patients have to be informed and give consent accordingly. The most frequent complications

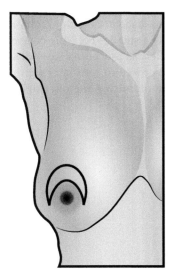
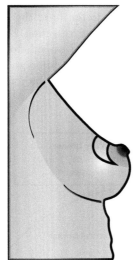

Figure 22.6 **Crescent mastopexy incision.**

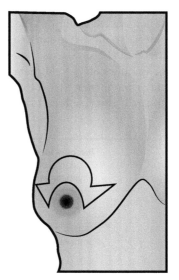
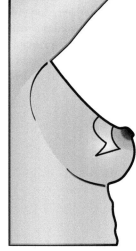

Figure 22.7 **Batwing mastopexy incision.**

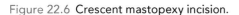
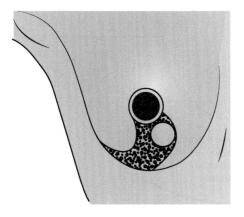
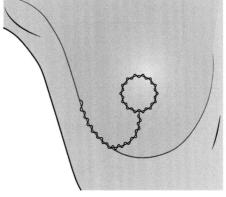

Figure 22.8 **Grissotti-type therapeutic mammoplasty.**

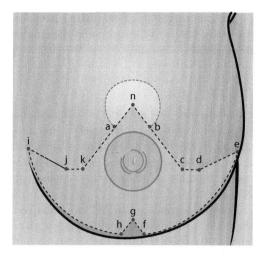

Figure 22.9 Wise pattern reduction which may be used with a variety of nipple pedicles depending on tumour location and breast size and shape.

are fat necrosis 25.9% vs. 9.5%, delayed wound healing (8.6% vs. 1.2%), nipple loss, sensitivity loss, nipple asymmetry, wound dehiscence and skin necrosis [107].

SURGERY FOR NON-PALPABLE BREAST LESIONS: OCCULT LESION LOCALIZATION

Clinically occult breast lesions represent screen-detected breast cancers (one-third of breast cancers) or lesions that are of uncertain significance or suspicious for malignancy and they need a surgical excision–biopsy. Wire-guided localization (WGL) is used as the standard procedure to identify these lesions and to guide the surgeon for the excision of the index lesion. The goal of any occult lesion localization technique is to perform an accurate and precise localization of a non-palpable breast lesion, to avoid excessive resection of surrounding healthy breast tissue, increase the free excision margin rate, decrease operative time and reduce patient discomfort.

Although the WGL offers an accurate localization, it has some disadvantages: it is difficult to perform in dense breasts, displacement may occur during surgery, there may be unnecessary extensive removal of healthy breast tissue and surgery may be difficult with a potentially compromised aesthetic outcome due to wire position.

Radioguided occult lesion localization (ROLL) is a relatively new method described and performed for more than 10 years in breast centres worldwide for the localization and facilitation of resection of non-palpable breast lesions. The method was developed at the European Institute of Oncology, Milan [108]. The method consists of injection of a small amount of radioactive substance (99m Tc–labelled colloidal serum albumin) peritumourally or directly into the lesion under US or stereotactic guidance. The accuracy of the localization is confirmed by imaging the needle tip position within the lesion (US or mammogram). The terms ROLL and sentinel node occult lesion localization (SNOLL) are also used to describe the procedure. The injection site ('hot area') is localized with a handheld gamma probe (the same device as used for the sentinel node identification), prior to incision [109]. The skin incision can be placed on the breast according to oncoplastic principles. After excising the 'hot spot' identified by using the gamma probe, the cavity walls are checked for residual radioactivity. The possible advantages of the method are precise localization and accurate removal of the lesion, reduced volume of excised breast tissue, improved rates of clear margins, better concentricity of the specimen, better cosmesis and increased patient comfort (no wire inserted into the breast).

The only RCT comparing WGL and ROLL [110] showed an increased volume of tissue excised with ROLL, but in this study unfortunately the investigators used an extremely high dose of 99m Tc nanocolloid, 120 MBq, which is 10–20 times higher than what has been used in other studies. This is a likely cause for the larger breast volume excised (to clear tissues of radioactivity). Ideal

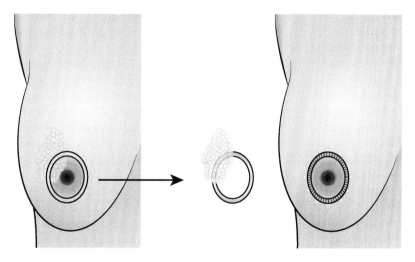
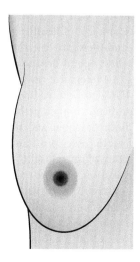

Figure 22.10 Round block or circumareolar approach for segmental resection.

colloids used for radioguided surgery (ROLL and SLNB) are different, with regard to their particle size: ideally for ROLL a larger particle size should be used in order for the particles to stay at the injection site and not to migrate too quickly through the lymphatic channels. This can be achieved by using a macro-aggregate of human serum albumin (99m Tc MAA, with a particle size of 10–90 µ), which is a 1000× larger particle size than that used for SLNB (Nanocoll). The studies presenting data following ROLL showed:

1. 99.6% localization rate, 91.6% negative margins [111]
2. Reduced localization time, subjective ease of procedure rated by the surgeon and radiologist and an 88.9% negative margin rate [112]
3. Localization rate 98.3%, negative margin 76% [113]
4. Significantly higher negative margins and lower re-excision rates for SNOLL with less cavity re-excisions needed during first surgery [114]
5. Significantly larger specimen volumes and higher re-excision rates (12% vs. 10%) for ROLL when using 120 MBq Nanocoll (small particle size) [110]

A systematic review of the ROLL literature concluded that the ROLL may be a superior technique to guide surgical resection for non-palpable breast lesions by achieving lower positive margin rates and fewer reoperations [115,116].

Other methods for occult lesion localizations are those which use radioactive seeds (titanium seed, I[125] labelled) and methods using iron particles and a handheld magnetometer (SentiMag, Endomagnetics UK) capable of detecting a magnetic dye (Sienna+, Endomagnetics UK) injected into the breast. This technology has already been successfully applied to sentinel lymph node biopsy (SLNB) in the SentiMag Multicentre Trial. Investigators are currently evaluating the use of the same magnetic dye (Sienna+) for simultaneous localization of non-palpable breast lesions and concurrent SLNB using the SentiMag handheld magnetometer [117].

IOUS can be safely used to localize and excise impalpable tumours with clear surgical margins. It can also reduce the amount of healthy breast tissue unnecessarily removed, and therefore can lead to a high negative margin rate at the first operation and optimal breast tissue resection rates. A systematic review and meta-analysis of the usage of IOUS to remove breast lesions showed a statistically significant higher pathologically negative margin rate, for both palpable and non-palpable lesions. IOUS can also lead to resections that reduce the total breast tissue resection volume close to what can be considered an optimal resection volume: this will lead to an improved cosmetic outcome of breast-conserving surgery (BCS). IOUS is cost-effective and could be performed by the breast surgeon during surgery. However, the method has a limitation in that it cannot be used for mammographically detected lesions (microcalcifications) which are not

visible on US scanning [118]. There is also a need for training in the use of US by the surgeon and the equipment is relatively expensive.

PREOPERATIVE SYSTEMIC THERAPY AND BREAST CONSERVATION

Preoperative systemic therapy (PST) is systemic treatment delivered prior to any surgical treatment being performed for breast cancer. PST is the first-line oncological treatment for inflammatory breast cancer and other locally advanced breast cancer. It is also used in early breast cancer to facilitate BCS.

There is overall agreement that PST can lead to downsizing of the breast primary and downstaging of the disease (metastatic axillary lymph nodes can be cleared of tumour cells), permitting breast conservation and avoidance of mastectomy in some cases. Several trials (NSABP B18) proved that chemotherapy delivered in the preoperative setting does not improve overall survival but can convert unresectable, locally advanced disease into resectable tumours. In case of resectable tumours PST can lead to an increase in BCS rates (from 7% to 12%) [119–121].

Tumour biology has an impact on the rate of possible breast conservation after preoperative chemotherapy: analyzing the data from the ACOSOG Z1071 trial, breast conservation rates were significantly higher in triple negative (46.8%) and HER-2 positive tumours (43.0%) than in the case of hormone receptor positive, HER-2 negative tumours (34.5%). This trial also shows that with current chemotherapy regimens the rates of pCR were 38.2% in triple negative and 45.4% in HER-2 positive cancers in contrast with the hormone receptor positive, HER-2 negative cancers, where the pCR was only 11.4% [122].

In conclusion, patients with triple negative and HER-2 positive breast cancers have the highest pCR and breast conservation rates after preoperative chemotherapy [122].

Despite the fact that PST does not improve overall survival compared with the treatment delivered in the adjuvant setting, the subgroup of patients with pCR do have improved disease-free and overall survival, a higher rate of BCS could be offered using oncoplastic techniques and it permits *in vivo* assessment of the disease response of a particular regimen.

Interestingly the Neo-ALTTO trial (comparing three regimens of targeted therapy and chemotherapy combinations) showed a pCR rate of 51.3% for the lapatinib–trastuzumab–paclitaxel arm, but the BCS rate still remained 41.4% [123]. The hypothesis to explain this included possible multiple factors: age, multicentricity, planned surgery prior to neoadjuvant treatment, preoperative imaging not conclusive or aggressive pathologic features.

The lesson learned from the trial is that the decision regarding surgical treatment post-PST is mainly based on the baseline tumour characteristics: type of planned surgery at original diagnosis, multicentricity and receptor status (ER negative is less likely to receive BCS) [123,124].

When deciding about PST there are factors to consider during decision making:

- The biological subtype (luminal B, HER-2 positive and triple negative) can indicate the likeliness of chemotherapy and targeted therapy efficacy [125].
- Detailed locoregional assessment of disease at diagnosis (lymph nodes, skin, chest wall, location of the tumour in the breast, distance from the NAC).
- Baseline MRI scan prior to any treatment with the assessment of extent of invasive and non-invasive component (extensive microcalcification, suggesting DCIS, multicentricity).
- If a mid-term clinical examination and MRI scan does not show measurable downsizing, the surgical approach should be reconsidered with a view to mastectomy.
- Patient preference should be included in the decision-making process.

Although PST can improve operability and BCS rates, postoperative adjuvant chemotherapy represents the standard of care for most patients who need chemotherapy [126].

To evaluate correctly the response to PST, pCR is defined as the absence of any residual invasive cancer on hematoxylin and eosin evaluation of the resected breast specimen and all sampled ipsilateral lymph nodes following completion of PST (i.e. ypT0, ypN0 in the current AJCC staging system) [127]. Neither DCIS nor LCIS is generally believed to regress with systemic therapy. The presence of residual DCIS or LCIS at the time of surgery should not be used to judge the effectiveness of PST [128].

Based on the outcome of PST assessed with a mid-term and final breast MRI scan the surgical options are different, but the surgical removal of the primary tumour site is necessary (and pretreatment insertion of marker clips, coils or radioactive seeds is a standard part of PST protocols to facilitate pathological assessment in case of pCR and pPR):

- *Tumour unchanged in size, no clinical regression of disease:* Proceed with mastectomy as originally planned.
- *Partial or complete radiological or clinical response:* Mastectomy or, if BCS possible, a localized excision of the area containing the marker should be performed.

To plan BCS, the post-chemotherapy tumour volume (based on presurgical clinical examination and post-PST imaging) should be assessed and the residual tumour resected with a margin of macroscopically healthy tissue. The extent of disease, including microcalcifications suggesting peritumoural DCIS, should be evaluated. The goal of surgery is to remove the residual disease or the original, marked tumour site in case of pCR, with microscopically clear surgical resection margins to reduce the risk of LR.

There is a higher LR rate after PST when breast radiotherapy is used without any surgical treatment. In case of more extensive disease, TMPL procedures (level 2 oncoplastic techniques) should be considered to increase the likeliness of clear resection margins at the first attempt. Moreover, marker clips should be left in the breast tumour bed to help precise radiotherapy planning. This is crucial in oncoplastic procedures when extensive glandular mobilization is performed.

Risk factors for locoregional recurrence after BCS in patients following PST are:

1. Larger original tumour size
2. Advanced nodal disease
3. Multifocal primary tumour pattern
4. Presence of lymphovascular invasion (LVI)
5. Residual disease after PST

A useful tool to select patients for BCS following PST is the MD Anderson Prognostic Index [129], which scores disease from 1 to 4, based on four statistically significant predictors of LR: clinical N2 or N3 disease, residual pathological tumour size >2 cm, multifocal or multicentric disease pattern and lymphovascular invasion. Patients with a low score (0–1) have low LR rates, and patients with a high score (representing 4% of patients) [129] might benefit from alternative local therapy (mastectomy).

Patients who have undergone PST can be divided into two groups according to their LR risk, based on their MD Anderson Prognostic Index:

- Score 0–1: 5-year LR rate 3% and 5-year locoregional recurrence rate 5% (84% of patients).
- Score 3–4: 5-year LR rate 18% and 5-year locoregional recurrence rate 42%; however, only 4% of patients were in the high-risk group [129].

BCS should be avoided in patients with a poor response to PST, if the residual tumour remains larger than 5 cm, if there is residual direct skin involvement or chest wall fixation and in multicentric disease. Inflammatory cancer should not be treated with BCS even after a good response. Aesthetics should never compromise oncological principles: if the post-BCS margin is highly likely to be compromised, a mastectomy with or without immediate reconstruction is a better option. Consideration should then be given to the indications for post-mastectomy radiotherapy when considering the optimal type of reconstruction bearing in mind the increased risks of implant reconstruction failure in irradiated cases.

Mastectomy: indications, contraindications and techniques

The conventional modified radical mastectomy as described by Madden [130] is still performed as a standard procedure on a large scale for the surgical treatment of locally extensive disease [131]. The most frequent indications for mastectomy currently are:

1. Multicentric disease (tumours in different quadrants or more than 4 cm apart)
2. Extensive DCIS >4 cm
3. Recurrence after BCS and radiotherapy
4. Relatively large tumour size to breast size which may compromise aesthetic outcome with BCS
5. Contraindications for radiotherapy following BCS
6. Patient preference

Contralateral prophylactic mastectomy (CPM) (for women who have unilateral breast cancer) has significantly increased in the past decade mainly in the US. The main reason that patients are asking for this is the fear of developing a second, CBC. Although CPM can reduce the risk of a contralateral second primary by around 90%, the overall survival benefit is not clear.

The Early Breast Cancer Trialists' Collaborative Group reported the annual rate of CBC was about 6 per 1000 women [132]; therefore, the 10-year cumulative risk of CBC is approximately 6%. This increases to 2% per year in women who are known BRCA gene carriers. The risk of CBC may be even lower with the routine use of 5 years of adjuvant aromatase inhibitor therapy or extended tamoxifen endocrine therapy compared to when these data were published [133].

The survival and potential life expectancy (LE) benefit of a CPM also depends on the mortality of the index breast cancer: the LE gain is lower in patients with high stage tumours [134].

Based on a Markov simulation model of survival outcomes, it seems that CPM could be more beneficial among younger women with stage I and ER negative disease, and a maximum 20-year survival difference with CPM is only 1.45%. In this study model, the absolute 20-year survival benefit from CPM was less than 1% [134]. It seems that there is a substantial overestimation of the risk of developing breast cancer among patients with newly diagnosed breast cancer and that there are unrealistic expectations regarding the LE benefits of CPM. This estimated survival data can help physicians to make more evidence-based decisions about CPM for individual women [135,136].

TECHNICAL CONSIDERATIONS FOR MASTECTOMY

During modified radical mastectomy without reconstruction the breast glandular tissue, nipple–areolar complex and overlying skin are all removed. A flat chest wall, with a relatively tight skin closure and no excessive skin, should remain after surgery.

Factors and technical details to be considered are careful preoperative marking of skin incisions, skin incision orientation according to tumour location (transversal or oblique), dissection of the inframammary fold (IMF) toward the abdominal wall and no redundant skin folds left in order to facilitate comfortable prosthesis fitting. The boundaries of dissection and glandular excision should follow the anatomical boundaries of the breast gland: superior, the lower border of the clavicle or second rib; inferior, 2–3 cm below the IMF; medial, sternal border; and lateral, latissimus dorsi (LD) muscle anterior border. To have a mastectomy flap that can be considered adequate, we should remove enough breast tissue to meet oncologic goals (reduce to a minimum the risk of LR) and maintain the viability and blood supply of the flap. This can be achieved by following the marked breast boundaries, dissecting at the breast glandular tissue surface at the superficial fascia level and leaving a layer of subdermal fatty tissue on the skin flap, preserving the subdermal vascular network. The thickness of the flap will vary depending on the degree of adiposity of the patient. This principle can be applied for any type of mastectomy; the difference is only in the length and thickness of the mastectomy skin flaps.

It is controversial whether the removal (dissection through) of the IMF is necessary. This boundary is situated at the pectoral muscle inferior insertion level and it is the zone of adherence of the superficial fascia to the chest wall. Cancer is rare at this level and it seems that preserving it during skin-sparing mastectomies leaves only minimal glandular tissue and does not affect the completeness of the mastectomy [137].

Prospective randomized trials have shown a LR rate of 4–12% at 6–10 years for stage I and II disease after conventional mastectomy. Most LRs occurred in the first 5 years. Young age, extensive nodal involvement (more than four nodes), extracapsular extension, margin status (positive pectoral – deep margin), high grade, lymphovascular invasion and negative ER status were significant risk factors for local chest wall failure [138,139].

SKIN-SPARING MASTECTOMY

With the high demand for offering immediate reconstruction for patients needing a mastectomy and to improve the aesthetic outcomes of immediate reconstruction, the skin-sparing mastectomy was introduced for breast cancer in 1991 by Toth and Lappert [140]. The benefits of the procedure are the reduction in post-mastectomy deformity, allowing a better breast shape after reconstruction, minimized scaring and reducing the need for contralateral symmetrization surgery.

By definition skin-sparing mastectomy is the procedure where most of the breast glandular tissue and the NAC are removed by dissection above the superficial fascia. The epidermis, dermis and a small amount of subdermal fatty tissue are left behind. The natural skin envelope of the breast and IMF is preserved. The primary goal of the procedure is improving the cosmetic outcome of mastectomy and the facilitation of immediate reconstruction, without compromising the long-term oncological outcome (LR rates are comparable with conventional mastectomy) [139,141].

Based on the incision type, there are four SSM types: I, periareolar with lateral extension; II, periareolar with 'en bloc' excision of the previous biopsy scar excision; III, periareolar with separate excision of the previous biopsy scar; and IV, wise pattern incision with lower pole skin reduction (Figures 22.11 and 22.12). The ideal skin flap thickness is controversial. The 'ultra-thin' versus the thicker flaps [142] have comparable recurrence and survival rates, but the ultra-thin flaps have an increased incidence of wound complications, lymphedema and prolonged hospital stay [142]. Therefore dissection at the superficial fascial level is advisable, with a flap thickness usually of 7–8 mm, but variable according to the level of adiposity of the patient.

The blood supply to the skin flaps can be assessed clinically (thickness, colour, bruising, presence of capillary bleeding) or by more objective methods (intraoperative indocyanine green angiography, fluorescein dye, laser Doppler).

In order to be oncologically safe, SSM should leave only extremely small amounts of breast tissue behind and it should have clear superficial resection margins.

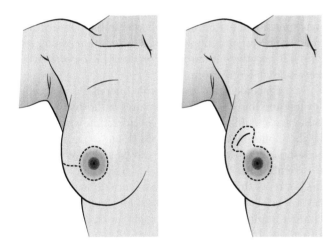

Figure 22.11 **SSM types I and II.**

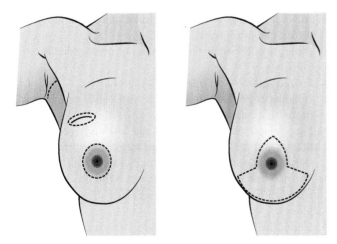

Figure 22.12 **SSM types III and IV.**

Analyzing the amount of residual breast tissue left behind after SSM, it was found that 59.5% of skin flap specimens contained residual breast tissue and that 9.5% of skin flaps had residual disease [143]. Another study [144] found that 23% of the analyzed skin flaps were involved with residual tumour, and this was mainly located in the skin flap directly over the area. The independent risk factors for positive margins in SSM are smaller specimen weight, smaller skin excision, extensive DCIS, multifocal or multicentric disease, palpable superficial tumours and tumour location (upper-inner quadrant) [145–147].

Despite these studies showing a relatively high incidence of residual breast tissue or even close or involved superficial margins, several studies in the past decades have shown that the LR rates are similar to those of non-skin-sparing mastectomies and that the procedure is oncologically safe. The LR rates after non-SSM in tumours up to 4 cm were 10% at 20 years [88] and the LR after SSM ranged between 0% and 7% [148,149]. For T3 tumours Carlson and colleagues [137,150] found a LR rate of 11%. However, these pro- and retrospective studies are difficult to compare due to differences in follow-up time, sample size, tumour characteristics, adjuvant treatment and stage of disease. The most significant predictors of LR after SSM are tumour size, nodal status, high grade, poor differentiation and presence of LVI, with an overall LR rate of 5–7% (follow-up period of 26, 65 and 73 months, respectively) [150–152].

Risk factors for complications after SSM are smoking, previous radiotherapy to the breast, large and ptotic breasts (high BMI, diabetes) and immediate reconstruction with fixed volume implants (due to tension on the overlying skin) [137,139,141].

In conclusion SSM is an oncologically safe procedure with LR rates comparable to those of conventional mastectomy for small and low-grade tumours.

Careful patient selection based on imaging, histology and clinical examination is crucial to keep the LR rates low.

NIPPLE-SPARING MASTECTOMY

Nipple-sparing mastectomy (NSM) has been used for risk reduction and recently also for therapeutic mastectomies. The procedure entails keeping the nipple–areolar complex, removing the nipple–areolar ducts and leaving only epidermis and dermis behind. The NAC flap thickness is usually 2–3 mm and best results are achieved by sharp dissection behind the NAC, always requesting targeted retro-areolar histology if the procedure is performed for cancer [153].

Multicentre studies have demonstrated that NSM can be performed with low recurrence and complications rates: NAC sensitivity will return in 48% of patients and there is higher patient satisfaction, improved aesthetic outcome and a positive impact on body image compared to non-nipple-sparing surgery [139,153].

The concerns around nipple-sparing mastectomies are related to the surgical risk (predominantly nipple necrosis) and the oncological safety of the procedure.

The most frequently used incision types are inframammary, radial (lateral or vertical at 6 o'clock position) and periareolar with lateral radial extension (Figure 22.13). There is no agreement on the optimal approach and there are different rates of NAC loss reported with different incision types [153].

Surgeons should use an approach that they are familiar with for achieving an optimal outcome.

The reported total nipple loss rates in larger series vary between 0% and 4.7% and partial nipple loss rates of between 6% and 19.5%. It has also been noted that periareolar incisions have higher nipple loss rates than radial or inframammary incisions [154–158].

The originally recommended selection criteria for NSM were tumour size less than 4.5 cm diameter, distance from the nipple 4 cm (clinical and radiological) and no NAC involvement (Paget's, blood-stained nipple discharge) [159]. The LR rates noticed in the breast were between 1.3% and 5.4%, but the recurrence at the preserved NAC level was only 0–2% in large series [154–157,160,161].

For comparison the LR rates in between modified radical mastectomy, skin-sparing mastectomy and nipple-sparing mastectomy were 11.5%, 10.4% and 11.7%, respectively, with a 0.9% nipple recurrence [160].

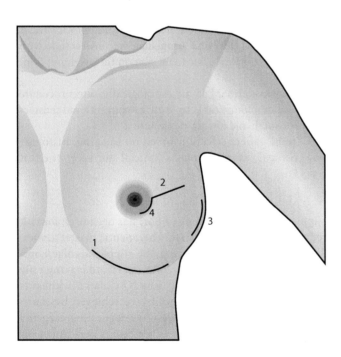

Figure 22.13 Nipple-sparing mastectomy incision types: 1, inframammary; 2, periareolar with or without lateral extension; 3, lateral; and 4, periareolar (which may also be used to lift nipple position in cases of mild ptosis).

It is reassuring of the safety of modern NSM that a consecutive series of 934 NSMs were presented by Petit et al., with a 50-month follow-up, where they had a 5-year cumulative LR rate of 3.6% (breast) and 0.8% nipple recurrence for 772 invasive cancers and a LR of 4.9% breast and 2.9% nipple recurrence rate for 162 non-invasive cancers [156].

All patients had retro-areolar intraoperative frozen sections performed and 70 patients were negative on frozen sections and positive on definitive histology. Out of these patients none developed nipple recurrence [156].

Ten out of the 11 patients with nipple recurrence had pure DCIS or invasive cancer with extensive DCIS and all 11 had negative frozen sections originally. Fifty-four patients out of the 70 with positive margins on definitive histology had DCIS not noticed by the intraoperative frozen section. This raises the question of how reliable the intraoperative frozen sections are to detect *in situ* disease. Although in this study the majority of the patients received intraoperative radiotherapy (ELIOT), the results could not objectively confirm that ELIOT decreases the risk of LR on the NAC.

What they could prove is that the significant risk factors for breast LR in the invasive group were grade, HER-2 overexpression and luminal B subtype. In the non-invasive group the breast and nipple LR risk factors were young age (<45), ER negative tumours and grade, HER-2 overexpression and high Ki-67 expression.

They concluded that the LR rate after NSM is acceptably low and that the biological features of the disease and a young age should be taken into consideration when deciding about offering the patients NSM [156].

Based on the literature NSM can be selectively offered to patients with breast cancer as an oncologically safe procedure as the LR rates are comparable with those of SSM (2–11%) and NAC recurrences are rare (0–2%). Even if larger multicentric tumours were included in series with a high LR rate (20%), the NAC LR rates were kept at 0% [162].

Based on the literature data optimal practice may be:

● MRI scan can give further information regarding the tumour distance from the NAC.
● A biopsy of the subareolar tissue is recommended in all NSMs.
● Frozen sections can miss *in situ* disease.
● If biopsy is positive on definitive histology, a re-excision of the NAC is recommended.
● Surgical risks are increased (nipple loss) in large, ptotic breasts and periareolar incisions longer than 30% of the areola circumference have higher risk of nipple loss.
● The plane of mastectomy dissection is the superficial fascia with preservation of the subdermal vascular plexus.
● Under the NAC sharp dissection is recommended [139,153,156].

Contraindications of NSM in breast cancer are:

- Tumours at less than 2 cm from the NAC (radiological distance)
- Multicentric disease
- Positive subareolar histology
- Presence of extensive DCIS

Biological features such as HER-2 overexpression or triple negative phenotype and high grade should be considered during decision making as markers of increased risk of LR [139,153,156].

Principles of breast reconstruction

For the majority of patients who need a mastectomy, a discussion about reconstruction should ideally be part of the breast cancer management plan. The 2009 UK NICE guidance recommends clinicians to 'discuss immediate breast reconstruction with all patients who are being advised to have a mastectomy, although comorbidities or decisions about adjuvant therapy may preclude this option'. A decision about the pros and cons for an immediate reconstruction should be taken together with the patient, and the responsible clinician should be able to provide detailed information regarding all reconstructive options, including implant and own tissue (autologous)-based reconstructions. Immediate reconstruction should never interfere with the oncological treatment of the breast cancer and should not cause delays in delivering surgery, adjuvant chemotherapy or radiotherapy.

Neoadjuvant chemotherapy should be considered in more aggressive tumours, where systemic treatment will be needed anyway: this will give time for the patient to make an informed decision about reconstructive options, and a more complex surgery will not cause delays in delivering cancer treatment.

Since women live longer after breast cancer treatment (between 2005 and 2009, 85% of women in England survived their breast cancer for 5 years or more), reconstruction has a key role in helping patients maintain their quality of life after treatment: it helps regain self-confidence, women feel more 'whole' and their body image is retained or rebuilt. In specialized breast units a range of different reconstructive methods should be available; the patients should make a choice under guidance and take a decision about their reconstruction after being fully informed. By reconstruction the surgical team should attempt to recreate a new breast that matches the healthy side in size and shape, and obtain acceptable symmetry (which may require contralateral symmetrization procedures to enlarge, reduce or lift the opposite breast), and the cleavage should ideally be rebuilt to allow confidence when wearing certain clothing styles and when leaning forward and to minimize potentially visible breast and donor site scars.

Patients should ideally be seen in specialist oncoplastic or reconstructive consultations. Counselling should aim to develop realistic expectations of outcomes for the patient and to indicate that reconstruction is a process rather than a single surgical intervention. Factors influencing the decision making for reconstruction are:

- Patient related: Preference for a certain procedure, general health and comorbidities, specific requirements (occupation, leisure activities)
- Disease related: Need for adjuvant chest wall radiotherapy (disadvantage of implant-based reconstruction due to increased capsule contraction), advanced disease (for increased risk of LR a delayed reconstruction might be a better choice)
- Surgical team related (preference, expertise)

IMPLANT-BASED RECONSTRUCTIONS

Implant-based reconstructions are the most widely used reconstructive procedures today and around 75% of breast reconstructions performed in the US are implant based, providing satisfactory results in the majority of the patients [163,164].

The patients who are the best candidates for implant-based reconstructions are those with small to medium breasts, slim, with minimal breast ptosis. Even patients with larger cup size breasts are suitable for implant-based reconstruction since the acellular dermal matrix (ADM) mesh lower pole support has been introduced or by using the skin-reducing wise pattern procedure with inferior dermal 'sling' support. Patients who choose implant-based reconstruction want a quicker recovery and simpler surgery, and they do not want to have donor site scars and morbidity.

There are a wide range of implants available: expandable, non-expandable, round or anatomic, gel or saline filled, and smooth or texture surfaced. The benefits and risks of each are listed in Table 22.6. Implant size selection requires careful measurements of dimensions and breast volume estimation which may be achieved by a variety of methods ranging from the use of sizer 'cups' to web-based apps to precise imaging calculation.

The two-stage implant-based reconstruction consists of placing a tissue expander in the submusculofascial pocket created under the pectoralis major muscle with progressive expansion until the desired volume is reached via either an integral filler port (Figure 22.14) or a subcutaneous injection port. An overexpansion of approximately 10–20% relative to the contralateral breast volume will allow the formation of a well-defined IMF and adequate ptosis. Independent risk factors for complications include smoking, obesity and age greater than 65 years [165].

Overall early complications are reported as 5.8% [165], such as haematoma (4%), infection (2.5%) and skin flap necrosis (2%). Chemotherapy administered during expansion or previous radiotherapy does not increase the incidence

Table 22.6 Differences between various types of breast implant

Implant type	Characteristics	Advantages	Disadvantages
Silicone (memory gel)	Set fill volume, cohesive gel	Keeps shape, more natural silhouette	Leakage
Anatomical	Teardrop shaped	More natural, mimicking breast silhouette	Risk of rotation
Round	Used mainly for augmentation	Less rotation	Less natural, breast looks fuller
Textured	Firmer	Less capsule contraction, less rotation	
Smooth	Softest feeling	More natural movements	More capsule contraction
Polyurethane	Outer layer of medical-grade polyurethane	Low rate of capsule contraction, no rotation	Needs accurate positioning, longer learning curve
Permanent expanders	35–50% set fill silicone compartment with flexible fill saline compartment	Textured, flexible fill volume	Firmer, harder, less natural feel
Saline	Flexible fill volume, sterile saline content	Less expensive, no silicone content	Firmer, less natural

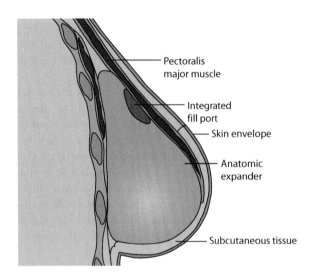

Figure 22.14 Submuscular placement of an expandable breast implant with an integral filler port.

of complications [164,165]. The overall late postoperative complications are mainly capsule contraction grade III/IV (10% in non-irradiated breasts or 20% in previously irradiated breasts) and implant rippling 6.6%, with a 4% implant exchange rate [165].

Implant-based reconstruction usually has high patient satisfaction scores (90–95% Breast-Q patient survey), but the satisfaction seems to decrease over time (compared with autologous reconstructions where satisfaction scores remain stable or increase with time) [165]. Post-reconstruction radiotherapy has a significantly negative impact on patient satisfaction, and this is mainly explained by the higher rate of capsule contraction. Patients report higher satisfaction scores with bilateral implant reconstructions – likely due to the better symmetry achieved.

In recent years one-stage implant-based reconstructions with ADMs for lower pole support have gained popularity.

These meshes are derived from processed human, porcine or bovine dermis that removes cells and significantly reduces the key component to play a major role in the xenogenic rejection response. The ADM has its extracellular matrix preserved and supports host tissue regeneration and integrates via revascularization and cellular repopulation [166–169].

Risk factors for SSM and immediate ADM and implant-based reconstructions are long-standing steroid treatment, BMI >30–32, diabetes, use of larger volume, definitive implants, C cup or greater breast volume, axillary clearance as part of the procedure (seroma), postoperative radiotherapy (fourfold higher risk of capsule contraction) [170,171] or psychologically unprepared patients.

Technically it gives greater inferior pole support than a fully submuscular technique as the ADM acts like a 'hammock' holding the implant which is covered by the pectoralis major muscle in the upper part and by the ADM in the lower.

In general, for small and medium-sized breasts, single-stage reconstruction gives good results using inframammary or lateral oblique skin incision, using breast mound recreation with an ADM and fixed volume anatomical cohesive gel silicone implants. Use of permanent expander implants is only necessary if the quality and quantity of overlying skin are not appropriate.

For larger breast where a skin-reducing mastectomy is needed, a wise pattern approach with lower pole de-epithelization (inferior dermal 'sling') or a transvertical approach with ADM can lead to satisfactory long-term outcomes.

The benefits of ADM-based reconstructions are that they give an extra layer of coverage for the implant (reduced palpability and visibility), behave like an 'internal bra' with lower pole support, create a hammock that allows more ptotic (naturally shaped) breasts, give control for implant location and help define the inframammary and lateral mammary folds. Also, larger implants can be used and the procedure can be done as a single-stage reconstruction. It also seems to reduce the capsule contraction if adjuvant radiotherapy has to be used on the reconstructed breast (4.4%, level III or IV evidence) (Figure 22.15) [172,173].

Overall complication rates after ADM and implant-based reconstructions are between 3.2% and 48.7% [174,175], and these can be skin flap necrosis (1.4–23.4%), seroma (7.2–14.1%), wound infection with implant rejection (3.3–8.9%) and implant loss (8.3–11.2%). Complications are usually higher when adjuvant radiotherapy or chemotherapy is given (13.7 vs. 30.7%) [174–178]. Recent studies using different types of ADM showed an explantation rate of 6.8–12.5% [163,179].

In 1990 Bostwick described the preservation of the lower de-epithelized skin flap during skin-sparing mastectomies, in order to give extra coverage for a submuscular implant (for prophylactic mastectomies) [180].

Later the method was developed for breast cancer [181,182], as the type IV skin-sparing mastectomy (final inverted T scar). The wise pattern mastectomy with skin envelope reduction is a suitable method in larger, more ptotic breasts for single-stage reconstruction with anatomical permanent implants. The implants are placed in a dermomuscular pouch with total implant coverage (superior, pectoralis; inferior, de-epithelized dermal flap). The additional dermal tissue layer at the lower pole reduces the risk of T junction complications and improves aesthetic outcomes. The nipple to IMF distance should be at least 10–12 cm to achieve sufficient lower pole coverage (inferior dermal 'sling'), and the internal mammary perforators ideally should be preserved

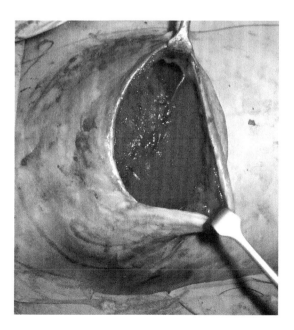

Figure 22.15 Intraoperative photograph showing an ADM-based reconstruction with a sheet of ADM sutured to the pectoralis muscle to form a fully submuscular pocket.

to avoid skin flap ischemic changes (native skin flap necrosis 10–22%) [183]. Smoking and previous radiation therapy can increase the skin flap necrosis rate (20.3% and 23.8%) [183].

AUTOLOGOUS TISSUE-BASED RECONSTRUCTIONS

Own tissue-based reconstructions were developed in the 1970s with the rediscovery by Olivari (1976) of the LD flap which can be used in combination with an implant to increase the breast volume or on its own, as an extended procedure where subcutaneous fatty tissue surrounding the peripheries of the muscle are left attached to the flap during harvesting in order to increase volume. The procedure can also be combined with immediate or delayed lipomodelling in order to avoid the use of an implant [184].

The LD flap can be used as a pedicled rotational flap; its blood supply comes from the thoracodorsal pedicle and accessory segmental pedicles from intercostal and lumbar arteries. The LD muscle normally functions to draw the arm backwards and causes internal rotation. Its removal has minimal effect on daily life or practice of amateur sports, causing some difficulty in cross-country skiing and rock climbing [184].

For autologous reconstruction fatty extensions of the LD muscle are used to increase flap volume: fat between the posterior aspect of the muscle and fascia superficialis, scapular hinge flap (upper LD margin), anterior hinge flap (lateral margin), suprailiac fat deposits ('love handles') and the adipose tissue anterior to the muscle surface. These areas are reliably vascularized by muscular perforators. The LD flap can be used for immediate or delayed reconstruction, and it is a reliable and surgically safe technique, even when adjuvant radiotherapy is needed.

Contraindications are rare: congenital absence of the muscle or neurovascular damage to the thoracodorsal pedicle. The autologous LD flap–based reconstruction gives high patient satisfaction rates (85% very good) and has low complication rates: donor site haematoma 1%, infection <1%, long-standing dorsal seroma formation 9%, flap loss extremely rare, dorsal skin flap necrosis (due to extensive dorsal undermining) 1%, shoulder stiffness and shoulder movement deficit (1%) [184].

Due to its excellent blood supply and in combination with a second stage fat transfer, this method is a versatile and reliable autologous breast reconstructive procedure with a low complication and morbidity rate and quick recovery.

Autologous tissue harvested from certain areas of the body including mainly skin, fatty tissue and some of the muscular elements can be transferred to the recipient site as a free flap, using microvascular techniques. This allows a safe transfer of significant amounts of the patient's own tissue, without the topographic limitations of a pedicled flap.

The reconstructed breast with free or autologous flaps gives a soft, natural-feeling, warm reconstructed breast;

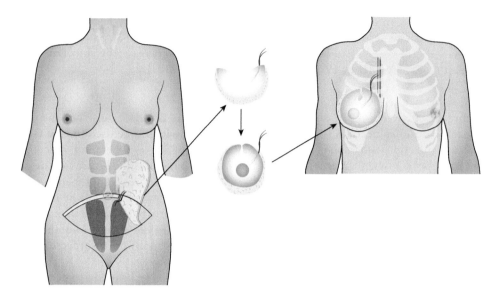

Figure 22.16 DIEP flap.

better symmetry is achieved which is not affected by postural position, even without a bra [185].

The procedures using free flaps necessitate special microvascular techniques, longer procedures that last usually 6–8 hours, with a longer hospital stay and recovery time, and it also has the risks of donor site morbidity.

Ideal candidates for autologous free flap–based reconstructions are patients with no major comorbidities that increase the risks of flap failure or systemic complications. Smoking, obesity, diabetes, previous history of deep vein thrombosis or other organ-related systemic disorders and the association of several of these risk factors increase significantly the failure rate and delayed recovery following free flap reconstruction.

Possible complications are flap-related (partial or complete flap loss 1–5%, fat necrosis 6–13%) or donor site (hernia – specially with myocutaneous flaps, delayed healing, scarring, indentation and flattening) complications.

When deciding about autologous free flap surgery patients have to be aware of the donor site morbidities and long-term effects of tissue harvesting [185].

Indications for autologous tissue-based reconstruction as a delayed or immediate procedure are:

- Risk-reducing mastectomy
- Large size, ptotic contralateral breast
- Previous complications or poor aesthetic outcome with implant-based reconstruction
- Any patients who would like to avoid an implant-based reconstruction or an autologous pedicled LD flap–based reconstruction

Contraindications for free flap reconstructions are significant systemic disorders that might interfere with postoperative recovery (cardiovascular, vasospastic disorders, significant mobility problems, psychologically unfit patients).

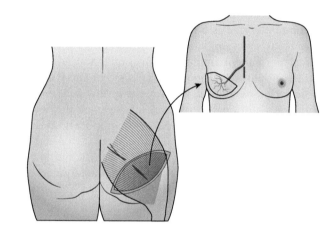

Figure 22.17 S-GAP flap.

As recipient vessels for a free flap microanastomosis, the internal thoracic, thoracodorsal, serratus, circumflex scapular and thoracic perforator vessels can be used.

The free perforator flaps are based on small perforator vessels feeding particular adipocutaneous areas and allow tissue harvest without muscular or fascia sacrifice, and they have the best outcomes with regard to donor site functional morbidity.

The most often used perforator flaps for breast reconstruction are:

- Free deep inferior epigastric perforator (DIEP) – muscle-sparing abdominal flap (Figure 22.16)
- Superior gluteal artery perforator (S-GAP) – upper third buttock flap (Figure 22.17)
- Inferior gluteal artery perforator (I-GAP) – lower third buttock flap
- Transverse upper gracilis flap (TUG) or anterolateral thigh flap (Figure 22.18) [185]

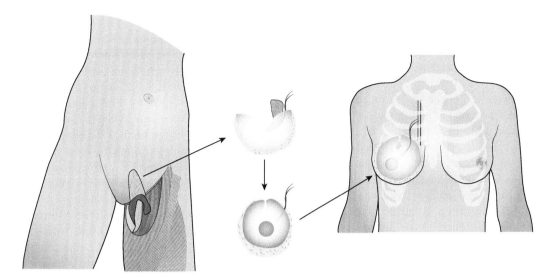

Figure 22.18 TUG flap.

When deciding about the type of reconstruction, patients should be helped in their choice by providing the necessary information in what regards immediate and late postoperative morbidities, recovery, long-term results, the need for further surgeries, donor site morbidities and long-term effect of tissue harvesting [185].

The patient's hobbies, lifestyle and expectations have to be explored before advising them toward a certain direction.

AXILLARY SURGERY

The status of the axillary nodes is the most significant prognostic factor in patients with breast cancer. The estimated benefits and role of axillary lymph node dissection (ALND) in the modern era have been influenced by the results of the randomized trial NSABP B04 that identified ALND as a staging procedure and for prevention of axillary recurrence with no impact in survival [186]. Although this was a landmark trial, it was underpowered to detect a small survival effect of axillary dissection. On the other hand, a meta-analysis combining six trials showed an average survival benefit of 5.4% of ALND [187].

Since the introduction of the sentinel lymph node biopsy (SNLB), the use of ALND has been reduced to patients with invasive breast cancer and a clinically positive axilla, to patients with inflammatory breast cancer, to those with an unsuccessful SNLB and to selected patients with a positive SNLB.

Axillary lymph node dissection

ANATOMY AND SURGICAL TECHNIQUE

The axilla is a space that is bounded anteriorly by the pectoralis major and minor; posteriorly by the subscapularis, teres major and latissimus dorsi (LD); medially by the serratus anterior muscle and the chest wall; laterally by the LD muscle; and cranially by the axillary vein. The axilla

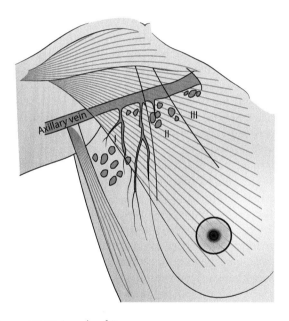

Figure 22.19 Levels of Berg.

has been divided anatomically into the three levels of Berg, based on the relationship of the tissue with the pectoralis minor muscle [188] (Figure 22.19).

Performing a level I and II ALND provides accurate staging for breast cancer when a minimum of 10 lymph nodes have been examined. Skip metastases, that is positive axillary nodes at level III with negative nodes in level II, are uncommon (< 1%) [189].

ALND can be carried out through the same incision as the mastectomy or with a different incision in breast-conserving surgery (BCS) and in some cases of skin-sparing or nipple-sparing mastectomy. Flaps are raised and the boundaries of the axilla are identified. Dissection is carried along the edge of the lateral border of the minor pectoralis muscle, identifying and preserving the lateral pectoral nerve bundle to reach the inferior edge of the axillary vein. The axillary contents are separated following the inferior aspect of the vein from medially to laterally and all superficial branches are ligated. The axillary specimen is then dissected from the LD muscle. Alternatively, dissection can be started from the lower later border of LD muscle and continued cranially and medially.

The long thoracic nerve lies 1 cm from the chest wall, deep in the axilla; care should be taken not to damage it to avoid a paresis of the serratus anterior muscle and a winged scapula. Lateral to the long thoracic nerve, the thoracodorsal bundle is identified, and axillary tissue beyond both is removed. During the dissection, branches of the intercostobrachial nerves are identified. If possible, preservation of the largest branches should be attempted.

If level III clearance is to be performed, dissection toward the apex to include the nodes medial to the pectoralis minor muscle is performed and facilitated by flexion of the draped arm at the shoulder.

POSTOPERATIVE MORBIDITY

In addition to common postoperative morbidity, such as infection, postoperative bleeding or haematoma, seroma formation is extremely common after axillary surgery. The prevalence ranges from 2.5% to 51% after ALND, although all breast surgery patients have some seroma formation. Several studies have examined whether closed low suction drainage is necessary after ALND. In a recent review from seven RCTs, there is limited evidence that insertion of a drain reduced the risk of developing a seroma or reduced the number of postoperative seroma aspirations [190].

Different techniques for avoiding seroma formation have been reported. Surgical manoeuvres as operative closure of the dead space using different types of sutures and techniques have been shown to reduce seroma formation, although the downside is the increased length of surgery [191]. The use of postoperative compression dressings does not appear to decrease seroma formation but increases postoperative discomfort. Electrocautery has been reported to increase seroma formation when compared to knife dissection. The electrothermal bipolar vessel sealing system may shorten surgical time and reduce seroma formation enabling early drain removal without increasing postoperative complications [192]. In terms of tissue sealants, fibrin sealants have not been shown to reduce seroma formation in large trials, although in some studies they have been shown to reduce drainage duration and overall drain output [193]. Octreotide is another agent that in a prospective randomized trial with 261 patients has been shown to reduce seroma formation, although larger studies are needed to clarify dose and duration of treatment [194].

Shoulder stiffness is usually a temporary and self-limiting side effect. Late complications include lymphedema, chronic postoperative pain, limitation of shoulder mobility, paresthesia and numbness of the upper arm [195].

ARM REVERSE MAPPING

The arm reverse mapping (ARM) procedure was developed to map and preserve arm lymphatic drainage in order to decrease rates of lymphedema in breast cancer patients with ALND or even with SLNB alone [196,197]. The technique consists of injecting 2.5 to 5 ml of blue dye subcutaneously in the upper inner arm along the medial intramuscular groove of the ipsilateral arm. Most lymphatics from the distal arm enter the axilla along the volar surface of the upper arm. However, there can be alternate anatomy; for example, a branch in the deltopectoral groove can completely bypass the axilla [198].

When the ARM procedure is used in conjunction with the SLNB, usually the radioactive tracer is injected in the breast and the blue dye in the arm. After injection, the site is massaged and the arm elevated for 5 minutes to facilitate drainage. When opening the axilla any blue lymphatics and blue nodes are identified (Figure 22.20).

The most consistent drainage is to the lymph node just below the vein and just on or lateral to the tendon of the LD muscle [199]. Rates of blue node identification are reported to be up to 90%.

However, in around 3.9–15% of patients, the blue ARM lymphatics have common lymphatic channels with the breast lymphatics, at the level of the breast sentinel node. In a small proportion of patients, the blue ARM node is the same as the breast sentinel node. Moreover, in approximately 40% of patients the blue ARM upper extremity lymphatics can be identified near the SLN.

Recent studies have reported very low rates of lymphedema when the blue ARM nodes have not been excised [199]. The decrease in the risk of lymphedema is more significant when ARM is performed in ALND patients, with rates from 9% in the preserved ARM group compared to 33% in the non-preserved group [200,201]. In patients with heavily involved axillas the blue ARM nodes may contain metastases. Therefore in these patients, preserving the blue ARM nodes should be done with caution [202].

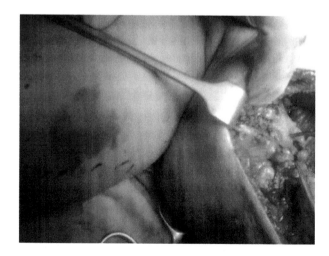

Figure 22.20 Intraoperative blue dye in an axillary lymphatic ARM procedure.

Also, subdermal injection of indocyanine green into the upper limb has been used, with the ARM node identification rate similar to that of the blue dye technique [203]. A limitation to the published studies is the short follow-up; longer follow-up is needed to confirm the safety and efficacy of the procedure.

Sentinel lymph node biopsy

The concept of SLNB was first studied in penile carcinoma and melanoma, and the sentinel node was defined as the first draining node of a tumour. In breast cancer SLNB was developed to provide accurate axillary staging but sparing patients from the morbidity of ALND. SLNB has become the standard of care in early breast cancer. It is currently the recommended procedure for axillary staging of early breast cancer with a clinically negative axilla. Randomized trials [204,205] have shown that ALND does not provide a survival advantage when the SLNB is negative. Shoulder abduction limitation, lymphedema and numbness are less in SLNB patients, reflecting the reduced morbidity of this procedure compared to ALND [195].

LYMPHATIC MAPPING

The SLNB technique has been described using radioisotope mapping with the use of a handheld gamma probe [206–208], blue dye [209,210] or a combination of both [211,212]. Different types of radioisotopes have been used (technetium 99m sulphur colloid or technetium 99m-colloidal albumin), as well as blue dye (isosulfan blue, patent blue or methylene blue). The doses of radioactive 99m Tc vary by institution and may range from 0.1 to 4 mCi. Higher identification rates can be reached and fewer sentinel nodes may be missed with the combination of blue dye and radioisotope than with single-agent mapping [211,212].

Disadvantages of the blue dye include 1–3% incidence of allergic reactions, higher with the use of isosulfan blue. Preoperative prophylaxis can decrease the rate of allergic reactions [213]. In addition, the blue discoloration may cause long-lasting skin staining which may be unsightly.

The diagnostic value of preoperative lymphoscintigraphy has also been discussed. Lymphoscintigraphy can identify the lymphatic drainage basin, being most helpful when extra-axillary nodal basins are explored. While studies have shown no additional benefit of lymphoscintigraphy for SLN identification in the axilla [214], others support its use (Figure 22.21) [215]. However, there is general agreement that lymphoscintigraphy should be performed when extra-axillary drainage is sought.

There is variation not only with regard to the mapping agents, but also in the optimal location of injection: subareolar, subdermal, peritumoural or intratumoural [216–219]. Studies comparing peritumoural radioactive tracer injection and intradermal blue dye injection, or subareolar injections of radioisotope to peritumourally injected blue dye, have shown a high concordance in lymphatic drainage pattern between the different methods [216–218]. With the introduction of the SLNB technique, several authors have studied the lymphatic drainage patterns of the breast. Most of them have concluded that although there is a high concordance rate between superficial and deep injections, deep tracer injections will more often visualize extra-axillary sentinel nodes, supporting the idea that deep lymphatics from the dorsal part of the breast drain to these nodes [220].

Superficial injections have the advantage of rapid migration of the mapping material in the lymphatics resulting in high sentinel node (SN) identification rates. In a recent meta-analysis, the pooled sentinel node identification rate was higher by the superficial injection technique than by the deep technique (94% vs. 91.2%). Combined deep and

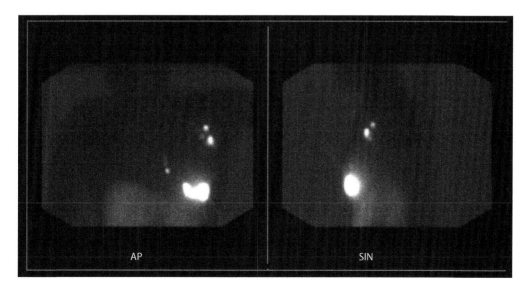

Figure 22.21 Lymphoscintigraphy showing lymphatic drainage to the axilla as well as to the internal mammary nodal basin.

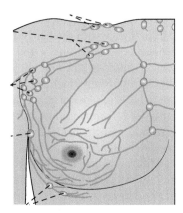

Figure 22.22 Major lymphatic drainage pathways from the breast.

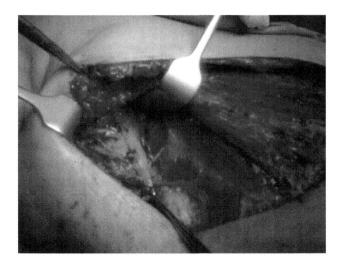

Figure 22.23 Blue node during a SLNB procedure with dual blue dye and radioisotope localization.

superficial injections had the highest pooled sentinel node detection rate (97.2%) [221]. Taking into consideration the different injection techniques, the preferential lymph drainage pathway from all quadrants is essentially toward the same axillary lymph nodes, although lymphatic drainage to the internal mammary nodes seems to be more common in medially located tumours [220,222].

The major lymphatic drainage pathway from the breast is toward the ipsilateral axilla, which comprises 75% of the entire lymphatic flow (Figure 22.22).

Extra-axillary drainage, mostly to the internal mammary chain, can be seen after peri- or intratumoural injection in 6–26% of patients. Internal mammary SLNB provides stage migration in patients with metastatic findings, accounting for 1–2% of all patients undergoing SLNB [222]. Patients with parasternal metastases and a node negative axilla represent approximately 1% of all breast cancer patients having a SLNB. In this group of patients, identification of parasternal nodal disease may alter the recommended adjuvant treatments offered, including chemotherapy and radiation therapy to target these nodes. However, the benefit of internal mammary node biopsy on survival seems small [223].

SURGICAL TECHNIQUE

The radioisotope is injected on the day of surgery or the day before surgery, while the blue dye is injected after induction of anaesthesia, at least 10 minutes before incision. During surgery, a handheld gamma probe is used to identify the hot nodes. When using blue dye, careful dissection is made to locate the blue lymphatic tract from the breast and follow it to the blue node (Figure 22.23).

There may be one or several sentinel nodes, but not all hot or blue nodes are true sentinel nodes. The tracer may spill from the sentinel node to second and third echelon nodes. During surgery, however, it is impossible to distinguish between true sentinel nodes and second echelon nodes.

In some institutions the 10% rule is applied, so all the radioactive nodes counting >10% of the higher radioactive node counts are excised to reduce false negative rates [189]. Several institutions still apply the 10% rule, showing that

the 10% rule identified 98.3% of positive nodes in patients with multiple nodes [207,224]. Multiple studies have demonstrated that removal of four or five nodes identifies almost 100% of patients with positive sentinel nodes [208,225].

In addition to harvesting blue or hot nodes, the open axilla should be carefully palpated and suspicious nodes harvested as well. Special attention should be paid to the lower medial part of the axilla, which is the most common location of the breast sentinel node. Trying to facilitate sentinel node identification at surgery, Clough et al. [226] have classified Berg's level I into four zones limited vertically by the lateral thoracic tributary of the axillary vein and horizontally by the second intercostobrachial nerve. In 98.2% of the 227 patients in this prospective study the axillary SLN was located alongside the lateral thoracic vein, either below (zone A, 86.8%) or above (zone B, 11.5%) the second intercostobrachial nerve, irrespective of the location of the tumour in the breast. So, whenever performing SLN, knowledge of the exact location of the sentinel node should help to focus the dissection and may reduce the morbidity of the procedure, as well as avoid false negative results. Moreover, the most common location of the ARM nodes is lateral to the thoracodorsal neurovascular bundle (see Arm Reverse Mapping section).

Nevertheless, several studies have shown that SLNB is a robust technique that can be successfully performed with different techniques with excellent results, with a false negative rate of less than 5% and an identification rate close to 100%. Also, axillary recurrence rates are low, usually less than 1% within 3–5 years [227,228]. In a meta-analysis with 48 studies that include 14,959 patients, axillary recurrence after a negative SLNB and no ALND was 0.3% after a median follow-up time of 34 months [229]. The majority of the axillary recurrences occurred in the first 2 years. The injection technique did not influence the axillary recurrence rate after negative SLNB. Randomized controlled trials with longer follow-up have shown similar, very low axillary recurrences rates [204].

One of the concerns in the first decade of the SLNB procedure was the wrong assumption that the false negative rate of the procedure was directly proportional to the rate of axillary recurrences. False negative rates in SLNBs have been reported to be from <5% to 10% [195,204,205,229], but axillary recurrences in this studies with follow-up between 3 and 8 years are <1%, which reinforces the knowledge that false negative results do not equate to recurrence rates.

However, the optimum technique for SLNB remains to be established. Therefore novel techniques have been studied in order to overcome the drawbacks of the current techniques. These novel techniques include mapping and fluorescent imaging with indocyanine green (ICG) [230], or mapping with superparamagnetic iron oxide [231–233]. These new techniques have been feasible with a non-inferior sentinel node detection rate when compared with the radio-isotope technique. As with other techniques, a learning curve is observed.

The method of lymphatic mapping ultimately should be selected based on those methods that have been proven safe, and on the technique that it is most familiar to the surgeon.

METHODS TO ASSESS SENTINEL NODE METASTASES

Not only the lymphatic mapping methods but also the assessment of sentinel node metastases vary greatly between institutions. The sentinel nodes can be evaluated during surgery using frozen section or imprint cytology. Instead of or in addition to intraoperative assessment, serial sectioning of the sentinel nodes is performed for definitive pathology. However, routine staining with immunohistochemistry to detect minimal involvement is not recommended. This recommendation is supported by the ACOSOG Z0010 trial [234].

Recently, molecular assessment of the sentinel node by one-step nucleic acid amplification (OSNA) assay (Sysmex Corporation, Kobe, Japan) has been reported as a detection procedure that analyzes lymph node metastasis by detection and amplification of cytokeratin 19 (CK19) mRNA [235]. Several studies have shown that OSNA can accurately detect sentinel node metastasis, and also that total tumour load detected by OSNA is a predictive factor for additional non-sentinel node metastasis [236,237].

INDICATIONS

SLNB is indicated in patients with invasive breast cancer and a clinically negative axilla regardless of the location of the tumour in the breast, previous surgery, age or gender. However, SLNB is not recommended in patients with inflammatory breast cancer.

Even though DCIS of the breast does not extend through the basal membrane, tumour positive sentinel node findings, most often micrometastases, have been detected in 1.4% of patients with pure DCIS [238]. Most guidelines recommend SLNB in patients with extensive DCIS undergoing mastectomy to avoid further surgery in case there is invasive tumour in the mastectomy specimen. In DCIS patients with breast conservation, routine SLNB is not recommended, but it may be performed when invasive cancer is suspected, such as with very large, high-grade disease or where microinvasion is seen [239].

In patients with Paget's disease of the breast, but without underlying cancer, SLNB is not recommended. In patients with Paget's disease and with invasive cancer or DCIS, the use of SNB is determined according to the underlying cancer and the planned type of breast surgery (breast conservation or mastectomy) [240].

Patients who undergo risk-reducing mastectomy have a risk of occult breast cancer of 1–5%. However, there is no evidence to recommend routine SLNB in patients undergoing risk-reducing mastectomy, especially as most will have had preoperative MRI screening [241].

Pregnancy is a contraindication for the use of blue dye but radiolabelled colloids can be safely used. Decisions should be taken individually regarding the stage of the pregnancy. When SLNB is performed in a pregnant patient, it may be preferable to use a low dose of radioisotope injected on the day of surgery [242].

Repeat SLNB in locally recurrent breast cancer is technically feasible but lymphatic drainage pathways may be altered and lymphscintigraphy may be helpful.

SENTINEL NODE BIOPSY IN PATIENTS UNDERGOING NEOADJUVANT TREATMENT

Neoadjuvant treatments (NATs) can downstage breast cancer and facilitate conservative breast surgery. The use of NAT may eradicate lymph node disease in up to 40% of node positive breast cancer patients. SNB can be offered to patients before or after NAT, but the timing of SLNB is under debate.

Proponents of performing SLNB prior to NAT argue that the SLNB is more accurate as it avoids the effects of NAT (fibrosis of tumour-involved lymphatics and obstruction of the lymphatics) and that sentinel node negative patients can avoid an ALND after NAT [243]. They also propose that knowing the original status of SLNB influences the treatment plan. The disadvantages of this approach include two surgeries, delayed initiation of chemotherapy and the loss of knowledge regarding nodal response to NAT as the positive sentinel node has been removed.

Proponents of SLNB after NAT argue that the response to NAT can be assessed providing even better prognostic information when compared with the original status of the sentinel node. Also, the need for ALND decreases in patients with a complete response in the axilla. Moreover, only one operation is needed [244,245].

Based on retrospective studies conducted on patients with a negative axilla before NAT, SLNB after NAT is considered acceptable, as the false negative rates are similar to those seen in patients who undergo SLNB prior to NAT or without NAT [246].

In those patients with a positive axilla, data from recent randomized trials of SLNB after NAT, ACOSOG Z0071 and SENTINA [247,248] has shown that false negative rates can be decreased in patients with cN1–2 who downstage to

N0 after PST when excising more than two sentinel nodes and using a dual technique. When considering these premises, SLNB after NAT correctly identified nodal status in 84–93% of all patients and was associated with a false negative rate of less than 10%.

Recently, in searching for new techniques for lowering the false negative results of SLNB after NAT, marking the axillary lymph node with radioactive iodine seeds (the MARI procedure) and selectively removing metastatic lymph nodes after NAT has shown a high identification rate and a low false negative rate [249].

More information on long-term data on the rate of axillary recurrence and survival in patients with SLNB after NAT is needed.

MANAGEMENT OF THE AXILLA IN SENTINEL NODE POSITIVE PATIENTS

ALND was the gold standard in the treatment of patients with a positive SNB for about 10 years. However, the role of routine ALND has been questioned after publication of three randomized trials. Data from the ACOSOG Z0011 trial suggest that ALND for SLN positive patients may no longer be justified for women who have early stage breast cancer and are treated with breast conservation including adjuvant radiation therapy and systemic therapy [250]. Although largely criticized as being underpowered, the Z0011 results are practice changing and are being incorporated into the recommendations of the American Society of Clinical Oncology [251].

Similarly, the IBCSG 23-01 study enrolled patients with micrometastasis in their sentinel nodes and found differences neither in locoregional recurrences nor on survival between the ALND and the observation groups. Patients in the IBCSG had a lower tumour burden, and they allowed patients with mastectomy (9%) and partial breast radiation (19%) [252].

The AMAROS trial in turn randomized sentinel node positive patients to axillary radiotherapy or ALND. Although the trial was underpowered for statistical assessment of the axillary recurrence rate, the 5-year axillary recurrence rates in both treatment arms were lower than expected. Moreover, there was less lymphedema associated with the radiotherapy arm [253].

Median follow-up in all these trials was 5 years or more. No substantial changes in axillary recurrence rates are expected to occur during longer follow-up, although for survival outcomes 5–6 years follow-up may be too short to draw meaningful conclusions.

The benefit of routine ALND for women with US-detected axillary disease is also not known. According to a recent meta-analysis [254], the number of involved axillary nodes was significantly higher in patients in whom axillary metastases were detected by ultrasound-guided biopsy than in patients with a positive SNB, reaffirming that these patients with a clinically positive axilla are not the same as the ones included in the Z0011. More data are needed to ascertain whether patients with positive axillary nodes on axillary ultrasound may avoid ALND and its associated morbidity.

PREDICTION TOOLS FOR NON-SENTINEL NODE METASTASES

Prediction tools or nomograms that predict probabilities of additional positive non-sentinel nodes in patients with a positive SNB are available. These nomograms usually perform best at the institutions where they were developed. When validated in other units, the performance has varied greatly due to differences in patient populations and histopathological methods used in the assessment sentinel node metastases, as well as in the use of and the sensitivity of axillary ultrasound [255–258]. Therefore, any predictive model or nomogram should be locally validated before applying it in clinical practice.

All the earlier predictive models rely on the histopathological assessment of sentinel node metastases. When the SLN is assessed by a molecular assay such as OSNA, a nomogram including five variables has been developed for predicting the probability of non-sentinel node metastases [259].

Conclusions and future perspectives for axillary surgery

Multimodal treatments have reduced the incidence of regional recurrences. The advances in targeted treatment and the results of the recent trials addressing axillary management in sentinel node positive patients indicate that for selected patients with ≤2 micrometastasis in the SLN no other axillary surgery is needed. In patients with SLN macrometastasis where more information on the probabilities of additional non-SLN metastasis is desirable, the nomograms may help in the decision-making process. And, in patients with SLN macrometastasis where an axillary intervention is recommended, ALND or axillary radiotherapy is equivalent in the prevention of regional relapse.

NO AXILLARY SURGERY

Investigators have searched for the subgroup of patients that do not benefit from axillary surgery at all. In a randomized setting, Martelli and colleagues compared ALND or no axillary surgery in patients 65 years and older and with T1N0 tumours treated with breast conservative surgery, radiotherapy and tamoxifen. After 15 years of follow-up, omission of ALND in this group of patients did not adversely affect overall outcome [260]. When they compared this group with the patients that were treated out of the trial, the outcomes were similar, concluding that these patients achieve excellent local–regional disease control without the need for axillary surgery [261]. The IBCSG 10-93 trial reached the same conclusions: patients older than 60 years old with a clinically negative axilla and receiving tamoxifen do not benefit from axillary surgery without compromising outcomes [262]. The ongoing SOUND trial compares SLB to observation in patients with a negative axillary ultrasound and who are candidates for BCS. This study will give insights into whether patients need any axillary surgery at all [263].

RADIATION THERAPY FOR BREAST CANCER

Radiation therapy (RT) is a critical part of the multidisciplinary care of women with breast cancer, facilitating the safe use of breast conservation surgery and the optimization of local control in high-risk cases after mastectomy and in the palliative therapy of locally advanced or metastatic disease. Breast cancer was one of the first types of cancer to be treated with RT shortly after its discovery more than 100 years ago. However, treatments are now more complex and sophisticated based on high-level research evidence and technological advances. These advances have not only improved rates of cancer control but also minimized the burden and toxicity of treatment, which is of paramount importance in the case of breast cancer, a disease site with a high long-term cure rate, for long-term quality of life and avoidance of side effects.

The quality of RT delivered across Europe is still variable. Even today some breast units in Europe do not properly delineate target volumes or continue to use rather basic RT techniques providing suboptimal outcomes.

ESTRO recently published a consensus guideline [264] for target volume delineation in breast cancer. The next step is to introduce volume contouring, in agreement with these guidelines, on a routine basis into all units across Europe. This will improve the quality of outcomes for the increasing number of women undergoing RT for breast cancer.

Below is a brief overview of the indications for RT in breast cancer.

Adjuvant radiation therapy after breast conservation therapy

Prior to 50 years ago, mastectomy was the norm for any woman with breast cancer regardless of the size of the cancer. The pioneering research of Fisher and Veronesi demonstrating breast conservation surgery combined with whole breast RT led to a revolution [265,266]. Local recurrence (LR) rates could be reduced from 35% following BCS alone to rates similar to those seen after mastectomy if RT was added. Initially RT was to the whole breast, often inducing cutaneous radiation injury, but current protocols ensure improved targeting of the tumour bed, minimizing the skin dose and the dose to the underlying lung and myocardium with corresponding reductions in toxicity (Figure 22.24) [267]. Initial regimes were until recently 25 doses of 2 Gy each, but both the recent START [268] and

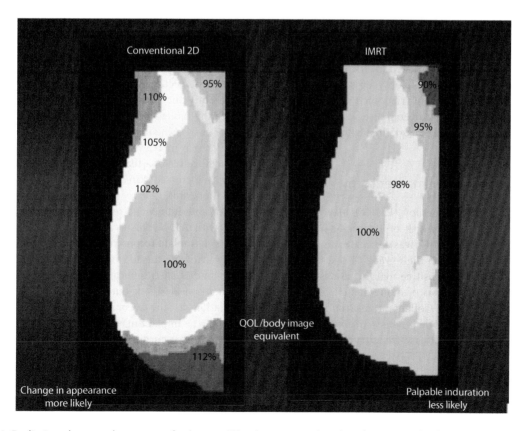

Figure 22.24 Radiation therapy dose zones for breast RT using conventional and IMRT methods. (Reproduced from Donovan, E, et al., *Radiother Oncol* 2007;82(3):254–64. With permission.)

Canadian [269] trials showed that hypofractionation with 15 to 16 doses has equivalent efficacy and side effects with reduced costs and time impact on the patient.

Recently interest in intraoperative RT (IORT) has been high and a number of techniques have been tested to compare outcomes with standard whole breast RT (WBRT). These include the TARGIT trial [270] evaluating IORT using a 50 kV system, the Milan ELIOT trial [271] evaluating IORT using an electron beam accelerator system and the GEC-ESTRO trial using interstitial brachytherapy [272]. With confirming results from other studies more recently reported but not yet published, it seems that the data from these studies with a follow-up up to 5 years (2.4 for TARGIT) suggests these approaches may have a quite comparable LR rate than standard WBRT and may be used in carefully selected patients with very good prognosis cancers.

In the era of oncoplastic surgery, the job of the radiation oncologist has become more complex as the primary tumour bed location has little or no relation to the skin scarring pattern and may be difficult to identify in preoperative CT-based contouring and treatment planning. It is vital that surgeons working with these more complex techniques liaise with their radiation oncologist colleagues to ensure a good understanding of the type of surgery, where the primary tumour originally was located and to mark the tumour bed consistently according to a clear protocol with clips at the time of surgery [273].

Axillary radiation therapy

Another area where the radiation oncologist is likely to have an increasing role is the treatment of the axilla. Historically axillary disease was primarily treated with axillary node clearance following positive core biopsy or sentinel node biopsy. However, recent data from trials such as AMAROS suggest that rates of regional and overall disease control may be similar with axillary RT and be associated with lower rates of long-term morbidity [253].

Radiation therapy after mastectomy

Post-mastectomy radiation therapy (PMRT) may also be used in women with a higher risk of locoregional recurrence. Until very recently, PMRT was advocated mainly in women with T3 or T4 disease or high-grade T2 disease with a heavy nodal burden or a positive margin after surgery. Recent data from meta-analysis of numerous trials by the Early Breast Cancer Trialists' Collaborative Group suggest that even for a lower nodal burden there is an advantage for locoregional control, overall disease-free survival and overall survival by delivering PMRT [274].

From a surgical perspective, in this era where rates of breast reconstruction are rising, this may impact on surgical treatment choices. It is well known that RT may impair the results of implant-based reconstructive surgery with higher rates of implant loss, fibrosis and capsule formation, as shown in Figure 22.25. Reconstruction where RT

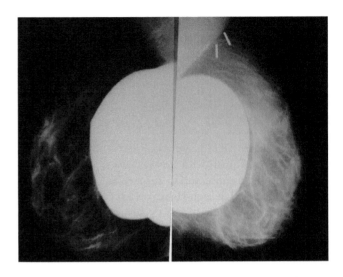

Figure 22.25 Bilateral mammography of a woman who has undergone breast conservation therapy to the left breast with implants *in situ* clearly showing fibrosis of the remaining breast tissue and capsule formation around the implant causing it to round up.

is predicted to be advised may be better performed as a delayed procedure and an autologous flap-based technique could be preferred [275]. Rates of capsule formation after RT to implant-based reconstructions are estimated to be increased 2.5-fold from about 16% to 40% [276].

Another impact of the rise of breast reconstruction is the increased complexity of irradiation planning and delivery of the chest wall with an immediate reconstruction *in situ*. Radiation oncologists are developing new ways of dealing with this, but it is important that the surgeon is aware of the potential need for RT when planning his reconstruction, especially when selecting implants, in trying to avoid those which may modify the breast shape in a way that RT excluding the healthy tissues like the other breast becomes difficult to achieve or by using materials that induce local radiation scatter which may increase the rate of local side effects (for example, metal valves of a tissue expander closely underneath the skin with increased skin changes after RT). There is undoubtedly a higher rate of early and especially late side effects from implant and autologous reconstruction surgery when combined with RT before or after breast reconstruction. Data relating to implant reconstructions suggest a 2.5-fold increase in the rate of late capsule formation [277,278] and a generally higher rate of all complications such as explantation, infection and poor aesthetic outcome [279]. There has been some speculation that the use of acellular dermal matrices (ADMs) alongside the implant may reduce this risk; however, the evidence for this is currently weak, with even some studies that showed that complications with ADM and RT are more frequent than without RT [280]. Many therefore recommend the use of autologous reconstruction in this setting, although even here, complications rates remain higher in patients undergoing RT either pre- or postoperatively [281] with higher rates of revision surgery. Overall, the indication for RT, which increases the risk for complications, should not be considered as an absolute contraindication for breast reconstruction as in the majority of the patients satisfactory results can be obtained. Careful multidisciplinary planning and timing is a pre-requisite for this, with many possible options available.

In the meantime, our knowledge about breast cancer and its treatment continues to increase, leading to changing attitudes toward the selection of the most appropriate target volumes which might be either smaller, like partial breast irradiation for low-risk patients, or quite more extended, like comprehensive locoregional irradiation including the internal mammary lymph nodes for patients with adverse risk factors. At the same time, dose prescription will follow the outcome of prospective clinical trials with hypofractionation with daily doses below 3 Gy already widely introduced in daily clinical practice and with higher daily doses or dose variation over the target volumes depending on the risk of recurrences being investigated. This can only go hand in hand with a continuing improvement of treatment delivery with a more homogeneous dose distribution overall and, if indicated, an intended dose variation like in the simultaneous integrated boost technique for high-risk volumes. For all of this, an optimal multidisciplinary collaboration is obviously indispensable.

PRIMARY SYSTEMIC AND ADJUVANT SYSTEMIC TREATMENT

The main indication for systemic therapies is to reduce the systemic recurrence rate and breast cancer mortality. Systemic therapies also reduce the risk of locoregional recurrence as well as contralateral breast cancer (CBC). Systemic postoperative adjuvant or preoperative systemic treatment (PST) is recommended if the 10-year recurrence risk is more than 10%. Systemic therapy is tailored according to tumour staging and biological profile (i.e. grade, proliferation index, hormone receptor status and HER-2 status) of the primary tumour. In the meta-analyses of the Early Breast Cancer Trialists' Collaborative Group adjuvant chemotherapy reduces the recurrence rates by 20–40% and mortality by 30%; trastuzumab by 40% and 30–40%, respectively; and endocrine treatment by 50% and 30%, respectively [282,283]. The sequential use of chemotherapy and endocrine treatment halves the mortality rate. Endocrine therapy reduces the isolated locoregional recurrence rate more than the distant recurrence rate (53% vs. 36%), whereas with chemotherapy the proportional reductions in local and distant recurrences are similar.

In the adjuvant setting the surgical tumour specimen determines the optimal treatment schedule, whereas neoadjuvant systemic therapy is tailored according to the biological profile of the core biopsy and imaging staging of the tumour. Online risk calculators like Adjuvant! OnLine or PREDICT or diagnostic tools like the Oncotype DX or MammaPrint tests may help in decision making in certain cases where the benefit of chemotherapy is borderline. The same systemic therapy regimens are used in both adjuvant and NAT for similar patients.

Neoadjuvant systemic treatment

Neoadjuvant systemic treatment is the initial treatment of locally advanced breast cancer (LABC). More recently neoadjuvant systemic therapy has increasingly been used both in clinical trials and in routine clinical practice for patients with operable breast cancer to reduce the size of the primary cancer to facilitate breast conservation surgery [284].

The use of neoadjuvant therapy also allows the assessment of response during treatment and regimen change if a poor response is seen. The prognosis is similar after neoadjuvant systemic treatment compared to the use of the same regimen in the adjuvant setting. Prognosis is better when complete response is achieved in patients with triple negative or HER-2 positive subtype tumours [285], but not in those with luminal subtype tumours.

Endocrine therapy

In patients with ER positive, low-risk disease only endocrine therapy is indicated. In higher-risk ER positive patients the initial treatment is chemotherapy with subsequent endocrine treatment once chemotherapy has finished.

For premenopausal patients the recommended endocrine therapy is tamoxifen for 5 or 10 years [286]. Ovarian suppression seems to benefit young women who remain premenopausal after adjuvant chemotherapy. Recent data also suggest that in premenopausal women exemestane plus ovarian suppression significantly reduces the recurrence rate when compared with tamoxifen plus ovarian suppression [287,288].

For postmenopausal patients aromatase inhibitors either for 5 years or sequentially with tamoxifen are recommended [289,290]. In high-risk node positive patients extension of endocrine therapy with aromatase inhibitors after 5 years of tamoxifen is recommended for the patients who are postmenopausal at this point in time.

Chemotherapy

Chemotherapy is indicated for higher-risk ER positive disease as well as in patients with HER-2 positive or triple negative disease. Chemotherapy usually consists of six or eight courses of treatment given over 5 or 6 months. Taxanes and anthracyclines given sequentially are the most efficient chemotherapy regimen, but other regimens like TC (docetaxel, cyclophosphamide), AC (doxorubicin, cyclophosphamide) or CMF (cyclophosphamide, methotrexate, 5-fluorouracil) may also be chosen. In HER-2 positive disease anti-HER-2 therapy, i.e. trastuzumab, is combined with taxanes and continued after chemotherapy for 1 year.

In triple negative breast cancer, chemotherapy is the only possible systemic treatment. The adjuvant regimens used do not differ from the ones used in other subtypes. In the neoadjuvant setting there is increasing evidence that these patients might benefit from platinum-based regimens, however.

Toxicities of systemic treatment

The most common acute toxicities of chemotherapy include nausea, fatigue, alopecia, neutropenia, infections, mucositis and peripheral neuropathy. In premenopausal women chemotherapy generally causes permanent or transient amenorrhoea, and this suppression of ovarian function accounts for some of its efficacy in ER positive disease. Moreover, taxane and anthracycline-based regimens advance menopause by approximately 5 years. A small percentage of women suffer from long-lasting cognitive disorders.

Endocrine treatment is better tolerated but causes menopausal symptoms in most patients. Additionally, tamoxifen increases the risk for thromboembolic complications (risk approximately 1 in 100 patients) and 5 years of tamoxifen is associated with a small increase in endometrial cancer (risk approximately 1 in 1000 patients). Tamoxifen should be stopped preferably 4 weeks before any surgery due to this increased risk of thromboembolic complications and worse microsurgical outcomes. On the other hand, tamoxifen produces favorable lipid profile changes and increases bone mineral density in postmenopausal women. Aromatase inhibitors (AIs) induce arthralgia and reduce the bone mineral density increasing the risk for osteoporosis. Bone density should therefore be monitored while on therapy and appropriate bone preservation measures taken if density is low or starts to fall on therapy. Use of calcium and vitamin D supplements is often advised and in some cases bisphosphonates. These measures have been shown to offset the potential effects of AIs on bone density.

Bisphosphonates

In a meta-analysis bisphosphonates achieved a significant reduction in the rates of distant recurrence, bone recurrence and mortality among postmenopausal women [291]. Both oral and intravenous bisphosphonates are associated with this benefit. The doses used in the treatment of osteoporosis seem adequate. However, there is still no consensus whether postmenopausal patients should be treated with bisphosphonates since most of the trials were not designed to answer these questions and a prospective randomized study is still pending. Taken together, it seems reasonable to use osteoporosis prophylaxis at least in high-risk patients.

LOCAL–REGIONAL RECURRENCE AND FOLLOW-UP

Local and regional recurrences are rare after modern multidisciplinary breast cancer treatment. Systemic recurrence is the most common form of first recurrence, even in T1 breast cancer.

The annual local recurrence (LR) rate after breast-conserving surgery (BCS) and radiotherapy in invasive breast cancer is 0.5% or even less. In DCIS, the LR rate is higher, 10-year LR rates being 13% in patients receiving radiotherapy. In DCIS, approximately 50% of the recurrences are invasive. The most important risk factors for LRs in both DCIS and invasive cancer include positive resection margins, omission of radiotherapy and young patient age. In invasive cancer, the risk of LR is twofold in patients with positive resection margins, when compared with patients with negative resection margins. Whole breast radiotherapy decreases the risk of LRs by 60–70% in invasive cancer and by 50% in DCIS.

LRs after mastectomy are also rare, approximately 0.5% in a year or less. Young age is also a risk factor for LRs after mastectomy. LRs are more common in node positive patients and in those with large primary tumours. Radiotherapy, in turn, decreases the LR rate, but remarkably only in node positive patients.

The 5-year axillary recurrence after negative sentinel node biopsy has been less than 1%. A rather similar, very low axillary recurrence rate has been observed in sentinel node positive patients, with axillary radiotherapy or even without further axillary treatment. In node positive patients with ALND the 5-year axillary recurrence rate has been less than 1%, but may be higher in patients with more extensive, that is N2–N3, nodal disease.

Recurrences in supraclavicular, contralateral axillary or supraclavical or in internal mammary nodal basins are rare as solitary, first events and even in connection with local or systemic relapses.

Aggressive tumour biology is a risk factor for local and regional recurrences, at least for early recurrences. The risk is also dependent on the systemic treatment available, like in HER-2 positive disease. In patients with biologically aggressive tumours, the most important recurrence to avoid is the systemic recurrence. No data support more extensive surgery in patients with biologically aggressive tumours.

The risk of contralateral breast cancer (CBC) during a 10-year follow-up is about 3%. Systemic adjuvant treatment of breast cancer is decreasing the risk, which on the other hand is slightly increased by breast radiotherapy. However, the risk, especially the lifelong risk, may be higher in young patients and especially in those with familial predisposition to breast cancer.

The local and regional recurrences are detected either during routine imaging, as a palpable lump or density by the patients, or, although rarely, in clinical examination during routine follow-up visits. LRs after breast conservation, detected in imaging or by the patient herself, may have better prognosis than LRs detected in clinical examination during routine follow-up visits.

Treatment of local and regional recurrences

After diagnosis of local or regional recurrence it is important to rule out distant disease by bone and CT scans or even by PET/CT.

Mastectomy with immediate breast reconstruction as an option is the gold standard in surgical treatment of patients with LRs after breast-conserving surgery (BCS) and whole breast radiotherapy. A second resection can be considered in highly selected patients as well as in those who have not received whole breast radiotherapy after primary surgery.

Wide local excision of the recurrent tumour is performed in LRs after mastectomy. In extensive LRs very wide resections or even thoracic wall resections with major reconstructive procedures are needed. Ruling out distant disease before surgery is of particular importance in these cases.

Second sentinel node biopsy can be performed in patients who experience a LR after breast conservation or even after mastectomy and with negative sentinel node biopsy. Sentinel node biopsy may be successful even after axillary lymph node dissection (ALND), showing drainage to other nodal basins than ipsilateral axilla. However, the influence of these procedures on patient survival and morbidity is obscure.

Salvage ALND is the procedure of choice in patients with axillary recurrences after either sentinel node biopsy or ALND. Solitary nodal metastases in supraclavicular basin or in neck can be removed in selected cases.

Patients with local or regional recurrences benefit from systemic treatment, in either an adjuvant or neoadjuvant setting. Systemic treatment is tailored according to tumour biology and patient features. Also, radiotherapy should be tailored according to the type of the recurrence and the possible previous radiotherapy.

The EBCTCG overview, published in 2005 in *Lancet*, showed that one patient can be saved from breast cancer death by preventing four LRs. The survival benefit may vary, however, according to primary tumour biology and the efficacy of available systemic treatment. Moreover, the site of recurrence may also influence. Patients with clinically overt nodal recurrences may have more adverse prognosis than patients with LR after mastectomy, not to talk about a late recurrence after breast conservation.

Follow-up

The aim of follow-up is to detect local and regional recurrences and CBC at a curable stage. The intensity and length of the follow-up have varied in different guidelines, however. In addition to routine follow-up visits, the patients should have an opportunity to contact the outpatient clinic, whenever they have symptoms or signs suspicious for disease recurrence. Nevertheless, the follow-up should include regular breast imaging, consisting of mammography and in selected cases also of breast ultrasound or MRI.

Routine imaging or blood tests to detect distant recurrences at a symptomatic phase are not beneficial, however.

Another important goal of follow-up is to monitor and treat treatment-associated long-time morbidities as well as to provide psychological support to the patient. Also encouraging the patients toward weight control, healthy diet and exercise is of value, in terms of both survival and quality of life.

LOCALLY ADVANCED BREAST CANCER

Locally advanced breast cancer (LABC) includes inflammatory breast cancer, cancer growing to the thoracic wall, primary tumour too large to allow primary wound closure after mastectomy or extensive nodal disease with matted nodes attached to axillary plexus. The disease is potentially curable and the treatment is started with neoadjuvant systemic treatment after excluding distant metastases.

The treatment of LABC is initiated with neoadjuvant systemic therapy. Before the start of therapy baseline radiologic imaging with breast ultrasound or MRI is needed as well as staging with whole body CT and bone scan. The bioprofile of the core biopsy specimen is needed to tailor the systemic therapy.

The same chemotherapy regimens that are used in the adjuvant therapy are usually chosen, i.e. taxanes and anthracyclines sequentially. In case of HER-2 positive disease anti-HER therapy, i.e. trastuzumab, is combined with taxanes and continued postoperatively for 1 year. Pertuzumab is used in combination with trastuzumab and chemotherapy in the first-line treatment of metastatic HER-2 positive breast cancer and is most likely beneficial in the treatment of locally advanced disease as well.

Endocrine treatment can be considered the initial systemic therapy for luminal A disease as well as for elderly or fragile patients with ER positive disease. Response to treatment should be evaluated before every course. The radiologic breast imaging should be repeated at least every other cycle. In case of progressive disease the treatment is changed. All of the planned six to eight chemotherapy courses should be given preoperatively.

Mastectomy with ALND is the gold standard in the surgical treatment of LABC. However, breast conservation may be feasible in patients with extensive axillary disease, but with limited tumour in the breast. SNB, either before or after neoadjuvant therapy, can be considered in patients with non-inflammatory breast cancer and with negative nodes before neoadjuvant systemic therapy. The safety of SNB in LABC that turn node negative during systemic treatment is unproven, so far.

Skin-sparing mastectomy and immediate breast reconstruction procedure are regarded as oncologically safe in LABC, except for inflammatory disease. However, the evidence is based on a few, rather small retrospective cohort studies and complication rates are significantly higher than those with conventional mastectomy. These complications may cause delay in radiotherapy. Another option is to also give radiotherapy before surgery, but the complication rate may also be high after this option.

If LABC remains inoperable after systemic therapy and eventual radiation, palliative mastectomy should not be done, unless the surgery is likely to result in an overall improvement in quality of life.

Postoperative radiotherapy is planned according to the baseline stage before neoadjuvant systemic therapy.

METASTATIC BREAST CANCER

Although only 5% of breast cancer patients have metastatic disease at primary presentation, metastases will subsequently affect some 25% of women with breast cancer and result in their ultimate death. The most common sites are bone, lung (parenchymal and pleural deposits), liver, soft tissue and brain. Life expectancy after metastatic diagnosis depends on the predominant metastatic site, with bone metastases tending to have a more indolent pattern and median survival of several years, whereas liver and brain metastases have median survivals of only months [292]. In addition the metastasis-free interval, original tumour grade and receptor status all impact on metastatic survival duration [293].

Patients with metastatic breast cancer are not curable and will eventually die of the disease. The goal of treatment is to prolong survival, alleviate the symptoms of the disease and maintain quality of life for as long as possible. Biopsy and biological profiling of metastases are recommended if technically possible, as the metastatic disease may alter its hormone receptor or HER-2 status relative to the primary site. For example, ER positive disease may become ER negative or HER-2 status may change in 10–15% of cases which may have an important impact on therapy decisions and prognosis [294]. In case a metastatic biopsy is not possible, the treatment is tailored according to the biological profile of the primary tumour. The site and extent of metastatic disease, previous therapies and response to them, symptoms of the disease as well as the patient's wishes of anticipated side effects should be taken into account.

In the case of ER positive disease endocrine systemic treatment is recommended unless the metastases are life threatening or cause severe symptoms. Endocrine therapies include tamoxifen, ovarian suppression, aromatase inhibitors, fulvestrant and medroxyprogesterone acetate. Hormone resistance can be postponed with m-TOR inhibitors or cyclin-dependent kinase inhibitors. Chemotherapy is appropriate for patients who are clearly refractory to endocrine treatment or are unlikely to respond to it. Many chemotherapy regimens and lines of therapy are available. The treatment is continued as long as it is effective and not too toxic. In HER-2 positive disease anti-HER-2 therapy is combined with other systemic therapy and continued until disease progression.

The median survival with metastatic breast cancer is about 3 years. However, some patients survive essentially longer. Especially the prognosis of HER-2 positive subtype has become better with sequential use of novel anti-HER-2 therapies like the combination of trastuzumab and pertuzumab with chemotherapy, TDM1 (trastuzumab-emtansine) and lapatinib.

Bisphosphonates or denosumab is combined with other systemic therapy to reduce the risk of skeletal events in patients with bone metastases. Radiotherapy is also used to reduce pain or risk for fracture. Surgery is sometimes needed for the treatment of symptomatic intraspinal metastases and pathological fractures of limb bone metastases whose management may be quite technically challenging from an orthopaedic surgery perspective and a multidisciplinary bone MDT may be useful for complex cases.

Surgery may be considered for solitary brain metastases. Stereotactic radiotherapy is suitable for up to three metastases. Multiple or leptomeningeal metastases are treated with whole brain irradiation. Some small-molecule anticancer agents can penetrate through the blood–brain barrier.

Because metastatic breast cancer is considered an incurable disease, surgery has been indicated only for palliative purposes. However, results from several studies suggest that patients with elective surgery of the primary tumour as a part of their treatment live longer than those without surgical treatment. These studies are summarized in an excellent review article from Ruiterkamp and Ernst [295]. Longer survival has been observed after both removal of primary breast tumour and resection of liver or pulmonary metastases. However, all these studies are retrospective and the observed longer survival may be just due to selection bias. Currently there is not sufficient evidence to recommend elective surgical treatment in these patients outside trials, but a few randomized trials have been launched to evaluate if elective surgery really prolongs survival in these patients.

BREAST CANCER IN SPECIAL GROUPS

Male breast cancer

Male breast cancer is rare accounting for less than 1% of all BC. Risk factors include hormonal factors (Klinefelter's syndrome), liver disorders, prostate cancer and family history. Men who carry germ line mutations in the BRCA1/2 gene have a higher risk of developing BC, and BRCA2 represents about 15% of breast cancer in men. The cumulative risks of breast cancer by age 80 years in men are 1.5% (95% CI = 0.3–3.9%) for BRCA1 and 5.1% (95% CI = 2.0–11.0%) for BRCA2 [296].

The most common presentation of male BC is a palpable mass, usually painless, retro- or periareolar and ill defined, although the most common diagnosis in men presenting with a palpable mass is gynecomastia (usually diffuse enlarged bilateral and tender breast). Other symptoms include breast pain, nipple retraction and less common nipple discharge. Mammography and ultrasound are diagnostic tools to differentiate between gynecomastia and BC. Suspicious breast imaging includes mass, architectural distortion and microcalcifications. Pathologic evaluation of the mass should be performed with a core needle biopsy.

In a retrospective study of 1473 male BC patients, median age at diagnosis was 68.5 years, 87% were ductal carcinomas, 52% grade II, 92% ER positive, 35% PgR positive, 87% AR positive, 25% highly proliferative and 5% HER-2 positive. Thus, male breast cancer is similar to luminal breast cancer in female patients. Notably, also very young men <35 years old can have breast cancer, although this is extremely rare [297].

Surgical treatment has been modified radical mastectomy for decades. Breast conservative plus radiation therapy (RT) is becoming more usual as some reported studies have shown similar outcomes as mastectomy [298]. BCS may be offered if feasible due to breast size and no involvement of the nipple. Sentinel lymph node biopsy can be performed extrapolated from women BC [299]. The adjuvant radiotherapy and systemic treatment are planned according to the guidelines for female BC patients. The only exception is endocrine treatment. Tamoxifen is the primary drug of choice. Aromatase inhibitors are only to be used with gonadotropin-releasing hormone analogues since in men 20% of circulating oestrogens result from testicular production.

Breast cancer in young and elderly patients

BREAST CANCER IN YOUNG PATIENTS

Breast cancer in young patients (≤40 years old) is relatively uncommon and represents fewer than 7% of BC in developed countries. The incidence of BC in very young patients (<35 years) has not increased significantly during the last decades in indicating genomic predisposition.

Young BC patients have higher rates of LRs, distant recurrences and death after a diagnosis of BC [300]. Additionally, they have more frequently aggressive tumours, i.e. high-grade, triple negative or HER-2 positive tumours, so it is unclear which factors (age or aggressive subtypes) affect the prognosis more [301]. Most of the randomized studies that compared BCS versus mastectomy did not provide the impact of age on outcomes. The meta-analysis of the Early Breast Cancer Trialists' Collaborative Group (EBCTCG) of randomized trials of BCS ± RT demonstrated that young age was associated with the highest rates of recurrence following BCS and the absolute recurrence reduction varied according to age (36% in <40-year-olds to 9% in >70-year-olds) [302]. An additional radiotherapy boost to the site of local excision must be offered after BCS and whole breast irradiation to all young patients due to the high risk of LR.

Overall, the risk for LRs decreased remarkably over the last decades, as demonstrated in three consecutive prospective randomized clinical trials, to a level (2% at 5 years in the Dutch Young Boost Trial) that age in general should not be considered any more as a contraindication for breast conservation [303]. When combining age and molecular subtypes, Arvold et al., among 1434 consecutive women with early stage invasive BC who received BCS, found that increasing age was associated with decreased risk of LR independent of BC subtype. The 5.0% risk of LR at 5 years is considered acceptable and lower than in older series, meaning that multimodal treatment support the use of BCS in young patients [304]. When analyzing triple negative BC patients who have the highest rate of LR, this increased risk

is present after surgical treatment with BCS or mastectomy [302,304]. However, very young patients <35 years with triple negative disease more often have a genetic predisposition to breast cancer so more extensive surgery may be indicated anyway.

Taken together, BCS is an option for young patients, but they should be informed of the higher risk for LR. Mastectomy and skin-sparing mastectomy with immediate reconstruction are other choices of treatment. As young age is also a recognized risk factor of increased local relapse after mastectomy, post-mastectomy irradiation should be evaluated on an individualized basis balancing potential benefits, adverse cosmetic outcome and long-term side effects. Indications for SLNB and surgical management of patients with SLN involvement are the same as in older patients.

The adjuvant systemic treatment of young BC patients is tailored according to the bioprofile and staging of the tumour similarly as in other BC patients. The decision to extend tamoxifen beyond 5 years and combining GnRH analogues with either tamoxifen or aromatase inhibitors should be individualized balancing the estimated absolute benefit, the risk for late relapse, quality of life issues and personal preferences, especially when benefits may be modest.

Young women with BC have unique needs regarding fertility, psychosocial, sexual health and genetic issues. Infertility treatment should be discussed and the procedures needed initiated as soon as possible after the BC diagnosis before the start of chemotherapy. The most common regimens, i.e. anthracyclines in sequence with taxanes, advance menopause by approximately 5 years. Additionally, possible endocrine therapies postpone possible pregnancy.

BREAST CANCER IN ELDERLY PATIENTS

Most breast cancers develop in older women. Around 50% of BC occur in women ≥65 years old and >30% occur in women >70 years of age [305]. Life expectancy has increased over years, so 65- and 75-year-old women can be expected to live approximately 20 and 13 more years, respectively. Despite the incidence of BC, patients >70 years are usually not included in clinical trials and are often not treated in accordance with guidelines. The treatment in elderly patients with BC has been controversial. When choosing the appropriate treatment, additional factors such as life expectancy, functional status, comorbidities, geriatric assessment and the benefits and risks of treatments should be considered. Older women usually have less aggressive tumours than young women, although this does not mean that it is an indolent disease. If surgery is determined to be the appropriate treatment, patients should not be denied this option because of their age. There is increasing evidence that preoperative assessment of frail patients might decrease the rate of postoperative complications and increase survival. Surgery and adjuvant treatment may decrease the LR and improve the survival in elderly patients [306]. With adequate perioperative risk stratification, functional assessment and oncologic prognostication, elderly patients with breast cancer can do as well as younger patients.

Regarding breast RT, a phase III trial demonstrated that radiation after BCS provided no survival and limited local control benefit to women aged 70 years and older with stage I, oestrogen receptor positive cancers who receive endocrine therapy [307]. Also in other patient groups the benefit of the treatment should outweigh life expectancy due to other disease. Additionally, performance status should allow frequent visits to therapy. However, for most of those patients the delivery of RT might be the preferred option over 5 years of endocrine treatment, whereas the risk for LRs after neither of those treatments most often remains too high.

Web-based tools estimate life span and can assess in planning the treatment for elderly patients. The evidence-based data are scarce on the treatment of elderly BC patients. However, if chemotherapy is indicated and the patient is fit for that, similar regimens should be considered as for younger patients. Suboptimal regimens and doses are to be avoided. More studies on how to treat elderly BC patients are warranted.

PREGNANCY-ASSOCIATED BREAST CANCER

The definition of pregnancy-associated breast cancer (PABC) is that the diagnosis of BC is made during pregnancy or within 1 year afterward. It is diagnosed approximately once per 3000 pregnancies, and it is expected to become more frequent since there is an increasing trend for women to delay childbearing. No specific risk factors for breast cancer in pregnancy are known [308,309]. The most common presentation is a palpable mass, but delay in diagnosis is often due to masses being considered normal physiologic changes during pregnancy. Initial diagnosis is made by ultrasound and mammogram with the use of abdominal shielding performed if malignant changes are suspected. Gadolinium is contraindicated during pregnancy so magnetic resonance imaging is not recommended. Chest X-ray with abdominal shielding and abdominal ultrasound are acceptable staging examinations when the results change clinical management.

Treatment decisions in pregnant women with BC are complex and require a multidisciplinary team that should include obstetricians besides the BC team. The treatment is tailored individually according to the gestational stage and tumour characteristics. Surgery is usually the initial treatment and can be performed at any time during pregnancy, although in the third trimester it increases the risk of preterm labour. There does not appear to be survival advantage of mastectomy over breast conservation for PABC. Thromboprophylaxis with heparin is required because of the increased risk of thromboembolic events. Radiotherapy to the breast or to the chest wall should be delayed after delivery. Although small reports, SLNB for staging of the regional lymph nodes can be performed safely during pregnancy, with low-dose radioisotope [310]. Current guidelines do not recommend the use of blue dye in sentinel node mapping in pregnant patients due to the risk of anaphylaxis.

According to the German breast group and Belgian register data chemotherapy can be given during the second and third trimesters, from 14 weeks on. Anthracyclines and taxanes seem safe. Antiemetics and granulocyte-stimulating growth factors are allowed if indicated. The last chemotherapy course should be given latest at week 35 to avoid neutropenia during delivery and drug accumulation in the fetus. Trastuzumab and endocrine therapies are contraindicated during pregnancy. After delivery the patient is not able to breastfeed because chemotherapy is to be continued as soon as she has recovered from delivery. Cancer treatment during pregnancy decreases the need for early delivery and prematurity, which are considered a bigger risk for the fetus [311]. However, data on the long-term outcome of the children exposed to chemotherapy are needed especially regarding second malignancies and fertility.

Axillary metastases with occult primary breast cancer

Less than 1% of all breast cancer cases present with axillary nodal metastases, without primary tumour in the ipsilateral breast in clinical examination, mammography or breast ultrasound. Possible other sources of axillary metastases include lung, ovarian, thyroid, pancreas and urogenital tract cancers as well as melanoma. Immunohistochemical stainings may be of help when distinguishing between breast cancer and other malignancies.

In patients with axillary nodal metastases, MRI can detect otherwise occult breast cancer in about 40% of the cases [312].

Traditionally, mastectomy and ALND have been recommended in patients with occult breast cancer and axillary metastases. Another treatment alternative is breast RT, providing a better local disease control than observation [313]. Due to the rarity of the condition, no data exist to conclude if mastectomy provides benefit over RT, regarding neither local disease control nor survival.

Paget's disease of the breast

Paget's disease is an eczematous change of the nipple–areola complex (NAC), representing dermal *in situ* cancer, with typical histomorphological features. The diagnosis is confirmed by skin biopsy. Paget's disease is rather rare, diagnosed in approximately 1–2% of all breast cancer cases. However, in patients with Paget's disease an underlying DCIS or invasive carcinoma is detected in up to 90% of the patients [314]. The underlying breast cancer is not always central, but often peripheral or multicentric. Surgical and adjuvant treatments are planned largely according to the underlying carcinoma.

In patients without breast cancer detected in clinical examination, mammography and ultrasound, MRI may reveal an occult cancer. In patients with Paget's disease only, that is without underlying breast cancer, central resection including NAC and a rim of healthy skin around the areola is performed. RT to the remaining breast tissue can be considered, although no data about the possible benefits exist, due to rarity of the condition. Alternatively, RT with a boost to the NAC without surgery can be considered as well (E. van Limbergen, personal communication, data on file).

NON-CARCINOMA MALIGNANCIES OF THE BREAST

The non-carcinoma malignancies of the breast can be broadly categorized into phyllodes tumours, sarcoma group tumours, hematopoietic tumours and metastatic tumours to the breast. In addition, malignant skin tumours may also manifest primarily on the skin of the breast. The non-carcinoma breast malignancies account for approximately less than 1% of all malignant breast tumours [315]. Due to the rarity of these tumours, their classification and nomenclature is somewhat inconsistent with little conclusive evidence on their management strategies.

Malignant phyllodes tumour is the most frequent noncarcinoma breast malignancy. The majority of phyllodes tumours are benign with approximately 10–20% of them being malignant or borderline malignant. Surgical resection with clear margins, by either wide local excision or mastectomy, remains the mainstay of phyllodes tumour management. There is no strong consensus on the appropriate width of tumour-free margins or on the benefit of adjuvant treatments in malignant phyllodes tumours. Axillary lymph node staging is not routinely recommended in malignant phyllodes tumours as they mainly undergo hematogenous dissemination. Five-year disease-free survival rates of 60–90% have been reported in the literature for malignant and borderline phyllodes tumours of the breast [316–318].

Various sarcomas, including angiosarcoma, carcinosarcoma, fibrosarcoma, liposarcoma and myosarcoma, are the next most frequent group of non-epithelial breast malignancies. The majority of breast sarcomas are radiation associated and secondary to previous radiotherapy of the breast region. Angiosarcoma of the breast is the most common secondary sarcoma after previous breast cancer surgery and is associated with not only radiotherapy but also chronic lymphedema after axillary lymph node dissection (ALND). Sarcomas of the breast seem to have similar natural history, histology and prognosis as other soft-tissue sarcomas and, in fact, the management strategies are largely based on data from other sites of soft-tissue sarcomas. Surgery is the primary treatment option of all sarcomas of the breast, with type of surgery depending on the size of the tumour and of the breast. Routine axillary surgery is not recommended in breast sarcomas. Generally the prognosis of sarcomas of the breast is considerably inferior to that of breast carcinomas, although little data are available on the different sarcoma types. The 5-year overall survival rate of patients with radiation-associated angiosarcoma is reported at 43% by a recent review [319].

There is no consensus on the benefit of adjuvant treatments in patients with sarcomas of the breast, although both radiotherapy and systemic chemotherapy have been reportedly used [315,320].

Primary breast lymphoma is a distinct type of extranodal non-Hodgkin lymphoma, most commonly of diffuse large B-cell histology. Primary breast lymphoma manifests as a solitary breast tumour with or without ipsilateral lymph node involvement. The diagnosis of breast lymphoma is acquired from core needle biopsy or excisional biopsy. The treatment of primary breast lymphoma is systemic chemotherapy and possible radiotherapy. Surgery of primary breast lymphoma, other than excisional biopsy, should be avoided as it leads to inferior local control and overall survival [321].

Finally, many malignancies may manifest with metastatic spread to the breast. Malignant melanomas, neuroendocrine tumours, and ovarian, lung and renal carcinomas are the most frequently cited in the literature to metastasize to the breast [322].

SURVIVOR ISSUES

All breast cancer treatment modalities, surgery, radiotherapy and systemic treatment are associated with long-time morbidity. These long-time morbidities not only decrease quality of life but may, although rarely, cause additional mortality.

Psychological morbidity

Every third breast cancer patient experiences significant psychological symptoms, such as depression, anxiety or traumatic stress reactions. These symptoms vary in duration and severity and most often emerge at the time of diagnosis, when disease recurs or when patient has severe treatment-associated adverse events or complications. Rapid relieving of the symptoms is important to prevent chronic psychological morbidity. Cornerstones here include sufficient information about prognosis, treatment and its side effects, as well as psychological support by professionals. Also, voluntary peers from breast cancer patient advocacy groups may be of help.

Cognition

Chemotherapy or endocrine treatment may induce cognitive dysfunction. Postchemotherapy cognitive impairment is called chemobrain and 20–30% of the patients suffer from this decrease in mental 'sharpness'; i.e. they have difficulties in memory, concentration, finishing tasks or learning new skills. Usually these symptoms gradually disappear in months or in a small minority in a couple of years. Tamoxifen can cause similar but minor dysfunction, and usually the patients recover soon after stopping the endocrine treatment. Menopause and senescence itself may include similar symptoms.

Lymphedema

Chronic lymphedema is the most notorious long-time arm morbidity after breast cancer treatment. Lymphedema may also affect the breast after breast-conserving surgery. The most important risk factor for chronic lymphedema is axillary surgery, especially ALND. Selective ALND, sparing lymphatics and lymph nodes draining the arm and removing just nodes draining the breast may be feasible by reverse axillary mapping. However, the safety and efficacy of the method are still under evaluation.

Radiation therapy (RT) to the axilla and sub- and supraclavicular fields further increases the risk of lymphedema, namely when the part of the axilla that was removed by the ALND is included in the RT fields (for which only exceptionally an indication exists). The incidence of chronic arm edema is 5% or less after sole sentinel node biopsy, about 20–30% after ALND, 15% after SNB and axillary RT and up to 40% after ALND and RT. Lymphedema is more common in obese patients.

The conservative treatment of lymphedema consists of manual lymphatic draining and supportive sleeve or glove. Surgical treatment has included liposuction or excision of edematous areas. After these treatments, use of a supportive sleeve is warranted to prevent recurrent edema. None of these treatment modalities is curative.

Recent proceedings in the surgical treatment of lymphoma include lymphatic or lymph venous anastomoses or autotransplantation of lymph nodes to the axilla. The preliminary results have been encouraging, but these procedures are still experimental.

Chronic pain and sensory disorders

Persisting chronic pain has been reported in as many as 20–50% of patients after breast cancer surgery. Furthermore, the intensity of this chronic pain may be moderate to severe in more than half of the patients with persisting pain. Persistent pain in breast cancer survivors is often regarded as neuropathic, being due to damage to the intercostobrachial nerves during axillary surgery, although pathological mechanisms leading to persisting pain after breast cancer treatments are likely multiple.

Persistent pain may be also due to tissue damage and inflammation caused by surgery or radiotherapy. Other significant risk factors for chronic pain include any chronic pain before surgery, pain in the operation area before surgery and also depression and anxiety.

Paracetamol and NSAIDs are not effective against neuropathic pain. Weak opioids like tramadol or codeine are therefore preferable. Gabapentin or pregabalin as well as antidepressants such as nortriptyline have been used successfully. If the painful area is restricted topical anaesthetics in the form of a gel or adhesive may also be helpful. In patients with severe pain, a combination of different medications is needed and referral to a pain clinic or consulting a pain specialist is often necessary.

Up to 80% of patients experience sensory disorders after ALND, such as numbness, tingling, pricking, loss of sensation or hyperesthesia, in the arm, the axilla or the breast or thoracic wall. Sensory disorders also occur after sole SNB, but less frequently and are less severe.

Functional upper limb disorders

Axillary lymph node dissection or axillary radiotherapy can also lead to motion restriction of the shoulder joint or muscle weakness. Functional disorders may also occur, although less often, after sole sentinel node biopsy.

Body image and sexuality

Breast cancer treatments often affect body image making the patients feel less sexually appealing or can even cause difficulties in dressing. Oncoplastic and reconstructive breast surgery leading to more favorable aesthetic outcomes after breast conservation and mastectomy prevent these problems, at least in part. However, the aesthetic outcome can be suboptimal also after these procedures. Moreover in mastectomy, the NAC itself or, even when spared, its erotic function is lost.

Peripheral neuropathy

Chemotherapy with taxanes, i.e. docetaxel or paclitaxel, is the most common cause of peripheral neuropathy in women who have had breast cancer. Platinum and vinca alkaloids induce peripheral neuropathy as well. Nerve damage can cause symptoms such as pins and needles, numbness or pain in the hands and feet. This may lead to problems with balance and walking. In later stages muscular weakness may accompany.

After treatment is over, the nerves slowly recover during several months. For some patients, the nerves do not completely recover but despite this, the symptoms become less troublesome over time since the patients learn to cope with them. There is no treatment to repair damaged nerves and the above-mentioned drugs for neuropathic pain offer little or no relief in chemotherapy-induced peripheral neuropathy.

Endocrine and fertility issues including bone health

Taxane and anthracycline-based chemotherapy regimens advance menopause by approximately 5 years. The fertility of breast cancer patients is reduced due to this preterm menopause and the time delay for pregnancy due to long duration of endocrine treatment. However, the duration of endocrine treatment can individually be tailored according to the disease and the patient's wishes for pregnancy. Infertility issues should be discussed with every premenopausal patient before the start of chemotherapy and gynaecologist referred if fertility therapies may be needed. Available evidence suggests that pregnancy after breast cancer is safe and does not seem to adversely affect breast cancer outcome when carefully planned.

All endocrine treatments cause menopausal symptoms. The effect of endocrine therapy on bone health depends on both the menopausal status of the patient and the treatment itself. Tamoxifen increases bone mineral density in postmenopausal women, whereas it decreases it in premenopausal patients.

Aromatase inhibitors can only be used for postmenopausal patients and they reduce the bone mineral density increasing risk for osteoporosis. The favorable results of bisphosphonates regarding early breast cancer prognosis support a low threshold for osteoporosis prophylaxis with these drugs [291].

Cardiovascular and pulmonary morbidity

Anthracyclines carry a significant risk for cardiac toxicity, which is exponentially dose dependent. The incidence of congestive heart failure (CHF) reaches 5% for doxorubicin and epirubicin, with cumulative doses of 400 and 920 mg/m², respectively. In the adjuvant treatment of breast cancer the cumulative doses for these drugs remain below half of these safety levels. The main other risk factors for chemotherapy-induced CHF include old age, hypertension, pre-existing coronary artery disease and previous mediastinal radiotherapy.

Targeted anti-HER-2 drug trastuzumab is associated with a small-to-modest risk for cardiotoxicity, which is typically manifested by an asymptomatic decrease in left ventricular ejection fraction and less often by clinical heart failure. Due to cardiotoxicity anthracyclines and trastuzumab are usually given sequentially.

Tamoxifen is associated with a twofold increased risk of thromboembolic events, whereas in postmenopausal women it produces favorable lipid profile changes. Patients should be made aware of the symptoms of venous thromboembolism and instructed in case of these symptoms to contact health care immediately.

Radiation therapy for breast cancer often involves some incidental exposure of the heart to ionizing radiation, increasing the subsequent rate of ischemic heart disease. The increase is proportional to the mean dose to the heart, begins within a few years of exposure and continues for at least 20 years. Women with pre-existing cardiac risk factors have greater absolute increases in risk from radiation therapy than other women. However, recent studies suggest that cardiac mortality has not been greater for patients treated for left-sided breast cancer with modern radiation therapy techniques.

Asymptomatic radiation pneumonitis (RP) is quite common after adjuvant radiation therapy, whereas symptomatic RP is rare. RP is related to the dose of radiation and develops along the irradiated fields and may result in pulmonary fibrosis. It usually appears 1–3 months after radiotherapy with cough, mild fever, tiredness or dyspnoea and can be treated with corticosteroids when symptomatic. Most often, it is fully reversible with no or only limited pulmonary function tests on follow-up.

Secondary malignancies

It is estimated that 1 in every 20 patients will develop a secondary non–breast cancer in 10 years, which corresponds to a 22% increase in the relative risk. This risk is related to genetic predisposition (BRCA2 and p53 carriers), radiotherapy (e.g. risk for secondary lung cancer), hormonal therapy (e.g. risk for uterine cancer secondary to tamoxifen) and chemotherapy (e.g. risk for secondary acute myeloid leukemia [AML] and myelodysplastic syndrome [MDS]).

Irradiated breast cancer patients have an increased risk of second lung cancer. The risk of second lung cancer after breast cancer radiation therapy increases linearly with radiation doses and the treatment lag between breast cancer radiation and lung cancer diagnosis is 5 and 10 years or more. Smoking increases this risk with approximately 20% per delivered Gray to the lung, while for non-smokers the risk is not significantly increased above baseline.

Radiation-induced secondary angiosarcomas are rare clinical entities with a cumulative incidence of 0.9 per 1000 breast cancer cases over 15 years and usually a latency period of 4–8 years. Because of their rarity and often seemingly harmless presentation with painless and bruise-like skin lesions, both patients and doctors easily neglect the initial symptoms and diagnosis is delayed. Surgery is the mainstay of treatment. The risk of local recurrence and metastasis is high and the prognosis poor.

The estimated annual risk of endometrial cancer in tamoxifen-treated patients is approximately 2 per 1000 women. Most of these cancers will be detected at an early stage when they are highly curable. The potential benefit of tamoxifen treatment in breast cancer patients outweighs this risk; however, all patients receiving tamoxifen should undergo regular gynaecologic evaluations.

Of the chemotherapy drugs used in the treatment of early breast cancer alkylating agents (cyclophosphamide) and anthracyclines increase the risk for MDS and AML, but the incidence is less than 1%. Alkylating agent–related AML typically develops after an average latency of 5–7 years, and overt leukemia is often (up to 70% of cases) proceeded by a dysplastic phase, whereas the latency period between exposure to anthracyclines and the onset of leukemia is usually about 2 years, and generally there is no previous myelodysplastic phase.

REFERENCES

1. Torre LA, Bray F, Siegel RL, Ferlay J, Lortet-Tieulent J, and Jemal A. Global cancer statistics, 2012. *CA Cancer J Clin* 2015;65(2):87–108.
2. Forouzanfar MH, Foreman KJ, Delossantos AM, Lozano R, Lopez AD, Murray CJ, and Naghavi M. Breast and cervical cancer in 187 countries between 1980 and 2010: a systematic analysis. *Lancet* 2011;378:1461–84.

3. Neal L, Sandhu NP, Hieken TJ, Glazebrook KN, Mac Bride MB, Dilaveri CA, Wahner-Roedler DL, Ghosh K, and Visscher DW. Diagnosis and management of benign, atypical, and indeterminate breast lesions detected on core needle biopsy. *Mayo Clin Proc* 2014;89:536–47.

4. Miki Y, Swensen J, Shattuck-Eidens D, et al. A strong candidate for the breast and ovarian cancer susceptibility gene BRCA1. *Science* 1994;266:66–71.

5. Wooster R, Bignell G, Lancaster J, Swift S, Seal S, Mangion J, Collins N, Gregory S, Gumbs C, and Micklem G. Identification of the breast cancer susceptibility gene BRCA2. *Nature* 1995;378:789–92.

6. Apostolou P, and Fostira F. Hereditary breast cancer: the era of new susceptibility genes. *Biomed Res Int* 2013:747318.

7. Melchor L, and Benitez J, The complex genetic landscape of familial breast cancer. *Hum Genet* 2013;132:845–63.

8. McBride KA, Ballinger ML, Killick E, Kirk J, Tattersall MH, Eeles RA, Thomas DM and Mitchell G. Li-Fraumeni syndrome: cancer risk assessment and clinical management. *Nat Rev Clin Oncol* 2014;11:260–71.

9. Pilarski R, Burt R, Kohlman W, Pho L, Shannon KM, and Swisher E. Cowden syndrome and the PTEN hamartoma tumour syndrome: systematic review and revised diagnostic criteria. *J Natl Cancer Inst* 2013;105:1607–16.

10. Corso G, Figueiredo J, Biffi R, et al. E-cadherin germline mutation carriers: clinical management and genetic implications. *Cancer Metastasis Rev* 2014;33:1081–94.

11. Yiannakopoulou E. Etiology of familial breast cancer with undetected BRCA1 and BRCA2 mutations: clinical implications. *Cell Oncol (Dordr)* 2014;37:1–8.

12. Sakoda LC, Jorgenson E, and Witte JS. Turning of COGS moves forward findings for hormonally mediated cancers. *Nat Genet* 2013;45:345–8.

13. Milne RL, Herranz J, Michailidou K, et al. A large-scale assessment of two-way SNP interactions in breast cancer susceptibility using 46,450 cases and 42,461 controls from the breast cancer association consortium. Hum *Mol Genet* 2014;23:1934–46.

14. Michailidou K, Hall P, Gonzalez-Neira A, et al. Large-scale genotyping identifies 41 new loci associated with breast cancer risk. *Nat Genet* 2013;45:353–61, 61e1–2.

15. Evans DG, Gareth ED, Kesavan N, et al. MRI breast screening in high-risk women: cancer detection and survival analysis. *Breast Cancer Res Treat* 2014;145:663–72.

16. Pharoah PD, Antoniou A, Bobrow M, Zimmern RL, Easton DF, and Ponder BA. Polygenic susceptibility to breast cancer and implications for prevention. *Nat Genet* 2002;31:33–6.

17. Green VL. Breast cancer risk assessment, prevention, and the future. *Obstet Gynecol Clin North Am* 2013;40:525–49.

18. Cuzick J, Sestak I, Bonanni B, et al. Selective oestrogen receptor modulators in prevention of breast cancer: an updated meta-analysis of individual participant data. *Lancet* 2013;381:1827–34.

19. Goss PE, Ingle JN, Ales-Martinez JE, et al. Exemestane for breast-cancer prevention in postmenopausal women. *N Engl J Med* 2011;364:2381–91.

20. Cuzick J, Sestak I, Forbes JF, et al. Anastrozole for prevention of breast cancer in high-risk postmenopausal women (IBIS-II): an international, double-blind, randomised placebo-controlled trial. *Lancet* 2014;383:1041–8.

21. Ingham SL, Sperrin M, Baildam A, Ross GL, Clayton R, Lalloo F, Buchan I, Howell A, and Evans DG. Risk-reducing surgery increases survival in BRCA1/2 mutation carriers unaffected at time of family referral. *Breast Cancer Res Treat* 2013;142:611–8.

22. Heemskerk-Gerritsen BA, Rookus MA, Aalfs CM, et al. Improved overall survival after contralateral risk-reducing mastectomy in BRCA1/2 mutation carriers with a history of unilateral breast cancer: a prospective analysis. *Int J Cancer* 2015;136:668–77.

23. Cooper BT, Murphy JO, Sacchini V, and Formenti SC. Local approaches to hereditary breast cancer. *Ann Oncol* 2013;24(Suppl.8):viii54–60.

24. Degnim AC, and King TA. Surgical management of high-risk breast lesions. *Surg Clin North Am* 2013;93:329–40.

25. Menes TS, Rosenberg R, Balch S, Jaffer S, Kerlikowske K, and Miglioretti DL. Upgrade of high-risk breast lesions detected on mammography in the Breast Cancer Surveillance Consortium. *Am J Surg* 2014;207:24–31.

26. Middleton LP, Sneige N, Coyne R, Shen Y, Dong W, Dempsey P, and Bevers TB. Most lobular carcinoma in situ and atypical lobular hyperplasia diagnosed on core needle biopsy can be managed clinically with radiologic follow-up in a multidisciplinary setting. *Cancer Med* 2014;3:492–9.

27. Lakhani S, Ellis I, Schnitt S, Tan P, and van de Vijver M. *WHO Classification of Tumours of the Breast*. Lyon: IARC Press, 2012.

28. Rakha EA, and Ellis IO. Modern classification of breast cancer: should we stick with morphology or convert to molecular profile characteristics. *Adv Anat Pathol* 2011;18:255–67.

29. Sobin LH, Gospodarowicz MK, and Wittekind C, eds. *TNM Classification of Malignant Tumours*. Oxford: Wiley-Blackwell, 2009.

30. Elston CW, and Ellis IO. Pathological prognostic factors in breast cancer. I. The value of histological grade in breast cancer: experience from a large study with long-term follow-up. *Histopathology* 1991;19:403–10.

31. Viale G. The current state of breast cancer classification. *Ann Oncol* 2012;23(Suppl.10):x207–10.

32. Vaz-Luis I, Winer EP, and Lin NU. Human epidermal growth factor receptor-2-positive breast cancer: does estrogen receptor status define two distinct subtypes? *Ann Oncol* 2013;24:283–91.

33. Goldhirsch A, Winer EP, Coates AS, Gelber RD, Piccart-Gebhart M, Thürlimann B, Senn HJ, and Panel Members. Personalizing the treatment of women with early breast cancer: highlights of the St Gallen International Expert Consensus on the Primary Therapy of Early Breast Cancer 2013. *Ann Oncol* 2013;24:2206–23.

34. Sorlie T, Perou CM, Tibshirani R, et al. Gene expression patterns of breast carcinomas distinguish tumour subclasses with clinical implications. *Proc Natl Acad Sci USA* 2001;98:10869–74.

35. Engelhardt EG, Garvelink MM, de Haes JH, van der Hoeven JJ, Smets EM, Pieterse AH, and Stiggelbout AM. Predicting and communicating the risk of recurrence and death in women with early-stage breast cancer: a systematic review of risk prediction models. *J Clin Oncol* 2014;32:238–50.

36. Oakman C, Santarpia L, and Di Leo A. Breast cancer assessment tools and optimizing adjuvant therapy. *Nat Rev Clin Oncol* 2010;7:725–32.

37. Sparano JA. TAILORx: trial assigning individualized options for treatment (Rx). *Clin Breast Cancer* 2006;7:347–50.

38. Cardoso F, Van't Veer L, Rutgers E, Loi S, Mook S, and Piccart-Gebhart MJ. Clinical application of the 70-gene profile: the MINDACT trial. *J Clin Oncol* 2008;26:729–35.

39. Sparano JA, Gray RJ, Makower DF, et al. Prospective validation of a 21-gene expression assay in breast cancer. *N Engl J Med* 2015;373:2005–14.

40. Wishart GC, Bajdik CD, Dicks E, et al. PREDICT Plus: development and validation of a prognostic model for early breast cancer that includes HER-2. *Br J Cancer* 2012;107:800–7.

41. Wishart GC, Rakha E, Green A, Ellis I, Ali HR, Provenzano E, Blows FM, Caldas C, and Pharoah PD. Inclusion of KI67 significantly improves performance of the PREDICT prognostication and prediction model for early breast cancer. *BMC Cancer* 2014;14:908.

42. Tabar L, Fagerberg CJ, Gad A, et al. Reduction in mortality from breast cancer after mass screening with mammography. Randomised trial from the Breast Cancer Screening Working Group of the Swedish National Board of Health and Welfare. *Lancet* 1985;1:829–32.

43. Shen Y, Yang Y, Inoue LY, Munsell MF, Miller AB, and Berry DA. Role of detection method in predicting breast cancer survival: analysis of randomized screening trials. *J Natl Cancer Inst* 2005;97:1195–203.

44. Joensuu H, Lehtimaki T, Holli K, Elomaa L, Turpeenniemi-Hujanen T, Kataja V, Anttila A, Lundin M, Isola J, and Lundin J. Risk for distant recurrence of breast cancer detected by mammography screening or other methods. *JAMA* 2004;292:1064–73.

45. Bordas P, Jonsson H, Nystrom L, and Lenner P. Survival from invasive breast cancer among interval cases in the mammography screening programmes of northern Sweden. *Breast* 2007;16:47–54.

46. Paajanen H, Kyhala L, Varjo R, and Rantala S. Effect of screening mammography on the surgery of breast cancer in Finland: a population-based analysis during the years 1985–2004. *Am Surg* 2006;72:167–71.

47. Cortesi L, Chiuri VE, Ruscelli S, Bellelli V, Negri R, Rashid I, Cirilli C, Fracca A, Gallo E, and Federico M. Prognosis of screen-detected breast cancers: results of a population based study. *BMC Cancer* 2006;6:17.

48. Gotzsche PC, and Olsen O. Is screening for breast cancer with mammography justifiable? *Lancet* 2000;355:129–34.

49. Marmot MG, Altman DG, Cameron DA, Dewar JA, Thompson SG, and Wilcox M. The benefits and harms of breast cancer screening: an independent review. *Br J Cancer* 2013;108:2205–40.

50. Puliti D, Duffy SW, Miccinesi G, de Koning H, Lynge H, Zappa M, Paci E, and Euroscreen Working Group. Overdiagnosis in mammographic screening for breast cancer in Europe: a literature review. *J Med Screen* 2012;19(Suppl.1):42–56.

51. Paci E, and Euroscreen Working Group. Summary of the evidence of breast cancer service screening outcomes in Europe and first estimate of the benefit and harm balance sheet. *J Med Screen* 2012;19(Suppl.1):5–13.

52. Yen MF, Tabar L, Vitak B, Smith RA, Chen HH, and Duffy SW. Quantifying the potential problem of overdiagnosis of ductal carcinoma in situ in breast cancer screening. *Eur J Cancer* 2003;39:1746–54.

53. Duffy SW, Agbaje O, Tabar L, Vitak B, Bjurstam N, Bjorneld L, Myles JP, and Warwick J. Overdiagnosis and overtreatment of breast cancer: estimates of overdiagnosis from two trials of mammographic screening for breast cancer. *Breast Cancer Res* 2005;7:258–65.

54. Breast Screening Frequency Trial Group. The frequency of breast cancer screening: results from the UKCCCR Randomised Trial. United Kingdom Co-ordinating Committee on Cancer Research. *Eur J Cancer* 2002;38:1458–64.

55. Klemi PJ, Toikkanen S, Rasanen O, Parvinen I, and Joensuu H. Mammography screening interval and the frequency of interval cancers in a population-based screening. *Br J Cancer* 1997;75:762–6.

56. Magnus MC, Ping M, Shen MM, Bourgeois J, and Magnus JH. Effectiveness of mammography screening in reducing breast cancer mortality in women aged 39–49 years: a meta-analysis. *J Women's Health (Larchmt)* 2011;20:845–52.

57. Moss SM, Cuckle H, Evans A, Johns L, Waller M, Bobrow L, and Group Trial Management. Effect of mammographic screening from age 40 years on breast cancer mortality at 10 years' follow-up: a randomised controlled trial. *Lancet* 2006;368:2053–60.

58. Pisano ED. Current status of full-field digital mammography. *Radiology* 2000;214:26–8.

59. Pisano ED, and Yaffe MJ. Digital mammography. *Radiology* 2005;234:353–62.

60. Pisano ED, Gatsonis C, Hendrick E, et al. Diagnostic performance of digital versus film mammography for breast-cancer screening. *N Engl J Med* 2005;353:1773–83.

61. Andersson I, Ikeda DM, Zackrisson S, Ruschin M, Svahn T, Timberg P, and Tingberg A. Breast tomosynthesis and digital mammography: a comparison of breast cancer visibility and BIRADS classification in a population of cancers with subtle mammographic findings. *Eur Radiol* 2008;18:2817–25.

62. Ciatto S, Houssami N, Bernardi D, et al. Integration of 3D digital mammography with tomosynthesis for population breast-cancer screening (STORM): a prospective comparison study. *Lancet Oncol* 2013;14:583–9.

63. Skaane P, Bandos AI, Gullien R, Eben EB, Ekseth U, Haakenaasen U, Izadi M, Jebsen IN, Jahr G, Krager M, and Hofvind S. Prospective trial comparing full-field digital mammography (FFDM) versus combined FFDM and tomosynthesis in a population-based screening programme using independent double reading with arbitration. *Eur Radiol* 2013;23:2061–71.

64. Berg WA, Zhang Z, Lehrer D, et al. Detection of breast cancer with addition of annual screening ultrasound or a single screening MRI to mammography in women with elevated breast cancer risk. *JAMA* 2012;307:1394–404.

65. Leach MO, Boggis CR, Dixon AK, et al. Screening with magnetic resonance imaging and mammography of a UK population at high familial risk of breast cancer: a prospective multicentre cohort study (MARIBS). *Lancet* 2005;365:1769–78.

66. Blair S, McElroy M, Middleton MS, Comstock C, Wolfson T, Kamrava M, Wallace A, and Mortimer J. The efficacy of breast MRI in predicting breast conservation therapy. *J Surg Oncol* 2006;94:220–5.

67. Deurloo EE, Klein Zeggelink WF, Teertstra HJ, Peterse JL, Rutgers EJ, Muller SH, Bartelink H, and Gilhuijs KG. Contrast-enhanced MRI in breast cancer patients eligible for breast-conserving therapy: complementary value for subgroups of patients. *Eur Radiol* 2006;16:692–701.

68. Yeh E, Slanetz P, Kopans DB, Rafferty E, Georgian-Smith D, Moy L, Halpern E, Moore R, Kuter I, and Taghian A. Prospective comparison of mammography, sonography, and MRI in patients undergoing neoadjuvant chemotherapy for palpable breast cancer. *AJR Am J Roentgenol* 2005;184:868–77.

69. Londero V, Bazzocchi M, Del Frate C, Puglisi F, Di Loreto C, Francescutti G, and Zuiani C. Locally advanced breast cancer: comparison of mammography, sonography and MR imaging in evaluation of residual disease in women receiving neoadjuvant chemotherapy. *Eur Radiol* 2004;14:1371–9.

70. Pickles MD, Lowry M, Manton DJ, Gibbs P, and Turnbull LW. Role of dynamic contrast enhanced MRI in monitoring early response of locally advanced breast cancer to neoadjuvant chemotherapy. *Breast Cancer Res Treat* 2005;91:1–10.

71. Willems SM, van Deurzen CH, and van Diest PJ. Diagnosis of breast lesions: fine-needle aspiration cytology or core needle biopsy? A review. *J Clin Pathol* 2012;65:287–92.

72. van Rijk MC, Deurloo EE, Nieweg OE, Gilhuijs KG, Peterse JL, Rutgers EJ, Kroger R, and Kroon BB. Ultrasonography and fine-needle aspiration cytology can spare breast cancer patients unnecessary sentinel lymph node biopsy. *Ann Surg Oncol* 2006;13:31–5.

73. Ibrahim AE, Bateman AC, Theaker JM, Low JL, Addis B, Tidbury P, Rubin C, Briley M, and Royle GT. The role and histological classification of needle core biopsy in comparison with fine needle aspiration cytology in the preoperative assessment of impalpable breast lesions. *J Clin Pathol* 2001;54:121–5.

74. Hukkinen K, Kivisaari L, Heikkila PS, Von Smitten K, and Leidenius M. Unsuccessful preoperative biopsies, fine needle aspiration cytology or core needle biopsy, lead to increased costs in the diagnostic workup in breast cancer. *Acta Oncol* 2008;47:1037–45.

75. Pisano ED, Fajardo LL, Tsimikas J, Sneige N, Frable WJ, Gatsonis CA, Evans WP, Tocino I, and McNeil BJ. Rate of insufficient samples for fineneedle aspiration for nonpalpable breast lesions in a multicentre clinical trial: the Radiologic Diagnostic Oncology Group 5 Study. The RDOG5 investigators. *Cancer* 1998;82:679–88.

76. Liberman L. Centennial dissertation. Percutaneous imaging-guided core breast biopsy: state of the art at the millennium. *AJR Am J Roentgenol* 2000;174:1191–9.

77. Darling ML, Smith DN, Lester SC, Kaelin C, Selland DL, Denison CM, DiPiro PJ, Rose DI, Rhei E, and Meyer JE. Atypical ductal hyperplasia and ductal carcinoma in situ as revealed by large-core needle breast biopsy: results of surgical excision. *AJR Am J Roentgenol* 2000;175:1341–6.

78. Brenner RJ, Jackman RJ, Parker SH, et al. Percutaneous core needle biopsy of radial scars of the breast: when is excision necessary? *AJR Am J Roentgenol* 2002;179:1179–84.

79. Halsted WS. The results of radical operations for the cure of carcinoma of the breast. *Ann Surg*, 1907;46:1–19.

80. Fisher B. Biological and clinical considerations regarding the use of surgery and chemotherapy in the treatment of primary breast cancer. *Cancer* 1977;40(Suppl.1):574–87.

81. Hellman S, and Harris JR. The appropriate breast cancer paradigm. *Cancer Res* 1987;47:339–42.

82. Edge SB, Byrd DR, Compton CC, et al., eds. Breast. In *AJCC Cancer Staging Manual*, 7th ed., pp. 347–76. New York, NY: Springer, 2010.

83. Veronesi U, Viale G, Rotmensza N, and Goldhirsch A. Rethinking TNM: breast cancer TNM classification for treatment decision-making and research. *Breast* 2006;15:3–8.

84. Mittendorf EA, Ballman KV, and McCall LM. Evaluation of the stage IB designation of the American Joint Committee on Cancer staging system in breast cancer. *J Clin Oncol* 2015;33:1119–27.

85. Sardanelli F, Boetes C, Borisch B, et al. Magnetic resonance imaging of breast: recommendations from the EUSOMA working group. *Eur J Cancer* 2010;46:1296–316.

86. Cooper KL, Meng Y, Harnan S, Ward SE, Fitzgerald P, Papaioannou D, Wyld L, Ingram C, Wilkinson ID, and Lorenz E. Positron emission tomography (PET) and magnetic resonance imaging (MRI) for the assessment of axillary lymph node metastases in early breast cancer: systematic review and economic evaluation. *Health Technol Assess* 2011;15:iii–iv,1–134.

87. Gradishar WJ, Anderson BO, Blair SL, et al. Breast cancer version 3.2014. *J Natl Compr Canc Netw* 2014;12(4):542–90.

88. Fisher B, Anderson S, Bryant J, et al. Twenty-year follow-up of a randomized trial comparing total mastectomy, lumpectomy, and lumpectomy plus irradiation for the treatment of invasive breast cancer. *N Engl J Med* 2002;347:1233–1241.

89. Veronesi U, Cascinelli N, Mariani L, et al. Twenty-year follow-up of a randomized study comparing breast-conserving surgery with radical mastectomy for early breast cancer. *N Engl J Med* 2002;347:1227–1232.

90. Masetti R, Di Leone A, Franceschini G, et al. Oncoplastic techniques in the conservative surgical treatment of breast cancer: an overview. *Breast J* 2006;12(Suppl.2):S174–S180.

91. Valero VV, Buzdar UA, Hortobagyi GN. Locally advanced breast cancer. *Oncologist* 1996;1:8–17.

92. Makris A, Powles TJ, Ashley SE, et al. A reduction in the requirements for mastectomy in a randomized trial of neoadjuvant chemoendocrine therapy in primary breast cancer. *Ann Oncol* 1998;9(11):1179–1184.

93. Patani N, Carpenter R. Oncological and aesthetic considerations of conservational surgery for multifocal/multicentric breast cancer. *Breast J* 2010;16(3):222–232.

94. White J, Achuthan R, Turton P, Lansdown M. Breast conservation surgery: state of the art. *Int J Breast Cancer* 2011; article ID 107981: 1–10.

95. Feldman SM. Surgical margins in breast conservation. *Int J Surg Oncol* 2013; article ID 136387: 1–2.

96. Simone NL, Dan T, Shih J, et al. Twenty-five year results of the National Cancer Institute randomized breast conservation trial. *Breast Cancer Res Treat* 2012;132(1):197–203.

97. Singletary SE. Surgical margins in patients with early-stage breast cancer treated with breast conservation therapy. *Am J Surg* 2002;184(5):383–393.

98. Morrow M, Harris JR, Schnitt SJ. Surgical margins in lumpectomy for breast cancer, bigger not better. *N Engl J Med* 2012;367:79–82.

99. Moran MS, Schnitt SJ, Giuliano AE, et al. Society of Surgical Oncology–American Society for Radiation Oncology Consensus Guideline on margins for breast-conserving surgery with whole-breast irradiation in stages I and II invasive breast cancer. *Int J Radiat Oncol Biol Phys* 2014;88:553–5644.

100. Cochrane RA, Valasiadou P, Wilson AR, et al. Cosmesis and satisfaction after breast-conserving surgery correlates with the percentage of breast volume excised. *Br J Surg* 2003;90(12):1505–1509.

101. Waljee JF, Hu ES, Newman L, et al. Predictors of re-excision among women undergoing breast-conserving surgery for cancer. *Ann Surg Oncol* 2008;15(5):1297–1303.

102. Baildam A, Bishop H, Boland G, et al. Oncoplastic breast surgery – a guide to good practice. *Eur J Surg Oncol* 2007;33(Suppl.1):S1–S23

103. Clough KB, Thomas SS, Fitoussi AD, et al. Reconstruction after conservative treatment for breast cancer: cosmetic sequelae classification revisited. *Plast Reconstr Surg* 2004;14:1743–1753.

104. Clough KB, Lewis JS, Couturaud B, et al. *Ann Surg* 2003;237(1):26–34.

105. Clough KB, Kaufman GJ, Nos C, et al. Improving breast cancer surgery: a classification and quadrant per quadrant atlas for oncoplastic surgery. *Ann Surg Oncol* 2010;17(5):1375–1391.

106. Holmes D, Schooler W, Smith R. Oncoplastic approaches to breast conservation. *Int J Breast Cancer* 2011; article ID 303879: 1–16.

107. Tenofsky PL, Dowell P, Topalovski T, et al. Surgical, oncologic, and cosmetic differences between oncoplastic and nononcoplastic breast conserving surgery in breast cancer patients. *Am J Surg* 2014;207:398–402.

108. Luini A, Zurrida S, Paganelli G, et al. Comparison of radioguided excision with wire localization of occult breast lesions. *Br J Surg* 1999;86(4):522–525.

109. Nadeem R, Chagla LS, Harris O, et al. Occult breast lesions: a comparison between radioguided occult lesion localization (ROLL) vs. wire-guided lumpectomy (WGL). *Breast* 2005;14(4):283–289.

110. Postma EL, Verkooijen HM, Van Esser S, et al. Efficacy of radioguided occult lesion localisation (ROLL) versus wire guided localisation (WGL) in breast conserving surgery for non-palpable breast cancer: a randomized controlled multicentre trial. *Breast Cancer Res Treat* 2012;136(2):469–478.

111. Monti S, Galimberti V, Trifiro G, et al. Occult lesion localization plus sentinel node biopsy (SNOLL): experience with 959 patients at the European Institute of Oncology. *Ann Surg Oncol* 2007;14(10):2928–2931.

112. Medina-Franco H, Abarca-Perez L, Garcia-Alvarez MN, et al. Radioguided occult lesion localisation (ROLL) versus wire-guided lumpectomy for non-palpable breast lesions: a randomized prospective evaluation. *J Surg Oncol* 2008;97(2):108–111.

113. Sarlos D, Frey LD, Haueisen H, et al. Radioguided occult lesion localization (ROLL) for treatment and diagnosis of malignant and premalignant breast lesions combined with sentinel node biopsy: a prospective clinical trial with 100 patients. *Eur J Surg Oncol* 2009;35(4):403–408.

114. Giacalone PL, Bourdon A, Trinh PD, et al. Radioguided occult lesion localization plus sentinel node biopsy (SNOLL) versus wire guided localization plus sentinel node detection: a case control study of 129 unifocal pure invasive non-palpable breast cancers. *Eur J Surg Oncol* 2012;38(3):222–229.

115. Lovrics PJ, Goldsmith CH, Hodgson N, et al. A multicentred randomized controlled trial comparing radioguided seed localization to standard wire localization for nonpalpable, invasive and in situ breast carcinomas. *Ann Surg Oncol* 2011;18(12):3407–3414.

116. Ahmed M, van Hemelrijk M, Douek M. Systematic review of radioguided versus wire-guided localization in the treatment of non-palpable breast cancers. *Breast Cancer Res Treat* 2013;149:241–252.

117. Ahmed M, Anninga B, Pouw J, et al. Magnetic sentinel node and occult lesion localization (MagSNOLL) in an in vivo porcine model. *Eur J Surg Oncol* 2013;39(11):S81–S82.

118. Pan H, Wu N, Ding H, et al. Intraoperative ultrasound guidance is associated with clear lumpectomy margins for breast cancer: a systematic review and meta-analysis. *PLoS One* 2013;8(9):e74028.

119. Fisher B, Bryant J, Wolmark N, et al. Effect of preoperative chemotherapy on the outcome of women with operable breast cancer. *J Clin Oncol* 1998;16:2672–2685.

120. Mieog JS, van der Hage JA, van de Velde CJ. Neoadjuvant chemotherapy for operable breast cancer. *Br J Surg* 2007;94(10):1189–1200.

121. Semiglazov VF, Semiglazov VV. Neoadjuvant (preoperative) therapy in breast cancer. In *Neoadjuvant Chemotherapy – Increasing Relevance in Cancer Management*, edited by M Markman. Rijeka, Croatia: InTech, 2013. http://www.intechopen.com/books/neoadjuvant-chemotherapy-increasing-relevance-in-cancer-management/neoadjuvant-preoperative-therapy-in-breast-cancer.

122. Boughey JC, McCall LM, Ballman KV, et al. Tumour biology correlates with rates of breast-conserving surgery and pathologic complete response after neoadjuvant chemotherapy for breast cancer: findings from the ACOSOG Z1071 (Alliance) Prospective Multicentre Clinical Trial. *Ann Surg* 2014;260(4):608–614.

123. Baselga J, Bradbury I, Eidtmann H, et al. Lapatinib with trastuzumab for HER-2-positive early breast cancer (NeoALTTO): a randomized, open-label, multicentre phase 3 trial. *Lancet* 2012;379(9816):633–640.

124. Criscitiello C, Azim HA Jr, Agbor-tarth D, et al. Factors associated with surgical management following neoadjuvant therapy in patients with primary HER-2-positive breast cancer: results from the NeoALTTO phase III trial. *Ann Oncol* 2013;24(8):1980–1985.

125. Liedtke C, Mazouni C, Hess KR, et al. Response to neoadjuvant therapy and long-term survival in patients with triple-negative breast cancer. *J Clin Oncol* 2008;26(8):1275–1281.

126. Schott AF, Hayes DF. Defining the benefits of neoadjuvant chemotherapy for breast cancer. *J Clin Oncol* 2012;30(15):1747–1749.

127. Von Minckwitz G, Untch M, Blohmer UJ, et al. Definition and impact of pathologic complete response on prognosis after neoadjuvant chemotherapy in various intrinsic breast cancer subtypes. *J Clin Oncol* 2012;30:1796–1804.

128. Mazouni C, Peintinger F, Wan-Kau S, et al. Residual ductal carcinoma in situ in patients with complete eradication of invasive breast cancer after neoadjuvant chemotherapy does not adversely affect patient outcome. *J Clin Oncol* 2007;25(19):2650–2655.

129. Chen AM, Meric-Bernstam F, Hunt KK, et al. Breast conservation after neoadjuvant chemotherapy. A prognostic index for decision making. *Cancer* 2005;103(4):689695.

130. Madden JL. Modified radical mastectomy. *Surg Gynecol Obstet* 1965;121(6):1221–1230.

131. Zurrida S, Bassi F, Arnone P, et al. The changing face of mastectomy (from mutilation to aid to breast reconstruction). *Int J Surg Oncol* 2011; article ID 980158: 1–7.

132. Tamoxifen for early breast cancer. Early Breast Cancer Trialists' Collaborative Group. *Cochrane Database Syst Rev* 2001;(1).

133. Howell A, Cuzick J, Baum M, et al. Results of the ATAC (arimidex, tamoxifen alone or in combination) trial after completion of 5 years' adjuvant treatment for breast cancer. *Lancet* 2005;365(9453):60–62.

134. Portschy P, Kuntz KM, Tuttle TM. Survival outcomes after contralateral prophylactic mastectomy: a decision analysis. *J Natl Cancer Inst* 2014;106(8).

135. Abbott A, Rueth N, Pappas-Varco S, et al. Perceptions of contralateral breast cancer: an overestimation of risk. *Ann Surg Oncol* 2011;18(11)3129–3136.

136. Davies C, Godwin J, Gray R, et al. Early Breast Cancer Trialists' Collaborative Group. Relevance of breast cancer hormone receptors and other factors to the efficacy of adjuvant tamoxifen: patient-level metaanalysis of randomised trials. *Lancet* 2011;378(9793):771–784.

137. Carlson GW. Technical advances in skin sparing mastectomy. *Int J Surg Oncol* 2011; article ID 396901: 1–7.

138. Freedman GM, Fowble BL. Local recurrence after mastectomy or breast-conserving surgery and radiation. *Oncology* 2000;14:1561–1581.

139. Tokin C, Weiss A, Wang-Rodriguez J, et al. Oncologic safety of skin-sparing and nipple-sparing mastectomy: a discussion and review of the literature. *Int J Surg Oncol* 2012; article ID: 921821: 1–8.

140. Toth BA, Lappert P. Modified skin incisions for mastectomy: the need for plastic surgical input in preoperative planning. *Plast Reconstr Surg* 1991;87(6):1048–1053.

141. Carlson GW. Skin sparing mastectomy: anatomic and technical consideration. *Am Surg* 1996;62(2):151–155.

142. Krohn IT, Cooper DR, Bassett JG. Radical mastectomy: thick vs thin skin flaps. *Arch Surg* 1982;117(6):760–763.

143. Torresan RZ, Santos CCD, Okamura H, et al. Evaluation of residual glandular tissue after skin-sparing mastectomies. *Ann Surg Oncol* 2005;12(12):1037–1044.

144. Ho CM, Mak CKL, Lay Y, et al. Skin involvement in invasive breast carcinoma: safety of skin-sparing mastectomy. *Ann Surg Oncol* 2003;10(2):102–107.

145. Cao D, Tsangaris TN, Kouprina N, et al. The superficial margin of the skin-sparing mastectomy for breast carcinoma: factors predicting involvement and efficacy of additional margin sampling. *Ann Surg Oncol* 2008;15(5):1330–1340.

146. Sheikh F, Rebecca A, Pockaj B, et al. Inadequate margins of excision when undergoing mastectomy for breast cancer: which patients are at risk? *Ann Surg Oncol* 2011;18(4):952–956.

147. Lovrics PJ, Cornacchi SD, Farrokhyar F, et al. The relationship between surgical factors and margin status after breast-conservation surgery for early stage breast cancer. *Am J Surg* 2009;197(6):740–746.

148. Slavin SA, Schnitt SJ, Duda RB, et al. Skin-sparing mastectomy and immediate reconstruction: oncologic risks and aesthetic results in patients with early-stage breast cancer. *Plast Reconstr Surg* 1998;102(1):49–62.

149. Kroll SS, Khoo K. Local recurrence risk after skin-sparing and conventional mastectomy: a 6-year follow-up. *Plast Reconstr Surg* 1999;104(2):421–425.

150. Carlson GW, Styblo TM, Lyles RH, et al. Local recurrence after skin-sparing mastectomy: tumour biology or surgical conservatism? *Ann Surg Oncol* 2003;10(2):108–112.

151. Medina-Franco H, Vasconez LO, Fix RJ, et al. Factors associated with local recurrence after skin-sparing mastectomy and immediate breast reconstruction for invasive breast cancer. *Ann Surg* 2002;235(6);814–819.

152. Spiegel AJ, Butler CE. Recurrence following treatment of ductal carcinoma in situ with skin-sparing mastectomy and immediate breast reconstruction. *Plast Reconstr Surg* 2003;111(2):706–711.

153. Spear SL, Willey S, Feldman E, et al. Nipple-sparing mastectomy for prophylactic and therapeutic indications. *Plast Reconstr Surg* 2011;128(5):1005–1014.

154. Crowe JP, Patrick RJ, Yetman RJ, et al. Nipple-sparing mastectomy update: one hundred forty-nine procedures and clinical outcomes. *Arch Surg* 2008;143(11):1106–1110.

155. Sacchini V, Pinotti JA, Barros ACSD, et al. Nipple-sparing mastectomy for breast cancer and risk reduction: oncologic or technical problem? *J Am Coll Surg* 2006;203(5):704–714.

156. Petit JY, Veronesi U, Orecchia R, et al. Risk factors associated with recurrence after nipple-sparing mastectomy for invasive and intraepithelial neoplasia. *Ann Oncol* 2012;23(8):2053–2058.

157. De Alcantara Filho P, Capko D, Barry JM, et al. Nipple-sparing mastectomy for breast cancer and risk-reducing surgery: the Memorial Sloan-Kettering Cancer Centre experience. *Ann Surg Oncol* 2011;18(11)3117–3112.

158. Stolier AJ, Sullivan SK, Dellacroce FJ. Technical considerations in nipple sparing mastectomy: 82 consecutive cases without necrosis. *Ann Surg Oncol* 2008;15:1341–1347.

159. Voltura AM, Tsangaris TN, Rossion GD, et al. Nipple-sparing mastectomy: critical assessment of 51 procedures and implications for selection criteria. *Ann Surg Oncol* 2008;15:3396–3401.

160. Gerber B, Krause A, Dieterich M. The oncological safety of skin sparing mastectomy with conservation of the nipple-areola complex and autologous reconstruction: an extended follow-up study. *Ann Surg* 2009;249:461–468.

161. Caruso F, Ferrara G, Castiglione G, et al. Nipple-sparing subcutaneous mastectomy: sixty-six months follow-up. *Eur J Surg Oncol* 2006;32(9):937–940.

162. Benediktsson KP, Perbeck L. Survival in breast cancer after nipple-sparing subcutaneous mastectomy and immediate reconstruction with implants: a prospective trial with 13 years median follow-up in 216 patients. *Eur J Surg Oncol* 2008;34(2):143–148.

163. Spear SL, Parikh PM, Reisin E, et al. Acellular dermis-assisted breast reconstruction. *Aesth Plast Surg* 2008;32:418–425.

164. Spear SL, Meshabi AN. Implant based reconstruction. *Clin Plast Surg* 2007;34(1):63–73.

165. Cordeiro PG, McCarthy CM. A single surgeon's 12-year experience with tissue expander/implant breast reconstruction: parts I and II. *Plast Reconstr Surg* 2006;118:825–839.

166. Breuing KH, Warren SM. Immediate bilateral breast reconstruction with implants and inferolateral AlloDerm slings. *Ann Plast Surg* 2005;55:232–239.

167. Glasberg SB, Light D. AlloDerm and Strattice in breast reconstruction: a comparison and techniques for optimizing outcomes. *Plast Reconstr Surg* 2012;129(6):1223–1233.

168. Himsl I, Drinovac V, Lenhard M, et al. The use of porcine acellular dermal matrix in silicone implant-based breast reconstruction. *Arch Gynaecol Obstet* 2012;286(1):187–192.

169. Ho G, Nguyen TJ, Shahabi A, et al. A systematic review and meta-analysis of complications associated with acellular dermal matrix assisted breast reconstruction. *Ann Plast Surg* 2012;68:346–356.

170. Salzberg CA, Dunavant C, Nocera N. Immediate breast reconstruction using porcine acellular dermal matrix (Strattice): long-term outcomes and complications. *J Plast Reconstr Aesthet Surg* 2013;66(3):323–328.

171. Jeevan R, Cromwell D, Browne J, et al. Third annual report of the national mastectomy and breast reconstruction audit 2010. Leeds: NHS Information Centre, 2010. www.ic.nhs.uk/mbr

172. Johnson RK, Wright CK, Ghandi A, et al. Cost minimisation analysis of using acellular dermal matrix (Strattice) for breast reconstruction compared with standard techniques. *Eur J Surg Oncol* 2013;39:242–247.

173. Jones G. The use of acellular dermal matrices in implant-based breast reconstruction. In *Oncoplastic and Reconstructive Breast Surgery*, edited by C Urban, M Rietjens. Milan: Springer Verlag Italia, 2013.

174. Kim JYS, Long JN. Breast reconstruction with acellular dermis. Medscape, 2011. http://emedicine.medscape.com/article/1851090-overview.

175. Butterfield JL. 440 consecutive immediate, implant-based, single-surgeon breast reconstructions in 281 patients: a comparison of early outcomes and costs between SurgiMend fetal bovine and AlloDerm human cadaveric acellular dermal matrices. *Plast Reconstr Surg* 2012;131(5):940–951.

176. Martin L, O'Donoghue JM, Horgan K, et al. Acellular dermal matrix (ADM) assisted breast reconstruction procedures. Joint Guidelines from the Association of Breast Surgery and the British Association of Plastic, Reconstructive and Aesthetic Surgeons. *Eur J Surg Oncol* 2013;39:425–429.

177. Newman MI. Avoiding and managing complications with acellular dermal matrices in breast reconstruction. In *QMP's Plastic Surgery Pulse News*, vol. 3, no. 4. St. Louis: Quality Medical Publishing, 2009.

178. Nguyen TJ, Carey JN, Wong AK. Use of human acellular dermal matrix in implant based breast reconstruction: evaluating the evidence. *J Plast Reconstr Aesthet Surg* 2011;64:1553–1561.

179. Spear SL, Seruya M, Clemens MW, et al. Acellular dermal matrix for the treatment and prevention of implant-associated breast deformities. *Plast Reconstr Surg* 2011;127(3):1047–1058.

180. Goyal A, Wu JM, Chandran VP, et al. Outcome after autologous dermal sling assisted immediate breast reconstruction. *Br J Surg* 2011;98:1267–1272.

181. Nava MB, Cortinovis U, Ottolenghi J, et al. Skin-reducing mastectomy. *Plast Reconstr Surg* 2006;118:603–610.

182. Hammond DC, Capraro PA, Ozolins EB, et al. Use of skin-sparing reduction pattern to create a combination skin-muscle flap pocket in immediate breast reconstruction. *Plast Reconstr Surg* 2002;110:206–211.

183. Carlson G. Technical advances in skin sparing mastectomy. *Int J Surg Oncol* 2011; article ID 396901.

184. Delay E, Ho Quoc H. Autologous latissimus dorsi breast reconstruction. In *Oncoplastic and Reconstructive Breast Surgery*, edited by C Urban, M Rietjens, 267–275. Milan: Springer Verlag Italia, 2013.

185. Weiler-Mithoff EM, Chew BK. Free flaps. In *Oncoplastic and Reconstructive Breast Surgery*, edited by C Urban, M Rietjens, 295–304. Milan: Springer Verlag Italia, 2013.

186. Fisher B, Montague E, Redmond C, et al. Findings from NSABP protocol no. B-04-comparison of radical mastectomy with alternative treatments for primary breast cancer. I. Radiation compliance and its relation to treatment outcome. *Cancer* 1980;46(1):1–13.

187. Orr RK. The impact of prophylactic axillary node dissection on breast cancer survival – a Bayesian meta-analysis. *Ann Surg Oncol.* 1999;6(1):109–16.

188. Berg JW. The significance of axillary node levels in the study of breast carcinoma. *Cancer* 1955;8(4):776–8.

189. Rosen PP, Lesser ML, Kinne DW, et al. Discontinuous or skip metastasis in breast carcinoma. Analysis of 1228 axillary dissections. *Ann Surg* 1983;197(3):276–83.

190. Thomson DR, Sadideen H, Furniss D. Wound drainage after axillary dissection for carcinoma of the breast. *Cochrane Database Syst Rev* 2013;20:10.

191. Kuroi K, Shimozuma K, Taguchi T, et al. Effect of mechanical closure of dead space on seroma formation after breast surgery. *Breast Cancer* 2006;13(3):260–5.

192. Cortadellas T, Córdoba O, Espinosa-Bravo M, et al. Electrothermal bipolar vessel sealing system in axillary dissection: a prospective randomized clinical study. *Int J Surg* 2011;9(8):636–40.

193. Van Bemmel AJM, van de Velde CJH, Schmitz RF, et al. Prevention of seroma formation after axillary dissection in breast cancer: a systematic review. *Eur J Surg Oncol* 291;37(10):820–35.

194. Carcoforo P, Soliani G, Maestroni U, et al. Octreotide in the treatment of lymphorrhea after axillary node dissection: a prospective randomized controlled trial. *J Am Coll Surg* 2003;196(3):365–9.

195. Mansel RE, Fallowfield L, Kissin M, et al. Randomized multicentre trial of sentinel node biopsy versus standard axillary treatment in operable breast cancer: the ALMANAC trial. *J Natl Cancer Inst* 2006;98:599–609.

196. Thompson M, Korourian S, Henry-Tillman R, et al. Axillary reverse mapping (ARM): a new concept to identify and enhance lymphatic preservation. *Ann Surg Oncol* 2007;14:1890–95.

197. Nos C, Leiseur B, Clough KB, et al. Blue dye injection in the arm in order to conserve the lymphatic drainage of the arm in breast cancer patients requiring an axillary dissection. *Ann Surg Oncol* 2007;14:2490–6.

198. Bland K, Klimberg VS. *Axillary Reverse Mapping in Mastery Techniques in General Surgery: Breast Surgery.* Philadelphia: Lippincott, Williams & Wilkins, 2011: 201–8.

199. Ochoa D, Korourian S, Boneti C, et al. Axillary reverse mapping: five year experience. *Surgery* 2014;156(5):1261–8.

200. Gennaro M, Maccauro M, Sigari C, et al. Selective axillary dissection after axillary reverse mapping to prevent breast-cancer-related lymphoedema. *Eur J Surg Oncol* 2013;39:1341–45.

201. Tausch C, Baege A, Dietrich D, et al. Can axillary reverse mapping avoid lymphedema in node positive breast cancer patients? *Eur J Surg Oncol* 2013;39:880–6.

202. Rubio IT, Cebrecos I, Peg V, et al. Extensive nodal involvement increases the positivity of blue nodes in the axillary reverse mapping procedure in patients with breast cancer. *J Surg Oncol* 2012;106(1):89–93.

203. Noguchi M, Yokoi M, Nakano Y. Axillary reverse mapping with indocyanine fluorescence imaging in patients with breast cancer. *J Surg Oncol* 2010;101:217–21.

204. Krag DN, Anderson SJ, Julian TB, et al. Sentinel-lymph-node resection compared with conventional axillary-lymph-node dissection in clinically node-negative patients with breast cancer: overall survival findings from the NSABP B-32 randomised phase 3 trial. *Lancet Oncol* 2010;11(10):927–33.

205. Veronesi U, Viale G, Paganelli G, et al. Sentinel lymph node biopsy in breast cancer: ten-year results of a randomized controlled study. Ann Surg 2010;251(4):595–600.

206. Krag D, Weaver D, Ashikaga T, et al. The sentinel node in breast cancer – a multicentre validation study. *N Engl J Med* 1998;339(14):941–6.

207. Rubio I, Korourian S, Cowan C, et al. Sentinel lymph node biopsy for staging breast cancer. *Am J Surg* 1998;176(6):532–7.

208. Ledenius M, Krogerus L, Toivonen T. The sensitivity of axillary staging when using sentinel node biopsy in breast cancer. *Eur J Surg Oncol* 2003;29(10):849–53.

209. Giuliano AE, Jones RC, Brennan M, et al. Sentinel lymphadenectomy in breast cancer. *J Clin Oncol* 1997;15:2345–50.

210. Borgstein PJ, Meijer S, Pijpers RJ, et al. Functional lymphatic anatomy for sentinel node biopsy in breast cancer: echoes from the past and the periareolar blue method. *Ann Surg* 2000;232:81–89.

211. Albertini JJ, Lyman GH, Cox C, et al. Lymphatic mapping and sentinel node biopsy in the patient with breast cancer. *JAMA* 1996;276:1818–22.

212. Cody HS III, Fey J, Akhurst T, et al. Complementarity of blue dye and isotope in sentinel node localization for breast cancer: univariate and multivariate analysis of 966 procedures. *Ann Surg Oncol* 2001;8:13–9.

213. Raut CP, Hunt KK, Akins JS, et al. Incidence of anaphylactoid reactions to isosulfan blue dye during breast carcinoma lymphatic mapping in patients treated with preoperative prophylaxis: results of a surgical prospective clinical practice protocol. Cancer 2005;104(4):692–9.

214. McMasters KM, Wong SL, Tuttle TM, et al. Preoperative lymphoscintigraphy for breast cancer does not improve the ability to identify axillary sentinel lymph nodes. *Ann Surg* 2000;231(5):724–31.

215. Giammarile F, Alazraki N, Aarsvold JN, et al. The EANM and SNMMI practice guideline for lymphoscintigraphy and sentinel node localization in breast cancer. *Eur J Nucl Med Mol Imaging* 2013;40(12):1932–47.

216. Klimberg VS, Rubio IT, Henry R, et al. Subareolar versus peritumoural injection for location of the sentinel lymph node. *Ann Surg* 1999;229(6):860–5.

217. Rodier JF, Velten M, Wilt M, et al. Prospective multicentric randomized study comparing periareolar and peritumoural injection of radiotracer and blue dye for the detection of sentinel lymph node in breast sparing procedures: FRANSENODE trial. *J Clin Oncol* 2007;25(24):3664–9.

218. Martin RC, Derossis AM, Fey J, et al. Intradermal isotope injection is superior to intramammary in sentinel node biopsy for breast cancer. *Surgery* 2001;130:432–8.

219. Leppänen E, Leidenius M, Krogerus L, et al. The effect of patient and tumour characteristics on visualization of sentinel nodes after a single intratumoural injection of Tc99m labelled human albumin colloid in breast cancer. *Eur J Surg Oncol* 2002;28(8):821–6.

220. Estourgie SH, Nieweg OE, Olmos RA, et al. Lymphatic drainage patterns from the breast. *Ann Surg* 2004;239(2):232–7.

221. Sadeghi R, Asadi M, Treglia G, et al. Axillary concordance between superficial and deep sentinel node mapping material injections in breast cancer patients: systematic review and meta-analysis of the literature. *Breast Cancer Res Treat* 2014;144:213–22.

222. Leidenius MH, Krogerus LA, Toivonen TS, et al. The clinical value of parasternal sentinel node biopsy in breast cancer. *Ann Surg Oncol* 2006;13(3):321–6.

223. Hennequin C, Fourquet A. Controversy about internal mammary chain irradiation in breast cancer. *Cancer Radiother* 2004;18:351–5.

224. Chung A, Yu J, Stempel M, et al. Is the "10% rule" equally valid for all subsets of sentinel-node-positive breast cancer patients? *Ann Surg Oncol* 200815(10):2728–33.

225. Goyal A, Newcombe RG, Mansel RE. Axillary Lymphatic Mapping Against Nodal Axillary Clearance (ALMANAC) Trialists Group. Clinical relevance of multiple sentinel nodes in patients with breast cancer. *Br J Surg* 2005;92(4):438–42.

226. Clough KB, Nasr R, Nos C, et al. New anatomical classification of the axilla with implications for sentinel node biopsy. *Br J Surg* 2010;97(11):1659–65.

227. Galimberti V, Manika A, Maisonneuve P, et al. Long-term follow-up of 5262 breast cancer patients with negative sentinel node and no axillary dissection confirms low rate of axillary disease. *Eur J Surg Oncol* 2014;40(10):1203–8.

228. Naik AM, Fey J, Gemignani M, et al. The risk of axillary relapse after sentinel lymph node biopsy for breast cancer is comparable with that of axillary lymph node dissection: a follow-up study of 4008 procedures. *Ann Surg* 2004;240(3):462–8.

229. van der Ploeg IM, Nieweg OE, van Rijk MC, et al. Axillary recurrence after a tumour negative sentinel node biopsy in breast cancer patients: a systematic review and meta-analysis of the literature. *Eur J Surg Oncol* 2008;34(12):1277–84.

230. Ballardini B, Santoro L, Sangalli C, et al. The indocyanine green method is equivalent to the 99 mTc-labeled radiotracer method for identifying the sentinel node in breast cancer: a concordance and validation study. *Eur J Surg Oncol* 2013;39(12):1332–6.

231. Thill M, Kurylcio A, Welter R, et al. The Central European SentiMag study: sentinel lymph node biopsy with superparamagnetic iron oxide (SPIO) vs. radioisotope. *Breast* 2014;23(2):175–9.

232. Douek M, Klaase J, Monypenny I, et al. Sentinel node biopsy using a magnetic tracer versus standard technique: the SentiMAG Multicentre Trial. *Ann Surg Oncol* 2014;21(4):1237–45.

233. Rubio IT, Diaz-Botero S, Esgueva A, et al. The superparamagnetic iron oxide is equivalent to the Tc99 radiotracer method for identifying the sentinel lymph node in breast cancer. *Eur J Surg Oncol* 2015;41(1):46–51.

234. Hunt KK, Ballman KV, McCall LM, et al. Factors associated with local-regional recurrence after a negative sentinel node dissection: results of the ACOSOG Z0010 trial. *Ann Surg* 2012;256(3):428–36.

235. Tamaki Y, Akiyama F, Iwase T, et al. Molecular detection of lymph node metastases in breast cancer patients: results of a multicentre trial using the one-step nucleic acid amplification assay. *Clin Cancer Res* 2009;15(8):2879–84.

236. Espinosa-Bravo M, Sansano I, Pérez-Hoyos S, et al. Prediction of non-sentinel lymph node metastasis in early breast cancer by assessing total tumoural load in the sentinel lymph node by molecular assay. *Eur J Surg Oncol* 2013;39(7):766–73.

237. Peg V, Espinosa-Bravo M, Vieites B, et al. Intraoperative molecular analysis of total tumour load in sentinel lymph node: a new predictor of axillary status in early breast cancer patients. *Breast Cancer Res Treat* 2013;139(1):87–93.

238. Intra M, Rotmensz N, Veronesi P, et al. Sentinel node biopsy is not a standard procedure in ductal carcinoma in situ of the breast: the experience of the European Institute of Oncology on 854 patients in 10 years. *Ann Surg* 2008;247(2):315–9.

239. Meretoja TJ, Heikkila PS, Salmenkivi K, et al. Outcome of patients with ductal carcinoma in situ and sentinel node biopsy. *Ann Surg Oncol* 2012;19(7):2345–51.

240. Siponen E, Hukkinen K, Heikkilä P, Joensuu H, Leidenius M. Surgical treatment in Paget's disease of the breast. *Am J Surg* 2010;200(2):241–6.

241. Balmana J, Diez O, Rubio IT, Cardoso F. BRCA in breast cancer: ESMO clinical practice guidelines. *Ann Oncol* 2011;22(Suppl.6):31–34.

242. Gentilini O, Cremonesi M, Toesca A, et al. Sentinel lymph node biopsy in pregnant patients with breast cancer. *Eur J Nucl Med Mol Imaging* 2010;37:78–83.

243. Menard JP, Extra JM, Jacquemier J, et al. Sentinel lymphadenectomy for the staging of clinical axillary node-negative breast cancer before neoadjuvant chemotherapy. *Eur J Surg Oncol* 2009;35(9):916–20.

244. Hunt KK, Yi M, Mittendorf EA, Guerrero C, et al. Sentinel lymph node surgery after neoadjuvant chemotherapy is accurate and reduces the need for axillary dissection in breast cancer patients. *Ann Surg* 2009;250(4):558–66.

245. Boileau JF, Poirier B, Basik M, et al. Sentinel node biopsy after neoadjuvant chemotherapy in biopsy-proven node-positive breast cancer: the SN FNAC study. *J Clin Oncol* 2015;33(3):258–64.

246. Van Deurzen CH, Vriens BE, Tjan-Heijen VC, et al. Accuracy of sentinel node biopsy after neoadjuvant chemotherapy in breast cancer patients. *Eur J Cancer* 2009;45(18):3124–30.

247. Kuehn T, Bauerfeind I, Fehm T, et al. Sentinel-lymph-node biopsy in patients with breast cancer before and after neoadjuvant chemotherapy (SENTINA): a prospective, multicentre cohort study. *Lancet Oncol* 2013;14:609–18.

248. Boughey JC, Suman VJ, Mittendorf EA, et al. Sentinel lymph node surgery after neoadjuvant chemotherapy in patients with node-positive breast cancer: the ACOSOG Z1071 (Alliance) clinical trial. *JAMA* 2013;310:1455–61.

249. Donker M, Straver ME, Wesseling J, et al. Marking axillary lymph nodes with radioactive iodine seeds for axillary staging after neoadjuvant systemic treatment in breast cancer patients: the MARI procedure. *Ann Surg* 2015;261(2):378–82.

250. Giuliano AE, Hunt KK, Ballman KV, et al. Axillary dissection vs no axillary dissection in women with invasive breast cancer and sentinel node metastasis: a randomized clinical trial. *JAMA* 2011;305(6):569–75.

251. Lyman GH, Temin S, Edge SB, et al. Sentinel lymph node biopsy for patients with early-stage breast cancer: American Society of Clinical Oncology clinical practice guideline update. *J Clin Oncol.* 2014;32(13):1365–83.

252. Galimberti V, Cole BF, Zurrida S, et al. International Breast Cancer Study Group Trial 23-01 investigators. Axillary dissection versus no axillary dissection in patients with sentinel-node micrometastases (IBCSG 23–01): a phase 3 randomised controlled trial. *Lancet Oncol* 2013;14:297–305.

253. Donker M, van Tienhoven G, Straver ME, et al. Radiotherapy or surgery of the axilla after a positive sentinel node in breast cancer (EORTC 10981-22023 AMAROS): a randomised, multicentre, open-label, phase 3 non-inferiority trial. *Lancet Oncol* 2014;15:1303–10.

254. van Wely BJ, de Wilt JH, Francissen C, et al. Meta-analysis of ultrasound-guided biopsy of suspicious axillary lymph nodes in the selection of patients with extensive axillary tumour burden in breast cancer. *Br J Surg* 2015;102(3):159–68.

255. Mittendorf EA, Hunt KK, Boughey JC, et al. Incorporation of sentinel lymph node metastasis size into a nomogram predicting nonsentinel lymph node involvement in breast cancer patients with a positive sentinel lymph node. *Ann Surg* 2012;255:109–15.

256. Van Zee KJ, Manasseh DM, Bevilacqua JL, et al. A nomogram for predicting the likelihood of additional nodal metastases in breast cancer patients with a positive sentinel node biopsy. *Ann Surg Oncol* 2003;10:1140–51.

257. Coutant C, Olivier C, Lambaudie E, et al. Comparison of models to predict nonsentinel lymph node status in breast cancer patients with metastatic sentinel lymph nodes: a prospective multicenter study. *J Clin Oncol* 2009;27:2800–8.

258. Meretoja TJ, Leidenius MH, Heikkila PS, et al. International multicentre tool to predict the risk of nonsentinel node metastasis in breast cancer. *J Natl Cancer Inst* 2012;104(24):1888–96.

259. Rubio IT, Espinosa-Bravo M, Rodrigo M, et al. Nomogram including the total tumoural load in the sentinel nodes assessed by one step nucleic acid amplification as a new factor for predicting nonsentinel lymph node metastasis in breast cancer patients. *Breast Cancer Res Treat* 2014;147(2):371–80.

260. Martelli G, Boracchi P, Ardoino I, et al. Axillary dissection versus no axillary dissection in older patients with T1N0 breast cancer: 15-year results of a randomized controlled trial. *Ann Surg* 2012;256:920–4.

261. Martelli G, Boracchi P, Orenti A, Lozza L, Maugeri I, Vetrella G, Agresti R. Axillary dissection versus no axillary dissection in older T1N0 breast cancer patients: a 15- year results of trial and out trial patients *Eur J Surg Oncol* 2014;40(7):805–12.

262. Rudenstam CM, Zahrieh D, Forbes JF, et al. International Breast Cancer Study Group. Randomized trial comparing axillary clearance versus no axillary clearance in older patients with breast cancer: first results of International Breast Cancer Study Group Trial 10-93. *J Clin Oncol* 2006;24(3):337–44.

263. Gentilini O, Veronesi U. Abandoning sentinel lymph node biopsy in early breast cancer? A new trial in progress at the European Institute of Oncology of Milan (SOUND: Sentinel Node vs Observation after Axillary Ultrasound). *Breast* 2012;21(5):678–81.

264. Offersen BV, Boersma LJ, Kirkove C, et al. ESTRO consensus guideline on target volume delineation for elective radiation therapy of early stage breast cancer. *Radiother Oncol* 2015;114(1):3–10.

265. Fisher B, Bauer M, Margolese R, et al. Five-year results of a randomized clinical trial comparing total mastectomy and segmental mastectomy with or without radiation in the treatment of breast cancer. *N Engl J Med* 1985;312(11):665–73.

266. Veronesi U, Saccozzi R, Del Vecchio M, et al. Comparing radical mastectomy with quadran-tectomy, axillary dissection, and radiotherapy in patients with small cancers of the breast. *N Engl J Med* 1981;305(1):6–11.

267. Donovan E, Bleakley N, Denholm E, et al. Randomised trial of standard 2D radiotherapy (RT) versus intensity modulated radiotherapy (IMRT) in patients prescribed breast radiotherapy. *Radiother Oncol* 2007;82:254–64.

268. Haviland JS, Owen JR, Dewar JA, et al. The UK Standardisation of Breast Radiotherapy (START) tri-als of radiotherapy hypofractionation for treatment of early breast cancer: 10-year follow-up results of two randomised controlled trials. *Lancet Oncol* 2013;14(11):1086–94.

269. Whelan TJ, Pignol JP, Levine MN, et al. Long-term results of hypofractionated radiation therapy for breast cancer. *N Engl J Med* 2010;362(6):513–20.

270. Vaidya JS, Wenz F, Bulsara M, Tobias JS, et al. Risk-adapted targeted intraoperative radiotherapy versus whole-breast radiotherapy for breast cancer: 5-year results for local control and overall sur-vival from the TARGIT-A randomised trial. *Lancet* 2014;383(9917):603–13.

271. Veronesi U, Orecchia R, Maisonneuve P, et al. Intraoperative radiotherapy versus external radio-therapy for early breast cancer (ELIOT): a ran-domised controlled equivalence trial. *Lancet Oncol* 2013;14(13):1269–77.

272. Strnad V, Ott OJ, Hildebrandt G, et al. 5-year results of accelerated partial breast irradiation using sole inter-stitial multicatheter brachytherapy versus whole-breast irradiation with boost after breast-conserving surgery for low-risk invasive and in-situ carcinoma of the female breast: A randomised, phase 3, non-inferiority trial. *Lancet* 2016;387(10015):229–38.

273. Lansu JT, Essers M, Voogd AC, et al. The influence of simultaneous integrated boost, hypofractionation and oncoplastic surgery on cosmetic outcome and PROMs after breast conserving therapy. *Eur J Surg Oncol* 2015;41(10):1411–16.

274. EBCTCG McGale P, Taylor C, Correa C, et al. Effect of radiotherapy after mastectomy and axillary surgery on 10-year recurrence and 20-year breast cancer mortality: meta-analysis of individual patient data for 8135 women in 22 randomised trials. *Lancet*, 2014;383:2127–35.

275. Kelley BP, Ahmed R, Kidwell KM, Kozlow JH, Chung KC, and Momoh AO. A systematic review of morbidity associated with autologous breast reconstruction before and after exposure to radiotherapy: Are current practices ideal? *Ann Surg Oncol* 2014;21(5):1732–8.

276. Momoh AO, Ahmed R, Kelley BP, Aliu O, Kidwell KM, Kozlow JH, and Chung KC. A systematic review of complications of implant-based breast reconstruc-tion with prereconstruction and postreconstruction radiotherapy. *Ann Surg Oncol* 2014;21(1):118–24.

277. Reish RG, Lin A, Phillips NA, Winograd J, Liao EC, Cetrulo Jr. CL, Smith BL, Austen Jr. WG, and Colwell AS. Breast reconstruction outcomes after nipple-sparing mastectomy and radiation therapy. *Plast Reconstr Surg* 2015;135:959–66.

278. Behranwala KA, Dua RS, Ross GM, Ward A, A'Hern R, and Gui GP. The influence of radiotherapy on capsule formation and aesthetic outcome after immediate breast reconstruction using biodi-mensional anatomical expander implants. *J Plast Reconstr Aesthet Surg* 2006;59:1043–51.

279. Ribuffo D, Monfrecola A, Guerra M, Di Benedetto GM, Grassetti L, Spaziani E, Vitagliano T, and Greco M. Does postoperative radiation therapy represent a contraindication to expander-implant based immediate breast reconstruction? An update 2012–2014. *Eur Rev Med Pharmacol Sci* 2015;19:2202–7.

280. Valdatta L, Cattaneo AG, Pellegatta I, Scamoni S, Minuti A, and Cherubino M. Acellular dermal matrices and radiotherapy in breast reconstruction: a systematic review and meta-analysis of the literature. *Plast Surg Int* 2014:472604.

281. Schaverien MV, Macmillan RD, and McCulley SJ. Is immediate autologous breast reconstruction with postoperative radiotherapy good practice? A systematic review of the literature. *J Plast Reconstr Aesthet Surg* 2013;66:1637–51.

282. EBCTCG. Effects of chemotherapy and hormonal therapy for early breast cancer on recurrence and 15-year survival: an overview of the randomised tri-als. *Lancet* 2005;365:1687–717.

283. EBCTCG. Comparisons between different poly-chemotherapy regimens for early breast cancer: meta-analyses of long term outcome among 100 000 women in 123 randomised trials. *Lancet* 2012;379:432–44.

284. Kaufmann M, von Minckwitz G, Mamounas E, et al. Recommendations from an international consensus conference on the current status and future of neo-adjuvant systemic therapy in primary breast cancer. *Ann Surg Oncol* 2012;19:1508–16.

285. von Minckwitz G, Untch M, Blohmer JU, et al. Definition and impact of pathologic complete response on prognosis after neoadjuvant chemotherapy in various intrinsic breast cancer subtypes. *J Clin Oncol* 2012;30:1796–804.

286. Davies C, Pan H, Godwin J, et al. Long-term effects of continuing adjuvant tamoxifen to 10 years versus stopping at 5 years after diagnosis of oestrogen receptor-positive breast cancer: ATLAS, a randomised trial. *Lancet* 2013;381:805–16.

287. Francis PA, Regan MM, Fleming GF, et al. Adjuvant ovarian suppression in premenopausal breast cancer. *N Engl J Med* 2015;372(5):436–46.

288. Pagani O, Regan MM, Walley BA, et al. Adjuvant exemestane with ovarian suppression in premenopausal breast cancer. *N Engl J Med* 2014;371:107–118.

289. Dowsett M, Cuzick J, Ingle J, et al. Meta-analysis of breast cancer outcomes in adjuvant trials of aromatase inhibitors versus tamoxifen. *J Clin Oncol* 2010;28:509–18.

290. Regan MM, Neve P, Giobbie-Hurder A, et al. Assessment of letrozole and tamoxifen alone and in sequence for postmenopausal women with steroid hormone receptor-positive breast cancer: the BIG 1–98 randomised clinical trial at 8.1 years median follow-up. *Lancet Oncol* 2011;12:1101–8.

291. Coleman R, Gnant M, Paterson A, et al. Effects of bisphosphonate treatment on recurrence and cause-specific mortality in women with early breast cancer: a meta-analysis of individual patient data from randomized trials. Presented at 2013 San Antonio Breast Cancer Symposium, December 12, 2013, abstract S4-07.

292. Wyld L, Gutteridge E, Pinder SE, James JJ, Chan SY, Cheung SY, Robertson JF, and Evans AJ. Prognostic factors for patients with hepatic metastases from breast cancer. *Br J Cancer* 2003;89:284–90.

293. James JJ, Evans AJ, Pinder SE, Gutteridge E, Cheung KL, Chan S, and Robertson JF. Bone metastases from breast carcinoma: histopathological-radiological correlations and prognostic features. *Br J Cancer* 2003;89:660–5.

294. Dieci MV, Barbieri E, Piacentini F, et al. Discordance in receptor status between primary and recurrent breast cancer has a prognostic impact: a single-institution analysis. *Ann Oncol* 2013;24(1):101–8.

295. Ruiterkamp J, Voogd AC, Bosscha K, Tjan-Heijnen VC, and Ernst MF. Impact of breast surgery on survival in patients with distant metastases at initial presentation: a systematic review of the literature. *Breast Cancer Res Treat* 2010;120:9–16.

296. Tai YC, Domchek S, Parmigiani G, Chen S. Breast cancer risk among male BRCA1 and BRCA2 mutation carriers. *J Natl Cancer Inst* 2007;99(23):1811–4.

297. Cardoso F, Bartlett J, Slaets L, van Deurzen C, et al. Characterization of male breast cancer: first results of the EORTC10085/TBCRC/BIG/NABCG International Male BC Program. Presented at San Antonio Breast Cancer Conference 2014, abstract S6-05.

298. Fields EC, DeWitt P, Fisher CM, et al. Management of male breast cancer in the United States: a surveillance, epidemiology and end results analysis. *Int J Radiat Oncol Biol Phys* 2013;87(4):747–52.

299. Maráz R, Boross G, Pap-Szekeres J. The role of sentinel node biopsy in male breast cancer. *Breast Cancer* 2016;23(1):85–91.

300. Partridge AH, Pagani O, Abulkhair O, et al. First international consensus guidelines for breast cancer in young women (BCY1). *Breast* 2014;23:209–20.

301. Cardoso F, Loibl S, Pagani O, Graziottin A, et al. The European Society of Breast Cancer Specialists recommendations for the management of young women with breast cancer. *Eur J Cancer* 2012;48(18):3355–77.

302. Early Breast Cancer Trialists' Collaborative Group (EBCTCG), Darby S, McGale P, et al. Effect of radiotherapy after breast conserving surgery on 10-year recurrence and 15-year breast cancer death: meta-analysis of individual patient data for 10,801 women in 17 randomised trials. *Lancet* 2011;378(9804):1707–16.

303. Poortmans P, Aznar M, Bartelink H. Quality indicators for breast cancer: revisiting historical evidence in the context of technology changes. *Semin Radiat Oncol* 2012;22(1):29–39.

304. Arvold ND, Taghian AG, Niemierko A, et al. Age, breast cancer subtype approximation, and local recurrence after breast-conserving therapy. *J Clin Oncol* 2011;29(29):3885–91.

305. Adkins FC, Gonzalez-Angulo A, Lei X, et al. Triple negative breast cancer is not a contraindication for breast conservation. *Ann Surg Oncol* 2011;18:3164–73.

306. Biganzoli L, Wildiers H, Oakman C, et al. Management of elderly patients with breast cancer: updated recommendations of the International Society of Geriatric Oncology (SIOG) and European Society of Breast Cancer Specialists (EUSOMA). *Lancet Oncol* 2012;13(4):e148–60.

307. Hughes KS, Schnaper LA, Berry D, et al. Lumpectomy plus tamoxifen with or without irradiation in women 70 years of age or older with early breast cancer. *N Engl J Med* 2004;351:971–77.

308. Amant F, Deckers S, van Calsteren K, et al. Breast cancer in pregnancy: recommendations of an international consensus meeting. *Eur J Cancer* 2010;46:3158–68.

309. Amant F, Loibl S, Neven P, et al. Breast cancer in pregnancy. *Lancet* 2012;379:570–79.

310. Gentilini O, Cremonesi M, Toesca A, et al. Sentinel lymph node biopsy in pregnant patients with breast cancer. *Eur J Nucl Med Mol Imaging* 2010;37(1):78–83.

311. Loibl S, Han SN, von Minckwitz G, et al. Treatment of breast cancer during pregnancy: an observational study. *Lancet Oncol* 2012;13(9):887–96.

312. de Bresser J, de Vos B, van der Ent F, Hulsewé K. Breast MRI in clinically and mammographically occult breast cancer presenting with an axillary metastasis: a systematic review. *Eur J Surg Oncol* 2010 Feb;36(2):114–9.

313. Barton SR, Smith IE, Kirby AM, Ashley S, Walsh G, Parton M. The role of ipsilateral breast radiotherapy in management of occult primary breast cancer presenting as axillary lymphadenopathy. *Eur J Cancer* 2011;47(14):2099–106.

314. Siponen E, Hukkinen K, Heikkilä P, Joensuu H, Leidenius M. Surgical treatment in Paget's disease of the breast. *Am J Surg* 2010;200(2):241–6.

315. Young JL, Ward KC, Wingo PA, and Howe HL. The incidence of malignant non-carcinomas of the female breast. *Cancer Causes Control* 2004;15:313–9.

316. Onkendi EO, Jimenez RE, Spears GM, Harmsen WS, Ballman KV, and Hieken TJ. Surgical treatment of borderline and malignant phyllodes tumours: the effect of the extent of resection and tumour characteristics on patient outcome. *Ann Surg Oncol* 2014;21:3304–9.

317. Mituś J, Reinfuss M, Mituś JW, Jakubowicz J, Blecharz P, Wysocki WM, and Skotnicki P. Malignant phyllodes tumour of the breast: treatment and prognosis. *Breast J* 2014;20:639–44.

318. McCarthy E, Kavanagh J, O'Donoghue Y, McCormack E, D'ArcyC, and O'Keeffe SA. Phyllodes tumours of the breast: radiological presentation, management and follow-up. *Br J Radiol* 2014;87:20140239.

319. Depla AL, Scharloo-Karels CH, de Jong MA, et al. Treatment and prognostic factors of radiation-associated angiosarcoma (RAAS) after primary breast cancer: a systematic review. *Eur J Cancer* 2014;50:1779–88.

320. Chugh R, and Baker L. Nonepithelial malignancies of the breast. *Oncology (Williston Park)* 2004;18:665–73; discussion 73–6.

321. Cheah CY, Campbell BA, and Seymour JF. Primary breast lymphoma. *Cancer Treat Rev* 2014;40:900–8.

322. DeLair DF, Corben AD, Catalano JP, Vallejo CE, Brogi E, and Tan LK. Non-mammary metastases to the breast and axilla: a study of 85 cases. *Mod Pathol* 2013;26:343–9.

23

Lung and pleura

MICHAEL SHACKCLOTH

INCIDENCE AND AETIOLOGY OF LUNG CANCER

Introduction and incidence

Lung cancer is the leading cause of cancer deaths in the UK in both males and females. It is the second most common cancer in men and women after prostate and breast cancer, respectively. In Europe more than 410,000 new cases were diagnosed in 2012 [1]. The highest rates are in Hungary for men and Denmark for women [1]. Figure 23.1 shows the incidence of lung cancer within Europe. In the UK 1 in 14 men and 1 in 18 women will develop lung cancer.

The incidence of lung cancer increases with age. It rises steeply from the age of 40 years and peaks in those aged greater than 80 years. Forty percent of cases are diagnosed in patients over the age of 75 years and almost 90% occur in patients over the age of 60 years.

Lung cancer occurs more frequently in males, although the difference between males and females is closing. This almost certainly reflects trends in smoking habit over time. Over the last 10 years, the incidence of lung cancer in males is decreasing in the UK but has increased in females. This decrease in males is probably due to the prevalence of cigarette smoking in men peaking about two decades earlier than in women.

Lung cancer carries a poor prognosis with an overall survival rate of 10.9% at 5 years [2]. There is significant variation in the 5-year survival rates of lung cancer across Europe [2]. Survival rates are highest in Scandinavia, Belgium and Switzerland [2].

Non–small cell lung cancer (NSCLC) makes up about 87% of all lung cancers, small cell lung cancer (SCLC) 12% and carcinoid tumours 1% [3]. There are different types of non–small cell lung cancer. The main types are adenocarcinoma and squamous cell carcinoma. The incidence of

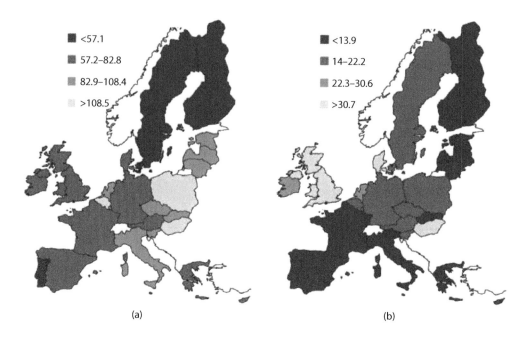

Figure 23.1 Age-standardized incidence rates (per 100,000 people) in the European Union (2000). (Reproduced with the permission of Cancer Research UK.)

adenocarcinoma is increasing and that of squamous cell carcinoma decreasing [4].

Surgery is generally accepted as offering the best chance of cure in patients with NSCLC where a complete resection of the tumour can be achieved, there is no evidence of metastatic disease and the patient is fit enough to tolerate the operation. SCLC is generally treated with chemotherapy and radiotherapy for limited disease, and chemotherapy for advanced disease.

Aetiology

The aetiology of lung cancer can be conceptualized as the interactions between an individual's exposure to aetiological agents and their susceptibility to these agents [4]. Most doctors have seen examples of this concept in clinical practice. On advising a patient to give up smoking one has heard the response 'my father smoked 60 cigarettes a day and he didn't get lung cancer', or on informing a patient of the diagnosis of lung cancer, hearing 'I only smoked 5 cigarettes a day'. There is a complex synergistic interaction between risk factors for lung cancer, often making it difficult to determine the effect an individual factor has on the incidence of lung cancer.

Cigarette smoking is the major cause of lung cancer. Eighty to ninety percent of cases are caused by lung cancer [4]. Other factors associated with lung cancer include pipe and cigar smoking [5,6], passive smoking [5,7], cannabis smoking [4], radon exposure [8] and exposure to chemicals such as asbestos [9], arsenic [10], silica [11], coal and coke fumes [12], beryllium [13] and nickel.

Smoking is by far the major cause of lung cancer. Both SCLC and NSCLC are caused by cigarette smoking [14]. The

duration of smoking and the number of cigarettes smoked affect an individual's risk of developing lung cancer [15]. Smoking 25 cigarettes per day increases the risk of lung cancer 25-fold. Smoking cessation is of benefit at any age; ex-smokers have a lower risk of lung cancer than current smokers [16]. As the time from quitting smoking increases the lung cancer risk decreases [17]. However, the risk of lung cancer remains elevated in ex-smokers even 40 years after giving up [17].

There has been a relative increase in adenocarcinoma of the lung compared with squamous cell carcinoma of the lung over the last few decades. This may be due to changes in cigarettes to low-yield filtered ones [18].

Passive smoking is a risk factor for developing lung cancer. It does not matter what the source of the smoke is; however, the evidence is strongest when a non-smoker lives with a smoker, where they have a 20–30% increased risk [17,19].

Lung cancer is the most common cancer caused by occupational exposure to carcinogens [20]. Asbestos exposure causes as many cases of lung cancer as it does mesothelioma. There is a fivefold increase in lung cancer in people exposed to asbestos; the greater the exposure to asbestos, the greater the risk [21]. The effect of asbestos exposure and cigarette smoking is synergistic [22].

Radon is an inert gas that is formed in the decay of uranium. When uranium decays, it releases particles which can damage DNA. Lung cancer has been found to have an increased incidence in uranium miners [23]. The effects of radon are synergistic with cigarette smoking [23]. Radon escapes from the ground and enters buildings causing indoor pollution. It has been shown that exposure to increased levels of radon in indoor air is associated with an increased incidence of lung cancer [24,25].

In addition to the aetiological factors discussed above, there are several intrinsic factors that make someone more susceptible to lung cancer. A family history is strongly associated with an increased risk of lung cancer [26].

The potential role of infections, especially TB, in the aetiology of lung cancer is well documented [27]. HIV infection may be a risk factor for lung cancer. Lung cancer is the third most common malignancy in patients with HIV behind lymphoma and Kaposi's sarcoma [28]. This appears to be additional to the increased risk caused by the increased incidence of smoking in patients with HIV.

A lot is known about the aetiology of lung cancer. Preventative strategies to reduce the risk of exposure to carcinogens, such as a ban on smoking in public places, are likely to have a much bigger impact on the number of deaths from lung cancer than any advances in surgery, chemotherapy or radiotherapy.

SCREENING FOR LUNG CANCER

In order for a screening programme for any cancer to be successful, the following criteria need to be met:

1. The disease must be common.
2. There must be a sensitive test to diagnose the cancer, i.e. few false negatives.
3. Any test must be specific to detect the cancer, i.e. low number of false positives.
4. The test must be safe and acceptable to patients.
5. The cancers detected must be treatable.
6. The programme must be cost-effective.

At first glance, screening for lung cancer fits most of these criteria; early-stage disease is curable by surgery, smoking is the major risk factor and a highly sensitive screening test is available. Low-dose CT scanning is recommended in the United States for screening patients at risk of lung cancer aged under 80 years [29]. The problems with screening are the physical harm the screening test may cause, the harm of further investigations of abnormal findings and the harm of treatment. There are also cost implications associated with any screening programme. In this section the various methods used for screening for lung cancer and the current literature will be reviewed.

Chest X-ray and sputum cytology

Several randomized studies have shown there is no benefit of screening for lung cancer with a chest X-ray (CXR) or sputum cytology [30–33].

In the Memorial Sloan Kettering study [32] and Johns Hopkins study [33], 10,040 male smokers and 10,387 patients, respectively, were randomized to either annual CXR or annual CXR and 4-monthly sputum cytology. The Mayo clinic study [31] randomized 9211 patients to annual CXR and sputum cytology or 4-monthly CXR and sputum cytology. None of these three studies showed a decrease in lung cancer mortality in the intervention group. In a study in high-risk males in the former Czechoslovakia, Kubik et al. [30] also found there was no benefit of CXR and sputum cytology screening compared with no intervention.

Nearly one-third of the lung cancers detected on first examination on the dual screen, and 14% of those on subsequent examinations, were found by cytological examination. However, there was no difference in survival [31,32]. This suggests that these cancers may be more indolent.

The Prostate, Lung, Colorectal and Ovarian Cancer (PLCO) Screening Trial [34] randomized 154,901 patients to annual CXR or usual care. This trial found that chest radiography screening did not reduce lung cancer mortality. This was also true when a subgroup analysis was carried out for patients that fit the criteria for the National Lung Cancer Screening Trial [35].

Computerized tomography

Data from the Early Lung Cancer Action Project (ELCAP) showed that in a high-risk population, CT scanning was superior to CXR at detecting lung nodules and early lung cancer [36]. These findings led to renewed interest in lung cancer screening, but with the use of CT scanning rather than CXR and sputum cytology. There have been several randomized trials investigating the use of low-dose CT for screening for lung cancer. The largest of these trials, the National Lung Cancer Screening Trial (NLST) [35], randomized 53,454 smokers or ex-smokers (<15 years) with at least a 30 pack-year history to yearly CT scan or CXR for 3 years. The trial was stopped a year early because the prespecified 20% reduction in lung cancer mortality had been reached in the low-dose CT arm. In this group there was a 6.7% reduction in all-cause mortality. Three hundred and twenty patients required screening to save one life.

Several European studies are underway and some have published interim results. The DANTE trial (Detection and Screening of Early Lung Cancer by Novel Imaging Technology and Molecular Essays) [37] randomized 2472 men with a greater than 20 pack-year smoking history to annual CT scan or clinic review. There was no difference in the lung cancer mortality or all-cause mortality in the two groups.

The Danish Lung Cancer Screening Trial (DLCST) [38] recruited 4104 patients with a greater than 20 pack-year smoking history to annual CT scan or usual care. The Multicentre Italian Lung Detection (MILD) study [39] randomized 4099 patients with a 20 pack-year history into three groups: annual CT, biennial CT or usual care. There was no difference in the lung cancer mortality or all-cause mortality in either study. All three European studies were underpowered to detect a difference in lung cancer mortality. There was also inadequate randomization, unclear allocation, differences in baseline demographic characteristics, differential follow-up or relatively short duration of follow-up in one or more of the studies [40].

One of the downsides of screening with low-dose CT scanning is its low positive predicted value. Subsequent procedures are often needed to obtain a diagnosis. These procedures are usually non-invasive, such as repeat CT and PET-CT scans; however, some may be invasive, such as CT-guided biopsy, bronchoscopy, endobronchial ultrasound scanning or surgery.

The risks of low-dose CT are very small. It has a radiation exposure similar to that of mammography [40]. Annual screening with low-dose CT is estimated to cause 1 radiation-induced lung cancer death for every 22 deaths it prevents [41].

Screening may cause psychological harm to those involved. In both the NELSON study [42] and DLCST [38], screening did not affect overall anxiety or quality of life. In the NELSON study anxiety was increased in patients who required further investigations following the screening CT but returned to baseline soon after the second screen [42].

Conclusions

Low-dose CT scanning can significantly reduce mortality from lung cancer in targeted populations. This has to be balanced against the risks associated with false positives. In the future, biomarkers from blood or exhaled breath may help predict individuals at high risk of lung cancer and aid in CT screening [43]. Smoking cessation will, however, remain the most important strategy in reducing lung cancer deaths.

DIAGNOSIS AND STAGING

Accurate diagnosis and staging of lung cancer is essential in order to provide the patient with the best possible treatment. Obtaining a histological diagnosis is necessary in patients fit enough to undergo treatment for lung cancer to ensure the most appropriate treatment is considered. The complexity of the process is increased by the need to also consider whether the patient is fit enough to undergo the proposed treatment.

TNM staging system

The 7th edition of the tumour, node, metastasis (TNM) staging system is currently used to treat NSCLC [44], SCLC [45] and neuroendocrine tumours of the lung [46]. This edition was based on the dataset of 68,463 patients with NSCLC and 13,032 with SCLC [47].

The main changes in the 7th edition include:

1. Tumours that were greater than 7 cm were reclassified from T2 to T3.
2. Tumour nodules in the same lobe, ipsilateral or contralateral lobes were changed to T3, T4 and M1a, respectively.
3. Pleural effusions were reclassified to M1a.

The TNM descriptors are shown in Table 23.1.

Stage groupings of TNM subsets

Various TNM groupings are classified into stages I–IV depending on survival [44]. These are shown in Table 23.1.

Stage IV disease is any T, any N with M1a or M1b (Table 23.1).

Symptoms and signs of lung cancer

One of the problems with diagnosing lung cancer is that symptoms and signs do not present until a late stage. This explains why 49% of patients present with stage IV disease [3]. With the increased usage of CT pulmonary angiograms, CT coronary angiograms and CT scanning to follow up other cancers, more lung cancers are being diagnosed at an earlier stage.

Like any cancer, the signs and symptoms can be divided into local symptoms, symptoms due to metastatic disease and constitutional symptoms. This section will concentrate on the local symptoms and the paraneoplastic symptoms that can be produced by certain histological types of lung cancers.

The local symptoms of lung cancer are varied and depend on the location of the tumour and the extent of spread. They include persistent cough, haemoptysis, chest or shoulder pain, dyspnoea, wheezing, stridor, hoarse voice, chest infection, weakness, pain and paraesthesia in the arm, and those of superior vena cava obstruction (oedema of the upper body and dilated veins on the upper chest wall).

Chest pain is one of the most accurate methods to assess whether a tumour involves the pleura or chest wall. Chest pain that is pleuritic in nature suggests that the tumour may be invading the parietal pleura and require an extrapleural strip at operation to remove the tumour. Pain that is constant in nature, and gradually becoming more severe, suggests probable chest wall invasion and may require a chest wall resection.

Pancoast's syndrome was described in 1924 [48]. It comprises Horner's syndrome (anhidrosis, meiosis and ptosis), arm pain and atrophy of the hand muscles. In 1929 Pancoast reported the link between this syndrome and superior sulcus tumours of the lung (Pancoast's tumours) [49]. Superior sulcus tumours account for between 3% and 5% of all lung cancers. The symptoms are caused by the invasion of the stellate ganglion of the sympathetic chain and the lower brachial plexus (Figure 23.2).

Paraneoplastic syndromes occur in 7–15% of patients with lung cancer [50]. They most often occur in SCLC. The most common ones are:

1. Hypercalcaemia due to tumours secreting parathyroid hormone–related protein, calcitriol or other cytokines including osteoclast-activating factors. One must remember that bony metastases remain the most common cause of hypercalcaemia in patients with lung cancer.
2. Finger clubbing or hypertrophic pulmonary osteoarthropathy is observed in 12% of patients with adenocarcinoma of the lung and less commonly in other cell types [51]. The exact pathogenesis is unknown.

Table 23.1 TNM staging of lung cancers

	Description
T stage	
T0	Primary tumour cannot be assessed, or cancer proven by the presence of malignant cells in sputum or bronchial washings but not visualized by imaging or bronchoscopy.
T_{is}	Carcinoma in situ.
T1	Tumour 3 cm or less in greatest dimension, surrounded by lung or visceral pleura, without bronchoscopic evidence of invasion more proximal than the lobar bronchus (e.g. not in the main bronchus).
T1a	Tumour 2 cm or less in greatest dimension.
T1b	Tumour more than 2 cm but 3 cm or less in greatest dimension.
T2	Tumour more than 3 cm but 7 cm or less or tumour with any of the following features (T2 tumours with these features are classified T2a if 5 cm or less): involves main bronchus, 2 cm or more distal to the carina; invades visceral pleura (PL1 or PL2); associated with atelectasis or obstructive pneumonitis that extends to the hilar region but does not involve the entire lung.
T2a	Tumour more than 3 cm but 5 cm or less in greatest dimension.
T2b	Tumour more than 5 cm but 7 cm or less in greatest dimension.
T3	Tumour more than 7 cm or one that directly invades any of the following: parietal pleural, chest wall (including superior sulcus tumours), diaphragm, phrenic nerve, mediastinal pleura, parietal pericardium; or tumour in the main bronchus less than 2 cm distal to the carina but without involvement of the carina; or associated atelectasis or obstructive pneumonitis of the entire lung or separate tumour nodule(s) in the same lobe.
T4	Tumour of any size that invades any of the following: mediastinum, heart, great vessels, trachea, recurrent laryngeal nerve, oesophagus, vertebral body, carina, separate tumour nodule(s) in a different ipsilateral lobe.
N stage	
N0	No regional lymph node metastases
N1	Metastasis in ipsilateral peribronchial and/or ipsilateral hilar lymph nodes and intrapulmonary nodes, including involvement by direct extension
N2	Metastasis in ipsilateral mediastinal and/or subcarinal lymph node(s)
N3	Metastasis in contralateral mediastinal, contralateral hilar, ipsilateral or contralateral scalene, or supraclavicular lymph node(s)
M stage	
M0	No distant metastasis
M1	Distant metastasis
M1a	Separate tumour nodule(s) in a contralateral lobe, tumour with pleural nodules or malignant pleural (or pericardial) effusion
M1b	Distant metastasis (outside the thorax)

3. Syndrome of inappropriate antidiuretic hormone (SIADH) production. Elevated levels of ADH can be found in 30–70% of patients with lung cancer [52]. Only a few of these patients will have symptoms. It is more common in SCLC but can occur in NSCLC.

4. Cushing's syndrome from ectopic adrenocorticotropic hormone (ACTH). ACTH is the most common hormone produced in lung cancer. This is most commonly associated with SCLC but can occur in bronchial carcinoids [53].

Diagnosis and staging investigations

There are a large number of investigations used to diagnose and stage lung cancer. The sequence of investigations varies depending on a number of factors including clinical features, prior radiological findings, patient's fitness, intended treatment, availability of the investigation, cost of the investigation and patient preference. The investigation carried out first should be the one that yields the most information with the least risk to the patient.

CXR

A CXR is usually the first investigation carried out in a patient with symptoms that may suggest lung cancer. However, once the decision has been made to proceed to a CT scan, a CXR has little to add. A lateral CXR is no longer required as it adds nothing additional to a CT scan.

CT SCAN

A CT scan is the investigation of choice in a patient with suspected lung cancer. It should be a contrast-enhanced CT scan of the lower neck (from vocal cords), chest and upper abdomen. It should include the liver and adrenals. The scan of the lower neck allows visualization of any N3 nodes, and

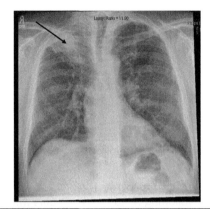

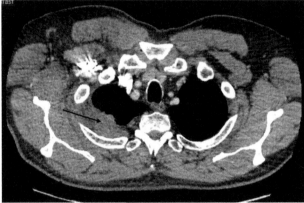

Figure 23.2 CXR and CT scan showing a superior sulcus tumour of the right lung (arrowed).

the adrenal glands should be included as metastases are present in 7% of lung cancer patients at presentation [54]. The CT scan should be performed prior to bronchoscopy in order to allow better-targeted bronchial washings and brushings [55].

CT scanning is very good at determining the T stage of a suspected lung cancer except where there is doubt over mediastinal invasion.

The size of mediastinal lymph nodes on CT scan is an important predictor of involvement with cancer, although it should be remembered that lymph nodes may be enlarged for other reasons such as distal atelectasis, pneumonia or other underlying pulmonary pathology. Lymph nodes less than 10 mm in short axis have less than a 15% chance of containing metastatic cancer, those 10–20 mm a 50% chance and those greater than 20 mm more than an 85% chance of containing metastatic cancer. This measurement should be used in combination with other investigations to determine the need for sampling of these lymph nodes. The site of lymph nodes should be documented according to the International Association for the Study of Lung Cancer (IALSC) study lymph node map (Figure 23.3) [56].

BRONCHOSCOPY

Fibre-optic bronchoscopy is one of the first diagnostic and staging investigations in a patient with a suspected lung cancer. Any visible tumour can be biopsied. Bronchial washing

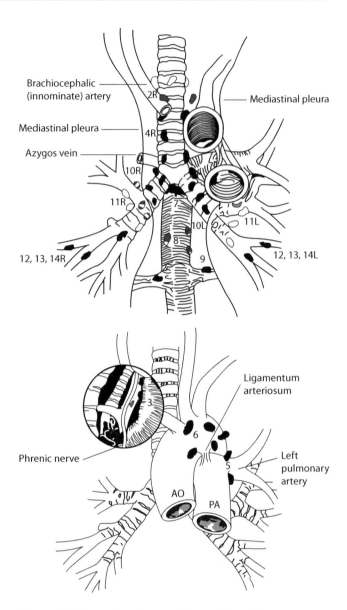

Figure 23.3 Lymph node map for staging of lung cancer. Single-digit stations represent mediastinal lymph nodes (N2) and double-digit N1 lymph nodes. PA, pulmonary artery; AO, aorta; R, right; L, left. (From Rusch VW, et al., *Journal of Thoracic Oncology*, 4(5), 568–77, 2009.)

and brushings can be taken from the bronchopulmonary segment containing the tumour on the CT scan to try to obtain a cytological diagnosis. Previously transbronchial needle aspiration could be performed at the same time to sample hilar and mediastinal lymph nodes; however, this has been replaced by endobronchial ultrasound scanning (EBUS).

PET-CT SCANNING

PET-CT scanning should be routinely used to assess the primary tumour, mediastinal lymph nodes and the presence or absence of distant metastasis in all patients potentially suitable for treatment with curative intent. The most common tracer used is ^{18}F-2-fluorodeoxyglucose (FDG), although gadolinium PET-CT is gaining popularity in neuroendocrine tumours.

Limitations of PET-CT are well recognized. False negatives may occur in tumours less than 8 mm, bronchioalveolar cell carcinomas and carcinoid tumours

A high systemic uptake value (SUV_{max}) of the tumour has been associated with a poor prognosis [57]. Therefore patients with a high SUV_{max} may warrant more detailed staging investigation including an MRI of the brain.

PET-CT is more accurate than CT scanning alone at assessing mediastinal lymph node status [58]. PET-CT is good at identifying adrenal metastasis with a sensitivity of 94–100% and specificity of 80–100% [59–64].

ENDOBRONCHIAL ULTRASOUND SCANNING

EBUS has largely replaced cervical mediastinoscopy in staging the mediastinum in patients prior to surgery for lung cancer. It is less invasive and can be carried out under local anaesthetic. Lymph node stations 2, 3, 4, 7, 10 and 11 can be sampled by EBUS. It has a sensitivity for staging the mediastinal nodes of 88–93% and a specificity of 100% [65,66].

Endo-oesophageal ultrasound (EUS) can be used to sample stations 7, 8 and 9.

Any lymph node that is greater than 10 mm in short axis or positive on PET scanning should be biopsied. Meta-analyses have shown that endosonographic mediastinal staging (EBUS and EUS) is equivalent to that of surgical staging.

MEDIASTINOSCOPY

There is currently debate about whether patients with a negative EBUS should undergo cervical mediastinoscopy. If the EBUS is to be solely relied upon, it is important to ascertain whether it is a negative EBUS (normal lymph node content), rather than a failed EBUS (bronchial mucosa or no lymphoid tissue). EBUS is operator dependent and whether a mediastinoscopy is required will depend on local results. The significance of a false negative EBUS is under debate as these patients have microscopic mediastinal lymph node involvement and may benefit from surgical treatment.

A cervical mediastinoscopy is performed under general anaesthesia with the patient supine and the neck extended. A 2–3 cm horizontal incision is made two fingerbreadths above the suprasternal notch. The superficial tissues are divided until the strap muscles are reached. The vertical raphe between the muscles is divided and they are retracted laterally. The pre-tracheal fascia is then divided. The video mediastinascope is inserted under the pre-tracheal fascia along the trachea. Lymph node stations 2, 4 and 7 can be biopsied. The lower lymph nodes should be biopsied first. Haemostasis can be achieved with diathermy and the wound closed in layers. If there is a possibility the pleura may have been opened, then a CXR should be carried out postoperatively to look for the presence of a pneumothorax. The procedure can be done as a day case. Complications specific to a cervical mediastinoscopy include bleeding due to major blood vessel damage, pneumothorax, recurrent laryngeal nerve injury and tracheal damage. Images from a mediastinoscopy are shown in Figure 23.4.

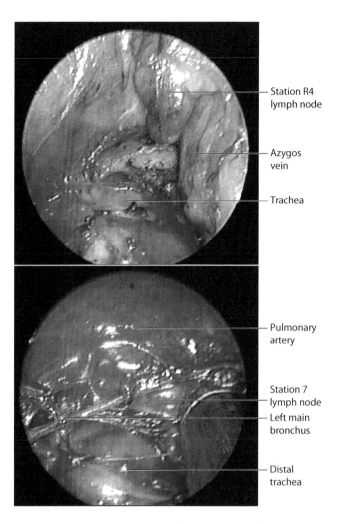

Figure 23.4 Operative views of station R4 and station 7 lymph nodes at mediastinoscopy.

ANTERIOR MEDIASTINOTOMY OR VIDEO-ASSISTED THORACIC SURGERY

Traditionally an anterior mediastinotomy (Chamberlain's procedure) has been used to stage patients with enlarged or PET-positive station 5 lymph nodes. The patient is positioned supine with a double-lumen endotracheal tube. A horizontal left parasternal incision, 5–6 cm in length overlying the second or third intercostal space, is made. The intercostal muscle is divided on the superior aspect of the rib taking care not to damage the neurovascular bundle. Resection of the rib is not usually necessary. The pleura then can be retracted laterally and the lymph nodes biopsied.

With advances in minimally invasive surgery, VATS is now being more commonly used to biopsy station 5 lymph nodes. Besides having the advantage of being minimally invasive, the whole pleural cavity can be assessed and lymph node stations 7, 8 and 9 can also be biopsied.

CT BIOPSY

This is performed for biopsy lesions not accessible via the bronchial tree. It is a relatively safe technique, but it does have complications. These include a 3–5% risk of pneumothorax

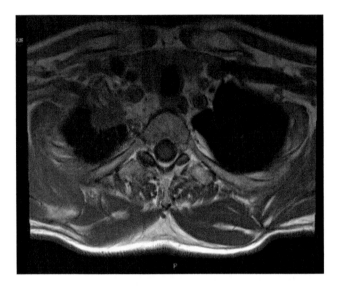

Figure 23.5 MRI scan of a superior sulcus tumour following neoadjuvant chemoradiotherapy.

and a 0.1% risk of death. It should only be used when a certain diagnosis would change treatment.

MRI SCANNING

MRI scans are not routinely used in the diagnosis and staging of lung cancer. They are sometimes used to look for cerebral metastasis in patients prior to radical surgery. The yield of a brain MRI is low in patients with early stage lung cancer, but in patients with a more advanced stage or a high SUV_{max} of the primary tumour on PET scanning, the yield is higher and it may be warranted as part of routine staging investigations.

The other indication for MRI scanning is to look for invasion of the brachial plexus and subclavian vessels in superior sulcus (Pancoast's) tumours (Figure 23.5).

SURGERY FOR LUNG CANCER

Introduction

It is generally accepted that surgery offers the best chance of cure for lung cancer provided this can be done with acceptable mortality and morbidity. Fundamentals of surgical management include obtaining a complete resection (R0) and systematic lymph node sampling or dissection. This is important to optimize the accuracy of the pathological stage and provides information to the surgeon and the patient on survival and the benefits of adjuvant chemotherapy.

Assessment of fitness for surgery

Lung cancer occurs most commonly in elderly patients who smoke. Smoking is also a major risk factor for chronic obstructive pulmonary disease (COPD) and cardiovascular disease. Consequently patients with lung cancer often have multiple comorbidities. It is important to fully assess these before embarking on surgery. The patient has to be fit enough to survive the operation, and have sufficient lung function remaining to have a reasonable quality of life.

All patients should have a full blood count, a biochemical profile, an electrocardiogram and full pulmonary function tests including a gas transfer factor (TLCO) to assess their fitness for surgery. Patients with a history of cardiac disease or a heart murmur should undergo an echocardiogram prior to surgery. Evidence for the routine use of cardiopulmonary exercise is lacking although it is recommended in the European Society of Thoracic Surgeons guidelines for the assessment of a patient's fitness for surgery.

A measure of a patient's operative risk and degree of postoperative breathlessness can be obtained by calculating the postoperative predicted forced expiratory volume in 1 second (FEV_1) and TLCO using the formula below:

$$PPV = FEV \times \frac{\left(\text{Total number of segments} - a\right) - b}{\left(\text{Total number of segments} - a\right)}$$

The total number of segments is usually 19 (3 right upper lobe, 2 right middle lobe, 5 right lower lobe, 5 left upper lobe and 4 left lower lobe) unless the patient has had a previous lung resection. a is the number of obstructed segments and b is the number of unobstructed segments to be resected.

MI or sudden cardiac death occurs in 1–5% of patients following surgery for lung cancer. The risk for cardiac complications should be assessed according to the 2007 American College of Cardiology guidelines [67]. Lung resection should be avoided within 30 days of a myocardial infarction and a cardiology review sort in patients with an active cardiac condition, three or more risk factors for a cardiac complication or poor cardiac functional capacity [68].

It is important for both surgeons and patients to be able to accurately estimate the in-hospital mortality rate of an operation for lung cancer. The mortality rate from a lobectomy is 2.3% and a pneumonectomy 5.8% [69]. Risk prediction models remain fairly rudimentary. Published literature has concentrated mainly on individual risk factors for mortality. These include type of resection, increased age, low FEV1, low transfer factor and high alcohol intake.

Thoracoscore is currently the best risk stratification available [70]. It was developed from the French Association of Thoracic and Cardiovascular Surgeons from a database of 30,000 patients with 336 deaths. It has nine variables: sex, age, American Society of Anaesthesiology grade, performance status, MRC dyspnoea score, priority for surgery, procedure (pneumonectomy or other), diagnosis (benign or malignant) and number of comorbidities. The risk of in-hospital mortality can be calculated using a logistic regression model. The model has a C statistic of 0.86. It has been validated in a North American population with a C statistic of 0.84 [71].

Patients should be encouraged to stop smoking prior to surgery. Cigarette smoking is associated with increased pulmonary complications. Stopping smoking reduces the incidence of pulmonary complications [72].

Lung cancer is associated with a decrease in quality of life. This is more so than other cancers [73]. Following lung resection quality of life deteriorates and takes approximately 6 months to return to baseline [74–77]. Where the patient has had a pneumonectomy, the quality of life does not return to baseline [77]. Bronchial and arterial sleeve resections should therefore be performed wherever possible to avoid the long-term decrease in quality of life associated with a pneumonectomy. Also, lower operative mortality and local recurrence rates have been reported following sleeve resections [78]. A lower operative mortality would be expected, as this is what is seen when comparing lobectomy to pneumonectomy. The difference in local recurrence is harder to explain and may be due to the non-randomized nature of this study.

Lobectomy is generally accepted as the gold standard operation for the treatment of lung cancer. Sub-lobar resections include wedge resection and segmentectomies. A wedge resection involves removing the tumour with a margin of normal lung surrounding it. It is non-anatomical. A segmentectomy involves formally dividing the segmental vein, artery and bronchus. It is anatomical and removes the draining veins and lymphatics. The most commonly performed segmentectomies are trisegmentectomy (apical, anterior and posterior segments) in the left upper lobe, lingulectomy or apical segmentectomy of the lower lobes. The only randomized trial comparing lobectomy with sub-lobar resection found that there was an increased local recurrence following sub-lobar resections [79]. These procedures should therefore be reserved for patients with limited pulmonary reserve where the surgeon wishes to preserve pulmonary function [68].

Open resections of the lung

Open lung resections are performed through an axillary, anterolateral or posterolateral thoracotomy depending on the preference of the surgeon. The patient is positioned laterally and intubated with a double-lumen endotracheal tube. Once the incision is made, any pleural adhesions are divided and the pleural cavity inspected for any evidence of metastatic deposits. The tumour is palpated to confirm which lobe(s) requires removal. The pulmonary vein, artery and bronchus to the section of lung to be removed are dissected free and divided with staples or in between ligatures. The fissures of the lung are then divided to remove the lobe of the lung.

Prior to closure of the chest the bronchial stump and lung parenchyma are submerged underwater and the remaining lung inflated, checking there is no air leak from the bronchial stump. Any air leak from the lung parenchyma can be sutured or a sealant applied.

One or two chest drains are inserted to prevent air and blood collecting in the pleural cavity and the wound is closed in layers. The patient is extubated at the end of the procedure. Analgesia is by both regional techniques and systemic opioids. Although epidural anaesthesia provides the best analgesia, there has been a move away from epidural analgesia to paravertebral blocks and catheters in recent years. Epidural analgesia can cause hypotension, fluid shifts and may limit early mobility. It is felt by some that these problems outweigh the benefits of superior pain relief.

VATS lobectomy

VATS lobectomy has been performed for more than 20 years, but its adoption has been slow and cautious despite an increasing body of evidence showing decreased complication rates and quicker recovery. One of the first studies was the CALGB 39802, a feasibility study of VATS lobectomy versus open lobectomy [80]. There were 111 patients who had T1N0 NSCLC, and 96 of these (86.5%) underwent successful VATS lobectomy. The median procedure length was 130 minutes with a median chest tube duration of 3 days. Perioperative mortality was 2.7%, and complication rates were also found to be lower than those reported for lobectomy via thoracotomy. This study therefore demonstrated the safety of VATS lobectomy as well as helping to develop a more standardized description of the procedure.

In a meta-analysis Whitson and colleagues [81] attempted to compare the VATS versus open lobectomy with respect to complication rates, length of stay and overall survival. In total the analysis involved 3256 thoracotomy and 3114 VATS lobectomy patients. The overall complication rate in the VATS patients was significantly lower than that in the thoracotomy patients ($p = 0.018$, 16.4% vs. 31.2%, respectively). VATS lobectomy also demonstrated statistically significant decreases in chest tube duration and length of stay. When overall annual survival rates were examined it was found VATS lobectomy showed an absolute survival advantage ranging from 5% at 1 year up to 17% at 4 years ($p = 0.003$). Obviously this study had several limitations, not least of which was the fact that it was essentially an observational study as only one of the studies it included was a randomized trial.

In a more recent meta-analysis of unmatched and matched patients undergoing VATS or open lobectomy, Cao and colleagues [82] found that mortality in the unmatched groups was significantly lower; however, this was not significant after propensity matching. In both the unmatched and matched group, there was a significantly lower morbidity rate and shorter hospital stay.

Some surgeons have questioned the oncologic efficacy of VATS lobectomy. In a large propensity-matched study, Paul and colleagues [83] showed that patients undergoing VATS lobectomy had similar overall, cancer-specific and disease-free survival as patients undergoing lobectomy.

Casali and Walker [84] looked at the cost-effectiveness of VATS lobectomy. The study population was made up of 346 patients undergoing lobectomy, 93 via VATS and 253 via thoracotomy. Though theatre costs were higher for VATS lobectomy versus thoracotomy, there was a decreased cost in the VATS group for high dependency unit care and hospital stay. This translated into an overall decrease in the cost of a VATS lobectomy (8023 ± 565 euros) compared with an open lobectomy (8178 ± 167 euros) ($p = 0.0002$).

SUPERIOR SULCUS TUMOURS

Although some authors have resected Pancoast tumours via VATS, open resection remains the norm. The tumour is usually approached via a high posterior thoracotomy (Paulson approach) [85] or an anterior approach (Dartevelle) [86,87]. Ribs, subclavian vessels and brachial plexus may need resecting. Most authors would advocate neoadjuvant chemoradiotherapy for Pancoast tumours. Five-year survival rates of between 20% and 30% have been reported with this treatment strategy.

The North American Lung Intergroup Trial 0160 [88] evaluated 110 eligible mediastinoscopy negative patients with induction chemoradiation (two cycles of cisplatin and etoposide with concurrent radiation [45 Gy] followed by resection of NSCLC of the superior sulcus, 3–5 weeks later). Of 88 cases (80%) who underwent thoracotomy, 83 (76%) had complete resection. Operative mortality was 1.8%. In all, 61 (56%) patients had complete or minimal microscopic disease remaining. Five-year survival was 44% overall and 54% in patients with complete resection.

CARINAL RESECTIONS

Tumours involving the carina (Figure 23.6) can be resected by way of carinal pneumonectomy or sleeve lobectomy with carinal resection. Right-sided procedures are easier to perform due to easier access to the carina on this side. On the left side the position of the aortic arch makes surgery difficult.

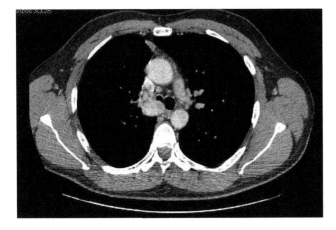

Figure 23.6 CT scan showing a mass invading the proximal right main bronchus and distal trachea (arrowed). Resection would require a right carinal pneumonectomy or right carinal sleeve resection.

Postoperative management

Pulmonary complications are the most common following lung resection. Postoperative care must include aggressive early mobilization, physiotherapy and good pain control to try to prevent them. Chest drains should be removed when there is no air leak and drainage is less than between 200 and 400 ml per day.

MESOTHELIOMA

Introduction

Malignant pleural mesothelioma (hereafter mesothelioma) is a malignant neoplasm of the pleura with a long latent period, but once it becomes clinically apparent it is often rapidly progressive. The median survival following diagnosis is 8.5 months with a 1- and 3-year survival rate of 40% and 8%, respectively [89]. There are approximately 2100 cases diagnosed per annum in the UK [89]. Mesothelioma most commonly affects the pleural cavity but can also develop in the peritoneal cavity. This section will concentrate on pleural mesothelioma.

Asbestos exposure is a strong risk factor in the development of mesothelioma. Ninety percent of cases of mesothelioma are caused by asbestos. The majority of asbestos fibres are either amphibole or serpentine. The amphibole fibres are more carcinogenic. They are typically found in brake linings, cement and the ship building industry. Mesothelioma is therefore most common in shipyard workers, pipe laggers, railway workers and other professions that use asbestos. There is a 20- to 50-year lag between asbestos exposure and the development of mesothelioma. As occupational exposure to asbestos is the main cause of mesothelioma, 83% of cases are male [89]. The median age at diagnosis is 73 years [89].

The effects of asbestos and cigarette smoking are synergistic.

Clinical features

Symptoms and signs of mesothelioma are usually nonspecific and can mimic those of many benign or malignant intrathoracic diseases. Mesothelioma usually presents with chest pain due to the tumour invading the chest wall, or shortness of breath due to the presence of a pleural effusion. The chest pain is usually constant, gradually increases in severity and may require opioid analgesia.

Diagnosis

CXR

A CXR is usually the first investigation a patient undergoes. This may reveal loss of volume on the effected side, pleural thickening or a pleural effusion (see Figure 23.7).

CT SCANNING

Any patient with any of the above features on a chest X-ray should have a CT scan of the lower neck and upper abdomen. Common findings on a CT scan are pleural

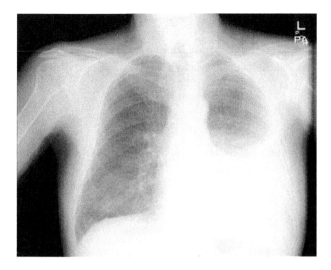

Figure 23.7 CXR showing a left pleural effusion in a patient with suspected mesothelioma.

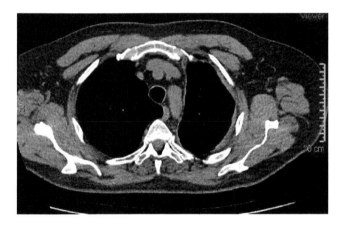

Figure 23.8 CT scan showing loss of volume in the left hemi-thorax and circumferential pleural thickening extending onto the mediastinal surface in a patient with mesothelioma.

thickening which extends onto the mediastinal surface (see Figure 23.8), volume loss in the affected hemi-thorax or a pleural effusion.

PET-CT SCANNING

Mesothelioma usually shows uptake of FDG. PET-CT is therefore useful in staging. It can also be used to assess response to treatment. PET-CT is not very accurate in determining the T stage but is very good at detecting N3 nodes and distant metastases [90].

MRI SCANNING

MRI scanning is useful in assessing invasion of the diaphragm, vertebra and mediastinal structures when considering radical surgery of tumours possibly invading these structures.

PLEURAL ASPIRATION

Any patient with suspected mesothelioma and a pleural effusion should undergo a diagnostic pleural aspiration.

This should be carried out under ultrasound guidance. The pleural fluid should be sent for biochemical analysis to see if it is an exudate or transudate as well as for cytology and microbiological culture.

VATS PLEURAL BIOPSY OR MEDICAL THORACOSCOPY

These are the procedures of choice to confirm the diagnosis in a patient who is symptomatic from a pleural effusion. They allow the pleural fluid to be drained completely, the pleural cavity to be inspected and multiple biopsies to be taken. A talc pleurodesis can be performed to try to prevent fluid recurrence. Medical thoracoscopy is performed under local anaesthetic.

A VATS pleural biopsy is performed under general anaesthesia with a double-lumen endotracheal tube so that the lung on the operative side can be collapsed. A bronchoscopy should be performed at the same time to help exclude a lung cancer. The patient is placed in the lateral position. A single port is made over the site of the effusion. If it is felt that the patient may be suitable for radical surgery if mesothelioma is confirmed then the port should ideally be positioned along the site where a future thoracotomy would be, so the port site can be excised. The telescope is introduced and any pleural fluid removed and sent for cytology. Multiple biopsies are then taken from all areas of the tumour by introducing the biopsy forceps alongside the telescope. Talc is then insufflated into the chest to try to achieve a pleurodesis. A chest drain is inserted at the end of the procedure. The chest drain is left in place until the drainage is less than 200 ml in 24 hours or 5 days depending on which is sooner.

CT BIOPSY

In patients with minimal pleural fluid and gross pleural thickening, a CT biopsy may be used to obtain a tissue diagnosis.

Staging of mesothelioma

Mesothelioma should be staged according to the International Mesothelioma Interest Group (ITMIG) staging system [91].

M0 means no distant metastasis and M1 means presence of distant metastasis. Various TNM groupings are classified into stages I–IV depending on survival. If M1 disease is present, then it is stage IV (see Tables 23.2 and 23.3).

Histological subtypes

There are three main histological subtypes of mesothelioma: epithelioid, sarcomatoid and mixed. Epithelioid carries the best prognosis and sarcomatoid the worst.

Treatment

SURGERY

Surgery for mesothelioma may be palliative or radical. The aim of palliative treatment is to restore the function

Table 23.2 TNM staging description for malignant pleural mesothelioma

	Description
T stage	
TX	Primary tumour cannot be assessed.
T0	No evidence of primary tumour.
T1a	No involvement of visceral pleura.
T1b	Tumour involves parietal and visceral pleura.
T2	Tumour involves each of the ipsilateral pleural surfaces (parietal, visceral, mediastinal and diaphragmatic) and invades at least one of the lung parenchyma or diaphragmatic muscle.
T3	Locally advanced but potentially resectable. Tumour involves each of the ipsilateral pleural surfaces (parietal, visceral, mediastinal and diaphragmatic) and invades at least one of the endothoracic fascia, mediastinal fat, non-transmural involvement of the pericardium and resectable focus of tissue extending into the soft tissues of the chest wall.
T4	Locally advanced, technically unresectable disease. Tumour involves each of the ipsilateral pleural surfaces (parietal, visceral, mediastinal and diaphragmatic) and invades at least one of the diffuse extension or multifocal masses of tumour in the chest wall, with or without associated rib destruction, direct transdiaphragmatic extension of tumour into the peritoneal cavity, direct extension of the tumour to the contralateral pleura, direct extension to the mediastinal organs, direct extension to the spine and tumour extending through to the internal surface of the pericardium.
N stage	
N0	No regional lymph nodes
N1	Metastasis in ipsilateral bronchopulmonary or hilar nodes
N2	Metastasis in the subcarinal, ipsilateral mediastinal, ipsilateral internal mammary or ipsilateral peridiaphragmatic nodes
N3	Metastasis in the contralateral mediastinal or contralateral internal mammary, ipsilateral or contralateral supraclavicular nodes

Table 23.3 Staging subgroup of mesothelioma

	N0	N1	N2	N3
T1a	IA	III	III	IV
T1b	IB	III	III	IV
T2	II	III	III	IV
T3	III	III	III	IV
T4	IV	IV	IV	IV

of the lung by removing the cancer that is entrapping it. The role of radical surgery for mesothelioma polarizes thoracic surgeons. The aims of radical surgery are to achieve macroscopic clearance of cancer. This has previously been achieved by an extrapleural pneumonectomy but now more commonly by an extended decortication. It is generally accepted that surgery alone does not produce a cure and will only do so as part of multimodality therapy including chemotherapy and radiotherapy.

An extrapleural pneumonectomy (EPP) involves removal of the pleura, lung, diaphragm and pericardium. The pericardium and diaphragm are then reconstructed. Although there are encouraging results from case series [92–95], there has only been one small randomized trial assessing the benefits of EPP, the Mesothelioma and Radical Surgery (MARS) trial [96]. In this trial, patients received three cycles of cisplatin-based chemotherapy and then were re-staged.

Patients were eligible for randomization if they had completed chemotherapy and had operable disease. They were randomized to no EPP or EPP followed by radiotherapy. Although not statistically significant there was a trend toward a worse survival and quality of life in the EPP group. The study concluded that a larger randomized trial was not feasible and suggests that EPP offers no benefit and possibly harms patients.

After the MARS trial there was a move toward surgeons performing an extended decortication. The aim of this operation is again to remove all visible tumour, but this time the lung is not removed. The term *extended decortication* is used rather than *radical decortication* as it was felt *radical* implied therapeutic benefit [97]. Results from a comparative study had found that patients undergoing an extended decortication had a better survival than those undergoing an EPP [98]. MARS 2 is a randomized trial which plans to evaluate the effects of extended decortication versus no surgery.

Palliative decortication is an operation used in patients with a trapped lung. The aim of the operation is not to remove all the tumour, but to get the lung to expand as much as possible, potentially improving the patient's quality of life. There is a lack of evidence to support this operation. In a randomized trial comparing VATS partial pleurectomy and talc pleurodesis [99], there were more complications and a longer hospital stay in the VATS partial pleurectomy group.

Quality of life was similar at baseline, 1, 3 and 6 months, but better in the VATS partial pleurectomy group at 12 months.

RADIOTHERAPY

Radiotherapy is potentially helpful in reducing chest pain in patients with mesothelioma [100]. It is recommended after radical surgery as part of trimodality therapy. Intensity-modulated radiotherapy (IMRT) allows more intense radiation delivery with greater accuracy. It has been used after EPP with encouraging results [101].

The role of radiotherapy in preventing recurrence at the site of any VATS, CT biopsy or chest drain is uncertain. Two ongoing clinical trials in the UK are investigating this subject.

CHEMOTHERAPY

Cisplatin is the backbone of most chemotherapy regimes in mesothelioma. A meta-analysis has shown it is the best single agent [102]. When used in combination with pemetrexed a response rate of 41.3% was seen compared with 16.7% for cisplatin alone. Median survival was increased from 9.3 months in the cisplatin group to 12.1 months in the cisplatin and pemetrexed group [103].

CONCLUSIONS

Mesothelioma is an uncommon but aggressive disease. Its incidence in Europe will peak over the next few years. It is important that good-quality clinical trials continue to determine the exact role of surgery and investigate novel biological agents.

PULMONARY METASTASECTOMY

Most deaths from cancer are due to metastatic disease. The most common sites of metastases are the regional lymph nodes, liver, brain, bone and lungs. Between 1.7% and 7.2% of patients with colorectal cancer will develop isolated lung metastasis [104]. The concept that removing these metastases will increase survival and potentially cure the patient is the basis behind pulmonary metastasectomy.

For at least 60 years, pulmonary metastasectomy has been used to treat lung metastasis from solid tumours. It is a very commonly performed operation for colorectal metastasis [105]. However, it is based on weak evidence [106]. Current evidence for all cancers comes from case series as no randomized clinical trials exist.

The first pulmonary metastasectomy was probably performed by Tudor Edwards in 1927 for a metastasis from a sarcoma of the leg [107]. The first reported excision of a pulmonary metastasis for a colonic metastasis was performed by Alfred Blalock in 1944 [108].

Metastatic disease often represents systemic and uncontrolled growth; however, some patients with cancer present with isolated metastases in the lung that are amenable to local treatment. This presumably represents more favourable tumour biology and therefore should not be viewed as untreatable.

Metastatic disease from any primary site can be onsidered for pulmonary metastasectomy. Colorectal metastases are the most commonly resected pulmonary metastases, followed by sarcoma, germ cell tumour and melanoma [109].

Pathology

Lung metastases mainly occur due to haematological spread. Tumour cells break away from the primary tumour and invade blood vessels or lymphatics. Tumour emboli then migrate to a distant site. Most tumour emboli will not survive. Occasionally one will survive and at some point multiplication and growth will occur until it develops into a detectable metastasis. The underlying tumour biology and host resistance mechanisms determine spread.

Pulmonary metastases can probably metastasize both haematologically and via lymphatics. Ten to thirty-two percent of patients undergoing pulmonary metastasectomy have hilar or mediastinal node involvement [110–114].

Imaging

CT scanning of the chest, abdomen and pelvis is now routinely performed in the follow-up of patients with previously resected colorectal cancer. There is little data to define the optimum type and protocol of CT imaging in pulmonary metastasis [115]. Helical scans detect up to 30% more nodules than conventional scans [116,117]. Images should be reviewed digitally by scrolling through them as this detects approximately 10–15% more nodules than plain, film-based reviewing [118,119].

With recent advances in CT scanners, the availability of 64-, 128-, and 256-slice CT has made chest CT possible using contiguous volumetric (<0.5 mm) thin sections. These sections can be viewed in multiple planes, with nodule detection software available. This has led to the detection of more and more nodules in patients with previously resected colorectal cancer. Nodules up to 2–3 mm can now be detected. Not all of these nodules will turn out to be malignant. Using 1 mm slice thickness multidetector row CT, Kang and colleagues did not find any more nodules at the time of surgery [120]. The CT scan should be performed within 4 weeks of surgery [115].

A ^{18}F-fluorodeoxyglucose (FDG) positron emission tomography (PET) scan should be carried out on all patients prior to performing a pulmonary metastasectomy for colorectal carcinoma to check for local control and look for other sites of metastatic disease [121]. Pasturino and colleagues found evidence of metastatic disease elsewhere that precluded surgery in 21% of patients with metastatic colorectal cancer [113].

One should also consider performing a magnetic resonance imaging (MRI) scan of the liver, as this is the most common site of metastases from colorectal cancer. MRI is better at picking up liver metastasis than a CT, ultrasound or PET scan.

Diagnosis

Pulmonary metastases may appear as solitary or multiple nodules and are usually well circumscribed. Five percent of patients with new nodules in previously treated breast or colon cancer are benign and up to 50% are new primaries [122,123]; however, this is considerably lower in non-smokers. Establishing a tissue diagnosis is important especially if one is to consider non-surgical options such as radiofrequency ablation, stereotactic radiotherapy or systemic therapy.

Obtaining a tissue diagnosis is fairly easy in some cancers but not others. Fine-needle aspiration (FNA) can often distinguish between lung cancer and a colonic or sarcoma metastasis, but it is much more difficult to distinguish between a metastasis from a squamous cell carcinoma of the head and neck and a primary lung cancer.

Indications

The indications for pulmonary metastasectomy are constantly evolving. Over the last decade, the development of new effective chemotherapy and targeted therapies has altered the indications for pulmonary metastasectomy [124].

A patient with a solitary metastasis with a long disease-free interval is probably still best treated surgically [124]. However, the role of surgery in a patient with multiple resectable lung and liver metastases with a relatively short disease-free interval is uncertain.

Analysis of case series has established well-accepted surgical selection criteria:

1. Primary disease is under control.
2. Metastases are limited to the lung (with the exception of hepatic lesions when it is possible to completely remove both hepatic and lung lesions).
3. Metastases can be completely excised.
4. Patient has the physiological reserve to tolerate the planned procedure.

Preoperative assessment

Most patients found to have pulmonary metastases are asymptomatic. They are usually picked up on routine surveillance CT scans. Few patients present with symptoms. Occasionally invasion of the parietal pleura or chest wall may cause chest pain; invasion or obstruction of an airway may cause haemoptysis or dyspnoea.

All patients undergoing a pulmonary metastasectomy should undergo physical examination, radiological examination and physiological testing. They should be assessed for surgery in a manner similar to that of patients undergoing a resection for primary lung cancer [68].

Patients with a pleural effusion should undergo thoracocentesis and cytological analysis. If this is negative, then a VATS examination of the thoracic cavity is advisable prior to surgical resection.

Surgical approach

The surgical approach to performing a pulmonary metastasectomy is very variable and is influenced more by the surgeon's preference than a sound evidence base [105,125]. A posterolateral thoracotomy is the standard approach for lung resections. It allows good access to all aspects of the lung. However, it can be very painful.

A median sternotomy allows access to both pleural cavities. Following the incision, each lung is sequentially deflated and palpated. Endoscopic staplers make the excision of nodules easier. Palpating the posteromedial aspects of the lower lobes can be difficult via a sternotomy, especially in obese patients or those with cardiomegaly. Hazelrigg and colleagues advocated combining a median sternotomy with VATS to increase exposure [126]. A clam shell incision allows good palpation of all areas of both thoracic cavities, but it is a large painful incision.

VATS has become increasingly popular for the diagnosis and treatment of pulmonary metastasis. However, its role remains controversial as it precludes bimanual palpitation of the lung. Whether a surgeon feels it is an acceptable technique depends on their beliefs, and possibly the quality of the CT scan. The European Society of Thoracic Surgeons working group survey showed potential inconsistencies between belief and practice in the treatment of colorectal metastasis. Palpation of the lung, impossible via VATS, was regarded as mandatory by 65% of surgeons, but 60% thought VATS was acceptable [105]. This implies that a third of surgeons feel the advantages of VATS are greater than the advantages of palpating the lung.

In earlier studies, surgeons have found more nodules at the time of thoracotomy than were detected on the CT scan [117,127,128]. In the most recent study published by Eckardt and Licht [129], patients underwent VATS resection followed by thoracotomy. Fifty-five nodules were identified on CT preoperatively, 51 were found by VATS and during thoracotomy an additional 29 nodules were found (6 of which were malignant). With CT scanners now detecting nodules as small as 2 mm, it is now becoming less common to find further nodules at the time of operation that were not seen on CT scanning. Using 1 mm slice thickness multidetector row CT, Kang and colleagues did not find any more nodules at the time of surgery [120]. The problem in fact has now become the reverse, finding some of the small nodules at operation seen on the CT scan.

Complications of VATS are rare and benefits include a shorter hospital stay. Mutsaerts and colleagues reported fewer complications in patients undergoing metastasectomy via VATS compared with thoracotomy [130]. VATS provides excellent visualization of the pleura enabling the surgeon to identify small pleural metastasis. Following VATS less adhesions will form between the lung and chest wall, making repeat resections easier.

One of the concerns regarding VATS is that of port site recurrence; however, data do not support the contention that it is a new problem unique to VATS [125]. To try to prevent port site recurrence all specimens should be removed in a retrieval bag or a wound protector used.

Results

Most studies in the literature report a postoperative mortality of 0% [131–137]. Ike and colleagues report a mortality of 2.4%, but in fact this is only one patient in their small series [138]. Postoperative morbidity and long-term sequelae of pulmonary metastasectomy such as the effect on pulmonary function and quality of life are poorly reported in the literature.

Five-year survival of patients following pulmonary metastasectomy for colorectal cancer is between 32% and 64% at 5 years [131–140].

Many case series in the literature have included a multivariate analysis to look for prognostic factors. However, we have to be very cautious reading too much into these studies as the range of variables entering any data analysis is severely limited by selection bias. Factors that have been shown to influence outcome in colorectal cancer include disease-free interval, number of metastases, a complete resection, carcinoembryonic (CEA) level, tumour doubling time and lymph node involvement (see Table 23.4).

A longer disease-free interval has been shown to have a better prognosis. The 5-year survival is improved if there is a metachronous presentation and the disease-free interval is greater than a year [139,141,142].

Although the number of metastases is not a contraindication to resection, it is an indication of the degree of dissemination of the cancer. The larger the number of metastases, the more likely that micrometastases are present. Van Halteran and colleagues found that patients with more than four metastasis all developed recurrence, compared

with 50% of those with less than four being disease free at 5 years [143]. Many authors report higher survival rates for patients with single lesions [109,139,142,144,145,146]. Others have not found a correlation between the number of lung metastases and survival [147,148].

Complete resection has repeatedly been shown to be a prognostic factor [146,149,150]. Melloni and colleagues found prognosis is significantly worse in patients with an incomplete resection [134]. A raised CEA has been found to be an adverse prognostic indicator in many [131,142,146,151,152] but not all studies [139]. Like all the factors discussed here, the conflicting results are most likely due to selection bias (see Table 23.5).

In an analysis of tumour doubling time in patients with a solitary pulmonary metastasis Tomimaru and colleagues [153] found that a shorter tumour doubling time was associated with a significant increase in intrapulmonary recurrence and a trend toward a shorter 5-year survival. However, in patients with multiple metastases there was a heterogeneous tumour doubling time for each metastasis [154].

Lymph node involvement has been shown to be a poor prognostic indicator following pulmonary metastasectomy in some studies [114,131,142,146,152,155], but not in others [132,137,138,140]. This is probably due to the small number of patients in these series.

PulMiCC trial

The effectiveness of pulmonary metastasectomy is now being questioned. The practice is widespread and increasing [105] and in spite of many follow-up studies claiming benefit [156], there are no randomized controlled trials. Many of these case series have combined metastasectomy from various cancer types including both carcinomas and sarcomas. The European Society of Thoracic Surgeons Lung Metastasectomy Working Group concluded that the evidence for metastasectomy was too low to set recommendations to guide its members. Patients are selected for surgery on the basis of characteristics well known to be favourable prognostic features as outlined above. Might this all be a matter of selection bias? Would these patients have survived as long (or longer) without a pulmonary metastasectomy? Utley and Treasure analyzed data from reported surgical follow-up studies and compared it with

Table 23.4 Staging subgroups of lung cancer

	N0	N1	N2	N3
T1a	IA	IIA	IIIA	IIIB
T1b	IA	IIA	IIIA	IIIB
T2a	IB	IIA	IIIA	IIIB
T2b	IIA	IIB	IIIA	IIIB
T3	IIB	IIIA	IIIA	IIIB
T4	IIIA	IIIA	IIIB	IIIB

Table 23.5 Indications for surgery

Universally accepted indications		Stage I and II lung cancer
Generally accepted indications		T3 N0–1 tumours requiring chest wall or diaphragm resection or tumours with satellite nodule in the same lobe
		T4 tumours requiring carinal resection or vertebral resection
		Superior sulcus tumours
Controversial indications		Single-station N2 disease
		T4 with satellite nodule in an adjacent lobe
		Oligometastatic disease T1–3 N0 M1b

how long similar patients recorded in the Thames Cancer Registry survived. Natural survival appeared to be as good as that following further surgery [157,158]. These doubts concerning the efficacy of this type of surgery have made the case for the Pulmonary Metastasectomy in Colorectal Cancer (PulMiCC) trial which is currently recruiting [159].

Image-guided ablative therapies

Percutaneous ablation of pulmonary metastases is becoming more popular. The attraction is the minimal invasiveness of the procedure and that it does not require a general anaesthetic. The disadvantage is that the margins cannot be examined histologically to confirm complete 'resection'. There are three types of thermoablative therapies currently available: radiofrequency ablation (RFA), microwave ablation or cryoablation.

Evidence of the beneficial symptomatic or prognostic effects for these techniques is extremely limited.

RADIOFREQUENCY ABLATION

Radiofrequency ablation (RFA) is performed by inserting an electrode into the lesion under CT guidance. The tip of the electrode has a non-insulated portion that generates medium-frequency electromagnetic waves of 400–500 kHz. Alternating radiofrequency current agitates ions in the tissue surrounding the needle creating frictional heat, which denatures and destroys tissue at predictable temperatures, in a relatively predictable volume.

Lung tumours are good targets for radiofrequency ablation because the surrounding air in the adjacent normal lung parenchyma provides an insulating effect, thus concentrating the energy within the tumour [160].

The procedure is well tolerated with a low complication rate. Potential complications include pneumothorax, haemorrhage, haemoptysis, reactive pleural effusion, damage to adjacent structures, and infections and abscess formation.

Petre and colleagues have reported a series of 45 patients undergoing RFA for colorectal pulmonary metastasis [161]. Three-year survival rates were 50%.

MICROWAVE ABLATION

Microwave ablation is a procedure that uses heat from microwave energy to destroy cancer cells by thermocoagulation. Similarly to RFA it is usually inserted percutaneously under CT guidance.

Stereotactic radiotherapy

Besides treating primary lung cancer, stereotactic radiotherapy has been used to treat lung metastases [162]. Have carried out a meta-analysis of stereotactic radiotherapy for pulmonary oligometastases. The techniques, doses and dose fraction schedules varied widely. The 2-year weighted local control was 77.9% and 2-year weighted overall survival was 53.7%.

Role of chemotherapy

The role of chemotherapy in the treatment of patients with lung metastasis is constantly evolving. The use of chemotherapy or other targeted therapies may assist in the control of micrometastases [151].

There is little data to assess the role of neoadjuvant and adjuvant chemotherapy in patients undergoing pulmonary metastasectomy. In subgroup analysis of patients with colorectal cancer, Lee and colleagues and Saito and colleagues could not find a significant impact of perioperative chemotherapy [131,133]. More recently, Younes and colleagues found a survival benefit in patients who had received neoadjuvant chemotherapy [149].

Conclusions

The current available evidence shows that pulmonary metastasectomy is a safe operation. With no randomized controlled trials, it is difficult to draw conclusions on the effectiveness of the operation. All patients with metastatic disease should be discussed at a multidisciplinary meeting which includes surgeons, oncologists and radiologists to determine what is believed to be the optimum treatment for that individual.

REFERENCES

1. Ferlay, J., et al. Cancer incidence and mortality patterns in Europe: estimates for 40 countries in 2012. *European Journal of Cancer* 49.6 (2013): 1374–403.
2. Verdecchia, A., et al. Recent cancer survival in Europe: a 2000–02 period analysis of EUROCARE-4 data. *Lancet Oncology* 8.9 (2007): 784–96. Erratum appears in *Lancet Oncology* 2008;9(5):416.
3. Health and Social Care Information Centre. National lung cancer audit report. Leeds, UK: Health and Social Care Information Centre, 2014a.
4. Alberg, A. J., et al. Epidemiology of lung cancer: ACCP evidence-based clinical practice guidelines (2nd edition). *Chest* 132.3:Suppl (2007): Suppl-55S.
5. Wingo, P. A., et al. Annual report to the nation on the status of cancer, 1973–1996, with a special section on lung cancer and tobacco smoking. *Journal of the National Cancer Institute* 91.8 (1999): 675–90.
6. Boffetta, P., et al. Cigar and pipe smoking and lung cancer risk: a multicenter study from Europe. *Journal of the National Cancer Institute* 91.8 (1999): 697–701.
7. Doll, R., and A. B. Hill. Lung cancer and other causes of death in relation to smoking. *British Medical Journal* 2.5001 (1956): 1071–81.
8. Samet, J. M. Radon and lung cancer. *Journal of the National Cancer Institute* 81.10 (1989): 745–57.
9. Blot, W. J., and J. F. Fraumeni Jr. Arsenical air pollution and lung cancer. *Lancet* 2.7926 (1975): 142–44.

10. Simonato, L., et al. A retrospective mortality study of workers exposed to arsenic in a gold mine and refinery in France. *American Journal of Industrial Medicine* 25.5 (1994): 625–33.

11. Simonato, L., and R. Saracci. Epidemiological aspects of the relationship between exposure to silica dust and lung cancer. *IARC Scientific Publications* 97 (1990): 1–5.

12. Lloyd, J. W. Long-term mortality study of steelworkers. V. Respiratory cancer in coke plant workers. *Journal of Occupational Medicine* 13.2 (1971): 53–68.

13. Saracci, R. Beryllium and lung cancer: adding another piece to the puzzle of epidemiologic evidence. *Journal of the National Cancer Institute* 83.19 (1991): 1362–63.

14. Khuder, S. A., and A. B. Mutgi. Effect of smoking cessation on major histologic types of lung cancer. *Chest* 120.5 (2001): 1577–83.

15. Doll, R., and R. Peto. Cigarette smoking and bronchial carcinoma: dose and time relationships among regular smokers and lifelong non-smokers. *Journal of Epidemiology & Community Health* 32.4 (1978): 303–13.

16. U.S. Department of Health and Human Services. Smoking and health: a national status report. Washington, DC: U.S. Department of Health and Human Services, 1987.

17. U.S. Department of Health and Human Services. The health benefits of smoking cessation: a report of the Surgeon General. Washington, DC: U.S. Department of Health and Human Services, 1990.

18. Wynder, E. L., and D. Hoffmann. Smoking and lung cancer: scientific challenges and opportunities. *Cancer Research* 54.20 (1994): 5284–95.

19. U.S. Department of Health and Human Services. The health consequences of involuntary tobacco smoke: a report of the Surgeon General. Atlanta GA: U.S. Department of Health and Human Services, 2006.

20. Doll, R., and R. Peto. The causes of cancer: quantitative estimates of avoidable risks of cancer in the United States today. *Journal of the National Cancer Institute* 66.6 (1981): 1191–308.

21. Newhouse, M. L., and G. Berry. Patterns of mortality in asbestos factory workers in London. *Annals of the New York Academy of Sciences* 330 (1979): 53–60.

22. Frost, G., A. Darnton, and A. H. Harding. The effect of smoking on the risk of lung cancer mortality for asbestos workers in Great Britain (1971–2005). *Annals of Occupational Hygiene* 55.3 (2011): 239–47.

23. Lubin, J. H., et al. Lung cancer in radon-exposed miners and estimation of risk from indoor exposure. *Journal of the National Cancer Institute* 87.11 (1995): 817–27.

24. Krewski, D., et al. Residential radon and risk of lung cancer: a combined analysis of 7 North American case-control studies. *Epidemiology* 16.2 (2005): 137–45.

25. Darby, S., et al. Radon in homes and risk of lung cancer: collaborative analysis of individual data from 13 European case-control studies. *BMJ* 330.7485 (2005): 223.

26. Lissowska, J., et al. Family history and lung cancer risk: international multicentre case-control study in eastern and central Europe and meta-analyses. *Cancer Causes & Control* 21.7 (2010): 1091–104.

27. Liang, H. Y., et al. Facts and fiction of the relationship between preexisting tuberculosis and lung cancer risk: a systematic review. *International Journal of Cancer* 125.12 (2009): 2936–44.

28. Mbulaiteye, S. M., et al. Immune deficiency and risk for malignancy among persons with AIDS. *Journal of Acquired Immune Deficiency Syndromes: JAIDS* 32.5 (2003): 527–33.

29. Moyer, V. A., and U.S. Preventive Services Task Force. Screening for lung cancer: U.S. Preventive Services Task Force recommendation statement. *Annals of Internal Medicine* 160.5 (2014): 330–38.

30. Kubik, A., et al. Lack of benefit from semi-annual screening for cancer of the lung: follow-up report of a randomized controlled trial on a population of high-risk males in Czechoslovakia. *International Journal of Cancer* 45.1 (1990): 26–33.

31. Fontana, R. S., et al. Lung cancer screening: the Mayo program. *Journal of Occupational Medicine* 28.8 (1986): 746–50.

32. Melamed, M. R., et al. Screening for early lung cancer. Results of the Memorial Sloan-Kettering study in New York. *Chest* 86.1 (1984): 44–53.

33. Tockman, Melvyn S. Survival and mortality from lung cancer in a screened population: the Johns Hopkins study. *Chest* 89.4:Suppl (1986): 324S–5S.

34. Oken, M. M., et al. Screening by chest radiograph and lung cancer mortality: the Prostate, Lung, Colorectal, and Ovarian (PLCO) randomized trial. *JAMA* 306.17 (2011): 1865–73.

35. National Lung Screening Trial Research Team, et al. Reduced lung-cancer mortality with low-dose computed tomographic screening. *New England Journal of Medicine* 365.5 (2011): 395–409.

36. Henschke, C. I., et al. Early Lung Cancer Action Project: overall design and findings from baseline screening. *Lancet* 354.9173 (1999): 99–105.

37. Infante, M., et al. A randomized study of lung cancer screening with spiral computed tomography: three-year results from the DANTE trial. *American Journal of Respiratory & Critical Care Medicine* 180.5 (2009): 445–53.

38. Saghir, Z., et al. CT screening for lung cancer brings forward early disease. The randomised Danish Lung Cancer Screening Trial: status after five annual screening rounds with low-dose CT. *Thorax* 67.4 (2012): 296–301.

39. Pastorino, U., et al. Annual or biennial CT screening versus observation in heavy smokers: 5-year results of the MILD trial. *European Journal of Cancer Prevention* 21.3 (2012): 308–15.

40. Humphrey, Linda L., et al. Screening for lung cancer with low-dose computed tomography: a systematic review to update the U.S. Preventive Services Task Force recommendation. *Annals of Internal Medicine* 159.6 (2013): 411–20.

41. de Koning, H. J., et al. Benefits and harms of computed tomography lung cancer screening strategies: a comparative modeling study for the U.S. Preventive Services Task Force. *Annals of Internal Medicine* 160.5 (2014): 311–20.

42. van den Bergh, K. A., et al. Long-term effects of lung cancer computed tomography screening on health-related quality of life: the NELSON trial. *European Respiratory Journal* 38.1 (2011): 154–61.

43. Tammemagi, M. C., and S. Lam. Screening for lung cancer using low dose computed tomography. *BMJ* 348 (2014).

44. Goldstraw, P., et al. The IASLC Lung Cancer Staging Project: proposals for the revision of the TNM stage groupings in the forthcoming (seventh) edition of the TNM classification of malignant tumours. *Journal of Thoracic Oncology* 2.8 (2007): 706–14. Erratum appears in *Journal of Thoracic Oncology* 2007;2(10):985.

45. Shepherd, F. A., et al. The International Association for the Study of Lung Cancer lung cancer staging project: proposals regarding the clinical staging of small cell lung cancer in the forthcoming (seventh) edition of the tumor, node, metastasis classification for lung cancer. *Journal of Thoracic Oncology* 2.12 (2007): 1067–77.

46. Travis, W. D., et al. The IASLC Lung Cancer Staging Project: proposals for the inclusion of bronchopulmonary carcinoid tumors in the forthcoming (seventh) edition of the TNM classification for lung cancer. *Journal of Thoracic Oncology* 3.11 (2008): 1213–23.

47. Rami-Porta, R., J. J. Crowley, and P. Goldstraw. The revised TNM staging system for lung cancer. *Annals of Thoracic & Cardiovascular Surgery* 15.1 (2009): 4–9.

48. Pancoast, H. K. Importance of careful roentgen-ray investigations of apical chest tumors. *Journal of the American Medical Association* 83.18 (1924): 1407–11.

49. Pancoast, H. K. Superior pulmonary sulcus tumor: tumor characterized by pain, Horner's syndrome, destruction of bone and atrophy of hand muscles. *Journal of the American Medical Association* 99.17 (1932): 1391–96.

50. Richardson, G. E., and B. E. Johnson. Paraneoplastic syndromes in lung cancer. *Current Opinion in Oncology* 4.2 (1992): 323–33.

51. Stenseth, J. H., O. T. Clagett, and L. B. Woolner. Hypertrophic pulmonary osteoarthropathy. *Diseases of the Chest* 52.1 (1967): 62–68.

52. Patel, A. M., D. G. Davila, and S. G. Peters. Paraneoplastic syndromes associated with lung cancer. *Mayo Clinic Proceedings* 68.3 (1993): 278–87.

53. Ejaz, S., et al. Cushing syndrome secondary to ectopic adrenocorticotropic hormone secretion: the University of Texas MD Anderson Cancer Center Experience. *Cancer* 117.19 (2011): 4381–89.

54. Silvestri, G. A., B. Littenberg, and G. L. Colice. The clinical evaluation for detecting metastatic lung cancer. A meta-analysis. *American Journal of Respiratory & Critical Care Medicine* 152.1 (1995): 225–30.

55. Laroche, C., et al. Role of computed tomographic scanning of the thorax prior to bronchoscopy in the investigation of suspected lung cancer. *Thorax* 55.5 (2000): 359–63.

56. Rusch, V. W., et al. The IASLC lung cancer staging project: a proposal for a new international lymph node map in the forthcoming seventh edition of the TNM classification for lung cancer. *Journal of Thoracic Oncology* 4.5 (2009): 568–77.

57. Berghmans, T., et al. Primary tumor standardized uptake value (SUVmax) measured on fluorodeoxyglucose positron emission tomography (FDG-PET) is of prognostic value for survival in non-small cell lung cancer (NSCLC): a systematic review and meta-analysis (MA) by the European Lung Cancer Working Party for the IASLC Lung Cancer Staging Project. *Journal of Thoracic Oncology* 3.1 (2008): 6–12.

58. Antoch, G., et al. Non-small cell lung cancer: dual-modality PET/CT in preoperative staging. *Radiology* 229.2 (2003): 526–33.

59. Gupta, N. C., et al. Clinical utility of PET-FDG imaging in differentiation of benign from malignant adrenal masses in lung cancer. *Clinical Lung Cancer* 3.1 (2001): 59–64.

60. Blake, M. A., et al. Adrenal lesions: characterization with fused PET/CT image in patients with proved or suspected malignancy – initial experience. *Radiology* 238.3 (2006): 970–77.

61. Yun, M., et al. 18F-FDG PET in characterizing adrenal lesions detected on CT or MRI. *Journal of Nuclear Medicine* 42.12 (2001): 1795–99.

62. Erasmus, J. J., et al. Evaluation of adrenal masses in patients with bronchogenic carcinoma using 18F-fluorodeoxyglucose positron emission tomography. *AJR American Journal of Roentgenology* 168.5 (1997): 1357–60.

63. Maurea, S., et al. Positron emission tomography (PET) with fludeoxyglucose F 18 in the study of adrenal masses: comparison of benign and malignant lesions [in Italian]. *Radiologia Medica* 92.6 (1996): 782–87.

64. Boland, G. W., et al. Indeterminate adrenal mass in patients with cancer: evaluation at PET with 2-[F-18]-fluoro-2-deoxy-D-glucose. *Radiology* 194.1 (1995): 131–34.

65. Adams, K., et al. Test performance of endobronchial ultrasound and transbronchial needle aspiration biopsy for mediastinal staging in patients with lung cancer: systematic review and meta-analysis. *Thorax* 64.9 (2009): 757–62.

66. Gu, P., et al. Endobronchial ultrasound-guided transbronchial needle aspiration for staging of lung cancer: a systematic review and meta-analysis. *European Journal of Cancer* 45.8 (2009): 1389–96.

67. Fleisher, L. A., et al. ACC/AHA 2007 guidelines on perioperative cardiovascular evaluation and care for noncardiac surgery: a report of the American College of Cardiology/American Heart Association Task Force on Practice Guidelines (Writing Committee to revise the 2002 guidelines on perioperative cardiovascular evaluation for noncardiac surgery). *Circulation* 116.17 (2007): e418–e500.

68. Lim, E., et al. Guidelines on the radical management of patients with lung cancer. *Thorax* 65 (2010): Suppl-27.

69. Health and Social Care Information Centre. National lung cancer audit. Leeds, UK: Health and Social Care Information Centre, 2007.

70. Falcoz, P. E., et al. The Thoracic Surgery Scoring System (Thoracoscore): risk model for in-hospital death in 15,183 patients requiring thoracic surgery. *Journal of Thoracic & Cardiovascular Surgery* 133.2 (2007): 325–32.

71. Chamogeorgakis, T. P., et al. Thoracoscore predicts midterm mortality in patients undergoing thoracic surgery. *Journal of Thoracic & Cardiovascular Surgery* 134.4 (2007): 883–87.

72. Bluman, L. G., et al. Preoperative smoking habits and postoperative pulmonary complications. *Chest* 113.4 (1998): 883–89.

73. Schag, C. A., et al. Quality of life in adult survivors of lung, colon and prostate cancer. *Quality of Life Research* 3.2 (1994): 127–41.

74. Dales, R. E., et al. Quality-of-life following thoracotomy for lung cancer. *Journal of Clinical Epidemiology* 47.12 (1994): 1443–49.

75. Zieren, H. U., et al. Quality of life after surgical therapy of bronchogenic carcinoma. *European Journal of Cardio-Thoracic Surgery* 10.4 (1996): 233–37.

76. Brunelli, A., et al. Quality of life before and after major lung resection for lung cancer: a prospective follow-up analysis. *Annals of Thoracic Surgery* 84.2 (2007): 410–16.

77. Balduyck, B., et al. Quality of life evolution after lung cancer surgery: a prospective study in 100 patients. *Lung Cancer* 56.3 (2007): 423–31.

78. Deslauriers, J., et al. Sleeve lobectomy versus pneumonectomy for lung cancer: a comparative analysis of survival and sites or recurrences. *Annals of Thoracic Surgery* 77.4 (2004): 1152–56.

79. Ginsberg, R. J., and L. V. Rubinstein. Randomized trial of lobectomy versus limited resection for T1 N0 non-small cell lung cancer. Lung Cancer Study Group. *Annals of Thoracic Surgery* 60.3 (1995): 615–22.

80. Swanson, S. J., et al. Video-assisted thoracic surgery lobectomy: report of CALGB 39802 – a prospective, multi-institution feasibility study. *Journal of Clinical Oncology* 25.31 (2007): 4993–97.

81. Whitson, B. A., et al. Surgery for early-stage non-small cell lung cancer: a systematic review of the video-assisted thoracoscopic surgery versus thoracotomy approaches to lobectomy. *Annals of Thoracic Surgery* 86.6 (2016): 2008–16.

82. Cao, C., et al. A meta-analysis of unmatched and matched patients comparing video-assisted thoracoscopic lobectomy and conventional open lobectomy. *Annals of Cardiothoracic Surgery* 1.1 (2012): 16–23.

83. Paul, S., et al. Long term survival with thoracoscopic versus open lobectomy: propensity matched comparative analysis using SEER-Medicare database. *BMJ* 349 (2014): g5575.

84. Casali, G., and W. S. Walker. Video-assisted thoracic surgery lobectomy: can we afford it? *European Journal of Cardio-Thoracic Surgery* 35.3 (2009): 423–28.

85. Paulson, D. L. Carcinomas in the superior pulmonary sulcus. *Journal of Thoracic & Cardiovascular Surgery* 70.6 (1975): 1095–104.

86. Macchiarini, P., et al. Technique for resecting primary and metastatic nonbronchogenic tumors of the thoracic outlet. *Annals of Thoracic Surgery* 55.3 (1993): 611–18.

87. Dartevelle, P., et al. Transcervical excision of bronchopulmonary cancers with apical invasiveness [in French]. *Revue de Pneumologie Clinique* 48.5 (1992): 211–16.

88. Rusch, V. W., et al. Induction chemoradiation and surgical resection for superior sulcus non-small-cell lung carcinomas: long-term results of Southwest Oncology Group Trial 9416 (Intergroup Trial 0160). *Journal of Clinical Oncology* 25.3 (2007): 313–18.

89. Health and Social Care Information Centre. Mesothelioma. National lung cancer report 2014. Report for the period 2008–2012. Leeds, UK: Health and Social Care Information Centre, 2014b.

90. Flores, R. M., et al. Positron emission tomography defines metastatic disease but not locoregional disease in patients with malignant pleural mesothelioma. *Journal of Thoracic & Cardiovascular Surgery* 126.1 (2003): 11–16.

91. Rusch, V. W. A proposed new international TNM staging system for malignant pleural mesothelioma. From the International Mesothelioma Interest Group. *Chest* 108.4 (1995): 1122–28.

92. Sugarbaker, D. J., W. G. Richards, and R. Bueno. Extrapleural pneumonectomy in the treatment of epithelioid malignant pleural mesothelioma: novel prognostic implications of combined N1 and N2 nodal involvement based on experience in 529 patients. *Annals of Surgery* 260.4 (2014): 577–80.

93. Rusch, V. W., et al. A phase II trial of surgical resection and adjuvant high-dose hemithoracic radiation for malignant pleural mesothelioma. *Journal of Thoracic & Cardiovascular Surgery* 122.4 (2001): 788–95.

94. Aziz, T., A. Jilaihawi, and D. Prakash. The management of malignant pleural mesothelioma; single centre experience in 10 years. *European Journal of Cardio-Thoracic Surgery* 22.2 (2002): 298–305.

95. Stewart, D. J., et al. The effect of extent of local resection on patterns of disease progression in malignant pleural mesothelioma. *Annals of Thoracic Surgery* 78.1 (2004): 245–52.

96. Treasure, T., et al. Extra-pleural pneumonectomy versus no extra-pleural pneumonectomy for patients with malignant pleural mesothelioma: clinical outcomes of the Mesothelioma and Radical Surgery (MARS) randomised feasibility study. *Lancet Oncology* 12.8 (2011): 763–72.

97. Rice, D., et al. Recommendations for uniform definitions of surgical techniques for malignant pleural mesothelioma: a consensus report of the International Association for the Study of Lung Cancer international staging committee and the international mesothelioma interest group. *Journal of Thoracic Oncology* 6.8 (2011): 1304–12.

98. Flores, R. M., et al. Extrapleural pneumonectomy versus pleurectomy/decortication in the surgical management of malignant pleural mesothelioma: results in 663 patients. *Journal of Thoracic & Cardiovascular Surgery* 135.3 (2008): 620–26.

99. Rintoul, R. C., et al. Efficacy and cost of video-assisted thoracoscopic partial pleurectomy versus talc pleurodesis in patients with malignant pleural mesothelioma (MesoVATS): an open-label, randomised, controlled trial. *Lancet* 384.9948 (2014): 1118–27.

100. Bissett, D., F. R. Macbeth, and I. Cram. The role of palliative radiotherapy in malignant mesothelioma. *Clinical Oncology (Royal College of Radiologists)* 3.6 (1991): 315–17.

101. Ahamad, A., et al. Promising early local control of malignant pleural mesothelioma following postoperative intensity modulated radiotherapy (IMRT) to the chest. *Cancer Journal* 9.6 (2003): 476–84.

102. Berghmans, T., et al. Activity of chemotherapy and immunotherapy on malignant mesothelioma: a systematic review of the literature with meta-analysis. *Lung Cancer* 38.2 (2002): 111–21.

103. Vogelzang, N. J., et al. Phase III study of pemetrexed in combination with cisplatin versus cisplatin alone in patients with malignant pleural mesothelioma. *Journal of Clinical Oncology* 21.14 (2003): 2636–44.

104. Tan, K. K., Gde L. Lopes Jr., and R. Sim. How uncommon are isolated lung metastases in colorectal cancer? A review from database of 754 patients over 4 years. *Journal of Gastrointestinal Surgery* 13.4 (2009): 642–48.

105. Internullo, E., et al. Pulmonary metastasectomy: a survey of current practice amongst members of the European Society of Thoracic Surgeons. *Journal of Thoracic Oncology* 3.11 (2008): 1257–66.

106. Treasure, T. Pulmonary metastasectomy for colorectal cancer: weak evidence and no randomised trials. *European Journal of Cardio-Thoracic Surgery* 33.2 (2008): 300–2.

107. Edwards, A. T. Malignant disease of the lung. *Journal of Thoracic Surgery* 4 (1934): 107–24.

108. Blalock, A. Recent advances in surgery. *New England Journal of Medicine* 231 (1944): 261–67.

109. Pastorino, U., et al. Long-term results of lung metastasectomy: prognostic analyses based on 5206 cases. *Journal of Thoracic & Cardiovascular Surgery* 113.1 (1997): 37–49.

110. Casali, C., et al. Prognostic factors and survival after resection of lung metastases from epithelial tumours. *Interactive Cardiovascular & Thoracic Surgery* 5.3 (2006): 317–21.

111. Ercan, S., et al. Prognostic significance of lymph node metastasis found during pulmonary metastasectomy for extrapulmonary carcinoma. *Annals of Thoracic Surgery* 77.5 (2004): 1786–91.

112. Loehe, F., et al. Value of systematic mediastinal lymph node dissection during pulmonary metastasectomy. *Annals of Thoracic Surgery* 72.1 (2001): 225–29.

113. Pastorino, U., et al. Fluorodeoxyglucose positron emission tomography improves preoperative staging of resectable lung metastasis. *Journal of Thoracic & Cardiovascular Surgery* 126.6 (2003): 1906–10.

114. Pfannschmidt, J., et al. Nodal involvement at the time of pulmonary metastasectomy: experiences in 245 patients. *Annals of Thoracic Surgery* 81.2 (2006): 448–54.

115. Detterbeck, F. C., et al. Imaging requirements in the practice of pulmonary metastasectomy. *Journal of Thoracic Oncology* 5.6:Suppl 2 (2010): Suppl-9.

116. Remy-Jardin, M., et al. Pulmonary nodules: detection with thick-section spiral CT versus conventional CT. *Radiology* 187.2 (1993): 513–20.

117. Margaritora, S., et al. Pulmonary metastases: can accurate radiological evaluation avoid thoracotomic approach? *European Journal of Cardio-Thoracic Surgery* 21.6 (2002): 1111–14.

118. Seltzer, S. E., et al. Spiral CT of the chest: comparison of cine and film-based viewing. *Radiology* 197.1 (1995): 73–78.

119. Tillich, M., et al. Detection of pulmonary nodules with helical CT: comparison of cine and film-based viewing. *AJR American Journal of Roentgenology* 169.6 (1997): 1611–14.

120. Kang, M. C., et al. Accuracy of 16-channel multi-detector row chest computed tomography with thin sections in the detection of metastatic pulmonary nodules. *European Journal of Cardio-Thoracic Surgery* 33.3 (2008): 473–79.

121. Lonneux, M., et al. FDG-PET improves the staging and selection of patients with recurrent colorectal cancer. *European Journal of Nuclear Medicine & Molecular Imaging* 29.7 (2002): 915–21.

122. Cahan, W. G., E. B. Castro, and S. I. Hajdu. Proceedings: the significance of a solitary lung shadow in patients with colon carcinoma. *Cancer* 33.2 (1974): 414–21.

123. McCormack, P. Surgical resection of pulmonary metastases. *Seminars in Surgical Oncology* 6.5 (1990): 297–302.

124. Rusch, V. W. Pulmonary metastasectomy: a moving target. *Journal of Thoracic Oncology* 5.6:Suppl 2 (2010): Suppl-1.

125. Molnar, T. F., C. Gebitekin, and A. Turna. What are the considerations in the surgical approach in pulmonary metastasectomy? *Journal of Thoracic Oncology* 5.6:Suppl 2 (2010): Suppl-4.

126. Hazelrigg, S. R., et al. Combined median sternotomy and video-assisted thoracoscopic resection of pulmonary metastases. *Chest* 104.3 (1993): 956–58.

127. Cerfolio, R. J., T. McCarty, and A. S. Bryant. Non-imaged pulmonary nodules discovered during thoracotomy for metastasectomy by lung palpation. *European Journal of Cardio-Thoracic Surgery* 35.5 (2009): 786–91.

128. Mutsaerts, E. L., et al. Outcome of thoracoscopic pulmonary metastasectomy evaluated by confirmatory thoracotomy. *Annals of Thoracic Surgery* 72.1 (2001): 230–33.

129. Eckardt, J., and P. B. Licht. Thoracoscopic versus open pulmonary metastasectomy: a prospective, sequentially controlled study. *Chest* 142.6 (2012): 1598–602.

130. Mutsaerts, E. L., et al. Long term survival of thoracoscopic metastasectomy vs metastasectomy by thoracotomy in patients with a solitary pulmonary lesion. *European Journal of Surgical Oncology* 28.8 (2002): 864–68.

131. Saito, Y., et al. Pulmonary metastasectomy for 165 patients with colorectal carcinoma: a prognostic assessment. *Journal of Thoracic & Cardiovascular Surgery* 124.5 (2002): 1007–13.

132. Shiono, S., et al. Histopathologic prognostic factors in resected colorectal lung metastases. *Annals of Thoracic Surgery* 79.1 (2005): 278–82.

133. Lee, W. S., et al. Pulmonary resection for metastases from colorectal cancer: prognostic factors and survival. *International Journal of Colorectal Disease* 22.6 (2007): 699–704.

134. Melloni, G., et al. Prognostic factors and analysis of microsatellite instability in resected pulmonary metastases from colorectal carcinoma. *Annals of Thoracic Surgery* 81.6 (2006): 2008–13.

135. Welter, S., et al. Long-term survival after repeated resection of pulmonary metastases from colorectal cancer. *Annals of Thoracic Surgery* 84.1 (2007a): 203–10.

136. Dahabre, J., et al. Surgical management in lung metastases from colorectal cancer. *Anticancer Research* 27.6C (2007): 4387–90.

137. Chen, F., et al. Prognostic factors of pulmonary metastasectomy for colorectal carcinomas. *World Journal of Surgery* 33.3 (2009): 505–11.

138. Ike, H., et al. Results of aggressive resection of lung metastases from colorectal carcinoma detected by intensive follow-up. *Diseases of the Colon & Rectum* 45.4 (2002): 468–73.

139. Onaitis, M. W., et al. Prognostic factors for recurrence after pulmonary resection of colorectal cancer metastases. *Annals of Thoracic Surgery* 87.6 (2009): 1684–88.

140. Watanabe, I., et al. Prognostic factors in resection of pulmonary metastasis from colorectal cancer. *British Journal of Surgery* 90.11 (2003): 1436–40.

141. Lin, B. R., et al. Pulmonary resection for colorectal cancer metastases: duration between cancer onset and lung metastasis as an important prognostic factor. *Annals of Surgical Oncology* 16.4 (2009): 1026–32.

142. Gonzalez, M., et al. Risk factors for survival after lung metastasectomy in colorectal cancer patients: a systematic review and meta-analysis. *Annals of Surgical Oncology* 20.2 (2013): 572–79.

143. van Halteren, H. K., et al. Pulmonary resection for metastases of colorectal origin. *Chest* 107.6 (1995): 1526–31.

144. Inoue, M., et al. Benefits of surgery for patients with pulmonary metastases from colorectal carcinoma. *Annals of Thoracic Surgery* 78.1 (2004): 238–44.

145. Girard, P., et al. Should the number of pulmonary metastases influence the surgical decision? *European Journal of Cardio-Thoracic Surgery* 12.3 (1997): 385–91.

146. Iida, T., et al. Prognostic factors after pulmonary metastasectomy for colorectal cancer and rationale for determining surgical indications: a retrospective analysis. *Annals of Surgery* 257.6 (2013): 1059–64.

147. McCormack, P. M., et al. Lung resection for colorectal metastases. 10-year results. *Archives of Surgery* 127.12 (1992): 1403–6.

148. Pfannschmidt, J., et al. Prognostic factors and survival after complete resection of pulmonary metastases from colorectal carcinoma: experiences in 167 patients. *Journal of Thoracic & Cardiovascular Surgery* 126.3 (2003): 732–39.

149. Younes, R. N., F. Abrao, and J. Gross. Pulmonary metastasectomy for colorectal cancer: long-term survival and prognostic factors. *International Journal of Surgery* 11.3 (2013): 244–48.

150. Schule, S., et al. Long-term results and prognostic factors after resection of hepatic and pulmonary metastases of colorectal cancer. *International Journal of Colorectal Disease* 28.4 (2013): 537–45.

151. Pfannschmidt, J., H. Hoffmann, and H. Dienemann. Reported outcome factors for pulmonary resection in metastatic colorectal cancer. *Journal of Thoracic Oncology* 5.6:Suppl 2 (2010): Suppl-8.

152. Hirosawa, T., et al. Prognostic factors in patients undergoing complete resection of pulmonary metastases of colorectal cancer: a multi-institutional cumulative follow-up study. *Surgery Today* 43.5 (2013): 494–99.

153. Tomimaru Y., et al. Metastatic tumor doubling time is an independent predictor of intrapulmonary recurrence after pulmonary resection of solitary pulmonary metastasis from colorectal cancer. *Dig Surg.* 2008;25(3):220–5 doi: 10.1159/000140693. Epub 2008 Jun 23.

154. Chojniak, R., and R. N. Younes. Pulmonary metastases tumor doubling time: assessment by computed tomography. *American Journal of Clinical Oncology* 26.4 (2003): 374–77.

155. Welter, S., et al. Prognostic impact of lymph node involvement in pulmonary metastases from colorectal cancer. *European Journal of Cardio-Thoracic Surgery* 31.2 (2007b): 167–72.

156. Fiorentino, F., et al. Pulmonary metastasectomy in colorectal cancer: a systematic review and quantitative synthesis. *Journal of the Royal Society of Medicine* 103.2 (2010): 60–66.

157. Utley, M., and T. Treasure. The use of scoring systems in selecting patients for lung resection: work-up bias comes full-circle. *Thoracic Surgery Clinics* 18.1 (2008): 107–12.

158. Utley, M., and T. Treasure. Interpreting data from surgical follow-up studies: the role of modeling. *Journal of Thoracic Oncology* 5.6 (2010): S200–2.

159. Treasure, T., L. Fallowfield, and B. Lees. Pulmonary metastasectomy in colorectal cancer: the PulMiCC trial. *Journal of Thoracic Oncology* 5.6:Suppl 2 (2010): Suppl-6.

160. Goldberg, S. N., et al. Radiofrequency tissue ablation in the rabbit lung: efficacy and complications. *Academic Radiology* 2.9 (1995): 776–84.

161. Petre, E. N., et al. Treatment of pulmonary colorectal metastases by radiofrequency ablation. *Clinical Colorectal Cancer* 12.1 (2013): 37–44.

162. Siva, S., M. MacManus, and D. Ball. Stereotactic radiotherapy for pulmonary oligometastases: a systematic review. *Journal of Thoracic Oncology* 5.7 (2010): 1091–99.

24

Esophageal cancer

FRANCO ROVIELLO, KAROL POLOM AND DANIELE MARRELLI

INTRODUCTION

Esophageal cancer (EC) is the eighth most common malignancy worldwide causing nearly 456,000 new cases in 2012 and is the sixth most common cause of cancer-related deaths worldwide. The highest incidence rates are observed in eastern Asia, and the lowest in western Africa. The two main types are squamous cell carcinoma (SCC) and adenocarcinoma (AC). The incidence of EC continues to rise with 17,460 new cases in 2012 in the US, and about 45,900 cases in Europe in 2012 [2]. Among European countries the highest age-standardized incidence rates for EC were observed in the Netherlands for men and in the UK for women. The lowest rates were observed in Macedonia for men and the Republic of Moldova for women [1,2].

The highest incidence of EC is observed in the Asian belt with countries like Turkey, Iran, Kazakhstan and northern–central China. The incidence of SCC in this region is more than 100 cases per 100,000 population per year.

European age-standardized incidence rates for males increased by 65% between 1975–1977 and 1999–2001. For females the increased number is smaller, ~26% between 1975–1977 and 1999–2001, and since then has fallen by 10% [3]. This phenomenon might be associated with changing exposure to known risk factors which include tobacco, insufficient fruit and vegetables intake, obesity and alcohol consumption [4].

SCC is the predominant form of EC worldwide, but an epidemiological shift has been observed in the US, UK, Australia and some European countries (e.g. Finland, France and the Netherlands) where more esophageal ACs than SCCs are now diagnosed.

The other less common types of EC are melanoma, leiomyosarcoma and small-cell carcinoma.

The tumour-type distribution varies among races in the US: ~64% of ECs among Caucasians is AC, and among the African American population 82% are SCC. The number of new cases among Caucasians doubled while in the same period the number of new cases among African Americans has decreased by about 50% [5]. The majority of the increase of EC in the US population is due to the massive 463% increase in esophageal AC.

The most common risk factors for EC are smoking and alcohol abuse. The combination of both these factors can increase the risk of esophageal SCC from 25- to 100-fold. The most common risk factors for both types of EC are tobacco use and a history of mediastinal radiation [6]. Alcohol consumption is a risk factor for SCC but not for AC [7]. Other known risk factors for AC are obesity, gastroesophageal reflux disease (GERD), Barrett's esophagus, a diet low in vegetables and fruits, increased age, male sex, medications that relax the lower esophageal sphincter and a familial history (rare) [6,8]. A high-grade dysplastic Barrett's esophagus is considered a premalignant condition as in half of the cases during biopsy an occult malignancy is seen. Another risk factor is familial keratosis palmaris and plantaris (tylosis). For SCC other risk factors are all conditions that lead to chronic irritation of the esophagus and inflammation – alcohol abuse, mutations of the enzymes that metabolize alcohol, achalasia, esophageal diverticula and frequent consumption of extremely hot beverages. Other environmental and nutritional factors for both EC types are zinc or nitrosamine exposure, malnutrition, vitamin deficiencies, anaemia, poor oral hygiene and dental caries and previous gastric surgery. Some esophageal conditions may also be associated with an increased risk of EC: achalasia, GERD, Barrett's esophagus, radiation esophagitis, caustic burns, Plummer–Vinson syndrome, leukoplakia, esophageal diverticula and ectopic gastric mucosa. Interestingly the risk of esophageal AC might be decreased by history of *Helicobacter pylori* infection [9] (Table 24.1).

One of the strongest risk factors of esophageal AC is symptomatic GERD. The symptoms are present in about 60% of patients. Additionally obesity is a known risk factor. These two factors might be responsible for the increasing number of new cases of AC in Western societies where obesity rates are rising rapidly [10]. The frequency of Barrett's syndrome is estimated at about 1.6% of the population, with up to 15% of those who undergo endoscopic procedures for reflux syndrome being diagnosed. The factors associated with Barrett's syndrome are GERD, bile reflux and obesity. The risk of an EC in Barrett's syndrome varies from 0.12% to 0.5% per year [11].

In case of high-grade dysplasia in Barrett's syndrome progression into AC occurs in 16–59% of patients [12].

Recently genetic biomarker studies have been shown to be useful for diagnosis and prognosis of EC. Certain genetic polymorphisms and micro-RNA expression may also influence susceptibility to EC [13].

PATHOLOGICAL SUBTYPES, STAGING AND PROGNOSIS

EC is an aggressive cancer from the perspective of both local spread and the development of metastatic disease. From an anatomical point of view the esophagus is the only part of the gastrointestinal (GI) tract without a serosal layer. This favours local infiltration of the surrounding tissues. In addition the disease metastasizes via extensive submucosal lymphatics and blood vessels.

Cancers of the cervical part of the esophagus drain into deep cervical, paraesophageal, posterior mediastinal and tracheobronchial lymph nodes. They can also infiltrate the trachea, aorta and left recurrent laryngeal nerve. In the distal third of the esophagus – where the majority of ACs are seen, the lymphatics drain into paraesophageal, celiac and splenic hilar lymph nodes. They can infiltrate the diaphragm, pericardium, stomach, lungs or liver. Mediastinal lymphatic drainage is complicated and extensive and metastatic spread into mediastinal, supraclavicular or celiac lymph nodes is often seen.

SCC is located mainly in the thoracic part of the esophagus, with 60% of cases seen in the middle third, and 30% in the distal third.

The main gross pathological divisions of SCC are fungating, ulcerating, infiltrating and polypoid. The best outcome

Table 24.1 Risk factors associated with EC and its main subtypes SCC and AC

SCC	AC
Smoking	Smoking
Alcohol consumption	Obesity
Familial keratosis palmaris and plantaris (tylosis)	Gastroesophageal reflux disease (GERD)
Conditions that lead to chronic irritation of the esophagus and inflammation	Barrett's esophagus
Mutations of the enzymes that metabolize alcohol	Diet low in vegetables and fruits
Achalasia	Increased age
Esophageal diverticula	Male sex
Frequent consumption of extremely hot beverages	Medications that relax the lower esophageal sphincter
Caustic injury	Familial history
Low socioeconomic status	
Zinc or nitrosamine exposure	
Malnutrition	
Vitamin deficiencies	
Anaemia	
Poor oral hygiene and dental caries	
Previous gastric surgery	
History of thoracic radiation	

is seen in the polypoid form with 5-year survivals of about 70%; the other three forms present a poor prognosis with 5-year survival seen in less than 15%. The current TNM classification of EC and the histologic-grade definitions for esophagus and esophagogastric junction cancer together with division into SCC and AC are presented in Tables 24.2 and 24.3.

In Western countries the most common type of EC is AC. In the majority of cases it is situated at the gastro-esophageal junction. It is four times more common among Caucasians than African Americans, and eight times more common among males than females. The prognosis for the majority of patients is strongly linked to tumour size. The TNM staging and survival by stage are shown in Table 24.3.

The overall 5-year survival rate for all patients diagnosed with EC ranged from 15% to 20% in 1980. It has improved largely as a result of using preoperative chemotherapy and chemoradiotherapy by 38% for chemotherapy and up to 60% for combined chemoradiotherapy [14,30,90].

Table 24.2 TNM status with histologic-grade definitions for esophagus and esophagogastric junction cancer

T status	N status	M status	Histologic grade
Tis: High-grade dysplasia	N0: No regional lymph node metastases	M0: No distant metastases	G1: Well differentiated
T1: Invasion into the lamina propria, muscularis mucosae or submucosa	N1: 1–2 positive regional lymph nodes	M1: Distant metastases	G2: Moderately differentiated
T2: Invasion into muscularis propria	N2: 3–6 positive regional lymph nodes		G3: Poorly differentiated
T3: Invasion into adventitia	N3: 7 or more positive regional lymph nodes		G4: Undifferentiated
T4a: Invades resectable adjacent structures (pleura, pericardium, diaphragm)			
T4b: Invades unresectable adjacent structures (aorta, vertebral body, trachea)			

Source: With kind permission from Springer Science+Business Media: AJCC Cancer Staging Manual, 7th ed, 2010, 103–15, Edge SB, Byrd DR, Compton CC.

Table 24.3 Stage groupings for esophagus and esophagogastric junction cancer and 5-year survival rates according to stage of the disease

Stage	Adenocarcinoma				Squamous cell carcinoma					5-year survival (%)
	T	N	M	Grade	T	N	M	G	Location	
0	Tis	0	0	1	Tis	0	0	1	Any	
IA	1	0	0	1–2	1	0	0	1	Any	50–94
IB	1	0	0	3	1	0	0	2–3	Any	
	2	0	0	1–2	2–3	0	0	1	Lower	
IIA	2	0	0	3	2–3	0	0	1	Upper, middle	15–65
					2–3	0	0	2–3	Lower	
IIB	3	0	0	Any	2–3	0	0	2–3	Upper, middle	
	1–2	1	0	Any	1–2	1	0	Any	Any	
IIIA	1–2	2	0	Any	1–2	2	0	Any	Any	6–23
	3	1	0	Any	3	1	0	Any	Any	
	4a	0	0	Any	4a	0	0	Any	Any	
IIIB	3	2	0	Any	3	2	0	Any	Any	
IIIC	4a	1–2	0	Any	4a	1–2	0	Any	Any	
	4b	Any	0	Any	4b	Any	0	Any	Any	
	Any	3	0	Any	Any	3	0	Any	Any	
IV	Any	Any	1	Any	Any	Any	1	Any	Any	<4

Source: With kind permission from Springer Science+Business Media: AJCC Cancer Staging Manual, 7th ed, 2010, 103–15, Edge SB, Byrd DR, Compton CC.
Note: Definitions of the cancer localization: upper thoracic, 20–25 cm from incisors; middle thoracic, 25–30 cm from incisors; lower thoracic, 30–40 cm from incisors.

CLINICAL PRESENTATION

The most common clinical presentation of EC is dysphagia, but the number of asymptomatic patients diagnosed by endoscopy has increased recently. Other significant symptoms include vomiting, weight loss and GI bleeding. Less common symptoms include odynophagia, retrosternal pain, constant hiccups, hypersalivation, halitosis and regurgitation [15]. There are significant differences in the clinical presentation of SCC versus AC. In SCC patients the most common presentation is dysphagia, accompanied by weight loss often linked with a strong history of smoking and drinking alcohol. In AC patients the average patient is a white man with a GERD history and recent onset dysphagia with minimal or no weight loss [16].

DIAGNOSIS

To cause dysphagia two-thirds of the esophageal lumen has to be obstructed. Initially patients complain of 'food sticking' at the level of the tumour. Dysphagia is the chief symptom of EC in 80–90% of cases, so any adult patient presenting with such a symptom must have endoscopy ± biopsy of any stricture identified.

Esophagogastroduodenoscopy and biopsy are the main tools in the diagnosis of EC, to both confirm the diagnosis and establish the location of the tumour (Figure 24.1). In distal esophageal tumours it is important to determine whether there is cardial and gastric involvement. In proximal esophageal tumours relations to the cricopharyngeus can be established. In proximal and middle esophageal tumours, bronchoscopy may be needed. Biopsy of abnormalities in the esophageal wall and also adjacent structures under ultrasound guidance may be helpful.

Radiological investigations routinely used in the assessment of disease extent include chest X-ray, barium swallow, CT, MRI and PET scanning. Plain chest X-ray is abnormal only in 50% of patients. An air-fluid level may be seen in an obstructed esophagus, or a dilated esophagus, mediastinal adenopathy or tracheal deviation may be seen. Double-contrast barium swallow shows the tumour location, length, degree of luminal narrowing, ulceration and strictures. Using CT and endoscopic ultrasound tumour location and adjacent lymphadenopathy can be assessed. MRI adds little additional information over that provided by CT. In case of difficulties in biopsying the tumour during standard endoscopy, endoscopic ultrasound-guided fine-needle aspiration (EUS-FNA) may be helpful. In Western countries, because of the low incidence of EC, a screening program is not cost-effective (Figures 24.1 through 24.9).

To enhance the accuracy of staging PET scanning has been shown to be valuable. It can help in assessing both the T and N statuses with a superior performance in comparison to CT scan [17]. PET scan is also widely used in assessing for distant metastases. In a paper by Duong and colleagues the usage of PET scanning was responsible for changed clinical management in 27 of 68 (40%) patients [18]. In 12 patients therapy intent was changed from curative to palliative, in 3 from palliative to curative and in 12 patients a different treatment modality or delivery was performed but with the same treatment intent. Therefore a PET scan is very valuable in proper treatment planning for patients. PET scanning may also have value for follow-up for recurrence and to evaluate response during and after chemoradiotherapy [19].

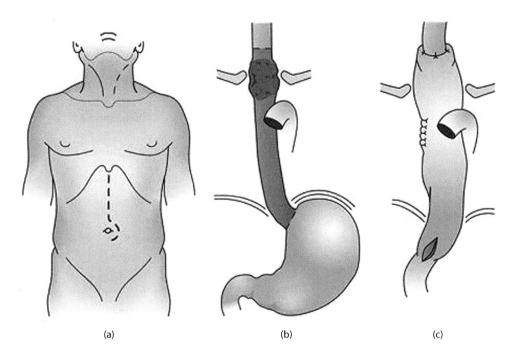

(a)   (b)   (c)

Figure 24.1 Transhiatal esophagectomy with gastric mobilization and gastric pull-up cervical anastomosis.

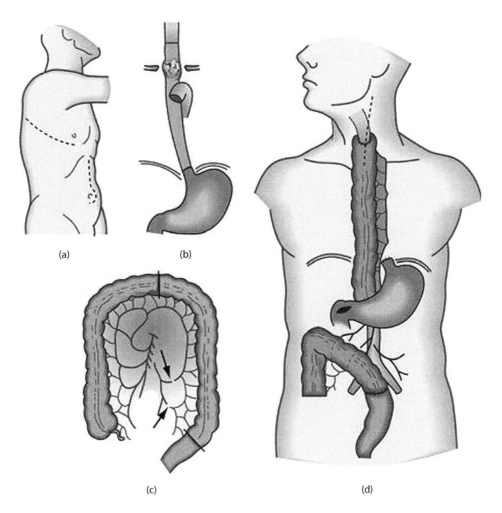

(a)   (b)

(c)   (d)

Figure 24.2 Esophagectomy with interposition of antiperistaltic segment of left colon.

STAGING

EC is staged using the TNM system. The 7th edition of the *AJCC Cancer Staging Manual* for esophageal and esophagogastric junction cancers is shown in Tables 24.2 and 24.3 [20,21]. In this classification gastroesophageal junction cancers and gastric cancers in the first 5 cm of the stomach and which extend to the gastroesophageal junction are classified alongside EC. Different classifications are made for SCC and AC (Tables 24.2 and 24.3).

In stage I cancer 5-year survival rates are 50–94%, in stage II 15–65%, in stage III 6–23% and in stage IV less than 4%.

Lymph node staging

The lymphatic drainage network of the esophagus is one of the most complex as it drains via three pathways: the neck, thoracic cavity and abdominal cavity. To evaluate lymph node status a range of imaging modalities may be used: EUS, CT, MRI and PET. Additional information may be gained from video-assisted thoracic surgery (VATS) or diagnostic laparoscopy. However, it is difficult to discriminate between enlarged lymph nodes due to hyperplasia or

metastatic disease with these imaging modalities [21,22]. Accuracy increases if EUS-FNA is also performed [22]. Useful prognostic information regarding recurrence risk may also be obtained by genetic mapping in node negative patients which may be of value in the future [23].

Staging for distant metastases

EUS is highly accurate for the estimation of T status (accuracy 80–92%) and N status (accuracy 45–100%) [24], and the metastatic status is usually determined by CT scanning. In patients with cancer in the upper and medial part of the esophagus a bronchoscopy should be performed for synchronous or metachronous malignancies in the pharynx, larynx and bronchial tree. Additional procedures like MRI, bone scans and staging mediastinoscopy should be performed only in symptomatic cases [25]. MRI is helpful in the assessment of T4 stage disease and for a more detailed assessment of metastatic disease (especially in the liver), but this procedure may over stage lymph node involvement. PET scanning is routinely used in all patients being considered for surgical resection to rule out metastases if other modalities are negative. PET scanning may change the stage of the disease in up to 20% of patients and may identify

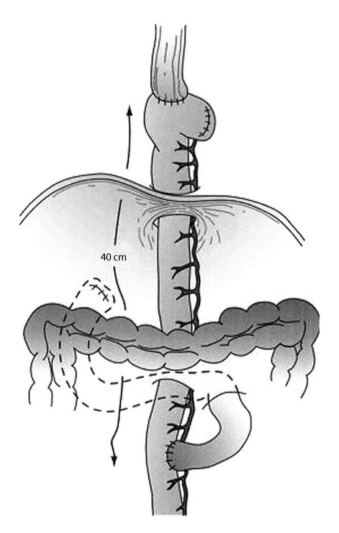

Figure 24.3 Roux-en-Y reconstruction after distal esophagectomy with total gastrectomy because of distal esophagus and cardiac cancer.

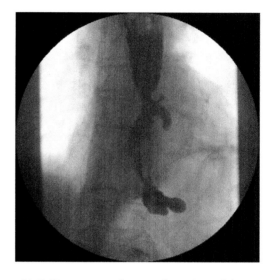

Figure 24.5 Contrast swallow confirmation of the tumour rupture after primarily chemoradiotherapy treatment.

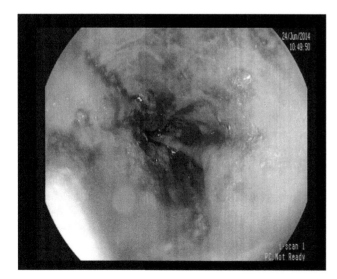

Figure 24.4 Endoscopic visualization of esophageal cancer.

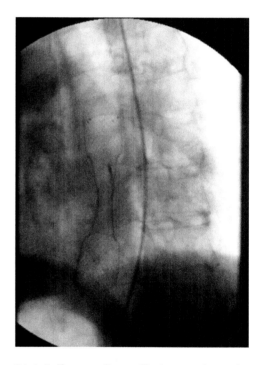

Figure 24.6 Self-expanding palliative esophageal stent visualization on X-ray.

occult metastatic disease in up to 15% of cases including M1 nodal metastases [25].

PET scanning is also of great value in assessing the response to neoadjuvant chemotherapy whereby early responders may complete their full course of preoperative chemotherapy, while non-responders proceed to surgery without further delay. The difference between responders and non-responders in event-free survival is 29.7 months versus 14.1 months ($p = 0.002$) [26]. The value of PET scanning in response evaluation in cases undergoing chemoradiotherapy is smaller. In AC the PET response does not

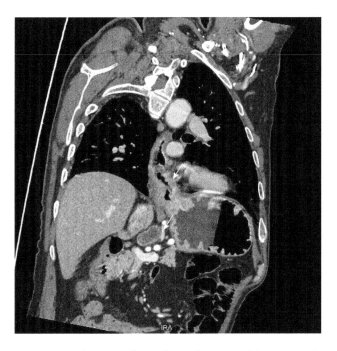

Figure 24.7 CT scan of esophageal cancer with metastatic lymph node.

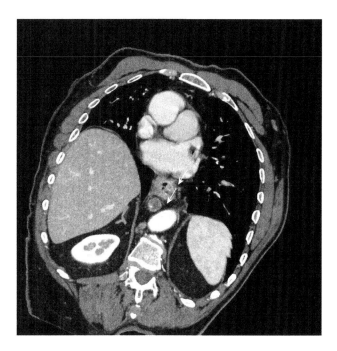

Figure 24.8 CT scan of esophageal cancer with metastatic lymph node.

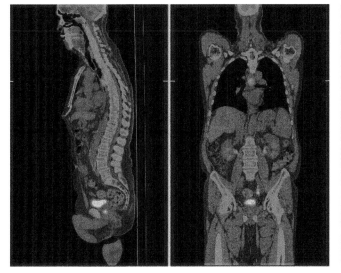

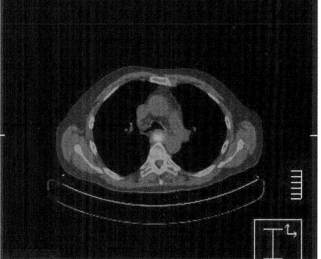

Figure 24.9 PET scan of a patient with esophageal cancer.

correlate with pathological response to neoadjuvant therapy, but in SCC this correlation is much stronger [27].

Minimally invasive staging

Minimally invasive staging (MIS) using laparoscopy or thoracoscopy is used only in selected patients. Laparoscopy improves the accuracy of staging offered by CT and ultrasound scan. It improves the detection rate for hepatic, peritoneal and lymph node metastases. Bronchoscopy should be used to evaluate upper- and middle-third tumours if there is a suspicion of local invasion or impending tracheoesophageal

fistulation. In comparison with PET, MIS shows a higher accuracy in the diagnosis of distant metastases, especially when the diameter of the lesion is less than 1 cm [28].

TREATMENT OF EC

Patients with early stage tumours (T1/2, N0, M0) have a good chance of being cured by surgery. Locally advanced disease (T3/4, N0/1, M0) is usually treated with multimodal treatment schedules, often including surgery if possible. In metastatic disease or in case of local recurrence the treatment is based on palliative chemotherapy and radiotherapy plus palliative stenting and laser ablation to control dysphagia. All have similar efficacy. Survival times are short and with a mean survival of about 140 days [29] so priority must be given to maintenance of quality of life (QoL).

Curative surgery

Early EC is a rare finding but if it is diagnosed in this stage (cancer invading the mucosa or submucosa) we can use less invasive methods with curative intent. Superficial EC can be treated endoscopically by mucosal resection, but in some cases ablative methods only, where no specimen is taken, such as laser therapy, argon plasma coagulation and photodynamic therapy, may be used.

As the cancer invades into deeper layers of the esophageal wall multimodal treatment gives superior results and must be tailored for each patient. In the CROSS trial, surgery alone achieved an R0 resection rate of 69% and a median survival of 24.2 months. In the neoadjuvant chemoradiotherapy arm an R0 resection was achieved in 92% ($p < 0.001$), with a complete pathological response seen in 29% of patients and a median survival of 49.4 months ($p = 0.003$). The 5-year survival rate was also significantly increased from 34% to 47%. Rates of locoregional recurrence were also significantly lower (34% vs. 14%; $p < 0.001$), and there was a reduced rate of peritoneal carcinomatosis (14% to 4%; $p < 0.001$). In patients with primarily operable gastric and lower esophageal AC, use of preoperative chemotherapy (epirubicin, cisplatin and fluorouracil) resulted in a reduced tumour size and stage and improved overall survival (MAGIC trial) [31].

Surgical planning requires careful consideration of patient fitness for what is major surgery. Fitness may be further compromised by malnutrition and the effects of chemotherapy and radiotherapy.

For those considered suitable for surgery there are four main techniques for esophagectomy depending on the site of the tumour, the experience of the surgeon and the fitness of the patient [32]:

- Transhiatal
- Transthoracic
- En bloc
- Video assisted

All have comparable morbidity and mortality rates and are described in more detail below.

Preoperative management

In cases presenting with significant esophageal stenosis or significant malnutrition preoperative endoscopic dilatation and stent insertion may be valuable. In some cases passage of a fine-bore feeding tube may be indicated and in more severe cases, total parenteral nutrition may be beneficial. The indications for preoperative enteral and parenteral support are generally still the subject of intense research. Even patients with premorbid obesity or overweight (with a body mass index [BMI] of more than 25 kg/m^2) have evidence of significant weight loss in 57% of cases in the months before diagnosis [33]. Commercial formulas given by tube feeding may help in delivering appropriate amounts of macro- and micronutrients in cases when oral feeding is not possible. A nasogastric tube, percutaneous endoscopic gastrostomy (PEG) or jejunostomy may all be used. Optimized nutritional status in patients undergoing major abdominal surgery, by use of enteral or parenteral nutritional support, has been shown to reduce postoperative complications and length of hospital stay. However, the results from clinical trials specifically on EC patients are not clear-cut [34]. The best results are observed in patients undergoing chemo- and radiotherapy, where nutritional support is beneficial. Globally the preferential use of enteral nutrition compared with parenteral nutrition may reflect the lower costs and fewer technical considerations of use rather than implying superiority of one over the other [34].

Transhiatal esophagectomy

Esophageal resection without thoracotomy is known as a transhiatal procedure [35] which was developed to avoid pulmonary complications as well as intrathoracic anastomotic leakage. The esophagus is blindly mobilized from below via the diaphragmatic hiatus and is reconstructed in the neck by anastomosis of the stomach to the cervical esophagus. The technique is contraindicated in the presence of direct tumour invasion of the aorta, pericardium or tracheobronchial tree due to the blind nature of the dissection.

Transhiatal esophagectomy (THE) is associated with reduced blood loss and lower rates of pulmonary complications but has a much higher rate of cervical leakage of the anastomosis. However, leakage in the neck will heal spontaneously or with local drainage in most cases without the major systemic risks of intrathoracic sepsis [36].

Transthoracic esophagectomy

The advantage of transthoracic esophagectomy (TTE) is the ability to perform a thoracic lymph node dissection under direct visualization and resection of the tumour mass with any adjacent tissues. However, the cost is an increased postoperative morbidity. After stomach mobilization excellent access and visualization of the thoracic contents are provided by right thoracotomy (in proximal esophageal tumours) or left thoracotomy (in the case of distal tumours). The problem is that opening two cavities – abdominal and thoracic – in weakened patients is responsible for pulmonary complications often necessitating prolonged mechanical ventilation and associated with a higher morbidity and mortality [37,38]. Anastomotic leakage occurs less frequently, but when it does occur inside the thoracic cavity it is associated with mediastinitis and sepsis which may be fatal in more than 50% of cases. Other disadvantages associated with TTE include reflux esophagitis because of surgical interruption of the lower esophageal sphincter mechanism, and if recurrence develops above the anastomosis it is technically very difficult to treat.

En bloc esophagectomy

EC has a high rate of lymph node metastases, and en bloc esophagectomy (EBE) permits careful and radical dissection of the regional lymph node stations en bloc with adjacent tissues. The tissue is resected along with the spleen, celiac nodes, posterior pericardium, azygos vein, thoracic duct and adjacent diaphragm. Oncologically very rigorous, this procedure is unfortunately associated with a higher rate of operative mortality of up to 11%. [39] due primarily to anastomotic leakage and pulmonary complications.

Minimally invasive esophagectomy

Minimally invasive techniques have progressed greatly in recent years. Currently it is estimated that ~30% of all operations are done using this technique [40]. Minimally invasive esophagectomy (MIE) may be a mix of different surgical techniques: a hybrid technique, a full MIE or a robotic technique. Each type of technique should be chosen carefully with respect to tumour position, general health status of the patient and the technical skills of the operator. The biggest problem associated with esophagectomy historically has been a relatively high mortality rate of up to 23% [41]. In a series of 1011 consecutive esophagectomies performed using laparoscopic and thoracoscopic techniques the operative mortality was only 1.7% with oncological results similar to those from a historical series of open esophagectomies [42]. The advantages of using this procedure are a lower number of pulmonary complications, reduced blood loss and reduced hospital stay [43–45]. The disadvantage is the prolonged operative time. In meta-analysis based on 16 studies it was found that MIE was able to retrieve a significantly greater number of lymph nodes than open techniques, probably because of better operation field visualization. However, this did not translate into an improvement in survival in comparison with open techniques [46].

Another important issue is QoL after surgery. Early studies showed that QoL after surgery worsened in the first 6 weeks but had returned to preoperative levels by 9 months in patients who survived 2 years or more [43]. MIE does improve QoL in comparison with classic open techniques.

TECHNIQUES OF RECONSTRUCTION AFTER ESOPHAGECTOMY

After esophageal resection a new conduit has to be created. The most commonly used manner of conduit placement is in the posterior mediastinum in the space left by the resected esophagus. In most cases the conduit is created from the stomach, but the colon or a Roux-en-Y loop of small intestine may also be used [44,45]. The popularity of the gastric conduit relates to its easy mobilization and robust blood supply. A colonic conduit is associated with a slightly higher rate of anastomotic leakage because of the necessity of performing three anastomoses. Use of the colon as a conduit is usually indicated in patients who have undergone previous gastric surgery or if the esophageal tumour extends into the stomach such that a minimum 5 cm margin cannot be achieved.

Some surgeons prefer to use a non-anatomical route for the new esophagus, for example in a substernal position, to reduce the likelihood of a local recurrence and problems with obstruction. It may avoid radiotherapy exposure to the new conduit. The route is technically more challenging as the substernal route is longer.

For very proximally located tumours reconstruction may be more challenging. In some cases not only the esophagus but also the pharynx may need to be resected. In these cases complex skin tubes, myocutaneous flaps and free microsurgical transfer of segments of jejunum may be required. In cases of cervicothoracic tumours the best option is laryngopharyngectomy with THE. Use of the colon as a conduit in this situation, rather than the stomach, may give more satisfactory results because of problems with regurgitation after pharyngogastric anastomosis.

Multimodal treatment

With the exception of patients with very early stage EC surgery alone is inadequate to cure the disease and tailored multimodal treatment is required. This must take into account not just disease stage, type and location but also the health status of the patient.

Neoadjuvant chemoradiotherapy

In case of locally advanced EC neoadjuvant chemoradiotherapy prior to surgery is the optimal form of multimodal treatment. Many studies have compared chemoradiotherapy followed by surgery versus surgery alone. The results have been heterogeneous with some showing no significant benefit and others a benefit [8,47–49]. One large multicentre study showed a benefit of neoadjuvant chemoradiotherapy with a greater effect in SCC patients. Overall review of the studies by meta-analysis has confirmed the beneficial effect of neoadjuvant chemoradiotherapy in EC patients [50].

Surgery with adjuvant chemotherapy, radiotherapy or chemoradiotherapy

The goal of postoperative radiotherapy is to destroy residual malignant cancer cells after surgery, especially in cases with positive surgical margins. In a prospective randomized trial survival was significantly improved in the group having surgery with postoperative radiotherapy versus surgery alone [51]. Other studies state that postoperative radiotherapy may play an important role in reducing the number of local recurrences but has no influence on improvement in overall survival [52].

Radiotherapy alone for EC should be selectively used with palliative intent, in patients who are not good candidates for surgery or chemotherapy [53]. Radiotherapy alone is associated with a low morbidity and improvement in obstruction in patients suffering from dysphagia usually within 7 days. This beneficial effect is short-lived, however, and symptoms usually recur within 6 months [54]. Radiotherapy is not suitable for patients presenting with a transesophageal fistula and indeed may cause this serious complication.

Postoperative radiotherapy alone (64 Gy) in comparison to radiotherapy (50 Gy) plus chemotherapy has shown that chemoradiotherapy results in significantly better rates of local control even at the lower radiotherapy dose used in the chemoradiotherapy regime [55]. Indeed in further studies to assess whether higher-dose RT is superior to lower (64.8 Gy in comparison with 50.4 Gy) as part of a chemoradiotherapy regime, the higher dose did not show any benefits in overall survival or local recurrence but was associated with a higher morbidity [56]. Currently chemoradiotherapy is standard procedure and radiotherapy alone is just warranted for those patients who are not fit for chemotherapy.

In the last decade or so investigators have focused on discovering the optimal multimodal combination of chemotherapy, radiotherapy and surgery. The new challenge is to discover what role new biological agents may have in improving cure rates. Cure rates have advanced with multimodal regimes compared with surgery alone in patients with stage I–III disease. Overall survival has improved to 39% with multimodal therapy versus 16% with surgery alone [57]. Adjuvant chemotherapy may significantly benefit patients, especially node positive patients. The ECOG E 8296 trial proved that using adjuvant cisplatin and paclitaxel after complete surgical resection in node positive patients is advantageous in AC patients. Trials performed by the Japan Clinical Oncology Group (JCOG) on SCC patients have shown significantly better outcomes with postoperative chemotherapy or chemoradiotherapy [58,59].

In addition better-targeted radiotherapy techniques such as intensity-modulated radiation therapy (IMRT) improve dose delivery to the target area and reduce damage to surrounding structures such as the lung, reducing the risk of pneumonitis, pericarditis, myocarditis, stricture, fistula formation and spinal cord damage [60].

Prognosis and follow-up

Today EC is one of the least studied forms of cancer with one of the highest mortality rates. The overall 5-year survival rate is about 17% [61] largely due to the late stage at diagnosis. At the time of diagnosis more than 50% of patients already have metastatic spread and 30% have locally advanced disease. Only 20% have localized, early stage disease where cure is likely [61,62]. For patients presenting with stage 0 and IA disease, based on the Worldwide Esophageal Cancer Collaboration, 5-year survival rates of between 70% and 80% may be achieved, with better outcome for AC than SCC [63]. For the 30% presenting with locally advanced disease a surgical procedure alone is sub-optimal and is associated with 5-year survival rates of between 10% and 30%. Multimodal therapy will increase this rate significantly.

Centralization of treatment

EC surgery is one of the most technically challenging and is associated with a high rate of postoperative complications with rates ranging between 26% and 41%, and high rates of postoperative mortality [6]. Acute surgical outcomes have improved recently, due to a combination of factors including a move toward centralization of such surgery to high-volume centres and high-volume surgeons. This has been shown to have a positive impact on postoperative complications, early postoperative mortality and health economics. The evidence of benefit for long-term survival and QoL is lacking, however. There is still no consensus on the ideal number of esophagectomies annually to optimize outcomes. A meta-analysis tried to answer the question about the number of cases treated in very low-volume hospitals (VLVHs) and very high-volume hospitals (HVHs), and defined a VLVH as fewer than 5 esophagectomies per year and HVH as more than 20 esophagectomies per year [64]. Comparison of outcomes between such units showed postoperative mortality in VLHV as 18% and HVH as 4.9%. It has to be pointed out that modern treatment of EC is not just related to surgical skills and patient volume, but to multidisciplinary teamwork, preoperative patient selection and preparation, the experience of the surgeon, anaesthetist and nursing staff, and the early diagnosis of and ability to manage complications [65].

Surgical approaches

The most commonly used surgical approaches to EC are THE, TTE (Ivor Lewis) and the McKeown (three-incision) esophagectomy (McKE). In case of THE, the following sequence is performed: abdominal exploration, stomach mobilization and preparation, lymph node dissection, hiatus enlargement, thoracic esophageal mobilization, lymph node dissection, left cervical exploration and finally cervical anastomosis. In case of TTE (Ivor Lewis) the following sequence has to be done: abdominal exploration, stomach mobilization and preparation, lymph node dissection, thoracic exploration, thoracic esophageal mobilization, lymph node dissection and anastomosis. The advantages of this technique are the lower number of postoperative strictures, a reduced anastomotic leak rate and reduced aspiration rates. When performing a McKE esophagectomy the following sequence is performed: thoracic exploration, thoracic esophageal mobilization, lymph node dissection, ligation of the thoracic duct, abdominal exploration, stomach mobilization and preparation, lymph node dissection and left cervical exploration for anastomosis. The advantages of McKE are a lower rate of local recurrences and easier treatment of cervical leakage from the anastomosis. Choice of technique will depend on the preoperative extension and location of the tumour. McKE is feasible for Siewert I and II tumours, as well as for the whole esophagus up to the clavicle. TTE by Ivor Lewis is also suitable for Siewert I and II tumours and other parts of the esophagus but not those located above the carina.

Lymphadenectomy

Currently two-field lymphadenectomy is a standard component of EC surgery. In the only phase III trial that compared THE and TTE for AC esophagectomy 5-year survival rates were 29% and 39%, respectively, but this was not statistically significant [66]. Another study (for SCC) did not show any significant survival improvement when comparing three-field versus two-field lymphadenectomy [67]. Another study comparing two-field lymphadenectomy versus lymph node sampling showed significant survival benefit for two-field lymphadenectomy (36% vs. 25%) [68]. Some authors still advocate three-field lymphadenectomy as the best way to improve the 5-year survival rate [69]. There are some problems associated with routine three-field lymphadenectomy in the case of EC. First, those with proven positive high mediastinal or cervical nodes in many cases also have nodal involvement elsewhere [70]. Pathologically proven metastases in the cervical nodes are found in about 15–30% of cases, but in the case of two-field lymphadenectomy a cervical node recurrence is a rare entity [71]. Using immunohistochemistry for nodal analysis rather than just standard H&E staining up to 50% of pathologically (H&E) node negative patients have micrometastases [72]. The presence of skip metastases to the cervical lymph nodes from lower-third EC is a rare entity [73]. The most commonly involved lymph nodes in cases of upper-third EC are the superior mediastinal nodes, so in this position of the tumour three-field lymphadenectomy should be considered [74]. Radical lymph node dissection in the cervical compartment in cases of three-field lymphadenectomy was associated with higher rates of postoperative morbidity like recurrent laryngeal nerve palsy, which can be associated with a higher rate of pulmonary complications, as well as anastomotic leakage [75]. In the new age of neoadjuvant chemotherapy it seems that two-field lymphadenectomy may be the preferred option for the majority of patients [76].

Sentinel node biopsy

Another minimally invasive technique that may be used in EC treatment is sentinel node biopsy (SNB) for lymphatic mapping and limited lymph node dissection. SNB is currently well established in the treatment of breast cancer and melanoma [77,78] with interest in its use in gastric, prostate and colon cancers, where it has shown that lymphatic networks are much more complicated than in the case of breast cancer or cutaneous melanoma [79–81]. The lymphatic network of the esophagus is complex with lots of lymphatic capillary networks, especially in the submucosal layer, that lead to longitudinal lymphatic drainage and are responsible for the phenomenon of skip metastases [82]. Lymphatic flow between the cervical esophagus and the abdomen is anatomically possible. Use of blue dye may be confounded because of the presence of mediastinal anthracitic lymph nodes in some patients. Use of radiocolloids is made technically challenging by the 'shine-through phenomenon' when in the region of the colloid injection site. Using SNB techniques during EC resections more tailored lymphadenectomy may be planned in patients with T2 or T3 stage disease and the optimal resection technique suggested for those with T1 stage disease. In patients with tumours located in the mediastinum, SNs were found from the cervical regions to the abdominal cavity [83,84]. For the upper mediastinal esophagus SNs were found to be situated in recurrent nodes to the cervical areas; in the middle esophagus the SNs were found in regions closely associated with the tumour (right recurrent, bifurcational, main bronchus lymph nodes) [83,84]. For the gastroesophageal junction tumours the SNs were mainly biopsied in the lower paraesophageal, paracardial, para-aortic and left gastric nodes [83,84]. Siewert I tumours showed a high rate of lower esophageal SNs, and Siewert II tumours drained into abdominal SNs.

Salvage esophagectomy

Salvage esophagectomy (SE) is one performed either for locoregional recurrence after definitive chemoradiotherapy where no surgery was planned (dCXRT), or sometimes for esophagectomies done more than 3 months after induction neoadjuvant chemoradiotherapy. In the case of those recurring after dCXRT and in whom there is no evidence of metastatic disease, there are few therapeutic alternatives to surgery. Further radiotherapy may exceed normal tissue tolerances and the tumour may be relatively radioresistant. Early diagnosis by undertaking regular follow-up every 4 months in the first 2 years and every 6–12 months later is important. All patients should undergo full re-staging before surgery is considered. Resection will depend on tumour location and extent but should be accompanied by two-field lymphadenectomy. The biggest challenge with this type of operation is conduit necrosis which is observed in up to 25% of cases [85], possibly due to radiation-induced impairment of tissue vascularity and fibrosis. There is also a higher rate of anastomotic leak if the anastomosis is performed using previously irradiated tissue; therefore such an anastomosis should be performed using non-radiated tissue if possible. The surgeon should also consider use of other organs to create the conduit such as the colon, or even the small intestine (±microvascular anastomosis). In cases of salvage resection the rate of R1 or R2 resections is high – from 10% to 70% of cases [86]. Patients that undergo SE have higher rates of in-hospital mortality, longer hospital stay, longer stay on intensive care unit, higher rates of complications and more blood transfusion [87]. The final outcome in patients for whom an R0 resection is achieved is good and 5-year survival rates may be as high as 60% in some studies, but this ranges from 0% to 35% in others [88–91]. The biggest available series presents 5-year survival in only 32% of patients [87].

BENIGN ESOPHAGEAL TUMOURS AND CYSTS

Benign tumours of the esophagus are rare [91,92]. They constitute 0.5–0.8% of all esophageal tumours. The most common tumour type is gastrointestinal stromal tumour (GIST) (60%), followed by cysts and polyps (20% and 5%) [93].

Esophageal GISTs

GISTs are the most common benign submucosal neoplasm of mesenchymal origin located in the esophagus. They may be benign or of borderline or overt malignancy. The majority of esophageal GISTs are observed in patients between 20 and 50 years old with an equal male and female distribution. The predominant location is in the middle and lower thirds of the esophagus. In the majority they present as a single lesion, very rarely as multiple tumours. A more detailed description of the biology of GISTs is included in Chapter 26.

DIAGNOSIS

Clinical presentation is with dysphagia or retrosternal pain in patients with tumours larger than 5 cm [94]. On esophagograms the tumour is often seen as a well-localized non-circumferential mass, smooth surfaced and well demarcated. The majority are now diagnosed during endoscopy where there is liminal narrowing associated with intact mucosa. Endoscopic ultrasonography shows a hypoechic tumour in the muscularis propria or submucosal layer.

TREATMENT

In most cases, benign tumours of the esophagus are treated with minimally invasive techniques. In those cases in a mucosal or submucosal location endoscopic resection techniques are usually preferred and have been shown to be safe. Some also advocate these techniques in deeper tumours in the muscular layer, but this is associated with a higher rate of perforation. For tumours in the muscular layer minimally invasive techniques such as laparoscopic or robotic excision, combined endoscopic and laparoscopic (rendezvous) techniques and abdominothoracic approaches are used [95].

Polyps

Esophageal polyps are usually sited in the proximal esophagus and are covered by normal epithelium with a fibroelastic core. The treatment is endoscopic resection or electrocoagulation or in some cases open surgical resection usually through a cervical incision.

REFERENCES

1. Siegel R, Naishadham D, Jemal A. Cancer statistics, 2012. *CA Cancer J Clin* 2012;62:10–29.
2. Ferlay J, Soerjomataram I, Dikshit R, Eser S, Mathers C, Rebelo M, Parkin DM, Forman D, Bray F. Cancer incidence and mortality worldwide: sources, methods and major patterns in GLOBOCAN 2012. *Int J Cancer* 2015;136(5):E359–86.
3. Rutegård M, Nordenstedt H, Lu Y, et al. Sex-specific exposure prevalence of established risk factors for oesophageal adenocarcinoma. *Br J Cancer* 2010;103(5):735–40.
4. Parkin DM, Boyd L, Walker LC. 16. The fraction of cancer attributable to lifestyle and environmental factors in the UK in 2010. Summary and conclusions. *Br J Cancer* 2011;105(S2):S77–81.
5. Horner M, Ries L, Krapcho M, et al. SEER cancer statistics review, 1975–2006. Bethesda, MD: National Cancer Institute. Available at http://seer.cancer.gov/csr/1975_2006/ (based on November 2008 SEER data submission posted to the SEER website, 2009).
6. Enzinger PC, Mayer RJ. Esophageal cancer. *N Engl J Med* 2003;349:2241–52.
7. Lee CH, Wu DC, Lee JM, et al. Carcinogenetic impact of alcohol intake on squamous cell carcinoma risk of the oesophagus in relation to tobacco smoking. *Eur J Cancer* 2007;43:1188–99.
8. Pennathur A, Gibson MK, Jobe BA, Luketich JD. Oesophageal carcinoma. *Lancet* 2013;381:400–12.
9. Islami F, Kamangar F. *Helicobacter pylori* and esophageal cancer risk: a meta-analysis. *Cancer Prev Res (Phila)* 2008;1:329–38.
10. Whiteman DC, Sadeghi S, Pandeya N, et al. Combined effects of obesity, acid reflux and smoking on the risk of adenocarcinomas of the oesophagus. *Gut* 2008;57:173–80.
11. Parameswaran R, Blazeby JM, Hughes R, Mitchell K, Berrisford RG, Wajed SA. Health-related quality of life after minimally invasive oesophagectomy. *Br J Surg* 2010;97:525–31.
12. Schnell TG, Sontag SJ, Chejfec G, et al. Long-term nonsurgical management of Barrett's esophagus with high-grade dysplasia. *Gastroenterology* 2001;120:1607–19.
13. Wang AH, Liu Y, Wang B, He YX, Fang YX, Yan YP. Epidemiological studies of esophageal cancer in the era of genome-wide association studies. *World J Gastrointest Pathophysiol* 2014;15;5(3):335–43.

14. Takagi I, Karasawa K. Growth of squamous cell esophageal carcinoma observed by serial esophagectomies. *J Surg Oncol* 1982;21:57–60.

15. Zwischenberger JB, et al. Esophagus. In Townsend CM Jr, Beauchamp RD, Evers BM, Mattox KL, eds., *Sabiston Textbook of Surgery*, 17th ed. Philadelphia: Elsevier, 2004: 1120, 1123.

16. Rice TW. Diagnosis and staging of esophageal cancer. In Pearson FG, Patterson GA, eds., *Pearson's Thoracic and Esophageal Surgery*, 3rd ed. Philadelphia: Churchill Livingstone/Elsevier, 2008: 454–63.

17. Kato H, Kuwano H, Nakajima M, et al. Comparison between positron emission tomography and computed tomography in the use of the assessment of esophageal carcinoma. *Cancer* 2002;94:921–8.

18. Duong CP, Demitriou H, Weih L, et al. Significant clinical impact and prognostic stratification provided by FDG-PET in the staging of oesophageal cancer. *Eur J Nucl Med Mol Imaging* 2006;33:759–69.

19. Kato H, Nakajima M. The efficacy of FDG-PET for the management of esophageal cancer: review article. *Ann Thorac Cardiovasc Surg* 2012;18(5):412–9.

20. Edge SB, Byrd DR, Compton CC, eds. *AJCC Cancer Staging Manual*, 7th ed. New York, NY: Springer, 2010: 103–15.

21. Rice TW, Blackstone EH, Rusch VW. 7th edition of the *AJCC Cancer Staging Manual*: esophagus and esophagogastric junction. *Ann Surg Oncol* 2010;17:1721–4.

22. Parmar KS, Zwischenberger JB, Reeves AL, et al. Clinical impact of endoscopic ultrasound-guided fine needle aspiration of celiac axis lymph nodes (M1a disease) in esophageal cancer. *Ann Thorac Surg* 2002;73:916–21.

23. Aloia TA, Harpole DH Jr, Reed CE, et al. Tumor marker expression is predictive of survival in patients with esophageal cancer. *Ann Thorac Surg* 2001;72:859–66.

24. Patel AN, Preskitt JT, Kuhn JA, et al. Surgical management of esophageal carcinoma. *Proc (Bayl Univ Med Cent)* 2003;16:280–4.

25. Levine MS, Chu P, Furth EE, Rubesin SE, Laufer I, Herlinger H. Carcinoma of the esophagus and esophagogastric junction: sensitivity of radiographic diagnosis. *AJR Am J Roentgenol* 1997;168:1423–26.

26. Lordick F, Ott K, Krause BJ, et al. PET to assess early metabolic response and to guide treatment of adenocarcinoma of the oesophagogastric junction: the MUNICON phase II trial. *Lancet Oncol* 2007;8:797–805.

27. Molena D, Sun HH, Badr AS, et al. Clinical tools do not predict pathological complete response in patients with esophageal squamous cell cancer treated with definitive chemoradiotherapy. *Dis Esophagus* 2014;27(4):355–9.

28. Luketich JD, Schauer P, Landreneau R, et al. Minimally invasive surgical staging is superior to endoscopic ultrasound in detecting lymph node metastases in esophageal cancer. *J Thorac Cardiovasc Surg* 1997;114:817–21, discussion 821–23.

29. Gee DW, Rattner DW. Management of gastroesophageal tumors. *Oncologist* 2007;12:175–85.

30. van Hagen P, Hulshof MC, van Lanschot JJ, et al. Preoperative chemoradiotherapy for esophageal or junctional cancer. *N Engl J Med* 2012;366(22):2074–84.

31. Cunningham D, Allum WH, Stenning SP, et al. Perioperative chemotherapy versus surgery alone for resectable gastroesophageal cancer. *N Engl J Med* 2006;355:11–20.

32. Bousamra M 2nd, Haasler GB, Parviz M. A decade of experience with transthoracic and transhiatal esophagectomy. *Am J Surg* 2002;183:162–7.

33. Ryan AM, Rowley SP, Healy LA, Flood PM, Ravi N, Reynolds JV. Post-oesophagectomy early enteral nutrition via a needle catheter jejunostomy: 8-year experience at a specialist unit. *Clin Nutr* 2006;25:386–93.

34. Bozzetti F. Nutritional support in patients with oesophageal cancer. *Support Care Cancer* 2010;18(Suppl. 2):S41–50.

35. Orringer MB, Sloan H. Esophagectomy without thoracotomy. *J Thorac Cardiovasc Surg* 1978;76:643–54.

36. Hulscher JB, Tijssen JG, Obertop H, et al. Transthoracic versus transhiatal resection for carcinoma of the esophagus: a metaanalysis. *Ann Thorac Surg* 2001;72:306–13.

37. Fok M, Law SY, Wong J. Operable esophageal carcinoma: current results from Hong Kong. *World J Surg* 1994;18:355–60.

38. Omloo JM, Lagarde SM, Hulscher JB, et al. Extended transthoracic resection compared with limited transhiatal resection for adenocarcinoma of the mid/distal esophagus: five-year survival of a randomized clinical trial. *Ann Surg* 2007;246(6):992–1000.

39. Anderson KD, Rouse TM, Randolph JG. A controlled trial of corticosteroids in children with corrosive injury of the esophagus. *N Engl J Med* 1990;323:637–40.

40. Boone J, Livestro DP, Elias SG, et al. International survey on esophageal cancer: part I surgical techniques. *Dis Esophagus* 2009;22:195–202.

41. Birkmeyer JD, Siewers AE, Finlayson EV, et al. Hospital volume and surgical mortality in the United States. *N Engl J Med* 2002;346:1128–37.

42. Luketich JD, Pennathur A, Awais O, et al. Outcomes after minimally invasive esophagectomy: review of over 1000 patients. *Ann Surg* 2012;256:95–103.

43. Pennathur A, Zhang J, Chen H, Luketich JD. The "best operation" for esophageal cancer? *Ann Thorac Surg* 2010;89:S2163–67.

44. Ikeda Y, Tobari S, Niimi M, et al. Reliable cervical anastomosis through the retrosternal route with stepwise gastric tube. *J Thorac Cardiovasc Surg* 2003;125:1306–12.

45. Davis PA, Law S, Wong J. Colonic interposition after esophagectomy for cancer. *Arch Surg* 2003;138:303–8.

46. Dantoc M, Cox MR, Eslick GD. Evidence to support the use of minimally invasive esophagectomy for esophageal cancer: a meta-analysis. *Arch Surg* 2012;147:768–76.

47. Le Prise E, Etienne PL, Meunier B, et al. A randomized study of chemotherapy, radiation therapy, and surgery versus surgery for localized squamous cell carcinoma of the esophagus. *Cancer* 1994;73:1779–84.

48. Bosset JF, Gignoux M, Triboulet JP, et al. Chemoradiotherapy followed by surgery compared with surgery alone in squamous-cell cancer of the esophagus. *N Engl J Med* 1997;337:161–67.

49. Urba SG, Orringer MB, Turrisi A, Iannettoni M, Forastiere A, Strawderman M. Randomized trial of preoperative chemoradiation versus surgery alone in patients with locoregional esophageal carcinoma. *J Clin Oncol* 2001;19:305–13.

50. Khushalani NI, Leichman CG, Proulx G, et al. Oxaliplatin in combination with protracted-infusion fluorouracil and radiation: report of a clinical trial for patients with esophageal cancer. *J Clin Oncol* 2002;20:2844–50.

51. Xiao ZF, Yang ZY, Liang J, et al. Value of radiotherapy after radical surgery for esophageal carcinoma: a report of 495 patients. *Ann Thorac Surg* 2003;75:331–6.

52. Teniere P, Hay JM, Fingerhut A, et al. Postoperative radiation therapy does not increase survival after curative resection for squamous cell carcinoma of the middle and lower esophagus as shown by a multicenter controlled trial. French University Association for Surgical Research. *Surg Gynecol Obstet* 1991;173:123–30.

53. Minsky BD. Combined modality therapy for esophageal cancer. *Semin Oncol* 2003;30:46–55.

54. Hishikawa Y, Kurisu K, Taniguchi M, et al. High-dose-rate intraluminal brachytherapy (HDRIBT) for esophageal cancer. *Int J Radiat Oncol Biol Phys* 1991;21:1133–5.

55. Cooper JS, Guo MD, Herskovic A, et al. Chemoradiotherapy of locally advanced esophageal cancer: long-term follow-up of a prospective randomized trial (RTOG 85-01). Radiation Therapy Oncology Group. *JAMA* 1999;281:1623–7.

56. Minsky BD, Pajak TF, Ginsberg RJ, et al. INT 0123 (Radiation Therapy Oncology Group 94-05) phase III trial of combined modality therapy for esophageal cancer: high-dose versus standard dose radiation therapy. *J Clin Oncol* 2002;20:1167–74.

57. Koshy M, Greenwald BD, Hausner P, Krasna MJ, Horiba N, Battafarano RJ, Burrows W, Suntharalingam M. Outcomes after trimodality therapy for esophageal cancer: the impact of histology on failure patterns. *Am J Clin Oncol* 2011;34(3):259–64.

58. Ando N, Iizuka T, Kakegawa T, et al. A randomized trial of surgery with and without chemotherapy for localized squamous carcinoma of the thoracic esophagus: the Japan Clinical Oncology Group Study. *J Thorac Cardiovasc Surg* 1997;114:205–9.

59. Ando N, Iizuka T, Ide H, et al. Surgery plus chemotherapy compared with surgery alone for localized squamous cell carcinoma of the thoracic esophagus: a Japan Clinical Oncology Group Study – JCOG9204. *J Clin Oncol* 2003;21:4592–96.

60. Macdonald JS, Smalley SR, Benedetti J, et al. Chemoradiotherapy after surgery compared with surgery alone for adenocarcinoma of the stomach or gastroesophageal junction. *N Engl J Med* 2001;345:725–30.

61. Zhang Y. Epidemiology of esophageal cancer. *World J Gastroenterol* 2013;19:5598–606.

62. Hayeck TJ, Kong CY, Spechler SJ, et al. The prevalence of Barrett's esophagus in the US: estimates from a simulation model confirmed by SEER data. *Dis Esophagus* 2010;23:451–7.

63. Rice TW, Blackstone EH, Rusch VW. A cancer staging primer: esophagus and esophagogastric junction. *J Thorac Cardiovasc Surg* 2010;139:527–529.

64. Metzger R, Bollschweiler E, Vallbohmer D, Maish M, DeMeester TR, Holscher AH. High volume centers for esophagectomy: what is the number needed to achieve low postoperative mortality? *Dis Esophagus* 2004;17:310–4.

65. Rouvelas I, Lagergren J. The impact of volume on outcomes after oesophageal cancer surgery. *ANZ J Surg* 2010;80(9):634–41.

66. Hulscher JB, van Sandick JW, de Boer AG, et al. Extended transthoracic resection compared with limited transhiatal resection for adenocarcinoma of the esophagus. *N Engl J Med* 2002;347:1662–9.

67. Nishihira T, Hirayama K, Mori S. A prospective randomized trial of extended cervical and superior mediastinal lymphadenectomy for carcinoma of the thoracic esophagus. *Am J Surg* 1998;175:47–51.

68. Fang W, Chen W, Yong J, et al. Thoraco-abdominal two-field lymphadenectomy combined with adjuvant chemotherapy in the management of thoracic esophageal carcinoma. *Chin J Thorac Cardiovasc Surg* 2005;21:268–71.

69. Altorki NK, Zhou XK, Stiles B, et al. Total number of resected lymph nodes predicts survival in esophageal cancer. *Ann Surg* 2008;248:221–6.

70. Lagarde SM, Cense HA, Hulscher JB, et al. Prospective analysis of patients with adenocarcinoma of the gastric cardia and lymph node metastasis in the proximal field of the chest. *Br J Surg* 2005;92:1404–8.

71. Mariette C, Balon JM, Piessen G, Fabre S, Van Seuningen I, Triboulet JP. Pattern of recurrence following complete resection of esophageal carcinoma and factors predictive of recurrent disease. *Cancer* 2003;97:1616–23.

72. Mueller JD, Stein HJ, Oyang T, et al. Frequency and clinical impact of lymph node micrometastasis and tumor cell microinvolvement in patients with adenocarcinoma of the esophagogastric junction. *Cancer* 2000;89:1874–82.

73. Tachibana M, Kinugasa S, Yoshimura H, et al. Clinical outcomes of extended esophagectomy with three-field lymph node dissection for esophageal squamous cell carcinoma. *Am J Surg* 2005;189:98–109.

74. Akiyama H, Tsurumaru M, Udagawa H, Kajiyama Y. Radical lymph node dissection for cancer of the thoracic esophagus. *Ann Surg* 1994;220:364–72.

75. Fang WT, Chen WH, Chen Y, Jiang Y. Selective three-field lymphadenectomy for thoracic esophageal squamous carcinoma. *Dis Esophagus* 2007;20:206–11.

76. Mariette C, Piessen G. Oesophageal cancer: how radical should surgery be? *Eur J Surg Oncol* 2012;38(3):210–13.

77. Veronesi U, Paganelli G, Viale G, et al. A randomized comparison of sentinel-node biopsy with routine axillary dissection in breast cancer. *N Engl J Med* 2003;349(6):546–53.

78. Valsecchi ME, Silbermins D, de Rosa N, Wong SL, Lyman GH. Lymphatic mapping and sentinel lymph node biopsy in patients with melanoma: a meta-analysis. *J Clin Oncol* 2011;29(11):1479–87.

79. van der Pas MH, Meijer S, Hoekstra OS, Riphagen II, de Vet HC, Knol DL, van Grieken NC, Meijerink WJ. Sentinel-lymph-node procedure in colon and rectal cancer: a systematic review and meta-analysis. *Lancet Oncol* 2011;12(6):540–50.

80. Wang Z, Dong ZY, Chen JQ, Liu JL. Diagnostic value of sentinel lymph node biopsy in gastric cancer: a meta-analysis. *Ann Surg Oncol* 2012;19(5):1541–50.

81. Sadeghi R, Tabasi KT, Bazaz SM, Kakhki VR, Massoom AF, Gholami H, Zakavi SR. Sentinel node mapping in the prostate cancer. Meta-analysis. *Nuklearmedizin* 2011;50(3):107–15.

82. Dabbagh Kakhki VR, Bagheri R, Tehranian S, Shojaei P, Gholami H, Sadeghi R, Krag DN. Accuracy of sentinel node biopsy in esophageal carcinoma: a systematic review and meta-analysis of the pertinent literature. *Surg Today* 2014;44(4):607–19.

83. Thompson SK, Bartholomeusz D, Jamieson GG. Sentinel lymph node biopsy in esophageal cancer: should it be standard of care? *J Gastrointest Surg* 2011;15(10):1762–68.

84. Grotenhuis BA, Wijnhoven BP, van Marion R, et al. The sentinel node concept in adenocarcinomas of the distal esophagus and gastroesophageal junction. *J Thorac Cardiovasc Surg* 2009;138(3):608–12.

85. Amini A, Ajani J, Komaki R, et al. Factors associated with local-regional failure after definitive chemoradiation for locally advanced esophageal cancer. *Ann Surg Oncol* 2014;21:306–14.

86. Hofstetter W. Salvage esophagectomy. *J Thorac Dis* 2014;6(S3):S341–9.

87. Marks JL, Hofstetter W, Correa AM, et al. Salvage esophagectomy after failed definitive chemoradiation for esophageal adenocarcinoma. *Ann Thorac Surg* 2012;94:1126–32.

88. Swisher SG, Wynn P, Putnam JB, et al. Salvage esophagectomy for recurrent tumors after definitive chemotherapy and radiotherapy. *J Thorac Cardiovasc Surg* 2002;123:175–83.

89. Gardner-Thorpe J, Hardwick RH, Dwerryhouse SJ. Salvage oesophagectomy after local failure of definitive chemoradiotherapy. *Br J Surg* 2007;94:1059–66.

90. Ychou M, Boige V, Pignon JP, et al. Perioperative chemotherapy compared with surgery alone for resectable gastroesophageal adenocarcinoma: an FNCLCC and FFCD multicenter phase III trial. *J Clin Oncol* 2011;1715:29–21.

91. Paul S, Altorki N. Outcomes in the management of esophageal cancer. *J Surg Oncol* 2014;110(5):599–610.

92. van Hagen P, Hulshof MC, van Lanschot JJ, et al. CROSS Group preoperative chemoradiotherapy for esophageal or junctional cancer. *N Engl J Med* 2012;366(22):2074–84.

93. Shamji F, Todd TR. Benign tumors. In Pearson FG, Cooper JD, Deslauiers J, et al., eds., *Esophageal Surgery*, 2nd ed. Philadelphia: Churchill Livingstone, 2002: 636–48.

94. Seremetis MG, Lyons WS, deGuzman VC, Peabody JW Jr. Leiomyomata of the esophagus. An analysis of 838 cases. *Cancer* 1976;38:2166–77.

95. Eckardt AJ, Lang H, Gockel I. Diagnosis and therapy of benign tumors of the esophagogastric junction. *Chirurg* 2014;85(12):1073–80.

25

Gastric cancer

WILLIAM H ALLUM, YOUNG-WOO KIM, ELISA FONTANA, NAUREEN STARLING
AND BANG WOOL EOM

INTRODUCTION

Management of patients with gastric cancer has evolved markedly over the last 30 years not only in terms of treatment but also with greater understanding of the molecular biology of what is a very common cancer worldwide. In this chapter the epidemiology of gastric cancer is presented with current understanding of aetiology as well as detail of pathology. The standard approaches to diagnosis are described including staging investigations. Finally there is a detailed discussion of both surgical and non-surgical treatments highlighting the latest developments from trials as well as improvements in outcome.

INCIDENCE

The non-standardized, incomplete nature of cancer data collection, which is commonly retrospective, limits epidemiology studies. The efficiency of registration as well as the change in population demographics can affect the impression of changes in disease incidence. Cases may be registered with comprehensive detail including specific histology or simply as 'stomach cancer'. The ageing population increases the number at risk even though incidence may appear to be decreasing as the total population increases. These factors can confound interpretation of incidence statistics but recent standardized registration approaches have improved reliability.

In 2012 there were 952,000 new cases of gastric cancer worldwide with 723,000 deaths, making it the fifth most common malignancy [1]. The incidence has significantly decreased over the last 40 years as it was the most common cancer in 1975. More than 70% of cases occur in developing countries with more than half of cases occurring in eastern Asia, principally China. The age-standardized incidence rates for men are double those for women and this relationship is constant across the world.

In high-incidence countries carcinoma of the distal stomach is the most prevalent. By contrast there has been a migration in location to the proximal stomach in countries with lower incidence such that in parts of northern Europe cardia cancers predominate. This change has been implicated in the poorer outcome in countries such as the UK, the Netherlands and Norway where cardia cancers are more common [2].

There does appear to be a geographical variation in incidence such that more temperate or colder latitudes are associated with higher incidence. This can produce intra-country variations as for example the mortality rates are almost double in northern provinces in Japan and China in comparison to the south. This may reflect environmental and dietary factors in aetiology.

AETIOLOGY

The traditional understanding of gastric cancer has been challenged by the changes in incidence implying it is a heterogeneous disease. The division into the two main histological subtypes of Lauren, intestinal and diffuse, is consistent with these changes [3]. Intestinal type has traditionally affected the distal stomach and has been explained aetiologically by the Correa hypothesis [4]. Cardia cancer tends to be a more diffuse type and affects a different population of higher social class, is associated with obesity and younger age and may have a more genetic basis, although this remains poorly understood.

Correa hypothesis

The Correa hypothesis was developed to postulate the effect of environmental factors on a step-wise change from atrophic gastritis through intestinal metaplasia and dysplasia to cancer (Figure 25.1). The hypothesis demonstrates the timing of environmental stimuli to histological changes in the development of intestinal-type gastric cancer.

Gastric cancer is principally a disease of low socioeconomic groups. In the Correa hypothesis the adverse effects of poor diet, social habits such as smoking and occupational exposure are apparent. The use of salt preservation of food is likely to be the principal factor, which was responsible for the high rates in the Far East in the mid-twentieth century. The lack of fresh fruits and vegetables in foods was common in economically poorer communities. This factor, however, appeared to be minimized with the advent of refrigerators and the increased intake

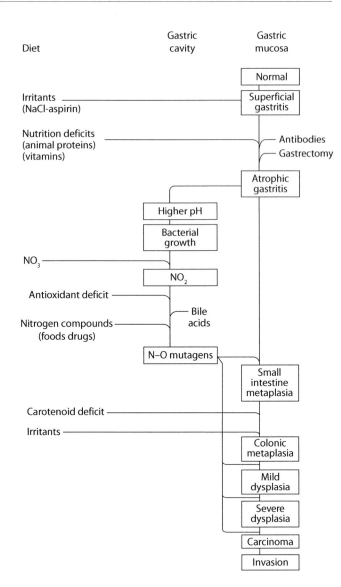

Figure 25.1 Correa hypothesis of gastric carcinogenesis.

of fresh foods [5]. Studies have attempted to determine the benefit of dietary intervention with high intake of vitamins A, C and E, as in theory these should protect against formation of nitrosamines and act as antioxidants. Such interventional studies have not shown a major effect, suggesting that it is more a balanced diet rather than one with enhanced supplements that is protective. Diets high in carbohydrates at the expense of protein intake, common in poorer communities, are implicated. Gastric mucosa protection and repair are impaired by protein deficiency. The established link between previous gastrectomy and gastric cancer is demonstrated by the adverse effect of excess bile salts.

The age of exposure to possible carcinogens seems to affect the risk of progression from gastric mucosal epithelial abnormality carcinogens to cancer. Migrants from Japan to the US had a lower rate of intestinal-type tumours than those who remained in Japan, reflecting their new environment and diet, although the diffuse types remained the same [6].

Helicobacter pylori

The effect of *H. pylori* in the development of gastric cancer has become a key area for intervention as a preventative strategy. *H. pylori* was designated a type I carcinogen by the International Agency for Research on Cancer in 1994 [7]. Evidence for its role includes epidemiological studies, which have demonstrated infection at a young age in communities with a high prevalence; many of these are poor socioeconomic communities. The decline in incidence in gastric cancer incidence has been paralleled by progressive reduction in rates of positive *H. pylori* serology.

The relationship between *H. pylori* and gastric cancer is apparent; however, not all those infected develop cancer. It is likely its effect is a reflection of bacterial virulence and host susceptibility. *H. pylori* initially causes an acute inflammation which untreated may induce a chronic gastritis and progress to mucosal atrophy, intestinal metaplasia and neoplasia. The infection reduces gastric ascorbic acid which suppresses N-nitroso compounds and free radicals [8]. This sets up an environment which supports proliferation of nitrosating bacteria. A specific genotype of the bacteria, *H. pylori* with cytotoxin-associated gene A (*cagA*), has been shown to carry the greatest risk [9]. In the West, 60% of *H. pylori* infections are *cagA* positive compared with 100% in Japan [10,11]. It is possible that inherited polymorphisms (normal variations in the genetic coding sequence of multiple genes) enhance susceptibility to *cagA* infection; first-degree relatives of those with intestinal-type gastric cancer have been shown to have higher rates of infection than controls.

H. pylori is also implicated in the development of diffuse-type gastric cancer. Polymorphisms associated with the production of variant proteins such as p53 have been identified more frequently in patients with diffuse gastric cancer than in matched controls [12]. DNA polymorphism in the interleukin-1 gene cluster appears to be a response to infection with *H. pylori*. As a result interleukin-1β production is increased, which as a proinflammatory cytokine inhibits gastric acid secretion and induces achlorhydria and gastric atrophy.

Hereditary diffuse gastric carcinoma

Hereditary diffuse gastric carcinoma (HDGC) is an autosomal dominantly inherited syndrome in which carriers have a 70% or more lifetime risk of diffuse gastric cancer. The inherited abnormality is a mutation in the *CDH1* tumour suppressor gene (the E-cadherin gene). Originally described in a series of Maori families in New Zealand, mutations have been detected in families of different ethnicities, all of whom have been shown to have mutations along the length of the gene rather than clustering as in sporadic cases.

HDGC families have been defined as those with two or more members younger than 50 years with diffuse gastric cancer or with three close relatives at any age [13]. Female carriers may also have a greater risk of lobular breast cancer. Clinical advice to these families requires

careful and experienced discussion. Although the risk of malignancy is high, a confounding finding is that 20–30% of *CDH1* mutations do not progress such that intramucosal disease remains quiescent analogous to prostatic cancer in elderly men.

The principal options are prophylactic total gastrectomy or endoscopic surveillance. Total gastrectomy is associated with both immediate perioperative morbidity and mortality and longer-term nutritional effects particularly as the surgery is undertaken at a young age. Endoscopy can be limited and falsely reassuring as in macroscopically normal stomach, intramucosal diffuse disease has been detected following resection [14,15]. Pathological studies have demonstrated patterns of mucosal abnormality allowing focusing of endoscopic biopsies. Improvements in targeting endoscopic biopsies with autofluorescence spectroscopy and chromoendoscopy may aid assessment. In practice most individuals undergo surgery between 20 and 30 years of age with endoscopy as the alternative depending on individual preference.

Hereditary cancer syndromes

The risk of developing gastric cancer is variably increased in a number of hereditary cancer syndromes [16]. This appears to reflect variations in the gene pool between different countries and populations and may be related to the underlying population incidence. For example in the Netherlands the risk of gastric cancer in association with Lynch syndrome, hereditary non-polyposis coli, is 2.1% compared with 30% in Korea. Other syndromes include Peutz–Jeghers syndrome, Li–Fraumeni syndrome, hereditary breast and ovarian cancer and familial adenomatous polyposis (FAP).

More recently a new syndrome has been described characterized by fundal gland polyps and gastric adenocarcinoma – gastric adenocarcinoma and proximal polyposis of the stomach [17]. It is an autosomal dominant syndrome in which polyps are restricted to the fundus with no evidence of colorectal or duodenal polyposis.

PATHOLOGY

Topographical pathology

EARLY AND ADVANCED GASTRIC CARCINOMA

Gastric cancer is classified as early (EGC) or advanced (AGC) combining both gross and microscopic features. EGC is defined as invasive carcinoma limited to the mucosa or submucosa, with or without lymph node metastases. Macroscopically EGC has been divided according to appearance (Figure 25.2) [18]. Commonly EGC is 2–5 cm in dimension, although it can be multifocal.

AGC is defined as penetration into and through the muscularis propria. The Borrmann classification has divided AGC according to gross appearance (Figure 25.3). Type IV includes linitis plastica in which tumour cells infiltrate submucosally and may be associated with minimal mucosal changes.

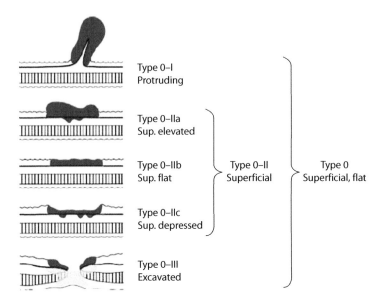

Figure 25.2 Classification of EGC.

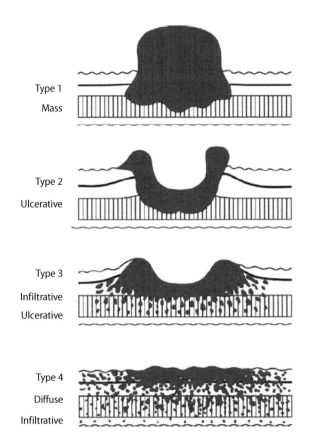

Figure 25.3 Macroscopic types of advanced gastric cancer.

Histopathology

A number of histological classifications have been described for gastric cancer. The Lauren classification [3] has been the most applied in routine practice. It divides tumours into intestinal (54% by proportion), diffuse (32%) and mixed or indeterminate (14%) types [19]. The intestinal type is associated with *H. pylori* infection [20,21] and the diffuse type is seen in younger and frequently female patients [3,22]. The degree of differentiation is a strong determinant of prognosis with poorly differentiated cancers having a poorer prognosis irrespective of local extent.

The WHO described a classification of the common histological findings of tubular, papillary, mucinous and poorly cohesive (including signet ring cell [SRC] carcinoma) cell types [23]. Tubular and papillary types are usually seen in EGC and are commonly well differentiated. An important differentiation is between intramucosal EGC and high-grade dysplasia which can be difficult with limited biopsy material as EGC has the potential to metastasize to lymph nodes. In AGC the papillary type is associated with a high rate of lymph node and liver metastasis. Mucinous adenocarcinoma is an unusual variant accounting for 10% of all cancers. The presence of SRCs is a pathognomonic feature of gastric cancer and the number of SRCs can vary from infrequent to extensive particularly in submucosal infiltration.

Patterns of spread

Gastric cancer exhibits four principal methods of spread: local infiltration, blood borne, lymphatic and transcoelomic. Blood-borne spread is usually via the portal venous system to the liver. Transcoelomic spread occurs once serosal penetration has occurred and cells are shed which commonly form deposits on peritoneal surfaces and classically into the pelvis as Krukenberg tumours of the ovary.

Lymphatic spread is particularly important as it has practical implications for treatment but also explains how gastric cancer spreads into the systemic circulation. Networks of lymphatics in all layers of the stomach have been demonstrated by electron microscopy studies. These lymphatics connect to extragastric lymph nodes, which drain to regional nodes.

The Japanese classification of gastric cancer (2011) [18] has divided the stomach into upper (C), middle (M) and lower (A) thirds, which determine the related lymph node stations either as the sole site or in combination. The regional nodal stations are considered anatomically according to the main vascular supply to the stomach: around the left gastric artery, around the splenic artery and around the common hepatic artery. Those around the left gastric artery drain lymphatics from the cardia and lesser curve nodes including anterior and posterior aspects of the upper third of the stomach. Those around the splenic artery drain both the upper greater curvature principally via the short gastric vessels and the left gastro-epiploic artery and the posterior proximal stomach and splenic hilum via the posterior gastric artery. The group around the common hepatic artery drains the distal third of the stomach via nodes associated with the right gastric artery and the right gastro-epiploic artery (the supra- and infra-pyloric nodes, respectively) and the lower greater curvature. Flow from the nodes along the hepatoduodenal ligament and the surface of the head of the pancreas also drains into the common hepatic group. These three major groups drain to the para-aortic nodes either via the coeliac axis nodes or via the superior mesenteric artery nodes or directly particularly from the splenic artery or retrohepatic and retropancreatic nodes. The para-aortic nodes drain via the cisterna chyli and thoracic duct and thus into the systemic circulation.

In previous TNM classifications of gastric cancer stage the anatomical sites were included as part of the staging

TNM stage (2009)

Depth of tumour invasion

TX   Depth of tumour unknown

T0   No evidence of primary tumour

T1   Tumour confined to the mucosa (M) (T1a) or submucosa (SM) (T1b)

T2   Tumour invades the muscularis propria (MP)

T3   Tumour invades the subserosa (SS)

T4   Tumour invasion is contiguous to or exposed beyond the serosa (SE) (T4a) or invades adjacent structures (SI) (T4b)

Lymph node metastasis

NX   Regional lymph nodes cannot be assessed

N0   No regional lymph node metastasis

N1   Metastasis in 1–2 regional lymph nodes

N2   Metastasis in 3–6 regional lymph nodes

N3   Metastasis in 7 or more regional lymph nodes

N3a Metastasis in 7–15 regional lymph nodes

N3b Metastasis in 16 or more regional lymph nodes

	N0	N1	N2	N3
T1a (M), T1b (SM)	IA	IB	IIA	IIB
T2 (MP)	IB	IIA	IIB	IIIA
T3 (SS)	IIA	IIB	IIIA	IIIB
T4a (SE)	IIB	IIIA	IIIB	IIIC
T4b (SI)	IIIB	IIIB	IIIC	IIIC
M1 (any T, any N)	IV			

Figure 25.4 TNM stage (2009).

system. Comparative studies have shown equivalent stage groupings with the number of nodes involved rather than the original tiers (Figure 25.4). Nevertheless, knowledge of the anatomy of the lymphatic drainage is important as this guides the approaches for radical lymph node excision as part of curative surgery.

TNM staging

The current TNM staging of gastric cancer [24] has made some significant changes to previous editions. The most significant was the classification of the location of tumours. Gastric cancers have been defined as tumours with an epicentre in the stomach greater than 5 cm from the oesophago-gastric junction or those within 5 cm of the oesophago-gastric junction without extension in the oesophagus. Tumours with an epicentre within 5 cm of the oesophago-gastric junction and

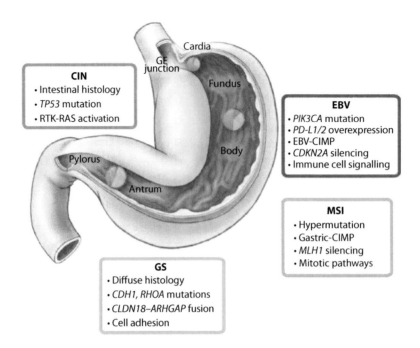

Figure 25.5 Molecular and genomic subtypes of gastric cancer: distribution according to regions of the stomach.

Molecular pathology

The heterogeneity of gastric cancer has become increasingly apparent with developments in molecular pathology. These have significant implications for the understanding of aetiology, natural history and treatment. Shah and colleagues [25] described differential gene expression data for proximal non-diffuse, diffuse and distal non-diffuse subtypes of gastric cancer. Recently The Cancer Genome Atlas (TCGA) [26] defined a molecular classification using gene expression or DNA sequencing. Four specific subtypes of gastric cancer were defined (Figure 25.5): tumours positive for Epstein–Barr virus (EBV), microsatellite unstable tumours (MSI), genomically stable tumours (GS) and tumours with chromosomal instability (CIN).

Such a classification provides far greater detail of an individual tumour for outcome comparisons and for design of further therapeutic interventions.

DIAGNOSIS AND STAGING

Symptomatic presentation

The common presentation of gastric cancer is with symptoms referable to the upper gastrointestinal tract. The difficulty with such symptoms is that they are non-specific, common and frequently ignored by the patient.

extending into the oesophagus are classified as oesophageal. These latter tumours include Siewert type III or true cardia cancers which many consider to be biologically gastric cancers. The other main change is the designation of lymph nodes already described.

- Upper abdominal mass consistent with stomach cancer
- Dysphagia
- Aged 55 and over with weight loss **and** any of the following:
  upper abdominal pain
  reflux
  dyspepsia.

Figure 25.6 Upper gastrointestinal cancers: guidelines for referral

As a result many patients present with established disease. Different countries have attempted to address the problem with initiatives to increase diagnosis rates. The size of the public health problem in Japan in the 1960s prompted a mass screening program (see below). Although this was aimed at the asymptomatic population approximately 50% with EGC had symptoms at diagnosis. Such approaches are not appropriate in countries with a lower incidence. However, public health proposals have tried to focus on those at risk. In the UK the National Health Service developed guidelines for urgent referral for suspicious symptoms (Figure 25.6) [27]. These were based on literature evidence and a desire to ensure a pragmatic approach. Although this has focused attention on the disease many of the symptoms are those of advanced disease and only modest numbers of cancers were diagnosed via this pathway.

Diagnostic investigations

Video endoscopy with biopsy for histological diagnosis is the investigation of choice for the diagnosis of gastric cancer. Conventional white light endoscopy can be supplemented with more advanced techniques if necessary including chromoendoscopy for equivocal findings or defining the extent of superficial EGC [28]. There is a variation in guidance for the number of biopsies required for diagnosis but most recommend a minimum of six taken from the edge of the macroscopic abnormality. Endoscopy reporting should be according to a standardized protocol to ensure an accurate description of lesions specifically in terms of location within the stomach, dimension and morphology.

Endoscopy practice should be carefully audited to ensure high quality of examinations. Approximately 10% of patients have had a 'normal' endoscopy in the 3 years prior to diagnosis and a further 10–20% require a second examination [29,30]. The principal factors associated with the need to re-endoscope are failure to suspect malignancy and (as a consequence) failure to take an adequate number of biopsies.

Staging

Staging of gastric cancer is based on cross-sectional and functional imaging in combination with interventional techniques to provide more detailed information.

CT scanning

Multidimensional CT (MDCT) scanning is principally intended to exclude metastatic disease once a histological diagnosis has been established. The combination of axial images with reformatted multiplanar images improves accuracy for discrimination of T3 and T4 disease [31,32].

MDCT has also been used for volumetric analysis which can be used as a 'virtual endoscopy', which in combination with axial images provides a three-dimensional view that has applications for EGC diagnosis [33,34].

PET-CT scanning

Although PET-CT scanning has the attraction of functional assessment of tumour biology, it is limited in mucinous and diffuse cancers [35], which do not take up the radiolabelled glucose. Nodal staging is variable with failure to identify peri-tumoural nodes in close proximity to avid tumours. However, the combination of PET-CT with CT is both accurate and sensitive for regional and distant nodes (sensitivity and specificity, 77% and 90%, respectively) [36]. The combination of PET-CT and CT is also useful for detection of metastatic disease (sensitivity 69–78%, specificity 82–88%).

Cross-sectional imaging has been evaluated as a method of determining the response to preoperative chemotherapy. There have been variable results reflecting the limitations of assessing viable and non-viable tumour. However, imaging is required to reassess a patient after completion of preoperative treatment to ensure that there has not been any occult disease progression.

Both techniques have their limitations in the detection of small-volume disease, particularly peritoneal seeding <5 mm. In addition specificity can be affected by uptake by foci of inflammation, particularly nodal sites. The risk of false positivity particularly with PET-CT implies histological or cytological confirmation to ensure accuracy for treatment decisions.

INTERVENTIONAL TECHNIQUES

Endoscopic ultrasound

The role of endoscopic ultrasound (EUS) in routine staging is mainly in the assessment of small T1a and T1b cancers to determine depth of penetration into submucosa in order to define appropriateness of endoscopic resection. EUS assessment of nodal disease is variable and operator dependent. Some reports cite a sensitivity of 91% for detecting nodal disease, although this decreases significantly in the assessment of regional nodal involvement because of the distance from the endoscopic probe to more distant nodes [37].

Laparoscopy

The inclusion of laparoscopy in staging algorithms is variable. In a systematic review of more than 20 studies Leake and colleagues [38] endorsed the use of laparoscopy for staging T3 and T4 tumours as it altered treatment decisions in 31–67% of cases. By contrast in T1 and T2 tumours there was a change in management in only 4% of patients. There was little benefit for nodal staging. However, there was a significant change in metastatic disease with approximately 60% of those staged M0 on cross-sectional imaging having small-volume metastases on laparoscopy. The addition of peritoneal lavage is also variable [39]. Cytology is likely to be positive in the presence of serosal or subserosal disease in otherwise operable tumours; nevertheless positive cytology is included in Japanese staging as evidence of more advanced disease. Such information is helpful in treatment planning and discussions with patients about prognosis.

SCREENING

Gastric cancer screening is commonly performed in countries with high disease prevalence, for example in Japan and Korea. Mass screening was started in 1960 and a nationwide program was established in 1983 under the Health Service Law for the Aged in Japan [40,41]. All individuals more than 40 years are recommended to have annual screening. According to the latest report in 2010, 3.8 million Japanese people (9.0%) underwent examination [42]. The screening rate increased to 32.3% after including other screening programs such as employer and self-referral. Screening methods include a questionnaire about risk factors of gastric cancer and a radiological contrast upper gastrointestinal series (UGIS) examination. When any abnormal findings are detected on UGIS, an endoscopy is performed. This mass screening achieved a remarkable reduction in mortality rates and consequently higher cure rates [43,44]. In the upcoming guidelines, currently in draft, endoscopy will be adopted as the screening method. In addition, the target population will be changed to individuals older than 50 years.

In Korea, a nationwide gastric cancer screening program was started in 1999 as a part of the National Cancer Screening Program (NCSP). Initially, the NCSP for gastric cancer invited Medical Aid recipients and National Health Insurance (NHI) beneficiaries in the lower-income brackets and aged 40 years or older. However, the target population was expanded to NHI beneficiaries in the lower 50% income bracket in 2005 [45]. Each participant undergoes either UGIS or endoscopy screening at a clinic, or hospital designated as a gastric cancer screening unit by the NHI Corporation. There has been debate on the optimal screening method as many recent studies showed better performance of endoscopy than UGIS [45,46]. Thus, endoscopy is now commonly used for screening in Korea. Further evaluation of the impact of these screening methods should be considered in Western and developing countries evaluating costs and reduction in mortality.

SURGERY FOR GASTRIC CANCER

Surgery is the mainstay for localized gastric cancer. The optimal treatment of gastric cancer must be tailored to the extent of disease (Figure 25.7). In early gastric cancer (EGC) localized tumours can be treated by endoscopic resection. The current criteria for endoscopic submucosal dissection are well-differentiated adenocarcinoma, T1a, no ulceration and size ≤2 cm [47]. This is possible because the risk of

nodal disease is <1% for such cancers [49]. Experience from large surgical series has demonstrated that these criteria can be extended because of the negligible risk of nodal disease to include:

1. No lymphatic or venous invasion
2. Differentiated type, intramucosal cancer regardless of size without ulceration
3. Differentiated type, intramucosa cancer <30 mm with ulceration
4. Undifferenteated type, intramucosal cancer <20 mm without ulceration
5. Differentiated type, minute submucosal penetration (sm1) and < 30 mm

More established cancers which do not fulfil these criteria or are locally advanced should be treated by radical surgery.

Extent of gastric resection

The key issues in surgical treatment for gastric cancer are curability, safety, conservation of physical function and maintenance of quality of life after operation. Too extensive surgery increases the risk of postoperative complications and poorer physical function, whereas too limited surgery can result in high recurrence and low survival rates.

The extent of gastric resection is determined by the need to obtain a microscopically free resection margin. Because gastric tumours spread intramurally, an adequate resection margin is necessary to ensure a low rate of anastomotic recurrence. Recent guidelines state that the required

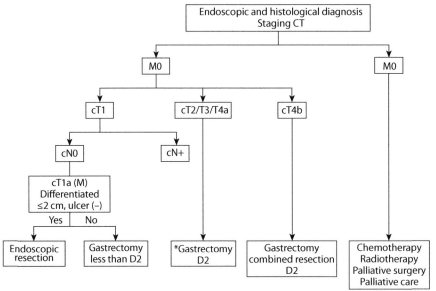

* The recommendations relating to D2 resection are based principally on expertise and physiological reasoning: current literature evidence does not conclusively demonstrate survival benefit for radical surgery.

Figure 25.7 Surgical treatment decision algorithm for gastric cancer, which is modified from the Japanese treatment guideline.

resection margin should be at least 2 cm in EGC, 3 cm or more in Borrmann types I and II, and 5 cm or more in Borrmann types III and IV [47,48]. Intraoperative frozen section histological examination is recommended to ensure a negative resection margin. Histological subtype is also important and an 8 cm margin is recommended in diffuse-type cancers. A tumour located in the middle or lower one-third should be treated by subtotal gastrectomy. If there is a tumour involvement more than 2 cm into the duodenum, pancreaticoduodenectomy may be necessary [50]. Total gastrectomy is required for tumours involving the proximal one-third or the entire stomach. Extended total gastrectomy is indicated for tumours involving the lower oesophagus which may require a transhiatal dissection or a thoracotomy.

Lymph node dissection

The extent of lymph node dissection in gastric cancer surgery has been a major topic of surgical controversy for several decades. Japanese surgeons developed the concept of the D2 gastrectomy, involving resection of not only the perigastric nodes in the vascular arcades along the curvatures but also the nodes along the main branches of the coeliac axis, to which the majority of the lymphatic flow from the stomach gravitates. In the guidelines of the Korean Gastric Cancer Association and the Japanese Gastric Cancer Association, D2 lymphadenectomy is the standard for all localized gastric cancers except clinical T1N0M0 [47,48]. In the West two trials have evaluated the role of D2 dissection and both showed an increased morbidity and mortality after D2 lymphadenectomy [51,52]. After long-term follow-up neither study showed there was a difference in survival rate between D2 and D1 lymphadenectomy [53,54]. However, after a median follow-up of 15 years, the Dutch trial showed that D2 lymphadenectomy was associated with reduced locoregional recurrence and improved cancer-specific survival [55].

The approach to cT1N0 cancers which are not appropriate for endoscopic therapy has been modified. The Japanese rules have recommended D1 + lymphadenectomy including common hepatic, coeliac axis and proximal splenic artery nodes for cT1N0 cancers according to the location in the stomach. Recently a large multicentre study has been set up to investigate whether D1 + lymphadenectomy is also possible in earlier advanced cancer of cT1N1, cT2N0, T2N1, T3N0 or T3N1 (ADDICT Trial, ClinicalTrials.gov, identifier: NCT02144727).

More extended lymphadenectomy has been evaluated in trials. In the Japanese JCOG 9501 trial para-aortic lymph node dissection did not provide better overall survival and recurrence-free survival rates in addition to standard D2 dissection, although there were no significant differences in complications and 30-day mortality [56]. There have been retrospective studies on extending dissection to include retropancreatic nodes and nodes along the superior mesenteric vein which have also shown no additional benefit.

The Italian group has shown some advantage for extended lymph node dissection in T3/4 tumours of diffuse type located in the proximal stomach [57].

Function-preserving surgery

Function-preserving gastrectomy was developed as the incidence of EGC increased with the screening programs in Japan and Korea. This includes pylorus-preserving gastrectomy (PPG), proximal gastrectomy (PG) and sentinel node navigation surgery.

In PPG, the tumour should be located at least 5 cm the pyloric ring, and the hepatic branch of the vagus nerve should be preserved. Although the supra- and infra-pyloric nodes may be incompletely dissected, studies have confirmed the oncological safety of PPG compared to subtotal gastrectomy, with the advantage over distal gastrectomy with respect to dumping syndrome and nutrition [58,59]. Retrospective studies of PG have also confirmed the oncological safety and nutritional advantages over total gastrectomy in clinical T1N0 gastric cancer [60,61]. However, there has been some debate about the reconstruction method because PG is more frequently complicated by reflux oesophagitis than total gastrectomy [62]. Sentinel node navigation surgery has been evaluated in EGC [63–65]; this is an investigational treatment, and results of trials are awaited although early results do suggest reliable detection of sentinel nodes, and when negative further nodal dissection is not required.

Palliative surgery

The role of surgery in palliating symptoms of gastric cancer has declined in recent years because of the improving results of non-surgical options such as stent insertion for obstruction or endoscopic treatment for bleeding. The principal symptoms which require treatment in patients with advanced gastric cancer are pain, vomiting, bleeding and anorexia. Gastrectomy has no role to play in correcting anorexia but can effectively deal with the other three symptoms in particular circumstances.

SPECIAL ISSUES

Reductive surgery in single-site metastatic disease

Reductive surgery in gastric cancer means reducing the volume of cancer by gastrectomy in patients with distant metastasis. Retrospective studies have shown the benefit of reductive surgery. The Dutch group reported an advantage to resection in those younger than 70 years with localized hepatic or peritoneal metastasis or N3 disease [66]. More recently however, in the randomized REGATTA trial the Japanese Clinical Oncology Group Study JCOG 0705 and Korean Gastric Cancer Association Study KGCA01 included patients with a single non-curable factor and demonstrated that gastrectomy followed by chemotherapy has no survival benefit over chemotherapy alone [67].

Conversion surgery

Conversion surgery, so-called salvage gastrectomy or secondary gastrectomy, has been performed in patients who have a good response to the chemotherapy despite distant metastases. Some retrospective studies have reported good results in selected patients [68,69]. A multidisciplinary approach with judicious monitoring of the patients could increase the chance of survival through conversion surgery. Future translational research on chemotherapy response and development of targeted immunotherapy could open a new paradigm for the treatment of metastatic gastric cancer.

Reconstruction

After subtotal gastrectomy, gastroduodenostomy (GD) with Billroth I anastomosis, gastrojejunostomy (GJ) with Billroth II anastomosis and gastrojejunostomy with Roux-en-Y anastomosis are all options for reconstruction. GD is more physiological than other reconstructions but is limited by the extent of gastric resection. GJ with Billroth II anastomosis is not limited by the extent of gastric resection but both GD and GJ can be limited by greater risk of biliary reflux. Most surgeons now reconstruct with a Roux-en-Y loop, which should be 55 cm in length to minimize biliary reflux; this is also the most favoured reconstruction after total gastrectomy.

Complications of surgery

Postoperative early complications include bleeding, abscess, obstruction and anastomosis leakage. Most can be managed non-operatively with endoscopic treatment of any bleeding point and radiological drainage of any intra-abdominal collections with appropriate antibiotics. Obstruction can occur because of oedema at the anastomosis site, and usually recovers with conservative management. Anastomotic leakage including duodenal stump leakage is usually the result of poor blood supply and tension at the anastomotic site. Although occasionally surgical exploration is necessary endoscopic closure is often successful, the main problem being control of local infection.

Late complications include dumping syndrome and anaemia. Dumping syndrome is classified as early with diarrhoea, nausea or palpitations or late with symptoms of hypoglycaemia. These symptoms can be difficult to manage although careful dietary advice is required. This can also reflect bile salt malabsorption and bacterial overgrowth, which requires appropriate treatment with broad-spectrum antibiotics. Anaemia frequently occurs after gastrectomy, usually from iron deficiency, although vitamin B12 deficiency occurs after total gastrectomy.

Minimal invasive gastrectomy

Laparoscopic distal gastrectomy was first reported in 1992 for benign ulcer and in 1994 for gastric cancer [70,71]. Laparoscopic gastrectomy has been enthusiastically practiced since the mid-1990s. According to the 10th national survey by the Japan Society of Endoscopic Surgery, 7341 laparoscopic gastrectomies were performed and this accounted for approximately 25% of gastric cancer surgery in 2009 [72]. Similar proportions (26%) of laparoscopic procedures for gastric cancer were also reported in the 2009 nationwide survey in South Korea [73]. Advances in surgical skill, development of laparoscopic instruments such as ultrasonic shears and surgeons' desire to improve the quality of life for patients contributed to this rapid adoption of laparoscopic surgery.

The feasibility and safety of laparoscopic gastrectomy have been demonstrated in many studies with reduced postoperative morbidity, intraoperative bleeding, postoperative analgesic consumption and hospital stay [74–76]. The long-term survival rate has been similar between laparoscopic and open distal gastrectomy. However, laparoscopic gastrectomy is still a technically difficult and time-consuming procedure.

The indications for laparoscopic gastrectomy are expanding. It is largely accepted as the procedure of choice for EGC in the Far East following a number of retrospective and prospective studies [77–80]. Two large-scale multicentre randomized trials have further evaluated the oncological safety of laparoscopic surgery for clinical stage I [81,82] and the results are awaited. It would appear from initial results that there is little difference between laparoscopic and open distal resection. There are also now three large-scale multicentre trials for advanced gastric cancer in three eastern Asia countries (Japan, Korea and China) [83,84].

Recently, robotic surgery has been introduced as this has advantages in terms of three-dimensional vision, correction of hand tremor and improved ergonomics. Comparable short-term outcomes and oncological feasibility of robotic gastrectomy compared to laparoscopic gastrectomy have been reported [85,86].

Early reports did not show any benefit with the robot. However, greater experience and improved technology may show the role of robotic gastrectomy [87]. Recent data from Korea, Japan and China have shown the benefit in N2 node dissection, in obese patients, in total gastrectomy with reduced morbidity [88–90]. Laparoscopic function-preserving surgery including PPG and PG has been described with similar overall and superior nutritional results compared to open procedures [91,92]. A systematic review and meta-analysis have demonstrated that laparoscopic sentinel node navigation surgery was technically feasible with an acceptable sensitivity [93–95]. A multicentre prospective phase III trial is ongoing in Korea (SENORITA), and laparoscopic sentinel navigation surgery could be an option for EGC in the near future.

In conclusion, recent evidence confirms feasible short- and long-term outcomes from minimally invasive surgery for gastric cancer. Further studies are expected to clarify the indications and oncological safety of minimally invasive gastric cancer surgery for the future.

NEO-ADJUVANT AND ADJUVANT THERAPIES

Poor survival outcomes after surgical resection alone as treatment for gastric cancer led to a global effort to define a better multidisciplinary or multimodality strategy to ameliorate these results. In addition to the heterogeneity in aetiology, incidence and clinical behaviour of this disease, different approaches across the world complicate the definition of standard treatment.

The aims of any adjunctive therapy in cancer treatment may be dual: when administered presurgically the target is that of downstaging the primary tumour in order to reach a microscopically radical resection. Moreover both neo-adjuvant and adjuvant approaches have as a primary objective the eradication of occult micro-metastatic disease. The use of adjuvant or perioperative chemotherapies or chemoradiation therapies varies regionally, but ultimately both have proven benefits in operable gastric cancer.

Perioperative chemotherapy

Based on two major European trials, the UK MRC MAGIC trial and the FNCLCC/FFCD French trial [96,97], a perioperative chemotherapy approach has become the treatment of choice for stage II and III gastric cancers in Europe and selected US centres (Table 25.1) [98].

A three-drug regimen (epirubicin, cisplatin and 5-fluorouracil in the UK trial) and a two-drug regimen (cisplatin and 5-fluorouracil in the French trial) administered perioperatively were compared to surgery alone in 503 and 224 patients, respectively. Overall survival, the primary end point in both trials, significantly improved with a hazard ratio for death of 0.75 (95% confidence interval 0.60–0.93) in the UK trial and of 0.69 (95% confidence interval 0.50–0.95) in the French trial. Moreover, in both studies the neo-adjuvant component of treatment significantly increased the percentage of curative resections, from 66.4% of the surgery alone arm to 69.3% in the experimental arm of the MAGIC trial and from 73% to 84% in the French trial. Similarly, a 35–37% reduction in disease recurrence, the majority of which were distant relapses, supports the utilization of systemic chemotherapy to treat occult micro-metastatic disease.

Having displayed comparable efficacy in the metastatic setting and with the advantage of not requiring a central venous access device, the orally available fluoropyrimidine capecitabine may replace the use of 5-fluorouracil in clinical practice [99]. In the UK NCRI ST03 study, perioperative ECX (epirubicin, cisplatin and capecitabine, three cycles pre- and post-surgery) was compared with the same with the addition of bevacizumab, an anti-vascular endothelial growth factor (VEGF) antibody, in patients with localized adenocarcinoma [100]. No significant survival benefit was demonstrated with the addition of bevacizumab (Hazard ratio 1.067; 95% Confidence interval 0.89–1.28; p=0.478). Of note, an increased risk of anastomotic leaks following oesophago-gastrectomy was demonstrated. Full publication of the results is awaited [101].

In terms of feasibility, these trials underline the increased difficulty in delivering a chemotherapy treatment after major surgery in this population. In MAGIC trial less than 50% of patients assigned to the perioperative chemotherapy treatment arm completed the postoperative component of treatment [96].

Conversely, the delay in surgical treatment caused by a neo-adjuvant approach must be taken into account: the risk of progression of the disease and the morbidity rate related to chemotherapy must be considered and accurately discussed with patients. In both trials, about 7–15% of patients randomized to the perioperative arm did not undergo surgery, for reasons including, but not limited to progression of the disease and rarely toxic death [96,97]. However, this might be also considered to be a method of sparing patients with an underlying aggressive disease biology undergoing an unnecessary operation with its associated morbidity.

Postoperative chemoradiation therapy

A treatment option more frequently adopted in North America is postoperative chemoradiation, mainly based on the INT0116 trial [102]. More than 550 patients were randomized to surgery alone or surgery followed by chemoradiation treatment, consisting of five cycles of 5-fluorouracil–leucovorin concomitant to 45 Gy in 25 fractions over 5 weeks during cycles 2 and 3. An updated analysis after 10 years of follow-up demonstrated a sustained long-term survival benefit for postoperative treatment compared to surgery alone, with a 5-year survival rate increased from 41% to 50% [103]. Criticisms of this study include the fact that more than 50% of patients received less than a D1 lymphadenectomy, difficulty delivering combination therapy following surgery and potential late toxic effects. Outside of the US, this approach is often considered in case of suboptimal surgery or R1 (microscopically incomplete) resection, as suggested by the retrospective analysis of the Dutch D1/D2 trial [104]. Further data on the role of postoperative chemoradiation therapy compared to adjuvant chemotherapy are awaited from the CRITICS trial, in which patients will receive preoperative chemotherapy followed by surgery and be subsequently randomized to adjuvant chemotherapy or chemoradiotherapy [105].

Adjuvant chemotherapy

In Asian patients two trials demonstrate the efficacy of postoperative chemotherapy in optimally resected patients. The Japanese ACTS-GC trial demonstrated a survival benefit for 1 year of oral S1 therapy in patients following D2

Table 25.1 Key randomized phase III trials of perioperative treatment in gastric adenocarcinoma

Authors	Years	Total no. of pts	Treatments	No.	Median age	Site of primary	Primary end point	% R0 resection	OS HR (95% CI)	p Value	Median OS (months)	3-Year survival %	% Postoperative mortality	Site of relapse (%)
Cunningham et al. [96]	1994–2002	503	Surgery	253	62	74% (G), 11% (OEO), 14% (OGJ)	OS	66.4	0.75 (0.60–0.93)	0.009	NR	23 (5 y)	5.9	20.6 (L) vs. 36.8 (D)
			ECF×3® Surgery® ECF×3	250	62	74% (G), 11% (OEO), 14% (OGJ)		69.3				36 (5 y)	5.6	14.4 (L) vs. 24.4 (D)
Ychou et al. [97]	1995–2003	224	Surgery	111	63	24% (G), 9% (OEO), 67% (OGJ)	OS	74	0.69 (0.50–0.95)	0.02	NR	24 (5 y)	4.6	8 (L) vs. 38 (D) vs. 18 (both)
			CF×3® Surgery® CF×3	113	63	25% (G), 13% (OEO), 62% (OGJ)		84				38 (5 y)	4.5	12 (L) vs. 30 (D) vs. 12 (both)
Sakuramoto et al. [106]	2001–2004	1059	Surgery	530	63	Gastric not further specified	OS	NA	0.66 (0.51–0.86)	0.002	NR	70.1	NR	2.8 (L) vs. 8.7 (LN) vs. 15.8 (per) vs. 11.3 (D)
			Surgery® S-1 for 1 year	529	63							80.1		1.3 (L) vs. 5.1 (LN) vs. 11.2 (per) vs. 10.2 (D)
Bang et al. [107]	2006–2009	1035	Surgery	515	56	98% (G), 2% (OGJ)	3 y DFS	NA	0.72 (0.52–1) (3 y OS)	0.049	Not available yet	78	NA	11 (per) vs. 8.5 (locoreg) vs. 15 (D)
			Surgery® CAPOX×8	520	56	97% (G), 3% (OGJ)						83		9 (per) vs. 4 (locoreg) vs. 9.4 (D)
MacDonald et al. [102]	1991–1998	556	Surgery	275	59	~80% (G), ~20% (OGJ)[a]	OS	NA	1.32 (1.10–1.60)[a]	0.0046[a]	27[a]	41	NA	8 (L) vs. 39 (reg) vs. 18 (D)[a]
			Surgery® CRT	281	60						35[a]	50		2 (L) vs. 22 (reg) vs. 16 (D)[a]
Lee et al. [132]	2004–2008	458	Surgery® adjuvant XP×6 (D2 dissection mandatory)	228	56	Gastric	DFS	NA	NR	NR	Not available yet	78.2 (DFS)	NA	8.3% (locoreg) vs. 24.6% (D)
			Surgery® adjuvant XP×2-XRT-XP×2	230	56							74.2 (DFS)		4.8% (locoreg) vs. 20.4% (D)

Note: CAPOX = capecitabine, oxaliplatin; CF = cisplatin, 5-fluorouracil; CRT = 5-fluorouracil, leucovorin concomitant to radiation therapy 45 Gy/25 lb; D = distant; DFS = disease-free survival; ECF = epirubicin, cisplatin, 5-fluorouracil; G = gastric; L = local; LN = lymph nodes; NA = not applicable; NR = not reported; OEO = lower oesophagus; OGJ = oesophago-gastric junction; OS = overall survival; per = peritoneal; reg = regional; XP = capecitabine, cisplatin; XRT = capecitabine concomitant to radiation therapy 45 Gy/25 lb.
[a] From the updated analysis after more than 10 years follow-up (7).

resection [106]. However, S1 is poorly tolerated in Western patients due to pharmacogenetic factors and therefore these results are not felt to be generalizable to Western patients. The CLASSIC trial compared adjuvant capecitabine plus oxaliplatin (6 months) to surgery alone in Asian patients that underwent D2 gastrectomy for stage II and III gastric cancer [107]. A recent report of 5-year follow-up data demonstrated an increase in estimated 5-year disease-free survival from 53% in the observation-only arm to 68% of the treatment arm. Similarly, the estimated 5-year overall survival improved from 69% to 78% [108]. The majority of trial data supportive of adjuvant chemotherapy are from trials in the Asian population: multiple studies in Western populations have been negative in this setting, although meta-analysis suggests a small benefit (6% at 5 years for 5-fluorouracil-based chemotherapy) [109]. Currently for Western patients, where tumour biology may differ and where a later stage at presentation is more common, the evidence base favours perioperative chemotherapy for its ability to downstage large tumours or postoperative chemoradiotherapy in the setting of suboptimal surgical resection. However, for a minority of highly selected patients following resection an adjuvant chemotherapy approach may be used.

Elderly population

Data from the Surveillance, Epidemiology and End Results (SEER) database show that more than 65% of gastric cancer patients are older than 65 years with a median age of 71 years at diagnosis and 74 at the time of death [110]. Data available from clinical trials in both early and advanced disease usually reflect selected populations with good performance status, a low prevalence of comorbidities and a lower median age. Therefore, all the evidence from randomized clinical trials must be extrapolated with caution to elderly patients in clinical practice.

To our knowledge, there are no trials specifically targeting an older population in the adjuvant or perioperative setting and the majority of data on the safety and outcomes of perioperative chemotherapy have been extrapolated by retrospective analysis of adjuvant trials and from phase II trials within the first-line metastatic setting [111–115]. The National Comprehensive Cancer Network (NCCN) guidelines consider the terms *medically fit* or *medically unfit* within the treatment algorithms, without any other definitive criteria [116]. Despite the fact the feasibility of such studies is extremely difficult, prospective trials designed to address these open questions are desirable.

LOCALLY ADVANCED AND METASTATIC DISEASE

The presence of locally advanced or metastatic disease is frequently related to a plethora of symptoms that might significantly impact on patients' general conditions and consequently on treatment decisions. A global assessment of the physical, mental and social condition of patients is crucial

before planning any action. Nutritional assessment is essential for the appropriate use of therapeutic strategies in the management of anorexia, cachexia and fatigue. A body mass index (BMI) of less than 18.5 kg/m^2, an unintentional weight loss of greater than 10% within the last 3–6 months or a BMI of less than 20 kg/m^2 concomitant to an unintentional weight loss of greater than 5% within the last 3–6 months is a clinical priority for consideration of nutritional support, as per UK NICE guidelines (https://www.nice.org.uk/guidance/CG32). Placement of palliative stenting or a by-pass surgery might be considered in order to facilitate control of gastrointestinal symptoms and enhance dietary intake.

In the absence of any active treatment, the overall survival is very poor, with a median survival of 3 months. Therefore, the identification of active treatment options is vital for this highly lethal disease. The use of chemotherapy demonstrates clear benefits not only in survival prolongation but also in symptom control and consequently in quality of life improvement [117,118]. Median overall survival for fit patients now approaches approximately 9–13 months within the context of clinical trials, in general with better outcomes for Asian patients than Western patients. A Cochrane meta-analysis including 5726 patients treated in 35 different clinical trials demonstrated that patients actively treated with chemotherapy have better survival than those managed with best supportive care only. Moreover, combination treatments seemed more beneficial than single-agent schedules [117]. Globally, there is no one universally accepted standard first-line palliative regimen. However, a platinum and fluoropyrimidine doublet is commonly used worldwide, with the addition of an anthracycline or a taxane in triplet regimens considered for fit patients. In the UK, triplets including epirubicin are commonly used based on several trials, including the UK NCRI REAL2 study [119]. This confirmed that oxaliplatin could replace cisplatin and capecitabine could replace 5-fluorouracil without loss of efficacy and with practical and toxicity benefits.

These results, together with those from an Asian study [120], have led to the licensing of capecitabine for gastric cancer. Several other trials including taxane-based and irinotecan-based combinations have also been reported (Table 25.2).

Although associated with a marginal benefit in survival, second-line treatments have been recently accepted as the standard approach after progressive disease with a fluoropyrimidine-based regimen. Quality of life benefits have also been clearly demonstrated for this approach in the UK COUGAR study [121]. Treatment options validated in clinical trials include either taxanes or irinotecan chemotherapy [122–124] (Table 25.3).

Although molecularly targeted agents have significantly improved outcomes across multiple tumour types, in gastric cancer treatment the monoclonal antibody trastuzumab still represents the only agent licensed in first-line setting in combination with chemotherapy. However, only 20% of

Table 25.2 Key randomized phase III trials of first-line chemotherapy for advanced gastric adenocarcinoma

Authors	Name of trial	Years	Total no. of pts	Treatments	No.	Median age	Site of primary	Primary end point	HR for primary end point (95% CI)	Response rate %	OS HR (95% CI)	p Value	Median OS (months)	Median PFS (months)
Van Cutsem et al. [133]	V325	1999–2003	457	DCF	227	55	81% (G), 19% (OGJ)	TTP	1.47 (1.19–1.82)	37	1.29 (1.0–1.6)	0.02	9.2	5.6 (TTP)
Cunningham et al. [99]	REAL-2	2000–2005	1002	CF	230	55	75% (G), 25% (OGJ)	Non-inferiority in OS	0.86 (0.80–0.99)	25	Ox vs. Cis 0.92 (0.80–1.10)	NR	8.6	3.7 (TTP)
				ECF	263	65	36.1% (G), 28.9% (OGJ) 34.9% (OEO)			40.7			9.9	6.2
				ECX	250	64	42.3% (G), 28.2% (OGJ), 29.5% (OEO)			46.4			9.9	6.7
				EOF	245	61	37% (G), 23.4% (OGJ), 39.6% (OEO)			42.4	X vs. 5FU 0.89 (0.77–1.02)	NR	9.3	6.5
				EOX	244	62	45.5% (G), 22.2% (OGJ), 34.3% (OEO)			47.9			11.2	7
Koizumi et al. [134]	SPIRITS	2002–2004	298	C S-1	148	62	Gastric not specified	OS	0.77 (0.61–0.98)	54	0.77 (0.61–0.98)	0.04	13	6
				S-1	150	62				31			11	4
Bang et al. [125]	ToGA	2005–2008	584	CF or CX + trastuzumab	294	59	80% (G), 20% (OGJ)	OS	0.74 (0.60–0.91)	47	0.74 (0.60–0.91)	0.004	13.8	6.7
				CF or CX	290	58	83% (G), 17% (OGJ)			35			11.1	5.5
Rao et al. [135]	MATRIX (phase II)	2005–2006	71	ECX	36	64	44% (G), 56% (OEO + OGJ)	Tumour response	NR (p = 0.994)	58	1.02 (0.61–1.70)	0.945	12.2	7.1
				ECX + matuzumab	35	59	40% (G), 60% (OEO + OGJ)			31			9.4	4.8
Ohtsu et al. [128]	AVAGAST	2007–2008	774	CX	387	59	87% (G), 13% (OGJ)	OS	0.87 (0.73–1.03)	37	0.87 (0.73–1.03)	0.1	10.1	5.3
				CX + bevacizumab	387	58	86% (G), 14% (OGJ)			46			12.1	6.7
Van Cutsem et al. [136]	GATE (phase II)	2006–2007	254	TE	79	59	90% (G), 37% (OGJ)	PFS	NR	23.1	NR	NR	9	4.5 (TTP)
				TEF	89	58	84% (G), 39% (OGJ)			46.6			14.5	7.7 (TTP)
				TEX	86	59	87% (G), 33% (OGJ)			25.6			11.3	5.6 (TTP)

(Continued)

Table 25.2 (Continued) Key randomized phase III trials of first-line chemotherapy for advanced gastric adenocarcinoma

Authors	Name of trial	Years	Total no. of pts	Treatments	No.	Median age	Site of primary	Primary end point	HR for primary end point (95% CI)	Response rate %	OS HR (95% CI)	p Value	Median OS (months)	Median PFS (months)
Waddell et al. [129]	REAL-3	2008–2011	553	EOX	275	62	32% (G), 27% (OGJ), 40% (OEO)	OS	1.37 (1.07–1.76)	42	1.37 (1.07–1.76)	0.013	11.3	7.4
				EOX + panitumumab	278	63	28% (G), 34% (OGJ), 38% (OEO)			46			8.8	6
Lordick et al. [130]	EXPAND	2008–2010	894	CX	449	59	83% (G), 16% (OGJ), 1% (unknown)	PFS	1.09 (0.92–1.29)	29	1 (0.87–1.17)	0.95	10.7	5.6
				CX + cetuximab	445	60	83% (G), 16% (OGJ), 2% (unknown)			30			9.4	4.4

Note: DCF = docetaxel, cisplatin, 5-fluorouracil; CF = cisplatin, 5-fluorouracil; ECF = epirubicin, cisplatin, 5-fluorouracil; ECX = epirubicin, cisplatin, capecitabine; EOF = epirubicin, oxaliplatin, 5-fluorouracil; EOX = epirubicin, oxaliplatin, capecitabine; C S-1 = cisplatin, S-1; CX = cisplatin, capecitabine; TE = docetaxel, oxaliplatin; TEF = docetaxel, oxaliplatin, 5-fluorouracil; TEX = docetaxel, oxaliplatin, capecitabine; G = gastric; OEO = lower oesophagus; OGJ = oesophago-gastric junction; TTP = time to progression; PFS = progression-free survival; OS = overall survival; NR = not reported.

Table 25.3 Key randomized phase III trials of salvage chemotherapy for advanced gastric adenocarcinoma

Authors	Years	Total no. of pts	Treatments	No.	Median age	Previous lines	ECOG Performance status	Primary end point	OS HR (95% CI)	p Value	Median OS (months)	Quality of life
Kang et al. [122]	2008–2010	202	Docetaxel or Irinotecan	133	56	1: 75% 2: 25%	0: 54% 1: 46%	OS	0.657 (0.485–0.891)	0.007	5.6	NR
			Best supportive care	69	56	1: 70% 2: 30%	0: 52% 1: 48%				3.8	
Thuss-Patience et al. [123]	2002–2006	40	Irinotecan	21	58	1: 100%	0–1: 81% 2: 19%	OS	0.48 (0.25–0.42)	0.012	4	NR
			Best supportive care	19	55	1: 100%	0–1: 74% 2: 26%				2.4	
Ford et al. [121]	2008–2012	168	Docetaxel	84	65	1: 100%	0: 28% 1: 55% 2: 17%	OS	0.67 (0.49–0.92)	0.01	5.2	p: 0.53; benefit in dysphagia and pain control
			Best supportive care	84	66	1: 100%	0: 26% 1: 60% 2: 14%				3.6	
Hironaka et al. [124]	2007–2010	223	Paclitaxel	111	64.5	1: 100%	0–1: 96.3% 2: 3.7%	OS	1.13 (0.86–1.49)	0.38	9.5	NR
			Irinotecan	112	65	1: 100%	0–1: 96.4% 2: 3.6%				8.4	
Fuchs et al. [126]	2009–2012	355	Ramucirumab	238	60	1: 100%	0: 28% 1: 72% 2: 0%	OS	0.776 (0.603–0.998)	0.047	5.2	No significant difference
			Best supportive care	117	60	1: 100%	0: 26% 1: 73% 2: 1%				3.8	
Wilke et al. [127]	2010–2012	665	Ramucirumab + paclitaxel	330	61	1: 100%	0: 35% 1: 65%	OS	0.807 (0.678–0.962)	0.017	9.6	No significant difference
			Placebo + paclitaxel	335	61	1: 100%	0: 43% 1: 57%				7.4	

Note: OS = overall survival; NR = not reported.

patients can benefit from its use, by virtue of overexpression of the target protein HER-2 or significant amplification of the target gene *HER-2/neu*. Trastuzumab has been licensed in combination with cisplatin and 5-fluorouracil after showing significant benefits in response rate, progression-free survival and overall survival in the phase III ToGA trial [125]. Median overall survival improved from 11.1 months for patients treated with the standard chemotherapy doublet to 13.8 months in the experimental arm. Moreover, in patients with HER-2 positivity defined as IHC 2+/FISH positive or IHC 3+, survival reached an unprecedented 16 months with the addition of the monoclonal antibody. Following these results, the determination of the HER-2 status should be mandatory before commencing any treatment for advanced disease.

In the second-line treatment of advanced gastric cancer another targeted drug has recently demonstrated efficacy. The anti-angiogenetic agent ramucirumab has received Food and Drug Administration approval in patients refractory to or with progressive disease following first-line therapy with platinum of fluoropyrimidine both as a single agent and in combination with paclitaxel [126,127]. That ramucirumab demonstrated such efficacy in this setting is somewhat surprising given the failure of the anti-VEGF monoclonal antibody bevacizumab in the first-line setting [128]; however, ramucirumab represents an important new addition to the therapeutic armamentarium for advanced gastric cancer patients.

HER-2 notwithstanding, the identification of biomarkers able to predict the beneficial use of high-cost targeted agents is mandatory and to date no other biomarker-selected novel agents have been developed for gastric cancer patients. In fact, several large randomized clinical trials targeting different pathways such as EGFR, PI3K/mTOR or VEGF have failed to demonstrate any survival benefit [129–131], and one common factor underlying these disappointing results is the lack of a selected target population. As discussed in the Pathology section, the results recently published in the TCGA project and ongoing molecular studies will be fundamental in patient stratification and in providing a scientific base for development of future therapeutic clinical trials [26].

REFERENCES

1. GLOBOCAN 2012. Estimated cancer incidence, mortality and prevalence worldwide in 2012 – stomach cancer. http://globocan.iarc.fr/old/FactSheets/cancers/stomach-new.asp.
2. De Angelis R, Sant M, Coleman MP, et al. Cancer survival in Europe 1999–2007 by country and age: results of EUROCARE-5 – a population based study. *Lancet Oncol* 2014; 15: 23–34.
3. Lauren P. The two histological main types of gastric carcinoma: diffuse and so-called intestinal-type carcinoma: an attempt at a histo-clinical classification. *Acta Pathol Microbiol Scand* 1965; 64: 31–49.
4. Correa P. A human model of gastric carcinogenesis. *Cancer Res* 1988; 48: 3554–3560.
5. Hirayama T. Actions suggested by gastric cancer epidemiological studies in Japan. In Reed PI, Hill MJ, eds., *Gastric Carcinogenesis*. Amsterdam: Excerpta Medica, 1988, pp. 209–28.
6. Correa P, Sasano N, Stemmerman N, et al. Pathology of gastric carcinoma in Japanese populations: comparisons between Miyagi prefecture, Japan, and Hawaii. *J Natl Cancer Inst* 1973; 51: 1449–59.
7. International Agency for Research on Cancer Working Group on the Evaluation of Carcinogenic Risks to Humans. Schistosomes, liver flukes and *Helicobacter pylori*. Lyon: International Agency for Research on Cancer, 1994, pp. 177–240.
8. Sobala GM, Schorah CJ, Shires S. Gastric ascorbic acid concentration and acute *Helicobacter pylori* infection. *Rev Esp Enf Digest* 1990; 78(Suppl. 1): 63.
9. Tomb JF, White O, Kerlavage AR, et al. The complete genome sequence of the gastric pathogen *Helicobacter pylori*. *Nature* 1997; 388: 539–47.
10. Vicari JJ, Peek RM, Falk GW, et al. The seroprevalence of cagA-positive *Helicobacter pylori*: strains in the spectrum of gastro-oesophageal reflux disease. *Gastroenterology* 1998; 115: 50–7.
11. Ito Y, Azuma T, Ito S, et al. Analysis and typing of the vacA gene from cagA-positive strains of *Helicobacter pylori* isolated in Japan. *J Clin Microbiol* 1997; 35: 1710–14.
12. Hiyama T, Tanaka S, Kitadai Y, et al. p53 codon 72 polymorphism in gastric cancer susceptibility in patients with *Helicobacter pylori* associated chronic gastritis. *Int J Cancer* 2002; 100: 304–8.
13. Fitzgerald RC, Hardwick R, Huntsman D, et al. (International Gastric Cancer Linkage Consortium). Hereditary diffuse gastric cancer: updated consensus guidelines for clinical management and directions for future research. *J Med Genet* 2010; 47: 436–44.
14. Huntsman DG, Carneiro F, Lewis FR, et al. Early gastric cancer in young asymptomatic carriers of germline E cadherin mutation. *N Engl J Med* 2001; 344: 1904–9.
15. Chun YS, Linder NM, Smyrk TC, et al. Germline E-cadherin germ mutations. Is prophylactic total gastrectomy indicated? *Cancer* 2001; 92: 181–7.
16. Keller G, Hofler H, Becker KF. Molecular mechanisms of gastric adenocarcinoma. *Expert Rev Mol Med* 2005; 7: 1–13.
17. Worthley DL, Phillips KD, Wayte N, et al. Gastric adenocarcinoma and proximal polyposis of the stomach (GAPPS): a new autosomal dominant syndrome. *Gut* 2012; 61: 774–9.
18. Japanese Gastric Cancer Association. Japanese classification of gastric carcinoma: 3rd English edition. *Gastric Cancer* 2011; 14: 101–12.

19. Polkowski W, van Sandick JW, Offerhaus GJ, et al. Prognostic value of Lauren classification and c-erbB-2 oncogene expression in adenocarcinoma of the oesophagus and gastroesophageal junction. *Ann Surg Oncol* 1999; 6: 290–7.

20. Kaneko S, Yoshimura T. Time trend analysis of gastric cancer incidence in Japan by histological types, 1975–1989. *Br J Cancer* 2001; 84: 400–5.

21. Parsonnet J, Vandersteen D, Goates, et al. *Helicobacter pylori* infection in intestinal and diffuse type gastric adenocarcinomas. *J Natl Cancer Inst* 1991; 83: 640–3.

22. Caldas C, Carneiro F, Lynch HT, et al. Familial gastric cancer: overview and guidelines for management. *J Med Genet* 1999; 36: 873–80.

23. Lauwers GY, Carneiro F, Graham DY. Gastric carcinoma. In Bosman FT, Carneiro F, Hruban RH, Thiese ND, eds., *WHO Classification of Tumours of the Digestive System*, 4th ed. Lyon: International Agency for Research on Cancer, 2010.

24. Sobin LH, Gospodarowicz MK, Wittekind C. TNM *Classification of Malignant Tumors*, 7th ed. Oxford: Wiley-Blackwell, 2009.

25. Shah MA, Khanin R, Tang L, et al. Molecular classification of gastric cancer: a new paradigm. *Clin Cancer Res* 2011; 17: 2693–701.

26. The Cancer Genome Atlas Research Network. Comprehensive molecular characterization of gastric adenocarcinoma. *Nature* 2014; 513: 202–9.

27. National Institute for Health and Care Excellence (NICE). Clinical guideline NG 12. Referral guidelines for suspected cancer. London: NICE, 2015.

28. Sakai Y, Eto R, Kasanuki J, et al. Chromoendoscopy with indigo carmine added to acetic acid in the diagnosis of gastric neoplasia: a prospective comparative study. *Gastrointest Endosc* 2008; 68: 635–41.

29. Bramble MG, Suvakovic Z, Hungin APS. Detection of upper gastrointestinal cancer in patients taking antisecretory therapy prior to gastroscopy. *Gut* 2000; 46: 464–7.

30. Yalamarthy S, Witherspoon P, McCole D, et al. Missed diagnosis in patients with upper gastrointestinal cancers. *Endoscopy* 2004; 36: 874–9.

31. Bhandari S, Shim CS, Kim JH, et al. Usefulness of three-dimensional, multidetector row CT (virtual gastroscopy and multiplanar reconstruction) in the evaluation of gastric cancer: a comparison with conventional endoscopy, EUS, and histopathology. *Gastrointest Endosc* 2004; 59: 619–26.

32. Fukuya T, Honda H, Kaneko K, et al. Efficacy of helical CT in T-staging of gastric cancer. *J Comput Assist Tomogr* 1997; 21: 73–81.

33. Hur J, Park MS, Lee JH, et al. Diagnostic accuracy of multidetector row computed tomography in T- and N staging of gastric cancer with histopathologic correlation. *J Comput Assist Tomogr* 2006; 30: 372–7.

34. Kim HJ, Kim AY, Oh ST, et al. Gastric cancer staging at multi-detector row CT gastrography: comparison of transverse and volumetric CT scanning. *Radiology* 2005; 236: 879–85.

35. Dassen AE, Lips DJ, Hoekstra CJ, et al. FDG-PET has no definite role in preoperative imaging in gastric cancer. *Eur J Surg Oncol* 2009; 35: 449–55.

36. Chowdhury FU, Bradley KM, Gleeson FV. The role of 18F-FDG PET/CT in the evaluation of oesophageal carcinoma. *Clin Radiol* 2008; 63: 1297–309.

37. Cardoso R, Coburn N, Seevaratnam R, et al. A systematic review and meta-analysis of the utility of EUS for preoperative staging for gastric cancer. *Gastric Cancer* 2012; 15(Suppl. 1): S19–26.

38. Leake P-A, Cardoso R, Seevaratnam R, et al. A systematic review of the accuracy and indications for diagnostic laparoscopy prior to curative-intent resection of gastric cancer. *Gastric Cancer* 2012; 15(Suppl. 1): S38–47.

39. Leake P-A, Cardoso R, Seevaratnam R, et al. A systematic review of the accuracy and utility of peritoneal cytology in patients with gastric cancer. *Gastric Cancer* 2012; 15(Suppl. 1): S27–37.

40. Hamashima C, Shibuya D, Yamazaki H, et al. The Japanese guidelines for gastric cancer screening. *Jpn J Clin Oncol* 2008; 38(4): 259–67.

41. Fukao A, Tsubono Y, Tsuji I, et al. The evaluation of screening for gastric cancer in Miyagi Prefecture, Japan: a population-based case-control study. *Int J Cancer* 1995; 60(1): 45–8.

42. Report on regional public health services and health promotion services 2012. Tokyo: Ministry of Health, Labour and Welfare, 2012.

43. Mizoue T, Yoshimura T, Tokui N, et al. Prospective study of screening for stomach cancer in Japan. *Int J Cancer* 2003; 106(1): 103–7.

44. Miyamoto A, Kuriyama S, Nishino Y, et al. Lower risk of death from gastric cancer among participants of gastric cancer screening in Japan: a population-based cohort study. *Prev Med* 2007; 44(1): 12–9.

45. Choi KS, Jun JK, Park EC, et al. Performance of different gastric cancer screening methods in Korea: a population-based study. *PLoS One* 2012; 7(11): e50041.

46. Choi KS, Jun JK, Suh M, et al. Effect of endoscopy screening on stage at gastric cancer diagnosis: results of the National Cancer Screening Programme in Korea. *Br J Cancer* 2015; 112: 608–12.

47. Japanese Gastric Cancer Association. Japanese gastric cancer treatment guidelines 2010 (ver. 3). *Gastric Cancer* 2011; 14(2): 113–23.

48. Korean Gastric Cancer Association, ed. *Gastric Cancer and Gastrointestinal Disease*. Seoul: Ilchokak, 2011.

49. Yamao T, Shirao K, Ono H, et al. Risk factors for lymph node metastasis from intramucosal gastric carcinoma. *Cancer* 1996; 77(4): 602–6.

50. Okagima K, Isozaki H. Principles of surgical treatment. In Nishi M, Ichikawa H, Nakajima T, et al., ed., *Gastric Cancer*. Tokyo: Springer-Verlag, 1993, pp. 280–92.

51. Bonenkamp JJ, Songun I, Hermans J, et al. Randomised comparison of morbidity after D1 and D2 dissection for gastric cancer in 996 Dutch patients. *Lancet* 1995; 345(8952): 745–8.

52. Cuschieri A, Fayers P, Fielding J, et al. Postoperative morbidity and mortality after D1 and D2 resections for gastric cancer: preliminary results of the MRC randomised controlled surgical trial. *Lancet* 1996; 347: 995–9.

53. Hartgrink HH, van de Velde CJ, Putter H, et al. Extended lymph node dissection for gastric cancer: who may benefit? Final results of the randomized Dutch gastric cancer group trial. *J Clin Oncol* 2004; 22(11): 2069–77.

54. Cuschieri A, Weeden S, Fielding J, et al. Patient survival after D1 and D2 resections for gastric cancer: long term results of the MRC randomised surgical trial. Surgical Co-operative Group. *Br J Cancer* 1999; 79: 1522–30.

55. Songun I, Putter H, Kranenbarg EM, et al. Surgical treatment of gastric cancer: 15-year follow-up results of the randomised nationwide Dutch D1D2 trial. *Lancet Oncol* 2010; 11(5): 439–49.

56. Sasako M, Sano T, Yamamoto S, et al. D2 lymphadenectomy alone or with para-aortic nodal dissection for gastric cancer. *N Engl J Med* 2008; 359(5): 453–62.

57. de Manzoni G, Di Leo A, Roviello F, et al. Tumour site and perigastric nodal status are the most important predictors of para-aortic involvement in advanced gastric cancer. *Ann Surg Oncol* 2011; 18: 2273–80.

58. Jiang X, Hiki N, Nunobe S, et al. Postoperative outcomes and complications after laparoscopy-assisted pylorus-preserving gastrectomy for early gastric cancer. *Ann Surg* 2011; 253(5): 928–33.

59. Morita S, Katai H, Saka M, et al. Outcome of pylorus-preserving gastrectomy for early gastric cancer. *Br J Surg* 2008; 95(9): 1131–5.

60. Katai H, Morita S, Saka M, et al. Long-term outcome after proximal gastrectomy with jejunal interposition for suspected early cancer in the upper third of the stomach. *Br J Surg* 2010; 97(4): 558–62.

61. Katai H, Sano T, Fukagawa T, et al. Prospective study of proximal gastrectomy for early gastric cancer in the upper third of the stomach. *Br J Surg* 2003; 90(7): 850–3.

62. An JY, Youn HG, Choi MG, et al. The difficult choice between total and proximal gastrectomy in proximal early gastric cancer. *Am J Surg* 2008; 196(4): 587–91.

63. Ryu KW, Eom BW, Nam BH, et al. Is the sentinel node biopsy clinically applicable for limited lymphadenectomy and modified gastric resection in gastric cancer? A meta-analysis of feasibility studies. *J Surg Oncol* 2011; 104(6): 578–84.

64. Kitagawa Y, Takeuchi H, Takagi Y, et al. Sentinel node mapping for gastric cancer: a prospective multicenter trial in Japan. *J Clin Oncol* 2013; 31(29): 3704–10.

65. Miyashiro I, Hiratsuka M, Sasako M, et al. High false-negative proportion of intraoperative histological examination as a serious problem for clinical application of sentinel node biopsy for early gastric cancer: final results of the Japan Clinical Oncology Group multicenter trial JCOG0302. *Gastric Cancer* 2014; 17(2): 316–23.

66. Hartgrink H, Putter H, Klein Kranenbarg E. Value of palliative resection in gastric cancer. *Br J Surg* 2002; 89: 1438–43.

67. Fujitani K, Yang HK, Mizusawa J, et. al. Gastrectomy plus chemotherapy versus chemotherapy alone for advanced gastric cancer with a single non-curable factor (REGATTA): a phase 3, randomised controlled trial. *Lancet Oncol.* 2016; 17(3): 309–18.

68. Kitayama J, Ishigami H, Yamaguchi H, et al. Salvage gastrectomy after intravenous and intraperitoneal paclitaxel (PTX) administration with oral S-1 for peritoneal dissemination of advanced gastric cancer with malignant ascites. *Ann Surg Oncol* 2014; 21(2): 539–46.

69. Novotny AR, Reim D, Friess HM, et al. Secondary gastrectomy for stage IV gastroesophageal adenocarcinoma after induction-chemotherapy. *Langenbecks Arch Surg* 2014; 399(6): 773–81.

70. Goh P, Tekant Y, Kum CK, et al. Totally intra-abdominal laparoscopic Billroth II gastrectomy. *Surg Endosc* 1992; 6(3): 160.

71. Kitano S, Iso Y, Moriyama M, et al. Laparoscopy-assisted Billroth I gastrectomy. *Surg Laparosc Endosc* 1994; 4(2): 146–8.

72. Japan Society for Endoscopic Surgery. Nationwide survey on endoscopic surgery in Japan. *J Jpn Soc Endosc Surg* 2010; 15: 557–679.

73. Jeong O, Park YK. Clinicopathological features and surgical treatment of gastric cancer in South Korea: the results of 2009 nationwide survey on surgically treated gastric cancer patients. *J Gastric Cancer* 2011; 11(2): 69–77.

74. Zeng YK, Yang ZL, Peng JS, et al. Laparoscopy-assisted versus open distal gastrectomy for early gastric cancer: evidence from randomized and nonrandomized clinical trials. *Ann Surg* 2012; 256(1): 39–52.

75. Vinuela EF, Gonen M, Brennan MF, et al. Laparoscopic versus open distal gastrectomy for gastric cancer: a meta-analysis of randomized controlled trials and high-quality nonrandomized studies. *Ann Surg* 2012; 255(3): 446–56.

76. Jiang L, Yang KH, Guan QL, et al. Laparoscopy-assisted gastrectomy versus open gastrectomy for resectable gastric cancer: an update meta-analysis based on randomized controlled trials. *Surg Endosc* 2013; 27(7): 2466–80.

77. Kitano S, Shiraishi N, Fujii K, et al. A randomized controlled trial comparing open vs laparoscopy-assisted distal gastrectomy for the treatment of early gastric cancer: an interim report. *Surgery* 2002; 131(1 Suppl.): S306–11.

78. Lee JH, Han HS, Lee JH. A prospective randomized study comparing open vs laparoscopy-assisted distal gastrectomy in early gastric cancer: early results. *Surg Endosc* 2005; 19(2): 168–73.

79. Kim YW, Baik YH, Yun YH, et al. Improved quality of life outcomes after laparoscopy-assisted distal gastrectomy for early gastric cancer: results of a prospective randomized clinical trial. *Ann Surg* 2008; 248(5): 721–7.

80. Kim YW, Yoon HM, Yun YH, et al. Long-term outcomes of laparoscopy-assisted distal gastrectomy for early gastric cancer: result of a randomized controlled trial (COACT 0301). *Surg Endosc* 2013; 27(11): 4267–76.

81. Kim HH, Han SU, Kim MC, et al. Prospective randomized controlled trial (phase III) to comparing laparoscopic distal gastrectomy with open distal gastrectomy for gastric adenocarcinoma (KLASS 01). *J Korean Surg Soc* 2013; 84(2): 123–30.

82. Nakamura K, Katai H, Mizusawa J, et al. A phase III study of laparoscopy-assisted versus open distal gastrectomy with nodal dissection for clinical stage IA/IB gastric cancer (JCOG0912). *Jpn J Clin Oncol* 2013; 43(3): 324–7.

83. Shinohara T, Satoh S, Kanaya S, et al. Laparoscopic versus open D2 gastrectomy for advanced gastric cancer: a retrospective cohort study. *Surg Endosc* 2013; 27(1): 286–94.

84. Park do J, Han SU, Hyung WJ, et al. Long-term outcomes after laparoscopy-assisted gastrectomy for advanced gastric cancer: a large-scale multicenter retrospective study. *Surg Endosc* 2012; 26(6): 1548–53.

85. Hyun MH, Lee CH, Kim HJ, et al. Systematic review and meta-analysis of robotic surgery compared with conventional laparoscopic and open resections for gastric carcinoma. *Br J Surg* 2013; 100(12): 1566–78.

86. Shen WS, Xi HQ, Chen L, et al. A meta-analysis of robotic versus laparoscopic gastrectomy for gastric cancer. *Surg Endosc* 2014; 28(10): 2795–802.

87. Kim HI, Han SU, Yang H-K, et al. Multicentre prospective comparative study of robotic versus laparoscopic gastrectomy for gastric adenocarcinoma. *Ann Surg* 2016 263: 103–9.

88. Kim YW, Reim D, Park JY, et al. Role of robot-assisted distal gastrectomy compared to laparoscopy-assisted distal gastrectomy in suprapancreatic nodal dissection for gastric cancer. *Surg Endosc* 2015; 1–6.

89. Suda K, Man IM, Ishida Y, et al. Potential advantages of robotic radical gastrectomy for gastric adenocarcinoma in comparison with conventional laparoscopic approach: a single institutional retrospective comparative cohort study. *Surg Endosc* 2015; 29: 673–85.

90. Shen W, Xi H, Wei B, et al. Robotic versus laparoscopic gastrectomy for gastric cancer: comparison of short-term surgical outcomes. *Surg Endosc* 2016; 30: 574–80.

91. Suh YS, Han DS, Kong SH, et al. Laparoscopy-assisted pylorus-preserving gastrectomy is better than laparoscopy-assisted distal gastrectomy for middle-third early gastric cancer. *Ann Surg* 2014; 259(3): 485–93.

92. Kinoshita T, Gotohda N, Kato Y, et al. Laparoscopic proximal gastrectomy with jejunal interposition for gastric cancer in the proximal third of the stomach: a retrospective comparison with open surgery. *Surg Endosc* 2013; 27(1): 146–53.

93. Wang Z, Dong ZY, Chen JQ, et al. Diagnostic value of sentinel lymph node biopsy in gastric cancer: a meta-analysis. *Ann Surg Oncol* 2012; 19(5): 1541–50.

94. Cardoso R, Bocicariu A, Dixon M, et al. What is the accuracy of sentinel lymph node biopsy for gastric cancer? A systematic review. *Gastric Cancer* 2012; 15(Suppl. 1): S48–59.

95. Symeonidis D, Koukoulis G, Tepetes K. Sentinel node navigation surgery in gastric cancer: current status. *World J Gastrointest Surg* 2014; 6: 88–93.

96. Cunningham D, Allum WH, Stenning SP, et al. Perioperative chemotherapy versus surgery alone for resectable gastro-esophageal cancer. *N Engl J Med* 2006; 355: 11–20.

97. Ychou M, Boige V, Pignon JP, et al. Perioperative chemotherapy compared with surgery alone for resectable gastroesophageal adenocarcinoma: an FNCLCC and FFCD multicenter phase III trial. *J Clin Oncol* 2011; 29: 1715–21.

98. Waddell T, Verheij M, Allum W, et al. (European Society for Medical Oncology [ESMO], European Society of Surgical Oncology [ESSO], European Society of Radiotherapy and Oncology [ESTRO]). Gastric cancer: ESMO-ESSO-ESTRO clinical practice guidelines for diagnosis, treatment and follow-up. *Eur J Surg Oncol* 2014; 40: 584–91.

99. Cunningham D, Starling N, Rao S, et al. (Upper Gastrointestinal Clinical Studies Group of the National Cancer Research Institute of the United Kingdom). Capecitabine and oxaliplatin for advanced esophagogastric cancer. *N Engl J Med* 2008; 358: 36–46.

100. Okines AF, Langley RE, Thompson LC, et al. Bevacizumab with peri-operative epirubicin, cisplatin and capecitabine (ECX) in localised gastro-oesophageal adenocarcinoma: a safety report. *Ann Oncol* 2013; 24: 702–9.

101. Cunningham D, Smyth E, Stenning S, Stevenson L, Robb C, Allum W, et al. Peri-operative chemotherapy +/- bevacizumab for resectable gastrooesophageal adenocarcinoma: Results from the UK Medical Research Council randomised STO3 trial (ISRCTN 46020948). *Eur J Cancer* 2015; 51(3):S400.

102. Macdonald JS, Smalley SR, Benedetti J, et al. Chemoradiotherapy after surgery compared with surgery alone for adenocarcinoma of the stomach or gastroesophageal junction. *N Engl J Med* 2001; 345: 725–30.

103. Smalley SR, Benedetti JK, Haller DG, et al. Updated analysis of SWOG-directed intergroup study 0116: a phase III trial of adjuvant radiochemotherapy versus observation after curative gastric cancer resection. *J Clin Oncol* 2012; 30: 2327–33.

104. Dikken JL, Jansen EP, Cats A, et al. Impact of the extent of surgery and postoperative chemoradiotherapy on recurrence patterns in gastric cancer. *J Clin Oncol* 2010; 28: 2430–6.

105. Randomized Phase III Trial of Adjuvant Chemotherapy or Chemoradiotherapy in Resectable Gastric Cancer (CRITICS). ClinicalTrials.gov. Identifier: NCT00407186 (accessed 1 February 2015).

106. Sakuramoto S, Sasako M, Yamaguchi T, et al. ACTS-GC Group: adjuvant chemotherapy for gastric cancer with S-1, an oral fluoropyrimidine. *N Engl J Med* 2007; 357: 1810–20. Erratum in *N Engl J Med* 2008; 358: 1977.

107. Bang YJ, Kim YW, Yang HK, et al. (CLASSIC trial investigators). Adjuvant capecitabine and oxaliplatin for gastric cancer after D2 gastrectomy (CLASSIC): a phase 3 open-label, randomised controlled trial. *Lancet* 2012; 379: 315–21.

108. Noh SH, Park SR, Yang HK, et al. (CLASSIC trial investigators). Adjuvant capecitabine plus oxaliplatin for gastric cancer after D2 gastrectomy (CLASSIC): 5-year follow-up of an open-label, randomised phase 3 trial. *Lancet Oncol* 2014; 15: 1389–96.

109. Paoletti X, Oba K, Burzykowski T, et al. (GASTRIC [Global Advanced/Adjuvant Stomach Tumor Research International Collaboration] Group). Benefit of adjuvant chemotherapy for resectable gastric cancer: a meta-analysis. *JAMA* 2010; 303: 1729–37.

110. Lichtman SM, Wildiers H, Chatelut E, et al. (International Society of Geriatric Oncology Chemotherapy Taskforce). International Society of Geriatric Oncology Chemotherapy Taskforce: evaluation of chemotherapy in older patients – an analysis of the medical literature. *J Clin Oncol* 2007; 25: 1832–43.

111. Trumper M, Ross PJ, Cunningham D, et al. Efficacy and tolerability of chemotherapy in elderly patients with advanced oesophago-gastric cancer: a pooled analysis of three clinical trials. *Eur J Cancer* 2006; 42: 827–34.

112. Choi IS, Oh DY, Kim BS, et al. Oxaliplatin, 5-FU, folinic acid as first-line palliative chemotherapy in elderly patients with metastatic or recurrent gastric cancer. *Cancer Res Treat* 2007; 39: 99–103.

113. Nardi M, Azzarello D, Maisano R, et al. FOLFOX-4 regimen as first-line chemotherapy in elderly patients with advanced gastric cancer: a safety study. *J Chemother* 2007; 19: 85–9.

114. Catalano V, Bisonni R, Graziano F, et al. A phase II study of modified FOLFOX as first-line chemotherapy for metastatic gastric cancer in elderly patients with associated diseases. *Gastric Cancer* 2013; 16: 411–19.

115. Fonck M, Brunet R, Becouarn Y, et al. Evaluation of efficacy and safety of FOLFIRI for elderly patients with gastric cancer: a first-line phase II study. *Clin Res Hepatol Gastroenterol* 2011; 35: 823–30.

116. Ajani JA, Bentrem DJ, Besh S, et al. (National Comprehensive Cancer Network). Gastric cancer, version 2.2013: featured updates to the NCCN Guidelines. *J Natl Compr Canc Netw* 2013; 11: 531–46.

117. Wagner AD, Unverzagt S, Grothe W, et al. Chemotherapy for advanced gastric cancer. *Cochrane Database Syst Rev* 2010 17; (3): CD004064.

118. Murad AM, Santiago FF, Petroianu A, et al. Modified therapy with 5-fluorouracil, doxorubicin, and methotrexate in advanced gastric cancer. *Cancer* 1993; 72: 37–41.

119. Cunningham D, Starling N, Rao S, Iveson T, Nicolson M, Coxon F, Middleton G, Daniel F, Oates J, Norman AR. Upper Gastrointestinal Clinical Studies Group of the National Cancer Research Institute of the United Kingdom. *N Engl J Med* 2008; 358: 36–46.

120. Kang YK, Kang WK, Shin DB, et al. Capecitabine/cisplatin versus 5-fluorouracil/cisplatin as first-line therapy in patients with advanced gastric cancer: a randomised phase III noninferiority trial. *Ann Oncol* 2009; 20: 666–73.

121. Ford HE, Marshall A, Bridgewater JA, et al. (COUGAR-02 Investigators). Docetaxel versus active symptom control for refractory oesophagogastric adenocarcinoma (COUGAR-02): an open-label, phase 3 randomised controlled trial. *Lancet Oncol* 2014; 15: 78–86.

122. Kang JH, Lee SI, Lim do H, et al. Salvage chemotherapy for pretreated gastric cancer: a randomized phase III trial comparing chemotherapy plus best supportive care with best supportive care alone. *J Clin Oncol* 2012; 30: 1513–8. Erratum in *J Clin Oncol* 2012; 30: 3035.

123. Thuss-Patience PC, Kretzschmar A, Bichev D, et al. Survival advantage for irinotecan versus best supportive care as second-line chemotherapy in gastric cancer – a randomised phase III study of the Arbeitsgemeinschaft Internistische Onkologie (AIO). *Eur J Cancer* 2011; 47: 2306–14.

124. Hironaka S, Ueda S, Yasui H, et al. Randomized, open-label, phase III study comparing irinotecan with paclitaxel in patients with advanced gastric cancer without severe peritoneal metastasis after failure of prior combination chemotherapy using fluoropyrimidine plus platinum: WJOG 4007 trial. *J Clin Oncol* 2013; 31: 4438–44.

125. Bang YJ, Van Cutsem E, Feyereislova A, et al. (ToGA Trial Investigators). Trastuzumab in combination with chemotherapy versus chemotherapy alone for treatment of HER2-positive advanced gastric or gastro-oesophageal junction cancer (ToGA): a phase 3, open-label, randomised controlled trial. *Lancet* 2010; 376: 687–97. Erratum in *Lancet* 2010; 376: 1302.

126. Fuchs CS, Tomasek J, Yong CJ, et al. (REGARD Trial Investigators). Ramucirumab monotherapy for previously treated advanced gastric or gastro-oesophageal junction adenocarcinoma (REGARD): an international, randomised, multicentre, placebo-controlled, phase 3 trial. *Lancet* 2014; 383: 31–9.

127. Wilke H, Muro K, Van Cutsem E, et al. (RAINBOW Study Group). Ramucirumab plus paclitaxel versus placebo plus paclitaxel in patients with previously treated advanced gastric or gastro-oesophageal junction adenocarcinoma (RAINBOW): a double-blind, randomised phase 3 trial. *Lancet Oncol* 2014; 15: 1224–35.

128. Ohtsu A, Shah MA, Van Cutsem E, et al. Bevacizumab in combination with chemotherapy as first-line therapy in advanced gastric cancer: a randomized, double-blind, placebo-controlled phase III study. *J Clin Oncol* 2011; 29: 3968–76.

129. Waddell T, Chau I, Cunningham D, et al. Epirubicin, oxaliplatin, and capecitabine with or without panitumumab for patients with previously untreated advanced oesophagogastric cancer (REAL3): a randomised, open-label phase 3 trial. *Lancet Oncol* 2013; 14: 481–9.

130. Lordick F, Kang YK, Chung HC, et al. (Arbeitsgemeinschaft Internistische Onkologie and EXPAND Investigators). Capecitabine and cisplatin with or without cetuximab for patients with previously untreated advanced gastric cancer (EXPAND): a randomised, open-label phase 3 trial. *Lancet Oncol* 2013; 14: 490–9.

131. Ohtsu A, Ajani JA, Bai YX, et al. Everolimus for previously treated advanced gastric cancer: results of the randomized, double-blind, phase III GRANITE-1 study. *J Clin Oncol* 2013; 31: 3935–43.

132. Lee J, Lim do H, Kim S, et al. Phase III trial comparing capecitabine plus cisplatin versus capecitabine plus cisplatin with concurrent capecitabine radiotherapy in completely resected gastric cancer with D2 lymph node dissection: the ARTIST trial. *J Clin Oncol* 2012; 30: 268–73.

133. Van Cutsem E, Moiseyenko VM, Tjulandin S, et al. (V325 Study Group). Phase III study of docetaxel and cisplatin plus fluorouracil compared with cisplatin and fluorouracil as first-line therapy for advanced gastric cancer: a report of the V325 Study Group. *J Clin Oncol* 2006; 24: 4991–7.

134. Koizumi W, Narahara H, Hara T, et al. S-1 plus cisplatin versus S-1 alone for first-line treatment of advanced gastric cancer (SPIRITS trial): a phase III trial. *Lancet Oncol* 2008; 9: 215–21.

135. Rao S, Starling N, Cunningham D, et al. Matuzumab plus epirubicin, cisplatin and capecitabine (ECX) compared with epirubicin, cisplatin and capecitabine alone as first-line treatment in patients with advanced oesophago-gastric cancer: a randomised, multicentre open-label phase II study. *Ann Oncol* 2010; 21: 2213–9.

136. Van Cutsem E, Boni C, Tabernero J, et al. Docetaxel plus oxaliplatin with or without fluorouracil or capecitabine in metastatic or locally recurrent gastric cancer: a randomized phase II study. *Ann Oncol* 2015; 26: 149–56.

26

Gastrointestinal stromal tumor

YOUNG-WOO KIM AND JI YEON PARK

INTRODUCTION

Gastrointestinal stromal tumor (GIST) is the most common mesenchymal tumor that typically arises from the alimentary tract. This tumor originates from the spindle cells present in the gut wall: the interstitial cells of Cajal (ICCs). Prior to the 1980s, stromal tumors of the gastrointestinal tract were thought to be neoplasms of smooth muscle origin and were therefore designated as leiomyomas, leiomyosarcomas or leiomyoblastoma depending on mitotic rate and morphology. Subsequently, it was found that GISTs were a separate entity with distinct ultrastructural features and a typical immunophenotype compared with smooth muscle tumors. For years, the only effective treatment available was surgery, but this was rarely curative for high-risk tumors. Postoperative recurrence and metastasis occurred in between 40% and 90% of all cases of GISTs treated surgically [1,2]. Surgery, in combination with conventional chemotherapy or radiation therapy, has largely been ineffective in treating the majority of patients with malignant GISTs.

The understanding of the pathobiology of GISTs expanded significantly since the landmark work by Hirota and colleagues in 1998 indicating that gain-of-function mutations in the *KIT* gene play an early and important role in the development of GISTs [3]. The subsequent work by Heinrich and colleagues in 2003 additionally uncovered intragenic activating mutations in the related receptor tyrosine kinase, platelet-derived growth factor receptor α

(PDGFRA) [4]. These mutations result in the constitutive activation of transmembrane receptor KIT or PDGFRA and their tyrosine kinase function, which leads to uncontrolled cell proliferation and resistance to apoptosis. The discovery of these tyrosine kinase receptor mutations in GISTs led to the remarkable development of the new molecularly targeted drug therapy with imatinib mesylate (Gleevec, Novartis Pharma, Basel, Switzerland), which targets and inhibits the activated KIT tyrosine kinase receptor. This drug has changed the therapeutic landscape of this previously treatment refractory tumor. Imatinib not only prolongs survival substantially but also improves quality of life with generally manageable side effects compared to conventional cytotoxic chemotherapeutic agents. Treatment of GISTs is currently regarded as the paradigm of molecular-targeted therapy in solid tumors.

EPIDEMIOLOGY

According to a population-based sample, the annual incidence of GISTs was estimated at 10–20 cases per million [5–9]. Of these, 20–30% cases are malignant tumors. GISTs demonstrate fairly similar distribution between genders, but some series showed a slight male predominance [1]. Although GISTs have been reported in patients of all ages, most of the people affected by the disease are between 40 and 80 years old at the time of diagnosis, with the median age of 63 to 69 years [5–7].

The majority of GISTs are sporadic, but there are several case reports of familial germline mutations in the *KIT* or *PDGFRA* proto-oncogenes [10–12]. These families have a predisposition to the early development of multiple gastric and small bowel GISTs, and in some cases, skin hyperpigmentation, dysphagia or GI autonomic nerve tumors such as paragangliomas.

Pediatric GISTs represent 1–2% of all GISTs and they tend to arise within defined syndromes, including Carney's triad and Carney–Stratakis syndromes [13]. GISTs occurring in children have distinct clinicopathologic features. In addition to a predilection in females, multifocal tumors and lymph node metastases are common, the histopathology is more likely to be epithelioid, and 85–90% of these pediatric GISTs are categorized as wild-type GISTs lacking *KIT* or *PDGFRA* mutations [13,14]. Although pediatric GIST is more prone to metastasis and local recurrences, it appears to have a more indolent course than adult GIST.

CLINICAL PRESENTATION

The majority (70%) of the patients diagnosed with GISTs have non-specific symptoms which vary depending on the size and site of involvement. The symptoms include bloating, early satiety or abdominal discomfort, which are related to mass effect, gastrointestinal bleeding from a mucosal erosion or an abdominal mass from a large-sized tumor [5]. Less frequently patients present with intestinal obstruction, possibly because the tumor serves as a lead point for intussusception. Patients with esophageal or duodenal GIST may rarely present with dysphagia or jaundice, respectively [15,16]. GISTs can also rupture into the peritoneum causing peritonitis or life-threatening intraperitoneal hemorrhage. Asymptomatic small GISTs are often detected incidentally during surgery or endoscopy for other conditions, during rectal examination, or occasionally as incidental radiologic findings. Ten percent of the cases are detected only at the time of autopsy.

GISTs occur throughout the GI tract from the esophagus to the anus. Approximately 40–60% of GISTs arise in the stomach, 25–30% in the jejunum or ileum, 5% in the duodenum, 5–15% in the colorectum and less than 5% in the esophagus [1,17]. Rarely, they can also develop in the omentum, mesentery, pancreas or other retroperitoneal organs, which are referred to as extra-gastrointestinal stromal tumors (EGISTs) [17,18].

GISTs frequently metastasize to the liver and peritoneum and rarely to regional lymph nodes. Metastasis to the lung or bone is uncommon [19].

DIAGNOSIS

Clinical diagnosis

Diagnostic protocols depend on the initial symptoms at presentation. Contrast-enhanced computed tomography (CT) of the abdomen and pelvis is useful to evaluate the primary tumor as well as to assess disease extent and whether metastatic disease is present. Oral as well as IV contrast should be administered to define the bowel margins. On CT scan, GISTs typically appear as hyperdense, enhancing masses, closely associated with the stomach or small intestine. Very large tumors may appear more complex due to necrosis, hemorrhage or degenerating components. It may difficult to identify the origin of a large mass because of exophytic growth. MRI or contrast-enhanced ultrasound may be an alternative. MRI may be preferred for GISTs at specific sites, such as the rectum or liver. Hypermetabolic uptake on fluorodeoxyglucose (FDG)–positron emission tomography (PET) is highly sensitive, but not specific enough for the diagnosis of GIST. PET can be useful for detecting an unknown primary site or resolving ambiguities from CT when the CT findings are inconclusive or inconsistent with the clinical findings (20). PET can also be used to monitor the clinical response of GISTs to imatinib treatment (Figure 26.1).

Endoscopy may be useful in the diagnosis of gastric GISTs. On endoscopy, a GIST appears as a submucosal mass with smooth margins and a normal overlying mucosa, since it originated from the bowel wall and not the mucosa. Central ulceration is occasionally seen. Endoscopic ultrasound (EUS) is useful for the diagnosis and preoperative assessment of gastric GISTs when the diagnosis or location is in doubt (Figure 26.2). EUS can also be used to guide fine-needle aspiration (FNA) for pathologic confirmation. Recent studies have shown that endoscopic FNA for the diagnosis of GISTs has a sensitivity as high as 80% [21]. However, biopsies by either percutaneous or endoscopic techniques theoretically can precipitate tumor rupture and lead to tumor dissemination or hemorrhage. Preoperative tissue diagnosis is not generally recommended for primary localized tumors unless the diagnosis is in doubt. Biopsy may be useful when another diagnosis, such as lymphoma, that would not benefit from surgical resection is entertained. Biopsy is also recommended for metastatic disease or in cases where the mass is marginally resectable and neoadjuvant imatinib is under consideration, both to confirm the diagnosis and to permit mutational analysis which may give guidance to the optimal medical therapy which may vary according to the underlying type of gene mutation.

Pathologic diagnosis

Pathologically, the diagnosis of GIST relies on morphology and immunohistochemistry. GISTs are monotonous tumors that can be divided into three principal subtypes depending on the microscopic morphology. The majority of GISTs (approximately 70% of cases) are spindle cell type, and about 20% of cases are composed of epithelioid cells, which are commonly seen in pediatric GISTs. The remaining 10% of GISTs have a mixed spindle and epithelioid cell morphology [2].

Immunohistochemical characteristics of GIST have proven very helpful in diagnosis. KIT (CD117) expression is a specific and sensitive marker for GIST, and approximately 95% of GISTs are immunoreactive for KIT. Most GISTs show

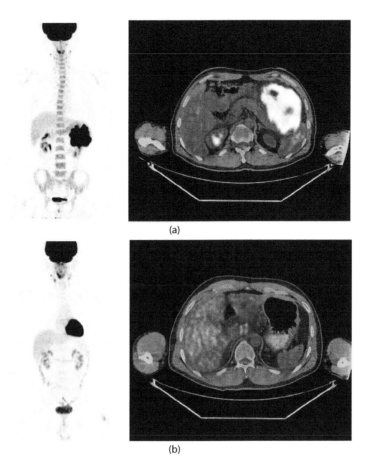

Figure 26.1 Therapeutic effect of imatinib on gastric GIST shown in positron emission tomography. (a) A hypermetabolic mass from the stomach was noticed at initial diagnosis before the imatinib treatment. (b) The size and metabolism of the lesion were markedly decreased after 6 months of imatinib treatment.

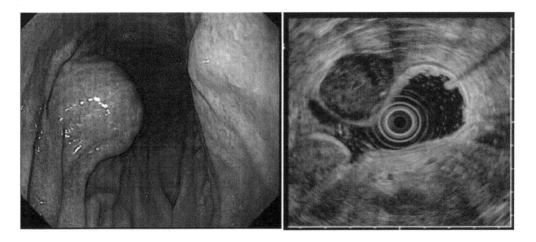

Figure 26.2 Appearance of gastric GIST on endoscopy and endoscopic ultrasound.

a strong and diffuse cytoplasmic staining for KIT, although there is variability in the level of KIT expression. KIT overexpression is usually related to mutations in the *KIT* gene, although *PDGFRA* mutations and other unknown mechanisms also appear to result in KIT overexpression without *KIT* gene mutation. Although KIT positivity is a major defining feature for GIST, KIT positivity alone may not be sufficient for diagnosis because there are non-GISTs that are positive for KIT. GIST can be confidently diagnosed if the morphology and immunophenotype are concordant; however, tumors with any unusual features should be sent to a referral institution with special expertise. In addition to KIT (CD117), 60–70% of GISTs express CD34, but several other mesenchymal neoplasms, which enter into the differential diagnosis of GISTs, stain with CD34. Thirty to forty percent of GISTs express smooth muscle actin (SMA), and nuclear and cytoplasmic positivity for S100 protein occurs in 5–10%, while small minorities of GISTs (2%) express desmin [22,23]. Another useful immunohistochemical stain is DOG-1 (discovered on GIST-1), which is expressed in nearly all GIST tumors, including KIT-negative *PDGFRA* mutant tumors [24,25].

Traditional microscopy and immunohistochemistry are usually sufficient to establish the diagnosis of GIST. However, in tumors where the diagnosis remains uncertain, real-time polymerase chain reaction (RT-PCR) testing for *KIT* or *PDGFRA* gene mutations may be useful. Gain-of-function mutations in the *KIT* gene are detectable in 75–80% of all GISTs. Most *KIT* gene mutations (approximately 75%) in GISTs affect exon 11 and result in ligand-independent receptor dimerization and activation. However, in some cases, a mutation is present in exon 9, 13 or 17, with a different structural biological mechanism that results in uncontrolled KIT signalling. *PDGFRA* mutations are present in a minority of GISTs (5–7%) and *PDGRFA* mutant GISTs are generally limited to the stomach, particularly with an epithelioid morphology, and are clinically less aggressive [4,26].

The diagnosis of KIT-negative GIST (in the 5% range of all GISTs) depends on tissue morphology as well as on genotyping the tumor for a *KIT* or *PDGFRA* mutation, as some tumors negative for KIT by immunohistochemistry have been shown to have either mutation [27,28]. A subset of 7–14% of GISTs are negative for detectable *KIT* and *PDGFRA* mutations. These are quite rare, but they are often localized to the stomach, multicentric in origin and can have an indolent clinical course. GISTs associated with Carney's triad (paraganglioma, pulmonary chondroma and gastric GIST) also appear to lack kinase gene mutations. Loss-of-function mutations in genes that encode subunits of the enzyme succinate dehydrogenase (SDH) have been identified in wild-type GIST lacking *KIT* and *PDGFRA* mutations; these findings have led to the use of the term *SDH-deficient GIST* for this subset of GIST [29]. Recently, the relevance of the mutational status of these genes for clinical prognosis, therapy decisions and prediction of response to treatment has been increasingly recognized. The current National Comprehensive Cancer Network (NCCN) and European Society of Medical Oncology (ESMO) guidelines recommend molecular genetic testing to identify mutations in the *KIT* and *PDGFRA* genes as useful in predicting sensitivity of molecularly targeted therapies. *SDH* gene mutational analysis for the identification of germline mutations in the *SDH* gene subunits should be considered for patients with KIT/PDFGRA wild-type GIST [20,30,31].

STAGING AND RISK ASSESSMENT

The best indicator of malignancy is the confirmation of metastatic disease. When there is no evidence of distant metastasis, the risk of relapse of operable disease is estimated on the basis of mitotic rate, tumor size, tumor location, surgical margins and whether tumor rupture occurred. Tumor size and mitotic count are considered by the 2002 consensus risk classification (Table 26.1) [22]. Importantly, neither small size nor low mitotic rate completely excludes the potential for malignant behaviour of the GIST.

Based on long-term follow-up of more than 1600 patients, Miettinen and colleagues proposed a risk partitioning scheme which incorporated primary tumor location in addition to the mitotic count and tumor size (Table 26.2) [32]. This classification is also named the NCCN classification. In particular, it reflects the fact that gastric GISTs have a better prognosis than small bowel or rectal GISTs. According to these guidelines, gastric GISTs that are 2 cm or smaller with a mitotic index of 5 or less per 50 high-power fields (HPF) can be regarded as essentially benign, but lesions larger than 2 cm with the same mitotic index have a risk for recurrence. Data are lacking on the prognosis of patients with GISTs smaller than 2 cm with a mitotic count of more than 5 per 50 HPF. Although the majority of GISTs can be classified by this system, GISTs without connection to the GI tract and esophageal GISTs are not included. Furthermore, the extreme adverse prognostic factor of tumor rupture is not recognized. Accordingly, Joensuu included tumor rupture into a modified risk assessment scheme in 2008 and called it the modified NCCN classification (Table 26.3) [33].

A nomogram utilizing the same criteria has been developed by Gold and colleagues to predict recurrence-free survival (RFS) after resection of localized primary GIST

Table 26.1 Risk of aggressive behaviour in GISTs

Risk	Size (cm)	Mitotic count (per 50 HPF)
Very low risk	<2	<5
Low risk	2–5	<5
Intermediate risk	<5	6–10
	5–10	<5
High risk	>5	>5
	>10	Any mitotic rate
	Any tumor	>10

Source: Adapted from Fletcher C et al., *Hum Pathol* 2002;33:459–65.

Table 26.2 Risk stratification of primary GIST by mitotic index, size and site

Tumor parameters		Risk for progressive disease (%), based on site of origin			
Mitotic index	Size (cm)	Stomach	Jejunum/ileum	Duodenum	Rectum
≤5 per 50 HPF	≤2	None	None	None	None
	>2, ≤5	Very low	Low	Low	Low
	>5, ≤10	Low	Moderate	Insufficient data	Insufficient data
	>10	Moderate	High	High	High
>5 per 50 HPF	≤2	None	High	Insufficient data	High
	>2, ≤5	Moderate	High	High	High
	>5, ≤10	High	High	Insufficient data	Insufficient data
	>10	High	High	High	High

Source: Adapted from Miettinen M, Lasota J, *Sem Diagn Pathol* 2006;23:70–83.

Table 26.3 Proposed modification of consensus classification for selecting patients with GIST for adjuvant therapy

Risk category	Tumor size (cm)	Mitotic index (per 50 HPF)	Primary tumor site
Very low risk	<2.0	≤5	Any
Low risk	2.1–5.0	≤5	Any
Intermediate risk	2.1–5.0	>5	Gastric
	<5.0	6–10	Any
	5.1–10.0	≤5	Gastric
High risk	Any	Any	Tumor rupture
	>10.0	Any	Any
	Any	>10	Any
	>5.0	>5	Any
	2.1–5.0	>5	Non-gastric
	5.1–10.0	≤5	Non-gastric

Source: Adapted from Joensuu H, *Hum Pathol* 2008;39:1411–19.

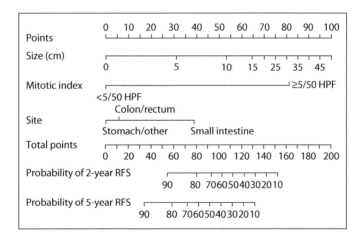

Figure 26.3 Nomogram to estimate 2- and 5-year recurrence-free survival after surgical resection of primary GIST in the absence of tyrosine kinase inhibitor therapy. (Adapted from Gold JS, et al., *Lancet Oncol* 2009;10:1045–52.)

(Figure 26.3) [34]. This nomogram was shown to accurately predict RFS after resection, and may be useful for patients' care, interpretation of trial results and selection of patients for postoperative imatinib therapy. Joensuu and colleagues generated novel prognostic contour maps estimating the risk of GIST recurrence after surgery through a pool of series of GIST patients not treated with adjuvant therapy [35]. This incorporates the mitotic index, tumor size and site, and tumor rupture is also considered. They have been validated against a reference series.

The added value of the TNM staging system developed by the American Joint Committee on Cancer (AJCC) and International Union Against Cancer (UICC) is still under debate [36].

It is not clear whether the presence or absence of *KIT* gene mutations per se is an important negative prognostic factor, but specific types of *KIT* mutations are associated with an aggressive phenotype, including those that affect exon 9 [37]. Tumor response to imatinib also correlates with the underlying kinase genotype. Patients with exon 11 mutations are more likely to respond to imatinib than are those with exon 9 mutations or who lack mutations altogether.

TREATMENT

The management of GISTs involving the GI tract depends on the level of confidence of the preoperative diagnosis, tumor location and size, extent of spread and clinical presentation. Successful treatment of GISTs requires the integration of surgery and molecular-targeted therapy. Thus, a multidisciplinary team that includes radiologists, medical oncologists, pathologists and surgeons is paramount for the effective care of these patients.

Primary localized GIST

SURGICAL RESECTION

Complete surgical resection is the mainstay of treatment for GISTs with no evidence of metastasis and should be initial therapy if the tumor is technically resectable with an acceptable morbidity risk. The objective of surgery is to achieve negative microscopic margins (R0 resection). Wide margins of uninvolved tissue have not been shown to be associated with a better prognosis. En bloc resection of the GIST and its pseudocapsule, if present, should be performed and adjacent organs densely adhered to the tumor should also be completely resected en bloc. At laparotomy, the abdomen should be thoroughly explored, with particular attention to the peritoneal surfaces and liver to exclude metastatic spread. Care should be exercised to avoid excessive tumor manipulation, which can disrupt what may be a friable tumor and lead to bleeding and intraperitoneal dissemination. Avoidance of tumor rupture is imperative. Segmental or wedge resection of the stomach or intestine should be performed, with the goal of achieving negative microscopic margins. In gastric GISTs, however, it may require total or subtotal gastrectomy, depending on tumor location and size. Lymphadenectomy is not routinely necessary unless loco-regional lymph nodes are enlarged, because regional lymph node involvement is rare in GIST.

Some patients may require extensive surgery for a poorly situated tumor. The operative risks and anticipated postoperative recovery must be weighed against the oncologic benefit of tumor resection. For instance, a tumor located near the gastroesophageal junction may require a proximal or total gastrectomy. Pancreaticoduodenectomy may be necessary to remove a duodenal GIST. Occasionally, an abdominoperineal resection is needed for a low rectal GIST. In these situations, preoperative multidisciplinary review is critical, because these patients may be spared radical resection after neoadjuvant imatinib.

The necessity of achieving negative microscopic margins is uncertain with large (>10 cm) GISTs. The management of a positive margin according to the final pathology report is not well defined and depends on whether the surgeon believes the findings accurately reflect the surgical procedure that was undertaken. Although patients who undergo a microscopically incomplete resection may be at a greater risk for a locoregional recurrence, other factors such as tumor grade and size may play a more significant role in determining the risk of recurrence. The risks and benefits of re-excision versus initiation of imatinib must be carefully considered [20].

In patients with persistent gross residual disease (R2 resection), it is recommended that postoperative imatinib be considered, including in patients who have received preoperative imatinib. Additional resection may be considered to remove residual disease. Imatinib treatment should be continued following re-resection, regardless of surgical margin, until progression.

All GISTs 2 cm or larger should be resected. Although a 2 cm cut-off is somewhat arbitrary, recent data suggest that it is reasonable [32]. However, the management of incidentally encountered GISTs smaller than 2 cm remains controversial. The natural history of these and other GISTs between 1 and 2 cm, including their growth rate and metastatic potential, remains unknown. Although these small GISTs may be followed endoscopically until they grow or become symptomatic, the optimal frequency of follow-up and specific risks of this strategy are uncertain. Successful endoscopic resection is reported, but it remains controversial because of the risk of positive margins, tumor spillage and perforation. For a subset of patients with very small gastric GISTs (<2 cm) with no high-risk EUS features, endoscopic surveillance at 6- to 12-month intervals may be considered [20]. When endoscopic assessment is not possible, excision is the standard approach.

Laparoscopic resection is a reasonably safe and feasible procedure for patients with low-risk smaller gastric GISTs. Gastric GISTs 5 cm or smaller may be removed through laparoscopic wedge resection. GISTs larger than 5 cm may be resected using a laparoscopic or laparoscopic-assisted technique with a hand port, depending on the location and shape. Successful use of laparoscopic techniques for the resection of small primary GISTs has been reported in small series, reporting technical feasibility with favorable oncologic outcomes when performed by skilled surgeon [38–42]. Intraoperative endoscopy or laparoscopic ultrasound may be used to assist the laparoscopic procedure as needed. Advantages of laparoscopic resection also include minimal manipulation of the tumor as well as better cosmesis. However, long-term data for patients who have undergone laparoscopic resection for GIST are generally lacking. Laparoscopic surgery could be feasible in other anatomic sites, such as smaller rectal GISTs. However, data on laparoscopic resection of GISTs at other sites are limited.

Complete gross resection of the tumor is the most significant factor for outcome and can be accomplished in 85% of patients with primary localized disease [43–45]. Prognosis of low-risk GISTs after complete resection is excellent. However, high-risk GISTs have a high rate of recurrence [45]. Without any further treatment, at least 50% of patients develop tumor recurrence and the 5-year survival rate is approximately 50% with the median survival ranging from 10 to 23 months [1,42].

TARGETED ADJUVANT THERAPY

Conventional adjuvant chemotherapy and radiation therapy are ineffective in treating the majority of patients with malignant GIST. The recognition of the mutational activation of the *KIT* or *PDGFRA* genes in GIST pathogenesis led to the development of effective systemic therapies in the form of tyrosine kinase inhibitors (TKIs) such as imatinib. Adjuvant

imatinib is provided in order to enhance the eradication of microscopic lesions after the complete gross resection, and proposed as an option for those patients with a high risk of recurrence. In a phase III trial by the American College of Surgeons Oncology Group (ACOSOG Z9001), 713 patients were randomized to imatinib 400 mg/day or placebo for 1 year after complete resection of primary localized GISTs (>3 cm) (Figure 26.4) [46]. At a median follow-up of 19.7 months, imatinib demonstrated a significant increase in RFS compared with a placebo (98% vs. 83%), although no difference in overall survival (OS) between the two treatment arms was noted. However, longer follow-up of the cohort will establish the impact of adjuvant imatinib on OS. In the subset analysis, the absolute benefit was greatest in those with high-risk (≥10 cm) and then with intermediate-risk tumors (≥6 and <10 cm). Results from another randomized controlled

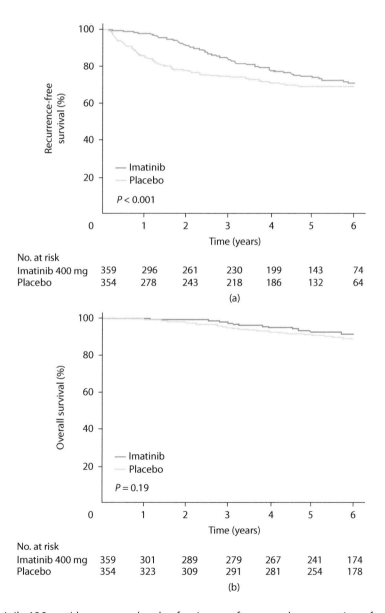

Figure 26.4 Effect of imatinib 400 mg/day versus placebo for 1 year after complete resection of primary localized GISTs larger than 3 cm. (a) Recurrence-free and (b) overall survival in entire population. (Adapted from Corless CL, et al., *J Clin Oncol* 2014;32:1563–70.)

trial, the Scandinavian Sarcoma Group XVIII (SSGXVIII/AIO) trial, suggested that adjuvant imatinib administered for 36 months improved RFS and OS, compared to adjuvant imatinib administered for 12 months (5-year RFS: 66% vs. 48%, respectively; 5-year OS: 92% vs. 82%, respectively), for patients with a high estimated risk of recurrence after surgery (mitotic count >5 mitoses/50 HPF, size >5 cm, non-gastric location and tumor rupture) at a median follow-up of 54 months [47]. Based on these results, use of adjuvant imatinib (400 mg) is recommended after complete resection of primary GIST with no preoperative imatinib in patients with intermediate or high risk of recurrence. It is recommended that postoperative imatinib is given for at least 36 months for patients with high-risk GISTs (tumor greater than 5 cm in size with high mitotic rate >5 mitoses/50 HPF), but the optimal duration of adjuvant imatinib treatment has yet to be determined [48].

Estimation of risk of recurrence is important in selecting patients who would benefit from postoperative imatinib after complete resection. Risk stratification after surgical resection should be based on tumor mitotic rate, size and location (33,34). In addition to risk assessment, mutational analysis may guide the selection of those patients who are more likely to benefit from the treatment. A daily dose of 400 mg/day is the usual approach, although if a *KIT* exon 9 mutation is identified, dose escalation to 800 mg/day may be considered, but there are no prospective data upon which to base a recommendation either for or against this practice [31,49].

In the case of tumor rupture at the time of surgery, where there has been spillage of tumor cells in the peritoneal cavity, occult peritoneal disease can be assumed. This puts the patients at a very high risk of peritoneal relapse [33]. Therefore, these patients should be considered for imatinib therapy in either the adjuvant setting or palliative setting. The optimal duration of treatment in these cases is unknown.

Refining the indications for adjuvant treatment remains a big task for future studies.

NEOADJUVANT THERAPY

The high response rates seen with imatinib in advanced disease have prompted interest in starting imatinib prior to surgery. The goals are to reduce the size of the tumor, thereby facilitating surgery or increasing the likelihood of organ preservation. Although there is no consensus as to the indications for neoadjuvant imatinib, patients with an unresectable or borderline resectable locally advanced tumor, or a potentially resectable tumor that requires extensive surgery or sacrifice of a large amount of normal tissue causing functional deficit, could be considered for initial therapy with imatinib. Patients with a GIST arising in the esophagus, esophagogastric junction, duodenum or distal rectum might also benefit from neoadjuvant treatment [50]. Preoperative imatinib might downstage the marginally resectable tumors and increase the likelihood of a complete (R0) resection, and permit a more conservative excision rather than radical surgery.

The initial dose of 400 mg/day of imatinib is the usual approach, unless the patient has documented *KIT* exon 9 mutations which may benefit from dose escalation up to 800 mg/day (given as 400 mg twice daily), as tolerated [48,49]. The optimal duration of neoadjuvant imatinib therapy is uncertain and the decision should be individualized based on treatment response. A careful pretreatment and frequent treatment response assessment by CT or PET scan should be performed in multidisciplinary discussion. Surgery should be performed after sufficient shrinkage of the tumors (typically between 4 and 6 months and up to 12 months) [38]. For patients who have undergone complete resection after neoadjuvant imatinib, continuation of imatinib following resection is warranted. Imatinib can be stopped right before the surgery and restarted as soon as the patient is able to tolerate oral medications.

Recurrent or metastatic GIST

A significant proportion of patients undergoing complete resection of primary GIST may develop tumor recurrence, and the median time to recurrence after surgery ranges from 18 to 25 months [1,38,44,51,52]. The most commonly involved site of recurrence is the liver, and peritoneal dissemination follows next. Metastases to extra-abdominal sites such as lung or bone sometimes occur with disease progression [1,51]. Local recurrence limited to the gastric wall of gastric GISTs is infrequent.

Because of the lack of any alternative therapies, surgical resection was considered for patients with recurrence after primary resection and for those with metastatic GIST in the pre-imatinib era. Patients with limited hepatic metastasis or isolated peritoneal recurrence were sometimes treated with surgical resection. The results of the surgical management for these patients have been variable depending on the factors such as tumor size, risk profile, completeness of tumor resection and the disease-free interval after initial surgery [52]. However, the outcome was usually very poor: the median survival of such patients only ranged from 6 to 19 months [1,52–54]. The literature in the era before the introduction of imatinib clearly demonstrates that surgery alone is not sufficient to provide long-term survival for high-risk GIST patients.

Imatinib is now the first-line treatment in patients who develop recurrent metastatic disease. Imatinib therapy has significantly improved the prognosis of patients with recurrent or metastatic GIST. Imatinib is reported to achieve partial tumor response or stable disease in approximately 80% of advanced GISTs [55,56]. Remarkably, the median survival has improved to nearly 5 years [57]. The majority of patients with metastatic GIST achieve a response within 6 months of imatinib therapy with a median time to response of approximately 3 months [55,56]. However, complete responses are only rarely achieved and positive responses are not maintained indefinitely after imatinib therapy alone in metastatic GIST, and the median interval to disease progression is less than 2 years [56]. Thus, a multimodal approach utilizing surgical resection in conjunction with imatinib therapy to treat recurrent and metastasis GIST in multidisciplinary teams is highly desirable.

Although imatinib benefits most patients with advanced GISTs, some develop resistance to the drug. Primary resistance is defined as evidence of clinical progression developing during the first 6 months of imatinib therapy and is most commonly seen in patients with *KIT* exon 9 mutations treated with imatinib 400 mg daily or patients with *PDGFRA* exon 18 D842V mutations, or those with SDH-deficient GIST [58]. Secondary resistance is seen in patients who have been on imatinib for more than 6 months with an initial response or disease stabilization followed by progression. It is well recognized that the clones of resistant tumor cells develop continuously after initiation of imatinib therapy, most commonly because of additional point mutation in the KIT kinase domains [59,60]. The risk of disease progression on imatinib and developing imatinib resistance seems to be proportional to the amount of residual viable tumor. Once maximal response to imatinib occurs (generally after 2–6 months of therapy), the disease should be evaluated again by a multidisciplinary team for further surgical treatment. Selected patients with metastatic GIST who have responsive disease or focal resistance to imatinib may benefit from elective cytoreductive surgery [61,62]. Imatinib therapy should be continued postoperatively, since treatment interruption is generally followed by rapid tumor re-growth in virtually all cases, even when lesions have been surgically excised [38,63]. However, surgery is generally not indicated in patients with generalized disease progression under imatinib treatment, unless to provide symptomatic relief [61,62]. In patients with overt diffuse progression, increasing the dose of imatinib or using other TKIs, such as sunitinib, is a more appropriate option [38].

In the case of confirmed progression or rare intolerance of imatinib (after attempts to manage side effects), standard second-line treatment is another TKI, sunitinib [30,31,64]. Sunitinib is a multikinase inhibitor active against a variety of tyrosine kinases, including KIT, PDGFR and vascular endothelial growth factor receptor (VEGFR). In randomized trials, sunitinib has resulted in a significant improvement in median time to progression and significantly greater estimated OS in patients with imatinib-resistant GIST than placebo [64]. At a median follow-up of 42 months, progression-free survival (PFS) was fourfold higher in the sunitinib

group than in the placebo group (27 vs. 6 weeks) [65]. The drug is effective with either a regimen of a 50 mg daily dose for 4 of every 6 weeks or continuous daily dosing with a lower daily dose (37.5 mg) [66].

Regorafenib is the third-line targeted therapy of choice for imatinib and sunitinib-refractory GISTs (30,31). Regorafenib was proven to significantly prolong PFS at the dose of 160 mg daily for 3 of every 4 weeks compared to placebo in patients (4.8 vs. 0.9 months) [67].

Limited data are available on the efficacy of other TKIs (i.e. sorafenib, dasatinib, motesanib, nilotinib, vatalanib, ponatinib and the experimental agent linsitinib) for imatinib and sunitinib-refractory GISTs. Patients with metastatic GIST should be considered for participation in clinical trials on new therapies or combinations. For patients who are refractory to multiple TKIs including imatinib and sunitinib, imatinib rechallenge is a preferred strategy to discontinuing a TKI altogether [68].

Response assessment

Traditional tumor response criteria such as Response Evaluation Criteria in Solid Tumors (RECIST) are based on unidimensional tumor size and do not take into account changes in tumor metabolism and density and decrease in the number of intratumoral vessels [69]. Radiographic response of GIST to TKIs is often indicated by an early decrease in tumor density, followed by slow tumor regression. This pattern of response is not well suited to the use of standard RECIST [70]. Likewise, disease progression in patients with GIST may also fail to be captured by standard RECIST. Tumor progression may manifest as new or enlarging tumor masses, as partial to complete filling in of previously hypodense lesions or as a hyperdense 'nodule-within-a-mass' patterns [71].

An alternative set of response evaluation criteria has been proposed by Choi and colleagues and these criteria use both tumor density and size to assess the response of GIST to TKI therapy (Table 26.4) [72]. These criteria correlate

Table 26.4 Modified CT response evaluation criteria

Response	Definition
CR	Disappearance of all lesions
	No new lesions
PR	A decrease in size[a] of ≥10% or a decrease in tumor density (HU) of ≥15% on CT
	No new lesions
	No obvious progression of non-measurable disease
SD	Does not meet the criteria for CR, PR or PD
	No symptomatic deterioration attributed to tumor progression
PD	An increase in tumor size of ≥10% and does not meet criteria of PR by tumor density (HU) on CT
	New lesions
	New intratumoral nodules or increase in the size of the existing intratumoral nodules

Source: Adapted from Choi H, et al., *J Clin Oncol* 2007;25(13):1753–9.
Note: CR, complete response; PR, partial response; HU, Hounsfield unit; SD, stable disease; PD, progression of disease.
[a] The sum of the longest diameters of target lesions as defined in RECIST.

much better with PET scan findings and are a better predictor of response to imatinib than RECIST.

An FDG-PET scan has proved to be highly sensitive in early assessment of tumor response and may be useful in cases where there is doubt, or when early prediction of the response is particularly useful (e.g. preoperative cytoreductive treatment) [73].

POSTOPERATIVE SURVEILLANCE

The median time to tumor recurrence ranges from 18 to 25 months in patients who have undergone surgical resection, and the most common sites for disease recurrence are the liver and peritoneum. Although there is no evidence that earlier detection of recurrent GIST improves survival, the consensus statements advocate intense surveillance during this period. Imatinib therapy may suspend tumor progression in most patients. Abdominal CT is an excellent imaging modality to monitor disease during the course of treatment and surveillance after surgery.

There are no evidence-based guidelines to indicate the optimal follow-up for surgically treated patients with localized GIST. The NCCN guidelines recommend CT scans should be obtained every 3 to 6 months for 3 to 5 years, then annually afterward for a completely resected tumor, while every 3 to 6 months for patients with residual tumor after resection (R2 resection) and receiving imatinib [48]. The guidelines from ESMO emphasize the value of risk assessment in choosing a routine follow-up policy [31]. For patients with low or very low-risk GISTs, less frequent surveillance with intervals of 6 to 12 months may be appropriate [31,48].

SUMMARY

In 2001, Joensuu and colleagues published their first experience with imatinib mesylate to treat metastatic GIST in a single patient who exhibited dramatic tumor regression [74]. Since then, numerous clinical trials have formally assessed the efficacy of imatinib in metastatic GIST, and they have reported approximately an 80% response rate, compared with a dismal 5% response to conventional chemotherapy. Imatinib mesylate has truly revolutionized the treatment of GIST. The treatment of GIST has evolved rapidly, and dramatic changes in clinical practice have been observed during the last decade. Nonetheless, treating GIST with a single agent alone carries many limitations, as resistance to imatinib has become a significant clinical problem.

Surgical resection still remains the only chance for a cure in GIST treatment. A key strategy for prolonging the survival of patients with GIST is to improve the outcome of surgery, and imatinib use in the management of GISTs may aid in attaining this objective successfully. It is clear that GIST is a complex disease. A multidisciplinary approach with close collaboration between the medical oncologist, the gastroenterologist, the radiologist and the surgeon is essential to optimize prognosis.

Some issues still require clarification; notably, the ideal duration of adjuvant imatinib after surgery is still unclear. It is difficult of determine the exact place of surgery in metastatic or recurrent GIST patients. It is also unclear whether surgery makes any difference to outcomes in patients with metastatic GIST. Future and ongoing studies will further delineate the feasibility of multimodal treatment for this disease.

REFERENCES

1. DeMatteo RP, Lewis JJ, Leung D, Mudan SS, Woodruff JM, Brennan MF. Two hundred gastrointestinal stromal tumors: recurrence patterns and prognostic factors for survival. *Annals of Surgery* 2000;231(1):51–8.
2. Sturgeon C, Chejfec G, Espat NJ. Gastrointestinal stromal tumors: a spectrum of disease. *Surgical Oncology* 2003;12(1):21–6.
3. Hirota S, Isozaki K, Moriyama Y, Hashimoto K, Nishida T, Ishiguro S, et al. Gain-of-function mutations of c-kit in human gastrointestinal stromal tumors. *Science* 1998;279(5350):577–80.
4. Heinrich MC, Corless CL, Duensing A, McGreevey L, Chen CJ, Joseph N, et al. PDGFRA activating mutations in gastrointestinal stromal tumors. *Science* 2003;299(5607):708–10.
5. Nilsson B, Bumming P, Meis-Kindblom JM, Oden A, Dortok A, Gustavsson B, et al. Gastrointestinal stromal tumors: the incidence, prevalence, clinical course, and prognostication in the preimatinib mesylate era – a population-based study in western Sweden. *Cancer* 2005;103(4):821–9.
6. Tran T, Davila JA, El-Serag HB. The epidemiology of malignant gastrointestinal stromal tumors: an analysis of 1,458 cases from 1992 to 2000. *American Journal of Gastroenterology* 2005;100(1):162–8.
7. Tryggvason G, Gislason HG, Magnusson MK, Jonasson JG. Gastrointestinal stromal tumors in Iceland, 1990–2003: the Icelandic GIST study, a population-based incidence and pathologic risk stratification study. *International Journal of Cancer* 2005;117(2):289–93.
8. Goettsch WG, Bos SD, Breekveldt-Postma N, Casparie M, Herings RM, Hogendoorn PC. Incidence of gastrointestinal stromal tumours is underestimated: results of a nation-wide study. *European Journal of Cancer* 2005;41(18):2868–72.
9. Tzen CY, Wang JH, Huang YJ, Wang MN, Lin PC, Lai GL, et al. Incidence of gastrointestinal stromal tumor: a retrospective study based on immunohistochemical and mutational analyses. *Digestive Diseases and Sciences* 2007;52(3):792–7.
10. Nishida T, Hirota S, Taniguchi M, Hashimoto K, Isozaki K, Nakamura H, et al. Familial gastrointestinal stromal tumours with germline mutation of the KIT gene. *Nature Genetics* 1998;19(4):323–4.

11. Chompret A, Kannengiesser C, Barrois M, Terrier P, Dahan P, Tursz T, et al. PDGFRA germline mutation in a family with multiple cases of gastrointestinal stromal tumor. *Gastroenterology* 2004;126(1):318–21.

12. Maeyama H, Hidaka E, Ota H, Minami S, Kajiyama M, Kuraishi A, et al. Familial gastrointestinal stromal tumor with hyperpigmentation: association with a germline mutation of the c-kit gene. *Gastroenterology* 2001;120(1):210–5.

13. Pappo AS, Janeway K, Laquaglia M, Kim SY. Special considerations in pediatric gastrointestinal tumors. *Journal of Surgical Oncology* 2011;104(8):928–32.

14. Janeway KA, Liegl B, Harlow A, Le C, Perez-Atayde A, Kozakewich H, et al. Pediatric KIT wild-type and platelet-derived growth factor receptor alpha-wild-type gastrointestinal stromal tumors share KIT activation but not mechanisms of genetic progression with adult gastrointestinal stromal tumors. *Cancer Research* 2007;67(19):9084–8.

15. Hatch GF 3rd, Wertheimer-Hatch L, Hatch KF, Davis GB, Blanchard DK, Foster RS Jr, et al. Tumors of the esophagus. *World Journal of Surgery* 2000;24(4):401–11.

16. Blanchard DK, Budde JM, Hatch GF 3rd, Wertheimer-Hatch L, Hatch KF, Davis GB, et al. Tumors of the small intestine. *World Journal of Surgery* 2000;24(4):421–9.

17. Liegl B, Hornick JL, Lazar AJ. Contemporary pathology of gastrointestinal stromal tumors. *Hematology/Oncology Clinics of North America* 2009;23(1):49–68, vii–viii.

18. Graadt van Roggen JF, van Velthuysen ML, Hogendoorn PC. The histopathological differential diagnosis of gastrointestinal stromal tumours. *Journal of Clinical Pathology* 2001;54(2):96–102.

19. Burkill GJ, Badran M, Al-Muderis O, Meirion Thomas J, Judson IR, Fisher C, et al. Malignant gastrointestinal stromal tumor: distribution, imaging features, and pattern of metastatic spread. *Radiology* 2003;226(2):527–32.

20. Demetri GD, von Mehren M, Antonescu CR, DeMatteo RP, Ganjoo KN, Maki RG, et al. NCCN Task Force report: update on the management of patients with gastrointestinal stromal tumors. *Journal of the National Comprehensive Cancer Network* 2010;8(Suppl. 2):S1–41; quiz S2–4.

21. Sepe PS, Moparty B, Pitman MB, Saltzman JR, Brugge WR. EUS-guided FNA for the diagnosis of GI stromal cell tumors: sensitivity and cytologic yield. *Gastrointestinal Endoscopy* 2009;70(2):254–61.

22. Fletcher CD, Berman JJ, Corless C, Gorstein F, Lasota J, Longley BJ, et al. Diagnosis of gastrointestinal stromal tumors: a consensus approach. *Human Pathology* 2002;33(5):459–65.

23. Parfitt JR, Streutker CJ, Riddell RH, Driman DK. Gastrointestinal stromal tumors: a contemporary review. *Pathology, Research and Practice* 2006;202(12):837–47.

24. Novelli M, Rossi S, Rodriguez-Justo M, Taniere P, Seddon B, Toffolatti L, et al. DOG1 and CD117 are the antibodies of choice in the diagnosis of gastrointestinal stromal tumours. *Histopathology* 2010;57(2):259–70.

25. Miettinen M, Wang ZF, Lasota J. DOG1 antibody in the differential diagnosis of gastrointestinal stromal tumors: a study of 1840 cases. *American Journal of Surgical Pathology* 2009;33(9):1401–8.

26. Corless CL, Schroeder A, Griffith D, Town A, McGreevey L, Harrell P, et al. PDGFRA mutations in gastrointestinal stromal tumors: frequency, spectrum and in vitro sensitivity to imatinib. *Journal of Clinical Oncology* 2005;23(23):5357–64.

27. Medeiros F, Corless CL, Duensing A, Hornick JL, Oliveira AM, Heinrich MC, et al. KIT-negative gastrointestinal stromal tumors: proof of concept and therapeutic implications. *American Journal of Surgical Pathology* 2004;28(7):889–94.

28. Tzen CY, Mau BL. Analysis of CD117-negative gastrointestinal stromal tumors. *World Journal of Gastroenterology* 2005;11(7):1052–5.

29. Janeway KA, Kim SY, Lodish M, Nose V, Rustin P, Gaal J, et al. Defects in succinate dehydrogenase in gastrointestinal stromal tumors lacking KIT and PDGFRA mutations. *Proceedings of the National Academy of Sciences of the United States of America* 2011;108(1):314–8.

30. von Mehren M, Randall RL, Benjamin RS, Boles S, Bui MM, Casper ES, et al. Gastrointestinal stromal tumors, version 2.2014. *Journal of the National Comprehensive Cancer Network* 2014;12(6):853–62.

31. Group TEESNW. Gastrointestinal stromal tumours: ESMO clinical practice guidelines for diagnosis, treatment and follow-up. *Annals of Oncology* 2014;25(Suppl. 3):iii21–6.

32. Miettinen M, Lasota J. Gastrointestinal stromal tumors: pathology and prognosis at different sites. *Seminars in Diagnostic Pathology* 2006;23(2):70–83.

33. Joensuu H. Risk stratification of patients diagnosed with gastrointestinal stromal tumor. *Human Pathology* 2008;39(10):1411–9.

34. Gold JS, Gonen M, Gutierrez A, Broto JM, Garcia-del-Muro X, Smyrk TC, et al. Development and validation of a prognostic nomogram for recurrence-free survival after complete surgical resection of localised primary gastrointestinal stromal tumour: a retrospective analysis. *Lancet Oncology* 2009;10(11):1045–52.

35. Joensuu H, Vehtari A, Riihimaki J, Nishida T, Steigen SE, Brabec P, et al. Risk of recurrence of gastrointestinal stromal tumour after surgery: an analysis of pooled population-based cohorts. *Lancet Oncology* 2012;13(3):265–74.

36. Edge S, Byrd D, Compton C, Fritz A, Greene F, Trotti A, American Joint Committee on Cancer. *AJCC Cancer Staging Manual*, 7th ed. New York: Springer, 2010.

37. Antonescu CR, Sommer G, Sarran L, Tschernyavsky SJ, Riedel E, Woodruff JM, et al. Association of KIT exon 9 mutations with nongastric primary site and aggressive behavior: KIT mutation analysis and clinical correlates of 120 gastrointestinal stromal tumors. *Clinical Cancer Research* 2003;9(9):3329–37.

38. Blay JY, Bonvalot S, Casali P, Choi H, Debiec-Richter M, Dei Tos AP, et al. Consensus meeting for the management of gastrointestinal stromal tumors. Report of the GIST Consensus Conference of 20–21 March 2004, under the auspices of ESMO. *Annals of Oncology* 2005;16(4):566–78.

39. Otani Y, Furukawa T, Yoshida M, Saikawa Y, Wada N, Ueda M, et al. Operative indications for relatively small (2–5 cm) gastrointestinal stromal tumor of the stomach based on analysis of 60 operated cases. *Surgery* 2006;139(4):484–92.

40. Nishimura J, Nakajima K, Omori T, Takahashi T, Nishitani A, Ito T, et al. Surgical strategy for gastric gastrointestinal stromal tumors: laparoscopic vs. open resection. *Surgical Endoscopy* 2007;21(6):875–8.

41. Huguet KL, Rush RM Jr, Tessier DJ, Schlinkert RT, Hinder RA, Grinberg GG, et al. Laparoscopic gastric gastrointestinal stromal tumor resection: the Mayo Clinic experience. *Archives of Surgery* 2008;143(6):587–90; discussion 91.

42. Sasaki A, Koeda K, Obuchi T, Nakajima J, Nishizuka S, Terashima M, et al. Tailored laparoscopic resection for suspected gastric gastrointestinal stromal tumors. *Surgery* 2010;147(4):516–20.

43. Miettinen M, Lasota J. Gastrointestinal stromal tumors – definition, clinical, histological, immunohistochemical, and molecular genetic features and differential diagnosis. *Virchows Archiv* 2001;438(1):1–12.

44. Pierie JP, Choudry U, Muzikansky A, Yeap BY, Souba WW, Ott MJ. The effect of surgery and grade on outcome of gastrointestinal stromal tumors. *Archives of Surgery* 2001;136(4):383–9.

45. Langer C, Gunawan B, Schuler P, Huber W, Fuzesi L, Becker H. Prognostic factors influencing surgical management and outcome of gastrointestinal stromal tumours. *British Journal of Surgery* 2003;90(3):332–9.

46. Dematteo RP, Ballman KV, Antonescu CR, Maki RG, Pisters PW, Demetri GD, et al. Adjuvant imatinib mesylate after resection of localised, primary gastrointestinal stromal tumour: a randomised, double-blind, placebo-controlled trial. *Lancet* 2009;373(9669):1097–104.

47. Joensuu H, Eriksson M, Sundby Hall K, Hartmann JT, Pink D, Schutte J, et al. One vs three years of adjuvant imatinib for operable gastrointestinal stromal tumor: a randomized trial. *JAMA* 2012;307(12):1265–72.

48. von Mehren M, Benjamin RS, Bui MM, Casper ES, Conrad EU 3rd, DeLaney TF, et al. Soft tissue sarcoma, version 2.2012: featured updates to the NCCN guidelines. *Journal of the National Comprehensive Cancer Network* 2012;10(8):951–60.

49. Gastrointestinal Stromal Tumor Meta-Analysis Group (MetaGIST). Comparison of two doses of imatinib for the treatment of unresectable or metastatic gastrointestinal stromal tumors: a meta-analysis of 1,640 patients. *Journal of Clinical Oncology* 2010;28(7):1247–53.

50. Jakob J, Mussi C, Ronellenfitsch U, Wardelmann E, Negri T, Gronchi A, et al. Gastrointestinal stromal tumor of the rectum: results of surgical and multimodality therapy in the era of imatinib. *Annals of Surgical Oncology* 2013;20(2):586–92.

51. Crosby JA, Catton CN, Davis A, Couture J, O'Sullivan B, Kandel R, et al. Malignant gastrointestinal stromal tumors of the small intestine: a review of 50 cases from a prospective database. *Annals of Surgical Oncology* 2001;8(1):50–9.

52. Ng EH, Pollock RE, Munsell MF, Atkinson EN, Romsdahl MM. Prognostic factors influencing survival in gastrointestinal leiomyosarcomas. Implications for surgical management and staging. *Annals of Surgery* 1992;215(1):68–77.

53. Gold JS, van der Zwan SM, Gonen M, Maki RG, Singer S, Brennan MF, et al. Outcome of metastatic GIST in the era before tyrosine kinase inhibitors. *Annals of Surgical Oncology* 2007;14(1):134–42.

54. Mudan SS, Conlon KC, Woodruff JM, Lewis JJ, Brennan MF. Salvage surgery for patients with recurrent gastrointestinal sarcoma: prognostic factors to guide patient selection. *Cancer* 2000;88(1):66–74.

55. Demetri GD, von Mehren M, Blanke CD, Van den Abbeele AD, Eisenberg B, Roberts PJ, et al. Efficacy and safety of imatinib mesylate in advanced gastrointestinal stromal tumors. *New England Journal of Medicine* 2002;347(7):472–80.

56. Verweij J, Casali PG, Zalcberg J, LeCesne A, Reichardt P, Blay JY, et al. Progression-free survival in gastrointestinal stromal tumours with high-dose imatinib: randomised trial. *Lancet* 2004;364(9440):1127–34.

57. Blanke CD, Demetri GD, von Mehren M, Heinrich MC, Eisenberg B, Fletcher JA, et al. Long-term results from a randomized phase II trial of standard- versus higher-dose imatinib mesylate for

patients with unresectable or metastatic gastrointestinal stromal tumors expressing KIT. *Journal of Clinical Oncology* 2008;26(4):620–5.

58. Heinrich MC, Maki RG, Corless CL, Antonescu CR, Harlow A, Griffith D, et al. Primary and secondary kinase genotypes correlate with the biological and clinical activity of sunitinib in imatinib-resistant gastrointestinal stromal tumor. *Journal of Clinical Oncology* 2008;26(33):5352–9.

59. Antonescu CR, Besmer P, Guo T, Arkun K, Hom G, Koryotowski B, et al. Acquired resistance to imatinib in gastrointestinal stromal tumor occurs through secondary gene mutation. *Clinical Cancer Research* 2005;11(11):4182–90.

60. Chen LL, Trent JC, Wu EF, Fuller GN, Ramdas L, Zhang W, et al. A missense mutation in KIT kinase domain 1 correlates with imatinib resistance in gastrointestinal stromal tumors. *Cancer Research* 2004;64(17):5913–9.

61. Raut CP, Posner M, Desai J, Morgan JA, George S, Zahrieh D, et al. Surgical management of advanced gastrointestinal stromal tumors after treatment with targeted systemic therapy using kinase inhibitors. *Journal of Clinical Oncology* 2006;24(15):2325–31.

62. DeMatteo RP, Maki RG, Singer S, Gonen M, Brennan MF, Antonescu CR. Results of tyrosine kinase inhibitor therapy followed by surgical resection for metastatic gastrointestinal stromal tumor. *Annals of Surgery* 2007;245(3):347–52.

63. Blay JY, Le Cesne A, Ray-Coquard I, Bui B, Duffaud F, Delbaldo C, et al. Prospective multicentric randomized phase III study of imatinib in patients with advanced gastrointestinal stromal tumors comparing interruption versus continuation of treatment beyond 1 year: the French Sarcoma Group. *Journal of Clinical Oncology* 2007;25(9):1107–13.

64. Demetri GD, van Oosterom AT, Garrett CR, Blackstein ME, Shah MH, Verweij J, et al. Efficacy and safety of sunitinib in patients with advanced gastrointestinal stromal tumour after failure of imatinib: a randomised controlled trial. *Lancet* 2006;368(9544):1329–38.

65. Demetri GD, Garrett CR, Schoffski P, Shah MH, Verweij J, Leyvraz S, et al. Complete longitudinal analyses of the randomized, placebo-controlled, phase III trial of sunitinib in patients with gastrointestinal stromal tumor following imatinib failure. *Clinical Cancer Research* 2012;18(11):3170–9.

66. George S, Blay JY, Casali PG, Le Cesne A, Stephenson P, Deprimo SE, et al. Clinical evaluation of continuous daily dosing of sunitinib malate in patients with advanced gastrointestinal stromal tumour after imatinib failure. *European Journal of Cancer* 2009;45(11):1959–68.

67. Demetri GD, Reichardt P, Kang YK, Blay JY, Rutkowski P, Gelderblom H, et al. Efficacy and safety of regorafenib for advanced gastrointestinal stromal tumours after failure of imatinib and sunitinib (GRID): an international, multicentre, randomised, placebo-controlled, phase 3 trial. *Lancet* 2013;381(9863):295–302.

68. Kang YK, Ryu MH, Yoo C, Ryoo BY, Kim HJ, Lee JJ, et al. Resumption of imatinib to control metastatic or unresectable gastrointestinal stromal tumours after failure of imatinib and sunitinib (RIGHT): a randomised, placebo-controlled, phase 3 trial. *Lancet Oncology* 2013;14(12):1175–82.

69. Eisenhauer EA, Therasse P, Bogaerts J, Schwartz LH, Sargent D, Ford R, et al. New response evaluation criteria in solid tumours: revised RECIST guideline (version 1.1). *European Journal of Cancer* 2009;45(2):228–47.

70. Benjamin RS, Choi H, Macapinlac HA, Burgess MA, Patel SR, Chen LL, et al. We should desist using RECIST, at least in GIST. *Journal of Clinical Oncology* 2007;25(13):1760–4.

71. Shankar S, vanSonnenberg E, Desai J, Dipiro PJ, Van Den Abbeele A, Demetri GD. Gastrointestinal stromal tumor: new nodule-within-a-mass pattern of recurrence after partial response to imatinib mesylate. *Radiology* 2005;235(3):892–8.

72. Choi H, Charnsangavej C, Faria SC, Macapinlac HA, Burgess MA, Patel SR, et al. Correlation of computed tomography and positron emission tomography in patients with metastatic gastrointestinal stromal tumor treated at a single institution with imatinib mesylate: proposal of new computed tomography response criteria. *Journal of Clinical Oncology* 2007;25(13):1753–9.

73. Van den Abbeele AD. The lessons of GIST – PET and PET/CT: a new paradigm for imaging. *Oncologist* 2008;13(Suppl. 2):8–13.

74. Joensuu H, Roberts PJ, Sarlomo-Rikala M, Andersson LC, Tervahartiala P, Tuveson D, et al. Effect of the tyrosine kinase inhibitor STI571 in a patient with a metastatic gastrointestinal stromal tumor. *New England Journal of Medicine* 2001;344(14):1052–6.

27

Small bowel and appendiceal tumors

SARAH T O'DWYER

INTRODUCTION

Despite accounting for 90% of the surface area of the gastrointestinal tract (GIT) tumors of the small bowel are rare, contributing in the order of 3% of all GIT neoplasms. True benign tumors including hamartomas and hyperplastic and inflammatory polyps account for approximately 20% of lesions; tumors with malignant potential such as low adenomatous polyps, gastrointestinal stromal tumors (GISTs) and non-invasive neuroendocrine (NEN) tumors (carcinoids) amount to 30% of the total, leaving 50% of small bowel tumors which are considered malignant at presentation. In the past, patients were rarely diagnosed preoperatively, but advances in imaging techniques have opened up opportunities for less invasive and more accurate diagnosis and staging. Taken alongside better organized specialist centres offering multimodality treatment, a more optimistic outcome for patients with small bowel and appendiceal tumors is now expected. In 2012 the European Neuroendocrine Tumor Society (ENETS) reported consensus guidelines for NEN neoplasms from the jejuno-ileum and the appendix [1]. In 2015 a consensus relating to the pathological classification of epithelial appendiceal neoplasms rationalized reporting of these tumors [2].

EPIDEMIOLOGY

Due to the rarity of these tumors very few large series have been reported with only one series reporting on greater than 100 patients [3–13] (Table 27.1). Cancer registers in the UK and US are a valuable source of information particularly for less common cancers. Interrogation of the US Surveillance, Epidemiology and End Results (SEER) database compiled from 11 tumor registries has revealed incidence rates for the most common major histological types of small bowel cancers. Over an 18-year registry the average annual incidence of small bowel cancer was almost 10 per million population with malignant carcinoid and adenocarcinomas of almost equal incidence of 3.8 and 3.7 per million, respectively [14]. Sarcomas and lymphomas occurred in 1.3 and 1.1 per million, respectively, and while the incidence of sarcoma remained static over the study period, the number of carcinoids and lymphomas slowly increased, the increase in lymphomas being more prominent. For all four histological subtypes rates were higher in men than women and over 90% of cases occurred in patients more than 40 years of age.

Similar UK incidence rates for small bowel cancers are documented as 12 per million population with a slightly higher rate in males of 14 versus 11 in females per million [15]. Valuable data have also been generated from the British Society of Gastroenterology (BSG) register of 395 small bowel tumors reported in 2003 [16]. The registry was compiled over 2 years (1998–2000) and identified adenocarcinoma in 44% of the cohort, lymphomas in 27% and carcinoid tumors in 20%. Evaluation of the other reported larger series from US, Europe and Australia demonstrates similar patterns of incidence by histological type [3–5,10]. Adenocarcinomas tend to be located more proximally in the duodenum and jejunum, NEN tumors or carcinoids in the ileum and appendix, and lymphomas evenly distributed throughout the small bowel.

Table 27.1 Published series of small bowel tumors: 1996–2005

Authors	Year	Number of cases	Length of series (year)
Cunningham et al. [3]	1997	73	21
Minardi et al. [4]	1998	89	10
Brucher et al. [5]	1998	71	—
Rodriguez et al. [6]	1998	42	—
O'Boyle et al. [7]	1998	25	10
Bozdag et al. [8]	2003	15	10
Torres-Maria et al. [9]	2003	13	2
Rangiah et al. [10]	2004	166	10
Mussi et al. [11]	2005	45	20
Catena et al. [12]	2005	34	10

Table 27.2 Risk factors for small bowel tumors

Family history	Immunological	Treatment related
FAP	Crohn's	Postradiotherapy
HNPCC	Celiac	Ileal conduits
Carcinoids	HIV/AIDS transplant recipients	

Note: FAP, familial adenomatous polyposis; HNPCC, hereditary non-polyposis colon cancer.

RISK FACTORS

The different histological types of small bowel malignancies are associated with individual predisposing conditions that increase the risk for an individual of developing a tumor (Table 27.2). The most recognized group are patients with celiac disease who have a greater incidence of both small bowel lymphoma and adenocarcinoma, and it is thought that treatment of the underlying condition seems to decrease their risk [15,16]. Adenocarcinomas are also associated with the gastrointestinal polyposis syndromes (familial polyposis) and hereditary non-polyposis colon cancer (HNPCC) families. Assessment of tumor incidence from an HNPCC registry revealed 42 individuals from 40 families who developed 42 primary and 7 metachronous small bowel tumors [17]. It is notable that the small bowel rather than the colon was the first site of carcinoma in 57% of cases and that in polyposis families the small bowel tumors presented at an earlier age (49 years) than those occurring in the general population (~60 years).

Genetic predisposition is also associated with neurofibromatosis and carcinoid tumors. Analysis of the Swedish family cancer database revealed that a history of carcinoids in first-degree relatives is associated with a relative risk of 3.6 over the population at large [18]. Furthermore, small bowel NEN tumors are more common in men and appendiceal NEN tumors are more common in women. Additional risk is dependent on chronic inflammatory bowel disease, particularly Crohn's disease and nodular lymphoid

hyperplasia, but is also recognized in patients with ileal conduits for urinary diversion. Immunodeficiency syndromes (e.g. HIV/AIDS), transplant recipients and previous radical abdominal radiotherapy also predispose to the generation of small bowel malignancies of varying histological types [19]. Awareness of these at-risk groups should generate enhanced vigilance and alert health care workers to the need for more intensive investigation of non-specific gastrointestinal symptoms.

SMALL BOWEL TUMORS

Clinical presentation, investigations and diagnosis

Small bowel neoplasms are notorious for their insidious presentation, vague symptoms and lack of physical signs which leads to a significant delay in reaching a definitive diagnosis. In a number of series the duration of symptoms is greater than 6 months. Abdominal pain, nausea and vomiting are the most common symptoms with anaemia and GI hemorrhage occurring in more benign tumors and obstruction in more malignant variants [12]. Emergency presentations include bleeding, commonly in GISTs, perforation in lymphomas, obstruction in adenocarcinomas and carcinoids, and intussusception in melanoma [10,12]. Earlier series note the few cases that have been satisfactorily diagnosed prior to surgery (~20%) [3], while more recently in a series of 166 cases a preoperative diagnosis was made in 77% [10].

Improved imaging using multi-thin-slice computed tomography (CT) scanning of the abdomen allows better definition of the small bowel, allowing evaluation of extrinsic and intrinsic disease (Figure 27.1). The use of CT has now superseded the need for standard contrast and fluoroscopic evaluation of the small bowel with CT enterography enhancing the appearance of mucosal and intramural lesions [20]. In the search for a primary tumor, cross-sectional imaging

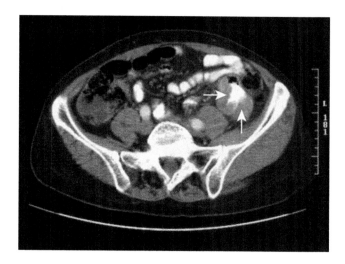

Figure 27.1 Arrows indicate soft tissue shadow adherent to small bowel causing partial obstruction in a patient previously diagnosed with malignant melanoma.

with CT or MRI is now recommended [1]. Additional value is obtained in staging the malignant tumors and assisting in planning treatment pathways that may include neoadjuvant treatments in adenocarcinoma and NEN tumors, and avoid unnecessary surgery in lymphoma. Improved planning allows decisions directed toward curative or palliative surgical approaches where appropriate. Functional techniques including positron emission tomography (PET) scanning can also assist in defining the extent of disease in adenocarcinoma and NEN staging should include somatostatin receptor imaging, ideally in combination with SPECT/CT. Gallium DOTATOC-PET is proving useful in defining the extent of metastases in NEN tumors. In more localized disease standard endoscopy, small bowel enteroscopy and wireless capsule enteroscopy have been successfully employed to achieve a diagnosis and may prove worthwhile in surveillance of polyposis syndromes and hopefully assist in early identification of progression to more aggressive disease [21,22].

Definitive diagnosis will usually require tissue sampling with adenocarcinomas being defined by differentiation, lymphatic and venous invasion. NEN tumors should be graded using mitoses and Ki-67, and secretory functional evidence may be useful to allow systemic treatment to be initiated. Serum chromogranin A and urinary hydroxyindoleacetic acid assessment (HIAA) alongside positive scanning is often diagnostic, although histological assessment remains the gold standard [1,26]. Elevation of circulating tumor markers including carcinoembryonic antigen (CEA) and CA 19-9 provides supporting evidence for adenocarcinomas, but surgical resection of the primary is usually undertaken unless there is obvious metastatic disease that lends itself to radiologically guided biopsy. Laparoscopy has its place, particularly where there is evidence of peritoneal involvement allowing more accurate staging than CT in these circumstances, with the added advantage of multiple-site biopsies to assist in planning treatment extent. There remain questions regarding port site implantation particularly for mucinous tumors, and if open surgery is contemplated at a later date during treatment excision of port site scars may be advisable (see the 'Appendiceal Tumors' section).

DEFINITIVE TREATMENT

For the majority of small bowel tumors surgical excision offers the best chance of cure, the notable exception being multifocal lymphoma which is best treated with minimal surgery and systemic chemotherapy. Benign lesions are usually easily resectable with minimal morbidity, while malignant tumors may be locally advanced rendering them unresectable or metastatic to lymph nodes, liver, peritoneum and occasionally extra-abdominal sites. Curative surgery is always recommended whenever feasible. Surgery of the primary should be performed as segmental resection with wide lymphadenectomy. In the case of lymph node involvement around the superior mesenteric artery, high lymph node dissection is recommended. In cases with severe desmoplastic reaction around the artery, radical tumor resection may not

be possible. Cholecystectomy may be performed during the initial session to prevent or treat cholelithiasis, which may in the case of later treatment cause cholecystitis, choledocholithiasis or cholangitis; the benefit of cholecystectomy has, however, never been prospectively proven. Overall at preoperative radiological staging extra gastrointestinal metastatic disease is present in around 45% of cases [10], and although in most reported series the majority of primary tumors are resectable (> 80%), curative resection is achieved in less than 65% of patients. Furthermore, where resection had been considered curative, recurrence occurred in 42% at a median time of 17 months [3]. Occasionally synchronous primary tumors occur of either similar or distinct histological types (e.g. adenocarcinomas and NEN) when multiple resections are appropriate, but more commonly multiple tumors reflect metastatic serosal deposits from a single primary. Careful histological and immunohistochemical evaluation using cytokeratin and neuronal and mesenchymal markers is often necessary to accurately define tumor types which will in turn guide the team in considering appropriate non-surgical adjuvant therapies.

The surgical management of metastatic disease is largely confined to liver lesions that may be suitable for resection, embolization or ablative treatment. Such an approach may be aimed at cure but even if palliative, these interventions can assist in decreasing tumor burden prior to the use of systemic therapy. Palliative procedures including the positioning of intraluminal stents can successfully allow relief of proximal small bowel obstruction and restoration of intestinal function [23]. Surgical by-pass procedures and limited resections for serosal deposits leading to obstruction or intussusception may be necessary but, where there is evidence of diffuse multifocal peritoneal disease, particularly if there is evidence of signet cell infiltration, surgery should be avoided and good supportive care employed (Figure 27.2). The insertion of a drainage gastrostomy may be a useful palliative manoeuvre to assist in keeping a terminal patient more comfortable.

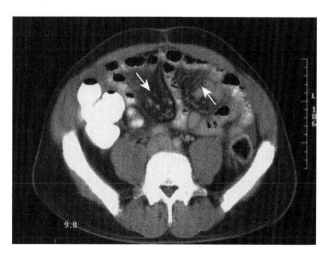

Figure 27.2 Multifocal intraperitoneal disease involving the serosa of the small bowel with tethering of bowel loops.

ADJUVANT TREATMENTS

Following surgery patients should be discussed by a multidisciplinary team and specialist advice sought for these rare tumors. While there is little place for radiotherapy except in the targeted palliation of pain, systemic therapies are now coming to the fore as neoadjuvant, adjuvant and supportive treatments. Examples of good response rates include the use of adjuvant immunotherapy in c-KIT positive GISTs [24] and downstaging tumors rendering resectability [25]. c-KIT negative sarcomas, however, have a less than 15% response rate to adjuvant treatment; hence an aggressive surgical approach with resection of multifocal disease is advised where possible [26] (Figure 27.3). After curative surgery for NEN tumors of the jejuno-ileum, there is no indication for specific medical treatment and there is no proven role for neoadjuvant or adjuvant medical treatment. The use of perioperative somatostatin analogues where there is definite metastatic disease is recommended to protect against haemodynamic fluctuation. Long-acting agents are employed in managing non-resectable metastases [27].

Outcome

In 2002 the number of deaths from small bowel cancer in the UK was recorded as 5 per million [14]. Taking the annual incidence as 12 per million the overall prognosis remains poor. Reported series are inevitably hindered by the length of time needed to acquire adequate numbers from which meaningful conclusions can be drawn. Furthermore, new and current treatments that may influence response rates and survival will not be reflected in such figures. The most accurate evaluation of overall survival in current practice emanates from the BSG registry that reported survival at 30 months as 78% for NEN tumors, 58% for adenocarcinoma and 45% for lymphoma [15]. Unfortunately, because of the rarity of these tumors and the indolent and diverse mode of presentation, patients may be treated by non-specialist groups. Improved organization of cancer services should lead to earlier referral to specialist units and allow improved access to appropriate treatment and entry into clinical trials.

APPENDICEAL TUMORS

The past two decades have seen a major shift in our knowledge and understanding regarding the origin and treatments for appendiceal tumors. While the most common tumor arising at this site is the NEN tumor, the majority of which are diagnosed incidentally and do not metastasize, epithelial adenomatous tumors are now known to be more pervasive, associated with the development of diffuse peritoneal neoplasia. When the tumor is mucinous in nature the features are best described as pseudomyxoma peritonei (PMP). The incidence of epithelial tumors that go on to generate the PMP syndrome is estimated as 1–2 per million of the population.

Epidemiology

Tumors of the appendix are rare accounting for 0.5% of GIT tumors. The principal tumor types are NEN tumors, adenomas and adenocarcinomas, and rarer pathologies include GISTs, mesenchymal tumors, metastatic carcinomas of colorectal origin and rarely melanomas. On analysis of appendicectomy specimens, removed largely for the presentation of appendicitis, <1% are found to have tumors and only one-tenth of these are primary malignant tumors [28]. Overall, 30–55% of tumors prove to be NEN tumors, 15% adenomas, 10% primary adenocarcinomas and 15% secondary malignancy, half of which were adenocarcinomas in patients with colorectal cancer. It is notable that in patients with appendiceal tumors of all histological types there is a high incidence of synchronous and metachronous colorectal cancer: NEN tumors 10%, adenomas 33% and secondary malignancy 55% [29]. Further support for an association between epithelial appendiceal tumors and colorectal cancer is provided from an observation of a 5% incidence of such tumors in appendices removed electively in patients undergoing rectal and colonic cancer surgery [30].

Clinical presentation, investigation and diagnosis

For most patients an appendiceal tumor is diagnosed following removal for incidental appendicitis. At operation the appendix may appear swollen and bulbous (Figure 27.3), but the majority of tumors are diagnosed coincidentally by the histopathologist. If extra-appendiceal mucus or other peritoneal disease is noted at operation this must be considered when planning further treatment (see the 'Outcome' section). NEN tumors are generally indolent and rarely perforate or metastasize, although the risk of progression increases with increasing size above 2 cm and with adenocarcinoid cellular differentiation [27]. Appendiceal NEN tumors are often diagnosed at an early age: 15–19 years in females and 20–29 years in males, and family history in

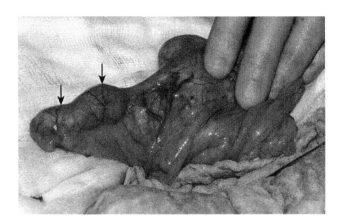

Figure 27.3 Macroscopic appearance of a distended swollen appendix containing tumor confined to the lumen.

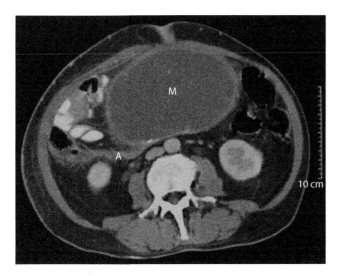

Figure 27.4 Appendix (A) with an extramural mucocele (M) following perforation. Classical appearance of very early localized pseudomyxoma peritonei.

Epithelial tumors and pseudomyxoma peritonei

In 2000 the pioneering work of Professor Sugarbaker from Washington, DC, was explored in a conference at the Royal College of Surgeons, London. At that time few surgeons and oncologists understood the pathophysiology of PMP and many patients were erroneously treated: women commonly for ovarian cancer and men misdiagnosed as gastric cancer or unknown GIT primaries. Although it is true that some mucin-producing tumors will mimic a PMP picture and produce a PMP syndrome (characterized by abundant production of mucinous ascites, gross abdominal distension, loss of peripheral lean body mass secondary to limited nutritional intake and GIT compression), it is now accepted that true PMP develops secondary to an epithelial adenomatous tumor of the appendix [34]. The spectrum of disease ranges from abundant production of mucin with very scant epithelial cell proliferation (diffuse peritoneal adenomucinosis) through peritoneal mucinous carcinoma of intermediate or discordant type (PMCA I/D) to peritoneal mucinous carcinomatosis (PMCA). Recent consensus has led to the publication and agreement of pathological description of appendiceal epithelial neoplasia [2]. The unique feature of PMP is the ability to develop surface peritoneal implants without progressing to intra-organal or lymph node metastases. Recent evaluation of adhesion molecules in PMP and colorectal cancer has demonstrated a distinct profile that may explain the pattern of disease and offer potential for molecular targeting to prevent invasion [35].

first-degree relatives increases the risk threefold [17]. Rarely patients present with a full-blown secretory carcinoid syndrome due to the systemic effects of 5-hydroxytryptamine (5HT): flushing, fever, diarrhoea, bronchospasm and cardiac dysfunction. Perforation of the appendix does occur with epithelial mucinous tumors and adenocarcinomas, both of which tend to reseal having disseminated cells into the peritoneal cavity (Figure 27.4). Adenomatous lesions of the appendix tend to generate mucinous PMP, while peritoneal carcinomatosis will follow perforated adenocarcinoma and progress rapidly with signs of multifocal peritoneal involvement.

Neuroendocrine tumors

Patients with diagnosed NEN tumor should be investigated for 5HT secretion using urinary 5HIAA analysis and chromogranin A is a useful serum marker. A CT scan of the thorax, abdomen and pelvis is required as synchronous primaries and metastatic disease needs to be determined. The majority of appendiceal NEN tumors do not metastasize. Debate remains regarding long-term follow-up as there are recorded cases of presentation with metastatic liver disease >10 years following excision of the primary. Metastatic NEN tumors may be diagnosed following identification of liver lesions on CT scan or occult lesions may be found using radionucleotide scanning. Recently more aggressive surgical excision and ablation has been adopted for control of systemic symptoms and the use of adjuvant chemotherapy and pharmacological manipulation with somatostatin helps palliate the disease [27]. Goblet cell carcinoid tumors run a more aggressive course progressing with peritoneal deposits [31]. Surgical approaches using cytoreductive surgery and hyperthermic intra-peritoneal chemotherapy have been adopted in specialist centres [32,33].

Many patients with PMP present to non-specialist centres and are misdiagnosed as having ovarian pathology [36]. Some are treated with repeated laparotomies, debulking of the tumor or removal of the mucin, while others receive systemic chemotherapy with minimal response. In men incidental presentation of peritoneal nodules or mucin in a hernial sac while undergoing hernia repair is often the case [37]. It is now recognized that repeat laparotomy is unlikely to achieve cure and the recommended treatment is an attempt at complete cytoreduction and administration of heated intraoperative intraperitoneal chemotherapy [38]. In the UK there are two centres designated for the treatment of tumors of appendiceal origin: North Hampshire Hospital, Basingstoke, and the Christie Hospital, Manchester. This approach is supported by the UK National Institute for Health and Care Excellence (NICE) whose recommendations for PMP treatment in designated centres were published in 2004 [39]. The concentration of patients to these treatment centres has allowed the teams to gain experience in the radical approach of cytoreductive surgery and intra-peritoneal chemotherapy leading to good outcomes and long-term survival [40,41].

Investigations include CT scanning that often demonstrates classical features of disease in the right and left upper quadrants, porta hepatus, omentum, right iliac fossa and pouch of Douglas (Figure 27.5). Tumor markers

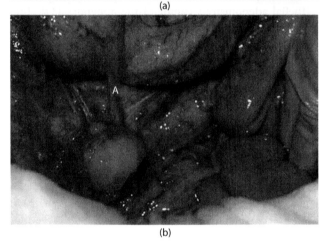

(a)

(b)

Figure 27.5 (a) Computed tomography (CT) scan demonstrating classical appearance of advanced pseudomyxoma peritonei: scalloping of liver (L) and involvement of spleen (S). (b) Large appendiceal mucocele (M) and appendix (A).

(CEA and CA 19-9) are helpful in determining disease activity, response to treatment and relapse during follow-up [42].

Unfortunately, some patients have severely advanced disease at presentation such that the more radical treatment cannot be offered. Palliative debulking has a place in these patients and systemic mitomycin and oral capecitabine have achieved tumor response and clinical benefit in one-third of 40 patients treated [43].

Outcome

The prognosis for patients diagnosed with tumors of the appendix is determined principally by the histological type but also by whether the disease is confined to the appendix. Low-grade NEN tumors are removed without long-term sequelae and overall appendicular NEN tumors have an 80–90% 5-year survival. For epithelial tumors the prognosis is dependent upon the ability to achieve

complete cytoreduction which is influenced by the histological variant and the distribution of the disease [44]. Debate continues regarding the need for right hemicolectomy for epithelial tumors confined to the appendix, but in the presence of peritoneal disease more extensive resection does not incur a survival advantage unless required for complete macroscopic cytoreduction [45]. The overall outlook for PMP patients is a 50–70% 5-year survival following cytoreduction and intraoperative chemotherapy [46]. The influence of histological type is also important as patients with intermediate or discordant features and PMCA do less well with 30% and 10% 3-year survival, respectively [47]. In all reported series the single most important factor that influences outcome is whether the surgeon can achieve complete macroscopic eradication of disease.

Advice regarding follow-up for patients with appendiceal tumors is difficult particularly when the tumor has been fully removed and confined to a non-perforated appendix. Unfortunately, there are reports of patients presenting with metastatic disease decades later; hence a healthy respect must be shown for early reinvestigation of occult symptoms in patients with a history of tumors of the appendix.

SUMMARY

Tumors of the small intestine and appendix are rare but can have devastating effects on individual patients as diagnosis is difficult and often delayed. The outcome for patients is influenced by their ability to access specialist teams that can offer multimodality treatment where appropriate. It is hoped that with increased knowledge and education about new treatment options patients will benefit from advances in both surgical and non-surgical treatments from designated specialist teams.

REFERENCES

1. Pape UF, Perren AF, Niederle BF, et al. ENETS Consensus Guidelines for the management of patients with neuroendocrine neoplasms from the jejuno-ileum and the appendix including goblet cell carcinomas. *Neuroendocrinology* 2012; 95: 135–56.
2. Carr N, Cecil T, Faheez M, et al. A consensus for classification and pathological reporting of pseudomyxoma peritonei and appendiceal neoplasia. *Am J Surg Pathol* 2015.
3. Cunningham JD, Aleali R, Aleali M, et al. Malignant small bowel neoplasms: histological determinants of recurrence and survival. *Ann Surg* 1997; 225: 300–6.
4. Minardi AJ Jr, Zibari GB, Aultman DF, et al. Small bowel tumours. *J Am Coll Surg* 1998; 186: 664–8.
5. Brucher BL, Roder JD, Fink U, et al. Prognostic factors in resected primary small bowel tumours. *Dig Surg* 1998; 15: 42–51.

6. Rodriguez BMA, Vasen HF, Lynch HT, et al. Characteristics of small bowel carcinoma in hereditary nonpolyposis colorectal carcinoma. *Cancer* 1998; 83: 240–4.

7. O'Boyle CJ, Kerin MJ, Feeley K, et al. Primary small bowel tumours: increased incidence of lymphoma and improved survival. *Ann R Coll Surg Engl* 1998; 80: 332–4.

8. Bozdag AD, Nazli O, Tansug T, et al. Primary tumours of the small bowel: diagnosis, treatment and prognostic factors. *Hepatogastroenterology* 2003; 50S2: 117–18.

9. Torres M, Matta E, Chinea B, et al. Malignant tumours of the small intestine. *J Clin Gastroenterol* 2003; 37: 372–80.

10. Rangiah DS, Cox M, Richardson M, et al. Small bowel tumours: a 10 year experience in four Sydney teaching hospitals. *ANZ J Surg* 2004; 74: 788–92.

11. Mussi C, Caprotti R, Sciani A, et al. Management of small bowel tumours: personal experience and new diagnostic tools. *Int Surg* 2005; 90: 209–14.

12. Catena F, Ansaloni L, Gazzotti F, et al. Small bowel tumours in emergency surgery: specificity of clinical presentation. *ANZ J Surg* 2005; 75: 997–9.

13. Chow JS, Chen CC, Ahsan H, et al. A population based study of the incidence of malignant small bowel tumours: SEER, 1973–1990. *Int J Epidemiol* 1996; 25: 722–8.

14. Toms JR. Cancer incidence survival and mortality in the UK and EU. CancerStats Monograph. London: Cancer Research UK, 2004.

15. Howdie PD, Jalal PK, Holmes GKT, et al. Primary small bowel malignancy in the UK and its association with coeliac disease. *QJM* 2003; 96: 345–53.

16. Ryan JC. Premalignant conditions of the small intestine. *Semin Gastrointest Dis* 1996; 7: 88–93.

17. Rossini FP, Risio M, Pennazio M. Small bowel tumours and polyposis syndromes. *Gastrointest Endosc Clin North Am* 1999; 9: 93–114.

18. Hemminki K, Li X. Incidence trends and risk factors of carcinoid tumours: a nationwide epidemiologic study from Sweden. *Cancer* 2001; 92: 2204–10.

19. Paulson SR, Huprich JE, Fletcher JG, et al. CT enterography as a diagnostic tool in evaluating small bowel disorders. *Radiographics* 2006; 26: 641–57.

20. Schwartz GD, Barkin JS. Small bowel tumours. *Gastrointest Endosc Clin North Am* 2006; 16: 267–75.

21. Ramage JK, Davies AHG, Ardill J, et al. Guidelines for the management of gastroenteropancreatic neuroendocrine (including carcinoid) tumours. *Gut* 2005; 54: 1–16.

22. Adler DG, Merwat SN. Endoscopic approaches for palliation of luminal gastrointestinal obstruction. *Gastroenterol Clin North Am* 2006; 35: 65–82.

23. Chiang KC, Chen TW, Yeh CN, et al. Advanced gastrointestinal stromal tumor patients with complete response after treatment with imatinib mesylate. *World J Gastroenterol* 2006; 12: 2060–4.

24. Sakakura C, Hagiwara A, Soga K, et al. Long-term survival of a case with multiple liver metastases from duodenal gastrointestinal stromal tumor drastically reduced by the treatment with imatinib and hepatectomy. *World J Gastroenterol* 2006; 12: 2793–7.

25. Guidelines for the management of Gastrointestinal stromal tumours (GISTs). Augis, 2005. www.augis.org/news/articles/gist.

26. Nowain A, Bhakta H, Pais S, et al. Isolated hepatic metastasis from a gastrointestinal stromal tumor (GIST) 17 years after initial resection: need for long-term surveillance. *J Clin Gastroenterol* 2005; 39: 925.

27. Pavel M, Baudin E, Couvelard A, et al. ENETS consensus guidelines for the management of patients with liver and other distant metastases from neuroendocrine tumors of foregut, midgut, hindgut, and unknown primary. *Neuroendocrinology* 2012; 95: 157–176.

28. Esmer-Sanchez DD, Martinez OJL, Roman ZP, et al. Appendiceal tumours: clinicopathologic review of 5,307 appendicectomies. *Cir Cir* 2004; 72: 375–8.

29. Connor SJ, Hanna GB, Frizelle FA. Appendiceal tumours: retrospective clinicopathologic analysis of appendiceal tumours from 7,970 appendicectomies. *Dis Colon Rectum* 1998; 41: 75–80.

30. Kjan J, Sexton R, Moran BJ. Five percent of patients undergoing surgery for left colon or rectal cancer have synchronous appendiceal neoplasia. *Colorectal Dis* 2006; 8S2: 20–1.

31. Lamarca A, Daisuke A, Nonaka B, et al. Appendiceal Goblet Cell Carcinoids: Management considerations from a reference peritoneal tumour service centre and ENETS centre of excellence. *Neuroendocrinology* 2015. doi: http://dx.doi.org/10.1159/000440725.

32. Mahteme H, Sugarbaker PH. Treatment of peritoneal carcinomatosis from adenocarcinoid of appendiceal origin. *Br J Surg* 2004; 91: 1168–73.

33. McConnell YJ, Mack LA, Gui XF, et al. Cytoreductive surgery with hyperthermic intraperitoneal chemotherapy: an emerging treatment option for advanced goblet cell tumors of the appendix. *Ann Surg Oncol* 2014; 21: 1975–82.

34. Sych C, Staebler A, Connolly DC, et al. Molecular genetic evidence supporting the clonality and appendiceal origin of pseudomyxoma peritonei in women. *Am J Pathol* 1999; 154: 1849–55.

35. Bibi R, Pranesh N, O'Dwyer ST, et al. A specific cadherin phenotype may characterise the disseminating yet non-metastatic behaviour of pseudomyxoma peritonei. *Br J Cancer* 2006; 95: 1258–64.

36. Esquival J, Sugarbaker PH. Clinical presentation of the pseudomyxoma peritonei syndrome. *Br J Surg* 2000; 87: 1414–8.
37. Esquival J, Sugarbaker PH. Pseudomyxoma peritonei in a hernia sac: analysis of 20 patients in whom mucoid fluid was found during hernia repair. *Eur J Surg Oncol* 2001; 27: 54–8.
38. Sugarbaker PH. New standard of care for appendiceal epithelial neoplasms and pseudomyxoma peritonei syndrome? *Lancet Oncol* 2006; 7: 69–76.
39. Complete cytoreduction for pseudomyxoma peritonei (Sugarbaker technique). 2004. www.nice.org.uk IPG056.
40. Moran BJ, Mukherjee A, Sexton R. Operability and early outcome in 100 consecutive laparotomies for peritoneal malignancy. *Br J Surg* 2006; 93: 100–4.
41. Rout S, Renehan A, Parkinson M, et al. Treatment and outcomes of peritoneal surface tumors through a centralized service. *Dis Colon Rectum* 2009; 52: 1705–15.
42. Carmifnani CP, Hampton R, Sugarbaker CE, et al. Utility of CEA and CA 19.9 tumour markers in diagnosis and prognostic assessment of mucinous epithelial cancers of the appendix. *J Surg Oncol* 2004; 87: 162–6.
43. Farquharson AL, Pranesh N, Witham G, et al. A phase 11 study evaluating the use of concurrent mitomycin C and capecitabine in patients with advanced unresectable PMP. *BJC* 2008. doi: http://dx.doi.org/10.1038/sj.bjc.6604522.
44. Ito H, Osteen RT, Bleday R, et al. Appendiceal adenocarcinoma: long term outcomes after surgical therapy. *Dis Colon Rectum* 2004; 47: 474–80.
45. Gonzalez MS, Sugarbaker PH. Right hemicoloectomy does not confer a survival advantage in patients with mucinous carcinoma of the appendix and peritoneal seeding. *Br J Surg* 2004; 91: 304–11.
46. Yan TD, Black D, Savady R, et al. A systematic review on the efficacy of cytoreductive surgery and perioperative intraperitoneal chemotherapy for pseudomyxoma peritonei. *Ann Surg Oncol* 2006; 10: 1245–58.
47. Ronnett BM, Yan H, Karman RJ, et al. Patients with pseudomyxoma peritonei associated with disseminated peritoneal adenomucinosis have a significantly more favourable prognosis than patients with peritoneal mucinous carcinomatosis. *Cancer* 2001; 92: 85–91.

RELEVANT WEBSITES

http://www.christie.nhs.uk/services/a-to-h/colorectal-and-peritoneal-oncology-centre/

28

Cancer of the colon and rectum

PETRA G BOELENS, PIETER J TANIS, GINA BROWN, NICHOLAS P WEST,
CORNELIS J H VAN DE VELDE AND HARM J T RUTTEN

INTRODUCTION TO COLORECTAL CANCER SURGERY

For most cases of colorectal cancer (CRC), surgery is the primary curative modality. Complete removal of the tumour 'en bloc' with the lymph nodes is crucial in most cases. This chapter gives a comprehensive overview of all aspects of CRC management including surgical anatomy and planes of dissection, laparoscopic surgery, innovative techniques, perioperative conditions, postoperative complications, pathologic tumour assessment and staging, recommended treatments and quality assurance of care.

Incidence and Mortality

- CRC third most common cancer site, CRC accounts for 13% of all cancers
- 1000 new CRC patients each day in Europe
- Highest incidence in males in Central Europe
- Highest incidence in females in the Netherlands and Denmark
- CRC second ranking in cancer mortality

EPIDEMIOLOGY OF CRC IN EUROPE

The large intestine is the third most common site of cancer in the European Union. After breast and prostate cancer, CRC constitutes 13% of all cancers [1]. New cancer cases diagnosed in 2012, in a cohort of 27 European countries, were estimated at a rate of 342,000 (nearly 1000 patients per day), of which males predominated (59%) [1]. The exact numbers of rectal cancers are variable depending on the exact definitions used for classifying rectosigmoid cancer to either the colon or rectum in the cancer registry, ranging from 27 to 58% [2]. After lung cancer, CRC ranks second in mortality. The estimated number of deaths caused by CRC in 2012 was 149,984, of which 53% were male and 47% female [1]. There is a considerable variation in the mortality of colorectal carcinoma among different EU countries, although the dissimilarities between countries for mortality are lower than for incidence; this could be related to differences in stage at the time of diagnosis and different patterns of treatment between countries. International comparisons of treatment deliver extremely valuable information about population-based cohorts, aiding optimization of cancer

care strategies and unravelling overtreatment or undertreatment issues [94].

Stage IV or metastatic CRC accounts for approximately 35% of all patients at diagnosis (stage IV). Their median survival is approximately 9 months. Patients treated with only supportive care have a median survival of about 5 months [3]. Stage IV patients undergoing potentially curative liver resection may have a 5-year overall survival rate of 44% and a 10-year overall survival rate of 33% [4].

The 10-year survival rate of colon cancer for all age groups and all stages in the Netherlands is 56% (increasing over time from 1989 when it was 50%). The 5-year survival rate is 62% for colon cancer based on a cohort of 43,089 patients from 2007 to 2012 [5,6].

- The incidence rate is the number of new cases per population at risk at a given time period.
- Prevalence is the proportion of cases in the population at a given time.
- Mortality rate is the number of deaths of a certain population.
- The age-specific mortality rate (ASMR) refers to the total number of deaths per year per 1000 people of a given age.

Hereditary CRC

Part of our role in assessing CRC patients is finding out the family history and recognizing persons at risk of familial predisposition to CRC. It is thought that 15%–30% of CRCs may have an hereditary component. About 5% of CRCs are due to an established familial genetic syndrome. Clinical suspicion is based on clinical criteria or on an abnormal molecular screen in the context of a suspicious personal or family history.

Lynch syndrome or HNPCC syndrome

Approximately 3% of all CRC cases occur in the setting of a Lynch syndrome or hereditary non-polyposis colorectal cancer (HNPCC) syndrome. If there is a clinical suspicion of polyposis or HNPCC, the patient should be referred to a specialist for genetic testing. HNPCC is formally defined by the presence of germline mutations in DNA mismatch repair (MMR) genes which are inherited in an autosomal dominant pattern and are associated with accelerated development of cancers. The lifetime risk for colorectal and endometrial cancers approaches 70%–80% and 40%–60%, respectively. At-risk family members who undergo screening colonoscopy have a reduced risk of developing HNPCC-related CRCs and lower mortality. Colonoscopies with polypectomies and transvaginal ultrasonography and endometrial biopsies repeated frequently are recommended. With surveillance intervals of 1–2 years, members of families with HNPCC have a lower risk of developing CRC than with surveillance intervals of 2–3 years.

Familial adenomatous polyposis

Familial adenomatous polyposis (FAP) syndrome is caused by a germline mutation in the adenomatous polyposis coli (APC) gene. In affected individuals, multiple adenomas in the rectum and colon will develop during life. Individuals with FAP carry a 100% lifetime risk of developing CRC. The main goals of managing FAP are cancer prevention and maintaining a good quality of life. Regular and systematic follow-up and supportive care should be offered to all FAP patients. There are still many areas of research in hereditary CRC syndromes such as the role of aspirin in polyp prevention, type and timing of surveillance modalities, ideal timing for surgery and type of surgery. In FAP patients, prophylactic surgery to prevent CRC is advocated in the late teens or early twenties. Total proctocolectomy, either with or without anal mucosectomy, with ileal pouch anal anastomosis (IPAA) is recommended for FAP patients. Subtotal colectomy with ileorectal anastomosis (IRA) may be considered in highly selected FAP patients. Desmoid tumours are rare non-metastasizing fibromatoses that may occur in association with FAP. Desmoids have a prevalence of 10%–26% in FAP and are usually a major source of morbidity and one of the most common causes of death in these patients. An interaction between female gender and early (<18 years) colectomy in patients developing desmoids has been observed (HR 2.5).

MUTYH-associated polyposis

MUTYH-associated polyposis (MAP) is a recently described hereditary cancer syndrome, transmitted in an autosomal recessive fashion. While the true incidence remains unknown, MAP may account for 0.5%–1% of all CRCs [14,52]. The colonic phenotype of MAP mimics that of attenuated FAP (AFAP), including a propensity for proximal colonic neoplasms. Extracolonic manifestations similar to those observed in FAP and AFAP have been reported. Patients with more than 10 polyps should be tested for MAP.

Hamartomatous polyposis

The hamartomatous polyposis syndromes are present with an overgrowth of cells native to the area in which they normally occur. Peutz–Jeghers syndrome (PJS) and juvenile polyposis syndrome (JPS) are the two main hamartomatous polyposis conditions, and are both inherited in an autosomal dominant way. Both syndromes carry an increased risk for developing CRC as well as other gastrointestinal and pancreatic cancers. The lifetime risk of CRC is 39% in patients with PJS (70%–90% lifetime risk of cancer) and 10%–38% in patients with JPS.

PJS has been associated with germline mutations or deletions in the LKB1 gene (STK11), a serine-threonine kinase that regulates p53-mediated apoptosis and the mammalian target of the rapamycin pathway, whereas JPS is caused by mutations in SMADH4, BMPR1A and ENG interacting within the transforming growth factor–beta (TGF-β)/SMAD pathway.

Polymerase proof-reading associated polyposis

Polymerase proofreading-associated polyposis (PPAP) is another polyposis syndrome characterized by multiple colorectal adenomas or early onset carcinoma, and shows an autosomal dominant inheritance. PPAP is associated with germline mutations in the proof-reading domains of two DNA polymerases, POLE and POLD1.

Hereditary mixed polyposis syndrome

Hereditary mixed polyposis syndrome (HMPS) is an autosomal dominantly inherited polyposis syndrome presenting with polyps of multiple and mixed morphologies including serrated lesions, Peutz–Jeghers polyps, juvenile polyps, conventional adenomas and CRC without any identifiable extracolonic features.

PATHOLOGY

Quality of pathological assessment

The pathologist plays an important role in examining resected tissue, describing its quality and producing a consistent and structured report describing all of the important prognostic features. Free text reporting has been shown to result in the absence of important information and therefore the use of proformas or structured lists is highly recommended to ensure complete data collection, international consistency and ease of understanding by the rest of the multidisciplinary team (MDT). Within the United Kingdom, the Royal College of Pathologists has recently updated its guidelines for reporting CRC and now includes separate datasets for major resections and local excision specimens [7]. European guidelines for the reporting of screen-detected lesions also exist and should be followed by all pathologists reporting cancers in a screening programme [8].

Specimens should ideally be received fresh and photographed prior to opening including views of the front and

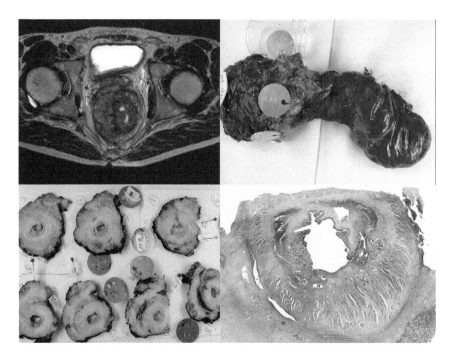

Figure 28.1 Example of the CORE study combining MRI, macroscopic, full transversal slides and whole mounted slides to evaluate the specimen.

back of the specimen to act as a permanent record of the quality of surgery. Fixation in formalin for at least 48 h should be undertaken to facilitate cross-sectional slicing of the tumour area at 3–4 mm intervals. Further photographs of the slices should be taken to allow correlation with radiology (Figure 28.1). Careful assessment of the slices is important as many high-risk features including circumferential resection margin (CRM) involvement, extramural venous invasion and peritoneal involvement can be identified macroscopically, allowing the most important areas to be blocked out for microscopic confirmation.

Quality of the specimen

Pathological judgement of specimen quality based on the integrity of the surgical planes is now well recognized to be of value (Figure 28.2).

RECTUM

Mesorectal grading was the first system to be introduced and categorizes the specimen as being in the *mesorectal plane* (intact mesorectum extensively covered by fascia with only minor defects), *intramesorectal plane* (significant defects in the mesorectum that do not extend down to the muscularis propria) or *muscularis propria plane* (significant defects that expose the muscularis propria or surgical perforations). This system was first used prospectively by local pathologists in the MRC CR07 trial and was shown to independently predict a higher rate of local disease recurrence in the muscularis propria plane group [9]. A recent meta-analysis of 18 studies including more than 4000 patients has confirmed this observation [10].

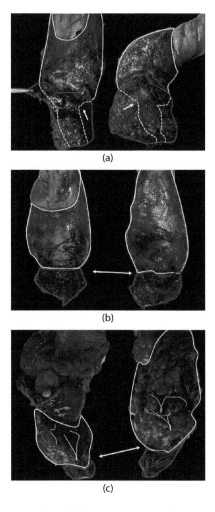

(a)

(b)

(c)

Figure 28.2 Quality of the specimen: (a) levator plane, (b) sphincteric plane and (c) intrasphincteric plane.

Abdomino-perineal excision (APE) of the rectum and anus is well recognized to be associated with poorer outcomes than restorative surgery for higher tumours. Recent evidence has shown that for locally advanced low rectal cancers, an extralevator APE is superior as it removes more tissue around the tumour leading to a lower CRM involvement and perforation rate [11–13]. Pathologists responded to this by developing a grading system that describes the plane of surgery around the sphincter complex and should be used in addition to mesorectal grading in APE specimens. The system includes the *levator plane* (levator muscles resected en bloc with the mesorectum and sphincter muscles), *sphincteric plane* (no levator resected but sphincters intact, resulting in a waisted specimen) and *intrasphincteric plane* (defects into the sphincter muscles or surgical perforations) (Figure 28.2). This grading system has been shown to be reproducible between pathologists and to provide immediate feedback on APE specimen quality [14,15]. It should be emphasized that for early low rectal tumours, perineal dissection in the intersphincteric and within the sphincteric plane is possible.

COLON

Recently, there has been an increasing focus on the quality of colon cancer resection following the observation that colon cancer outcomes have not improved similarly to rectal cancer. There are three important variables in colon cancer specimens that should be described by pathologists including [1]: the integrity of the mesocolon [2], the radicality of the central dissection (distance between the tumour and the high vascular tie) and [3] the extent of longitudinal resection. A mesocolic grading system was developed that closely mirrors the mesorectal grading system used for rectal cancer including the mesocolic plane (intact mesocolon extensively covered by peritoneum or fascia with only minor defects), intramesocolic plane (significant defects in the mesocolon that do not extend down to the muscularis propria) and muscularis propria plane (significant defects that expose the muscularis propria or surgical perforations). Studies have shown that this grading system similarly predicts patient outcome with a 15% difference in overall 5-year survival rising to 27% in stage III disease [16]. European surgeons undertaking complete mesocolic excision with central vascular ligation (CME with CVL) report some of the best outcomes in the literature to date [17]. These more radical specimens are more likely to be in the mesocolic plane and remove a significant amount of additional tissue between the tumour and the high vascular tie than conventional surgery [18]. The technique can be similarly undertaken laparoscopically [19], and can be easily adopted following surgical education programmes leading to an immediate improvement in the oncological quality of colon cancer specimens [20]. Surgeons who have adopted CME with CVL as a standard have recently reported significantly improved survivals compared to comparable centres with no significant increase in morbidity [21].

Pathological assessment of resection margins

Longitudinal resection margins are rarely involved in CRC and are not routinely sampled unless the tumour is located 3 cm or less from the margin. The importance of the CRM in rectal cancer was initially described in 1986 with tumour located 1 mm or less from the CRM predicting a higher rate of local disease recurrence [22]. A large meta-analysis including more than 17,500 patients has confirmed the importance of avoiding tumour involvement of the CRM [23]. There are various mechanisms by which a tumour can extend to the CRM including direct spread, discontinuous spread, intravenous, intralymphatic, perineural and intranodal. There is continued debate as to the importance of an involved CRM solely due to tumour within a lymph node, particularly if there is no evidence of extracapsular spread and the mesorectal fascia is intact. Isolated CRM involvement due to nodal disease is rare, being identified in only 1% of cases in the UK MERCURY study [24]. While the evidence in the literature is limited, small studies have suggested that the risk of recurrence is significantly less than that of the other methods of CRM involvement [25].

The evidence for the importance of tumour involvement of the retroperitoneal margin in colon cancer is significantly less. Studies have shown the rate of margin involvement in right-sided resections to be between 7% and 8%, but the independent prediction of local recurrence has not been demonstrated [26–28]. One study showed that involvement of the retroperitoneal margin in right-sided cancers was a marker of advanced disease with other high-risk features driving prognosis, including peritoneal involvement and distant metastases [28].

On the basis of the evidence of the importance of the CRM, TNM have recently revised their criteria for the assessment of completeness of excision. The R1 category (incomplete microscopic resection) previously required the tumour to extend right to the margin; however, this has now been subdivided into R1-dir (direct involvement of the margin) and R1 ≤ 1 mm [29].

TNM staging

The TNM staging system for CRC has been frequently criticized over recent years following serial changes to the way the disease is staged based on little evidence and poor assessment of reproducibility [30]. Some countries have opted to stay on the fifth version of TNM to ensure consistency until prospective randomized clinical trial evidence shows that any suggested changes offer additional value and are reproducible by pathologists around the world.

There are a number of issues that the TNM system currently does not address, including lymph node staging, the reversal of pT4a and pT4b, low rectal cancer staging and the assessment of perforations below the peritoneal reflection. TNM version 5 abolished the pN3 category and introduced the '3 mm rule' whereby any tumour deposit with no residual lymph node structure was counted as an involved lymph node. Version 6 abolished this rule and suggested that rounded deposits should be classed as involved nodes and irregular deposits as vascular invasion. This was shown to be poorly reproducible between pathologists and also flawed, as nodal deposits with extracapsular spread will be irregular and many vascular deposits show the rounded shape of the vessel wall. Version 7 abolished this rule and leaves it to individual pathologists to determine the origin of tumour deposits. They also introduced the pN1c category whereby any node negative cases with tumour deposits are classed as pN1c and therefore stage III disease. There is no guidance on how big deposits should be and how far away from the primary tumour, and therefore reproducibility will be poor [31].

Tumour perforation

Pathologists are recommended to state in text form whether the case shows peritoneal involvement, tumour perforation or involvement of surrounding organs. Surgical perforations below the peritoneal reflections are not recognized by TNM staging and therefore the United Kingdom has issued guidance in its reporting dataset that these cases should also be classed as pT4 due to their poor prognosis [7].

Low rectal cancer

Staging of low rectal cancers is problematic if they involve the anal canal and sphincter complex. TNM suggests that these should be staged like anal cancers on the basis of size; however, the biology of squamous cell carcinoma of the anus is very different from that of low rectal adenocarcinomas that behave more like higher rectal cancers. The pT staging criteria of the higher rectum cannot be easily applied to the anal sphincter complex due to anatomical differences in the layers of the bowel. The internal sphincter can be composed of multiple layers which often intermingle with the skeletal muscle fibres of the external sphincter and the intersphincteric space does not always exist. For this reason it is recommended that rather than applying a pT stage for these tumours, the maximum extent of invasion should be assessed above and within the sphincters separately using a description of the deepest layer of penetration, e.g. the outer layer of the muscularis propria above the sphincters and internal sphincter within the sphincters.

Lymph nodes and stage II high-risk features

It is critical that pathologists identify all of the high-risk features within the specimen that might be used to determine eligibility for adjuvant treatment. It is expected that all of the lymph nodes are identified and examined to determine the presence of nodal metastases. Many factors contribute to nodal yields including host immunity, tumour biology, extent of surgery and pathological diligence. For this reason nodal yields are complicated and appear to indicate

prognosis, even in the absence of lymph node metastases. This may reflect tumour biology with mismatch repair–deficient tumours having a better prognosis and higher yield, but it also reflects the quality of pathology. Pathologists with higher nodal yields are known to identify higher rates of other high-risk features including positive margins, extramural vascular invasion and peritoneal involvement, and nodal yields can therefore be used as a surrogate marker of the quality of pathology [32]. Pathologists should audit their nodal yields and ensure that on average in excess of 12 are identified; however, many specialist centres now find many more than this with some identifying 37 nodes on average with specialist techniques, leading to significant upstaging in early disease [33].

It is important that pathologists standardize their assessment for high-risk features in stage II disease as these are increasingly being used as indicators for adjuvant treatment. Evidence suggests that patients with high-risk stage II disease actually have a worse prognosis than early stage III disease [34]. Extramural venous invasion and peritoneal involvement are frequently missed by pathologists due to inadequate sampling of the specimen. The UK Royal College of Pathologists has suggested that at least 30% of specimens should contain venous invasion, and if individual pathologists fail to hit this target, then the use of supplementary stains to highlight vessel walls may be helpful [7]. There are similar targets for the frequency of peritoneal involvement in cancers of the colon (20%) and rectum (10%), and pathologists are encouraged to regularly assess for these standards across a series of at least 50 resections for symptomatic cancer that have not undergone preoperative treatment.

Assessment of specimens after preoperative treatment

It is important that a standardized approach is taken for the assessment of specimens after preoperative therapy so that an accurate indication can be given of the response to treatment (Figure 28.3). A number of subjective tumour regression grading systems exist in the literature, which causes confusion; hence it is important that pathologists describe exactly which system they are using. It is increasingly recognized that pathologists cannot separate mild regression from an absence of regressive changes due to the variable degree of desmoplastic stroma in untreated cases, and therefore four grade systems are considered to be more reproducible, e.g. complete pathological response (no viable tumour), near-complete response (scattered viable tumour cells), significant response (residual tumour but fibrosis predominates) and minimal or no regression (the tumour still predominates) [7]. Complete pathological response rates vary markedly in the literature and reflect a lack of standardization in pathological sampling. Many countries have now adopted the protocol used in the European CORE trial whereby the entire area of fibrosis should be blocked out and each block examined at three levels prior to calling

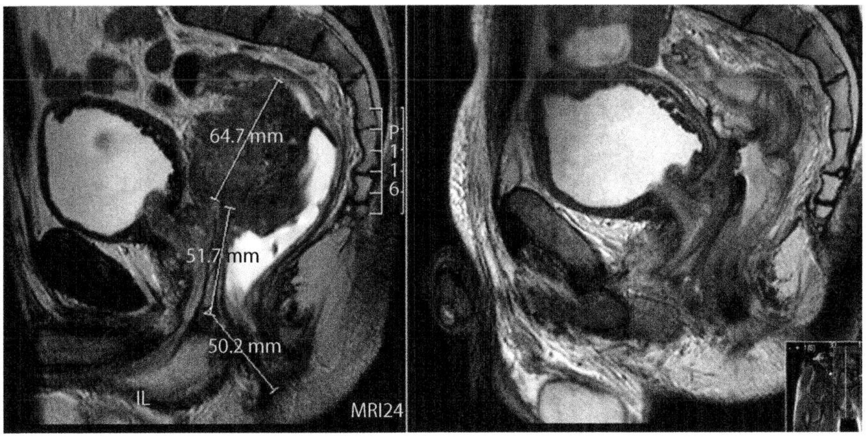

Figure 28.3 High-resolution preoperative imaging before and after neoadjuvant treatment and postoperative imaging is necessary to develop a final treatment plan.

a complete response. This is thought to represent a balance between adequate assessment and practicality and should allow comparability of trials if universally adopted [7].

Molecular pathology

Molecular testing of CRCs is now commonplace and is used routinely in metastatic disease to indicate whether patients may benefit from the addition of anti-epidermal growth factor receptor (EGFR) monoclonal antibodies. Cases with microsatellite instability often show poor differentiation but are known to be associated with a better prognosis [35]. For this reason poor differentiation should not be used as a high-risk feature in the absence of mismatch repair status, which can be easily determined by immunohistochemistry for the commonly involved genes and confirmed by sequencing. Many pathologists across Europe are now undertaking immunohistochemical screening as a prognostic tool and a way of identifying patients with Lynch syndrome.

KRAS mutations are known to predict the response to anti-EGFR monoclonal antibodies. Initially it was shown that mutations in codons 12 and 13 of the gene result in downstream activation of signalling independent of EGFR blockade [36]. For this reason KRAS mutated tumours are unlikely to respond to treatment. Further work has shown that codons 59, 61, 117 and 146 and NRAS codons 12, 13, 59 and 61 also predict response to these drugs and should be tested prior to treatment with such agents [37]. In addition to its predictive effect, KRAS is an independent prognostic marker with KRAS mutants having a poorer prognosis than wild-type tumours [35]. A similar effect is seen with BRAF mutations in stage IV disease, although this appears to disappear in early stage disease in cases with coexisting mismatch repair deficiency [35]. Newer biomarkers emerging from the EGFR pathway include PIK3CA which has been suggested to predict the risk of disease recurrence on aspirin treatment [38]. This exciting development requires validation but could provide an effective predictive test for a cheap and widely available agent. All of these mutations

can be detected using a variety of technologies with varying degrees of sensitivity. Many centres are now utilizing next-generation sequencing where it is possible to test the status of a number of genes simultaneously across a large number of samples, thus increasing the cost-effectiveness and allowing novel markers to be easily introduced into routine panels. Many other prognostic and predictive biomarkers have been suggested in the literature to date; however, none have yet been independently validated in at least two prospective studies and therefore their value remains unknown. Some biomarkers are referred to in Table 28.2.

PREOPERATIVE IMAGING OF COLON CANCER

The gold standard for screening and symptomatic cancer detection remains optical colonoscopy. Colonoscopy and CT colonography are important complementary diagnostic tools [39,40]. For diagnosing CRC, a tissue sample with histopathological confirmation of cancer should be obtained by colonoscopy. Colon cancer is optimally staged, when synchronous lesions are identified or ruled out, and distant metastases are searched for by abdominal CT and chest x-ray or CT. In case of synchronous metastatic disease, staging before and after treatment is mandatory for response evaluation after treatment (Table 28.1) [41,42].

Colonoscopy

A complete colonoscopy is recommended in all cases suspected of colon cancer. Visualization of the suspected lesion and the complete colon is necessary to rule out other polyps and lesions, facilitating biopsy of the lesions, polypectomy and tattooing for laparoscopic procedures [43–45]. Incomplete colonoscopies occur due to inadequate bowel preparation, patient discomfort, stenosis or other technical difficulties. Guidelines recommend a minimum colonoscopic completion rate (caecal intubation) of more than 90% [46,47], which suggests that a considerable proportion of patients will have an incomplete colonoscopy. In these cases

Table 28.1 Demonstrating the differences between TNM editions

	TNM 5th Edition			TNM 7th Edition		
Stage	TNM	Stage		TNM	Dukes	MAC
0	Tis N0 M0	0		Tis N0 M0		
I	T1 N0 M0	I		T1 N0 M0	A	A
	T2 N0 M0			T2 N0 M0	A	B1
II	T3 N0 M0	IIA		T3 N0 M0	B	B2
	T4 N0 M0	IIB		T4a N0 M0	B	B2
	T4 N0 M0	IIC		T4b N0 M0	B	B3
III	Any T N1	IIIA		T1–T2 N1/N1c M0	C	C1
	Any T N2			T1 N2a M0	C	C1
	Any T N2	IIIB		T3–T4a N1/N1c M0	C	C2
	Any T N2			T2–T3 N2a M0	C	C1/C2
	Any T N2			T1–T2 N2b M0	C	C1
	Any T N2	IIIC		T4a N2a M0	C	C2
	Any T N2			T3–T4a N2b M0	C	C2
	Any T N1/N2			T4b N1–N2 M0	C	C3
IV	Any T Any N M1	IVA		Any T Any N M1a	D	D
	Any T Any N M1	IVB		Any T Any N M1b	D	C

Note: MAC, modified Asler Coller. The TNM staging system tries to describe the extent of disease according to different prognostic variables, relating to tumour extent (T), lymph node involvement (N), and the presence of metastases (M) at the time of diagnosis. The staging system is modified when new significant knowledge within each group of variables becomes available. At this moment the TNM 7th edition is the latest variant. Variables T, N and M are pooled in different prognostic groups. Prefixes indicate whether the staging is based on clinical parameters (cTNM) or after pathology of the resected specimen (pTNM). The addition of y to the pTNM (ypTNM) signifies that between the clinical and pathological staging neoadjuvant treatment may have changed the original clinical staging. Furthermore, in the future other prefixes may be added, like mr, which indicates a clinical staging with an MRI scan after neoadjuvant treatment. The risk of changes to the TNM staging system is that it will be difficult to compare patients who were staged with different TNM additions.

CT colonography may be complementary [40,48], although CT colonography is less sensitive in a high-risk patient as it will miss smaller lesions [49,50].

CT colonography

CT colonography has been recognized as a highly sensitive and specific diagnostic modality for lesions > 9 mm [51]. For smaller lesions CT colonography (CTC) cannot compete with a colonoscopy [52]. In a recent meta-analysis CTC was compared with colonoscopy and showed a relative sensitivity of 96% for CRC [40]. The SIGGAR trial found that in up to 30% of cases CTC will detect a lesion that requires further evaluation by colonoscopy [51].

Air contrast barium enema

There is no place for contrast barium enema anymore as a primary diagnostic tool in detecting CRC, due to lower detection rates for smaller lesions and patient discomfort. The SIGGAR trial investigated patient tolerance and found a lower satisfaction and greater physical discomfort in patients undergoing contrast barium enema compared to CT colonography [51]. Both investigations require bowel preparation and insufflation, and the positional changes necessary for a barium enema are challenging for elderly patients [51,53].

Abdominal CT

All patients with newly diagnosed colon and rectal cancer should undergo preoperative staging using a multidetector CT. The scans are performed following the oral administration of 1 L of water and intravenous administration of iodinated contrast. Scans should be reviewed following multiplanar reconstruction which enables review in the coronal and sagittal planes in addition to the conventional axial plane. Scans are reviewed on 3–5 mm reconstructions.

Morphology

Tumours are classed as either mucinous or non-mucinous. Mucinous tumours show a distinct appearance on CT, characterized by a lack of enhancement due to mucin, and are of relatively low density compared with the bowel wall and non-mucinous tumours. These are more prevalent in right-sided colonic tumours, where the mucinous subtype can be notoriously difficult to diagnose on preoperative biopsy [54] and may carry a worse prognosis due to a more advanced stage at presentation, but also to the much higher risk of tumour spillage during surgery. Thus preoperative documentation of this subtype which has a 10%–15% prevalence will help with surgical planning. On the other hand, tumours with a polypoidal morphology have a better prognosis than annular ulcerating adenocarcinomas of the colon.

T stage assessment

In determining the local extent of the tumour in colon cancer, it is first important to establish the invasive borders of the malignancy. Such tumours will have an advancing front along the mesenteric or peritonealized border. The latter will have a high risk for T4 spread and intraperitoneal recurrence. Posteriorly, the retroperitoneal margin can be at risk of circumferential margin involvement from more advanced ascending and descending colon tumours and distal sigmoid tumours. In these cases, preoperative assessment will allow a plan for the surgical plane to be extended. Thus radiological documentation of the proximity to such margins, the risk of peritoneal spread and the degree of mesenteric infiltration will all assist with the subsequent surgical approach.

Depth of tumour invasion

The extent of tumour beyond the muscularis propria on CT can be assessed and studies have shown that CT is effective at distinguishing relatively early stage-good prognosis colon cancers from more advanced poor-prognosis T3 and T4 node positive cancers simply by using a 5-mm cut-off for depth of spread beyond the colonic wall. Patients identified with good prognostic features on imaging have a 3-year survival of 87% versus 53% in patients with poor prognostic features [55]. This has also been proven to be reproducible in the multicentre setting by radiologists and was evaluated as the entry criterion for patients to receive preoperative chemotherapy in the phase III randomized FOxTROT trial [56]. Analysis of the trial pilot study control arm (straight to surgery), of CT-identified high-risk patients, showed that 86% of patients with tumour spread > 5 mm on CT also had high-risk features on subsequent pathology [57].

Extramural venous invasion

Extramural venous invasion (EMVI) has been shown to be an independent prognostic indicator in colon cancer [58]. As with MRI identification of EMVI, this feature manifests as direct spread with expansion of vessels. CT has been able to identify gross evidence of venous invasion with >70% agreement with histopathology [57]. This feature is also strongly associated with the subsequent appearance of hepatic metastatic disease and on CT is the only independent preoperative variable associated with the development of liver-only metastatic disease.

Nodal status assessment by CT

CT scanning has an accuracy of 95% for the detection of distant metastases [59]. However, CT has been shown to be poor in identifying nodal disease. Nodal size measurements are too unreliable as a predictor for malignancy and should not be used for defining whether lymph nodes are involved [60,61]. Despite this it has been shown that CT T substaging enables better identification of high-risk patients preoperatively than assessing nodes on CT.

The ability of any imaging modality to identify nodal involvement is limited [60,62,63], and as highlighted above, there are more reliable features that can more accurately identify patients with poor prognosis (namely depth of spread > 5 mm and EMVI). The vast majority of studies evaluating the performance of CT in assessing nodal status have shown equally poor results. This is not surprising since CT can only depict the size of nodes and the studies confirm the lack of any association with nodal size and risk of malignancy [55,57,64,65]. Therefore CT is not recommended in preoperative staging of nodal status and its evaluation does not carry any prognostic value. Since there is a much higher correlation between lymph node metastases and EMVI and extramural spread of more than 5 mm, it is better to define such patients as likely or high risk for nodal involvement. When considering a stratification for preoperative therapy or more radical colonic surgery such patients would be most likely to benefit.

T4 invasion, obstruction and perforation

A significant proportion of colon cancer patients present with emergency obstruction or perforation. Emergency CT assessment plays an important role in these situations and will enable stratification and separation of patients with obstruction due to small obstructive tumours which can be readily resected versus a more extensive tumour which may need extended resection and in some instances may benefit from preoperative therapy.

***

Key message: Colon cancer diagnostic imaging

Colonoscopy and biopsy are the gold standard for diagnosing colorectal carcinoma.

In case of an incomplete colonoscopy, additional CT colonography or completion colonoscopy is indicated.

CT colonography is an acceptable alternative imaging tool to colonoscopy to detect colorectal lesions > 1 cm.

Preoperative radiological staging of colon cancer is based on CT chest and CT abdomen or pelvis.

Frail patients should primarily be considered for a CT colonography.

Air barium contrast enema has become obsolete for colorectal carcinoma.

***

The following should be routinely reported when assessing colon cancers using CT to help with surgical planning and prognostic stratification:

- Tumour morphology: Annular, semi-annular, mucinous, ulcerating.

- Site: Caecum, ascending, hepatic flexure, transverse, splenic flexure, descending, sigmoid.
- Border of infiltration: Mesenteric versus peritonealized.
- Diameter and thickness of tumour.
- T substage (good or poor): T3 < 5 mm or > 5 mm.
- Nodal and venous spread: Ileocolic, middle colic, left colic, sigmoidal veins. The risk of nodes identified being malignant will be most accurately predicted using the depth or EMVI stratification (extramural spread > 5 mm or CT detected EMVI = high risk of nodal metastasis).
- Adjacent organ infiltration/perforation/obstruction.
- Synchronous metastatic disease.

PREOPERATIVE IMAGING OF RECTAL CANCER

Accurate staging impacts on the quality of the treatment. Preoperative imaging of rectal cancer should be an MRI for local staging and a CT of the chest, abdomen and pelvis for detection of distant metastases [66,67].

High-resolution MRI facilitates distinct outlining of the tumour. Preoperative identification of prognostic features by MRI influences medical decision making for preoperative treatment. Prognostic features include the depth of tumour invasion into the mesorectum and beyond (T stage and T3 substage), nodal disease (N stage), the distance to the borders of the tumour in relation to the mesorectal fascia (MRF) and extramural venous invasion (EMVI). Cases with these features are associated with an increased risk of local recurrence or metastatic disease. These patients might benefit from neoadjuvant therapies, to downsize the tumour, increasing the potential for curative surgery. Therefore, rectal cancer should be visualized by MRI, with specific reference to evaluating the MRF, the T3 substage, nodal disease and the presence of EMVI. Figure 28.4 shows the distinct features of a mucinous rectal cancer.

Low rectal tumours

Low rectal tumours are a more complicated subgroup of rectal tumours as they have a higher risk of local recurrence and the outcome is worse than that for tumours in the middle and upper thirds of the rectum [14]. The aim of surgery should be to achieve a complete resection with a clear margin. It was shown that patients undergoing abdomino-perineal excision have a 30% higher rate of local recurrence than other cases [68]. The anatomy on preoperative MRI is of the utmost importance to planning surgical resection or whether neoadjuvant treatment would be beneficial. MRI can be used to define the relationship of the tumour to the sphincter complex and determine whether resection margins are likely to be involved if sphincter conservation is attempted [12].

Locoregional imaging

For early tumours (cT1), endorectal ultrasound is a useful assessment for depth of tumour invasion. Endoscopic ultrasound (EUS) in experienced hands permits discrimination of stage T1 from stage T2 tumours; however, others have shown that it fails to discriminate T1 substages (SM1–3) accurately [69]. For successful local excision, the latter is the most important.

Extramural spread is an independent prognostic factor in rectal cancer. Extramural extension of 5 mm or less is associated with a significantly improved 5-year cancer-specific survival compared with tumours showing extramural spread beyond 5 mm (85% vs. 54%, respectively) [70]. MRI is highly accurate in detecting extramural spread and in the identification of tumours with good (< 5 mm invasion) versus poor (> 5 mm invasion) prognostic characteristics [71].

Peritoneal involvement

Peritoneal involvement is an independent risk factor for intraperitoneal recurrence [72]. MRI enables preoperative detection of peritoneal involvement in rectal cancer [72,73]

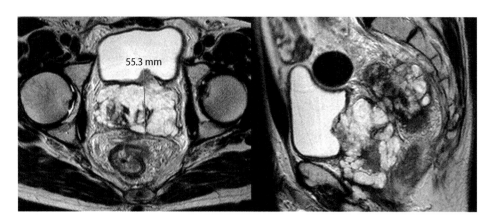

Figure 28.4 Images of mucinous rectal carcinoma.

Table 28.2 Molecular markers and their clinical consequences

Biomarker	Function	Impact of chemotherapeutic agent
Thymidylate-synthase (TS)	TS expression ↑	5-FU response ↓
	TS expression ↓	5-FU response ↑
Dihydropyrimidine-dehydrogenase (DPD)	DPD activity ↓	5-FU toxicity ↑↑
		5-FU response ↑
UDP-glucuronosyltransferase 1A1 (UGT1A1)	Glucuronidation SN-38 ↓	CPT-11 neutropenia ↑
ERCC1	ERCC1 – gene expression ↓	Oxaliplatin response ↑
		Oxaliplatin survival ↑
K-Ras	GTPase activity ↓ constitutive activation of downstream pathways	Resistance to anti-EGFR MoAb treatment (panitumumab or cetuximab)
B-Raf	Constitutive activation of downstream pathways	Survival ↓
COX2 gene	Promoter activity ↓	Cetuximab PFS ↑
IL-8 VEGF	VEGF expression ↑	Recurrence ↑
DCC	Apoptosis ↓	Survival ↓
Microsatellite instability	MMR function ↓	Prognosis ↑

Note: VEGF, vascular epidermal growth factor; PFS, progression-free survival; SNP, single nucleotide polymorphism; 5-FU, 5-fluorouracil; CPT-11, irinotecan; MoAb, monoclonal antibody; DCC, deleted in colon cancer; LOH, loss of heterozygosity; MSI-H, high level of microsatellite instability; MMR, mismatch repair.

which may facilitate cytoreductive surgery and hyperthermic intraperitoneal chemotherapy (HIPEC) in suitable patients by transferal of care to recognized centres.

Circumferential resection margin

It is widely accepted that a clear circumferential resection margin (CRM) is the most important factor in avoiding local recurrence and improving survival [74]. To accomplish complete removal of rectal cancer, preoperative imaging by MRI and a preoperative MDT discussion of the scan enable surgical planning of the resection to optimize the chance of a clear CRM [75] or advise on the need for neoadjuvant treatment to shrink the tumour to facilitate such radical surgery. On imaging, a CRM of > 1 mm, is considered sufficient [76]. The MERCURY Group demonstrated that MRI has a high specificity (92%) in assessing the likelihood of a clear CRM [68]. A prospective observational study reported a high negative predictive value (NPV) for the assessment of an involved mesorectal fascia in mid- to high rectal tumours at the expense of a lower positive predictive value (PPV). For low rectal tumours, CT is significantly less sensitive than MRI and cannot replace it [77–79].

Circumferential margin for low rectal cancers

First, there is the mesorectal dissection plane: the distal TME dissection leads to the intersphincteric plane which may be appropriate for tumours that are not infiltrating through the rectal wall at or just above the level of the puborectal sling. For more advanced tumours at this level,

such an approach runs a significant risk of tumour perforation and positive margins [80]. Second, there is the extralevator dissection plane, recommended for tumours located at or in the intersphincteric plane at or just above the puborectal sling. Using a low rectal staging classification, it is possible to give precise information to the surgeon about what planes of excision are likely to be clear of tumour and which are threatened. This allows preoperative decision making based on MRI-predicted planes of excision and clinical information [80,81].

Extramural venous invasion

Extramural venous invasion means extension of tumour into the extramural veins. EMVI is an independent prognostic factor for local and distant recurrence and for overall survival in rectal cancer [82,83], but histopathological reporting of venous invasion varies from 10% to 54% [84,85]. MRI is the imaging of choice for determining if tumour signal extends into the extramural vasculature (mrEMVI) which has been documented in 30%–40% of patients scanned. Systemic chemotherapy for patients exhibiting EMVI on MRI might improve disease-free survival. CT is not as reliable at identifying EMVI in CRC [57].

While nodal staging in rectal cancer lacks sensitivity in all imaging modalities, nodes in imaging reports might result in 'overtreatment' with (chemo)irradiation. Before the implementation of TME surgery, nodal involvement was associated with a higher risk of local recurrence, regardless of the number of lymph nodes involved. TME surgery, properly performed, changed this; only the presence of >4 lymph nodes seems to be associated with a higher risk of local recurrence [86], and this in turn is largely associated with tumours exhibiting increasing depth of spread (which is more readily identified preoperatively than N2 status). Endoscopic ultrasound is inferior to CT and MRI in identifying nodal involvement [87] and this relates to the lack of visualization of the entire mesorectum. High-resolution MRI is the most accurate imaging tool for identifying nodal disease. Mixed signal intensity and irregular edges are the factors on MRI predicting nodal involvement with a sensitivity of 85% and specificity of 97% [73]. Nodal size must not be relied upon to discriminate between benign and malignant lymph nodes [73,88].

This implies that we should recommend relying on MRI for T substage, mesorectal fascia (MRF) involvement and EMVI, as nodal staging is less reliable.

Summary of rectal cancer diagnostic imaging recommendations

- Preoperative MDT discussion of MRI rectal cancer findings leads to improved outcomes.
- MRI is the best modality to identify patients at risk of local recurrence based on potential involvement by tumour within 1 mm of mesorectal fascia.
- A low rectal cancer staging classification based on the relationship of the tumour to the distal TME plane at or just above the puborectal sling will prevent inadvertent surgical perforation of the tumour from the distal TME dissection and selective use of the extralevator APE.
- Other risk factors for outcome that are readily and reliably assessed using MRI include depth of extramural spread (mrT stage) and the presence or absence of extension of tumour signal into extramural veins (mrEMVI).
- EUS, CT and MRI have suboptimal accuracy for nodal staging. While nodes > 3 mm can be characterized as malignant or benign by signal and border features, on high-resolution MRI, nodes < 3 mm in diameter containing metastatic foci remain a challenge for identification.

CR07 showed that when TME surgery was performed and the circumferential margin was negative (which can be more readily predicted using MRI) there was no added risk of local recurrence if patients were node positive compared with node negative cases. There is some evidence that suggests that with good TME surgery, limited nodal involvement is no longer a risk factor for local recurrence [89]. Identifying nodal disease with imaging is difficult. Modern higher-resolution MRI can better assess nodal features such as border irregularity and heterogeneity. Improved sensitivities and specificities have been reported when using these features rather than size [19].

Imaging after radio(chemo)therapy: responders versus non-responders

The detection of subtle residual tumour remains problematic and a complete remission after chemoradiation cannot be reliably predicted with non-invasive imaging techniques [90]. Although EUS, CT and MRI can show downsizing of the tumour, they are not accurate if fibrotic thickening of the rectal wall is seen. Fibrosis makes it difficult to predict if downstaging has resulted in a ypT0, ypT1, ypT2 or ypT3 tumour. The accuracy is increased by the addition of diffusion-weighted imaging (DWI) to standard MR. Increased sensitivity in comparison to phased-array MRI was found in discriminating between ypT0–2 and ypT3. Therefore, diffusion-weighted MRI is more sensitive than MRI for prediction of a pathological complete response [91–93]. Post-radiation FDG-PET in responders versus non-responders seems promising, but again minimal residual disease is difficult to detect [91].

COLON CANCER TREATMENT BY STAGE

In situ and malignant polyps

The underlying rationale of colonoscopy with polypectomy is resecting the early potential of CRC [94]. In short, it begins with a small adenomatous polyp, followed by formation of a larger polyp with dysplasia, which finally leads to the development of invasive carcinoma. Vogelstein and colleagues proposed this model of colorectal tumourigenesis in which the steps required for the development of cancer often catch the mutational activation of oncogenes (K-Ras) combined with the loss of several genes that normally suppress tumourigenesis (APC, DCC, p53) [95]. This stepwise combination of molecular alterations occurs in parallel with a stepwise transformation in morphology [96].

To highlight their clinical relevance, during screening colonoscopies, polyps are present in 20%–40% of subjects and their occurrence is associated with an increased risk of future CRC [97]. During surveillance colonoscopy the adenoma detection rate was found to be 34.1% [97]. About 5% of adenomatous polyps are estimated to become malignant in a process that takes approximately 10 years. The risk of recurrent adenomas is dependent on the number (>3) and size (>1 cm) of the adenomas and the presence of high-grade dysplasia or villous morphology. These patients need surveillance colonoscopy more frequently to rule out new polyp growth or regrowth. In the case of hereditary polyps, colonoscopies are recommended annually.

During screening colonoscopy the adenocarcinoma detection yield is estimated around 0.8%–1%. After surveillance colonoscopy (after a previous cancer for example) the detection rate of cancer is 1.3% [97].

The treatment of colon cancer is dependent on stage: for most stages complete removal of the tumour with the draining lymph nodes is the best available option for cure. However, in very early stages such as in situ cancer, or malignant polyps, colectomy might be regarded as over-treatment. The risk of lymph node metastases is lower and endoscopic local resection may be possible. However, to avoid 'oops' situations, pathology examination needs to be performed impeccably, confirming a complete resection and a favourable grade. These patients should be scheduled for frequent endoscopic surveillance in the first 3 years as well as undergoing regular carcinoembryonic antigen (CEA) testing. To illustrate the arguments for both overtreatment or undertreatment in these cases, survival rates for pTis and pT1 at 5 years are 99% and at 10 years 97%, while in-hospital mortality following a colectomy might be around 3%–5%. Care should be taken to avoid incomplete or piecemeal resection: these patients are at risk of recurrence and metastasis and in such cases colectomy should be offered. Although endoscopic resection is performed as part of daily routines in some countries, no randomized data on long-term endpoints are available and the difficulty remains that interpretation of series from expert centres might be obscured by selection bias. Quality assurance after endoscopic resection in terms of oncologic outcomes has yet to be established.

cT1 Nx endoscopic, laparoscopic or open?

Laparoscopic or conventional colectomy is still the gold standard for cT1 N0 colon cancer. For pT1 N0 M0, the alternative of endoscopic resection could be discussed with the patient but keeping in mind that lymph node metastases are estimated at 11% (range 6.3–16.9%) in pT1 colon cancer, based on 17 studies including 3621 patients [98]. Predictors of low risk of lymph node metastasis are (1) absence of lymphatic invasion, (2) budding, (3) submucosal invasion ≥ 1 mm and (4) poor histological differentiation. Clear resection margins are associated with a good prognosis; piecemeal resection is not. Data are from a retrospective cohort study in which, after endoscopic resection of cT1 colon cancers, all patients underwent additional curative oncological colon resection. The 5-year overall survival rate was 96.3% in T1 colon cancer after additional oncological surgical treatment following endoscopic resection. Lymph node metastases occurred in approximately 8.2% [99]. For early colon cancer (Tis-T1), advanced endoscopic techniques such as endoscopic mucosal resection (EMR), endoscopic submucosal dissection (ESD) and even endoscopic mucosal ablation (EMA) can be considered as alternatives to colectomy [100]. The risk of lymph node metastasis should always be carefully discussed in a MDT meeting and with the patient. If the pathologic examination indicates incomplete resection, or high-risk features, colonic resection should be offered subsequently to avoid recurrence.

cT2–cT3 N0

Surgery remains the cornerstone treatment for cT2–cT3 colon cancers. Planning the extent of the colectomy is dependent on the blood supply of the tumour-bearing segment; moreover, it is of the utmost importance to remove the tumour en bloc with the lymph nodes located in the mesenteric pedicle (Figure 28.5), along the vessels (for more details see the section below on anatomy). A laparoscopic approach may be considered for T1–T3 tumours (for more information see the section, Laparoscopic surgery for colorectal cancer, on laparoscopic colectomy).

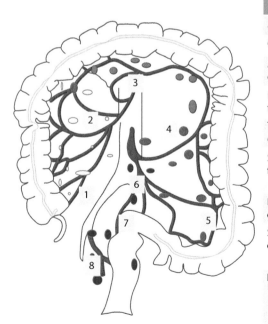

Site	Reginal lymph nodes	
Appendix	Ileocolic	1
Caecum	Ileocolic, right colic	1,2
Ascending colon	Ileocolic, right colic, middle colic	1,2,3
Hepatic flexure	Right colic, middle colic	2,3
Transverse colon	Right colic, middle colic (left colic)	2,3 [4]
Splenic flexure	Middle coilc, left colic (inferior mesenteric)	3,4 [5]
Descending colon	Left colic, inferior mesenteric, sigmoid	4,5,6
Sigmoid colon	Left colic, sigmoid, inferior mesenteric (superior rectal)	4,5,6,7
Rectum	Inferior mesenteric, superior, middle and inferior rectal, inferior iliac arteries	5,6,7,8

Figure 28.5 Regional lymph nodes and the vascular pedicle belonging to them determine the extent of the colorectal resection.

High-risk stage II

Patients with stage II colon cancer do worse than those staged at IIIa. High-risk stage II patients are without positive lymph nodes, but with other unfavourable pathologic characteristics such as a T4 tumour, lymphovascular invasion and poor differentiation. For these patients adjuvant chemotherapy may be advantageous (see the section on chemotherapy in CRC below) [101,102].

cT4

For a successful oncological colonic resection, important stages of the operation include:

1. Inspection of the abdominal cavity for peritoneal carcinomatosis. If this is present resection should be stopped and consideration given to whether the patient might be a candidate for cytoreductive surgery and HIPEC.
2. Palpation or intraoperative ultrasound of the liver, to rule out liver metastases, should be performed.
3. Inspection of the tumour for signs of perforation, which has a very unfavourable prognostic significance and needs to be described in the pathology and operative report.
4. Iatrogenic perforation during surgery, which also has an adverse effect on prognosis and needs to be reported.
5. Complete resection en bloc with any other invaded organs in cT4 disease.
6. Number of harvested lymph nodes counted (at least 12).
7. Formation of a tension-free anastomosis.
8. Careful observation of the vascularization to prevent ischemia of the anastomotic loops.

In most cases a stoma is not required for elective colon cancer surgery, unless patient factors suggest a high risk of anastomotic failure, such as frailty, advanced old age, malnutrition or significant comorbidities.

As is the case for rectal cancer, where patients may benefit from neoadjuvant treatment, the FOxTROT (Fluoropyrimidine, Oxaliplatin and Targeted Receptor Preoperative Therapy for patients with high-risk, operable colon cancer) collaborative group performed the first randomized feasibility study to assess the benefit of neoadjuvant chemotherapy in colon cancer. The study assessed whether neoadjuvant chemotherapy ± panitumumab followed by deferred surgery then completion of chemotherapy postoperatively was superior to standard surgery and postoperative chemotherapy. It also assessed whether adding panitumumab to neoadjuvant therapy for patients with KRAS/NRAS wild-type tumours increased antitumour activity as measured by tumour shrinkage. In the preoperative group more patients completed the chemotherapy cycles than the adjuvant patients. The FOxTROT trial showed benefits for patients undergoing neoadjuvant chemotherapy before colonic resection. There is now a need

for phase III trials to fully establish the equivalence or superiority of neoadjuvant chemotherapy in locally advanced colon cancer [56].

Stage III colon cancer

Stage III colon cancer is divided into three categories:

- IIIa: T1, N1 (1–3 nodes), M0 or T2, N1, M0
- IIIb: T3, N1, M0 or T4, N1, M0
- IIIc: Any T, N2 (4 or more nodes), M0

Consequently the number of nodes is important in stage allocation and this cannot be reliably done based on preoperative imaging and is usually indicated in the postoperative pathology report.

When nodal involvement is present, it is usual to offer chemotherapy postoperatively to fit patients. Adjuvant oxaliplatin plus capecitabine (CAPOX) or leucovorin–5-fluorouracil (XELOX/FOLFOX) is considered a standard treatment option. For more information about chemotherapy see the section, Adjuvant chemotherapy for CRC, below on chemotherapy for CRC. Despite the controversies in the prescription of adjuvant therapies to patients older than 80 years and with comorbidity, a recent pooled analysis of four randomized trials showed that this recommendation holds true for patients in all age groups or in those with comorbidities, consistent with those who were eligible for these clinical trials [103]. However, this information needs to be regarded cautiously at present, and large observational prospective studies would give a less biased insight into this debate.

If patients do not tolerate oxaliplatin or have comorbidities that are linked to cardiac failure, monotherapy with capecitabine is advised.

Advanced colon cancer and HIPEC

In advanced colonic cancer, tumour fixation to retroperitoneal structures is usually managed with neoadjuvant treatment, either systemic chemotherapy or radiotherapy [104,105]. However, the use of radiotherapy in the abdomen is limited by radio-sensitive structures like the small bowel or kidneys. In large tumours, the tumour itself can be used as a spacer and the irradiation volume limited to the area of fixation.

Another presentation of advanced colonic cancer is exfoliation of tumour cells into the abdominal cavity leading to peritonitis carcinomatosa (PC). PC occurs in 5% synchronously and 5% metachronously in colon cancer patients. Survival is poor and limited to 5–7 months even with systemic therapy [106,107].

Most often PC is missed on staging CT scans and is encountered while opening the abdomen (or when starting with a staging laparoscopic procedure) for the resection of the colon tumour. If the involvement of PC is present in five or less than five out of the seven abdominal regions and if cytoreductive surgery removing all macroscopic gross tumour burden is possible, the optimal approach would be to perform the cytoreductive surgery and administer hyperthermic intraperitoneal chemotherapy (HIPEC) during the same procedure [108]. However, this is a time-consuming procedure and even in specialized centres an ad hoc decision to do a HIPEC procedure is from a logistical point of view impractical. In these cases it is better to avoid further damage to the peritoneum, leave the colonic tumour untouched, if no obstruction is present, and refer the patient as soon as possible to a HIPEC centre. Sometimes PC is suspected on CT, and a diagnostic laparoscopy can be performed to stage the PC to see if it is limited to five or less than five out of seven regions and to decide whether cytoreductive surgery is possible. For example gross involvement of the small bowel and central mesentery is considered a contraindication for HIPEC.

In a randomized trial with patients without further distant metastatic disease cytoreductive surgery and HIPEC led to an improved median survival of 22 months [109], if the disease is limited to five of the seven abdominal regions and a near-complete surgical cytoreduction can be obtained. Median survival rates of up to 60 months have been reported with expected cure rates of 30% [110–112]. More details are given in the chapter on peritoneal surface oncology (Chapter 30).

MANAGING NON-METASTATIC COLON CANCER

Rectal cancer treatment

In rectal cancer, total mesorectal excision (TME) is still the gold standard and local recurrence rates of < 5% are achievable by meticulous surgery following the surgical planes. Considerable morbidity and loss of function are related to rectal resection (detailed in the section on postoperative complications and surgical performance). New techniques have been developed in early stage disease to preserve function and reduce the extent of surgery while retaining

oncological safety. In more advanced stages, aggressive and extensive surgery beyond the TME borders may be necessary.

cT1

For rectal cancer preoperatively staged cT1, N0, M0 TME surgery is still the gold standard resulting in excellent local recurrence rates and long-term survival. The local alternative is called transanal endoscopic microsurgery (TEM) (Figure 28.6) and may be performed with equal overall survival at 5 years [113–115]. Local recurrence rates are higher and the pathology examination might identify that completion or salvage TME will be necessary or not.

TEM is a minimally invasive procedure, using a transanal approach, using one rectal port of about 4 cm, CO_2 insufflation, a proctoscope and about three working channels in the rectal port for laparoscopic instruments. The idea is to cut a wide full-thickness specimen with negative margins from the rectal wall. A macroscopic margin of at least 5 mm from the tumour needs to be taken for both benign and malignant tumours. Excision is performed using monopolar cautery under general anaesthesia. TEM is safer in terms of blood loss, hospital stay, postoperative morbidity, less anorectal and genitourinary dysfunction and better quality of life than traditional surgery [113,116]. Of note, a higher local recurrence rate was found after TEM in comparison to TME surgery, in a patient population with negative resection margins [114]. In principle, the use of local excision requires that there is a non-obstructing tumour and its dimension is less than half of that of the lumen or with a size of less than 4 cm diameter [115]. As with any challenging new, complex surgical technique, learning curves must be acknowledged and supervised training provided [117].

The specimen after local excision has to be carefully analyzed to evaluate its completeness, the depth of invasion in the bowel wall, the absence of margin infiltration both laterally and deeply, and the presence of adverse pathologic factors: poor grade and blood or lymphatic vessel invasion [118,119].

After transanal excision, in those cases with a confirmed pathological stage pT1, Nx with low-risk features (sm1, low

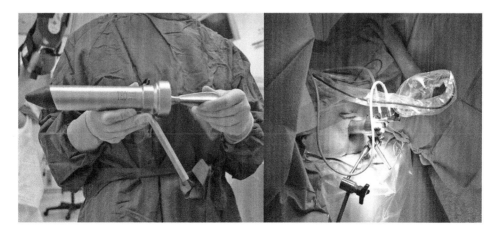

Figure 28.6 TEM scope.

grade, no lymphatic or blood invasion), local excision may remain the only treatment [101,102]. No formal agreement is available for T1sm2, so two possible treatment options are available: (1) 'close observation' or (2) proceed to TME surgery. If the pathology report shows a more extensive tumour (≥ pT1sm2) or other high-risk prognostic factors (i.e. high grade, blood or lymphatic vascular invasion, sm3) following local excision the patient should undergo TME surgery [101]. It is not recommended to administer postoperative chemoradiation after incomplete or prognostically unfavourable histology following a TEM procedure. Depending on tumour location, salvage or completion surgery after local excision may compromise the ability to perform a sphincter-sparing operation. After salvage TME surgery for cT1–2, if the pathologic stage confirms a pT1–2, N0 tumour the patient may be observed in follow-up [101,102].

In a retrospective case-matched study, with 25 patients in each group, early salvage or completion TME surgery after TEM appears to be safe when compared to patients undergoing primary TME; a good-quality TME specimen was associated with the best long-term results [120–124]. In the Dutch TME trial patients treated in the 5 × 5 Gy radiotherapy group, a subgroup of patients undergoing completion TME after initial TEM (n = 95) was studied in comparison to the 881 patients undergoing primary TME surgery, and a higher rate of colostomy and local recurrence (TEM completion group 10.2% versus TME 5.2%) was found [125].

Endoscopic mucosal resection (EMR) is another new technique performed endoscopically [100,126]. However, there is not enough evidence to recommend this procedure as standard treatment at present. After EMR, pathological analysis of submucosal infiltration is essential to assess the completeness of the resection, and further surgery is recommended if submucosal margins are inadequate or invaded [100,126].

Transanal minimally invasive surgery for TME (TAMIS), also called taTME, involves performing TME surgery through a single transanal port from caudal to cephalad. The benefit is the enhanced view of the distal rectum, which can be difficult to visualize at laparoscopy, for instance in the obese male with a bulky tumour and a narrow pelvis. It is a form of NOTES (natural orifice surgery) and can be performed with or without laparoscopic assistance. A transanal approach can be performed using the TEM (TEO) platform or the single-incision laparoscopic surgery (SILS) port, or even robotic-assisted transanal endoscopic proctectomy. Although trials have been undertaken since 2008 and results show its feasibility in experienced hands, it is too early to recommend this approach yet; its safety and non-inferiority will first have to be proven in properly designed trials, for instance in comparison to laparoscopic TME [127]. At this moment the COLOR III trial is assessing this comparison, using a clear CRM as the primary endpoint.

cT2

In T2 rectal cancer, as determined by MRI, TME surgery is also the gold standard. Because 10%–30% of patients have a complete response after chemoradiation, organ preservation is often anticipated with either a watch-and-wait policy or local excision. TEM after chemoradiation in comparison to TME surgery for patients staged T2 N0 M0 was investigated by Lezosche and colleagues [128]. A 30% complete response rate was found, with no differences in local recurrence or survival over 84 months of follow-up. If recurrences occurred, they did so in patients without a significant response to neoadjuvant chemoradiation. A more recent study (ACOSOG Z6041) included 90 patients with T2 N0 rectal cancer in a phase II trial, and found a 44% complete response rate and considerable downstaging, meaning local excision was often feasible. The authors stated that the toxicity of chemoradiation was considerable and patients should be warned about postoperative rectal pain when considering this alternative approach to TME surgery [129].

cT3

T3 rectal cancer includes a very heterogeneous range of presentations, depending on the extent and location of the tumour infiltration through the muscularis propria into the surrounding mesorectal fat. There is a huge difference in prognosis for posteriorly located tumours, just extending a few millimetres in the dorsal mesorectal fat compared to tumours which fill up the mesorectal space to the full extent of the circumferential resection margin. It was proposed to subclassify T3 tumours on the basis of the MR images. A T3a tumour would invade less than 1 mm into the mesorectal fat, a T3b 1–5 mm, a T3c 5–15 mm and T3d more than 14 mm [130].

However, this subclassification still does not relate to prognoses and does not give sufficient information for preoperative treatment planning. At present, MRI is the basis for the subclassification of T3 tumours, but not only based on penetration depth but rather on its relation to the circumferential resection margin. If the margin is less than 1 mm, circumferential resection margin positivity is very likely [76,89]. Tumours located on the posterior aspect of the rectum can extend into the mesorectal fat for many millimetres before they affect prognosis, whereas this is completely different for tumours at the level of the pelvic floor or on the ventral side of Denonvilliers' fascia, which only need to infiltrate a few millimetres to threaten the circumferential resection margin. Consensus exists that MRI is the single most important tool to tailor preoperative radiotherapy. Tumour infiltration into the surroundings of the mesorectum of more than 5 mm is also considered a poor prognostic omen, which predicts the likelihood of nodal metastasis. In northern European countries, like the Scandinavian countries, the Netherlands, Belgium and the UK, a tumour which infiltrates more than 5 mm into the mesorectal fat without threatening the circumferential resection margins, and therefore not requiring downstaging, is considered to be a candidate for 5 × 5 short-course radiotherapy, based on the Swedish and Dutch rectal cancer studies [131,132]. Tumours which do threaten the circumferential resection margins are candidates for long-course radiochemotherapy.

In some countries 5 × 5 Gy has not been accepted as widely as in northern European countries, and all patients that are at risk, either by infiltration of more than 5 mm into the mesorectum or by threatening the circumferential resection margins, will receive preoperative chemoradiotherapy. A Polish and Australian study did not show a difference between short-course radiotherapy and radiochemotherapy [133,134]. In the Stockholm II trial, the Dutch TME trial, and the UK CRO7 trial 5 × 5 Gy preoperative radiotherapy was followed by immediate surgery. The Stockholm III trial aims to find out whether immediate surgery versus delayed surgery should be done [135,136]. The interim results seem to show that delayed surgery results in downstaging and fewer complications. The final results of the Stockholm III trial are not available yet, but there seems to be an argument, especially in the elderly, to avoid the toxicity of immediate surgery and perform delayed surgery after 5 × 5 Gy [137]. After radiochemotherapy surgery is always delayed.

There is another point of discussion regarding the surgical treatment plan: If you have a locally advanced T3 tumour after radiochemotherapy, should an MRI be performed to judge the response to treatment and can it alter the final treatment plan? It was learned that response to treatment is an important prognostic variable [138,139]. Bulky tumours with a pushing boundary may exhibit a completely different topographical relation, when downsized. Therefore, in these patients the treatment plan can be altered. The opposite is equally true. If after radiochemotherapy a bulky tumour does not show a response, and if there is a chance of positive circumferential margins or at least margins that are less than 1 mm are likely to occur, one should consider referral of these patients to a pelvic surgery team, accustomed to doing more extended resections.

The final discussion point is about when to perform surgery after a long course of radiochemotherapy. The general opinion is that in responsive tumours a longer waiting period will also lead to a more pronounced downsizing and even downstaging. When response is strictly monitored by MRI or endorectal ultrasound it could be defended to continue waiting and individualize treatment based on the response.

Intensification of neoadjuvant treatment has been tried by combining different chemotherapeutic agents, like bevacizumab and 5-FU or capecitabine, or combining a 5-FU-based drug with oxaliplatin, but this kind of intensification has not led to better oncological outcomes [140,141]. However, research is now focusing on systemic neoadjuvant treatment with preoperative radiotherapy. The dose of the chemotherapy, which is combined with radiotherapy, is relatively low in comparison to true systemic treatment. Therefore, an intensification method could be to administer 5 × 5 Gy in combination with several courses of systemic chemotherapy in the usual dose. At this moment this is the subject of the multinational RAPIDO study [142] looking at preoperative 5 × 5 short-course radiotherapy followed by several courses of systemic chemotherapy in the usual dose versus neoadjuvant radiochemotherapy without any additional systemic treatment. As of yet no results are available.

PELVIC ADVANCED DISEASE

Differences between locally advanced and locally recurrent rectal cancer

Both T4 and locally recurrent rectal tumours are difficult to classify. The depth of invasion into the surrounding structures, location in the pelvis and previous pelvic surgery make them very heterogeneous tumours, requiring site-specific surgical and reconstructive approaches. For treatment planning a preoperative MRI will give the best anatomical information [76,143] (Figure 28.7). In T4 tumours MRI can also be used to assess response to treatment and possibly result in less extensive procedures [138,139,144]. It is difficult to determine the response to neoadjuvant treatment by MRI, due to reactive fibrosis. Fibrosis is frequently present in locally recurrent cases as a result of the primary resection [145]. In addition, a PET/CT can give useful information not only for confirming the diagnosis but also for response evaluation [146]. However, if recurrence is complicated by chronic infection PET/CT may be falsely positive and other indicators may be necessary, like elevated CEA levels, clinical symptoms or changes on repeated MRI scans. Pathologic biopsies cannot always be obtained to rule out viable tumour cells in the fibrosis. It is important to rule out metastatic disease by careful evaluation of the abdomen and lungs with a CT scan. If resectable metastases are present, these should be treated first, as their treatment is less demanding and does result in less loss of function than treatment of the pelvic disease. However, if metastatic disease is present it may also be a strong indicator of progressive incurable disease. In these cases systemic treatment may be indicated to observe response and gain more time to make a final decision if a surgical resection of both the metastases and the pelvic tumour is a reasonable approach [147].

The topographical anatomical relations of locally advanced and locally recurrent rectal cancer show major differences, which require a different surgical approach. In locally advanced rectal cancer the tumour invades through the mesorectal fascia into the surrounding organs or pelvic structures, but in the unaffected part of the pelvis normal topographical relations remain intact, allowing for a fairly standard surgical dissection along the interfascial spaces up to the affected area. In locally recurrent rectal cancer, on the other hand, surgery for the primary tumour has already opened these interfascial planes, exposing virtually the whole pelvic content to tumour invasion by the recurrence. In recurrent cases it may be necessary to pursue the dissection lateral of the endopelvic fascia in order to include the primary dissection field for the primary in the tumour specimen. At the site of the recurrence adjacent anatomical structures like vessels, the sacrum, internal genitals and the pelvic floor have to be removed en bloc with the regrowth. Rarely local recurrences present as a well-defined local problem. Even in centrally located recurrences or seemingly pure anastomotic recurrences, the tumour often spreads into the surrounding fibrosis and scar, which extend to the endopelvic fascia.

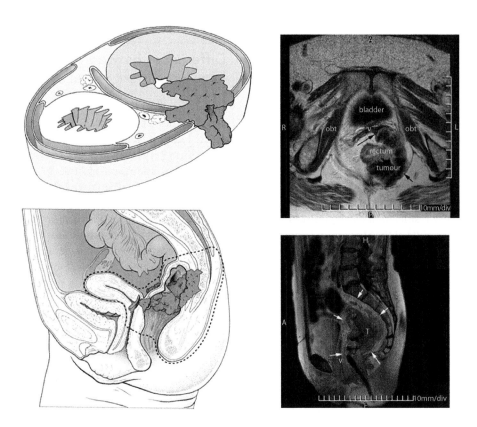

Figure 28.7 Advanced pelvic disease requiring extended, extra-anatomical and multivisceral resections.

The only chance for cure in both locally advanced T4 tumours and locally recurrent rectal cancers is to achieve a radical R0 resection [148]. One of the most important tools helping to achieve this goal is the use of neoadjuvant radio(chemo)therapy, which in locally advanced cancers may downsize and even downstage the tumour to facilitate the resection and allow for a less wide resection [149]. In contrast, in locally recurrent rectal cancer fibrosis and scar tissue most often harbour the tumour, and although a response after radio(chemo)therapy is likely to occur, downsizing of the fibrosis does not occur, and rarely can the surgical strategy be changed and the whole volume of fibrosis needs to be resected en bloc [150].

Another complicating factor in locally recurrent cancer surgery is that it is more frequent following treatment of more advanced primary tumours that have already been treated with radiotherapy or chemotherapy in their original treatment plan. These patients cannot be treated again with a full course of radio(chemo)therapy due to maximal tissue tolerance limitations. Some authors claim that re-irradiation to a limited dose of 30 Gy with concurrent chemotherapy is feasible [151,152]. Bosman describes almost equally good results after re-irradiation in combination with an intraoperative radiotherapy (IORT) boost compared to a full course of radio(chemo)therapy and IORT [153]. Even a limited dose of re-irradiation in combination with IORT can lead to an improved oncological outcome (Figure 28.8).

IORT can be used to apply an extra boost of irradiation to the area of risk. Radiotherapy-sensitive structures may be shielded or moved out of the target area for the boost [154]. By doing so, limitations to external beam radiotherapy of maximum dose tolerance can be overcome. A single intraoperative boost of 10 Gy delivered with electrons from a linear accelerator or with high-dose rate brachytherapy is biologically equivalent to 30 Gy fractionated external beam radiotherapy. Figure 28.9 shows the dose distribution from an intraoperative applicator from a linear accelerator. This boost comes on top of the preoperative external beam dose. IORT can be used in both T4 or locally recurrent rectal cancer. In a recent comprehensive review Mirnezami concluded that IORT is an effective treatment modality, despite missing evidence from randomized trials, which are very difficult to perform in these kind of relatively rare patients [155].

Depending on the extent of the resection, reconstructive surgery may be necessary. Large perineal defects or reconstruction of a posterior vaginal wall can be done with a vertical rectus abdominis transposition. If defects of the ureter are too large for a primary anastomosis, reimplantation into the bladder after mobilization of the bladder can be used to preserve normal urinary function. After total exenteration a urinary conduit is necessary. Lateral sidewall involvement can jeopardize vascularization to the leg and vascular reconstructions are necessary. Sacral resections lead to loss of innervation of the bladder and genital organs,

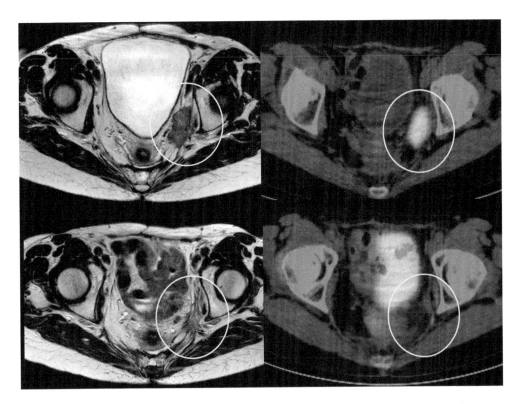

Figure 28.8 Lateral sidewall local recurrence before and after re-irradiation on MRI and corresponding PET scan. Normalization of PET, but residual of the fibrosis on MRI.

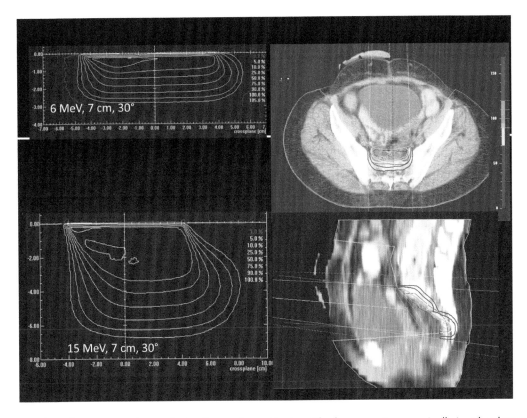

Figure 28.9 Principles of intraoperative radiation boost for patients with close or microscopically involved margins.

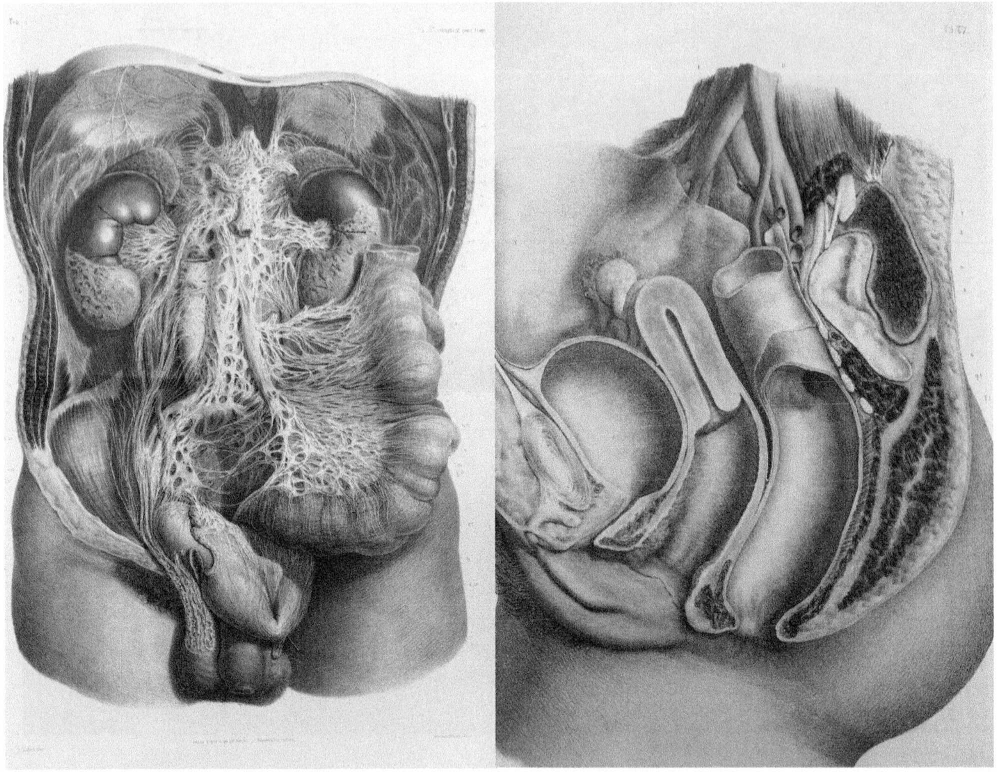

Figure 28.10 Anatomy and innervation of the rectum. (From Bourgery JM, *Traité complet de l'anatomie de l'homme, comprenant la médécine opératoire*, Paris: C. A. Delaunay, 1844.)

which require specific aftercare [Figure 28.10]. An expert group is trying to develop guidelines for these heterogeneous diseases [156].

Key message

- Locoregional pelvic disease can be treated curatively by aggressive surgery in specialized centres.
- Re-irradiation and intraoperative radiation add to an improved outcome.

Modern anatomical approach to CRC surgery

The basic principle of colon cancer surgery is to develop the retroperitoneal interfascial planes of the sections of the colon, which develop in a retroperitoneal position during embryological development. By doing so, the tumour-bearing segment and its lymphovascular pedicle can be fully exposed as far as its origin from the mesenteric base, so allowing removal of all the primary lymph nodes en bloc with the specimen. For a caecal or ascending colonic tumour a right colectomy is recommended, with the resection including from the first few centimetres of the terminal ileum and extending to the proximal half of the transverse colon. The vessels to be transected are the ileocolic, right colic and right branch of the middle colic artery. Steps in the dissection include mobilization of the caecum by incising the white line of Toldt, which is the peritoneal reflection of the paracolic groove, ensuring dissection in the plane above the renal fascia (of Gerota). Moving cranially and medially, the dissection should avoid harming the duodenum dorsal to the hepatic flexure, the right ureter and the superior mesenteric artery. Side-to-side ileotransverse anastomosis, aligning the antimesenteric side protecting its vascularization, can be performed using staplers [157]. Reinforcement of the staple line with some sutures is thought to limit adhesions to the staples. 'Closing the mesenteric defect' prevents internal herniation. The anastomosis should rest without tension and without torsion and be well perfused (as pink as the rest of the bowel loops).

The left colectomy is similar to the right in many aspects. Three practice points that need to be considered are:

1. Mobilizing of the splenic flexure needs to be carried out carefully to avoid iatrogenic harm to the spleen and pancreas when dissecting the splenocolic, phrenicocolic and pancreaticocolic ligaments.
2. Identify the left ureter.
3. Avoid injury to the duodenum which can be located very low, in close proximity to the origin of the inferior mesenteric artery or superior rectal artery.

Usually a mesenteric dissection above the caudal border of the pancreas is undesirable.

The danger points during sigmoid colectomy are similar to those of a left hemicolectomy. When entering the mesorectal plane distally injury to the sympathetic nerves (hypogastric, in proximity to the inferior mesenteric artery), parasympathetic nerves (pelvic splanchnic nerves) and left ureter crossing the iliac vessels just lateral of the promontory must be prevented.

Rectal cancer surgery

The first abdomino-perineal resection was tried unsuccessfully by Czerny in 1883 in an emergency situation during a perineal rectal resection. It took until 1895 for Quénu to perform the first successful abdomino-perineal resections and defeat the paradigm, which was formulated by Billroth in 1883 stating that rectal cancer was an incurable disease (Figure 28.11) [158]. Soon Miles published a successful series [159]. During their lifetimes they would witness that local recurrence, which was inevitable in purely perineal approaches, could be avoided and that cure rates of up to 40%–50% could be achieved. Despite some improvements in rectal cancer surgery, like the development of low and stapled anastomoses, which reduced the number of perineal amputations, oncologic outcomes did not improve until the end of the twentieth century, when the concept of rectal resection based on anatomical principles was introduced.

Since imaging (MRI), surgery and pathology are based on anatomical relations of the tumour in the pelvis, oncological outcome has improved and now at least equals the outcome of colonic surgery [160,161].

Heald was the first to describe the principle of removal of the complete rectum with its mesorectal fat enveloped in its mesorectal fascia: total mesorectal excision (TME) [162]. Quirke is to be credited for stressing that the pathologist should not only look at the tumour, but also describe the quality of the surgical specimen [22]. The quality of surgery, more specifically the status of the circumferential resection margin, turned out to be the most important prognostic factor for rectal cancer surgery and later also colon cancer surgery [163–165].

Rectal surgical anatomy

The anatomical bases for rectal resection are the fascial layers of the pelvis and the spaces between them. Most of the rectum and surrounding mesorectal fat which contain the main lymphovascular pedicles are enveloped in a visceral fascia called the mesorectal fascia. The parietal fascia surrounds the mesorectal fascia. Laterodorsal to the mesorectal fascia, the endopelvic fascia covers the iliac vessels, sacral neural and venous plexuses, pelvic muscles, gonadal vessels, ureters and sacral bone. Ventral to the sacral bone, the fascia is called the presacral fascia (Waldeyer's fascia) and covers the presacral veins, sympathic trunk, autonomous nervi erigentes from the sacral foramina, pudendal nerve and levator ani nerve (Figure 28.12). Between these two layers a virtual compartment exists filled with loose areolar tissue, where these layers can easily be separated. The dorsolateral part of this interfascial compartment

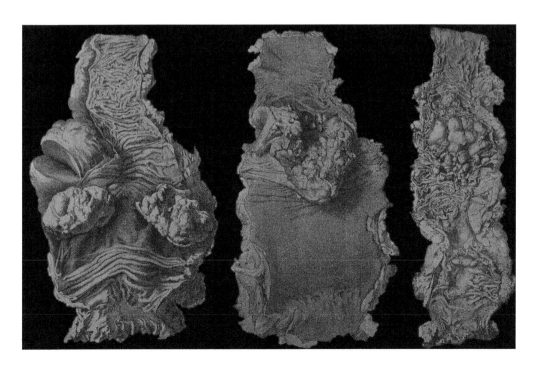

Figure 28.11 Drawings from the first successful abdomino-perineal resections done by Quénu in 1895.

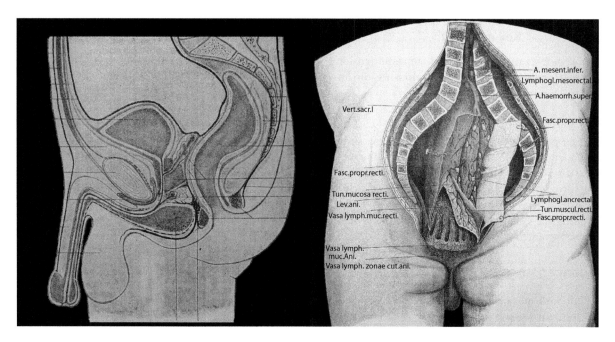

Figure 28.12 Waldeyer described the endopelvic fascia and the importance of these fascias for the anatomy of the pelvis in 1899. One of the first drawings of the mesorectal fascia enveloping the rectum (fascia propria recti). (From Waldeyer W, *Das Becken*, 1st ed., Bonn: Verlag von Friedrich Cohen, 1899.)

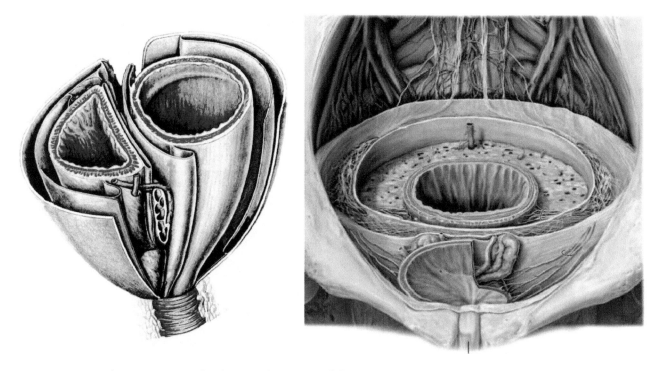

Figure 28.13 *Prometheus Anatomy Atlas* showing the nerves of the pelvis and their relation to the interfascial spaces. (From THIEME atlas Das Becken. In: von Lanz T, Wachsmuth W. Praktische Anatomie:T.8A. Berlin: Springer-Verlag; 1986.)

is called the presacral space and can easily be opened in the midline at the level of the promontory (Figure 28.13). Using sharp dissection the rectum, covered by its mesorectal fascia, can easily be mobilized. At the level of S3–S4 a dense longitudinal connection between the presacral fascia and the mesorectal fascia is encountered: the recto sacral ligament, which has to be cut. Blunt dissection of this structure can lead to disruption of the presacral fascia and damage to the underlying structures like the venous plexus, but also the autonomic nerves, or ventrally the mesorectal fascia can be torn exposing the mesorectal fat and even the tumour, resulting in an incomplete resection.

The ureters are located laterally in this interfascial compartment. On the mesorectal fascia the superior hypogastric nerve and plexus pass through this compartment and have to be dissected carefully from the mesorectal fascia to preserve their function. Just below the peritoneal reflection structures originating laterally and dorsally from the parietal fascia invaginate through the interfascial plane in the direction of the mesorectum; this lympho-neurovascular bundle is called the lateral ligament and contains the middle rectal artery (if present), but also autonomic innervation for the rectum. At this level the superior hypogastric plexus blends with the sympathetic fibres of the sympathetic trunk and the nervi erigentes from the sacral foramina to form the inferior hypogastric plexus. This plexus continues laterally from the genitourinary organs to innervate the bladder and genitals, but in the shape of a T junction it also gives branches to the rectum. During rectal resections it is important just to transect the nerves for the rectum and to preserve the rest of the plexus. More distally, the parietal fascia becomes denser and covers the pelvic floor muscles. Where the mesorectum becomes thin the mesorectal fascia blends with the parietal fascia and in the anorectal canal, the longitudinal muscle layer of the muscularis propria blends also with this combined fascia and continues as the corrugator ani muscle ending in the perianal skin. Anteriorly, the parietal fascia separates the genitourinary structures from the rectum. More proximally the interfascial space is made of Denonvilliers' fascia which can easily be separated from the vagina or prostate; more distally somatic fibres from the pelvic floor muscles and urogenital diaphragm intertwine with the smooth muscularis propria muscle and finally condense as an important anchoring point for muscles: the perineal body (Figure 28.14). For the perineal phase of a rectal resection it is important to realize that there is no interfascial space below Denonvilliers' fascia and dissection in this area may easily result in a false route entering the rectum or urethra in males and the vagina in females.

Surgical technique of TME

During embryological development part of the colon and sigmoid come to lie in a secondary retroperitoneal position. However, the visceral fascia and the parietal retroperitoneal fascia, which cover the retroperitoneal organs and ureter and gonadal vessels, do not fuse and can easily be divided again exposing the mesentery and lymphovascular pedicle, which is an important step in colonic surgery to remove the tumour-bearing segment of the colon. The mobilization of the retroperitoneal part of the sigmoid is not only important for the exposure of the inferior mesenteric artery and its first branch, the left colic artery, but also equally important for the identification of the parietal fascia and correct identification of the interfascial space, which opens the door to the posterolateral interfascial mobilization of the mesorectum and its mesorectal fascia. When the ureter and gonadal vessels seem to be tethered to the mesosigmoid, the dissection

is too lateral to the parietal fascia, and the correct interfascial plane should be looked for medially to the ureter and gonadal vessels.

When the mesosigmoid is mobilized correctly, the inferior mesenteric artery can be transected either 1 cm from its origin on the aorta or just distally from its first branch, the left colic artery. A transection flush at its origin could lead to substantial damage of the superior hypogastric plexus which lies on the aorta. If the left colic artery is preserved the afferent bowel loop for an anastomosis after rectal resection is less mobile. If a long afferent loop is required, the splenic flexure should be taken down and mobilized until the inferior mesenteric vein (IMV) is visible up to its vanishing point behind the inferior border of the pancreas. Transection of the IMV at the inferior border of the pancreas and the IMA 1 cm below its origin in the aorta will result in an optimally long and well-vascularized afferent bowel loop, which will allow any kind of anastomosis (side to end, J pouch or straight) of the descending colon or proximal sigmoid in the lower pelvis.

The incision of the pelvic peritoneum is lateral to the rectum and anterior of the deep peritoneal reflection, in male patients at the level of the arch of the vesicles, in female patients at the level of the posterior fornix. The deepest point of the peritoneal reflection is close to the anterior wall of the rectum and can be tethered to an anterior tumour and should be taken out en bloc with the rectum. In the midline the Denonvilliers' fascia which is part of the retroperitoneal part of the anterior mesorectum can be identified and mobilized.

When the retroperitoneal space is opened, the rectosacral ligament dissected, the neurovascular midrectal pedicle transected and Denonvilliers' fascia fully mobilized, the rectum is mobile until the pelvic floor and ready for transection. The level of transection includes at least 5 cm (if possible) of mesorectal fat and 1 cm of mucosal tube below the tumour. This results (in low and midrectal tumours) in an anastomosis at the pelvic floor (total mesorectal excision [TME]). The lower the anastomosis, the poorer the functional outcome, especially after preoperative radiotherapy. Some authors argue that it is better to preserve a small distal stump of the rectum to improve functional outcomes and to perform a partial mesorectal excision (PME), as it is unlikely, especially after preoperative radiotherapy, that there will be satellite tumour deposits more than 2 cm below the inferior border of the mesorectum [166,167]. The same is true for progression of tumour in the mucosa, and perhaps 5 mm is also acceptable. In higher tumours a PME is possible without compromising oncologic principles [168,169].

Surgical approach for low rectal tumours

The parietal fascia is funnel shaped at the level of the pelvic floor. It is closely adherent to the pelvic floor muscles and blends with the visceral fascia of the distal anorectum, which enters the narrow part of the funnel becoming the

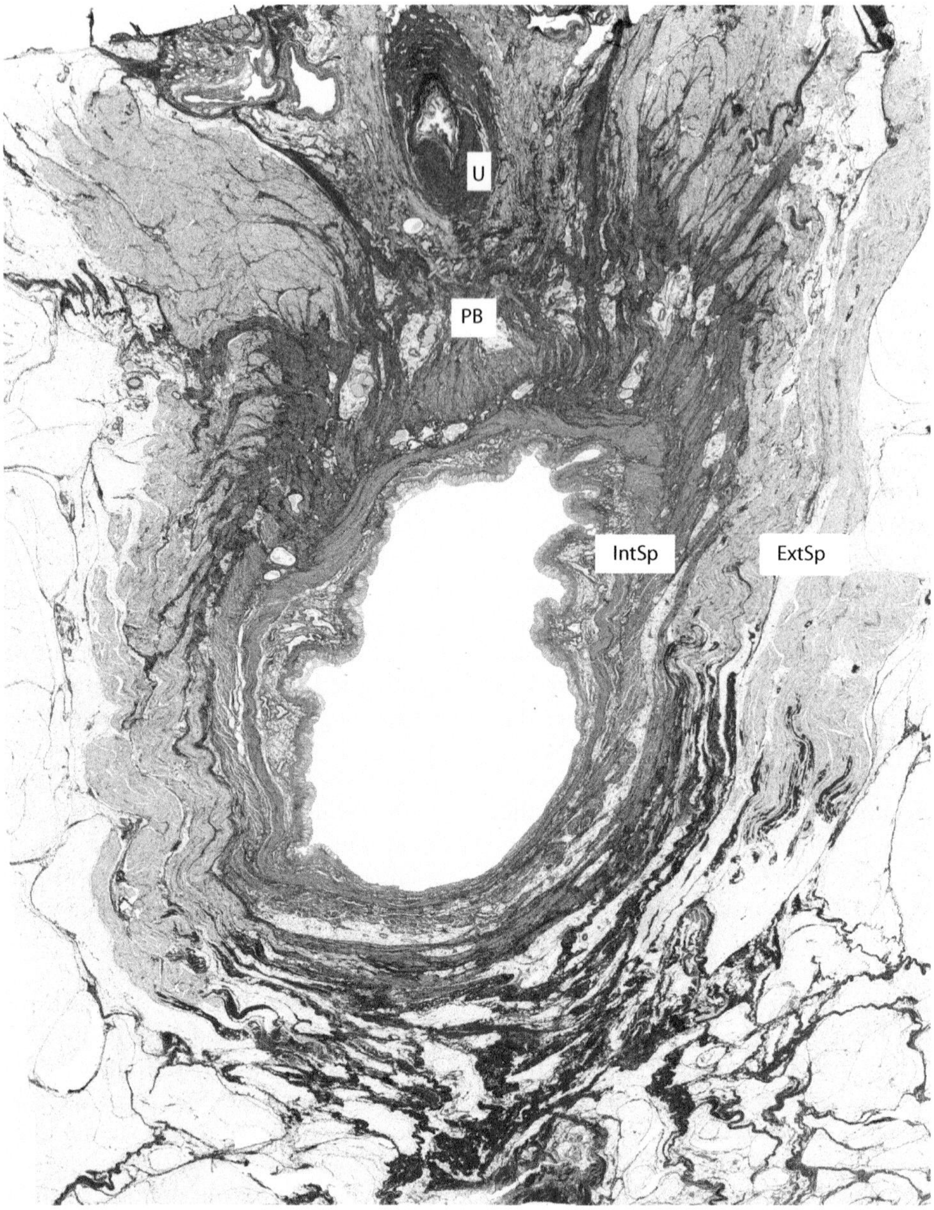

Figure 28.14 Whole mounted slide of distal rectum demonstrating complex relation of the perineal body (PB), internal sphincter (IntSp), external sphincter(ExtSp) and periuretheral muscles (U, urethra). (From http://slides.virtualpathology. leeds.ac.uk/Research_5/LIMM/Nick_West/GIFT/Gift_Rectums/Gift_03_14/extra_Stains/view.apml?.)

internal sphincter muscle, whereas the pelvic floor muscles become the external sphincter. Between the two sphincters the parietal fascia, visceral mesorectal fascia and smooth longitudinal muscle fuse and run farther between the two sphincters as the corrugator ani muscle and end in the perineal skin.

Laterally and dorsally the adherence between internal and external sphincters is slight and allows for the development of an intersphincteric resection plane. On the anterior side the somatic pelvic floor muscles, which distally join in a tendinous perineal body, are very adherent to the anterior part of the anal rectum. Therefore no such thing as an intersphincteric dissection plane is present anteriorly to the distal rectum [170]. This is a very important anatomical fact

which influences the way low rectal tumours can be dissected. An abdomino-perineal excision (APE) can be performed in one of three dissection planes:

1. The intersphincteric plane which is close to the internal sphincter and only suitable for tumours which are confined to the muscularis propria of the rectum.
2. The extra levator plane which follows the external fascia of the external sphincter continuously along the external fascia of the levator ani muscles and transects these muscles as laterally as possible before entering the abdomen.
3. The ischiorectal plane which also removes the ischiorectal fat and follows the external fascia of the pelvis

removing the ischiorectal fat en bloc with the levator ani muscles. Again, the abdomen is entered as laterally as possible at the level of the attachment of the levator ani muscles to the pelvic wall (see Figure 28.16).

In most distal rectal carcinomas the extralevator abdomino perineal excision (ELAPE) is recommended to achieve a complete resection with a negative circumferential resection margin (CRM) [171]. The patient may be either operated on in the supine position with the legs in movable stirrups or turned to the prone position for a perineal approach [172]. When the operation is performed in the supine position the patient does not need to be turned and the procedure can start with either the perineal phase or the abdominal phase.

SUPINE

In the supine position the dissection starts with an incision around and subsequent closure of the anus [173,174] (Figure 28.15). The external perineal fascia which covers the external sphincter can be followed until the lateral attachment of the levator muscle to the pelvic sidewall. At this level the levator ani can be cut exposing the mesorectum. Dorsally, the anococcygeal ligament has to be transected. Depending on the location of the tumour, the presacral space may be entered ventral to the coccyx, or in dorsally located tumours, the coccyx may be removed to enter the presacral space. After transection of the levators on both sides, exposing the mesorectum and opening the presacral space exposing the dorsal part of the distal mesorectum, the anterior dissection may commence. The anterior part of the levator ani muscle encloses the internal genital organs

and needs to be transected at the level of Denonvilliers' fascia. After exposing Denonvilliers' fascia the dissection continues distally. Retracting the specimen dorsally helps to identify the somatic perineal muscles, which are closely adherent to the anorectum. The transection takes place in the somatic muscles avoiding a *fausse route* (French, meaning 'false passage') into the bowel. If the operation was not started with the abdominal phase, the abdomen is opened now. Dissection is according to TME principles avoiding nerve damage. As the pelvic floor muscles are already transected, taking out the specimen is a relatively uncomplicated procedure.

PRONE

If the operation is performed in the prone position the procedure most often starts with the abdominal phase with the patient lying in the supine position [175] (Figure 28.16). Again, care must be taken not to push the dissection too deep down at the risk of coning in, resulting in dissection of the pelvic floor off the mesorectum and subsequent waist formation in the specimen. However, it is important to develop the presacral space until the coccyx is exposed. On the lateral side the low hypogastric plexus has to be dissected off the mesorectum and the lateral pillars also have to be transected. Denonvilliers' fascia has to be exposed before the abdominal phase can be completed and the patient can be turned to the prone position for the perineal phase.

In the prone position a teardrop-like incision is made around the anal skin and extended proximally above the anococcygeal joint. After closure of the anus, the deep perineal fascia is followed from the external sphincter until the lateral attachments of the levator ani. After cutting the

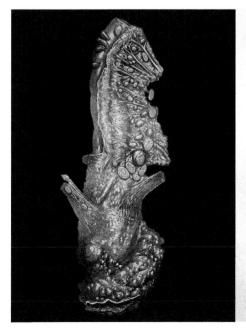 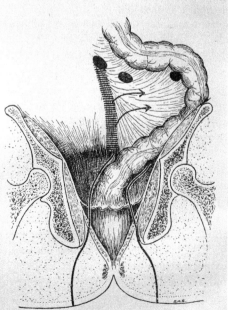

Figure 28.15 Extralevatoric approach described by Miles. (From Miles WE, *Cancer of the Rectum*, London: Harrison and Sons, 1926.)

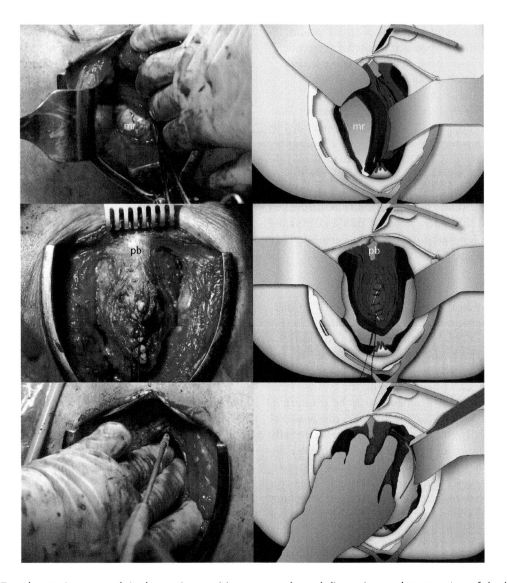

Figure 28.16 Extralevatoric approach in the supine position: posterolateral dissection and transection of the levator ani muscles exposing the mesorectum (mr). Anteriorly the specimen is attached at the level of the perineal body (pb). Subsequently downward traction and working from inside out facilitates the anterior dissection. (From Orsini RG, et al., *Eur J Cancer Suppl* 2013, 11(2), 60–71.)

coccyx the already opened presacral space is entered and the lateral attachments of the levator ani can be cut. After arriving at the level of Denonvilliers' fascia, the specimen can be everted through the perineal wound and the dissection of the anterior plane of the specimen commences under direct vision. First, the puborectal sling has to be cut, as must also the deep perineal muscles which are closely adherent to the anterior part of the anorectum. Again the dissection is carried out from proximally to distally. Cutting the perineal body is the last part of the operation before taking out the specimen. Care must be taken not to damage the urethra and the neural bundles of Walsh, which are very close to this dissection plane.

In both positions a complete extralevator abdominoperineal excision can be performed. In the prone position visibility of the perineal operating field is improved at the cost of a longer incision, which requires closure with a (biological) mesh or musculocutaneous flap [176]. In the supine position simultaneous access to the tumour from the abdomen and perineum may be an advantage in more advanced tumours. An intersphincteric or ischiorectal approach is more commonly performed in the supine position. In both positions, the abdominal phase may also be performed laparoscopically.

After exposing the coccyx and the lateral attachment of the levator ani muscle, the coccyx is transected likewise the levator ani muscle is transected starting dorsally and continuing in ventral direction. Next, the rectum is everted allowing for the dissection of the anterior plane exposing the prostate and vesiculae seminales (vs) [177].

LAPAROSCOPIC SURGERY FOR CRC

Introduction

Minimally invasive surgery for cancer of the colon and rectum is increasingly performed in daily surgical practice. Of note is the highly variable degree of implementation between and within European countries [178,179]. This is mainly related to the availability of well-trained laparoscopic surgeons and adequate equipment, as well as residual scepticism about the advantages among some surgeons. The main area of concern for sceptics of laparoscopic cancer surgery was oncological safety (complete resection, sufficient lymph node harvest and port site recurrences). These fears are now outdated by the increasing body of evidence showing superiority of short-term results [180]. Supervised training in laparoscopic techniques is necessary to perform laparoscopic resection of CRC. For the principles of training refer to the website of the European Association for Endoscopic Surgery (EAES) (www.eaes-eur.org) and www.websurg.com.

In 1902 the first laparoscopic procedure was described in dogs and in 1910 in humans. Minimally invasive surgery was implemented in gastrointestinal surgery in 1990. Cholecystectomy was the first laparoscopic procedure recommended over an open approach. Most laparoscopic colon and rectal resections can be performed with between three and six ports or trocars. Open-insertion techniques for the first access port for creation of the pneumoperitoneum are thought to be safest compared to use of the Veress needle [181,182]. Tilting the patient on the table in the opposite direction of the working field will move the intestines away and improve exposure.

One of the difficulties in performing laparoscopic surgery for CRC is that not every patient is equally suitable for minimally invasive surgery, mostly due to abdominal adhesions or advanced disease, although this is only the minority of patients in experienced hands. Dissection can also be problematic in the obese, leading to longer operation times, using more ports and sometimes a higher conversion rate [183].

The early advantages of laparoscopic resection of colon cancer include reduced postoperative pain and blood loss, earlier return of bowel function and shorter length of hospital stay [184–187]. Laparoscopic total mesorectal excision (TME) is associated with less blood loss ($p < 0.05$; two studies), earlier return to normal dietary intake, reduced postoperative pain and reduced analgesics use in a Cochrane review including 48 studies ($n = 4224$ patients) [188]. In the update of the Cochrane review published in 2014, 14 randomized controlled studies were included analyzing 3528 patients with rectal cancer. Benefits were reported on short- and long-term outcomes; local recurrence, 5-year disease-free survival and overall survival rates were similar [189]. Postoperative complications, anastomotic leakage and mortality were similar between open and laparoscopic

rectal cancer surgery; moreover, laparoscopy reduced hospital stay by an average of 2 days [12]. The COLOR II trial, a non-inferiority phase III trial randomizing 1103 patients to laparoscopic rectal surgery or open surgery, showed improved recovery with similar short-term results with respect to margins, completeness of resection, 28-day mortality, anastomotic leaks and re-interventions [190]. The laparoscopic approach in a fast-track setting showed the shortest length of hospital stay [191]. A meta-analysis of five randomized controlled trials (RCTs) revealed that in laparoscopic colorectal surgery, ERAS was associated with fewer complications (RR 0.67) than traditional perioperative care [192].

Laparoscopic surgery long-term results

No significant differences in overall survival, local recurrence and distant metastasis rates between laparoscopic and open surgery were found in a Cochrane review based on 12 studies, for both colon and rectal cancer [193]. Two trials reported survival rates per tumour stage and no significant differences in survival between laparoscopic and open surgery among stages I, II and III were found [194,195]. However, heterogeneity of follow-up and missing actuarial survival data in five studies may have influenced the results of the meta-analyses.

Potential long-term advantages of laparoscopic surgery for CRC are a reduction in the rates of incisional hernias and adhesive small bowel obstruction. A population-based study from the UK demonstrated a significant reduction in admission or re-intervention for adhesions [196], although data from Swedish patients participating in the COLOR I trial showed no difference in readmission due to adhesions or small bowel obstruction [195]. Long-term results from the Dutch LAFA study showed that open resection was associated with a significantly higher rate of incisional hernia (OR 2.44) and adhesion-related small bowel obstruction (OR 3.70) compared to laparoscopic surgery [197].

Learning curve in laparoscopic surgery

Miskovic and colleagues studied the learning curve for different outcome factors using cumulative sum charts [198]. The learning curve in days stretched from 87 for blood loss to 152 for conversion. Once again, the need for training of laparoscopic colorectal surgery under supervised conditions is underlined here [199]. The quality of laparoscopic colorectal surgery needs to be monitored using nationwide clinical auditing [178].

Conversion in laparoscopic surgery

Conversion rates in laparoscopic colorectal surgery are approximately 15%–18% [178,189,200]. Subgroup analyses of the randomized trials suggested negative outcomes of conversion from laparoscopic to open surgery, due to more blood loss, longer operating time, longer hospital stay and higher risk of recurrence without an impact on survival [26,200–202]. A methodological limitation of this study was that the converted laparoscopy group was compared to completed laparoscopic procedures, while comparison to open surgery would be more appropriate.

Conversion can be either pre-emptive (early) or reactive (late) [203]. Pre-emptive conversion can be considered a laparoscopic exploration followed by open resection in less suitable cases. Reactive conversion is the result of complications intraoperatively. As expected, reactive conversion has a negative impact on outcome.

Cost-effectiveness

Laparoscopic procedures were thought to be more expensive since they have a lengthier operation time and frequently use expensive disposables and specific equipment. Nevertheless, laparoscopic resection is cost-effective due to its short-term advantages and shorter hospital stay [204,205]. A prospective study from the UK demonstrated that the operative costs were higher for laparoscopic surgery than for the open approach (£2049 vs. £1263), due to the costs of disposable instruments. On the contrary, laparoscopy was accompanied by a reduction of hospital stay resulting in reduced hospital costs (£1807 vs. £3468) [206]. Another cost-effectiveness study showed a benefit of £699 in hospital bed days [207].

PERIOPERATIVE CONDITIONS AND THEIR MANAGEMENT IN THE CRC PATIENT

Nutrition is of vital importance to the CRC surgery patient. Further details of the role of nutrition in cancer surgery are given in chapter 11.

Fast-track or ERAS protocols

Enhanced Recovery After Surgery (ERAS) protocols promote an oral diet after surgery as soon as tolerated [208]. Fast-track protocols in surgery were developed to reduce surgical complications by implementing a multimodal protocol of 'as good as possible' evidence-based tools to accomplish early recovery after surgery [209]. This was first done for patients undergoing colectomy and later was also implemented for the care of patients undergoing total mesorectal resection or liver surgery. ERAS focuses on the following standardized protocol elements: improving patient education, reducing pain, reducing nausea and vomiting, stimulating normal dietary intake and early patient mobilization [208]. Implementation of fast-track projects has resulted in large reductions in length of hospital stay [210]. The main challenge to optimize perioperative care remains a constant team effort on the part of the patient, surgeon, anaesthesiologists, general practitioner and nurses.

Prevention of postoperative ileus is achieved by implementing several components of the protocol, such as maintaining adequate pain control, prescribing antiemetic drugs, minimizing surgical trauma, maintaining normotension by optimization of intravenous fluids [211] and promoting early mobilization and early nutrition.

Postoperative ileus

After surgical procedures, a temporary postoperative ileus is present in most patients varying in severity according to the manipulation [212] or transection of viscera and the implementation of ERAS protocol components [213]. Postoperative ileus is defined as the inability to have normal intake or stool due to symptoms of anorexia, nausea, vomiting or absent bowel movements and defecation. Postoperative ileus results in increased health care costs, due to longer duration of hospital stay, more prescribed drugs and prescribed artificial nutrition [213]. Artificial nutrition such as enteral feeds and parenteral formulas is known for its route-dependent complications, such as tube dislodgement, accidental removal and occlusion and line infections [214]. Both can adequately supply calories and proteins relevant for recovery after surgery. Randomizing early enteral versus early parenteral in a group of patients undergoing surgery for locally advanced or recurrent rectal malignancies, a reduction of postoperative ileus, anastomotic dehiscence and hospital stay was observed in the post-pylorically fed patients [214].

POSTOPERATIVE COMPLICATIONS AND SURGICAL PERFORMANCE

Anastomotic leakage and protective stoma

In CRC surgery, the most feared complication is anastomotic leakage causing abdominal sepsis, usually leading to one or more reoperations and formation of a stoma or even to death. Patients with leaks have a worse long-term outcome than patients who do not leak [215]. Anastomotic leakage is seen in restorative CRC surgery at rates ranging from 5% to 19% of cases. The causes and risk factors are variable [215–218].

In a systematic review and meta-analysis, it was concluded that anastomotic leakage is associated with higher rates of local recurrences and a reduced long-term cancer-specific survival [216]. This finding was confirmed by a more recent nationwide cohort study of the Danish Colorectal Cancer Group (*n* = 9333), showing an anastomotic leakage rate of 6.4%, which also led to reduced use of adjuvant chemotherapy in stage III colon cancer [217].

A pelvic abscess is variably classified as a leak; however, it might not always lead to a reoperation. If possible a percutaneous radiological drainage and antibiotics may result in resolution. A CT scan is recommended when leakage is suspected based on clinical and biochemical parameters; however, it should be remembered that a false negative CT scan does not rule out anastomotic leakage fully [219].

Factors impacting on leaks

The anastomosis is formed by connecting the afferent and efferent loops of the ileum, colon and rectum and is formed by staplers, hand sewn or using mixed techniques. The healing (or otherwise) of the intestine is dependent on numerous factors in the perioperative period. For example, the volume of fluid resuscitation matters (normovolemia is optimal); use of vasopressors intraoperatively, perioperative oxygen supply (oxygen saturations of more than 97% are thought to be beneficial for the anastomosis), careful tissue handling, reduction of blood loss, accurate stapling and tying during operation and, lastly, no torsion or tension on the bowel loops contribute to the anastomosis [220,221]. Adequate pain control (pain negatively impacts on the levels of inflammatory mediators [cytokines]), preventing postoperative ileus, and an inadequate intake of nutrients are all associated with worse clinical outcomes, especially infectious complications. Nutritional status (malnutrition before and during the postoperative period) and patient comorbidities (diabetes, obesity, smoking alcoholism, cardiovascular diseases) may impact on anastomotic healing [214,220,221]. Even NSAIDs are thought to influence the rate of anastomotic leaks and the inflammatory status postoperatively in animal models and might be associated with anastomotic leakage in humans [222,223].

To prevent or protect against anastomotic leakage in high-risk cases a double-loop ileostomy or colostomy is formed. This is advisable in high-risk patients such as in ultra-low rectal cancers or due to patient factors such as old age (frequently accompanied by frailty, poor appetite, sarcopenia and malnutrition [224]).

Some schools advise a protective stoma in all, since it reduces the occurrence in anastomotic leaks in relatively high-incidence populations [218]; however, considerable morbidity and leakage of stoma repair surgeries should be anticipated in the postoperative course of temporary stomas.

There is no proof of superiority of an ileostomy over a colostomy: both have their complications which need to be considered in conjunction with the wishes of the patient [225]. Ileostomies are known for their high fluid outputs and risk of dehydration, which may ultimately lead to renal failure if not correctly managed, while colostomies are known to lead to prolapse and wound closure infections [226].

In ileocolic stapled anastomosis does better than a hand-sewn anastomosis and the same holds true for closure of loop ileostomies [157,227,228]. No superiority could be found in the techniques of stapling versus hand sewn for colorectal anastomosis in the Cochrane systematic review examining nine trials [229].

Postoperative complications of CRC surgery

In random order:

1. Infectious – anastomotic leakage, central line infection, thrombophlebitis, pneumonia, intra-abdominal abscess, sepsis and peritonitis, urinary tract infection, wound infection
2. Postoperative ileus and malnutrition – transient hyperglycemia, neo-diabetes
3. Decompensation cordis, arrhythmias, myocardial infarction, electrolyte disturbances
4. Pulmonary atelectasis and pneumothorax, secondary pleural effusion
5. Intestinal ischemia
6. Pulmonary embolus, deep vein thrombosis
7. Compartment syndrome of lower leg
8. Bleeding, iatrogenic splenic injury
9. Necrosis of ostomy, dermatitis, adjacent abscess, retraction or prolapse of stoma

Symptoms of anastomotic leaks

Symptoms of an anastomotic leak are very wide ranging and sometimes non-specific; therefore, it may be difficult to diagnose an anastomotic leak and this can lead to an unfavourable delay in treatment.

The symptoms of an early leak are quite often those of abdominal sepsis, while leaks occurring later may be more vague: a patient who is not recovering as anticipated, presenting with anorexia, nausea, vomiting, absence of bowel sounds and flatus, sometimes abdominal pain and sometimes fever.

The air leak test could be used during surgery to reduce the risks and a postoperative C-reactive protein (CRP) on day 3 or 4 may be indicative. Clinical algorithms may reduce the time to diagnosis and a CT with rectal contrast is advised to confirm the suspicion of a leak [230,231].

Quality of life and functional loss after rectal surgery

In rectal cancer surgery, the technique of total mesorectal resection (TME) has improved locoregional relapse and survival [132,232]. At diagnosis, the main focus for rectal cancer patients is treatment of and long-term cure of their cancer. However, cancer survivors need to live with the impact of the treatment on their quality of life and bowel functioning [233]. This frequently includes dealing with urinary and faecal urgency, clustering, incontinence or living with an ileostomy or colostomy and sexual dysfunction.

Both rectal cancer surgery and radiotherapy can have a negative impact on the pelvic nerves. The Low Anterior Resection Syndrome (LARS) Score is a five-item instrument for evaluation of bowel function and is very appropriate for patients after rectal surgery [234]. Scandinavian studies have reported frequent, long-term functional problems in patients receiving neoadjuvant treatment compared to patients having TME surgery alone [235–237]. Faecal incontinence is described in 15% of patients having surgery alone versus 49% of patients having preoperative radiotherapy. Urgency is admitted to by 16% and 44%, and sanitary pads are needed by 13% and 52% of the same two groups. Nine or more daily bowel movements are reported by 3% versus 19%, and urinary incontinence increases from 2% to 9% following radiotherapy. Dyspareunia is seen in 11% of patients having surgery alone versus 35% for women also having radiotherapy, and the erectile dysfunction score is reduced from 14 to 7 by radiotherapy. A restricted social life is reported by 7% of patients treated by surgery alone versus 35% of patients treated by radiotherapy and surgery. Hip fracture occurs in 1% of the patients after surgery alone versus 5% for rectal surgery and radiotherapy, and the rate of a second cancer is doubled by radiotherapy, from 4.3% to 9.5% [238].

Follow-up after CRC

Follow-up schemes are different at different sites. A practical combination is to measure CEA levels preoperatively for a baseline value and postoperatively, four times during the first 2 years, then biannually or yearly. In addition, once a year an abdominal CT should be performed to rule out liver metastasis, in combination with an annual chest x-ray which is comparable informatively to a chest CT. A complete colonoscopy in the first 3 years is necessary to rule out metachronous invasive neoplasia and polyps. In case of symptoms other imaging could be indicated to perform.

Lifestyle recommendations to prevent CRC include increasing dietary fibre, reducing red and processed meat consumption, reducing alcoholic drinks and engaging in regular physical exercise.

Time trends

Using population-based analysis of relative survival, which can be explained by the use of a correction for the average mortality at any age and sex [2], in the countries analyzed in the EUROCARE project, survival of CRC has markedly improved since the 1980s. From 1980 until 2000–2002, 5-year survival for all patients increased from 51% to 60% in northern Europe, from 52 to 62% in western European registries and from 45% to 58% in southern European registries. Some groups did not see the improvement, such as elderly patients and patients with stage IV disease [2]. Moreover, it was observed that improvements in survival took place during the 1990s and were more important for rectal than for colon cancer patients, with the exception of eastern European countries, levelling 5-year survival for patients with colon and rectal cancer [2].

Population-based studies describe the incidence (new cases), prevalence (all cases) and mortality of all cases in a certain predefined area.

Overall survival represents the proportion of people alive with a certain diagnosis.

Disease-specific survival estimates the proportion of people.

Relative survival analyzes deaths due to the disease in a single time period and equals the total number of deaths (overall number of deaths) minus the expected number of deaths in the general population.

Changeable risk factors for CRC

The risk for CRC can be modified, especially in males. The most recent, systematic review of the evidence concluded that there is convincing evidence that increased consumption of red and processed meat and alcoholic drinks (especially among males) and body and abdominal fatness all increase the risk for CRC, especially in taller people [239]. There is substantial evidence that foods containing dietary fibre reduce the risk of CRC [100]. Regular physical activity reduces the risk for colon cancer as well [240].

Smoking has also been associated with an increased risk of CRC with long latency times [241]. Some drugs have been related to CRC risk, such as statins, although no consistent evidence was found in a meta-analysis [242]. Oral contraceptive was found protective regarding CRC risk [243]. Aspirin might also be a chemopreventive agent, especially among patients with Lynch syndrome. Notwithstanding without consensus about the dose and the long-term balance between risk and benefit further prospective research is being initiated [244].

EFFECT OF AGEING AND COMORBIDITY ON CRC TREATMENT

The physiologic changes of ageing vary widely among individuals. All bodily functions become weaker, but not necessarily in the same range. For major abdominal surgery the impact of different physiological changes differs. Therefore it is obvious that calendar age is not an appropriate measure for decision making [245]. In elderly comorbidity is often present, even multiple comorbidities. Again, different comorbidities also have different impacts on treatment [246]. Figure 28.17 represents the patterns of different comorbid diseases in Dutch CRC patients according to age. In this population-based sample 30% of patients < 60 years suffered from comorbidities compared to 71% of the patients aged > 80 years [247]. In addition, a rising prevalence of comorbidities in all age groups was found during the study period. Regardless of age, having comorbidity is associated with adverse outcome after colorectal surgery (Figure 28.18) [248,249]. In the elderly,

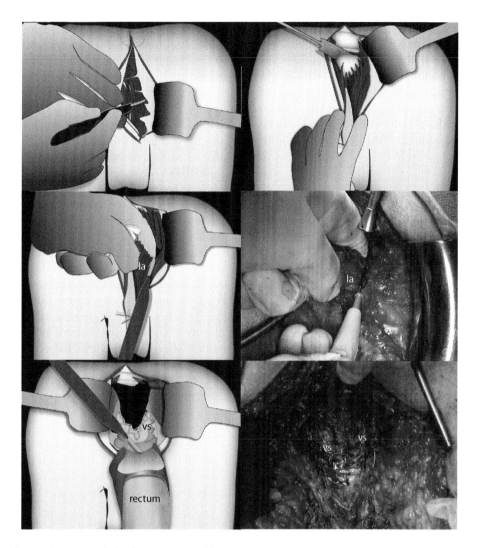

Figure 28.17 Extralevatoric approach in the prone position.

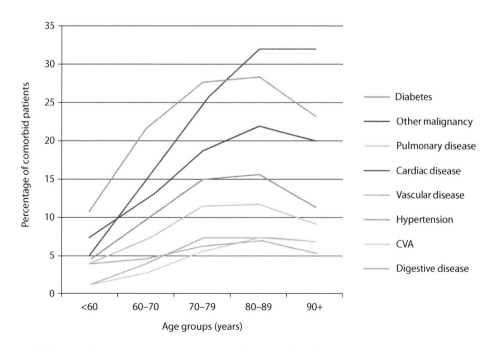

Figure 28.18 Comorbidity in relation to age. (Courtesy Dutch Surgical Colorectal Audit.)

acute presentations of CRC have more impact on physiology and outcome than in younger patients [250].

Frailty or absence of frailty refers to the functional reserve, necessary to undergo multimodality treatment for CRC. The limited functional reserve results in poor coping with complications resulting in a high postoperative mortality. In the elderly, risk for postoperative mortality can be protracted as long as 6 to 12 months [251,252].

Key message

Functional reserve is more compromised in the elderly, due to physiologic ageing and the prevalence of multiple comorbidities, especially in the acute situation.

Thirty-day postoperative mortality is not a good measure for true postoperative mortality in the elderly.

During the last decades cancer registry data show a steady improvement in overall survival of CRC patients. However, when these data are split according to age it is clear that only the younger patients seem to benefit from better imaging and treatment. In the elderly patients overall survival did not improve significantly [251,253,254]. Excess mortality related to the treatment compromises their results. However, if corrected for age and first year excess mortality, older patients seem to have the same prognosis as their younger counterparts [255]. Paradoxically better treatment improving oncological outcome is also responsible for an increase in the mortality rate.

The complexity of the health condition of elderly CRC patients requires a tailor-made individualized approach. A more comprehensive assessment, including non-typical oncologic disciplines like a cardiologist, pulmonologist or geriatrician, may be the base for the discussion in a multidisciplinary team before any oncologic treatment is started, which in turn can help to counsel the patient and his family and result in a well-informed shared decision about the treatment plan [117–119].

Often life expectancy of an elderly patient is underestimated; i.e. an 80-year-old has a median life expectancy of 9 years [256]. In curable CRC, a palliative approach certainly would be undertreatment. The challenge is to find a less toxic alternative curative approach.

Surgery remains the cornerstone of CRC treatment. Alternatives for surgery are limited: in rectal cancer, neoadjuvant treatment can lead to a complete response, which would allow for a wait-and-see approach. Unfortunately, only the minority of patients will experience a complete response. In the future intensification of neoadjuvant treatment may lead to more complete responders. Promising research is looking at intensification of irradiation with endorectal brachytherapy or endorectal irradiation with the Papillon technique to increase the rate of complete responders [257–260]. As long as response is observed, surgery

may be postponed; it may take several months to achieve a complete response. The interim results of the Stockholm III trial, comparing short-course radiotherapy followed by immediate surgery, short-course radiotherapy followed by delayed surgery and long-course radiotherapy and delayed surgery, show that delay in surgery results in good downsizing and less postoperative complications [261]. The lessons learned from this trial could be that sufficient waiting time between treatment modalities should be allowed for, especially in the elderly. In view of the small differences in outcome between chemoradiation, this may be replaced by long- or short-course radiotherapy avoiding the systemic toxicity of chemotherapy.

The use of adjuvant chemotherapy can be debated. The elderly are underrepresented in chemotherapy trials and on a population-based level the limited advantage of the widespread use of chemotherapy must be counterbalanced against the increased morbidity in elderly patients [262,263]. In most population-based studies survival is better after adjuvant chemotherapy, but this could also be the result of selection bias [264]. The best approach could be not to advocate chemotherapy except in the fit elderly patient.

In colon cancer major surgery in acute situations may be too demanding for the physiological reserve of the patient. In these cases, the smallest intervention would be the safest. Stenting should be considered to bridge the symptoms of acute obstruction and to allow for prehabilitation before the final resection [265]. If surgery is unavoidable, a double-barrel, right-sided colostomy for a left-sided obstruction or an ileotransversostomy for a right-sided obstruction is the safer alternative. If resection of the tumour is performed, an anastomosis can be avoided by creating a double-barrel stoma of the afferent and efferent loops in proximal tumours, or a Hartmann's procedure in distal colonic tumours.

If still necessary, major surgery can be performed in a fully optimized patient.

Key message

Avoid major surgery in the acute situation in the suboptimally prepared patient.

OBSTRUCTIVE COLON CANCER, ACUTE SURGERY OR COLONIC STENTING

About 10%–15% of patients with colon cancers present with obstructive symptoms. The clinical presentation of obstructive disease can be mild abdominal distension with an absence of stools, resolving after conservative management using enemas and laxatives, a complete obstruction requiring a decompressing intervention, or an acute abdomen with signs of abdominal sepsis in case of a blowout of the caecum requiring emergency surgery. Obstructive colon cancer is associated with substantial morbidity and mortality. In addition, obstruction impairs oncological outcomes [266].

It is still a matter of debate how to treat left-sided obstructing colon cancer. The mortality rate of emergency surgery for obstructive CRC was nearly 15% in a British dataset [267]. Minimally invasive decompression by using a metal stent in the acute setting followed by elective resection after decompression appeared a more successful strategy. The alternative treatment for decompression is formation of a diverting colostomy for acute management; unfortunately this is accompanied by stoma-related morbidity. If curative intent is a possibility, diverting colostomy may be followed by elective resection with closing of the colostomy (two-stage procedure), or stoma closure in a third procedure (three-stage procedure). In the palliative setting, a diverting colostomy often becomes a permanent stoma, and stenting seems to be a more attractive approach.

Diverting colostomy versus acute resection

To answer the question whether we should remove the obstructing tumour in the acute setting, only one randomized controlled trial (RCT) has been published, in 1995. Kronborg and colleagues randomized 58 patients to first a colostomy via laparotomy and second removal of the tumour and anastomosis, and 63 patients to an acute resection with either a Hartmann's procedure or anastomosis [268]. A permanent colostomy was less often observed in patients undergoing staged resection (3/35 vs. 14/50, $p < 0.05$). Postoperative mortality or cancer-specific survival was similar between the groups. A more recent study observed a lower mortality rate after initial decompressing colostomy through a small transverse incision compared to acute resection (1% vs. 8%) [269].

Stent versus emergency surgery

Using a stent to settle the bowel wall before resection of the tumour and formation of the anastomosis for left-sided obstructive colon cancer initially looked very promising [265,270]. Several RCTs comparing stenting and acute resection were designed to test the hypothesis of superiority; however, most of them were underpowered and four RCTs prematurely stopped because of stent-related problems in three trials. The overall technical success rate of stent placement is about 70%, but ranges from 47% to 100% among the individual studies. Stent-related perforations within 30 days have been observed in up to 13% [271,272] and long-term perforations in up to 40% [272]. Two trials reported occult perforations that were identified during pathological examination of the resected specimen with a stent in place. The overall occult perforation rate in these two trials was 11/45 (24%).

Several meta-analyses have been published, all concluding quite similarly on this topic.

Tan and colleagues [273] found no difference in in-hospital mortality, anastomotic leakage and 30-day reoperation rates based on four RCTs [272,274,275]. Though early stoma formation was significantly lower in the stent group, there was a trend in favour of the stent group with respect to the number of permanent stomas.

Stent versus diverting colostomy

Two RCTs compared stenting with elective diverting colostomy in palliative patients [276,277]. In the trial of Xinopoulos and colleagues 6 of 15 patients developed tumour ingrowth into the stent, which was treated by laser [278]. In a prospective cohort (2005–2013) all consecutive patients with palliative endoscopic placement of self-expanding metal stents (SEMSs) for obstructive colon cancer were selected. The clinical success rate was 85%; however, stent-related mortality was 13%, all related to perforation of the stent. The eventual rate of stoma formation in this group was 15% [279].

Clinical decision making

After the original enthusiasm about colorectal stenting, this procedure has now become controversial due to serious complications of which perforation is the most important. Stenting has been associated with a negative impact on oncological outcomes in the curative setting [280–282]. Colonic stenting is implemented differently in Europe. In the UK, stenting is considered the standard of care by many surgeons who often perform the stent placement themselves, but the results of the recently completed CREST trial will probably influence practice in the UK. In contrast, stenting has been practically abandoned in France, Sweden, Norway and the Netherlands. The European Society of Gastrointestinal Endoscopy (ESGE) initiated an evidence-based multidisciplinary guideline on endoscopic stenting for left-sided malignant colonic obstruction. This guideline has been recently published and was endorsed by the American Society for Gastrointestinal Endoscopy (ASGE). Based on the available evidence, it was concluded that use of a stent as a bridge to surgery in the curative setting is not recommended as standard treatment, but may be considered in patients with an increased risk of postoperative mortality (i.e. age > 70 years, ASA > II) [283].

It seems that in patients with a reduced life expectancy stenting could be considered a good palliative care option. Of note, late perforations can occur if anti-angiogenic agents like bevacizumab are administered in the palliative setting [284]. A diverting colostomy, on the other hand, has its stoma-related morbidity. To aid in medical decisions, CT staging in the acute setting is very important to assess locoregional involvement of the tumour and the presence of intra-abdominal metastasis. Bowel perforation seen as free abdominal air can be adequately identified by CT, even without contrast.

Treatment of left-sided colonic obstruction should be a patient-tailored approach. The elderly frail patient with a short stenosis that is technically considered to be a 'stentable' lesion is probably a good candidate for a stent as a bridge to surgery in the curative setting, rather than acute resection [285]. In healthy patients (i.e. below 70 years of age without significant co-morbidities), acute resection should be considered as the standard of care. For patients not suitable for stenting and with a high operative risk, a diverting colostomy is a suitable treatment option. This procedure does not have the disadvantages of a laparotomy in the acute setting. A diverting transverse colostomy as a bridge to elective (laparoscopic) resection of the primary tumour, also referred to as a 'blow hole', is a very effective surgical approach [286,287]. Finally, given the clinical problems associated with obstruction, early detection and treatment are of utmost importance. This may be achieved by reducing the symptom-to-diagnosis and symptom-to-treatment intervals [288].

ADJUVANT CHEMOTHERAPY FOR CRC

Cancer surgeons with a special expertise in the treatment of CRC should have a good understanding of the fundamentals of the most frequently prescribed medicines in medical oncology for neoadjuvant, adjuvant and palliative therapies for colorectal carcinoma. Traditional chemotherapeutic agents are cytotoxic and act by killing rapidly dividing cells, also harming healthy cells with a normally rapid turnover, such as bone marrow, intestinal cells, skin and hair. This results in the most common side effects of chemotherapy: myelosuppression (decreased production of blood cells, also called immunosuppression), mucositis (inflammation of the lining of the digestive tract) and in some cases alopecia (hair loss). Hair loss does not occur with the first-line chemotherapeutics used for CRC.

Most chemotherapy regimens for CRC combine the fluoropyrimidine *5-FU* or its oral prodrug *capecitabine* with *oxaliplatin* or *irinotecan*, both in the adjuvant (high-risk stage II colon cancer and node positive colon cancer [289]) and palliative (stage IV colon and rectal cancer) settings. At this moment several studies have shown that adjuvant chemotherapy for rectal cancer does not result in clear benefits for disease-free survival or overall survival (Table 28.3) [290,291].

The antitumour activity of the fluoropyrimidines was first reported by Charles Heidelberger in his report in *Nature* of 1957 [292]. Response rates increase by around 10% when a combination is given. Of note, one-half of the patients treated with chemotherapeutic agents do not benefit from antineoplastic agents. Systemic toxicity, including neutropenia, stomatitis, diarrhoea and hand–food syndrome, can lead to dose reduction or noncompliance [293].

Pooled analysis of patients completely resected for stage II colon cancer receiving adjuvant chemotherapy did not show a benefit in overall survival. However, disease-free survival was significantly better [294].

Capecitabine and 5-FU

Capecitabine (Xeloda) is an orally administered chemotherapeutic agent, which is a prodrug, which is enzymatically converted to 5-fluorouracil (5-FU) in the body. Both are from the chemotherapy group called antimetabolites.

The single-agent response rates of 5-FU are around 20% to 25% of patients with advanced stage CRC. 5-FU is an anticancer prodrug that is converted intracellularly into three leading active metabolites, and one of these nucleotides form thymine. Thymine is a nucleic acid in DNA. The beneficial effect of 5-FU-based chemotherapy is associated with expression levels of more than a few genes including thymidylate synthase (TS) and dihydropyrimidine dehydrogenase (DPD). 5-FU is a TS inhibitor.

Inhibition of TS blocks thymidylate production and therefore rapidly stops DNA synthesis and repair and prompts apoptosis. Though inconsistent results on TS protein and mRNA expression have been reported, a number of independent studies constantly agreed that low levels of intratumoural TS protein and mRNA expression are robust prognostic markers for response to 5-FU-based chemotherapy regimens in CRC.

DPD deficiency

Dihydropyrimidine dehydrogenase (DPD) is involved in pyrimidine degradation; it catalyzes the reduction of uracil and thymine. Around 8% of the population have inherited at least partial DPD deficiency; total DPD deficiency is thought to be present in 0.2% of the population [295]. These patients are at risk for severe and lethal toxicity when encountering 5-FU and capecitabine. Patients should be informed about this potentially serious side effect.

Oxaliplatin

Oxaliplatin (Eloxatin) is a platinum-based antineoplastic agent. Its mechanism of action is to damage the DNA of tumours in a non-targeted way by forming DNA strand cross links which prevent replication and transcription and ultimately result in cell death.

The side effects of oxaliplatin treatment can potentially include neurotoxicity (leading to chemotherapy-induced peripheral neuropathy), hand–foot syndrome, fatigue, nausea, vomiting, diarrhoea, neutropenia (low number of a type of white blood cells), ototoxicity and persistent hiccups, and some patients may experience an allergic reaction to platinum-containing drugs [297].

Irinotecan

Irinotecan (Camptosar, CPT-11) is thought to work by blocking the action of an enzyme in cells called topoisomerase I. In chemical terms, it is a semisynthetic analogue of the natural alkaloid camptothecin. Blocking this enzyme leads to breaks in the DNA, which leads to cell death. Its main use is in colon cancer, in combination with other antineoplastic agents, for instance, the treatment FOLFIRI, which is a combination of intravenous 5-fluorouracil, leucovorin and irinotecan. Not all patients benefit from adding irinotecan to the schedule [305].

Table 28.3 Recent phase III randomized trials on adjuvant chemotherapy including resected colon cancer patients stage II, III or both

Study acronym First author Journal Year	Patient population	Study arm	Control arm	Third or fourth study arm	Design	Primary end point	Follow-up (years)	Results
X-ACT Twelves Ann Oncol 2012 [296]	Resected Stage III colon	Oral capecitabine N = 1004	Bolus 5-FU/FA N = 983		Multicentre Randomized Open label Phase III	DFS	4.3	Oral capecitabine is effective alternative to 5-FU
XELOXA Haller J Clin Oncol 2011 [297]	Resected Stage III colon	XELOX N = 938	FU/FA N = 926		Multinational Open label Randomized Phase III	DFS	5.9	XELOX 31% relapse vs. 37.5% in the control HR 0.8, DFS benefit OS ns
MOSAIC Andre J Clin Oncol 2009 [298]	Resected Stage II and III colon N = 2407	FOLFOX4 N = 1123 59.8% stage 3	LV-5-FU-2 N = 1123 60.1% stage 3		Multicentre Randomized Phase III	DFS	5 6	Improved 5 y DFS and 6 y OS in the study arm 73.3% vs. 67.4% DFS
NSABP-C07 Kuebler J Clin Oncol 2007 [299]	Resected Stage II and III colon	FULV N = 1207	FLOX N = 1200		Multicentre Randomized Phase III	DFS	3.5	Adding oxaliplatin or FLOX can be recommended
NSABP-C08 Allegra J Clin Oncol 2011, 2013 [300,301]	Resected Stage II and III colon	FOLFOX6 N = 1356 75.2% stage 3	FOLFOX6 + bevacizumab N = 1354 75% stage 3		Multinational Randomized Phase III	DFS	> 5	Use of bevacizumab cannot be recommended
AVANT De Gramont Lancet Oncol 2012 [302]	Resected Stage III and high-risk II colon	Bevacizumab FOLFOX4 N = 960 stage 3 N = 194 stage 2	Bevacizumab XELOX N = 952 stage 3 N = 187 stage 2	FOLFOX4 N = 955 stage III N = 192 stage II	Multinational Open label Randomized Phase III	DFS	4	Bevacizumab does not improve DFS in stage III OS worse effect of oxaliplatin combined with bevacizumab
PETACC-3 Van Cutsem J Clin Oncol 2009 [303]	Resected Stage II and III colon	LV-5-FU2 N = 1497	LV-5-FU2 + irinotecan N = 1485	Comparison of AIO + irinotecan (N = 135) vs. AIO alone (N = 124)	Multicentre Open label Randomized Phase III	DFS	5.6	More toxicity No benefit on DFS or OS of irinotecan
CABLG 89803 Saltz J Clin Oncol 2007 [304]	Resected Stage III colon	Irinotecan–FU-LV N = 635	LV-5-FU N = 629		Multicentre Randomized controlled	OS DFS RFS	4.8	Weekly bolus irinotecan + FU + LV Not recommended in stage III colon

Bevacizumab

Bevacizumab (Avastin) is a recombinant humanized monoclonal antibody that stops angiogenesis by inhibiting vascular endothelial growth factor A (VEGF-A). VEGF-A is a chemical signal that stimulates angiogenesis in cancer. Bevacizumab was approved by the FDA in February 2004 for use in metastatic CRC when used with standard chemotherapy treatment (as first-line treatment) and with 5-fluorouracil-based therapy for second-line metastatic CRC. This recommendation was based on the E3200 trial – addition of bevacizumab to oxaliplatin, 5-FU and leucovorin (FOLFOX4) therapy [306]. In adjuvant colon cancer treatment, data from two large randomized studies have shown no significant benefit and a potential to cause harm in this setting [302].

Cetuximab

Cetuximab is an epidermal growth factor receptor (EGFR) inhibitor. Its efficacy is not proven in the adjuvant setting in CRC. The PETACC-8 study randomized patients with resected stage III CRC to 12 cycles of FOLFOX4 twice a week with or without cetuximab. The addition of cetuximab to FOLFOX4 did not improve DFS compared with FOLFOX4 alone in patients with KRAS exon 2 wild-type resected stage III colon cancer [307]. Another phase III randomized trial also concluded that cetuximab did not seem to add to disease-free survival [308].

Panitumumab

A human monoclonal antibody to the epidermal growth factor receptor, panitumumab targets KRAS. Lack of the RAS mutation was associated with a reduced benefit in a prospective–retrospective analysis [309]. More studies are needed to establish its efficacy and role in treatment.

ROLE OF RADIOTHERAPY IN THE MANAGEMENT OF CRC

Radiotherapy is an integral part of the management of rectal cancer, whereas it is not part of the guidelines of the management of colon cancer, and is limited to use in exceptional cases, where the tumour is fixed to the surrounding structures and an individualized approach is necessary. In rectal cancer there is currently no role for postoperative radiotherapy, as has been demonstrated in several randomized controlled trials. There is still some ongoing discussion about which preoperative radiotherapy regime should be used for rectal cancer. In patients at risk of lymph node metastases 5 × 5 short-course RT may suffice to irradicate lymph nodes, which are being left behind by the surgeon. However, if downstaging and downsizing of the tumour are necessary, there is agreement that long-course radiotherapy with concomitant chemotherapy is the better option and will ultimately facilitate surgical resection and enhanced rates of radical margins.

Some studies have investigated the role of concomitant chemotherapy as a radio-sensitizing agent. However, multiple drugs used as concomitant chemotherapy have been trialled and abandoned including several studies which looked at the combination of a 5-FU derivate with oxaliplatin or a biological agent. A theoretical advantage of short-course radiotherapy is that surgery can be performed immediately after the completion of radiotherapy, thereby leading to a reduced overall treatment time. However, the Stockholm III trial, comparing short-course radiotherapy with immediate surgery versus short-course radiotherapy and late surgery, or long-course radiotherapy and delayed surgery, showed that 5 × 5 Gy also has a downstaging and downsizing effect, but above all of the complication rate seems to be lower after delaying surgery. So increasingly, institutions using both short-course and long-course therapy are also now waiting longer after short-course therapy.

The focus of radiotherapy in the management of rectal cancer patients is shifting. Several authors have shown that radiotherapy, especially in combination with chemotherapy, is able to downsize and downstage the tumour in such a way that the organ can be preserved and major surgery can be omitted. Especially in smaller tumours organ preservation can be achieved by radiotherapy. The paradox with this approach is that small tumours, which do not require any preoperative radiotherapy, can be cured by radiotherapy, especially when used in combination with chemotherapy. However, not all patients achieve organ preservation after radiotherapy. So those who do not need radiotherapy and who do not achieve complete downstaging still have the jeopardy of both treatments. They have the complications from the radiotherapy, but also the complications of surgery, which may be even more prominent than after surgery without preoperative radiotherapy. Therefore, future research will focus on intensification of the preoperative radiotherapy regime, resulting in a higher chance of a complete response for more patients and facilitating an organ-preserving approach.

Intensification of radiotherapy can be done either by combining radiotherapy with systemic chemotherapy before and after the radiotherapy or after the radiotherapy, as is being investigated in the RAPIDO study. Another approach is to intensify the radiotherapy treatment itself by delivering a separate boost to the tumour itself. Several promising rectal brachytherapy approaches have been reported and even endoluminal kilovolt radiotherapy, as propagated by Papillon almost half a century ago, is currently experiencing a revival.

FUTURE PERSPECTIVES

The two important challenges that have to be solved in the near future are how to improve the treatment for CRC in elderly patients and reverse the widening gap in outcomes between elderly and younger patients [254] and how we can provide patients with the tools to understand treatment options and reach a well-balanced and well-informed shared decision. Technical developments and new fundamental insight in the prognostic and predictive factors can help us to achieve these goals.

In the last decades there has been a spectacular change in our understanding of the molecular profile of CRC and the subsequent molecular pathways which determine all aspects of the development, course and outcome of CRC. In the foreseeable future molecular profiles will probably narrow down the treatment options for patients by showing which patients are at risk for local recurrence or not, allowing for a more individualized approach. Drugs, interfering with these molecular pathways, have been developed, although the majority still need to be tested. In stage IV disease, they seem to prolong life effectively, but their use in early CRC is still not clearly defined. Hopefully, unravelling the molecular signature will also lead to a more selective use of adjuvant chemotherapy. Despite the massive increase in the use of both biologicals and chemotherapy in colon and rectal cancer, the improvement in outcomes of especially colon cancer has only been very modest and may also be contributed to by better perioperative care [310,311]. In rectal cancer, for which chemotherapy doesn't play such a prominent role, the improvement in outcomes in some countries of more than 10% can be entirely attributed to better diagnostic work-up with the introduction of MRI, better neoadjuvant treatment with the introduction of preoperative radiotherapy or radiochemotherapy, and of course a better anatomically based surgical approach [2,312]. So, in the near future it is not likely that chemotherapy and molecular-based therapy will replace surgery.

However, organ preservation may also become a very important issue in coming years. It was noticed that with the introduction of neoadjuvant radiochemotherapy a substantial number of patients had a complete response, and the question was raised whether these patients could be left alone or should still undergo surgical resection of their tumour. The smaller the tumour, the more complete responders will be found [313,314]. Thanks to the early work of the Habr-Gama group in São Paulo we know that patients can be cured without any surgery if they have achieved complete response [315–317].

The criticism that had been raised against the Habr-Gama approach has opened a debate about the optimal selection of patients in whom complete response is likely [318]. The problem with inducing complete remissions is that the best responders will be patients who have small tumours. But even in these cases the majority of patients will not experience a complete response, and the downside is that these patients have received a possibly toxic treatment without having any benefit from it, because these patients could otherwise be operated on without neoadjuvant treatment and without the attendant toxicity.

Either identification of patients who are likely to undergo complete response has to improve, or neoadjuvant treatment will have to be intensified to increase the number of complete responders. One of the most promising results is presented by researchers who use endorectal brachytherapy on top of external radiotherapy [259,260,319,320]. As mentioned earlier combining multiple drugs during radiochemotherapy has not led to a significantly higher rate of complete response.

Individualization of treatment and the use of evidence-based guidelines seem to be mutually exclusive. Multidisciplinary tumour boards are necessary to reconcile these two disparate concepts, although this simply reflects the fact that our protocols are not yet sophisticated enough. The best approach is to discuss patients in a multidisciplinary team meeting, when all the diagnostic procedures have been performed, and before commencement of any therapy. Only by discussing the results in a multidisciplinary team will a well-informed consultation with the patient be possible, weighing all the different treatment options against each other. Especially in elderly people it is important to discuss these patients before commencement of any treatment, as the consequences of treatment in terms of toxicity and the final outcome are amplified in this group of patients.

Individualization presumes knowledge about patients' preferences, and in turn the patient has to be informed about what influence cancer treatment will have on their functioning and well-being.

The oncological outcome for CRC patients has improved steadily over recent decades as randomized trial data show how stepwise improvements can be made in outcomes with different treatment patterns. However, randomized trials have limitations related to the fact that very few cases are conducted within trials, which are not 'real world' and may not be representative of actual practice and outcomes. Less than 1%, or even 0.1% on a global scale, of cases are included in randomized controlled trials. The danger is that the results of these trials in a limited, possibly biased, group of patients may not always reflect what is going on in real life.

Only population-based registries catching data on outcomes comprehensively can validate the findings of RCTs. A good example is the Dutch TME trial which included early rectal cancer patients and randomized them between preoperative short-course radiotherapy or not. The conclusion was that preoperative radiotherapy reduced the chance of local recurrence at least by 50% [132]. It was learned many years later that high-quality surgery was the most important factor to reduce the numbers of local recurrences and that for only patients in stage III or more locally advanced rectal cancer was preoperative radiotherapy necessary [321]. It was also demonstrated on a population level that the introduction of selective use of radiotherapy and modern anatomical TME surgery led to an improvement in survival of at least 10% in many countries [2,321]. This is an example of stage migration, which does not truly reflect better outcomes, just more detailed stage analysis. If stage migration occurs as the result of better diagnostic imaging, all stages will have a better prognosis irrespective of the intervention performed after the improvement in staging. An example is the introduction of laparoscopic surgery in elderly colon cancer patients which has been reported to lead to fewer complications and better oncological outcomes [322]. However, the significant differences in observational studies are still not reflected in improved population-based outcomes and possibly selection bias may play a role [254,323]. The same is true for the increased use of adjuvant chemotherapy in the last decade, which resulted in only a modest population-based effect on survival [324].

Survival data for specific cancers in different countries from the national cancer registries are collected by EUROCARE, which can be used to identify poor-performing countries, which may help to drive change [2,324]. However, cancer registries work differently in different countries; the coverage is different and sometimes registration is mandatory and other times voluntarily [325].

The complexity of CRC management with many interacting variables and lack of standardization makes it difficult to develop a representative dataset, which also can react to changes in the guidelines over time. However, the multinational EURECCA group is trying to define a dataset based on the best evidence or expertise available, which can be used in different national or local registries. The knowledge available is updated on a regular basis. If a comprehensive unbiased objective database is available it can be used to assess differences between countries, hospitals and even individual teams [326]. But even if this dataset could be acquired, the evaluation will remain difficult, as many variables interact and case mix may be different due to referral patterns, the introduction of patients' preferences, which can lead to deviations from the standard, and the presence of significant but unknown or unregistered variables. Registries will be excellent tools to investigate differences, but are less suitable to single out one variable as a quality indicator.

CONCLUSION

The management of CRC is a multidisciplinary business. Input from different disciplines has made progress possible and will continue to do so in the future. Multidisciplinary working groups recruiting the most experienced specialists and researchers are able to disentangle the information that accumulates from numerous studies and observations. In this way, guidelines for treatment may be put together and the direction for future research can be prioritized. This chapter reflects the output from the colorectal EURECCA group and the 'Beyond TME working group' [156,327–334].

This interdisciplinary collaboration should also be reflected on an institutional level through multidisciplinary tumour board meetings, in which all CRC patients are being discussed, preferably before the start of any treatment.

Most CRC patients can be cured by high-quality surgery. However, surgery can have unwanted side effects and complications, and therefore other treatment options have to be explored. Selection of patients for individualized treatment

plans will become important. More and more patients will have a better prognosis if different treatment modalities are to be combined. In an ageing world, special attention must be given to elderly CRC patients, as they have not been able to benefit from new insights and treatment modalities as their younger counterparts.

REFERENCES

1. Ferlay J, Steliarova-Foucher E, Lortet-Tieulent J, et al. Cancer incidence and mortality patterns in Europe: estimates for 40 countries in 2012. *Eur J Cancer* 2013, 49(6), 1374–1403.
2. Brenner H, Bouvier AM, Foschi R, et al. Progress in colorectal cancer survival in Europe from the late 1980s to the early 21st century: the EUROCARE study. *Int J Cancer* 2012, 131(7), 1649–1658.
3. Scheithauer W, Rosen H, Kornek GV, Sebesta C, Depisch D. Randomised comparison of combination chemotherapy plus supportive care with supportive care alone in patients with metastatic colorectal cancer. *BMJ* 1993, 306(6880), 752–755.
4. Cucchetti A, Ferrero A, Cescon M, et al. Cure model survival analysis after hepatic resection for colorectal liver metastases. *Ann Surg Oncol* 2015, 22(6), 1908–1914.
5. Integraal Kankercentrum Nederland. Dutch cancer figures. 2015. Available at http://www.cijfersoverkanker.nl/
6. van Erning FN, van Steenbergen LN, Lemmens VE, et al. Conditional survival for long-term colorectal cancer survivors in the Netherlands: who do best? *Eur J Cancer* 2014, 50(10), 1731–1739.
7. Loughrey MB, Quirke P, Shepherd NA. Standard and datasets for reporting cancers. In *Dataset for Colorectal Cancer Histopathology Reports*, 3rd ed. London: Royal College of Pathologists, 2014.
8. Von Karsa L, Patnick J, Segnan N, et al. European guidelines for quality assurance in colorectal cancer screening and diagnosis: overview and introduction to the full supplement publication. *Endoscopy* 2013, 45(1), 51–59.
9. Quirke P, Steele R, Monson J, et al. Effect of the plane of surgery achieved on local recurrence in patients with operable rectal cancer: a prospective study using data from the MRC CR07 and NCIC-CTG CO16 randomised clinical trial. *Lancet* 2009, 373(9666), 821–828.
10. Bosch SL, Nagtegaal ID. The importance of the pathologist's role in assessment of the quality of the mesorectum. *Curr Colorectal Cancer Rep* 2012, 8(2), 90–98.
11. West NP, Finan PJ, Anderin C, Lindholm J, Holm T, Quirke P. Evidence of the oncologic superiority of cylindrical abdominoperineal excision for low rectal cancer. *J Clin Oncol* 2008, 26(21), 3517–3522.

12. Holm T, Ljung A, Haggmark T, Jurell G, Lagergren J. Extended abdominoperineal resection with gluteus maximus flap reconstruction of the pelvic floor for rectal cancer. *Br J Surg* 2007, 94(2), 232–238.

13. West NP, Anderin C, Smith KJ, Holm T, Quirke P. Multicentre experience with extralevator abdominoperineal excision for low rectal cancer. *Br J Surg* 2010, 97(4), 588–599.

14. Nagtegaal ID, van de Velde CJ, Marijnen CA, van Krieken JH, Quirke P. Low rectal cancer: a call for a change of approach in abdominoperineal resection. *J Clin Oncol* 2005, 23(36), 9257–9264.

15. Martijnse IS, Dudink RL, West NP, et al. Focus on extralevator perineal dissection in supine position for low rectal cancer has led to better quality of surgery and oncologic outcome. *Ann Surg Oncol* 2012, 19(3), 786–793.

16. West NP, Morris EJ, Rotimi O, Cairns A, Finan PJ, Quirke P. Pathology grading of colon cancer surgical resection and its association with survival: a retrospective observational study. *Lancet Oncol* 2008, 9(9), 857–865.

17. Hohenberger W, Weber K, Matzel K, Papadopoulos T, Merkel S. Standardized surgery for colonic cancer: complete mesocolic excision and central ligation – technical notes and outcome. *Colorectal Dis* 2009, 11(4), 354–364.

18. West NP, Hohenberger W, Weber K, Perrakis A, Finan PJ, Quirke P. Complete mesocolic excision with central vascular ligation produces an oncologically superior specimen compared with standard surgery for carcinoma of the colon. *J Clin Oncol* 2010, 28(2), 272–278.

19. West NP, Kennedy RH, Magro T, et al. Morphometric analysis and lymph node yield in laparoscopic complete mesocolic excision performed by supervised trainees. *Br J Surg* 2014, 101(11), 1460–1467.

20. West NP, Sutton KM, Ingeholm P, Hagemann-Madsen RH, Hohenberger W, Quirke P. Improving the quality of colon cancer surgery through a surgical education program. *Dis Colon Rectum* 2010, 53(12), 1594–1603.

21. Bertelsen CA, Neuenschwander AU, Jansen JE, et al. Disease-free survival after complete mesocolic excision compared with conventional colon cancer surgery: a retrospective, population-based study. *Lancet Oncol* 2015, 16(2), 161–168.

22. Quirke P, Durdey P, Dixon MF, Williams NS. Local recurrence of rectal adenocarcinoma due to inadequate surgical resection. Histopathological study of lateral tumour spread and surgical excision. *Lancet* 1986, 2(8514), 996–999.

23. Nagtegaal ID, Quirke P. What is the role for the circumferential margin in the modern treatment of rectal cancer? *J Clin Oncol* 2008, 26(2), 303–312.

24. Shihab OC, Quirke P, Heald RJ, Moran BJ, Brown G. Magnetic resonance imaging-detected lymph nodes close to the mesorectal fascia are rarely a cause of margin involvement after total mesorectal excision. *Br J Surg* 2010, 97(9), 1431–1436.

25. Birbeck KF, Macklin CP, Tiffin NJ, et al. Rates of circumferential resection margin involvement vary between surgeons and predict outcomes in rectal cancer surgery. *Ann Surg* 2002, 235(4), 449–457.

26. Guillou PJ, Quirke P, Thorpe H, et al. Short-term endpoints of conventional versus laparoscopic-assisted surgery in patients with colorectal cancer (MRC CLASICC trial): multicentre, randomised controlled trial. *Lancet* 2005, 365(9472), 1718–1726.

27. Bateman AC, Carr NJ, Warren BF. The retroperitoneal surface in distal caecal and proximal ascending colon carcinoma: the Cinderella surgical margin? *J Clin Pathol* 2005, 58(4), 426–428.

28. Scott N, Jamali A, Verbeke C, Ambrose NS, Botterill ID, Jayne DG. Retroperitoneal margin involvement by adenocarcinoma of the caecum and ascending colon: what does it mean? *Colorectal Dis* 2008, 10(3), 289–293.

29. Wittekind C, Compton C, Quirke P, et al. A uniform residual tumor (R) classification: integration of the R classification and the circumferential margin status. *Cancer* 2009, 115(15), 3483–3488.

30. Quirke P, Cuvelier C, Ensari A, et al. Evidence-based medicine: the time has come to set standards for staging. *J Pathol* 2010, 221(4), 357–360.

31. Nagtegaal ID, Tot T, Jayne DG, et al. Lymph nodes, tumor deposits, and TNM: are we getting better? *J Clin Oncol* 2011, 29(18), 2487–2492.

32. Maughan NJ, Morris E, Forman D, Quirke P. The validity of the Royal College of Pathologists' colorectal cancer minimum dataset within a population. *Br J Cancer* 2007, 97(10), 1393–1398.

33. Jepsen RK, Ingeholm P, Lund EL. Upstaging of early colorectal cancers following improved lymph node yield after methylene blue injection. *Histopathology* 2012, 61(5), 788–794.

34. Morris EJ, Maughan NJ, Forman D, Quirke P. Who to treat with adjuvant therapy in Dukes B/stage II colorectal cancer? The need for high quality pathology. *Gut* 2007, 56(10), 1419–1425.

35. Hutchins G, Southward K, Handley K, et al. Value of mismatch repair, KRAS, and BRAF mutations in predicting recurrence and benefits from chemotherapy in colorectal cancer. *J Clin Oncol* 2011, 29(10), 1261–1270.

36. Van Cutsem E, Kohne CH, Hitre E, et al. Cetuximab and chemotherapy as initial treatment for metastatic colorectal cancer. *N Engl J Med* 2009, 360(14), 1408–1417.

37. Wong NA, Gonzalez D, Salto-Tellez M, et al. RAS testing of colorectal carcinoma – a guidance document from the Association of Clinical Pathologists Molecular Pathology and Diagnostics Group. *J Clin Pathol* 2014, 67(9), 751–757.

38. Domingo E, Church DN, Sieber O, et al. Evaluation of PIK3CA mutation as a predictor of benefit from nonsteroidal anti-inflammatory drug therapy in colorectal cancer. *J Clin Oncol* 2013, 31(34), 4297–4305.

39. Kim DH, Pickhardt PJ, Taylor AJ, et al. CT colonography versus colonoscopy for the detection of advanced neoplasia. *N Engl J Med* 2007, 357(14), 1403–1412.

40. Pickhardt PJ, Hassan C, Halligan S, Marmo R. Colorectal cancer: CT colonography and colonoscopy for detection – systematic review and meta-analysis. *Radiology* 2011, 259(2), 393–405.

41. FOxTROT Collaborative Group. Feasibility of preoperative chemotherapy for locally advanced, operable colon cancer: the pilot phase of a randomised controlled trial. *Lancet Oncol* 2012, 13(11), 1152–1160.

42. Evans J, Patel U, Brown G. Rectal cancer: primary staging and assessment after chemoradiotherapy. *Semin Radiat Oncol* 2011, 21(3), 169–177.

43. Barret M, Boustiere C, Canard JM, et al. Factors associated with adenoma detection rate and diagnosis of polyps and colorectal cancer during colonoscopy in France: results of a prospective, nationwide survey. *PLoS One* 2013, 8(7), e68947.

44. Conaghan PJ, Maxwell-Armstrong CA, Garrioch MV, Hong L, Acheson AG. Leaving a mark: the frequency and accuracy of tattooing prior to laparoscopic colorectal surgery. *Colorectal Dis* 2011, 13(10), 1184–1187.

45. Kaminski MF, Regula J, Kraszewska E, et al. Quality indicators for colonoscopy and the risk of interval cancer. *N Engl J Med* 2010, 362(19), 1795–1803.

46. Rabeneck L, Rumble RB, Axler J, et al. Cancer Care Ontario colonoscopy standards: standards and evidentiary base. *Can J Gastroenterol* 2007, 21(Suppl. D), 5D–24D.

47. Valori R, Rey JF, Atkin WS, et al. European guidelines for quality assurance in colorectal cancer screening and diagnosis. First edition – quality assurance in endoscopy in colorectal cancer screening and diagnosis. *Endoscopy* 2012, 44(Suppl. 3), SE88–105.

48. Pullens HJ, van Leeuwen MS, Laheij RJ, Vleggaar FP, Siersema PD. CT-colonography after incomplete colonoscopy: what is the diagnostic yield? *Dis Colon Rectum* 2013, 56(5), 593–599.

49. Regge D, Laudi C, Galatola G, et al. Diagnostic accuracy of computed tomographic colonography for the detection of advanced neoplasia in individuals at increased risk of colorectal cancer. *JAMA* 2009, 301(23), 2453–2461.

50. Yee J, Rosen MP, Blake MA, et al. ACR appropriateness criteria on colorectal cancer screening. *J Am Coll Radiol* 2010, 7(9), 670–678.

51. Atkin W, Dadswell E, Wooldrage K, et al. Computed tomographic colonography versus colonoscopy for investigation of patients with symptoms suggestive of colorectal cancer (SIGGAR): a multicentre randomised trial. *Lancet* 2013, 381(9873), 1194–1202.

52. Rosman AS, Korsten MA. Meta-analysis comparing CT colonography, air contrast barium enema, and colonoscopy. *Am J Med* 2007, 120(3), 203–210.

53. Taylor SA, Halligan S, Burling D, Bassett P, Bartram CI. Intra-individual comparison of patient acceptability of multidetector-row CT colonography and double-contrast barium enema. *Clin Radiol* 2005, 60(2), 207–214.

54. Hyngstrom JR, Hu CY, Xing Y, et al. Clinicopathology and outcomes for mucinous and signet ring colorectal adenocarcinoma: analysis from the National Cancer Data Base. *Ann Surg Oncol* 2012, 19(9), 2814–2821.

55. Smith NJ, Bees N, Barbachano Y, Norman AR, Swift RI, Brown G. Preoperative computed tomography staging of nonmetastatic colon cancer predicts outcome: implications for clinical trials. *Br J Cancer* 2007, 96(7), 1030–1036.

56. Foxtrot Collaborative Group. Feasibility of preoperative chemotherapy for locally advanced, operable colon cancer: the pilot phase of a randomised controlled trial. *Lancet Oncol* 2012, 13(11), 1152–1160.

57. Dighe S, Swift I, Magill L, et al. Accuracy of radiological staging in identifying high-risk colon cancer patients suitable for neoadjuvant chemotherapy: a multicentre experience. *Colorectal Dis* 2012, 14(4), 438–444.

58. Sternberg A, Amar M, Alfici R, Groisman G. Conclusions from a study of venous invasion in stage IV colorectal adenocarcinoma. *J Clin Pathol* 2002, 55(1), 17–21.

59. Leufkens AM, van den Bosch MA, van Leeuwen MS, Siersema PD. Diagnostic accuracy of computed tomography for colon cancer staging: a systematic review. *Scand J Gastroenterol* 2011, 46(7–8), 887–894.

60. Bipat S, Glas AS, Slors FJ, Zwinderman AH, Bossuyt PM, Stoker J. Rectal cancer: local staging and assessment of lymph node involvement with endoluminal US, CT, and MR imaging – a meta-analysis. *Radiology* 2004, 232(3), 773–783.

61. Brown G, Richards CJ, Bourne MW, et al. Morphologic predictors of lymph node status in rectal cancer with use of high-spatial-resolution MR imaging with histopathologic comparison. *Radiology* 2003, 227(2), 371–377.

62. Dighe S, Blake H, Koh MD, et al. Accuracy of multidetector computed tomography in identifying poor prognostic factors in colonic cancer. *Br J Surg* 2010, 97(9), 1407–1415.

63. Dighe S, Purkayastha S, Swift I, et al. Diagnostic precision of CT in local staging of colon cancers: a meta-analysis. *Clin Radiol* 2010, 65(9), 708–719.

64. Burton S, Brown G, Bees N, et al. Accuracy of CT prediction of poor prognostic features in colonic cancer. *Br J Radiol* 2008, 81(961), 10–19.

65. Ashraf K, Ashraf O, Haider Z, Rafique Z. Colorectal carcinoma, preoperative evaluation by spiral computed tomography. *J Pak Med Assoc* 2006, 56(4), 149–153.

66. Poston GJ, Tait D, O'Connell S, Bennett A, Berendse S. Diagnosis and management of colorectal cancer: summary of NICE guidance. *BMJ* 2011, 343, d6751.

67. Torkzad MR, Pahlman L, Glimelius B. Magnetic resonance imaging (MRI) in rectal cancer: a comprehensive review. *Insights Imaging* 2010, 1(4), 245–267.

68. MERCURY Study Group. Diagnostic accuracy of preoperative magnetic resonance imaging in predicting curative resection of rectal cancer: prospective observational study. *BMJ* 2006, 333(7572), 779.

69. Zorcolo L, Fantola G, Cabras F, Marongiu L, D'Alia G, Casula G. Preoperative staging of patients with rectal tumors suitable for transanal endoscopic microsurgery (TEM): comparison of endorectal ultrasound and histopathologic findings. *Surg Endosc* 2009, 23(6), 1384–1389.

70. Merkel S, Mansmann U, Siassi M, Papadopoulos T, Hohenberger W, Hermanek P. The prognostic inhomogeneity in pT3 rectal carcinomas. *Int J Colorectal Dis* 2001, 16(5), 298–304.

71. MERCURY Study Group. Extramural depth of tumor invasion at thin-section MR in patients with rectal cancer: results of the MERCURY study. *Radiology* 2007, 243(1), 132–139.

72. Shepherd NA, Baxter KJ, Love SB. Influence of local peritoneal involvement on pelvic recurrence and prognosis in rectal cancer. *J Clin Pathol* 1995, 48(9), 849–855.

73. Brown G, Richards CJ, Bourne MW, et al. Morphologic predictors of lymph node status in rectal cancer with use of high-spatial-resolution MR imaging with histopathologic comparison. *Radiology* 2003, 227(2), 371–377.

74. Wibe A, Rendedal PR, Svensson E, et al. Prognostic significance of the circumferential resection margin following total mesorectal excision for rectal cancer. *Br J Surg* 2002, 89(3), 327–334.

75. Burton S, Brown G, Daniels IR, Norman AR, Mason B, Cunningham D. MRI directed multidisciplinary team preoperative treatment strategy: the way to eliminate positive circumferential margins? *Br J Cancer* 2006, 94(3), 351–357.

76. Taylor FG, Quirke P, Heald RJ, et al. One millimetre is the safe cut-off for magnetic resonance imaging prediction of surgical margin status in rectal cancer. *Br J Surg* 2011, 98(6), 872–879.

77. Maizlin ZV, Brown JA, So G, et al. Can CT replace MRI in preoperative assessment of the circumferential resection margin in rectal cancer? *Dis Colon Rectum* 2010, 53(3), 308–314.

78. Vliegen R, Dresen R, Beets G, et al. The accuracy of multi-detector row CT for the assessment of tumor invasion of the mesorectal fascia in primary rectal cancer. *Abdom Imaging* 2008, 33(5), 604–610.

79. Wolberink SV, Beets-Tan RG, de Haas-Kock DF, van de Jagt EJ, Span MM, Wiggers T. Multislice CT as a primary screening tool for the prediction of an involved mesorectal fascia and distant metastases in primary rectal cancer: a multicenter study. *Dis Colon Rectum* 2009, 52(5), 928–934.

80. Salerno GV, Daniels IR, Moran BJ, Heald RJ, Thomas K, Brown G. Magnetic resonance imaging prediction of an involved surgical resection margin in low rectal cancer. *Dis Colon Rectum* 2009, 52(4), 632–639.

81. Shihab OC, Taylor F, Salerno G, et al. MRI predictive factors for long-term outcomes of low rectal tumours. *Ann Surg Oncol* 2011, 18(12), 3278–3284.

82. Shirouzu K, Isomoto H, Kakegawa T, Morimatsu M. A prospective clinicopathologic study of venous invasion in colorectal cancer. *Am J Surg* 1991, 162(3), 216–222.

83. Talbot IC, Ritchie S, Leighton M, Hughes AO, Bussey HJ, Morson BC. Invasion of veins by carcinoma of rectum: method of detection, histological features and significance. *Histopathology* 1981, 5(2), 141–163.

84. Dresen RC, Peters EE, Rutten HJ, et al. Local recurrence in rectal cancer can be predicted by histopathological factors. *Eur J Surg Oncol* 2009, 35(10), 1071–1077.

85. Messenger DE, Driman DK, Kirsch R. Developments in the assessment of venous invasion in colorectal cancer: implications for future practice and patient outcome. *Hum Pathol* 2012, 43(7), 965–973.

86. Hermanek P, Merkel S, Fietkau R, Rodel C, Hohenberger W. Regional lymph node metastasis and locoregional recurrence of rectal carcinoma in the era of TME [corrected] surgery. Implications for treatment decisions. *Int J Colorectal Dis* 2010, 25(3), 359–368.

87. Puli SR, Reddy JB, Bechtold ML, Choudhary A, Antillon MR, Brugge WR. Accuracy of endoscopic ultrasound to diagnose nodal invasion by rectal cancers: a meta-analysis and systematic review. *Ann Surg Oncol* 2009, 16(5), 1255–1265.

88. Kim JH, Beets GL, Kim MJ, Kessels AG, Beets-Tan RG. High-resolution MR imaging for nodal staging in rectal cancer: are there any criteria in addition to the size? *Eur J Radiol* 2004, 52(1), 78–83.

89. Taylor FG, Quirke P, Heald RJ, et al. Preoperative high-resolution magnetic resonance imaging can identify good prognosis stage I, II, and III rectal cancer best managed by surgery alone: a prospective, multicenter, European study. *Ann Surg* 2011, 253(4), 711–719.

90. Barbaro B, Fiorucci C, Tebala C, et al. Locally advanced rectal cancer: MR imaging in prediction of response after preoperative chemotherapy and radiation therapy. *Radiology* 2009, 250(3), 730–739.

91. Curvo-Semedo L, Lambregts DM, Maas M, Beets GL, Caseiro-Alves F, Beets-Tan RG. Diffusion-weighted MRI in rectal cancer: apparent diffusion coefficient as a potential noninvasive marker of tumor aggressiveness. *J Magn Reson Imaging* 2012, 35(6), 1365–1371.

92. Kim SH, Lee JM, Hong SH, et al. Locally advanced rectal cancer: added value of diffusion-weighted MR imaging in the evaluation of tumor response to neo-adjuvant chemo- and radiation therapy. *Radiology* 2009, 253(1), 116–125.

93. Lambregts DM, Vandecaveye V, Barbaro B, et al. Diffusion-weighted MRI for selection of complete responders after chemoradiation for locally advanced rectal cancer: a multicenter study. *Ann Surg Oncol* 2011, 18(8), 2224–2231.

94. Winawer SJ, Zauber AG, Ho MN, et al. Prevention of colorectal cancer by colonoscopic polypectomy. The National Polyp Study Workgroup. *N Engl J Med* 1993, 329(27), 1977–1981.

95. Vogelstein B, Fearon ER, Hamilton SR, et al. Genetic alterations during colorectal-tumor development. *N Engl J Med* 1988, 319(9), 525–532.

96. Vogelstein B, Papadopoulos N, Velculescu VE, Zhou S, Diaz LA Jr, Kinzler KW. Cancer genome landscapes. *Science* 2013, 339(6127), 1546–1558.

97. Fairley KJ, Li J, Komar M, Steigerwalt N, Erlich P. Predicting the risk of recurrent adenoma and incident colorectal cancer based on findings of the baseline colonoscopy. *Clin Transl Gastroenterol* 2014, 5, e64.

98. Bosch SL, Teerenstra S, de Wilt JH, Cunningham C, Nagtegaal ID. Predicting lymph node metastasis in pT1 colorectal cancer: a systematic review of risk factors providing rationale for therapy decisions. *Endoscopy* 2013, 45(10), 827–834.

99. Kobayashi H, Higuchi T, Uetake H, et al. Resection with en bloc removal of regional lymph node after endoscopic resection for T1 colorectal cancer. *Ann Surg Oncol* 2012, 19(13), 4161–4167.

100. Kim MN, Kang JM, Yang JI, et al. Clinical features and prognosis of early colorectal cancer treated by endoscopic mucosal resection. *J Gastroenterol Hepatol* 2011, 26(11), 1619–1625.

101. van de Velde CJ, Boelens PG, Tanis PJ, et al. Experts reviews of the multidisciplinary consensus conference colon and rectal cancer 2012: science, opinions and experiences from the experts of surgery. *Eur J Surg Oncol* 2014, 40(4), 454–468.

102. van de Velde CJ, Boelens PG, Borras JM, et al. EURECCA colorectal: multidisciplinary management: European consensus conference colon & rectum. *Eur J Cancer* 2014, 50(1), 1.

103. Haller DG, O'Connell MJ, Cartwright TH, et al. Impact of age and medical comorbidity on adjuvant treatment outcomes for stage III colon cancer: a pooled analysis of individual patient data from four randomized controlled trials. *Ann Oncol* 2015.

104. Arredondo J, Pastor C, Baixauli J, et al. Preliminary outcome of a treatment strategy based on perioperative chemotherapy and surgery in patients with locally advanced colon cancer. *Colorectal Dis* 2013, 15(5), 552–557.

105. Norgaard A, Dam C, Jakobsen A, Ploen J, Lindebjerg J, Rafaelsen SR. Selection of colon cancer patients for neoadjuvant chemotherapy by preoperative CT scan. *Scand J Gastroenterol* 2014, 49(2), 202–208.

106. Segelman J, Granath F, Holm T, Machado M, Mahteme H, Martling A. Incidence, prevalence and risk factors for peritoneal carcinomatosis from colorectal cancer. *Br J Surg* 2012, 99(5), 699–705.

107. Lemmens VE, Klaver YL, Verwaal VJ, Rutten HJ, Coebergh JW, de Hingh IH. Predictors and survival of synchronous peritoneal carcinomatosis of colorectal origin: a population-based study. *Int J Cancer* 2011, 128(11), 2717–2725.

108. Koh JL, Yan TD, Glenn D, Morris DL. Evaluation of preoperative computed tomography in estimating peritoneal cancer index in colorectal peritoneal carcinomatosis. *Ann Surg Oncol* 2009, 16(2), 327–333.

109. Verwaal VJ, Bruin S, Boot H, van SG, van TH. 8-Year follow-up of randomized trial: cytoreduction and hyperthermic intraperitoneal chemotherapy versus systemic chemotherapy in patients with peritoneal carcinomatosis of colorectal cancer. *Ann Surg Oncol* 2008, 15(9), 2426–2432.

110. Elias D, Gilly F, Boutitie F, et al. Peritoneal colorectal carcinomatosis treated with surgery and perioperative intraperitoneal chemotherapy: retrospective analysis of 523 patients from a multicentric French study. *J Clin Oncol* 2010, 28(1), 63–68.

111. Piso P, Dahlke MH, Ghali N, et al. Multimodality treatment of peritoneal carcinomatosis from colorectal cancer: first results of a new German centre for peritoneal surface malignancies. *Int J Colorectal Dis* 2007, 22(11), 1295–1300.

112. Shen P, Hawksworth J, Lovato J, et al. Cytoreductive surgery and intraperitoneal hyperthermic chemotherapy with mitomycin C for peritoneal carcinomatosis from nonappendiceal colorectal carcinoma. *Ann Surg Oncol* 2004, 11(2), 178–186.

113. Doornebosch PG, Tollenaar RA, Gosselink MP, et al. Quality of life after transanal endoscopic microsurgery and total mesorectal excision in early rectal cancer. *Colorectal Dis* 2007, 9(6), 553–558.

114. De Graaf EJ, Doornebosch PG, Tollenaar RA, et al. Transanal endoscopic microsurgery versus total mesorectal excision of T1 rectal adenocarcinomas with curative intention. *Eur J Surg Oncol* 2009, 35(12), 1280–1285.

115. Guerrieri M, Baldarelli M, Organetti L, et al. Transanal endoscopic microsurgery for the treatment of selected patients with distal rectal cancer: 15 years experience. *Surg Endosc* 2008, 22(9), 2030–2035.

116. Wu Y, Wu YY, Li S, et al. TEM and conventional rectal surgery for T1 rectal cancer: a meta-analysis. *Hepatogastroenterology* 2011, 58(106), 364–368.

117. Barendse RM, Dijkgraaf MG, Rolf UR, et al. Colorectal surgeons' learning curve of transanal endoscopic microsurgery. *Surg Endosc* 2013, 27(10), 3591–3602.

118. Quirke P. *Minimum Dataset for Colorectal Cancer Histopathology Reports*. London: Royal College of Pathologists, 1998.

119. Quirke P, Palmer T, Hutchins GG, West NP. Histopathological work-up of resection specimens, local excisions and biopsies in colorectal cancer. *Dig Dis* 2012, 30(Suppl. 2), 2–8.

120. Doornebosch PG, Ferenschild FT, de Wilt JH, Dawson I, Tetteroo GW, De Graaf EJ. Treatment of recurrence after transanal endoscopic microsurgery (TEM) for T1 rectal cancer. *Dis Colon Rectum* 2010, 53(9), 1234–1239.

121. Stipa F, Giaccaglia V, Burza A. Management and outcome of local recurrence following transanal endoscopic microsurgery for rectal cancer. *Dis Colon Rectum* 2012, 55(3), 262–269.

122. Levic K, Bulut O, Hesselfeldt P, Bulow S. The outcome of rectal cancer after early salvage surgery following transanal endoscopic microsurgery seems promising. *Dan Med J* 2012, 59(9), A4507.

123. Levic K, Bulut O, Hesselfeldt P, Bulow S. The outcome of rectal cancer after early salvage TME following TEM compared with primary TME: a case-matched study. *Tech Coloproctol* 2013, 17(4), 397–403.

124. Hompes R, McDonald R, Buskens C, et al. Completion surgery following transanal endoscopic microsurgery: assessment of quality and short- and long-term outcome. *Colorectal Dis* 2013, 15(10), e576–e581.

125. van GW, Brehm V, de GE, et al. Unexpected rectal cancer after TEM: outcome of completion surgery compared with primary TME. *Eur J Surg Oncol* 2013, 39(11), 1225–1229.

126. Bories E, Pesenti C, Monges G, et al. Endoscopic mucosal resection for advanced sessile adenoma and early-stage colorectal carcinoma. *Endoscopy* 2006, 38(3), 231–235.

127. Araujo SE, Crawshaw B, Mendes CR, Delaney CP. Transanal total mesorectal excision: a systematic review of the experimental and clinical evidence. *Tech Coloproctol* 2015, 19(2), 69–82.

128. Lezoche E, Baldarelli M, Lezoche G, Paganini AM, Gesuita R, Guerrieri M. Randomized clinical trial of endoluminal locoregional resection versus laparoscopic total mesorectal excision for T2 rectal cancer after neoadjuvant therapy. *Br J Surg* 2012, 99(9), 1211–1218.

129. Garcia-Aguilar J, Shi Q, Thomas CR Jr, et al. A phase II trial of neoadjuvant chemoradiation and local excision for T2N0 rectal cancer: preliminary results of the ACOSOG Z6041 trial. *Ann Surg Oncol* 2012, 19(2), 384–391.

130. Taylor FG, Swift RI, Blomqvist L, Brown G. A systematic approach to the interpretation of preoperative staging MRI for rectal cancer. *AJR Am J Roentgenol* 2008, 191(6), 1827–1835.

131. Swedish Rectal Cancer Trial. Improved survival with preoperative radiotherapy in resectable rectal cancer. *N Engl J Med* 1997, 336(14), 980–987.

132. Kapiteijn E, Marijnen CA, Nagtegaal ID, et al. Preoperative radiotherapy combined with total mesorectal excision for resectable rectal cancer. *N Engl J Med* 2001, 345(9), 638–646.

133. Bujko K, Nowacki MP, Nasierowska-Guttmejer A, et al. Sphincter preservation following preoperative radiotherapy for rectal cancer: report of a randomised trial comparing short-term radiotherapy vs. conventionally fractionated radiochemotherapy. *Radiother Oncol* 2004, 72(1), 15–24.

134. Ngan SY, Burmeister B, Fisher RJ, et al. Randomized trial of short-course radiotherapy versus long-course chemoradiation comparing rates of local recurrence in patients with T3 rectal cancer: Trans-Tasman Radiation Oncology Group trial 01.04. *J Clin Oncol* 2012, 30(31), 3827–3833.

135. Pettersson D, Cedermark B, Holm T, et al. Interim analysis of the Stockholm III trial of preoperative radiotherapy regimens for rectal cancer. *Br J Surg* 2010, 97(4), 580–587.

136. Pettersson D, Glimelius B, Iversen H, Johansson H, Holm T, Martling A. Impaired postoperative leucocyte counts after preoperative radiotherapy for rectal cancer in the Stockholm III trial. *Br J Surg* 2013, 100(7), 969–975.

137. Bujko K. Timing of surgery following preoperative therapy in rectal cancer: there is no need for a prospective randomized trial. *Dis Colon Rectum* 2012, 55(3), e31–e32.

138. Patel UB, Taylor F, Blomqvist L, et al. Magnetic resonance imaging-detected tumor response for locally advanced rectal cancer predicts survival outcomes: MERCURY experience. *J Clin Oncol* 2011, 29(28), 3753–3760.

139. Patel UB, Brown G, Rutten H, et al. Comparison of magnetic resonance imaging and histopathological response to chemoradiotherapy in locally advanced rectal cancer. *Ann Surg Oncol* 2012, 19(9), 2842–2852.

140. Gerard JP, Azria D, Gourgou-Bourgade S, et al. Clinical outcome of the ACCORD 12/0405 PRODIGE 2 randomized trial in rectal cancer. *J Clin Oncol* 2012, 30(36), 4558–4565.

141. van Dijk TH, Tamas K, Beukema JC, et al. Evaluation of short-course radiotherapy followed by neoadjuvant bevacizumab, capecitabine, and oxaliplatin and subsequent radical surgical treatment in primary stage IV rectal cancer. *Ann Oncol* 2013, 24(7), 1762–1769.

142. Nilsson PJ, van EB, Hospers GA, et al. Short-course radiotherapy followed by neo-adjuvant chemotherapy in locally advanced rectal cancer – the RAPIDO trial. *BMC Cancer* 2013, 13, 279.

143. Shihab OC, Heald RJ, Rullier E, et al. Defining the surgical planes on MRI improves surgery for cancer of the low rectum. *Lancet Oncol* 2009, 10(12), 1207–1211.

144. Trakarnsanga A, Gonen M, Shia J, et al. What is the significance of the circumferential margin in locally advanced rectal cancer after neoadjuvant chemoradiotherapy? *Ann Surg Oncol* 2013, 20(4), 1179–1184.

145. Dresen RC, Kusters M, Daniels-Gooszen AW, et al. Absence of tumor invasion into pelvic structures in locally recurrent rectal cancer: prediction with preoperative MR imaging. *Radiology* 2010, 256(1), 143–150.

146. Maas M, Rutten IJ, Nelemans PJ, et al. What is the most accurate whole-body imaging modality for assessment of local and distant recurrent disease in colorectal cancer? A meta-analysis: imaging for recurrent colorectal cancer. *Eur J Nucl Med Mol Imaging* 2011, 38(8), 1560–1571.

147. Chau I, Brown G, Cunningham D, et al. Neoadjuvant capecitabine and oxaliplatin followed by synchronous chemoradiation and total mesorectal excision in magnetic resonance imaging-defined poor-risk rectal cancer. *J Clin Oncol* 2006, 24(4), 668–674.

148. Bhangu A, Ali SM, Darzi A, Brown G, Tekkis P. Meta-analysis of survival based on resection margin status following surgery for recurrent rectal cancer. *Colorectal Dis* 2012, 14(12), 1457–1466.

149. Battersby NJ, Moran B, Yu S, Tekkis P, Brown G. MR imaging for rectal cancer: the role in staging the primary and response to neoadjuvant therapy. *Expert Rev Gastroenterol Hepatol* 2014, 8(6), 703–719.

150. Heriot AG, Byrne CM, Lee P, et al. Extended radical resection: the choice for locally recurrent rectal cancer. *Dis Colon Rectum* 2008, 51(3), 284–291.

151. Mohiuddin M, Marks G, Marks J. Long-term results of reirradiation for patients with recurrent rectal carcinoma. *Cancer* 2002, 95(5), 1144–1150.

152. Valentini V, Morganti AG, Gambacorta MA, et al. Preoperative hyperfractionated chemoradiation for locally recurrent rectal cancer in patients previously irradiated to the pelvis: a multicentric phase II study. *Int J Radiat Oncol Biol Phys* 2006, 64(4), 1129–1139.

153. Bosman SJ, Holman FA, Nieuwenhuijzen GA, Martijn H, Creemers GJ, Rutten HJ. Feasibility of reirradiation in the treatment of locally recurrent rectal cancer. *Br J Surg* 2014, 101(10), 1280–1289.

154. Dresen RC, Gosens MJ, Martijn H, et al. Radical resection after IORT-containing multimodality treatment is the most important determinant for outcome in patients treated for locally recurrent rectal cancer. *Ann Surg Oncol* 2008, 15(7), 1937–1947.

155. Mirnezami R, Chang GJ, Das P, et al. Intraoperative radiotherapy in colorectal cancer: systematic review and meta-analysis of techniques, long-term outcomes, and complications. *Surg Oncol* 2013, 22(1), 22–35.

156. Beyond TME Collaborative. Consensus statement on the multidisciplinary management of patients with recurrent and primary rectal cancer beyond total mesorectal excision planes. *Br J Surg* 2013, 100(8), E1–E33.

157. Choy PY, Bissett IP, Docherty JG, Parry BR, Merrie AE. Stapled versus handsewn methods for ileocolic anastomoses. *Cochrane Database Syst Rev* 2007, 3, CD004320.

158. Quenu E, Hartmann H. *Chirurgie du rectum*. Paris: Steinheil, 1899.

159. Miles WE. *Cancer of the Rectum*. London: Harrison and Sons, 1926.

160. Van Gijn W, van de Velde CJ. Quality assurance through outcome registration in colorectal cancer: an ECCO initiative for Europe. *Acta Chir Iugosl* 2010, 57(3), 17–21.

161. Waldeyer W. *Das Becken*, 1st ed. Bonn: Verlag von Friedrich Cohen, 1899.

162. Heald RJ, Husband EM, Ryall RD. The mesorectum in rectal cancer surgery – the clue to pelvic recurrence? *Br J Surg* 1982, 69(10), 613–616.

163. Sondenaa K, Quirke P, Hohenberger W, et al. The rationale behind complete mesocolic excision (CME) and a central vascular ligation for colon cancer in open and laparoscopic surgery: proceedings of a consensus conference. *Int J Colorectal Dis* 2014, 29(4), 419–428.

164. Moran B, Heald RJ. *Manual of Total Mesorectal Excision*. London: CRC Press, 2013.

165. von Lanz T, Wachsmuth W. *Praktische Anatomie: T.8A*. Berlin: Springer-Verlag, 1986.

166. Williams NS, Dixon MF, Johnston D. Reappraisal of the 5 centimetre rule of distal excision for carcinoma of the rectum: a study of distal intramural spread and of patients' survival. *Br J Surg* 1983, 70(3), 150–154.

167. Pahlman L, Bujko K, Rutkowski A, Michalski W. Altering the therapeutic paradigm towards a distal bowel margin of < 1 cm in patients with low-lying rectal cancer: a systematic review and commentary. *Colorectal Dis* 2013, 15(4), e166–e174.

168. Brown CJ, Fenech DS, McLeod RS. Reconstructive techniques after rectal resection for rectal cancer. *Cochrane Database Syst Rev* 2008, 2, CD006040.

169. Liao C, Gao F, Cao Y, Tan A, Li X, Wu D. Meta-analysis of the colon J-pouch vs transverse coloplasty pouch after anterior resection for rectal cancer. *Colorectal Dis* 2010, 12(7), 624–631.

170. Stelzner S, Holm T, Moran BJ, et al. Deep pelvic anatomy revisited for a description of crucial steps in extralevator abdominoperineal excision for rectal cancer. *Dis Colon Rectum* 2011, 54(8), 947–957.

171. Stelzner S, Koehler C, Stelzer J, Sims A, Witzigmann H. Extended abdominoperineal excision vs. standard abdominoperineal excision in rectal cancer – a systematic overview. *Int J Colorectal Dis* 2011, 26(10), 1227–1240.

172. Holm T. Abdominoperineal resection revisited: is positioning an important issue? *Dis Colon Rectum* 2011, 54(8), 921–922.

173. Martijnse I, West N, Quirke P, Heald R, van de Velde C, Rutten HJ. Will extralevator abdominoperineal excision become the new gold standard? In Valentini V, Schmoll H-J, van de Velde C, eds., *Multidisciplinary Management of Rectal Cancer*, 1st ed. New York: Springer, 2012, pp. 261–274.

174. Martijnse IS, Dudink RL, West NP, et al. Focus on extralevator perineal dissection in supine position for low rectal cancer has led to better quality of surgery and oncologic outcome. *Ann Surg Oncol* 2012, 19(3), 786–793.

175. Shihab OC, Heald RJ, Holm T, et al. A pictorial description of extralevator abdominoperineal excision for low rectal cancer. *Colorectal Dis* 2012, 14(10), e655–e660.

176. Holm T, Ljung A, Haggmark T, Jurell G, Lagergren J. Extended abdominoperineal resection with gluteus maximus flap reconstruction of the pelvic floor for rectal cancer. *Br J Surg* 2007, 94(2), 232–238.

177. Orsini RG, Wiggers T, DeRuiter MC, et al. The modern anatomical surgical approach to localised rectal cancer [conference paper]. *Eur J Cancer Suppl* 2013, 11(2), 60–71.

178. Kolfschoten NE, van Leersum NJ, Gooiker GA, et al. Successful and safe introduction of laparoscopic colorectal cancer surgery in Dutch hospitals. *Ann Surg* 2013, 257(5), 916–921.

179. Schwab KE, Dowson HM, Van DJ, Marks CG, Rockall TA. The uptake of laparoscopic colorectal surgery in Great Britain and Ireland: a questionnaire survey of consultant members of the ACPGBI. *Colorectal Dis* 2009, 11(3), 318–322.

180. Lorenzon L, La TM, Ziparo V, et al. Evidence based medicine and surgical approaches for colon cancer: evidences, benefits and limitations of the laparoscopic vs open resection. *World J Gastroenterol* 2014, 20(13), 3680–3692.

181. Sangrasi AK, Memon AI, Memon MM, Abbasi MR, Laghari AA, Qureshi JN. A safe quick technique for placement of the first access port for creation of pneumoperitoneum. *JSLS* 2011, 15(4), 504–508.

182. Ahmad G, O'Flynn H, Duffy JM, Phillips K, Watson A. Laparoscopic entry techniques. *Cochrane Database Syst Rev* 2012, 2, CD006583.

183. Makino T, Shukla PJ, Rubino F, Milsom JW. The impact of obesity on perioperative outcomes after laparoscopic colorectal resection. *Ann Surg* 2012, 255(2), 228–236.

184. Stage JG, Schulze S, Moller P, et al. Prospective randomized study of laparoscopic versus open colonic resection for adenocarcinoma. *Br J Surg* 1997, 84(3), 391–396.

185. Schwenk W, Bohm B, Haase O, Junghans T, Muller JM. Laparoscopic versus conventional colorectal resection: a prospective randomised study of postoperative ileus and early postoperative feeding. *Langenbecks Arch Surg* 1998, 383(1), 49–55.

186. Lacy AM, Garcia-Valdecasas JC, Delgado S, et al. Laparoscopy-assisted colectomy versus open colectomy for treatment of non-metastatic colon cancer: a randomised trial. *Lancet* 2002, 359(9325), 2224–2229.

187. Reza MM, Blasco JA, Andradas E, Cantero R, Mayol J. Systematic review of laparoscopic versus open surgery for colorectal cancer. *Br J Surg* 2006, 93(8), 921–928.

188. Breukink S, Pierie J, Wiggers T. Laparoscopic versus open total mesorectal excision for rectal cancer. *Cochrane Database Syst Rev* 2006, 4, CD005200.

189. Vennix S, Pelzers L, Bouvy N, et al. Laparoscopic versus open total mesorectal excision for rectal cancer. *Cochrane Database Syst Rev* 2014, 4, CD005200.

190. van der Pas MH, Haglind E, Cuesta MA, et al. Laparoscopic versus open surgery for rectal cancer (COLOR II): short-term outcomes of a randomised, phase 3 trial. *Lancet Oncol* 2013, 14(3), 210–218.

191. Vlug MS, Wind J, Hollmann MW, et al. Laparoscopy in combination with fast track multimodal management is the best perioperative strategy in patients undergoing colonic surgery: a randomized clinical trial (LAFA-study). *Ann Surg* 2011, 254(6), 868–875.

192. Zhao JH, Sun JX, Gao P, et al. Fast-track surgery versus traditional perioperative care in laparoscopic colorectal cancer surgery: a meta-analysis. *BMC Cancer* 2014, 14, 607.

193. Kuhry E, Schwenk WF, Gaupset R, Romild U, Bonjer HJ. Long-term results of laparoscopic colorectal cancer resection. *Cochrane Database Syst Rev* 2008, 2, CD003432.

194. Leung KL, Kwok SP, Lam SC, et al. Laparoscopic resection of rectosigmoid carcinoma: prospective randomised trial. *Lancet* 2004, 363(9416), 1187–1192.

195. Clinical Outcomes of Surgical Therapy Study Group. A comparison of laparoscopically assisted and open colectomy for colon cancer. *N Engl J Med* 2004, 350(20), 2050–2059.

196. Burns EM, Currie A, Bottle A, Aylin P, Darzi A, Faiz O. Minimal-access colorectal surgery is associated with fewer adhesion-related admissions than open surgery. *Br J Surg* 2013, 100(1), 152–159.

197. Bartels SA, Vlug MS, Hollmann MW, et al. Small bowel obstruction, incisional hernia and survival after laparoscopic and open colonic resection (LAFA study). *Br J Surg* 2014, 101(9), 1153–1159.

198. Miskovic D, Ni M, Wyles SM, Tekkis P, Hanna GB. Learning curve and case selection in laparoscopic colorectal surgery: systematic review and international multicenter analysis of 4852 cases. *Dis Colon Rectum* 2012, 55(12), 1300–1310.

199. Miskovic D, Ni M, Wyles SM, et al. Is competency assessment at the specialist level achievable? A study for the national training programme in laparoscopic colorectal surgery in England. *Ann Surg* 2013, 257(3), 476–482.

200. Clancy C, O'Leary DP, Burke JP, et al. A meta-analysis to determine the oncological implications of conversion in laparoscopic colorectal cancer surgery. *Colorectal Dis* 2015, 17(6), 482–490.

201. Kaiser AM, Kang JC, Chan LS, Vukasin P, Beart RW Jr. Laparoscopic-assisted vs. open colectomy for colon cancer: a prospective randomized trial. *J Laparoendosc Adv Surg Tech A* 2004, 14(6), 329–334.

202. Curet MJ, Putrakul K, Pitcher DE, Josloff RK, Zucker KA. Laparoscopically assisted colon resection for colon carcinoma: perioperative results and long-term outcome. *Surg Endosc* 2000, 14(11), 1062–1066.

203. Yang C, Wexner SD, Safar B, et al. Conversion in laparoscopic surgery: does intraoperative complication influence outcome? *Surg Endosc* 2009, 23(11), 2454–2458.

204. da Luz Moreira A, Kiran RP, Kirat HT, et al. Laparoscopic versus open colectomy for patients with American Society of Anesthesiology (ASA) classifications 3 and 4: the minimally invasive approach is associated with significantly quicker recovery and reduced costs. *Surg Endosc* 2010, 24(6), 1280–1286.

205. Vaid S, Tucker J, Bell T, Grim R, Ahuja V. Cost analysis of laparoscopic versus open colectomy in patients with colon cancer: results from a large nationwide population database. *Am Surg* 2012, 78(6), 635–641.

206. Dowson HM, Gage H, Jackson D, Qiao Y, Williams P, Rockall TA. Laparoscopic and open colorectal surgery: a prospective cost analysis. *Colorectal Dis* 2012, 14(11), 1424–1430.

207. Jordan J, Dowson H, Gage H, Jackson D, Rockall T. Laparoscopic versus open colorectal resection for cancer and polyps: a cost-effectiveness study. *Clinicoecon Outcomes Res* 2014, 6, 415–422.

208. Fearon KC, Ljungqvist O, Von MM, et al. Enhanced recovery after surgery: a consensus review of clinical care for patients undergoing colonic resection. *Clin Nutr* 2005, 24(3), 466–477.

209. Kehlet H. Multimodal approach to control postoperative pathophysiology and rehabilitation. *Br J Anaesth* 1997, 78(5), 606–617.

210. Kehlet H, Mogensen T. Hospital stay of 2 days after open sigmoidectomy with a multimodal rehabilitation programme. *Br J Surg* 1999, 86(2), 227–230.

211. Lobo DN, Bostock KA, Neal KR, Perkins AC, Rowlands BJ, Allison SP. Effect of salt and water balance on recovery of gastrointestinal function after elective colonic resection: a randomised controlled trial. *Lancet* 2002, 359(9320), 1812–1818.

212. Boeckxstaens GE, de Jonge WJ. Neuroimmune mechanisms in postoperative ileus. *Gut* 2009, 58(9), 1300–1311.

213. Iyer S, Saunders WB, Stemkowski S. Economic burden of postoperative ileus associated with colectomy in the United States. *J Manag Care Pharm* 2009, 15(6), 485–494.

214. Boelens PG, Heesakkers FF, Luyer MD, et al. Reduction of postoperative ileus by early enteral nutrition in patients undergoing major rectal surgery: prospective, randomized, controlled trial. *Ann Surg* 2014, 259(4), 649–655.

215. Nachiappan S, Askari A, Malietzis G, et al. The impact of anastomotic leak and its treatment on cancer recurrence and survival following elective colorectal cancer resection. *World J Surg* 2015, 39(4), 1052–1058.

216. Mirnezami A, Mirnezami R, Chandrakumaran K, Sasapu K, Sagar P, Finan P. Increased local recurrence and reduced survival from colorectal cancer following anastomotic leak: systematic review and meta-analysis. *Ann Surg* 2011, 253(5), 890–899.

217. Krarup PM, Nordholm-Carstensen A, Jorgensen LN, Harling H. Anastomotic leak increases distant recurrence and long-term mortality after curative resection for colonic cancer: a nationwide cohort study. *Ann Surg* 2014, 259(5), 930–938.

218. Matthiessen P, Hallbook O, Rutegard J, Simert G, Sjodahl R. Defunctioning stoma reduces symptomatic anastomotic leakage after low anterior resection of the rectum for cancer: a randomized multicenter trial. *Ann Surg* 2007, 246(2), 207–214.

219. Kornmann VN, van RB, Smits AB, Bollen TL, Boerma D. Beware of false-negative CT scan for anastomotic leakage after colonic surgery. *Int J Colorectal Dis* 2014, 29(4), 445–451.

220. Frasson M, Flor-Lorente B, Ramos Rodriguez JL, et al. Risk factors for anastomotic leak after colon resection for cancer: multivariate analysis and nomogram from a multicentric, prospective, national study with 3193 patients. *Ann Surg* 2014, 262(2), 321–330.

221. Sultan R, Chawla T, Zaidi M. Factors affecting anastomotic leak after colorectal anastomosis in patients without protective stoma in tertiary care hospital. *J Pak Med Assoc* 2014, 64(2), 166–170.

222. Bhangu A, Singh P, Fitzgerald JE, Slesser A, Tekkis P. Postoperative nonsteroidal anti-inflammatory drugs and risk of anastomotic leak: meta-analysis of clinical and experimental studies. *World J Surg* 2014, 38(9), 2247–2257.

223. Subendran J, Siddiqui N, Victor JC, McLeod RS, Govindarajan A. NSAID use and anastomotic leaks following elective colorectal surgery: a matched case-control study. *J Gastrointest Surg* 2014, 18(8), 1391–1397.

224. Santilli V, Bernetti A, Mangone M, Paoloni M. Clinical definition of sarcopenia. *Clin Cases Miner Bone Metab* 2014, 11(3), 177–180.

225. Chen J, Wang DR, Zhang JR, Li P, Niu G, Lu Q. Meta-analysis of temporary ileostomy versus colostomy for colorectal anastomoses. *Acta Chir Belg* 2013, 113(5), 330–339.

226. Rondelli F, Reboldi P, Rulli A, et al. Loop ileostomy versus loop colostomy for fecal diversion after colorectal or coloanal anastomosis: a meta-analysis. *Int J Colorectal Dis* 2009, 24(5), 479–488.

227. Sajid MS, Craciunas L, Baig MK, Sains P. Systematic review and meta-analysis of published, randomized, controlled trials comparing suture anastomosis to stapled anastomosis for ileostomy closure. *Tech Coloproctol* 2013, 17(6), 631–639.

228. Choy PY, Bissett IP, Docherty JG, Parry BR, Merrie A, Fitzgerald A. Stapled versus handsewn methods for ileocolic anastomoses. *Cochrane Database Syst Rev* 2011, 9, CD004320.

229. Neutzling CB, Lustosa SA, Proenca IM, da Silva EM, Matos D. Stapled versus handsewn methods for colorectal anastomosis surgery. *Cochrane Database Syst Rev* 2012, 2, CD003144.

230. den DM, Noter SL, Hendriks ER, et al. Improved diagnosis and treatment of anastomotic leakage after colorectal surgery. *Eur J Surg Oncol* 2009, 35(4), 420–426.

231. Daams F, Wu Z, Lahaye MJ, Jeekel J, Lange JF. Prediction and diagnosis of colorectal anastomotic leakage: a systematic review of literature. *World J Gastrointest Surg* 2014, 6(2), 14–26.

232. Birgisson H, Talback M, Gunnarsson U, Pahlman L, Glimelius B. Improved survival in cancer of the colon and rectum in Sweden. *Eur J Surg Oncol* 2005, 31(8), 845–853.

233. Chen TY, Emmertsen KJ, Laurberg S. Bowel dysfunction after rectal cancer treatment: a study comparing the specialist's versus patient's perspective. *BMJ Open* 2014, 4(1), e003374.

234. Emmertsen KJ, Laurberg S. Low anterior resection syndrome score: development and validation of a symptom-based scoring system for bowel dysfunction after low anterior resection for rectal cancer. *Ann Surg* 2012, 255(5), 922–928.

235. Bruheim K, Tveit KM, Skovlund E, et al. Sexual function in females after radiotherapy for rectal cancer. *Acta Oncol* 2010, 49(6), 826–832.

236. Bruheim K, Guren MG, Dahl AA, et al. Sexual function in males after radiotherapy for rectal cancer. *Int J Radiat Oncol Biol Phys* 2010, 76(4), 1012–1017.

237. Bruheim K, Guren MG, Skovlund E, et al. Late side effects and quality of life after radiotherapy for rectal cancer. *Int J Radiat Oncol Biol Phys* 2010, 76(4), 1005–1011.

238. Birgisson H, Pahlman L, Gunnarsson U, Glimelius B. Late adverse effects of radiation therapy for rectal cancer – a systematic overview. *Acta Oncol* 2007, 46(4), 504–516.

239. Continuous Update Project. Colorectal cancer report, 2011: Food, nutrition, physical activity and the prevention of colorectal cancer. Washington, DC: World Cancer Research Fund/American Institute for Cancer Research. 2011.

240. Simons CC, Hughes LA, van EM, Goldbohm RA, van den Brandt PA, Weijenberg MP. Physical activity, occupational sitting time, and colorectal cancer risk in the Netherlands cohort study. *Am J Epidemiol* 2013, 177(6), 514–530.

241. Liang PS, Chen TY, Giovannucci E. Cigarette smoking and colorectal cancer incidence and mortality: systematic review and meta-analysis. *Int J Cancer* 2009, 124(10), 2406–2415.

242. Browning DR, Martin RM. Statins and risk of cancer: a systematic review and metaanalysis. *Int J Cancer* 2007, 120(4), 833–843.

243. Fernandez E, La VC, Balducci A, Chatenoud L, Franceschi S, Negri E. Oral contraceptives and colorectal cancer risk: a meta-analysis. *Br J Cancer* 2001, 84(5), 722–727.

244. Chan AT, Arber N, Burn J, et al. Aspirin in the chemoprevention of colorectal neoplasia: an overview. *Cancer Prev Res (Phila)* 2012, 5(2), 164–178.

245. Clegg A, Young J, Iliffe S, Rikkert MO, Rockwood K. Frailty in elderly people. *Lancet* 2013, 381(9868), 752–762.

246. Lemmens VE, Janssen-Heijnen ML, Houterman S, et al. Which comorbid conditions predict complications after surgery for colorectal cancer? *World J Surg* 2007, 31(1), 192–199.

247. van Leersum NJ, Janssen-Heijnen ML, Wouters MW, et al. Increasing prevalence of comorbidity in patients with colorectal cancer in the South of the Netherlands 1995–2010. *Int J Cancer* 2013, 132(9), 2157–2163.

248. Dekker JW, Gooiker GA, van der Geest LG, et al. Use of different comorbidity scores for risk-adjustment in the evaluation of quality of colorectal cancer surgery: does it matter? *Eur J Surg Oncol* 2012, 38(11), 1071–1078.

249. Janssen-Heijnen ML, Maas HA, Houterman S, Lemmens VE, Rutten HJ, Coebergh JW. Comorbidity in older surgical cancer patients: influence on patient care and outcome. *Eur J Cancer* 2007, 43(15), 2179–2193.

250. Kolfschoten NE, Wouters MW, Gooiker GA, et al. Nonelective colon cancer resections in elderly patients: results from the Dutch surgical colorectal audit. *Dig Surg* 2012, 29(5), 412–419.

251. Dekker JW, Gooiker GA, Bastiaannet E, et al. Cause of death the first year after curative colorectal cancer surgery; a prolonged impact of the surgery in elderly colorectal cancer patients. *Eur J Surg Oncol* 2014, 40(11), 1481–1487.

252. Rutten HJ, den DM, Lemmens VE, van de Velde CJ, Marijnen CA. Controversies of total mesorectal excision for rectal cancer in elderly patients. *Lancet Oncol* 2008, 9(5), 494–501.

253. Quaglia A, Tavilla A, Shack L, et al. The cancer survival gap between elderly and middle-aged patients in Europe is widening. *Eur J Cancer* 2009, 45(6), 1006–1016.

254. van den Broek CB, Dekker JW, Bastiaannet E, et al. The survival gap between middle-aged and elderly colon cancer patients. Time trends in treatment and survival. *Eur J Surg Oncol* 2011, 37(10), 904–912.

255. Dekker JW, van den Broek CB, Bastiaannet E, van de Geest LG, Tollenaar RA, Liefers GJ. Importance of the first postoperative year in the prognosis of elderly colorectal cancer patients. *Ann Surg Oncol* 2011, 18(6), 1533–1539.

256. Walter LC, Covinsky KE. Cancer screening in elderly patients: a framework for individualized decision making. *JAMA* 2001, 285(21), 2750–2756.

257. Gerard JP, Benezery K, Doyen J, Francois E. Aims of combined modality therapy in rectal cancer (M0). *Recent Results Cancer Res* 2014, 203, 153–169.

258. Lindegaard J, Gerard JP, Sun MA, Myerson R, Thomsen H, Laurberg S. Whither Papillon? Future directions for contact radiotherapy in rectal cancer. *Clin Oncol (R Coll Radiol)* 2007, 19(9), 738–741.

259. Sun MA, Lee CD, Snee AJ, Perkins K, Jelley FE, Wong H. High dose rate brachytherapy as a boost after preoperative chemoradiotherapy for more advanced rectal tumours: the Clatterbridge experience. *Clin Oncol (R Coll Radiol)* 2007, 19(9), 711–719.

260. Sun MA, Mukhopadhyay T, Ramani VS, et al. Can increasing the dose of radiation by HDR brachytherapy boost following pre operative chemoradiotherapy for advanced rectal cancer improve surgical outcomes? *Colorectal Dis* 2010, 12(Suppl. 2), 30–36.

261. Pettersson D, Glimelius B, Iversen H, Johansson H, Holm T, Martling A. Impaired postoperative leucocyte counts after preoperative radiotherapy for rectal cancer in the Stockholm III trial. *Br J Surg* 2013, 100(7), 969–975.

262. Townsley CA, Selby R, Siu LL. Systematic review of barriers to the recruitment of older patients with cancer onto clinical trials. *J Clin Oncol* 2005, 23(13), 3112–3124.

263. Zulman DM, Sussman JB, Chen X, Cigolle CT, Blaum CS, Hayward RA. Examining the evidence: a systematic review of the inclusion and analysis of older adults in randomized controlled trials. *J Gen Intern Med* 2011, 26(7), 783–790.

264. Abraham A, Habermann EB, Rothenberger DA, et al. Adjuvant chemotherapy for stage III colon cancer in the oldest old: results beyond clinical guidelines. *Cancer* 2013, 119(2), 395–403.

265. Watt AM, Faragher IG, Griffin TT, Rieger NA, Maddern GJ. Self-expanding metallic stents for relieving malignant colorectal obstruction: a systematic review. *Ann Surg* 2007, 246(1), 24–30.

266. Cortet M, Grimault A, Cheynel N, Lepage C, Bouvier A, Faivre J. Patterns of recurrence of obstructing colon cancers after surgery for cure: a population-based study. *Colorectal Dis* 2013, 15(9), 1100–1106.

267. Morris EJ, Taylor EF, Thomas JD, et al. Thirty-day postoperative mortality after colorectal cancer surgery in England. *Gut* 2011, 60(6), 806–813.

268. Kronborg O. Acute obstruction from tumour in the left colon without spread. A randomized trial of emergency colostomy versus resection. *Int J Colorectal Dis* 1995, 10(1), 1–5.

269. Jiang JK, Lan YT, Lin TC, et al. Primary vs. delayed resection for obstructive left-sided colorectal cancer: impact of surgery on patient outcome. *Dis Colon Rectum* 2008, 51(3), 306–311.

270. Tilney HS, Lovegrove RE, Purkayastha S, et al. Comparison of colonic stenting and open surgery for malignant large bowel obstruction. *Surg Endosc* 2007, 21(2), 225–233.

271. Pirlet IA, Slim K, Kwiatkowski F, Michot F, Millat BL. Emergency preoperative stenting versus surgery for acute left-sided malignant colonic obstruction: a multicenter randomized controlled trial. *Surg Endosc* 2011, 25(6), 1814–1821.

272. van Hooft JE, Bemelman WA, Oldenburg B, et al. Colonic stenting versus emergency surgery for acute left-sided malignant colonic obstruction: a multi-centre randomised trial. *Lancet Oncol* 2011, 12(4), 344–352.

273. Tan CJ, Dasari BV, Gardiner K. Systematic review and meta-analysis of randomized clinical trials of self-expanding metallic stents as a bridge to surgery versus emergency surgery for malignant left-sided large bowel obstruction. *Br J Surg* 2012, 99(4), 469–476.

274. Alcantara M, Serra-Aracil X, Falco J, Mora L, Bombardo J, Navarro S. Prospective, controlled, randomized study of intraoperative colonic lavage versus stent placement in obstructive left-sided colonic cancer. *World J Surg* 2011, 35(8), 1904–1910.

275. Cheung HY, Chung CC, Tsang WW, Wong JC, Yau KK, Li MK. Endolaparoscopic approach vs conventional open surgery in the treatment of obstructing left-sided colon cancer: a randomized controlled trial. *Arch Surg* 2009, 144(12), 1127–1132.

276. Fiori E, Lamazza A, De CA, et al. Palliative management of malignant rectosigmoidal obstruction. Colostomy vs. endoscopic stenting. A randomized prospective trial. *Anticancer Res* 2004, 24(1), 265–268.

277. Fiori E, Lamazza A, Schillaci A, et al. Palliative management for patients with subacute obstruction and stage IV unresectable rectosigmoid cancer: colostomy versus endoscopic stenting: final results of a prospective randomized trial. *Am J Surg* 2012, 204(3), 321–326.

278. Xinopoulos D, Dimitroulopoulos D, Theodosopoulos T, et al. Stenting or stoma creation for patients with inoperable malignant colonic obstructions? Results of a study and cost-effectiveness analysis. *Surg Endosc* 2004, 18(3), 421–426.

279. van den Berg MW, Ledeboer M, Dijkgraaf MG, Fockens P, Ter BF, van Hooft JE. Long-term results of palliative stent placement for acute malignant colonic obstruction. *Surg Endosc* 2015, 29(6), 1585–1585.

280. Sabbagh C, Chatelain D, Trouillet N, et al. Does use of a metallic colon stent as a bridge to surgery modify the pathology data in patients with colonic obstruction? A case-matched study. *Surg Endosc* 2013, 27(10), 3622–3631.

281. Sabbagh C, Browet F, Diouf M, et al. Is stenting as "a bridge to surgery" an oncologically safe strategy for the management of acute, left-sided, malignant, colonic obstruction? A comparative study with a propensity score analysis. *Ann Surg* 2013, 258, 107–115.

282. Sloothaak DA, van den Berg MW, Dijkgraaf MG, et al. Oncological outcome of malignant colonic obstruction in the Dutch Stent-In 2 trial. *Br J Surg* 2014, 101(13), 1751–1757.

283. van Hooft JE, van Halsema EE, Vanbiervliet G, et al. Self-expandable metal stents for obstructing colonic and extracolonic cancer: European Society of Gastrointestinal Endoscopy (ESGE) clinical guideline. *Gastrointest Endosc* 2014, 80(5), 747–761.

284. Manes G, de BM, Fuccio L, et al. Endoscopic palliation in patients with incurable malignant colorectal obstruction by means of self-expanding metal stent: analysis of results and predictors of outcomes in a large multicenter series. *Arch Surg* 2011, 146(10), 1157–1162.

285. Guo MG, Feng Y, Liu JZ, et al. Factors associated with mortality risk for malignant colonic obstruction in elderly patients. *BMC Gastroenterol* 2014, 14, 76.

286. Kasten KR, Midura EF, Davis BR, Rafferty JF, Paquette IM. Blowhole colostomy for the urgent management of distal large bowel obstruction. *J Surg Res* 2014, 188(1), 53–57.

287. Yang HY, Wu CC, Jao SW, Hsu KF, Mai CM, Hsiao KC. Two-stage resection for malignant colonic obstructions: the timing of early resection and possible predictive factors. *World J Gastroenterol* 2012, 18(25), 3267–3271.

288. Esteva M, Leiva A, Ramos M, et al. Factors related with symptom duration until diagnosis and treatment of symptomatic colorectal cancer. *BMC Cancer* 2013, 13, 87.

289. Wilkinson NW, Yothers G, Lopa S, Costantino JP, Petrelli NJ, Wolmark N. Long-term survival results of surgery alone versus surgery plus 5-fluorouracil and leucovorin for stage II and stage III colon cancer: pooled analysis of NSABP C-01 through C-05. A baseline from which to compare modern adjuvant trials. *Ann Surg Oncol* 2010, 17(4), 959–966.

290. Breugom AJ, van GW, Muller EW, et al. Adjuvant chemotherapy for rectal cancer patients treated with preoperative (chemo)radiotherapy and total mesorectal excision: a Dutch Colorectal Cancer Group (DCCG) randomized phase III trial. *Ann Oncol* 2015, 26(4), 696–701.

291. Breugom AJ, Swets M, Bosset JF, et al. Adjuvant chemotherapy after preoperative (chemo)radiotherapy and surgery for patients with rectal cancer: a systematic review and meta-analysis of individual patient data. *Lancet Oncol* 2015, 16(2), 200–207.

292. Heidelberger C, Chaudhuri NK, Danneberg P, et al. Fluorinated pyrimidines, a new class of tumour-inhibitory compounds. *Nature* 1957, 179(4561), 663–666.

293. Gustavsson B, Carlsson G, Machover D, et al. A review of the evolution of systemic chemotherapy in the management of colorectal cancer. *Clin Colorectal Cancer* 2015, 14(1), 1–10.

294. Figueredo A, Coombes ME, Mukherjee S. Adjuvant therapy for completely resected stage II colon cancer. *Cochrane Database Syst Rev* 2008, 3, CD005390.

295. Caudle KE, Thorn CF, Klein TE, et al. Clinical Pharmacogenetics Implementation Consortium guidelines for dihydropyrimidine dehydrogenase genotype and fluoropyrimidine dosing. *Clin Pharmacol Ther* 2013, 94(6), 640–645.

296. Twelves C, Scheithauer W, McKendrick J, et al. Capecitabine versus 5-fluorouracil/folinic acid as adjuvant therapy for stage III colon cancer: final results from the X-ACT trial with analysis by age and preliminary evidence of a pharmacodynamic marker of efficacy. *Ann Oncol* 2012, 23(5), 1190–1197.

297. Haller DG, Tabernero J, Maroun J, et al. Capecitabine plus oxaliplatin compared with fluorouracil and folinic acid as adjuvant therapy for stage III colon cancer. *J Clin Oncol* 2011, 29(11), 1465–1471.

298. Andre T, Boni C, Navarro M, et al. Improved overall survival with oxaliplatin, fluorouracil, and leucovorin as adjuvant treatment in stage II or III colon cancer in the MOSAIC trial. *J Clin Oncol* 2009, 27(19), 3109–3116.

299. Kuebler JP, Wieand HS, O'Connell MJ, et al. Oxaliplatin combined with weekly bolus fluorouracil and leucovorin as surgical adjuvant chemotherapy for stage II and III colon cancer: results from NSABP C-07. *J Clin Oncol* 2007, 25(16), 2198–2204.

300. Allegra CJ, Yothers G, O'Connell MJ, et al. Phase III trial assessing bevacizumab in stages II and III carcinoma of the colon: results of NSABP protocol C-08. *J Clin Oncol* 2011, 29(1), 11–16.

301. Allegra CJ, Yothers G, O'Connell MJ, et al. Bevacizumab in stage II-III colon cancer: 5-year update of the National Surgical Adjuvant Breast and Bowel Project C-08 trial. *J Clin Oncol* 2013, 31(3), 359–364.

302. de Gramont A, Van CE, Schmoll HJ, et al. Bevacizumab plus oxaliplatin-based chemotherapy as adjuvant treatment for colon cancer (AVANT): a phase 3 randomised controlled trial. *Lancet Oncol* 2012, 13(12), 1225–1233.

303. Van Cutsem E, Labianca R, Bodoky G, et al. Randomized phase III trial comparing biweekly infusional fluorouracil/leucovorin alone or with irinotecan in the adjuvant treatment of stage III colon cancer: PETACC-3. *J Clin Oncol* 2009, 27(19), 3117–3125.

304. Saltz LB, Niedzwiecki D, Hollis D, et al. Irinotecan fluorouracil plus leucovorin is not superior to fluorouracil plus leucovorin alone as adjuvant treatment for stage III colon cancer: results of CALGB 89803. *J Clin Oncol* 2007, 25(23), 3456–3461.

305. Klingbiel D, Saridaki Z, Roth AD, Bosman FT, Delorenzi M, Tejpar S. Prognosis of stage II and III colon cancer treated with adjuvant 5-fluorouracil or FOLFIRI in relation to microsatellite status: results of the PETACC-3 trial. *Ann Oncol* 2015, 26(1), 126–132.

306. Giantonio BJ, Catalano PJ, Meropol NJ, et al. Bevacizumab in combination with oxaliplatin, fluorouracil, and leucovorin (FOLFOX4) for previously treated metastatic colorectal cancer: results from the Eastern Cooperative Oncology Group Study E3200. *J Clin Oncol* 2007, 25(12), 1539–1544.

307. Taieb J, Tabernero J, Mini E, et al. Oxaliplatin, fluorouracil, and leucovorin with or without cetuximab in patients with resected stage III colon cancer (PETACC-8): an open-label, randomised phase 3 trial. *Lancet Oncol* 2014, 15(8), 862–873.

308. Alberts SR, Sargent DJ, Nair S, et al. Effect of oxaliplatin, fluorouracil, and leucovorin with or without cetuximab on survival among patients with resected stage III colon cancer: a randomized trial. *JAMA* 2012, 307(13), 1383–1393.

309. Douillard JY, Oliner KS, Siena S, et al. Panitumumab-FOLFOX4 treatment and RAS mutations in colorectal cancer. *N Engl J Med* 2013, 369(11), 1023–1034.

310. Breugom AJ, Swets M, Bosset JF, et al. Adjuvant chemotherapy after preoperative (chemo)radiotherapy and surgery for patients with rectal cancer: a systematic review and meta-analysis of individual patient data. *Lancet Oncol* 2015, 16(2), 200–207.

311. van den Broek CB, Bastiaannet E, Dekker JW, et al. Time trends in chemotherapy (administration and costs) and relative survival in stage III colon cancer patients – a large population-based study from 1990 to 2008. *Acta Oncol* 2013, 52(5), 941–949.

312. de Angelis R, Sant M, Coleman MP, et al. Cancer survival in Europe 1999–2007 by country and age: results of EUROCARE-5 – a population-based study. *Lancet Oncol* 2014, 15(1), 23–34.

313. Maas M, Nelemans PJ, Valentini V, et al. Long-term outcome in patients with a pathological complete response after chemoradiation for rectal cancer: a pooled analysis of individual patient data. *Lancet Oncol* 2010, 11(9), 835–844.

314. Maas M, Beets-Tan RG, Lambregts DM, et al. Wait-and-see policy for clinical complete responders after chemoradiation for rectal cancer. *J Clin Oncol* 2011, 29(35), 4633–4640.

315. Habr-Gama A, Perez RO, Proscurshim I, et al. Patterns of failure and survival for nonoperative treatment of stage c0 distal rectal cancer following neoadjuvant chemoradiation therapy. *J Gastrointest Surg* 2006, 10(10), 1319–1328.

316. Habr-Gama A. Assessment and management of the complete clinical response of rectal cancer to chemoradiotherapy. *Colorectal Dis* 2006, 8(Suppl. 3), 21–24.

317. Habr-Gama A, Perez RO. Non-operative management of rectal cancer after neoadjuvant chemoradiation. *Br J Surg* 2009, 96(2), 125–127.

318. Glynne-Jones R, Hughes R. Critical appraisal of the 'wait and see' approach in rectal cancer for clinical complete responders after chemoradiation. *Br J Surg* 2012, 99(7), 897–909.

319. Gerard JP, Ortholan C, Benezery K, et al. Contact x-ray therapy for rectal cancer: experience in Centre Antoine-Lacassagne, Nice, 2002–2006. *Int J Radiat Oncol Biol Phys* 2008, 72(3), 665–670.

320. Gerard JP, Myint AS, Croce O, et al. Renaissance of contact x-ray therapy for treating rectal cancer. *Expert Rev Med Devices* 2011, 8(4), 483–492.

321. van Gijn W, Marijnen CA, Nagtegaal ID, et al. Preoperative radiotherapy combined with total mesorectal excision for resectable rectal cancer: 12-year follow-up of the multicentre, randomised controlled TME trial. *Lancet Oncol* 2011, 12(6), 575–582.

322. Zeng WG, Zhou ZX, Hou HR, et al. Outcome of laparoscopic versus open resection for rectal cancer in elderly patients. *J Surg Res* 2015, 193(2), 613–618.

323. Lemmens V, van SL, Janssen-Heijnen M, Martijn H, Rutten H, Coebergh JW. Trends in colorectal cancer in the south of the Netherlands 1975–2007: rectal cancer survival levels with colon cancer survival. *Acta Oncol* 2010, 49(6), 784–796.

324. van den Broek CB, Bastiaannet E, Dekker JW, et al. Time trends in chemotherapy (administration and costs) and relative survival in stage III colon cancer patients – a large population-based study from 1990 to 2008. *Acta Oncol* 2013, 52(5), 941–949.

325. van den Broek CB, van GW, Bastiaannet E, et al. Differences in pre-operative treatment for rectal cancer between Norway, Sweden, Denmark, Belgium and the Netherlands. *Eur J Surg Oncol* 2014, 40(12), 1789–1796.

326. Vermeer TA, Orsini RG, Rutten HJ. Surgery for rectal cancer – what is on the horizon? *Curr Oncol Rep* 2014, 16(3), 372.

327. Breugom AJ, Boelens PG, van den Broek CB, et al. Quality assurance in the treatment of colorectal cancer: the EURECCA initiative. *Ann Oncol* 2014, 25(8), 1485–1492.

328. van de Velde CJ, Aristei C, Boelens PG, et al. EURECCA colorectal: multidisciplinary mission statement on better care for patients with colon and rectal cancer in Europe. *Eur J Cancer* 2013, 49(13), 2784–2790.

329. van Gijn W, van den Broek CB, Mroczkowski P, et al. The EURECCA project: Data items scored by European colorectal cancer audit registries. *Eur J Surg Oncol* 2012, 38(6), 467–471.

330. Tudyka V, Blomqvist L, Beets-Tan RG, et al. EURECCA consensus conference highlights about colon and rectal cancer multidisciplinary management: the radiology experts review. *Eur J Surg Oncol* 2014, 40(4), 469–475.

331. Quality assurance in surgical oncology: the EURECCA platform. *Eur J Surg Oncol* 2014, 40(11), 1387–1390.

332. Boelens PG, Taylor C, Henning G, et al. Involving patients in a multidisciplinary European consensus process and in the development of a 'patient summary of the consensus document for colon and rectal cancer care'. *Patient* 2014, 7(3), 261–270.

333. Valentini V, Glimelius B, Haustermans K, et al. EURECCA consensus conference highlights about rectal cancer clinical management: the radiation oncologist's expert review. *Radiother Oncol* 2014, 110(1), 195–198.

334. Quirke P, West NP, Nagtegaal ID. EURECCA consensus conference highlights about colorectal cancer clinical management: the pathologists expert review. *Virchows Arch* 2014, 464(2), 129–134.

Anal cancer

PER J NILSSON

INTRODUCTION

The anal canal has several definitions but for clinical purposes the puborectalis muscle ring and the intersphincteric groove can be used to determine cranial and caudal boundaries, respectively. In the upper part the epithelial lining initially consists of colorectal glandular epithelium that, approximately 1.5 cm above the dentate line, becomes the anal transitional zone (ATZ). The ATZ displays a variety of cell types including cells with various epithelial differentiation, e.g. columnar, flat and squamous, as well as endocrine cells and melanocytes. Below the dentate line cell lining is more consistently composed of non-keratinized squamous epithelium [1]. The perianal area, usually defined as within a 5 cm radius from the anus, is covered by keratinized squamous epithelium with hair follicles and apocrine appendages, i.e. perianal skin.

Many different neoplastic lesions can occur in the anal canal and perianal area, most being uncommon or rare, and a thorough knowledge of anatomy and tumour characteristics is crucial in management of these different tumours. The treatment of squamous cell carcinoma of the anus (SCCA) has undergone a paradigmatic change over the past 40 years and may serve as a model for therapeutic evolvement in other tumour forms.

INCIDENCE AND AETIOLOGY

Carcinoma of the anus is an uncommon disease accounting for 1–2% of digestive tract tumours. SCCA has an annual incidence of 1 in 100,000, is more common among women and has an increasing incidence [2]. Data from the UK and Scandinavian countries show incidence increase in both sexes, and temporal trends indicate a gradually increasing risk among individuals born from 1940 and onward [3]. SCCA is associated with human papillomavirus (HPV), in particular HPV16 and HPV18, as is its precursor lesion anal intraepithelial neoplasia (AIN). Host response to HPV, with virus DNA integration leading to genomic change, appears to be necessary but not sufficient for malignant transformation [4]. Other risk factors identified include smoking [5], sexual behaviour and immunosuppression including solid organ transplant recipients and affliction with autoimmune disorders. Markedly increased incidence figures have been reported in HIV positive individuals but whether this may be changed by the introduction of highly active anti-retroviral therapy (HAART) is unclear [6].

DIAGNOSIS AND PRE-TREATMENT IMAGING

Anal tumours commonly present with bleeding but may also display symptoms of itching, discharge or a palpable mass. The unspecific nature of symptoms may lead to patient's delay as well as doctor's delay in diagnosis as symptoms can wrongly be attributed to haemorrhoids. Only rarely the presenting symptom is enlarged inguinal lymph nodes.

When the patient seeks medical advice diagnosis can be obvious by palpation and rigid proctoscopy. However, in some patients symptoms necessitate an examination under general anaesthesia. Biopsy is mandatory to confirm diagnosis and besides a full medical history and clinical body exam a CT scan of the thorax and abdomen and a pelvic MRI should be performed. Assessment of genital tract in females to exclude other HPV-associated malignancies should be considered as should a HIV test in all patients.

Fine-needle aspiration should be performed when palpable inguinal nodes are present and PET/CT may be performed.

PATHOLOGY AND STAGING

AIN, also known as anal squamous intraepithelial lesion (ASIL), is a squamous cell dysplastic lesion, analogous to cervical intraepithelial neoplasia (CIN), which can be a precursor to invasive SCCA. Anal cytology with a brush technique can be used for screening and, in the case of positive findings, further mapping can be performed with high-resolution anoscopy. Depending on depth of lesion AIN is subdivided into AINs I–III. The more superficial AINs I and II only rarely progress into cancer, whereas a substantial risk appears to exist for AIN III, in particular among immunocompromised and HIV positive individuals [7].

SCCA constitutes the vast majority of anal canal cancers. Previously used histological division into various sub-types of SCCA (e.g. basaloid, cloacogenic) has generally been abandoned as they have no bearing on management. Adenocarcinomas occur in the anal canal and can be of rectal type, from glands and ducts, or associated with long-standing fistula [8]. Anorectal melanomas are rare and carry poor prognosis. For anorectal melanomas radiotherapy and chemotherapy are of limited importance, and surgery with uninvolved margins appears to offer the best chance of cure [9].

Also among tumours of the anal margin SCCA is the dominating histology with sub-types such as Bowen's disease (intraepithelial squamous cell cancer of the anal margin) and verrucous carcinoma, also known as Buschke–Löwenstein tumour, which generally carry a more favourable prognosis. Perianal Paget's disease is an intraepithelial adenocarcinoma that may be associated with a synchronous rectal or other adenocarcinoma.

Following proper diagnostic work-up including digital rectal examination, MRI and possibly endo-anal ultrasound, anal canal cancers are staged according to the TNM system used by AJCC/UICC (Tables 29.1 and 29.2) [10]. Tumours of the anal margin are also classified according to the TNM system but slightly different as staging should be done as with skin tumours. In contrast to colorectal cancer, it is the size of the lesion, not depth of invasion, that determines T-stage.

TREATMENT OF PREMALIGNANT LESIONS

AIN appears to be uncommon in the general population but occurs more often in certain risk populations. HIV positive men who have sex with men (MSM) are a high-risk population, but also HIV negative MSM and HIV positive non-MSM; in particular women with a previous history of other HPV-associated neoplasia have an increased risk. Other immunocompromised patients such as solid organ transplant recipients may also have an elevated risk, and screening programmes have been suggested for different

Table 29.1 TNM staging of anal canal cancer

T – Primary Tumour

T0	No evidence of primary tumour
Tis	Carcinoma in situ, Bowen's disease, high-grade squamous intraepithelial lesion (HSIL), anal intraepithelial neoplasias II–III (AIN II-III)
T1	Tumour 2 cm or less in greatest dimension
T2	Tumour more than 2 cm but not more than 5 cm in greatest dimension
T3	Tumour more than 5 cm in greatest dimension
T4	Tumour of any size invades adjacent organ(s), e.g. vagina, urethra, bladder

N – Regional Lymph Nodes

N0	No regional lymph node metastasis
N1	Metastasis in perirectal lymph node(s)
N2	Metastasis in unilateral internal iliac and/or unilateral inguinal lymph node(s)
N3	Metastasis in perirectal and inguinal lymph nodes and/or bilateral internal iliac and/or bilateral inguinal lymph nodes

M – Distant Metastasis

M0	No distant metastasis
M1	Distant metastasis

Source: Adapted from Sobin LH, et al., eds., *TNM Classification of Malignant Tumours*, 7th ed., Oxford: Wiley-Blackwell, 2009, pp. 106–109.

Table 29.2 Stage grouping anal canal cancer

Stage	T	N	M
Stage 0	Tis	N0	M0
Stage I	T1	N0	M0
Stage II	T2, T3	N0	M0
Stage IIIA	T1, T2, T3	N0	M0
	T4	N0	M0
Stage IIIB	T4	N1	M0
	Any T	N2, N3	M0
Stage IV	Any T	Any N	M1

Source: Adapted from Sobin LH, et al., eds., *TNM Classification of Malignant Tumours*, 7th ed., Oxford: Wiley-Blackwell, 2009, pp. 106–109.

risk populations [11]. When AIN is detected it is of great importance to determine whether it is an AIN I or II or an AIN III and whether the affected patient belongs to a risk population. There are few evidence-based guidelines for the treatment and follow-up of AIN, but different algorithms have been proposed [12]. In individuals with an elevated risk surgery in the form of local excision should be undertaken at least for AIN III lesions. Wide margins are generally not indicated and healing by secondary intention is often an acceptable alternative.

NON-SURGICAL TREATMENT

SCCA was treated with primary surgery until the mid-1980s, but primary surgery has since become obsolete following the publications on combined modality therapy from the 1970s. The introduction of radiation therapy combined with 5-FU and mitomycin C (MMC) proved to offer complete clinical and pathological response in a substantial proportion of patients, rendering surgery unnecessary [13]. Although primary radical surgery and chemoradiotherapy (CRT) have never been compared in a randomized trial, comparative data suggest favourable outcome with non-surgical therapy [14].

During the 1990s three large randomized trials (EORTC 22861, UKCCCR ACT I and RTOG 87-04) determined that chemoradiation was superior to radiotherapy alone and that the combination of 5-FU and MMC was superior to 5-FU alone in terms of cancer-specific survival. In a second generation of randomized trials (RTOG 98-11, ACCORD-03 and CRUK ACT II), the role of cisplatin, as an alternative to MMC and as a neo-adjuvant prior to CRT, and the potential benefit of maintenance or consolidation therapy after CRT were explored. In brief, results indicate that neo-adjuvant chemotherapy is non-beneficial, cisplatin is not superior to MMC and maintenance therapy has no impact on local control or survival [15–20].

Recent European guidelines recommend concomitant MMC and 5-FU with external beam radiotherapy to a dose of at least 45–50 Gy without a treatment gap as the primary therapeutic option in SCCA [21]. Inclusion of inguinal nodes in the radiation field and non-reduced treatment protocols for frail or elderly patients are recommended. However, increasingly the long-term side effects of CRT (i.e. effects on quality of life and faecal incontinence [22]) are being studied. Most probably side effects of CRT can be reduced when more sophisticated ways of delivering irradiation (e.g. intensity-modulated radiation therapy) are deployed.

Although a vast majority of patients are planned for primary non-surgical treatment, the surgeon is a key player in the multidisciplinary team (MDT) around the anal cancer patient. Clinical tumour assessment (basically determining the T-stage) is often the surgeon's task and may need general anaesthesia to be performed properly. Pre-treatment stomas are unusual but may be necessary because of symptoms (e.g. pain, fistula, incontinence) and should sometimes be considered a pre-emptive measure to avoid radiotherapy interruptions that may compromise the radiotherapy effect. Generally, a loop sigmoidostomy is the preferred option for anal cancer patients, and in patients planned for CRT this procedure can be combined with implantation of a subcutaneous venous port.

SURGERY

Only in small (<2 cm) lesions, preferably highly differentiated and on the anal margin, is primary surgery in the form of a local excision recommended, provided that excision can be performed with adequate margins and without compromising sphincter function. Primary abdominoperineal excision (APE) may be offered to patients having undergone previous pelvic irradiation or, uncommonly, patients having a preference.

Despite the advances in non-surgical therapy for SCCA, a substantial proportion of patients eventually will be candidates for an APE. Data from published series and from the randomized trials indicate that about a quarter to a third of patients with intended curative non-surgical therapy suffer a local treatment failure either immediately as a residual tumour or later as a recurrence [18–20,23]. Following CRT, timing and methods used for response evaluation are of importance. Digital rectal examination, often under general anaesthesia, is a cornerstone but should be complemented by radiological methods (e.g. MRI, CT or possibly PET/CT). The effects of CRT on tumour regression can be difficult to assess and in patients where clinical and radiological complete response is under question, the time for a definitive decision on salvage surgery can be extended to 26 weeks after termination of CRT. Post-treatment biopsies can be difficult to interpret because of radiation effects on tissues, and may also cause pain and slowly healing ulcerations. However, a decision to proceed to salvage surgery must be based on histological confirmation of viable tumour cells.

When a local disease failure is suspected or detected, proper work-up and assessment for the appropriateness of salvage surgery in a designated multidisciplinary tumour board (MDT) is mandatory. If assessment is at an experienced anal cancer tumour board >70% of potential candidates can be offered surgery with curative intention [23,24], in comparison to about 50% observed in the randomized trials. MRI of the pelvis offers an excellent way to define local tumour growth and a CT scan of the thorax and abdomen (or possibly a PET/CT) should be used to exclude distant metastases.

Surgery generally includes at least an APE. When performing this operation for an anal cancer the surgeon must be aware that the procedure differs from the same operation when performed on a rectal cancer patient. First, the irradiated field and the dose given are both larger; second, potential directions of spread are different; and third, overgrowth onto adjacent organs (e.g. posterior vaginal wall) occurs more often. These differences put together, and given the relative rarity of the disease, indicate that surgery for SCCA should preferably be centralized to units with experience of multi-visceral excisions and access to plastic reconstructive surgeons and other surgical oncologists including urologists and gynaecology tumour surgeons.

The extra-levator APE (elAPE) described for rectal cancer does not meet all demands faced in SCCA. Given the differences outlined above, the operation in an anal cancer patient requires a wider excision of perianal skin and excision of ischioanal fat which leads to a wide perineal defect and risk of healing problems. The use of musculocutaneous flaps (e.g. vertical rectus abdominis flap or gluteal flap) can reduce the rate of perineal complications and is strongly recommended [25]. In addition, clearance of nodes in the iliac or obturator area may be necessary, as can be inguinal clearance. In a proportion of patients a formal posterior or full pelvic exenteration is necessary to achieve clear resection margins (R0).

Overall survival rates of 30–60% following salvage surgery in SCCA are reported in several case series. Since achievement of R0 has a significant impact on surgical outcomes [26], the sequence of clinical patient assessment, tumour extent definition with high-quality MRI, tailoring surgery and performing the necessary resection and reconstruction for each patient should be uncontroversial.

LOCALLY ADVANCED AND METASTATIC DISEASE

Distant spread of SCCA occurs in 10–20% and most common locations include para-aortic lymph nodes, lungs, liver and skin. Distant relapses are often detected in conjunction with a local failure and are associated with poor prognosis. However, in patients with limited metastatic disease, evaluation by an appropriate MDT with the aim of offering potentially curative surgical or chemoradiation options should be included. Locally recurrent tumours after previous salvage surgery are extremely challenging and surgery attempting radical resection can be an option only exceptionally. A palliative sigmoidostomy and sometimes urinary deviation with pyelostomas may be best options.

There is no consensus regarding optimal palliative chemotherapy. Choice of treatment can depend on chemotherapy used during CRT and experience, and a number of agents have been reported to be active. More recently, the epidermal growth factor receptor (EGFR) inhibitor has been used in combination with chemotherapy.

Palliative care of an anal cancer patient with a local disease failure is difficult and demanding also when the faecal and urinary streams have been deviated. Meticulous skin care is important, pain management often requires specialist care and re-irradiation can sometimes reduce symptoms. Symptoms from a local failure can include odour which puts further emphasis to the need of professional support for patient and close relatives in the terminal palliative phase.

REFERENCES

1. Fenger C, The anal transitional zone. *Acta Pathol Microbiol Immunol Scand* 95 (1987): Suppl. 289.
2. Jemal A, Simard EP, Dorell C, et al. Annual report to the nation on the status of cancer, 1975–2009, featuring the burden and trends in human papillomavirus (HPV)-associated cancer and HPV vaccination coverage levels. *J Natl Cancer Inst* 105 (2013): 175–201.
3. Robinson D, Coupland V, and Møller H. An analysis of temporal and generational trends in the incidence of anal and other HPV-related cancers in southeast England. *Br J Cancer* 100 (2009): 527–531.
4. Gervaz P, Hirschel B, and Morel P. Molecular biology of squamous cell carcinoma of the anus. *Br J Surg* 93 (2006): 531–538.
5. Nordenvall C, Nilsson PJ, Weimin Y, et al. Smoking, snus use and risk of right- and left-sided colon, rectal and anal cancer: a 37-year follow-up study. *Int J Cancer* 128 (2011): 157–165.
6. Sunesen KG, Nørgaard M, Thorlacius-Ussing O, et al. Immunosuppressive disorders and risk of anal squamous cell carcinoma: a nationwide cohort study in Denmark, 1978–2005. *Int J Cancer* 127 (2010): 675–684.
7. Scholefield JH, Castle MT, and Watson NFS. Malignant transformation of high-grade anal intraepithelial neoplasia. *Br J Surg* 92 (2005): 1133–1136.
8. Garrett K and Kalady MF. Anal neoplasms. *Surg Clin N Am* 90 (2010): 147–161.
9. Nilsson PJ and Ragnarsson-Olding BK. Importance of clear resection margins in anorectal malignant melanoma. *Br J Surg* 97 (2010): 98–103.
10. Sobin LH, Gospodarowicz MK, and Wittekind Ch, eds. *TNM Classification of Malignant Tumours*, 7th ed. Oxford: Wiley-Blackwell, 2009, pp. 106–109.
11. Salit IE, Lytwyn A, Raboud J, et al. The role of cytology (Pap tests) and human papillomavirus testing in anal cancer screening. *AIDS* 24 (2010): 1307–1313.
12. Simpson JD and Scholefield JH. Diagnosis and management of anal intraepithelial neoplasia and anal cancer. *Br Med J* 348 (2011): d6818.
13. Nigro ND. An evaluation of combined therapy for squamous cell cancer of the anal canal. *Dis Colon Rectum* 27 (1984): 763–766.
14. Goldman S, Glimelius B, Glas U, et al. Management of anal epidermoid carcinoma – an evaluation of treatment results in two population-based series. *Int J Colorectal Dis* 4 (1989): 234–243.
15. Bartelink H, Roelofsen F, Eschwege F, et al. Concomitant radiotherapy and chemotherapy is superior to radiotherapy alone in treatment of locally advanced anal cancer: results of a phase III randomized trial of the European Organization for Research and Treatment of Cancer Radiotherapy and Gastrointestinal Cooperative Groups. *J Clin Oncol* 15 (1997): 2040–2049.
16. Epidermoid anal cancer: results from the UKCCR randomised trial on radiotherapy alone versus radiotherapy, 5-fluorouracil, and mitomycin. UKCCR Anal Cancer Trial Working Party. UK Co-ordinating Committee on Cancer Research. *Lancet* 348 (1996): 1049–1054.
17. Flam M, John M, Pajak TF, et al. The role of mitomycin in combination with fluorouracil and radiotherapy, and of salvage chemoradiation in the definitive nonsurgical treatment of epidermoid carcinoma of the anal canal: results of a phase III randomized intergroup study. *J Clin Oncol* 14 (1996): 2527–2539.

18. Ajani JA, Winter KA, Gunderson LL, et al. Fluorouracil, mitomycin, and radiotherapy vs fluorouracil, cisplatin, and radiotherapy for carcinoma of the anal canal: a randomized controlled trial. *JAMA* 299 (2008): 1914–1921.

19. Peiffert D, Tournier-Rangeard L, Gérard JP, et al. Induction chemotherapy and dose intensification of the radiation boost in locally advanced anal canal carcinoma: final analysis of the randomized UNICANCER ACCORD 03 trial. *J Clin Oncol* 30 (2012): 1941–1948.

20. James RD, Glynne-Jones R, Meadows HM, et al. Mitomycin or cisplatin chemoradiation with or without maintenance chemotherapy for treatment of squamous-cell carcinoma of the anus (ACT II): a randomised, phase 3, open-label, 2×2 factorial trial. *Lancet Oncol* 14 (2013): 516–524.

21. Glynne-Jones R, Nilsson PJ, Aschele C, et al. Anal cancer: ESMO-ESSO-ESTRO clinical practice guidelines for diagnosis, treatment and follow-up. *Radiother Oncol* 111 (2014): 330–339.

22. Bentzen AG, Balteskard L, Wanderås EH, et al. Impaired health-related quality of life after chemoradiotherapy for anal cancer: late effects in a national cohort of 128 survivors. *Acta Oncol* 52 (2013): 55–60.

23. Renehan AG, Saunders MP, Schofield PF, et al. Patterns of local disease failure and outcome after salvage surgery in patients with anal cancer. *Br J Surg* 92 (2005): 605–614.

24. Nilsson PJ, Svensson C, Goldman S, et al. Salvage abdominoperineal resection in anal epidermoid cancer. *Br J Surg* 89 (2002): 1488–1493.

25. Sunesen KG, Buntzen S, Tei T, et al. Perineal healing and survival after anal cancer salvage surgery: 10-year experience with primary perineal reconstruction using the vertical rectus abdominis myocutaneous (VRAM) flap. *Ann Surg Oncol* 16 (2009): 68–77.

26. Schiller DE, Cummings BJ, Rai S, et al. Outcomes of salvage surgery for squamous cell carcinoma of the anal canal. *Ann Surg Oncol* 10 (2007): 2780–2789.

30

Peritoneal surface malignancies

SANTIAGO GONZÁLEZ-MORENO, PAUL H SUGARBAKER, GLORIA ORTEGA-PÉREZ,
OSCAR ALONSO-CASADO, DOMINIQUE ELIAS, MARCELLO DERACO, POMPILIU PISO
AND KURT VAN DER SPEETEN

INTRODUCTION

Peritoneal metastases (PMs) represent a route of cancer dissemination as significant as lymphatic or hematogenous spread, which has attracted much attention in the last decades. Malignant peritoneal disease can derive from tumors arising in organs located within the abdomen and pelvis (peritoneal carcinomatosis) or from the peritoneal lining itself (primary peritoneal neoplasms). A radical approach that combines cytoreductive surgery (CRS) and perioperative intraperitoneal chemotherapy (PIC), complemented by systemic chemotherapy, has been extensively investigated and currently has clear indications in the management of selected patients and disease processes. Hyperthermic intraperitoneal chemotherapy (HIPEC) is the most commonly used form of PIC.

Peritoneal surface oncology (PSO) is a rapidly expanding field, with a growing demand for specific education and training. Although expert treatment centres have materialized around the world, additional ones are needed since the percentage of patients who can benefit from an expert evaluation of malignant peritoneal disease within a dedicated multidisciplinary team is still limited.

ETIOLOGY AND INCIDENCE

Primary malignant peritoneal diseases are quite infrequent compared with peritoneal carcinomatosis (PC) secondary to gastrointestinal or gynaecologic cancers.

Primary peritoneal neoplasms

Diffuse malignant peritoneal mesothelioma (DMPM) accounts for approximately 25% of all mesotheliomas. In the United States the incidence is 300–400 new cases per year. It has been etiologically linked to asbestos exposure, although this fact is less commonly identified in peritoneal than in pleural mesothelioma patients. Its incidence in Europe is rising.

Serous primary peritoneal carcinoma (SPPC) is a peritoneal papillary serous neoplasm clinically defined by predominant peritoneal tumor load, with scant or no ovarian involvement. It accounts for around 20% of all serous papillary carcinomas. A possible origin in residual Müllerian epithelium remaining in the peritoneum after embryologic development can be inferred. Its management does not differ from that of epithelial ovarian or tubal cancer.

Desmoplastic small round cell tumor is a very rare disease of uncertain origin (100 new cases per year worldwide), invariably presenting with peritoneal masses. Its cells show a pathognomonic translocation involving the WT1 and EWSR1 genes, which is diagnostic. It affects adolescents and young adults.

Peritoneal carcinomatosis (secondary malignant peritoneal neoplasms)

PC occurs in the natural history of locally advanced tumors of the gastrointestinal or gynaecologic tracts, or as a common form of recurrence after primary curative intent resection. When cancer cells gain access to the free peritoneal cavity they efficiently seed in the parietal or visceral peritoneal surfaces and give rise to tumor implants in predictable sites and recesses determined by peritoneal fluid circulation [1].

Overall, the incidence of PC in colorectal cancer (including appendiceal neoplasms) is greater than 15%, in gastric cancer 40%, in pancreatic cancer 25% and in epithelial ovarian cancer 60% [2]. Pseudomyxoma peritonei (PMP) is a specific example of secondary peritoneal spread of mucus and cells from a ruptured mucinous appendiceal neoplasm. Although its incidence is quite low (one to two new cases

per million per year), it represents a paradigm in peritoneal dissemination and in the development of PSO [2].

All origins considered, it has been estimated that approximately 1.5 million new cases of PSM occur yearly worldwide [3].

PATHOLOGY AND STAGING

An accurate pathological evaluation of peritoneal surface malignancy (PSM) is critical to establish an accurate tissue diagnosis, its histopathological variants and a precise staging. These provide crucial prognostic information for therapeutic decision making, including the indications for CRS and HIPEC or of perioperative systemic therapies. Therefore, an expert pathologist is a key member of the multidisciplinary team for PSM.

The pathway for the differential pathological diagnosis of PSMs using morphologic and immunohistochemical markers is outlined in Figure 30.1.

Peritoneal mesothelioma (PMe) includes two major subsets:

1. Favorable prognosis: Well-differentiated papillary PMe and multicystic PMe
2. Unfavorable prognosis, also known as diffuse malignant peritoneal mesothelioma (DMPM): Epithelioid, biphasic and sarcomatoid

Definitive diagnosis of DMPM is challenging and requires specific immunohistochemical assessment [4] (Figure 30.1).

Epithelial appendiceal tumors span a wide variety of morphological entities. The majority of them are low

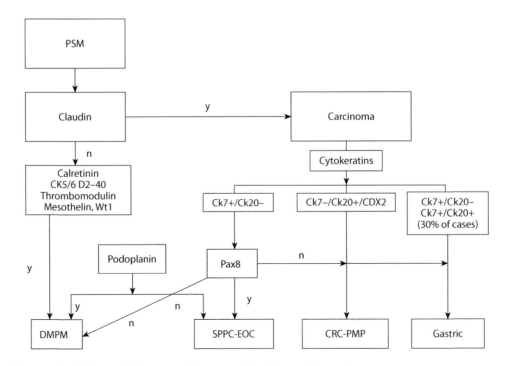

Figure 30.1 Differential pathological diagnosis of peritoneal surface malignancies. y = yes, n = no.

grade and mucinous type. The nomenclature and characterization of PMs from appendiceal mucinous neoplasms (including the entity known as pseudomyxoma peritonei) and those of the primary tumors are topics of heated debate, but their prognostic impact is unquestionable [5]. A panel of international PSM experts under the auspices of the Peritoneal Surface Oncology Group International (PSOGI) are working to achieve a consensus on the optimal system [6].

The World Health Organization (WHO) classification for colorectal carcinomas is in common use [7]. Of note, mucinous adenocarcinoma (with more than 50% of the tumor volume composed of extracellular mucin) and signet-ring cell (with more than 50% of its cells with this morphology) are variants associated with an increased risk of developing PC and carry a worse prognosis.

In gastric cancer the Lauren classification is still valid and useful. It divides gastric cancers into (1) intestinal type and (2) diffuse type (includes signet-ring carcinoma). The indeterminate type was included to describe all uncommon histologies. The most common is the intestinal type; the diffuse type is characterized by a high tendency to metastasize in the peritoneum.

Surface epithelial ovarian cancers (EOCs) account for approximately 90% of ovarian malignancies. Studies on the application of CRS and HIPEC have been mostly conducted in this tumor type, which includes five major subtypes: serous, mucinous, endometrioid, clear cell and transitional cell.

Serous primary peritoneal carcinoma (SPPC) is histologically similar to advanced stage epithelial ovarian carcinoma. Recently, the Gynecologic Oncology Group (GOG) developed a standardized set of criteria to diagnose SPPC.

Staging

In the TNM staging system for the various gastrointestinal cancers, PC means stage IV by definition.

According to the new FIGO classification of ovarian, fallopian tube and SPPC, PC from these gynaecological neoplasms is classified as IIIA2, IIIB or IIIC [8].

A TNM-based staging system for DMPM has been described; further studies are necessary for its external validation [9].

DIAGNOSIS AND PREOPERATIVE IMAGING

Imaging studies play an important role in the assessment of peritoneal tumor spread and help select those patients who will benefit from CRS and PIC. For this purpose a close correlation between radiological and surgical findings would be desirable, but the reality is that, despite significant advances, accuracy of peritoneal tumor detection by the current imaging studies is still challenging. The role of imaging in patient selection is aimed at ruling out

extraperitoneal disease, assessing peritoneal disease volume and distribution as a guide for surgical planning and evaluating possible signs that may preclude a complete cytoreduction [10]. Quantitative scoring systems such as the Peritoneal Cancer Index (PCI), explained below, are useful tools employed for this assessment.

International consensus achieved in Milan in 2006 was unanimous in considering contrast-enhanced, multidetector CT scan of the thorax, abdomen and pelvis the procedure of choice in the evaluation of PSM patients for CRS and PIC [11]. This statement remains valid today. Indications for MRI with diffusion-weighted imaging (DWI) sequences and PET-CT are currently under investigation [12]. In a study correlating the findings of CT, PET-CT and surgery, the correlation between CT and surgical findings was moderate, while that of PET-CT and surgery was low [13].

The assessment of peritoneal disease by CT scan needs to be done in a systematic fashion, based on knowledge of the pathobiology of the disease and of the mechanisms of peritoneal spread [1]. CT scan underestimates peritoneal disease burden in up to 70% of cases [13], especially in lesions less than 5 mm in size and for invasive, non-mucinous tumors. In these cases, a high peritoneal disease burden on CT scanning is an indicator for caution when considering the indication for CRS. This is not the case in non-invasive processes such as PMP, where widespread, voluminous disease can be completely cytoreduced.

Disease in the small bowel and its mesentery constitutes a key limiting criterion for successful CRS. Therefore, its evaluation is a crucial component in the preoperative imaging assessment of PC. Nodules associated with the bowel surface, irregularities or wall thickening, air-fluid levels, diffuse loss of mesenteric fat clarity, mesenteric retraction and loss of the normal mesenteric vessel configuration are all signs of small bowel involvement, which is also largely underestimated by CT scan. Although with less spatial contrast, MRI has been reported to be superior to CT scan in the assessment of the intestinal tract and mesenteric involvement because of its superior soft-tissue constrast [14]. Further development of MRI with the use of DWI sequences and the standardization of its use may represent the next revolution in the evaluation of these patients.

Another potential contraindication for the procedure in cases of PC with invasive features is disease located in and around the porta hepatis.

In conclusion, with CT scanning as the first choice, limitations of currently available imaging modalities do not allow us to accurately predict in which patients with PSM a complete cytoreduction will be possible, but provide crucial information to help us decide which patient should be offered a surgical exploration with a cytoreductive intent. Close interaction and cooperation between surgical oncologists and radiologists is of the utmost importance in this regard. Dedicated, motivated radiologists are required to obtain the most precise and clinically useful imaging interpretation [10].

PREVENTION AND EARLY DETECTION

Prevention

It has been said that 'it is better to prevent than to cure', and this is also true for PM. In this regard, three basic rules must be honoured:

1. Detection and early treatment of the primary tumor at the earliest possible stage will diminish the number of patients presenting at high risk of development of PM. This is the responsibility of national cancer detection campaigns.
2. Adequate performance of surgical resection of primary localized tumors according to well-established onco-logic rules: wide excision margins around the tumor and en bloc resection, avoiding tumor rupture.
3. Administration of appropriate adjuvant therapy, which decreases the risk of recurrence.

Early detection and early treatment of PM

PC of colorectal origin is the best scenario to illustrate this topic. Currently, a curative approach for colorectal PM using complete CRS and HIPEC renders a 72% 5-year overall survival in patients presenting with a PCI between 1 and 5, better than that of patients presenting with one liver metastasis [15]. Therefore, it appears that CRS and HIPEC are most efficient and less aggressive if the peritoneal disease burden is minimal.

However, the problem is that early detection of minimal PC is not possible because it causes no clinical symptoms, shows no signs on imaging and has no biological markers. Only a planned second-look surgical exploration is able to detect it. This reason justifies the proposal of a systematic second-look surgery to asymptomatic patients at high risk of developing PM, so that they can be treated at an early stage [16]. In our opinion, the very difficult 're-exposure' of every previous dissection plane and the impossibility of pal-pating tissue abnormalities disqualify laparoscopy for this purpose.

This aggressive and resource-consuming procedure should be exclusively reserved for a selected population of high-risk patients. Elias and colleagues [16] defined this high-risk PM-prone population as patients presenting with one or several of the following three criteria: limited, synchronous PM completely resected with the primary tumor, ovarian metastasis (synchronous or metachro-nous) and spontaneous or iatrogenic perforation of the primary tumor. A systematic literature review confirmed these criteria [17]. The risk of developing PM in the con-text of positive peritoneal cytology, pT4 lesions and muci-nous type or signet-cell tumors was considered moderate (20–25%).

The mentioned high-risk features were used as selection criteria to include 29 patients in the first prospective trial that addressed this question [16]. Second-look surgery was planned for asymptomatic patients after a negative work-up including CT scan and tumor markers, 6 months after final-ization of adjuvant chemotherapy and 12 months after the primary tumor resection. Macroscopic PC was discovered in 55% of the entire group. Synchronous PC, ovarian metas-tasis and perforated tumor led to the detection of perito-neal recurrence in 63%, 75% and 33% of cases, respectively. Complete CRS (CCRS) plus HIPEC did not cause any mortality in this group. The morbidity rate was 14%. The preliminary survival data were encouraging, with a 2-year disease-free survival higher than 50%. In this study, only patients with initially synchronous PM or PC discovered during second-look surgery received HIPEC. The subse-quent peritoneal recurrence rates were far lower in the subgroup of peritoneal recurrence-free patients when the treatment involved HIPEC than when it did not (17% vs. 43%, respectively). This led to a second prospective trial that included 47 similar patients [18]. The protocol was modi-fied from the initial study in order to treat every patient with HIPEC, with either a curative or prophylactic intent. The incidence of peritoneal recurrence was consistent with the previous study (56%). The 5-year overall survival rate was 90% and the 5-year disease-free survival rate was 44%. Importantly, only 17% of the patients had recurrence in the peritoneum. Unfortunately, one patient died in the postop-erative period.

These studies served as scientific background for a multicentre randomized trial opened for enrolment in France in 2011 (PROPHYLOCHIP, NCT01226394). Patients with a negative work-up after 6 months of adjuvant systemic FOLFOX were randomized between standard surveillance (control group) and second-look laparotomy with systematic HIPEC performed 8 months after the initial surgery. The primary endpoint is the peritoneal recurrence rate at 3 years. The objective is to increase 3-year disease-free survival from 40% to 65%. As of September 2014, enrolment of the planned 130 patients was complete.

At the present time, the addition of HIPEC to the resec-tion of a primary colorectal cancer should be proposed only to patients presenting with synchronous PM or ovarian metastasis identified on preoperative imaging studies. If PM or ovarian metastasis is incidentally found during a pri-mary colorectal cancer resection (8% of cases), the absence of informed consent would prevent the surgical team from performing CCRS plus HIPEC.

CYTOREDUCTIVE SURGERY

CRS involves peritonectomy procedures [19] (Figure 30.2) and visceral resections. The required goal of this surgery is the complete removal of all visible evidence of cancer within the abdomen and pelvis ('complete cytoreduc-tion'). CRS is followed by PIC (HIPEC or EPIC or both), as described later in this chapter. This is highly complex and time-consuming and demands extensive experience if the goal of complete cytoreduction is to be met.

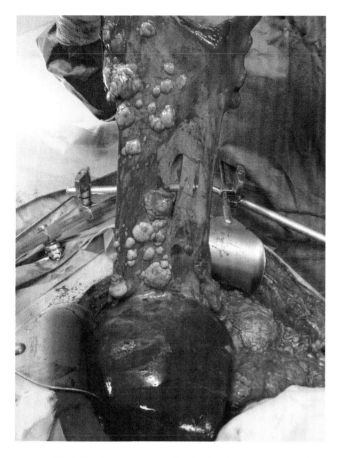

Figure 30.2 Peritonectomy effectively clears peritoneal surface tumor deposits. The photograph shows a right subphrenic peritonectomy specimen still attached to its reflection onto the liver peritoneal surface at the umbilical fissure.

Indications and contraindications

The ideal patient must have a complete cytoreduction of isolated progression of PM in the absence of extensive lymph nodal disease, liver metastases or systemic metastases.

In general, as the extent of disease increases, the requirement for a minimally invasive, low-grade histology increases. One is unlikely to achieve a complete cytoreduction with an aggressive large-volume disease process. In contrast, a large volume of a low-grade minimally invasive malignancy (adenomucinosis from an appendiceal primary malignancy, low-grade PMe and low malignant potential ovarian malignancy) may be an excellent candidate for a curative approach.

Contraindications to CRS include systemic disease, liver metastases or extensive lymph nodal disease within the abdomen and pelvis. If the patient will not be made clinically disease free as a result of the CRS, the patient is less likely to experience long-term benefits. Exceptions to this requirement for complete cytoreduction are primary advanced ovarian cancer with involvement of visceral peritoneal surfaces and epithelioid DMPM.

Main technical aspects of CRS

A xipho-pubic midline abdominal incision is required. If the diaphragms are to be stripped, a xiphoidectomy will greatly improve the exposure. Skin edges are elevated on the frame of a self-retaining retractor in order to ensure a clean resection of any disease in periumbilical port sites or an old abdominal incision. A peritoneal window is used to explore the parietal peritoneum and the small bowel regions. Assessment of the small bowel and its possibility for complete cytoreduction is important before proceeding with the extended cytoreductive procedure. After clearing the anterior parietal peritoneum the fixed retractor is positioned to provide wide exposure of all four quadrants of the abdomen simultaneously. Oftentimes, removal of the greater omentum is a first step in order to clear a large volume of disease from the operative field. Then, stripping of the undersurface of the right hemidiaphragm and stripping of the undersurface of the left hemidiaphragm are completed. With the peritonectomy of the left hemidiaphragm completed the spleen becomes mobile and can be elevated into the operative field for a safe resection without damage to the tail of the pancreas. Usually, the right and left paracolic sulcus must be stripped and at the lower aspect of the dissection, the ureter is identified. The peritoneum is stripped away from the lower aspect of the abdominal incision and a search for the urachus is necessary. Strong traction on the urachus will facilitate the peritonectomy required on the surface of the bladder. This peritonectomy proceeds into the depths of the pelvis and beneath the right and left pararectal fossa.

At this point the surgeon must make a decision regarding the need for resecting the rectosigmoid colon or whether a cul-de-sacectomy will clear disease from the anterior aspect of the mid-rectum. If the rectosigmoid colon is to be spared, one moves ahead with the cul-de-sacectomy. Oftentimes, the hysterectomy precedes the cul-de-sacectomy. Traction on the posterior aspect of the transected vagina can greatly facilitate the removal of the disease from the anterior rectum without damage to this structure.

If the disease is attached to the anterior rectum and invasive into it then a rectosigmoid colon resection is performed. A linear cutter is used to divide the colon at the junction of the sigmoid and descending colon (Figure 30.3). Centripetal surgery is used to isolate the rectum and circumferentially remove as much of the perirectal fat as possible. The rectum is divided with a stapling device leaving the rectal stump as long as possible.

Oftentimes, a right colon resection is necessary because of the tendency of disease to accumulate in the distal small bowel, in and around the ileocecal valve, and on the ascending colon.

Combination with PIC (HIPEC, EPIC or both)

Microscopic residual disease is treated with the PIC. It is important that this is used prior to the cancer cells being

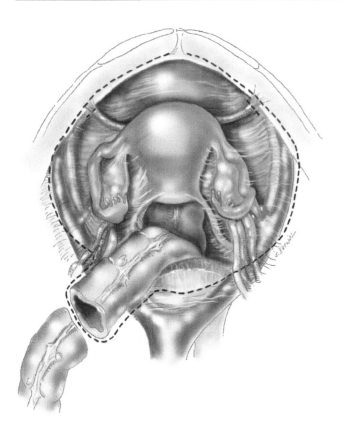

Figure 30.3 Boundaries of a regular pelvic peritonectomy with rectosigmoid resection. (Reproduced with permission of PH Sugarbaker, copyright owner.)

embedded within fibrosis. The PIC will not penetrate scar tissue to destroy cancer cells within. Therefore, HIPEC is a planned part of the surgical procedure. There is great theoretical advantage of HIPEC prior to intestinal reconstruction or closure of the abdominal incision in order to prevent suture line or abdominal incision recurrence. EPIC follows in the 4 or 5 days immediately after the surgical procedure before adhesions have formed.

Learning curve for CRS and HIPEC

There is definitely a learning curve for the surgeon, for the anaesthesiologist and for all of the support personnel taking care of the patient. This learning curve will be most prominent in those diseases that require extensive peritonectomy and visceral resections. With the difficult cytoreductions the team may need experience with more than a hundred procedures in order to minimize any unnecessary morbidity or mortality.

Surgical palliation

The proper use of HIPEC in patients who have an incomplete cytoreduction but have a complete clearing of the abdomen and pelvis of all disease down to 2.5 cm in diameter with complete mobility of all of the intra-abdominal structures is controversial. The answer has never been subjected to a

critical investigation. Further pharmacologic studies are necessary in this group of patients.

In patients with debilitating ascites that is not responsive to systemic chemotherapy, limited CRS (removal of an omental cake and other deposits of tumor that would significantly palliate the patient in terms of long-term gastrointestinal function) and HIPEC (using doxorubicin as one of the agents) can be of great value. We have also found it extremely helpful to use EPIC paclitaxel for its marked local–regional effect but little systemic toxicity.

NEOADJUVANT AND ADJUVANT THERAPIES

Perioperative chemotherapy (intraperitoneal [IP] and intravenous [IV]) is administered to preserve the surgical complete response by eradicating microscopic residual disease that would at a later time progress. The IP route of delivering chemotherapy is logistically convenient but technologically more challenging than conventional IV chemotherapy. The perioperative timing of administration (intra- or early postoperative) adds numerous advantages.

Principles of perioperative intraperitoneal chemotherapy

PHARMACOKINETIC RATIONALE: THE DEDRICK DIFFUSION MODEL

The pharmacokinetic rationale of PIC is based on the dose intensification provided by the peritoneal–plasma barrier [20]. From peritoneal dialysis research, Dedrick and colleagues [21] concluded that the peritoneal permeability of a number of hydrophilic anticancer drugs may be considerably less than the plasma clearance of the same drug after IP administration. The peritoneal clearance is inversely proportional to the square root of its molecular weight and results in a higher concentration in the peritoneal cavity than in the plasma after IP administration. A simplified mathematical diffusion model considers the plasma to be a single compartment separated from another single compartment, the peritoneal cavity, by an effective membrane (Figure 30.4).

The simple conceptual model does not reveal anything about the specific penetration of the chemotherapy drug into the tissue or tumor nodule. After CRS, this concentration difference increases the possibility of exposing residual tumor cells to high doses of chemotherapeutic agents with reduced systemic concentrations and lower systemic toxicity. This advantage is expressed by the area under the curve (AUC) ratios of IP versus IV exposure.

BIDIRECTIONAL INTRAOPERATIVE CHEMOTHERAPY

By the combination of intraoperative IV and intraoperative IP cancer chemotherapy, a bidirectional diffusion gradient is created through the intermediate tissue layer containing the cancer nodules. This bidirectional approach offers the possibility of optimizing chemotherapy delivery to

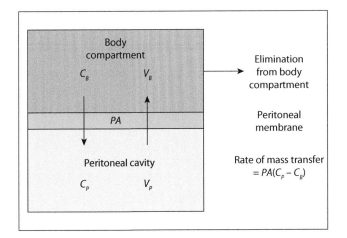

Figure 30.4 The traditional two-compartment model of peritoneal transport. Transfer of a drug from the peritoneal cavity to the blood occurs across the 'peritoneal membrane'. The permeability–area product (PA) governs this transfer. PA is calculated by measuring the rate of drug disappearance from the cavity, which is divided by the overall concentration difference between the peritoneal cavity and the blood (or plasma). C_B = free drug concentration in the blood (or plasma), V_B = volume of distribution of the drug in the body, C_p = free drug concentration in the peritoneal fluid, V_p = volume of the peritoneal cavity. (Adapted from Dedrick RL, *J Natl Cancer Inst* 1997;89[7]:480–7.)

effectively target the peritoneal tumor nodules. Most current protocols advocate bidirectional intraoperative chemohyperthermia (BIC).

Cancer chemotherapy drugs for intraperitoneal application

Table 30.1 summarizes the pharmacologic properties of the chemotherapy drugs most frequently selected for IP application. The rationale for their administration is mostly based on the combination of extrapolation of data of systemic chemotherapy and perceived beneficial pharmacologic properties such as high molecular weight.

Timing of cancer chemotherapy in relation to the surgical intervention

The administration of chemotherapy in PC patients can occur at four time points. The greatest benefit will probably result from a combination of the four treatment strategies.

Induction (neoadjuvant) chemotherapy is given before CRS with the aim to reduce cancer dissemination to the extra-abdominal space, test the tumor biology and reduce the extent of peritoneal disease. Theoretically, this approach may facilitate definitive CRS not indicated at initial exploratory laparoscopy or laparotomy.

The most common route for administration of induction chemotherapy for PC is IV. A combined IV and IP option,

called neoadjuvant intraperitoneal and systemic (NIPS) chemotherapy, has been described mainly for gastric cancer [22], but is also attractive to explore for other forms of PC. Fibrosis as a response to induction chemotherapy may occur and render judgments concerning the extent of PC difficult or impossible to assess during definitive CRS.

HIPEC is administered intraoperatively after a complete cytoreduction has been achieved. It constitutes the most widely explored PIC modality, having shown consistently improved outcomes in many phase II trials and several phase III trials. It uses cell cycle non-specific drugs. Inflow and outflow catheters are placed and a continuous flow of the chemotherapy solution is established by a heater circulator that maintains moderate hyperthermia (41–43°C) within the abdomen and pelvis (Figure 30.5). Intraoperative administration optimizes chemotherapy distribution since no adhesions exist.

Open- and closed-abdomen techniques for HIPEC administration have been described. Both have potential advantages and disadvantages in terms of perceived (but unreal) occupational hazards [23] or optimization of the cytotoxic solution distribution or tissue penetration. No differences in treatment outcomes have ever been demonstrated between the open or closed methods [24].

Hybrid open–closed techniques have been described, which attempt to combine the optimal distribution of the open technique with the improved occupational safety of the closed technique.

Early postoperative intraperitoneal chemotherapy (EPIC) is administered after CRS at the time of minimal residual tumor burden and before wound healing and intra-abdominal adhesions occur, maximizing uniform drug distribution by gravity (changing patient position). It employs cell cycle–specific drugs such as 5-fluorouracil and taxanes. EPIC is administered on postoperative day 1 through day 4 or 5, via drains inserted at the time of CRS. Each administration dwells for 23 hours and is then drained. It can be applied with or without HIPEC.

Adjuvant postoperative chemotherapy is started several weeks after complete CRS. Therefore, it is not a perioperative use by definition.

Long-term combined intraperitoneal and systemic chemotherapy combines IV and IP chemotherapy administered through an IP port. Concerns about adequate IP drug distribution in the presence of postoperative adhesions and increased morbidity have been raised. It is mostly employed in advanced ovarian cancer.

The indication of standard IV adjuvant chemotherapy after complete CRS and HIPEC, especially if induction therapy was successfully used, is much debated and specific studies to address this issue are warranted. Multivariate analysis of a large multicentric series suggests that it may provide an additional survival advantage in PC of colorectal origin [25]. The biological behaviour of the disease to be treated is a key factor in this decision, to be discussed in a multidisciplinary committee. The choice of drugs and the use of biological agents in this context also deserve consideration.

Table 30.1 Pharmacologic properties of the chemotherapy drugs most frequently selected for IP application

Drug name	Drug family	Molecular weight (Da)	Dose (mg/m²)	Exposure time	AUC ratio (IP/IV)	Penetration depth	Thermal augmentation	Remarks
Cisplatin	Alkylator	300.1	50–250	30 minutes–20 hours	7.8–21	1–5 mm	Yes	Dose-limiting nephrotoxicity
Carboplatin	Alkylator	371.25	200–800	30 minutes–20 hours	1.9–10	0.5–9 mm	Yes	
Oxaliplatin	Alkylator	397.3	360–460	30 minutes–20 hours	3.5–16	1–2 mm	Yes	Dextrose-based carrier solution
Melphalan	Alkylator	305.2	50–70	90–120 minutes	93		Yes	Rapid degradation
Mitomycin C	Antitumor antibiotic	334.3	15–35	90–150 minutes	10–23.5	2 mm	Yes	
Doxorubicin	Antitumor antibiotic	579.99	15–75	90 minutes	162–579	4–6 cell layers	Yes	
Docetaxel	Antimicrotubuli agent	861.9	45–150	30 minutes–23 hours	552	NA	Conflicting data	Cell cycle specific
Paclitaxel	Antimicrotubuli agent	853.9	20 mg/m²–180 mg total dose	30 minutes–23 hours	1000	>80 layers	Conflicting data	Cell cycle specific
5 Fluorouracil	Antimetabolite	130.08	650 for 5 days (EPIC)	23 hours	250	0.2 mm	Yes, mild	Cell cycle specific
Gemcitabine	Antimetabolite	299.5	50–1000	60 minutes–24 hours	500	NA	NA	Cell cycle specific
Pemetrexed	Antimetabolite	471.4	500	24 hours	19.2	NA	NA	Cell cycle specific

Note: NA = Not available.

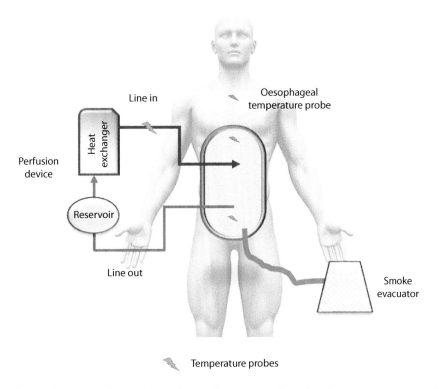

Figure 30.5 For the delivery of HIPEC inflow and outflow catheters are placed and a continuous flow of the chemotherapy solution is established by a heater circulator that maintains moderate hyperthermia (41–43°C) within the abdomen and pelvis.

PROGNOSTIC FACTORS, INDICATIONS AND PATIENT SELECTION FOR CRS AND HIPEC

Selected patients with PSMs can be treated by a multimodal approach including CRS, HIPEC, systemic chemotherapy and targeted therapy, with improved survival compared to past treatment strategies. However, selection of the appropriate patients is very challenging and associated with a long learning curve. The multidisciplinary team lies at the very centre of these decisions and needs to analyze a multitude of parameters (Figure 30.6) with the intention to define a prognostic benefit that will justify the morbidity and mortality related to the procedure.

Resectability and peritoneal disease extension

Assessing resectability in these patients is one of the central challenges, and this is directly related to the actual extension and distribution of the peritoneal lesions. As previously explained in this chapter, preoperative assessment of PSM by all the currently available imaging modalities is generally difficult, has limitations and requires a very experienced radiologist working in close collaboration with the surgical oncologist [10]. When making treatment decisions we count on the fact that the disease extent on CT scan is usually lower than the one to be found at surgical exploration. To some extent, this has improved by adding laparoscopy

to the diagnostic tools. It is also important to carefully read previous operative notes to know where exactly small deposits have been described. Knowing the actual extension of disease, one can assess the probability of achieving a complete macroscopic cytoreduction, which is the main goal. Therefore, peritoneal disease volume and extension (as quantified by the PCI; Figure 30.7) and the outcome of CRS (as categorized by the Completeness of Cytoreduction [CC] Score) are the two most important prognostic factors for any PSM treated by this combined strategy [26].

The PCI is determined at the time of the surgical exploration of the abdomen. When feasible, it can also be assessed by exploratory laparoscopy prior to CRS or HIPEC. The higher the PCI, in every disease process, the less likely is the patient to achieve a long-term disease-free status within the abdomen and pelvis. It should be noted that the PCI has independent prognostic significance even though the cytoreduction is complete. The highest score is 39; a PCI of more than 20 in PC of colorectal origin or higher than 10 in gastric origin is mostly regarded as an exclusion criterion for CRS and HIPEC. There is, however, no clear cut-off and the critical number may vary depending on the tumor type.

The CC Score is determined at the end of CRS. The surgeon always aims for a CC-0 score, meaning no visible remaining tumor. However, a CC-1 score, with residual tumor nodules smaller than 2.5 mm, seems acceptable and also qualifies as a complete cytoreduction in low-to-moderate-grade processes when using HIPEC, given its penetration depth

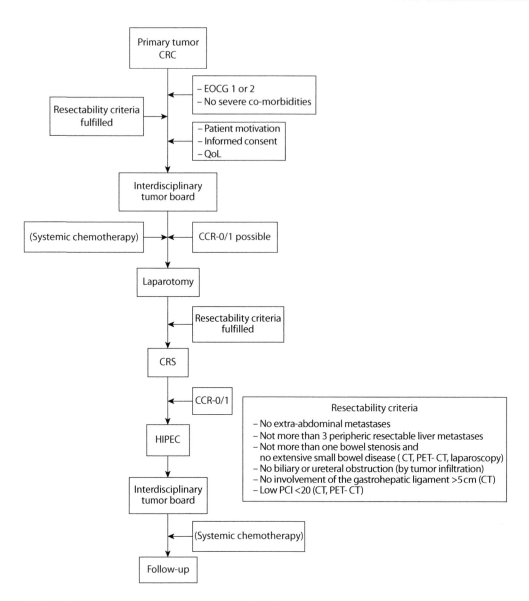

Figure 30.6 Multidisciplinary decision making in peritoneal surface oncology.

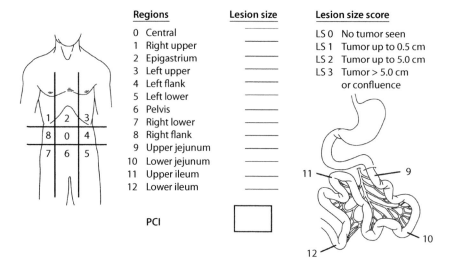

Figure 30.7 The Peritoneal Cancer Index (PCI) results from the addition of the lesion size scores assigned to all 13 regions. It is a key prognostic factor in peritoneal surface oncology.

of up to 2.5–3.0 mm. Incomplete cytoreduction is defined as residual disease between 2.5 mm and 2.5 cm (CC-2) or greater than 2.5 cm or confluent lesions (CC-3).

In most diseases, a complete cytoreduction (CC-0 or CC-1) is necessary for long-term benefit. This includes appendiceal malignancy, colorectal cancer and gastric malignancy. However, a near-complete cytoreduction (CC-2) may result in benefit with primary advanced ovarian malignancy and with peritoneal mesothelioma when additional chemotherapy is given.

Tumor type and biology

Oncological criteria are also of great importance in patient selection. It is reasonable to treat patients with limited disease when tumor type and biological behaviour are favorable. Colorectal, gastric, appendiceal and ovarian cancer as well as DMPM (especially epithelioid type and low-grade varieties) are appropriate indications for CRS and HIPEC. It is important to consider that PC from rectal cancer behaves in a more aggressive fashion than PC of colonic origin. The tumor biology can be assessed by the response to a prior, neoadjuvant chemotherapy treatment, by the metastasizing pattern (e.g. liver metastases, extra-abdominal metastases, lymph node metastases) or by the histological subtype, with signet-ring cell carcinomas being among the most aggressive tumors.

Other selection factors

Regarding indications for CRS and HIPEC for PC of colorectal origin in the presence of liver metastases there is no clear recommendation, but there are data that suggest that a limited number (mostly stated with up to three) of peripheral liver metastases is no contraindication for CRS and HIPEC if the patient can be resected CC-0/CC-1 [27].

Other factors are patient-related ones (patient's motivation, informed consent, acceptable quality of life predictable, comorbidities and general state of health) as well as the experience of the centre where the patient is treated [28].

Recently the Peritoneal Surface Disease Severity Score (PSDSS) has been proposed by the American Society of Peritoneal Surface Malignancies (ASPSM). This score integrates three readily available preoperative variables (symptoms, extent of peritoneal dissemination assessed by imaging or laparoscopy and histology). Esquivel and colleagues state that PSDSS can predict long-term survival after CRS and HIPEC in patients suffering from colorectal PC [29], holding potential for integration in the multidisciplinary therapeutic decision-making process. This study, however, is a retrospective analysis and has to be validated by further prospective data.

After having assessed all the mentioned selection factors together, treatment options have to be discussed interdisciplinarily for each patient. If a CC-0 or CC-1 cytoreduction is likely to be achieved, CRS and HIPEC should be performed at a specialized centre [28]. Postoperatively, it seems that adjuvant systemic chemotherapy would prolong the disease-free interval and overall survival in some patients, at least in PC of colorectal origin [25,28].

In conclusion, the multiple factors that are taken into consideration during the selection process (resectability, biological, patient related) lead to a real tailored approach for each patient [30]. In the future molecular factors will further refine this process.

RADICAL TREATMENT RESULTS

Table 30.2 shows the overall outcome figures for complete CRS combined with PIC in landmark studies for various PSMs.

ACKNOWLEDGEMENTS

The authors acknowledge and appreciate the work and contributions of Diane Goéré, MD and Charles Honoré, MD (Villejuif, France), Liesselotte Lemoine, MSc (Genk, Belgium), and L März, MD and BMJ Lampl, MD (Regensburg, Germany) in the preparation of this chapter.

Table 30.2 Outcome figures for complete CRS combined with PIC

Disease	Median survival (months)	5-year survival (%)	Source
Peritoneal carcinomatosis of appendiceal origin (mucinous type)	Not reached	85	PSOGI multi-institutional registry, 2012 (n = 2298) [5]
Peritoneal carcinomatosis of colorectal origin	48	45	Pivotal Dutch randomized trial (Netherlands Cancer Institute), 2008 (n = 105) [31]
Peritoneal carcinomatosis of gastric origin	15	23	French multi-institutional registry, 2010 (n = 159) [32]
Diffuse malignant peritoneal mesothelioma	53	47	PSOGI multi-institutional registry, 2009 (n = 405) [33]
Desmoplastic small round cell tumor	63.4	NA	MD Anderson Cancer Center, 2014 (n = 26) [34]

REFERENCES

1. Sugarbaker PH. Observations concerning cancer spread within the peritoneal cavity and concepts supporting an ordered physiopathology. *Cancer Treat Res* 1996;82:79–100.

2. González-Moreno S. Pseudomyxoma peritonei: a rare disease and a disease model in peritoneal surface oncology. *Clin Transl Oncol* 2011;13:211–2.

3. Nisan A, Stojadinovic A, Garofalo A, Esquivel J, Piso P. Evidence-based medicine in the treatment of peritoneal carcinomatosis. Past, present and future. *J Surg Oncol* 2009; 100:335–344.

4. Cao S, Jin S, Cao J, Shen J, et al. Advances in malignant peritoneal mesothelioma. *Int J Colorectal Dis* 2014;30(1):1–10.

5. Chua TC, Moran BJ, Sugarbaker PH, et al. Early- and long-term outcome data of patients with pseudomyxoma peritonei from appendiceal origin treated by a strategy of cytoreductive surgery and hyperthermic intraperitoneal chemotherapy. *J Clin Oncol* 2012;30:2449–56.

6. Carr NJ. Current concepts in pseudomyxoma peritonei. *Ann Pathol* 2014;34:9–13.

7. Bosman FT, Carneiro F, Hruban RH, et al., eds. *WHO Classification of Tumors of the Digestive System.* Lyon: International Agency for Research on Cancer, 2010: 122e5.

8. Zeppernick F, Meinhold-Heerlein I. The new FIGO staging system for ovarian, fallopian tube, and primary peritoneal cancer. *Arch Gynecol Obstet* 2014; 290:839–4.

9. Yan TD, Deraco M, Elias D, et al. A novel tumor-node-metastasis (TNM) staging system of diffuse malignant peritoneal mesothelioma using outcome analysis of a multi-institutional database. *Cancer* 2011;117:1855–63.

10. González-Moreno S, González-Bayón L, Ortega-Pérez G, González-Hernnado C. Imaging of peritoneal carcinomatosis. *Cancer J* 2009;15:184–9.

11. Yan TD, Morris DL, Kusamura S, et al. Preoperative investigations in the management of peritoneal surface malignancy with cytoreductive surgery and perioperative intraperitoneal chemotherapy: expert consensus statement. *J Surg Oncol* 2008;98:224–7.

12. Schwenzer NF, Schmidt H, Gatidis S, et al. Measurement of apparent diffusion coefficient with simultaneous MR/positron emission tomography in patients with peritoneal carcinomatosis: comparison with 18F-FDG-PET. *J Magn Reson Imaging* 2014;40:1121–8.

13. Dromain C, Leboulleux S, Auperin A, et al. Staging of peritoneal carcinomatosis: enhanced CT vs PET/CT. *Abdom Imaging* 2008;33:87–93.

14. Low RN, Barone RM, Lucero J. Comparison of MRI and CT for predicting the Peritoneal Cancer Index (PCI) preoperatively in patients being considered for cytoreductive surgical procedures. *Ann Surg Oncol.* 2014;22(5):1708–15.

15. Elias D, Lefebre JH, Chevalier J, et al. Complete cytoreductive surgery plus intraperitoneal chemohyperthermia with oxaliplatin for peritoneal carcinomatosis of colorectal origin. *J Clin Oncol* 2009;27:681–5.

16. Elias D, Goéré D, Di Pietrantonio D, et al. Results of systematic second-look surgery in patients at high risk of developing colorectal peritoneal carcinomatosis. *Ann Surg* 2008;247:445–50.

17. Honoré C, Goéré D, Souadka A, et al. Definition of patients presenting a high risk of developing peritoneal carcinomatosis after curative surgery for colorectal cancer: a systematic review. *Ann Surg Oncol* 2013;20:183–92.

18. Elias D, Honoré C, Dumont F, et al. Results of systematic second-look surgery plus HIPEC in asymptomatic patients presenting a high risk of developing colorectal peritoneal carcinomatosis. *Ann Surg* 2011;254:289–93.

19. Sugarbaker PH. Peritonectomy procedures. *Surg Oncol Clin N Am* 2003;12:703–27.

20. Ceelen WP, Flessner MF. Intraperitoneal therapy for peritoneal tumors: biophysics and clinical evidence. *Nat Rev Clin Oncol* 2010;7:108–15.

21. Dedrick RL, Myers CE, Bungay PM, Jr. Pharmacokinetic rationale for peritoneal drug administration in the treatment of ovarian cancer. *Cancer Treat Rep* 1978;62:1–11.

22. Yonemura Y, Bandou E, Sawa T, et al. Neoadjuvant treatment of gastric cancer with peritoneal dissemination. *Eur J Surg Oncol* 2006;32:661–5.

23. Konate A, Poupon J, Villa A, et al. Evaluation of environmental contamination by platinum and exposure risks for healthcare workers during a heated intraperitoneal perioperative chemotherapy (HIPEC) procedure. *J Surg Oncol* 2010;103(1):6–9.

24. Ortega-Deballon P, Facy O, Jambet S, et al. Which method to deliver hyperthermic intraperitoneal chemotherapy with oxaliplatin? An experimental comparison of open and closed techniques. *Ann Surgl Oncol* 2010;17:1957–63.

25. Elias D, Gilly F, Boutitie F, et al. Peritoneal colorectal carcinomatosis treated with surgery and perioperative intraperitoneal chemotherapy: retrospective analysis of 523 patients from a multicentric French study. *J Clin Oncol* 2010;28:63–8.

26. Jacquet P, Sugarbaker PH. Clinical research methodologies in diagnosis and staging of patients with peritoneal carcinomatosis. *Cancer Treat Res* 1996;82:359–74.

27. Elias D, Benizri E, Pocard M, et al. Treatment of synchronous peritoneal carcinomatosis and liver metastases from colorectal cancer. *Eur J Surg Oncol* 2006;32:632–6.

28. Piso P, Glockzin G, von Breitenbuch P, et al. Patient selection for a curative approach to carcinomatosis. *Cancer J* 2009;15:236–42.

29. Esquivel J, Lowy AM, Markman M, et al. The American Society of Peritoneal Surface Malignancies (ASPSM) multiinstitution evaluation of the Peritoneal Surface Disease Severity Score (PSDSS) in 1,013 patients with colorectal cancer with peritoneal carcinomatosis. *Ann Surg Oncol* 2014;21:4195–201.

30. González-Moreno S, Ortega-Perez G, Gonzalez-Bayón L. Indications and patient selection for cytoreductive surgery and perioperative intraperitoneal chemotherapy. *J Surg Oncol* 2009;100:287–92.

31. Verwaal VJ, Bruin S, Boot H, et al. 8-Year follow-up of randomized trial: cytoreduction and hyperthermic intraperitoneal chemotherapy versus systemic chemotherapy in patients with peritoneal carcinomatosis of colorectal cancer. *Ann Surg Oncol* 2008;15:2426–32.

32. Glehen O, Gilly FN, Arvieux C, et al. Peritoneal carcinomatosis from gastric cancer: a multi-institutional study of 159 patients treated by cytoreductive surgery combined with perioperative intraperitoneal chemotherapy. *Ann Surg Oncol* 2010;17:2370–7.

33. Yan TD, Deraco M, Baratti D, et al. Cytoreductive surgery and hyperthermic intraperitoneal chemotherapy for malignant peritoneal mesothelioma: multi-institutional experience. *J Clin Oncol* 2009;27:6237–42.

34. Hayes-Jordan A, Green HL, Lin H, et al. Complete cytoreduction and HIPEC improves survival in desmoplastic small round cell tumor. *Ann Surg Oncol* 2014;21:220–4.

31

Pancreatic and ampullary cancer

KULBIR MANN, TIMOTHY GILBERT, FRANCES OLDFIELD AND PAULA GHANEH

INCIDENCE AND AETIOLOGY INCLUDING HEREDITY

Pancreatic cancer remains a devastating malignancy with 331,000 deaths per year worldwide, making it the seventh most common malignant cause of death in both sexes [1]. In 2011, the incidence and mortality of pancreatic cancer were 9.7 and 9.1 per 100,000, respectively, in the United Kingdom, a total of 8773 cases [2,3]. The male-to-female ratio almost equates to 1:1 with respect to incidence and mortality. The incidence has increased by 4% in men and 11% in women since 2002 [2]. Latest figures from the United Kingdom have shown it to be the 13th most common malignancy in men and 9th in females, becoming more prevalent in patients over the age of 75 [2].

The European trends are not dissimilar with estimated age-standardized rates of incidence of 8.3 and 5.5 in men and women per 100,000, in 2012. The age-standardized rates of mortality are 8.2 in men and 5.3 in women per 100,000. This confers a cumulative risk of 0.6% male and 0.4% female worldwide and 1.0% male and 0.6% female in Europe. This small variation between Europe and the rest of the world is likely to be due to poor diagnosis and reporting [1]. The overall survival rate remains at less than 5% over 5 years, which has not changed for the last quarter of a century [4].

There is less epidemiological information available with regard to carcinoma of the ampulla of Vater. A total of 3,258 patients were diagnosed between 1998 and 2007 in the UK and represent 6–8% of all tumours found at the pancreatic head and 0.2–0.5% of all gastrointestinal malignancies [5]. Age-standardized incidence rates are 0.6 and 0.4 per 10,000 in men and women, respectively, and the 1-year and 5-year survival rates after diagnosis are 35.9% and 20.8% [6]. There are few European registries quoting data on ampullary cancer, but a recent paper gathered information from a French registry and gave an incidence of 0.83 and 0.75 per 100,000 in men and woman, respectively. They quoted a 1-year and 3-year survival rate of 60.5% and 27.7% based on 256 patients in a 33-year period in Burgundy [7]. Due to its rarity detailed data collection is required from large cancer databases to truly elicit its prevalence, especially on a larger scale.

Modifiable risk factors

Multiple modifiable risk factors have been suggested for developing pancreatic cancer and many recent reviews and meta-analyses have provided further information on clarifying these risk factors. Table 31.1 summarizes these aetiological factors.

Table 31.1 Aetiological factors in pancreatic cancer

	Predisposing factors			Protective factors	
Inflammation	Tobacco		Immunity	Allergies	
	Alcohol			O blood group	
	Pancreatitis				
	Cholecystectomy				
	Gastrectomy				
	Helicobacter pylori				
	Hepatitis B and C				
Resistance	Fructose		DNA repair	Dietary folate	
	Hyperglycaemia			Fruits	
	Diabetes				
	Obese/central adiposity/poor fitness				
	Adiponectin levels				
	Metabolic syndromes				
Susceptibility	Family history		Glycaemic control	Metformin	
	Germline mutations				
	Single nucleotide polymorphisms				
Haemostasis	Non-O blood group				
	Venous thrombosis				
DNA damage	Tobacco				
	Red meat				
	Chlorinated hydrocarbon (CHC) compounds				

Source: Maisonneuve P, Lowenfels AB, *International Journal of Epidemiology* 2015;44(1):186–98.

TOBACCO USE

There is a significant risk of pancreatic cancer in patients who smoke tobacco. This has been shown in multiple cohort and case-control studies over the past 10 years from the Americas, Europe and Southeast Asia. Iodice in 2008 performed a meta-analysis of 82 published studies and concluded that there is an overall risk of 1.74 and 1.2 of developing pancreatic cancer in smokers and former smokers, respectively. For pipe and cigar smokers the overall risk was 1.47 and 1.29, respectively. These risks persist for up to 20 years post smoking cessation but may persist for an additional decade [8,9]. The strength of these findings is supported by multiple studies from Japan suggesting relative risk rates of 1.6–2.2 in smokers and 1.1–1.2 in non-smokers [10]. It is worth noting that a study conducted in 2004 found a relative risk rate of 1.21 in those patients exposed to tobacco though having never smoked [11].

CHRONIC PANCREATITIS

Chronic pancreatitis has been linked to the development of pancreatic cancer and a meta-analysis from 2010 has shown a relative risk rate of 13.3. This factors in the potential lag between episodes of pancreatitis and the development of cancer, which may be up to 20 years [12]. The chronic inflammatory effects on the pancreas are thought to cause disruption to the protective anti-proliferation pathways. The most common cause of chronic pancreatitis is alcohol abuse and is certainly a modifiable risk of malignancy. Other causes of pancreatitis such as hereditary predisposition prove more difficult to control [13].

OBESITY

There have been a number of studies describing the increased risk of pancreatic malignancy with a BMI greater than 30 kg/m^2 [14]. This has been corroborated by two recent meta-analyses giving a relative risk per 5 kg/m^2 increase in BMI, of between 1.12 [15] and 1.19 [16]. The mechanisms of obesity-induced carcinogenesis are pancreatic hypertrophy and hyperplasia, increasing the risk of uncontrolled pancreatic cellular proliferation [9]. The metabolic conditions associated with obesity such as hyperglycaemia and insulin resistance all contribute to increasing the risk of developing pancreatic malignancy [9].

DIABETES

The development of diabetes has been extensively reviewed as a risk factor for pancreatic cancer, if not a manifestation of early disease. Prediabetes has been suggested as a risk factor for multiple malignancies and a recent meta-analysis showed a relative risk of 1.15 with significant increases in the risk of stomach, colonic, liver and pancreatic malignancy [17]. A further meta-analysis focused on pancreatic cancer specifically and found a relative risk of 1.14 for development of the disease for every increase in serum glucose of 0.56 mmol/L [18]. A pooled analysis of a pancreatic cancer cohort consortium in the US showed a relative risk of 1.4 in the development of malignancy in patients with self-reported diabetes, with the highest risk in patients suffering for 2–8 years (RR = 1.79) [19]. Interestingly the treatment of diabetes has also been reviewed with regard to risk of malignancy and the use of metformin has been shown to be a protective agent against the disease. A meta-analysis reviewing 13 cohort studies showed the use of this oral hypoglycaemic drug leads to a relative risk of 0.63 of developing pancreatic cancer [20].

DIET

Larsson and colleagues have published numerous meta-analyses on the risks of red meat consumption on many health conditions. The consumption of all red meat and processed meat has an all-cause mortality of 1.23 and 1.29, respectively [21]. They found the relative risk of pancreatic cancer when consuming 50 g of processed red meat a day to be 1.19, but this finding was not reproducible in females [22]. In 2013 the Ohsaki Cohort Study reviewed vegetable and fruit consumption of almost 33,000 patients with 11 years of follow-up. The hazard ratio for the development of pancreatic cancer with fruit consumption was 0.89 in men and 0.67 in women and for vegetable consumption, 0.89 in men and 0.67 in women. They concluded that consumption of fruits and vegetables was not associated with an increased risk of pancreatic cancer [23]. Similar findings were found in a meta-analysis of 14 cohort studies from Koushik and colleagues in 2012 [24].

There are very few studies reviewing the aetiology and risk factors of ampullary carcinoma. One of the largest studies from China reviewed 1086 patients in a 5-year period and found that the conditions of diabetes, hyperlipidaemia, chronic pancreatitis and gallstones have associations with ampullary tumour development. This is the only case-controlled study for ampullary carcinoma of its kind [25].

Hereditary risk factors

Multiple studies have shown hereditary associations of pancreatic cancer over the years, but poor data collection and confounding factors prevent definitive conclusions. A meta-analysis from 2009 collated nine case-control and cohort studies to ascertain a relative risk factor that demonstrated

a significant genetic link. They found a significant cancer risk in patients with an affected first-degree relative with a relative risk of 1.8 and similar figures for early and late onset disease. It has been estimated that 5–10% of pancreatic malignancy patients have a genetic component [26]. The ultimate aim for delineating the key genetic mutations is to identify and stratify patients into a high-risk category and afford the opportunity for early detection, screening and gene-specific treatment [9,27]. Table 31.2 highlights the genetic predisposing conditions for pancreatic cancer.

At present there are no uniformly defined non-syndromic familial pancreatic cancers, but it is expected that as more discoveries are made classifications will appear as they have for breast cancers and colorectal cancer syndromes (Lynch syndrome) that predispose to malignancy (HNPCC and FAP) [28]. Family registries are the key to these discoveries and the National Familial Pancreas Tumour Registry (NFPTR) is one of the largest based at Johns Hopkins Hospital, and the European Registry of Familial Pancreatic Cancer and Hereditary Pancreatitis (EUROPAC) in Europe. The long-term follow-up and close observations afford opportunities for highlighting genetic trends, especially in families that develop malignancy that were registered disease-free [27].

Several genes have been identified that are associated with pancreatic cancer. The BRCA2 gene has been shown by a number of studies to be implicated. Ten to twelve percent of families with two or more first-degree relatives with pancreatic cancer have BRCA2 mutations. A more recent study looking at 1072 known BRCA2 carriers showed significantly higher observed versus expected rates of pancreatic cancer, with a standardized incidence ratio (SIR) of 2.7. This association is not seen with BRCA1 mutations [29]. This finding follows a recent trend of studies showing no link between BRCA1 and pancreatic cancer after initial associations [27]. CDKN2A is a gene that has been characterized in malignant melanoma and this mutation confers a 60–90% risk

Table 31.2 Inherited predisposition to pancreatic malignancy

Setting of inherited syndrome	Gene	Risk of pancreatic cancer up to 70 years [153]
Hereditary Tumour Predisposition Syndrome		
Peutz–Jeghers syndrome	LKB1	36
Familial atypical multiple mole melanoma syndrome (FAMMM)	CDKN2A, CDK4	17
Hereditary breast–ovarian cancer (HBOC)	BRCA1, BRCA2	3–8
Li–Fraumeni syndrome	TP53	<5
Hereditary non-polyposis colorectal carcinoma (HNPCC)	MLH1, MSH2	<5
Familial adenomatous polyposis (FAP)	APC	<5
Syndromes with Chronic Inflammation of the Pancreas		
Hereditary pancreatitis	PRSS1, SPINK1	40
Cystic fibrosis	CFTR	<5
Familial pancreatic cancer (FPC) syndrome	BRCA2, PALB2, ATM	2 first-degree relatives: 8–12% >3 first-degree relatives: 16–38%

Source: Rustgi AK, *Genes & Development* 2014;28(1):1–7.

of developing pancreatic cancer. This is a tumour suppressor gene coding for the p16 protein which regulates the cell cycle [9]. Patients with colorectal familial syndromes have a high association with pancreatic cancer. Patients with Lynch syndrome have a 3.68% lifetime risk of pancreatic cancer, which is an 8.6-fold increase compared to patients without the mutation [30]. FAP is caused by a mutation in another tumour suppressor gene, APC. This condition manifests with hundreds of colorectal adenomatous polyps and results in a 4.5- to 6-fold risk of developing pancreatic cancer [9]. Another gastrointestinal polyposis familial syndrome, Peutz–Jegers, is associated with a mutation in the STK11 gene and has a 132-fold increased risk of pancreatic malignancy [27]. Given the increased risk associated with chronic pancreatitis, it is important to note that hereditary pancreatitis is an important genetic risk factor for pancreatic carcinoma. Germline mutations in PRSS1, CFTR and SPINK1 are key mutations to hereditary pancreatitis and the lifetime risk of developing pancreatic cancer is 30–44% [27,28].

A familial pancreatic cancer syndrome has been described with two first-degree relatives affected with pancreatic malignancy that does not match with other tumour syndromes, but is associated with an increased risk of cancer. The exact genetic defect has yet to be elucidated, but the NFPTR has described a nine fold increased risk in developing pancreatic cancer with patients who have a first-degree relative affected with familial pancreatic cancer gene, compared to those with sporadic pancreatic malignancy. Further genomic analysis is needed to highlight the key genetic mutations underlying this syndrome [9,31].

Ampullary carcinoma can occur sporadically (0.04–0.12%) or as part of a familial polyposis syndrome (40–90%) [25,32]. Familial adenomatous polyposis (FAP) is autosomal dominant and is commonly associated with colonic polyps and the development of carcinoma. It is believed that the pathology of ampullary cancer follows the adenoma–carcinoma sequence as found in malignant colorectal disease. Duodenal polyps are often found in asymptomatic FAP patients undergoing surveillance endoscopy. The duodenum represents the second most common location for polyps and ampullary cancer is the second most common cause of death from malignancy in FAP [33].

PATHOLOGY AND STAGING

Histological classification of pancreas tumours

Tumours can be broadly classified into two groups focusing on the type of pancreas cell they arise from, endocrine or exocrine. The most common exocrine tumour is adenocarcinoma most commonly known as pancreatic ductal adenocarcinoma (PDAC), which arises from the ductal epithelium evolving from a precursor pancreatic intraepithelial neoplasia. Intraductal papillary mucinous neoplasms (IPMNs) are cells that grow within the pancreatic duct and secrete a thick mucinous fluid. They are graded depending on their degree of dysplasia and have the potential to grow into invasive ductal cancer [34,35]. The histological classifications of exocrine tumours are shown in Table 31.3.

Table 31.3 WHO histological classification of tumours of the exocrine pancreas

Benign	Serous cystadenoma	
	Mucinous cystadenoma	
	Intraductal papillary mucinous adenoma	
	Mature teratoma	
Borderline (uncertain malignant potential)	Mucinous cystic neoplasm with moderate dysplasia	
	Intraductal papillary mucinous adenoma with moderate dysplasia	
	Solid-pseudopapillary neoplasm	
Malignant	Ductal adenocarcinoma	Mucinous non-cystic carcinoma
		Signet ring cell carcinoma
		Adenosquamous carcinoma
		Undifferentiated (anaplastic) carcinoma
		Undifferentiated carcinoma with osteoclast-like giant cells
		Mixed ductal–endocrine carcinoma
	Serous cystadenoma	
	Mucinous cystadenocarcinoma	Non-invasive
		Invasive
	Intraductal papillary mucinous carcinoma	Non-invasive
		Invasive (papillary mucinous carcinoma)
	Acinar cell carcinoma	Acinar cell cystadenocarcinoma
		Mixed acinar–endocrine carcinoma
	Pancreatoblastoma	
	Solid-pseudopapillary carcinoma	

Source: Bosman FT, et al., *WHO Classification of Tumours of the Digestive System*, 4th ed., Lyon: International Agency for Research on Cancer, 2010.

Tumours with acinar differentiation include acinar cell carcinoma, pancreatoblastoma and mixed cellular differentiation. They are clinically unique tumours with genetic alterations and histological characteristics distinct from PDAC. They comprise 1–2% of pancreas tumours and a poor prognosis is often associated with lesions of this type [36]. Other malignant tumours include serous or mucinous cystadenocarcinoma and solid-pseudopapillary carcinoma [37].

Those lesions arising from endocrine cells are called neuroendocrine tumours (NETs) and comprise 1–2% of all pancreas tumours. They can be sporadic in nature or comprise part of a familial genetic syndrome such as von Hippel-Lindau, neurofibromatosis and tuberous sclerosis. They have an improved prognosis and long-term survival compared to exocrine tumours and run a slower, more insidious course. They are further divided by whether the lesion has ectopic secretions of a biochemically active substance [38].

Histological classification of ampullary tumours

Periampullary lesions are distinct tumours arising from the epithelium of the pancreatic duct (66%), distal bile duct (12%), ampulla (16%) and duodenum (6%) and may have starkly different 5-year survival rates [39]. Ampullary cancer has a better prognosis than pancreatic because of its location-increased likelihood of clinical symptoms. It is also more distant from mesenteric and coeliac vessels increasing the chances of an R0 resection [5]. Kimura initially described the histology of ampullary tumours in 1994, finding an intestinal type, resembling stomach or colon tubular adenocarcinoma, and a pancreatobiliary type, characterized by papillary projections. The prognosis varied with intestinal-type lesions having little invasive potential but pancreatobiliary lesions were more likely to infiltrate surrounding tissue [5,40].

TMN staging of pancreatic and ampullary tumours

The current staging is taken from the Union for International Cancer Control (UICC) which periodically updates and revises this classification [41,42] (Table 31.4). It is a tumour–node–metastasis classification based on preoperative imaging via contrast-enhanced CT scan. Table 31.4 demonstrates the TNM classification of pancreas and ampullary cancer. It is important that there are consistency and recognized standards for pathological reporting of resection specimens. The UK Royal College of Pathologists has developed a dataset for reporting pancreatic and ampullary cancer which is widely used internationally [43]. The definition of R0 and R1 staging is classified by the degree of tumour involvement at the margin of the resection specimen. A recent retrospective histological review determined that even microscopic involvement of tumour within a centimetre of the margin confers a poorer survival and should be deemed an incomplete excision [44].

DIAGNOSIS AND PREOPERATIVE IMAGING

Clinical symptoms and signs

Due to the retroperitoneal position and relationship to other organs, pancreatic cancer often has a vague clinical presentation. Patients may describe an insidious abdominal discomfort that can localize to a dull gnawing pain at the location of the tumour. Systemic symptoms include nausea, decreased appetite and weight loss. The location of the tumour may manifest in specific complications, such as a lesion at the head of the pancreas may invade or compress the bile duct and cause obstructive jaundice, or occlusion of the pancreatic duct may lead to pancreatitis. The development of diabetes may be attributed to a lesion in the pancreas, but suspicion should be further aroused in conjunction with other symptoms. A recent case-control study identified the triad of back pain, lethargy and new onset diabetes as highly indicative of PDAC in the year prior to diagnosis [45]. Ampullary carcinoma has a very similar clinical presentation but due to the location of the lesion, is more likely to have jaundice as a presenting symptom than pancreatic cancer. Rare presentations for both conditions include gastric outlet obstruction or bleeding from the upper gastrointestinal tract [34,46].

On physical examination systemic signs may be apparent such as cachexia and muscle wasting. Patients may also have scleral jaundice, peripheral lymphadenopathy, hepatomegaly and ascites. Abdominal examination may reveal an epigastric mass or fullness, and a palpable gallbladder in the absence of abdominal pain is suspicious [34].

Serum analysis often provides vague indications of chronic disease such as mildly deranged liver function tests (in the absence of jaundice), normocytic or microcytic anaemia and hyperglycaemia. CA 19-9 is the only biomarker used in current practice for therapeutic monitoring and early detection of recurrent disease. Unfortunately it is not a specific maker as it can also be elevated in cholestasis and pancreatitis [34].

Investigations and preoperative work-up

Both pancreatic and ampullary tumours employ the same set of investigations in diagnosis and staging. As mentioned above, the importance of preoperative imaging has become key to the devising of an appropriate management plan, especially regarding tumour identification, staging, vessel involvement and distant metastases [47]. As technology increases the detail available has become all the more informative, with the current standard imaging modality being multidetector computed tomography (MDCT). However, ultrasound (US), endoscopic ultrasound (EUS), magnetic resonance imaging (MRI) and positron emission tomography (PET) all have their place. Endoscopic retrograde cholangiopancreatography (ERCP) is commonly used as a therapeutic measure for jaundiced patients.

Table 31.4 TNM clinical staging of pancreas and ampullary cancer [42]

Stage	TNM	PDAC	Ampullary
0	Tis, N0, M0	Tis = Carcinoma in situ (includes PanIN-III classification)	Tis = Carcinoma in situ
		N0 = No regional lymph node metastasis	N0 = No regional lymph node metastasis
		M0 = No distant metastasis	M0 = No distant metastasis
IA	T1, N0, M0	T1 = Tumour limited to the pancreas, ≤2 cm in greatest dimension	T1 = Tumour limited to ampulla of Vater or sphincter of Oddi
		N0 = No regional lymph node metastasis	N0 = No regional lymph node metastasis
		M0 = No distant metastasis	M0 = No distant metastasis
IB	T2, N0, M0	T2 = Tumour limited to the pancreas, >2 cm in greatest dimension	T2 = Tumour invades duodenal wall
		N0 = No regional lymph node metastasis	N0 = No regional lymph node metastasis
		M0 = No distant metastasis	M0 = No distant metastasis
IIA	T3, N0, M0	T3 = Tumour extends beyond the pancreas but without involvement of the coeliac axis or the superior mesenteric artery	T3 = Tumour invades pancreas
		N0 = No regional lymph node metastasis	N0 = No regional lymph node metastasis
		M0 = No distant metastasis	M0 = No distant metastasis
IIB	T1–3, N1, M0	T1–3 = Tumour limited to the pancreas, ≤2 cm in greatest dimension up to tumour extending beyond the pancreas not involving coeliac axis or SMA	T1–3 = Tumour limited to ampulla of Vater, invades duodenal wall, invades pancreas
		N1 = Regional lymph node metastasis	N1 = Regional lymph node metastasis
		M0 = No distant metastasis	M0 = No distant metastasis
III	T4, any N, M0	T4 = Tumour involves the coeliac axis or the superior mesenteric artery	T4 = Tumour invades peri-pancreatic soft tissues or adjacent organs or structures
		NX, 0, 1 = Regional lymph nodes cannot be assessed/no involvement/regional involvement	NX, 0, 1 = Regional lymph nodes cannot be assessed/no involvement/regional involvement
		M0 = No distant metastasis	M0 = No distant metastasis
IV	Any T, any N, M1	TX, is, 1–4 = Primary tumour cannot be assessed, no evidence of primary tumour, carcinoma in situ, tumour limited to pancreas <2 cm to extending beyond and involving coeliac axis and SMA	TX, is, 1–4 = Primary tumour cannot be assessed, no evidence of primary tumour, carcinoma in situ, tumour invading duodenal wall, pancreas, peri-pancreatic soft tissues or other adjacent organs
		NX, 0, 1 = Regional lymph nodes cannot be assessed/no involvement/regional involvement	NX, 0, 1 = Regional lymph nodes cannot be assessed/no involvement/regional involvement
		M1 = Distant metastasis	M1 = Distant metastasis

Source: Faris JE, Wo JY, Oncologist 2013;18(9):981–5.
Note: pTNM is a pathological category and corresponds to T and N. pN0 is defined as histological examination of a regional lymphadenectomy specimen and will ordinarily include 10 or more nodes. If the nodes are negative but the number ordinarily examined is not met, it is classified as pN0.

ULTRASOUND

Often patients will undergo an US as a first-line investigation for upper abdominal pain and derangement in liver function tests. This is essentially to rule out gallstone disease as a cause of symptoms but in the presence of malignancy, ultrasound can be equivocal. Common findings include a dilated common bile and pancreatic duct and potentially a hyperechoic mass, but often bowel gas can obscure views of the pancreas [47]. It has been suggested that slight dilatation of the pancreatic duct and small pancreatic cysts are important predictive signs of early disease [48]. However, overall US is a poorly sensitive diagnostic test for pancreatic cancer [47].

COMPUTED TOMOGRAPHY

This modality provides good spatial and temporal resolution and anatomical coverage allowing a single visit to potentially stage the malignancy. Vascular involvement can be readily studied using arterial or portovenous contrast. A recent study reported that the sensitivity and specificity were 100% and 71% with positive and negative predictive values of 85% and 100% [49]. For lesions smaller than 10 mm the sensitivity can drop to 33–44% [48]. CT is not always able to detect liver or peritoneal metastases and iso-attenuating pancreatic tumours [47–49].

MAGNETIC RESONANCE IMAGING

Advances in MRI scanners have resulted in improvements in images and diagnostic accuracy, with certain situations where MRI is more useful than CT. Magnetic Resonance Cholangiopancreatography (MRCP) is commonly used in the diagnosis of choledocholithiasis, but MRI has been shown to be useful in patients with small tumours, a hypertrophied pancreatic head, iso-attenuating lesions and fatty infiltration of the parenchyma. It is a very helpful modality for characterizing tumours, especially when analyzing the parenchyma and the pancreatic duct [47].

POSITRON EMISSION TOMOGRAPHY

PET is a functional imagining technique and identifies malignant tissue by visually representing areas of abnormally high metabolic activity through the uptake of radiolabeled glucose analogues such as 18F-2-fluoro-2-deoxy-D-glucose (18 FDG) [47,48]. More recently techniques have developed to allow the collection of both PET and CT imaging, enabling the merger of anatomical and functional data into a single image. Several studies have shown that PET/CT is superior to PET alone in the diagnosis of solid tumours [50]. In relation to pancreatic cancer studies report PET/CT to have a sensitivity and specificity in the region of 85–97% and 61–94%, respectively [51]. The strengths of PET/CT lie in its ability to characterize iso-attenuating pancreatic masses, the detection of small-volume metastases and the identification of recurrence [51,52]. Its ability to distinguish between mass-forming chronic pancreatitis and pancreatic cancer is debated and its additional benefit in determining local resectability and nodal involvement is limited [51,53,54].

ENDOSCOPIC ULTRASOUND

EUS has a wide range of diagnostic and therapeutic applications in pancreatitis, masses and cystic lesions [55]. The sensitivity of EUS in detecting solid pancreas masses is 81.2%, but it supersedes other investigations in specificity at 93.2%. For lesions less than 3 cm reported sensitivity rates reach 99%, which is greater than for CT (50–89%) [56]. A high negative predictive value has led to the suggestion that EUS can effectively exclude pancreatic malignancy [55,57]. In the context of nodal staging EUS has reported accuracies of 64–82% and may be helpful in assessing tumour size and vascular invasion, especially with the use of novel oral contrast agents [55–57]. In the case of neuroendocrine tumours, EUS has been found to be reliable in detecting size and localization, but also in the monitoring of lesions for patients with MEN1 [56,58]. However, this procedure remains an invasive investigation with complication rates of 1.1–3.0% [57]. The diagnostic and therapeutic interventions afforded by EUS include

fine-needle aspiration (FNA), cyst drainage and biliary access and decompression [55].

Endoscopic ultrasound has been advocated for staging in ampullary lesions. It has been reported to be superior to helical CT in assessment of tumour size, detecting regional metastatic disease and major vessel involvement. The development of an intraductal probe has brought increased accuracy to mucosal layer imaging. In combination with ERCP, there is scope for detecting intraductal extension before considering endoscopic treatment [59].

FINE-NEEDLE ASPIRATION

FNA via endoscopic ultrasound has a sensitivity of 95%, specificity of 100%, positive predictive value of 100% and negative predictive value of 85%. For patients with chronic pancreatitis there exists a lower sensitivity of 73.9%, but no differences in specificity or accuracy. Extensive research has gone into the size of needles used for FNA, the potential of a core biopsy, the number of passes versus the yield of pancreatic cells and the use of suction. Having access to immediate on-site cytopathology provides accurate assessment and may reduce the number of passes of the needle [55,56,60]. This may be advantageous in reducing the complication rate of pancreatitis which is usually quoted at 0.64–2% [56]. There are still other complications of FNA including bleeding, infection, potential tumour seeding and duodenal perforation that are reported at 5% [61].

The incidence of a benign histology after surgery is 5–13%, with autoimmune pancreatitis being the most commonly associated diagnosis. Interestingly those patients operated on for chronic pancreatitis will have a 5–9% incidence of malignancy. The use of ERCP brushings has traditionally been employed for a cytological diagnosis from a biliary stricture because patients may require the insertion of a drainage stent for decompression. Unfortunately the sensitivity of this technique is reported to be only 33–54% with specificity at 90–100% and a poor accuracy level of 43–75%. The development of EUS FNA has significantly improved the chances of a histological diagnosis, but the essential consideration is a patient with a high suspicion of malignancy yet negative histology or cytology. Despite the improvement in diagnostic accuracy there are no papers that suggest this type of patient should not be operated on [61,62]. Given the unnecessary risks and costs of an invasive diagnostic procedure the International Study Group of Pancreatic Surgery (ISGPS) has recommended that patients with a solid pancreatic mass and a low suspicion of autoimmune pancreatitis do not require biopsies before proceeding to pancreatoduodenectomy [61].

ENDOSCOPIC RETROGRADE CHOLANGIOPANCREATOGRAPHY

Obstructive jaundice is a common presenting complaint for malignancy at the ampulla or pancreatic head. The role of preoperative biliary stenting has been examined in a number of studies and recent meta-analyses have demonstrated that the complication rate from preoperative ERCP and plastic stenting is higher than that for patients proceeding directly to resection. van der Gaag and colleagues performed a multicentre randomized control trial of 202 patients who underwent either preoperative biliary drainage or surgery alone. They found significant differences in morbidity with a complication rate of 74% in the preoperative drainage group and 39% in the early surgery group. There was a trend toward significance in surgery-related complications, 47% in those stented and 37% in those undergoing early surgery ($p = 0.14$). There was no difference in mortality [63]. A recent Cochrane database review took this study and five others and concluded that there may be an increased risk of adverse events with preoperative biliary drainage but not with respect to mortality. They do not advocate the use of biliary drainage outside of a randomized trial setting [64]. One of the drawbacks to those studied was the use of plastic stents and current standard practice has progressed to use covered metal stents. There have been numerous studies which have demonstrated the superior safety and efficacy of this approach compared with plastic stents [65–67]. A meta-analysis of this subgrouping suggested that there is a lower overall mortality when utilizing metal stents, though the evidence base is weak [68].

ENDOSCOPIC PAPILLECTOMY

Many papers have recommended the therapeutic use of endoscopy to excise ampullary adenomas, with high success and low recurrence rates. Techniques such as snare polypectomy, submucosal injections, electrocautery, ablative therapy and prophylactic pancreatic and biliary stenting have all been utilized, but there is no standardized technique for this procedure. Successful excision has been reported from 46% up to 92% from a variety of studies. The complication rates vary from 8% to 35% and include pancreatitis (5–15%), bleeding (2–15%), perforation and cholangitis. Mortality is rare and reported between 0% and 7% [59,69]. It has been suggested that complete excision of polyps with low- to high-grade dysplasia may not warrant a pancreatoduodenectomy but regular endoscopic follow-up. In cases of incomplete excision

of high-grade dysplastic lesions and carcinoma, surgery is mandatory. In the absence of prospective randomized studies there are no accepted safe techniques or guidelines for endoscopic papillectomy [32,59,69–71].

SURGERY FOR PRIMARY OPERABLE PANCREATIC AND AMPULLARY CANCER

When considering an operation for pancreatic and ampullary malignancies, there are many factors that need to be addressed. Many centres have advocated a preoperative assessment with an anaesthetist to determine if a patient is suitable for a pancreatoduodenectomy, with the ability to carry out cardiorespiratory investigations such as pulmonary function tests and echocardiography. All decisions for management of pancreas and ampullary lesions are discussed at a multidisciplinary team (MDT) meeting, where the investigations are reviewed and appropriate recommendations are made whether they are for an operation, further imaging or a consultant outpatient review. Table 31.5 highlights the radiological criteria for determining resectability.

Resectable lesions of the ampulla and pancreatic head

The current standard operation for ampullary and pancreatic tumours of the head of the pancreas is a pancreatoduodenectomy [72]. There are two techniques employed. The first is the classic Kausch–Whipple (KW) originally developed by Kausch in 1912 and improved upon by Whipple in 1935 (Figure 31.1). This involves an en bloc resection of the pylorus, duodenum, head of the pancreas, gallbladder and common bile duct. The second technique conserves the pylorus and is called a pylorus preserving Kausch–Whipple pancreatoduodenectomy (PPKW). This was originally performed by Watson in 1944 and became popularized by Traverso and Longmire in 1980. The fundamental difference is the

Table 31.5 Definition of resectable, borderline and unresectable pancreatic adenocarcinoma

Resectable	• No distant metastases
	• No radiological evidence of superior mesenteric vein (SMV) or portal vein (PV) distortion
	• Clear fat planes around coeliac axis, hepatic artery and superior mesenteric artery (SMA)
Borderline resectable	• No distant metastases
	• Venous involvement of the SMV, PV with distortion or narrowing of the vein or occlusion of the vein with suitable vessel proximal and distal, allowing for safe resection and replacement
	• Gastroduodenal artery encasement up to the hepatic artery with either short-segment encasement or direct abutment of the hepatic artery without extension to the coeliac axis
	• Tumour abutment of the SMA not to exceed greater than 180° of the circumference of the vessel wall
Unresectable	• Distant metastases
	• Greater than 180° SMA encasement, any coeliac abutment
	• Unreconstructible SMA/portal occlusion
	• Aortic invasion or encasement

Source: Bockhorn M, et al., *Surgery* 2014;155(6):977–88.

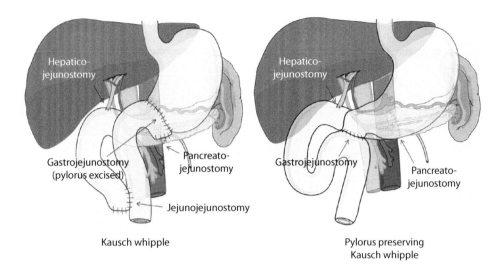

Figure 31.1 Pictorial representation of the Kausch–Whipple and pylorus preserving Kausch–Whipple resection.

formation of a gastrojejunostomy without utilizing a Roux limb, meaning there is one less anastomosis and theoretical advantages in gastric emptying and reduced risk of dumping syndrome leading to improved weight gain [73].

A recent Cochrane meta-analysis reviewed six randomized control trials comparing these two techniques. Neither operation was superior from an oncological perspective nor was there a long-term difference in overall survival. There were no significant differences between mortality and morbidity, especially not in pancreatic fistulation, bile leaks or postoperative bleeding. There is a significantly shorter operative time by 68 minutes, but the clinical implications of this are unclear. Overall the reviewers reported that no differences existed between these two procedures and that a PPKW may be beneficial because of the shorter operative time [73].

The morbidity of a KW or PPPD has been reported at 35–60% and the important complications of pancreatoduodenectomy (5–20%) are a pancreatic fistula and delayed gastric emptying (7–37%). An intra-abdominal collection may develop into an abscess and cause life-threatening sepsis. Intra-abdominal haemorrhage is a less common complication at 2–8% but may require immediate intervention [74]. There have been various trials to reduce these complications from an intraoperative perspective and use of medications postoperatively. Operative techniques to reduce pancreatic fistula formation include a pancreaticogastrostomy versus pancreaticojejunostomy, and a duct-to-mucosa anastomosis with a one-layer end to side pancreaticojejunostomy, and with or without a pancreatic duct stent. The lack of randomized control trials with clear selection criteria makes conclusions difficult [74]. The use of somatostatin in reducing pancreatic fistulas has also not been fully elucidated, as a recent meta-analysis has shown it reduces morbidity rates but not necessarily pancreatic fistula rates [75]. With regard to delayed gastric emptying, it has been found that a retrocolic gastrojejunostomy has higher rates of delayed emptying than the antecolic anastomosis. The evidence for the location of

the pancreatic anastomosis is less clear, and it seems unlikely that it has an impact on the emptying of the stomach [74].

The optimal degree of lymphadenectomy has yet to be elucidated and extended procedures have failed to provide better outcomes, and have caused higher rates of morbidity. The International Study Group of Pancreatic Surgery (ISGPS) reviewed the current literature in order to define the levels of lymph nodes and their optimal clearance. The Japanese Pancreas Society nomenclature of peri-pancreatic lymph nodes has been recommended as the standard definitions of lymph node stations. The definition of the standard lymphadenectomy should include lymph nodes 13 and 17 found in the pancreaticoduodenal groove, 14a and 14b of the right side of the superior mesenteric artery (SMA), and nodes 5, 6, 8a, 12b and 12c of the hepatoduodenal ligament (Figure 31.2). The distal pancreatectomy should include node 10 at the hilum of the spleen, 11 at the splenic artery and 18 along the inferior border of the body and tail of the pancreas. Dissection is also recommended for nodes that are adjacent to the resection that are easily incorporated into the procedure. The extended lymphadenectomy has not been shown to be beneficial with respect to patient outcomes and increased the risk of complications [72,76].

Laparoscopic and robotic-assisted laparoscopic techniques have been described and employed for this operation. Given the proven success of these new technologies in other specialities, the impact on a pancreatoduodenectomy has yet to be established. A meta-analysis of 11 studies was published last year. Unsurprisingly there is a statistically significant longer operating time given the reduced access and exposure, but there were lower rates of wound infection and length of stay. Mortality and morbidity rates were similar but the selection criterion for robotic or laparoscopic surgery is currently not established and is at the discretion of the operating surgeon. This makes open and minimally invasive surgery not directly comparable at baseline. It is clear that the learning curve for these procedures will have a large impact on early outcomes, but there is not enough

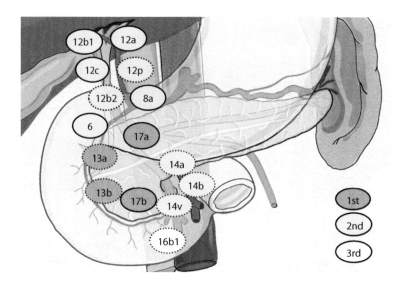

Figure 31.2 Japanese Pancreas Society classification of regional lymph nodes around the pancreas. Colours represent the hierarchical order of nodes for malignancy. First order: 13 – Posterior pancreatoduodenal (PPD). a. Superior to ampulla of Vater. b. Inferior to ampulla of Vater. 17 – Anterior pancreatoduodenal (APD). a. Superior to ampulla of Vater. b. Inferior to ampulla of Vater. Second order: 6 – Infrapyloric. 8a – Superior to common hepatic artery. 12 – Hepatoduodenal ligament. a. Hepatic artery. b1. Superior to bile duct. b2. Inferior to bile duct. c. Around cystic duct. p. Portal vein. 14 – Superior mesenteric artery (SMA). a. Origin of SMA. b. Origin of inferior pancreatoduodenal artery. v. Superior mesenteric vein. Third order: 16b1 – Left renal artery and inferior mesenteric artery. (From Jones L, et al., *Digestive Surgery* 1999;16(4):297–304.)

evidence at present to comment on the future role of minimally invasive pancreatoduodenectomy [77].

Resectable pancreatic cancer of the body and tail

A distal pancreatectomy is employed for resectable pancreatic tumours of the body and tail, but is not as frequently performed as pancreatoduodenectomy because tumours are often diagnosed at a late stage and are already unresectable. This is often because of metastatic disease or the lesion involves the middle colic vessels [46]. A conventional distal pancreatectomy for malignancy includes a splenic resection for oncological clearance, but the spleen is preserved for the more common chronic pancreatitis procedure. A recent retrospective article reviewed the progress made with distal pancreatectomy over the past 15 years, noting that there was an absence of robust studies looking at the specific postoperative morbidity and long-term survival [78]. The complication rate of the procedure is 34.5%, which includes a major complication rate (Clavien–Dindo Grade 3 or more) of 16.2%, development of a pancreatic fistula at 27.3% and bleeding from a preserved or non-preserved spleen and subsequent sup-phrenic abscess at 4.3% [78,79]. These results compared favourably to previous studies especially with regard to re-laparotomy rates and long-term survival (29.5% at 5 years). Note the incidence of pancreatic fistula has not changed and remains at the above rate [78]. With the advent of minimally invasive surgery and the often benign nature of the open distal pancreatectomy, it has become quite popular to perform laparascopically [80].

Laparoscopic surgery is inherently difficult in pancreatic surgery compared to other specialties, because of the proximity of major blood vessels, retroperitoneal position and potential complications. A recent meta-analysis reviewed 18 studies comparing laparoscopic and open distal pancreatectomy procedures for a variety of conditions; none of them featured a randomized control trial. The laparoscopic procedure had significantly less blood loss by 355 ml, a reduced median length of stay of 4 days and a reduced incidence of complications (33.9% vs 44.2%, OR = 0.73). There were no significant differences with regard to operative time, pancreatic fistula occurrence or mortality. Only 11 studies included malignant lesions, meaning they could not make accurate oncological conclusions [81]. A further systematic review of 13 studies noted that open procedures were performed for statistically significant larger lesions and malignant masses: this makes direct comparisons of open versus laparoscopic surgery very difficult in these retrospective studies [82]. The Sloan Kettering Centre performed such a study of 805 patients and compared laparoscopic (131 cases), robotic (37 cases) and open procedures (637 cases). They found pancreatic ductal adenocarcinoma in 39% of the open group, 15% in the laparoscopic group and 11% in the robotic group. There was significantly less blood loss and a reduction in median length of stay with no differences in morbidity or mortality rates in the minimally invasive group. The R0 resection rate was 100% in the laparoscopic and robotic groups and 88% in the open group, though this was not significant. Lymph node yields were significantly higher in the open group but positive nodal disease was not [83]. There are only a handful of papers published on case series that cite laparoscopic procedures for distal pancreatic carcinoma, and for those that do there is coherence in the fact that there are equal R0 resections in open and laparoscopic groups. Numbers of lymph nodes resected remain inconsistent, especially for procedures where the spleen is preserved, and these cases are often benign or low risk of malignancy. There is a degree of selection bias involved in these patients and it is for this reason that a well-constructed prospective study is required to compare laparoscopic versus open surgery for distal pancreatic cancer [80]. It is worth noting that despite the cost of surgical material, the financial implications of a laparoscopic operation are as cost-effective as those of an open procedure, mainly because of the reduced length of stay [80]. There is mounting evidence for the benefits of laparoscopic distal pancreatectomy, especially as centres become more experienced and the learning curve becomes less steep.

As mentioned above the incidence of a pancreatic fistula postoperatively has not changed and is significantly higher than with a pancreaticoduodenectomy. The leakage of pancreatic digestive enzymes from the pancreatic ductal system or from the pancreaticojejunostomy can lead to abdominal pain, ileus, sepsis, abscess and haemorrhage [84]. The fistula part of the definition refers to the abnormal connection of the pancreatic ducts to the peri-pancreatic space, peritoneal cavity, other cavities and skin. There are many risk factors for fistula occurrence that include endogenous, operative and perioperative categories [85]. It is often diagnosed from high-output postoperative or percutaneous drain outputs and raised drain fluid amylase levels [84]. In 2005 a review was published on pancreatic fistulation and noted that there was variability in the definition of postoperative pancreatic fistula, leading to incomparable datasets. They set out to focus on two essential aspects before defining the complication: daily volume output and duration of fistula [86].

The use of drains is commonplace in pancreatic procedures as they have an essential place in the management of postoperative leaks and collections. There have been many reported studies looking at whether amylase levels on day 1 may be a predictor of a pancreatic fistula and subsequently guiding the removal of drains. A recent study reviewed the predictability of surgical drain amylase levels. If the amylase levels, of a persistent volume of drain fluid on day 3, were three times above the serum levels, then it was defined as a fistula and the drain was left *in situ* as well as further imaging or drainage conducted. They found a strong correlation between a drain fluid amylase of 90 U/L and a pancreatic fistula, meaning that the drain can be removed early if the level is lower than this which may potentially improve morbidity rates [87]. This supports previous data suggesting early drain removal reduces the incidence of a fistula and intra-abdominal infections [88,89].

Closure of the pancreatic stump is the key step in reducing fistula rates, with the two main techniques being stapled closure of the pancreatic parenchyma and a suture closure of the pancreatic duct [84]. It was initially thought that the latter technique significantly reduced postoperative fistula rates because of direct visualization and closure of the duct [90]. A prospective multicentre study called DISPACT was performed involving 352 patients that were randomized into stapler and hand-sewn closure groups. They found no significant difference between techniques with 32% in the stapled group and 28% in the hand-sewn group [91]. A more recent meta-analysis reviewed 31 studies that compared closure techniques and found a significant difference in favour of stapled closure. They also found that anastomotic closure combined with stapled closure was more effective than suture closure alone. One form of stapling therefore appears to be the most effective technique of reducing postoperative pancreatic fistulas [92].

Other methods have been suggested such as the use of a pancreatic duct stent to divert secretions into the duodenum, but this was also deemed ineffectual [93]. Techniques of distal reinforcements such as a falciform ligament patch, absorbable buttress sleeve sutures or an absorbable mesh buttress have been suggested [84,94]. The mesh buttress has been shown to have significantly fewer leaks than no mesh controls and may be a suitable adjunct [84]. There is a lack of multi-institutional prospective trials in this area, but it is without question that the fundamentals of fistula reduction are meticulous surgical technique, close clinical observation and early suspicion [84].

Borderline resectable pancreatic and ampullary cancer

There are a proportion of patients who present with borderline resectable disease due to involvement of vascular structures. The outcomes following surgery for these patients can be poor and they may have an unresectable tumour at the time of surgery. It is important that there is a widely accepted definition of borderline resectable so that outcomes can be compared between study groups to improve care for these patients. There have been advances in technology and practices to enable a higher resection rate, be it involving a portal vein resection or en bloc excisions involving arterial vessels. A mass involving the mesentericoportal and arterial axis is deemed a borderline resectable lesion and has posed certain questions with respect to oncological clearance despite being technically resectable.

The criteria for resectability should be assessed from a specialized pancreatic protocol CT within 1 month of the planned surgery date. The decision should be made using a multidisciplinary approach according to established international guidelines highlighted in Table 31.5. A recent meta-analysis involving 19 studies and including almost 3000 patients found no significant difference between patients who had venous resections and those who did not, with respect to 5-year survival rates (12.3%) [95]. Other high-volume centres have reproduced these findings and if an R0 resection is possible, then the added postoperative morbidity risks can be justified. The ISGPS recommended that these complex resections be performed by experienced surgical teams in high-volume centres [96]. With regard to arterial involvement, a solid institutional experience base is essential before considering this operative undertaking, and exploration may be advocated to verify the arterial involvement prior to resection and reconstruction. Palliative treatment is then advocated as the standard of care for patients with arterial invasion [96]. Further operative dilemmas exist when the tumour appears locally advanced or borderline resectable with obvious spread to lymph nodes and potentially other organs. An extensive resection is technically feasible but unlikely to provide oncological clearance. This is covered in the next section. The more difficult situations arise when tumours are borderline or locally advanced and the degree of lymph node excision.

Total and extended pancreatectomy

A total pancreatectomy incorporates both elements of a pancreatoduodenectomy and distal pancreatectomy. The indications for this operation have changed over the years as the understanding of tumour biology has increased. Decisions for a total pancreatectomy over a pancreatoduodenectomy or distal pancreatectomy are whether there is disease at the neck of the pancreas and an R0 resection is feasible. There may be spread across the pancreas or a further isolated lesion that is suspicious. The improved recognition of multifocal parenchymal diseases such as IPMNs, NETs and renal cell metastases has led to an increased frequency of total pancreatectomy. This operation has also been performed for patients at increased hereditary risk with suspicions of intraepithelial neoplasia. A completion pancreatectomy has been utilized for persistent fistulation or secondary bleeding postoperatively, but with the advent of advanced interventional radiology techniques this has become less frequent [35,97]. The morbidity of the procedure has reduced but remains high with reported complication rates of 32–54%. This is attributed to improved peri- and postoperative care and regular specialist diabetes care to reduce the impact of 'brittle' diabetes [97,98].

The ISGPS definition of extended pancreatectomy is a pancreatoduodenectomy that incorporates the resection of adjacent organs or vascular structures, incorporating those having neoadjuvant chemotherapy. The standard pancreatoduodenectomy and distal pancreatectomy are defined as above but may also incorporate Gerota's fascia and elements of the transverse mesocolon. The extended versions of these procedures may involve the resection of more than the distal half of the stomach, colon, jejunum, coeliac trunk, splenoportal axis, either the adrenal gland or kidney, liver and diaphragmatic crura. These procedures are indicated when a macroscopic clearance is achievable in the absence of metastatic disease. These procedures are often associated with higher blood loss, longer operating times with higher level of care required, increased morbidities and longer hospital stays. Morbidity is increased when an arterial resection is performed; however, perioperative mortality remains equal.

The median survival and 5-year mortality are improved compared to palliative treatment for locally advanced disease. It is emphasized once again that high-volume centres with experienced surgeons are recommended for the performance of an extended pancreatectomy [99].

Preoperative preparation, peri- and postoperative care

Enhanced recovery after surgery (ERAS) is a structured, multimodal, perioperative strategy to reduce surgical stress and encourage a rapid return to normal function. Given the improvement in survival rates at high-volume centres and the evidence base for ERAS in other general surgical specialties, there have been analyses and recommendations applying these principles to pancreatoduodenectomy. Table 31.6 summarizes the recommendations of the ERAS Society [100]. There may be specific advantages in utilizing minimally invasive surgery, but inconsistency in the utilization of ERAS principles negates these operative benefits [101].

Minimally invasive surgery has proved to be a fundamental aspect to enhanced recovery, especially in bariatric and colorectal surgery. These procedures have yet to be commonplace in pancreas surgery, though distal pancreatectomy employs these techniques more frequently. A few Italian studies have reported a high number of institutions performing robotic and laparoscopic procedures without uniform perioperative care. One Italian study of 115 patients undergoing pancreatoduodenectomy employed the ERAS principles and recorded significant improvements against a control group in days to passing flatus, tolerating diet and the proportion of patients mobilizing on day 1 postoperatively. Adherence to the recommendations is more difficult compared to other specialties due to the complexity of pancreatic surgery and the significant complications that may arise. There was no significant difference in morbidity or mortality and the patients that had minimal complications (Clavien–Dindo Grade 0–2) had significantly faster rehabilitation duration and a shorter length of stay (11 vs 13 days). There was enough evidence that, for patients without serious complications, the ERAS protocol proved beneficial [102].

A meta-analysis in 2013 reviewed the majority of studies utilizing ERAS protocols. They considered a report to be ERAS if it included four of the measures in Table 31.6. Of the four trials analyzed, there was no change in mortality but a significant reduction in morbidity in the ERAS groups stating an absolute risk of 8.2. Interestingly, although there was no significant difference with regard to delayed gastric emptying or pancreatic fistula between the two groups, rates did vary considerably from 13% to 57% and 2% to 15%, respectively. They also noted difficulties in adherence to the ERAS protocol, especially with carbohydrate preloading and early introduction of fluids and diet [103].

Enhanced recovery is at an early stage in pancreatic surgery and adherence is far from consistent. There is enough

Table 31.6 Pancreatoduodenectomy perioperative care guidelines

Item	Recommendation
Preoperative counselling	Patients should receive dedicated counselling routinely.
Perioperative biliary drainage	This should be undertaken routinely in patients with a serum bilirubin <250 μmol/L.
Preoperative smoking and alcohol consumption	For alcohol abusers, 1 month of abstinence before is beneficial and should be attempted. For daily smokers, 1 month of abstinence before surgery is beneficial. For appropriate group, both should be attempted.
Preoperative nutrition	Routine use is not warranted but significantly malnourished patients should be optimized orally or enterally.
Perioperative oral immunonutrition (IN)	Balance of evidence suggests that IN for 5–7 days perioperatively may be considered to reduce infectious complications.
Oral bowel preparation	Extrapolating from colorectal studies, this should not be used.
Preoperative fasting and treatment with carbohydrates	Intake of clear fluids up to 2 hours before anaesthesia does not increase gastric residual volume. Extrapolating data from colorectal studies suggests oral carbohydrate therapy be used in patients without diabetes.
Pre-anaesthetic medication	No clinical benefit from preoperative use of long-acting sedatives; short-acting anxiolytics may be used for smaller anaesthetic procedures.
Anti-thrombolytic prophylaxis	Low-molecular-weight heparin reduces risk of thromboembolic complications and should be continued for 4 weeks after hospital discharge.
Antimicrobial prophylaxis and skin preparation	Prevents surgical site infections and used in a single-dose manner 30–60 minutes before skin incision.
Epidural analgesia	Mid-thoracic epidurals are recommended based on evidence that they are superior to intravenous opioids with a reduced incidence of respiratory complications.
Transverse abdominis plane block/infusions	Conflicting and variable results but some evidence is in support of this procedure.
Postoperative nausea and vomiting	There are benefits to using multimodal pharmacological agents depending on patient's history.
Incision	At the discretion of surgeon.
Avoiding hypothermia	Intraoperative patient warming should be used by forced air or circulating water garments.
Postoperative glycaemic control	Insulin resistance and hyperglycaemia are strongly associated with morbidity and mortality. Intravenous insulin may be used, but close monitoring as to avoid hypoglycaemia is essential.
Nasogastric intubation	Does not improve outcomes, not warranted routinely.
Fluid balance	Near-zero fluid balance and avoiding overload of electrolytes and water improve outcomes. Intraoperative monitoring of stroke volume with a transoesophageal Doppler is recommended. Balanced crystalloid solutions are preferred to 0.9% saline.
Perianastomotic drain	Early removal after 72 hours in patients that are low risk for developing a pancreatic fistula (drain amylase <5000 U/L).
Somatostatin analogues	Somatostatin and its analogues show no benefit on outcomes.
Urinary drainage	Transurethral catheters can be removed safely on postoperative day 1 or 2 unless otherwise indicated.
Delayed gastric emptying	No acknowledged strategy.
Stimulation of bowel movement	Oral laxatives and chewing gum given postoperatively are safe, and may accelerate gastrointestinal transit.
Postoperative artificial nutrition	Allow a normal diet after surgery without restrictions. Begin carefully and increase intake depending on tolerance. Enteral feeding should be given for specific indications and parenteral should not be used routinely.
Early and scheduled mobilization	Mobilize actively from morning of first postoperative day and encourage to meet daily targets.
Audit	Systematically improves compliance and clinical outcomes.

Source: Lassen K, et al., Clinical Nutrition 2012;31(6):817–30.

evidence to suggest that there is no detriment to the patient in following the protocol and that it is quite likely to result in a faster initiation of rehabilitation and a shorter length of stay postoperatively. The impact of complications from a pancreatoduodenectomy is unlikely to be improved by enhanced recovery guidelines.

NEOADJUVANT AND ADJUVANT THERAPIES

Adjuvant chemotherapy in pancreatic and ampullary cancer

The European Study Group for Pancreatic Cancer has performed a number of important clinical trials focusing on differing regimens for the management of pancreatic cancer. The first adequately powered randomized trial was initiated in 2001 and recruited 541 patients across 61 international centres over a 6-year period. It assessed the roles of surgery, adjuvant chemotherapy in the form of 5-fluorouracil (5-FU) and folinic acid (FA) and chemoradiotherapy on overall survival. Median survival was 20.1 months for those who had chemotherapy and 15.5 months for those who had surgery alone. It was recommended that adjuvant chemotherapy provided significant overall survival benefit but chemoradiotherapy did not [104–106]. This study was not powered adequately to provide a comparison with open surgery alone; however, different iterations of this trial and a subsequent ESPAC-3 trial afford the opportunity to make these comparisons. They reported a significant reduction in the risk of death of 30% when utilizing 5-FU and FA compared with just operating alone [105].

The CONKO-001 trial in 2008 was a randomized study of 368 patients with median follow-up of 53 months, comparing adjuvant gemcitabine with observation alone in patients following a curative pancreatic resection. Median disease-free survival was 13.4 months in the gemcitabine group, compared to 6.9 months in the observation group. Interestingly they found no significant difference between patients with an R0 or an R1 resection. There was a 5-year overall survival rate of 20.7% in the gemcitabine group and 10.4% in the observation group, concluding that gemcitabine is the preferred adjuvant chemotherapeutic agent [106,107].

The JASPAC-01 trial in Japan enrolled 385 patients to compare adjuvant gemcitabine and fluorinated pyridimine S-1 for resected pancreatic cancer. They found improved survival in the S-1 group at 2 years compared to gemcitabine (70% vs 53%, respectively), and better recurrence-free survival (49% vs 29%). The metabolic differences between Asian and Caucasian populations allow higher doses in the former, meaning that the gastrointestinal complications would prevent such a dose in Caucasians [106]. Further trials have been performed using S-1 and gemcitabine in conjunction with overall survival at 54% at 2 years and 33% at 5 years [108]. There are still concerns that there are gastrointestinal complications in Western populations, but S-1

certainly has a prominent role in the treatment of pancreatic cancer in Japanese populations [109].

The ESPAC-3 version 2 cohort of 1088 patients were divided into two treatment arms, those receiving 5-FU plus FA and those treated with gemcitabine. Though the overall survival did not improve (23 vs 23.6 months, respectively) the serious adverse events did with 14% in the 5-FU and FA group and 7.5% in the gemcitabine group [110]. These positive findings were also found in patients with R1 resections and node positive disease. Therefore it has been recommended that surgical resection followed by chemotherapy offers the best chance of a long-term cure, with gemcitabine being the current gold standard agent. The optimal duration of chemotherapy was reviewed and whether it commenced at 6 or 12 weeks postoperatively, it was the completion of six cycles that significantly improved patient survival. This affords patients time to recover from their procedures, especially those with major complications [111]. Currently gemcitabine remains the standard adjuvant chemotherapy agent for pancreatic cancer, but further trials and drugs are showing promise for the future.

There are very few studies looking specifically at adjuvant treatment of periampullary cancer. Retrospective series from France and the United States have shown no real benefit to the use of adjuvant chemotherapy, but there has only been one prospective randomized trial to date [112]. ESPAC-3 reviewed 434 patients with periampullary cancers randomly allocated into three arms, 5-FU and FA, gemcitabine and observation alone. They reported median survival times of 38.9, 45.7 and 35.2 months, respectively. There was a significant difference between surgery alone and adjuvant chemotherapy, especially with regard to gemcitabine [113]. At present, similarly to pancreatic cancer, gemcitabine is the best adjuvant chemotherapy agent for ampullary cancer. The development of the ESPAC-4 trial will hopefully provide further evidence for adjuvant therapy in both pancreatic and ampullary cancer. It is a phase III, multicentre randomized control trial comparing gemcitabine and gemcitabine combined with capecitabine chemotherapy.

Adjuvant chemoradiotherapy in pancreatic and ampullary cancer

Adjuvant radiotherapy has had conflicting reports over the years, to the point where it was even suggested that it had deleterious effects on survival [114]. It has been noted that there may have been poor adherence to protocols that may have skewed results [115]. Adjuvant radiotherapy has had disappointing results in patients with locally advanced pancreatic tumours and has shown very little benefit outside of palliation and pain relief. The large stromal component of PDAC makes it less likely to shrink radiologically, even if cells are responding to treatment. A recent meta-analysis reviewed the role of radiotherapy as a neoadjuvant treatment as well as in combination with chemotherapy. Of the 111 studies, there was a large degree of heterogeneity between patients that were resectable and non-resectable as well as varying chemotherapy agents. The conclusions derived were that combination therapies significantly improved resection probabilities in those initially non-resectable patients. There was less of an important finding with patients who had initially resectable tumours [116]. Unfortunately many of the study methodologies did not involve randomization and were not powered individually, thus making combined conclusions hazardous. Newer technical advances are being assessed, for example improved anatomically refined clinical target volumes, three-dimensional conformal radiotherapy, intensity-modulated radiation therapy, photon beam and stereotactic body radiation therapy [117,118]. At the present time there is no evidence for the standard use of adjuvant chemoradiotherapy and further assessment of its role should be undertaken in the context of clinical trials [119].

There is very little evidence for the use of adjuvant chemotherapy in ampullary tumours and even less with respect to chemoradiotherapy and radiotherapy alone. A recent retrospective review of a US population of 329 resected patients showed no survival benefit for adjuvant radiotherapy. They stated that their patients were comparable at baseline, in that adjuvant therapy was not given to those with adverse tumour characteristics [120]. A further study from the United States reviewed the usage of adjuvant chemoradiotherapy in 61 resected ampullary carcinoma patients and suggested a trend to improved overall 3-year survival of 62% (vs. 46% who did not receive adjuvant treatment), but this did not reach significance [121]. The Johns Hopkins Hospital retrospectively reviewed 186 patients with resected ampullary cancer, of whom 66 had adjuvant chemoradiation and 120 surgery alone. They found that patients with node positive disease had a survival advantage with chemoradiation (medial overall survival 32.1 months vs. 15.7 months for surgery only), but the patients receiving this therapy had a significantly higher stage of tumour [122]. The heterogeneity and rarity of patients with ampullary cancer in these retrospective reviews deems their conclusions unreliable [120,123]. There is a clear need for randomized prospective trials.

Neoadjuvant therapy in pancreatic and ampullary cancer

Neoadjuvant treatment is defined as any preoperative treatment aimed to enable a non-resectable lesion to become resectable with a view to microscopic tumour clearance [124]. There have been many phase II trials that suggest that median survival in pancreatic cancer may be longer in patients with resectable lesions post neoadjuvant treatment. The borderline resectable patient may have a higher probability of resection and microscopically clear margins with neoadjuvant treatment. There have been few randomized prospective trials, and the bulk have been retrospective, opening them to accusations of selection bias in a heterogeneous cohort of patients [124].

One of the first groups to suggest preoperative treatment may improve outcomes and resectability in pancreatic cancer was that of Delpero in France. They performed a retrospective review of 1399 consecutive patients from 2004 to 2009, with 402 of these patients requiring some form of venous resection. They found that the median survival for those requiring this complexity of operation was 8 months less than that of a cleanly resected specimen, but that adjuvant and neoadjuvant treatment were associated with improved long-term survival [125,126]. In 2011 they published their results of 173 consecutive patients, divided into two non-randomized cohorts depending on whether patients had neoadjuvant treatment or primary surgery. They found significant differences in that the chemoradiation group had a 43% resection rate compared to a 79% resection rate in the primary surgery group. From a histopathological perspective, the chemoradiation group had smaller tumours, less perineural and lymphatic invasion, fewer positive lymph nodes and fewer positive margins. There was a significant increase in the rate of locoregional recurrence of the primary surgery group compared to chemoradiation but no significant differences with respect to mortality or median survival. The patients that were not suitable for resection developed local or distant metastatic spread, indicating that neoadjuvant treatment may reduce local tumour development but not systemic spread [127].

There have been three recent meta-analyses reviewing 10 to 111 neoadjuvant chemotherapy trials. Laurence and colleagues reported that 40% of patients who were deemed non-resectable before neoadjuvant therapy went on to have resections at operation. They found patients who had neoadjuvant treatment at less risk of having a positive resection margin, and no higher risk of major complications but a higher risk of perioperative mortality [128]. Gillen and colleagues divided studies into two groups: those that were deemed resectable at onset and those that were borderline or non-resectable. They discerned that patients in the first group that went on to have neoadjuvant treatment only had 73.6% of patients amenable to resection compared to 33.2% in the second group. They found a higher rate of complications in the second group, 26.7% versus 39%, and a higher rate of mortality, 3.9% versus 7.1%. The implications of this are important: patients being resectable after being deemed non-resectable is a valuable finding, but having patients not suitable for surgery after being assessed as resectable is deleterious [116]. Festa and colleagues analyzed borderline resectable patients and noted that only 16% of them had downstaging of their lesion and 69% had no change at all, with the remainder showing progression despite treatment. They concluded that preoperative chemoradiation may have a role to play in the treatment of locally advanced non-resectable lesions, but not for those resectable at the time of staging [129].

It was noted in every meta-analysis that there was a high degree of heterogeneity with respect to the trials, which all authors tried to compensate for. They all also reported the lack of a prospective trial with randomized arms.

This leads to selection bias and makes it difficult to manage the trials on an intention-to-treat basis. There is also a lack of a universal definition of a borderline resectable tumour, meaning the decision to operate or give neoadjuvant treatment is open to further bias. This makes the results of these meta-analyses truly difficult to interpret. There has been one randomized prospective phase II trial from Germany that compared preoperative gemcitabine–cisplatin and primary surgery for patients with resectable tumours. Sadly they recruited only 73 patients and then the trial stopped because of slow recruitment and their results were deemed non-significant [130]. From all these papers the role of neoadjuvant therapy appears to lie in the patients unlikely to have an R0 resection. There is clearly a need for a multicentre prospective trial with suitable randomization methodology and a consensus on selection criteria [124].

There are very few studies reviewing neoadjuvant treatment of ampullary cancer, and a study described by Palta and colleagues from North Carolina reviewed 18 patients following neoadjuvant chemoradiotherapy. Sixty-seven percent of these patients were downstaged and 28% had a complete pathological response. There was no discussion regarding the type of ampullary tumour but a suggestion was made that this type of tumour is more receptive to neoadjuvant treatment [121].

LOCALLY ADVANCED AND METASTATIC DISEASE

Palliative procedures

The decision to not offer surgical intervention is based on the criteria that deem a lesion unresectable on up-to-date CT imaging, as shown in Table 31.1. Given the high proportion of patients that are not amenable for surgical resection, the palliation of pancreatic carcinoma is well studied and reported. Locally advanced ampullary cancer may be difficult to distinguish from malignancy of the head of the pancreas and thus susceptible to the same type of complications. There are common complications that need to be pre-empted for depending on the location of the tumour: biliary tree obstruction, which is quite commonplace (70–90%), and gastric outlet obstruction. Patients may suffer symptoms of malnourishment, persistent vomiting, liver failure and biliary sepsis. Both of these conditions potentially can shorten an already limited life expectancy and need appropriate management [131].

BILIARY OBSTRUCTION

Open biliary bypass surgery is a feasible option in that recurrent jaundice is unlikely (2–5%) but there are significant morbidity and mortality rates (up to 56% and 24%, respectively) [131]. The development of endoscopic and fluoroscopic interventions has significantly improved these risks with the advent of a biliary luminal stent. There are few studies that directly compare open and

endoscopic biliary bypass but endoscopic stent placement has become the standard palliative procedure. A recent study advocated the use of open bypass procedures for those able to tolerate surgery. They reviewed 69 patients over an 8-year period and noted no in-hospital death, and no change in overall survival compared to endoscopic stenting. It was recommended that the open procedure may have a role in prophylaxis with a view to palliative chemotherapy [132].

In 2006 a meta-analysis reviewed 21 trials and recommended that biliary obstruction be managed with an endoscopic stent. They suggested a 10 Fr polyethylene stent for patients with a short expected survival and a metal expandable stent for those likely to survive past 6 months [131]. Over the past decade there have been many advances from the placement of a plastic prosthesis, which was prone to blockage and migration. Two recent multicentre studies have recommended the use of a fully covered self-expanding metal stent in patients with malignant biliary strictures. Both studies noted successful decompression with median patency rates of 219 and 328 days and complication rates of 8.8% and 23% [67,133,134]. The stent-specific complications include migration, occlusion from tumour overgrowth and cholangitis. The procedural complications focus around pain, pancreatitis, perforation and post-sphincterotomy bleeding. A recent meta-analysis found that covered metal stents have longer patency rates but similar dysfunction rates compared to the uncovered prosthesis [135]. It seems clear that these procedures have high technical success levels and low morbidity rates, but ultimately their patency is essential to palliate patients with a relatively short life expectancy.

GASTRIC OUTLET OBSTRUCTION

Anatomical imaging is essential in elucidating the exact mechanism of obstruction, prior to planning intervention because the tumour may be invading the duodenum or duodenojejunal junction or causing extrinsic compression. Endoscopic management focuses around the self-expanding metal stent that extends over a length of 6–12 cm. It has a high success rate of 92–100% and symptomatic relief is often within 24 hours [136]. Complications include perforation, haemorrhage, aspiration pneumonia and compression of the common bile duct or pancreatic duct. Occluded stents may require replacing or insertion of a new stent by telescoping the original. If a bile duct stent is also required, this is performed first, though stenting through a duodenal stent has been possible [136].

Surgical relief of obstruction is feasible in the form of a gastrojejunal side-to-side anastomosis, or a Roux-en-Y bypass. Nutritional recovery can be quite slow as symptoms may take a few days to resolve and delayed emptying has been reported from 9% to 26%. A recent systematic review covered 13 studies that compared endoscopic, open and laparoscopic measures to relieve gastric outlet obstruction. They found significantly shorter mean times to symptom resolution and length of stay, a difference of 6.9 and

11.8 days in the endoscopic and open, respectively. There were no differences in complication or mortality rates. There have been too few studies to make conclusions on laparoscopic surgery [137,138].

The advent of biliary obstruction may predict the development of gastric outlet obstruction and so if a laparotomy is performed, then a double bypass may be considered. The 30-day mortality rate of laparotomy alone is 5% compared to 6.5% of patients having a palliative bypass [139]. If the patient has an attempt at curative resection and it is established that it is not resectable, then a double bypass is indicated because the mortality from a laparotomy is significant enough in itself. They may have a longer length of stay and higher morbidity risk, but it is a palliation measure, especially in the context of further treatment such as chemotherapy [136,139].

As alluded to above the precise anatomical details are necessary to predict the palliative outcomes of the disease and plan management. A study of 1126 patients from Pennsylvania found that gastrojejunostomy was performed in 33%, hepatico- or cholecystectojejunostomy in 36% and both were performed in 31% of cases. They reported a morbidity rate of 20% and a mortality rate of 6.5% and advocated risk stratification in order to select the right procedures for a palliative patient [139].

Palliative therapy

Given the difficulty in distinguishing locally infiltrative and advanced pancreatic and ampullary cancer, most trials have been performed on both tumours without distinguishing them. There does not exist any separate study reviewing palliative chemotherapy, chemoradiotherapy or radiotherapy for ampullary cancer in isolation.

The research base for chemoradiation for locally advanced pancreatic cancer remains turbulent with few studies showing solid evidence for radiotherapy. One of the problems encountered included dosing of radiotherapy leading to treatment-related toxicity and poor compliance to additional chemotherapy [140,141]. Evidence favours chemotherapy or chemoradiation but nil suggest radiotherapy in the first instance as an isolated therapy, as occult metastatic disease would not be treated at the risk of radiotherapy-related complications [142]. Theoretically induction chemotherapy as a first line may improve local control of the tumour and the subsequent chemoradiation can potentially reduce tumour size further. A French group carried out a randomized phase III study, LAP 07, and randomized 442 locally advanced pancreatic cancer patients into chemotherapy arms of gemcitabine and gemcitabine with erlotinib as induction chemotherapy treatments. Those with stable disease went on to a second randomization to receive either continued chemotherapy or capecitabine-based chemoradiation. The trial was halted after 3 years because there was no significant difference in overall survival or progression-free survival [142].

5-FU was the mainstay of treatment for locally advanced disease for a long period of time, until it was then used in combination with gemcitabine. The current body of research has trialled new chemotherapeutic agents and multiple combinations with gemcitabine in patients with locally advanced or metastatic disease. There have been some very promising results. A phase III study from the UK randomized 533 advanced pancreatic cancer patients into a gemcitabine arm (Gem) and a gemcitabine plus capecitabine arm (GEM-CAP). They found an improved response rate in the GEM-CAP group and a trend toward improved survival, 6.2 months and 7.1 months, Gem versus GEM-CAP, respectively. This did not reach significance until these results were pooled with three further phase III trials as a meta-analysis [143]. A phase II trial from Germany combined the GEM-CAP combination with oxaliplatin (GEMOXEL) and compared it to gemcitabine alone in 67 randomized patients with metastatic cancer. They found significantly improved median survival of 11.9 and 7.1 months, respectively, with no significant change in severe adverse complications [144]. Interestingly S-1 has been used in combination with gemcitabine for local advanced pancreatic cancer in multiple Asian studies. A recent meta-analysis has found that the patients receiving combination therapy had a higher proportion live for more than a year, 43.4% compared to 31.4% in the gemcitabine group. Unfortunately there were higher toxic haematological complications [145]. Multiple other drugs have been used with gemcitabine including cisplatin, irinotecan, erlotinib and cetuximab. There are two combinatorial chemotherapy regimens that have shown more promise than those described above [146].

The ACCORD trial in 2011 found overall survival to increase in patients with metastatic disease when treated with the FOLFIRINOX chemotherapy combination of fluorouracil, leucovorin, oxaliplatin and irinotecan. Conroy and colleagues randomized 342 metastatic pancreatic cancer patients to receive FOLFIRINOX or gemcitabine. They found a significantly higher median overall survival between the two groups in favour of FOLFIRINOX (11.1 vs. 6.8 months). Unfortunately there was an increased risk of adverse events, 5.4% had febrile neutropenia, and there was a high incidence of gastrointestinal toxicity. Therefore this drug combination has been recommended in the very fit younger population group with a high performance status [147,148]. Faris and colleagues then took these findings and trialled this combination in patients with locally advanced tumours. They paid particular attention to the diagnosis and staging of lesions and incorporated four national oncology associations. There were two groups: 87 patients were deemed resectable and had no neoadjuvant treatment and 47 had FOLFIRINOX prior to explorative surgery. The latter group had a significant downstaging of median tumour size from 3.6 to 2.2 cm. Seven of these patients had locally advanced and metastatic disease. Patients in the neoadjuvant group had significantly longer operative times, five venous resections and more blood loss. There was no significant change in postoperative morbidity, length of stay, mortality or readmissions.

The pathological findings were encouraging with 35% of patients having positive lymph nodes in the neoadjuvant groups compared to 79% in the primary surgery group. There was a higher R0 resection with 92% in the neoadjuvant group compared to 86% in the primary surgery group, but this was not statistically significant. The FOLFIRINOX group had a significant longer overall survival. They did report that radiologically they were unable to differentiate fibrosis and a viable tumour and that patients should be explored with a view to serial frozen section to investigate vessel involvement [149].

There were some early phase trials utilizing docetaxel, which had limited numbers of patients and variable clinical activity. Paclitaxel was developed and shown to have a higher bioavailability, and further improved when bound to human serum albumin: nab-paclitaxel. Promising early phase trials led to the first phase III trial in advanced pancreatic cancer by Von Hoff et al. [150]. A total of 861 patients were divided evenly between a nab-paclitaxel–gemcitabine group and a gemcitabine group; all patients had metastatic pancreatic cancers. They found a significant overall survival of 8.5 and 6.7 months, respectively, with significantly increased 1-year mortalities of 35% versus 23%, respectively. There were also significantly increased morbidities in the nab-paclitaxel–gemcitabine group including febrile neutropenia (38% vs. 27%), fatigue (17% vs. 7%) and neuropathy (17% vs. 1%). Considerations of these complications are essential to the conclusions that nab-paclitaxel with gemcitabine offers improved overall survival, progression-free survival and response rates [150].

Long-term results from this trial have recently been published and followed suit, in that the median overall survival is statistically longer with similar figures of 8.7 versus 6.6 months favouring the nab-paclitaxel group. They also noticed the usefulness of CA 19-9 and neutrophil-to-lymphocyte ratio as prognostic markers. There is a clear indication that nab-paclitaxel has a survival benefit to patients with metastatic disease, and further prospective randomized trials must be performed to validate these results and progress to patients with less advanced disease [151].

It has become well established that gemcitabine alone is not as effective as it is in doublets or in three or four drug combinations, with statistically significant increased overall survivals. Future experiments are likely to involve multicentre prospective randomized trials, but rigorous methodological control is essential to enable comparative effectiveness [146].

FUTURE ADVANCES

Throughout the whole of this chapter there have been multiple trials and meta-analyses in all aspects of pancreatic and ampullary malignancy. Unfortunately the 5-year survival has changed little over the years. There have been significant advances in the staging and imaging of these lesions, the strategy and extent of surgery, the peri- and postoperative care of these patients and the chemotherapy agents available as adjuvant therapy. This only provides a potential cure in a small proportion of patients with pancreatic and ampullary cancer because many are diagnosed too late. This has become a hallmark of pancreas research, the detection of biomarkers and genetic screening strategies. Identifying not only those at risk of developing malignancy but also those who are susceptible to specific chemotherapy agents is directing the management of pancreatic and ampullary cancer to a personalized approach. As the understanding of tumour biology increases we are finding new metabolic, cell signaling and immunological targets for drug therapy but also the patients that are likely to find benefit from them [152].

REFERENCES

1. Ferlay J, Soerjomataram I, Dikshit R, Eser S, Mathers C, Rebelo M, et al. Cancer incidence and mortality worldwide: sources, methods and major patterns in GLOBOCAN 2012. *International Journal of Cancer* 2015;136(5):E359–86.
2. Cancer Research UK. Statistics report: cancer incidence in the UK in 2011. London: Cancer Research UK, 2014.
3. Cancer Research UK. UK cancer incidence 2011 and mortality 2012 summary. London: Cancer Research UK, 2014.
4. Khan ICK. In *Hepatobiliary and Pancreatic Surgery: A Companion to Specialist Surgical Practice*, 4th ed., Garden J, ed. Philadelphia: Saunders Ltd., 2009.
5. Perysinakis I, Margaris I, Kouraklis G. Ampullary cancer – a separate clinical entity? *Histopathology* 2014;64(6):759–68.
6. Coupland VH, Kocher HM, Berry DP, Allum W, Linklater KM, Konfortion J, et al. Incidence and survival for hepatic, pancreatic and biliary cancers in England between 1998 and 2007. *Cancer Epidemiology* 2012;36(4):e207–14.
7. Rostain F, Hamza S, Drouillard A, Faivre J, Bouvier AM, Lepage C. Trends in incidence and management of cancer of the ampulla of Vater. *World Journal of Gastroenterology* 2014;20(29):10144–50.
8. Iodice S, Gandini S, Maisonneuve P, Lowenfels AB. Tobacco and the risk of pancreatic cancer: a review and meta-analysis. *Langenbeck's Archives of Surgery* 2008;393(4):535–45.
9. Becker AE, Hernandez YG, Frucht H, Lucas AL. Pancreatic ductal adenocarcinoma: risk factors, screening, and early detection. *World Journal of Gastroenterology* 2014;20(32):11182–98.
10. Maisonneuve P, Lowenfels AB. Risk factors for pancreatic cancer: a summary review of meta-analytical studies. *International Journal of Epidemiology* 2015;44(1):186–98.

11. Villeneuve PJ, Johnson KC, Mao Y, Hanley AJ, Canadian Cancer Registries Research G. Environmental tobacco smoke and the risk of pancreatic cancer: findings from a Canadian population-based case-control study. *Canadian Journal of Public Health* 2004;95(1):32–7.

12. Raimondi S, Lowenfels AB, Morselli-Labate AM, Maisonneuve P, Pezzilli R. Pancreatic cancer in chronic pancreatitis; aetiology, incidence, and early detection. *Best Practice & Research Clinical Gastroenterology* 2010;24(3):349–58.

13. Pandol SJ, Raraty M. Pathobiology of alcoholic pancreatitis. *Pancreatology* 2007;7(2–3):105–14.

14. Donohoe CL, O'Farrell NJ, Doyle SL, Reynolds JV. The role of obesity in gastrointestinal cancer: evidence and opinion. *Therapeutic Advances in Gastroenterology* 2014;7(1):38–50.

15. Larsson SC, Orsini N, Wolk A. Body mass index and pancreatic cancer risk: a meta-analysis of prospective studies. *International Journal of Cancer Journal* 2007;120(9):1993–8.

16. Berrington de Gonzalez A, Sweetland S, Spencer E. A meta-analysis of obesity and the risk of pancreatic cancer. *British Journal of Cancer* 2003;89(3):519–23.

17. Huang Y, Cai X, Qiu M, Chen P, Tang H, Hu Y, et al. Prediabetes and the risk of cancer: a meta-analysis. *Diabetologia* 2014;57(11):2261–9.

18. Liao WC, Tu YK, Wu MS, Lin JT, Wang HP, Chien KL. Blood glucose concentration and risk of pancreatic cancer: systematic review and dose-response meta-analysis. *BMJ* 2015;349:g7371.

19. Elena JW, Steplowski E, Yu K, Hartge P, Tobias GS, Brotzman MJ, et al. Diabetes and risk of pancreatic cancer: a pooled analysis from the pancreatic cancer cohort consortium. *Cancer Causes & Control* 2013;24(1):13–25.

20. Wang Z, Lai ST, Xie L, Zhao JD, Ma NY, Zhu J, et al. Metformin is associated with reduced risk of pancreatic cancer in patients with type 2 diabetes mellitus: a systematic review and meta-analysis. *Diabetes Research and Clinical Practice* 2014;106(1):19–26.

21. Larsson SC, Orsini N. Red meat and processed meat consumption and all-cause mortality: a meta-analysis. *American Journal of Epidemiology* 2014;179(3):282–9.

22. Larsson SC, Wolk A. Red and processed meat consumption and risk of pancreatic cancer: meta-analysis of prospective studies. *British Journal of Cancer* 2012;106(3):603–7.

23. Shigihara M, Obara T, Nagai M, Sugawara Y, Watanabe T, Kakizaki M, et al. Consumption of fruits, vegetables, and seaweeds (sea vegetables) and pancreatic cancer risk: the Ohsaki Cohort Study. *Cancer Epidemiology* 2014;38(2):129–36.

24. Koushik A, Spiegelman D, Albanes D, Anderson KE, Bernstein L, van den Brandt PA, et al. Intake of fruits and vegetables and risk of pancreatic cancer in a pooled analysis of 14 cohort studies. *American Journal of Epidemiology* 2012;176(5):373–86.

25. He XD, Wu Q, Liu W, Hong T, Li JJ, Miao RY, et al. Association of metabolic syndromes and risk factors with ampullary tumors development: a case-control study in China. *World Journal of Gastroenterology* 2014;20(28):9541–8.

26. Permuth-Wey J, Egan KM. Family history is a significant risk factor for pancreatic cancer: results from a systematic review and meta-analysis. *Familial Cancer* 2009;8(2):109–17.

27. Klein AP. Identifying people at a high risk of developing pancreatic cancer. *Nature Reviews Cancer* 2013;13(1):66–74.

28. Rustgi AK. Familial pancreatic cancer: genetic advances. *Genes & Development* 2014;28(1):1–7.

29. Mersch J, Jackson MA, Park M, Nebgen D, Peterson SK, Singletary C, et al. Cancers associated with BRCA1 and BRCA2 mutations other than breast and ovarian. *Cancer* 2015;121(2):269–75.

30. Kastrinos F, Mukherjee B, Tayob N, Wang F, Sparr J, Raymond VM, et al. Risk of pancreatic cancer in families with Lynch syndrome. *JAMA* 2009;302(16):1790–5.

31. Bartsch DK, Gress TM, Langer P. Familial pancreatic cancer – current knowledge. *Nature Reviews Gastroenterology & Hepatology* 2012;9(8):445–53.

32. Laleman W, Verreth A, Topal B, Aerts R, Komuta M, Roskams T, et al. Endoscopic resection of ampullary lesions: a single-center 8-year retrospective cohort study of 91 patients with long-term follow-up. *Surgical Endoscopy* 2013;27(10):3865–76.

33. Ma T, Jang EJ, Zukerberg LR, Odze R, Gala MK, Kelsey PB, et al. Recurrences are common after endoscopic ampullectomy for adenoma in the familial adenomatous polyposis (FAP) syndrome. *Surgical Endoscopy* 2014;28(8):2349–56.

34. Hidalgo M. Pancreatic cancer. *New England Journal of Medicine* 2010;362(17):1605–17.

35. Kulu Y, Schmied BM, Werner J, Muselli P, Buchler MW, Schmidt J. Total pancreatectomy for pancreatic cancer: indications and operative technique. *HPB* 2009;11(6):469–75.

36. Wood LD, Klimstra DS. Pathology and genetics of pancreatic neoplasms with acinar differentiation. *Seminars in Diagnostic Pathology* 2014;31(6):491–7.

37. Bosman FT, World Health Organization, International Agency for Research on Cancer. *WHO Classification of Tumours of the Digestive System*, 4th ed. Lyon: International Agency for Research on Cancer, 2010.

38. Rustagi T, Farrell JJ. Endoscopic diagnosis and treatment of pancreatic neuroendocrine tumors. *Journal of Clinical Gastroenterology.* 2014;48(10):837–44.

39. He J, Ahuja N, Makary MA, Cameron JL, Eckhauser FE, Choti MA, et al. 2564 resected periampullary adenocarcinomas at a single institution: trends over three decades. *HPB* 2014;16(1):83–90.

40. Kimura W, Futakawa N, Yamagata S, Wada Y, Kuroda A, Muto T, et al. Different clinicopathologic findings in two histologic types of carcinoma of papilla of Vater. *Japanese Journal of Cancer Research* 1994;85(2):161–6.

41. Edge SB, Compton CC. The American Joint Committee on Cancer: the 7th edition of the *AJCC Cancer Staging Manual* and the future of TNM. *Annals of Surgical Oncology* 2010;17(6):1471–4.

42. Sobin LH, Gospodarowicz MK, Wittekind C, International Union Against Cancer. *TNM Classification of Malignant Tumours*, 7th ed. Chichester: Wiley-Blackwell, 2010.

43. Pathologists TRCo. Standards and datasets for reporting cancers: dataset for the histopathological reporting of carcinomas of the pancreas, ampulla of Vater and common bile duct. London: Pathologists TRCo, 2010. Available from https://www.rcpath.org/resourceLibrary/dataset-for-the-histopathological-reporting-of-carcinomas-of-the-pancreas–ampulla-of-vater-and-common-bile-duct.html.

44. Campbell F, Smith RA, Whelan P, Sutton R, Raraty M, Neoptolemos JP, et al. Classification of R1 resections for pancreatic cancer: the prognostic relevance of tumour involvement within 1 mm of a resection margin. *Histopathology* 2009;55(3):277–83.

45. Keane MG, Horsfall L, Rait G, Pereira SP. A case-control study comparing the incidence of early symptoms in pancreatic and biliary tract cancer. *BMJ Open* 2014;4(11):e005720.

46. Garden OJ, Parks RW. *Hepatobiliary and Pancreatic Surgery*, 5th ed. Edinburgh: Saunders Elsevier, 2014.

47. Lee ES, Lee JM. Imaging diagnosis of pancreatic cancer: a state-of-the-art review. *World Journal of Gastroenterology* 2014;20(24):7864–77.

48. Hanada K, Okazaki A, Hirano N, Izumi Y, Teraoka Y, Ikemoto J, et al. Diagnostic strategies for early pancreatic cancer. *Journal of Gastroenterology* 2015;50(2):147–54.

49. Kaneko OF, Lee DM, Wong J, Kadell BM, Reber HA, Lu DS, et al. Performance of multidetector computed tomographic angiography in determining surgical resectability of pancreatic head adenocarcinoma. *Journal of Computer Assisted Tomography* 2010;34(5):732–8.

50. Antoch G, Saoudi N, Kuehl H, Dahmen G, Mueller SP, Beyer T, et al. Accuracy of whole-body dual-modality fluorine-18-2-fluoro-2-deoxy-D-glucose positron emission tomography and computed tomography (FDG-PET/CT) for tumor staging in solid tumors: comparison with CT and PET. *Journal of Clinical Oncology* 2004;22(21):4357–68.

51. Wang XY, Yang F, Jin C, Fu DL. Utility of PET/CT in diagnosis, staging, assessment of resectability and metabolic response of pancreatic cancer. *World Journal of Gastroenterology* 2014;20(42):15580–9.

52. Kitajima K, Murakami K, Yamasaki E, Kaji Y, Shimoda M, Kubota K, et al. Performance of integrated FDG-PET/contrast-enhanced CT in the diagnosis of recurrent pancreatic cancer: comparison with integrated FDG-PET/non-contrast-enhanced CT and enhanced CT. *Molecular Imaging and Biology* 2010;12(4):452–9.

53. Asagi A, Ohta K, Nasu J, Tanada M, Nadano S, Nishimura R, et al. Utility of contrast-enhanced FDG-PET/CT in the clinical management of pancreatic cancer: impact on diagnosis, staging, evaluation of treatment response, and detection of recurrence. *Pancreas* 2013;42(1):11–9.

54. Strobel K, Heinrich S, Bhure U, Soyka J, Veit-Haibach P, Pestalozzi BC, et al. Contrast-enhanced 18F-FDG PET/CT: 1-stop-shop imaging for assessing the resectability of pancreatic cancer. *Journal of Nuclear Medicine* 2008;49(9):1408–13.

55. Teshima CW, Sandha GS. Endoscopic ultrasound in the diagnosis and treatment of pancreatic disease. *World Journal of Gastroenterology* 2014;20(29):9976–89.

56. Fusaroli P, Kypraios D, Caletti G, Eloubeidi MA. Pancreatico-biliary endoscopic ultrasound: a systematic review of the levels of evidence, performance and outcomes. *World Journal of Gastroenterology* 2012;18(32):4243–56.

57. Gonzalo-Marin J, Vila JJ, Perez-Miranda M. Role of endoscopic ultrasound in the diagnosis of pancreatic cancer. *World Journal of Gastrointestinal Oncology* 2014;6(9):360–8.

58. Puli SR, Kalva N, Bechtold ML, Pamulaparthy SR, Cashman MD, Estes NC, et al. Diagnostic accuracy of endoscopic ultrasound in pancreatic neuroendocrine tumors: a systematic review and meta analysis. *World Journal of Gastroenterology* 2013;19(23):3678–84.

59. De Palma GD. Endoscopic papillectomy: indications, techniques, and results. *World Journal of Gastroenterology* 2014;20(6):1537–43.

60. Chen J, Yang R, Lu Y, Xia Y, Zhou H. Diagnostic accuracy of endoscopic ultrasound-guided fine-needle aspiration for solid pancreatic lesion: a systematic review. *Journal of Cancer Research and Clinical Oncology* 2012;138(9):1433–41.

61. Asbun HJ, Conlon K, Fernandez-Cruz L, Friess H, Shrikhande SV, Adham M, et al. When to perform a pancreatoduodenectomy in the absence of

positive histology? A consensus statement by the International Study Group of Pancreatic Surgery. *Surgery* 2014;155(5):887–92.

62. Eloubeidi MA, Varadarajulu S, Desai S, Shirley R, Heslin MJ, Mehra M, et al. A prospective evaluation of an algorithm incorporating routine preoperative endoscopic ultrasound-guided fine needle aspiration in suspected pancreatic cancer. *Journal of Gastrointestinal Surgery* 2007;11(7):813–9.

63. van der Gaag NA, Rauws EA, van Eijck CH, Bruno MJ, van der Harst E, Kubben FJ, et al. Preoperative biliary drainage for cancer of the head of the pancreas. *New England Journal of Medicine* 2010;362(2):129–37.

64. Fang Y, Gurusamy KS, Wang Q, Davidson BR, Lin H, Xie X, et al. Pre-operative biliary drainage for obstructive jaundice. *Cochrane Database of Systematic Reviews* 2012;9:CD005444.

65. Wasan SM, Ross WA, Staerkel GA, Lee JH. Use of expandable metallic biliary stents in resectable pancreatic cancer. *American Journal of Gastroenterology* 2005;100(9):2056–61.

66. Soderlund C, Linder S, Bergenzaun PE, Grape T, Hakansson HO, Kilander A, et al. Nitinol versus steel partially covered self-expandable metal stent for malignant distal biliary obstruction: a randomized trial. *Endoscopy* 2014;46(11):941–8.

67. Kitano M, Yamashita Y, Tanaka K, Konishi H, Yazumi S, Nakai Y, et al. Covered self-expandable metal stents with an anti-migration system improve patency duration without increased complications compared with uncovered stents for distal biliary obstruction caused by pancreatic carcinoma: a randomized multicenter trial. *American Journal of Gastroenterology* 2013;108(11):1713–22.

68. Sun C, Yan G, Li Z, Tzeng CM. A meta-analysis of the effect of preoperative biliary stenting on patients with obstructive jaundice. *Medicine* 2014;93(26):e189.

69. De Palma GD, Luglio G, Maione F, Esposito D, Siciliano S, Gennarelli N, et al. Endoscopic snare papillectomy: a single institutional experience of a standardized technique. A retrospective cohort study. *International Journal of Surgery* 2015;13:180–3.

70. Kim HK, Lo SK. Endoscopic approach to the patient with benign or malignant ampullary lesions. *Gastrointestinal Endoscopy Clinics of North America* 2013;23(2):347–83.

71. Tsuji S, Itoi T, Sofuni A, Mukai S, Tonozuka R, Moriyasu F. Tips and tricks in endoscopic papillectomy of ampullary tumors: single-center experience with large case series (with videos). *Journal of Hepato-Biliary-Pancreatic Sciences* 2015;22(6):E22–7.

72. Tol JA, Gouma DJ, Bassi C, Dervenis C, Montorsi M, Adham M, et al. Definition of a standard lymphadenectomy in surgery for pancreatic ductal adenocarcinoma: a consensus statement by the International Study Group on Pancreatic Surgery (ISGPS). *Surgery* 2014;156(3):591–600.

73. Diener MK, Fitzmaurice C, Schwarzer G, Seiler CM, Huttner FJ, Antes G, et al. Pylorus-preserving pancreaticoduodenectomy (pp Whipple) versus pancreaticoduodenectomy (classic Whipple) for surgical treatment of periampullary and pancreatic carcinoma. *Cochrane Database of Systematic Reviews* 2014;11:CD006053.

74. Kawai M, Yamaue H. Analysis of clinical trials evaluating complications after pancreaticoduodenectomy: a new era of pancreatic surgery. *Surgery Today* 2010;40(11):1011–7.

75. Connor S, Alexakis N, Garden OJ, Leandros E, Bramis J, Wigmore SJ. Meta-analysis of the value of somatostatin and its analogues in reducing complications associated with pancreatic surgery. *British Journal of Surgery* 2005;92(9):1059–67.

76. Jones L, Russell C, Mosca F, Boggi U, Sutton R, Slavin J, et al. Standard Kausch-Whipple pancreatoduodenectomy. *Digestive Surgery* 1999;16(4):297–304.

77. Qin H, Qiu J, Zhao Y, Pan G, Zeng Y. Does minimally-invasive pancreaticoduodenectomy have advantages over its open method? A meta-analysis of retrospective studies. *PloS One* 2014;9(8):e104274.

78. Paye F, Micelli Lupinacci R, Bachellier P, Boher JM, Delpero JR, on behalf of the French Surgical A. Distal pancreatectomy for pancreatic carcinoma in the era of multimodal treatment. *British Journal of Surgery* 2015;102(3):229–36.

79. Kirk RM. *General Surgical Operations*, 5th ed. Edinburgh: Churchill Livingstone/Elsevier, 2006.

80. Bjornsson B, Sandstrom P. Laparoscopic distal pancreatectomy for adenocarcinoma of the pancreas. *World Journal of Gastroenterology* 2014;20(37):13402–11.

81. Venkat R, Edil BH, Schulick RD, Lidor AO, Makary MA, Wolfgang CL. Laparoscopic distal pancreatectomy is associated with significantly less overall morbidity compared to the open technique: a systematic review and meta-analysis. *Annals of Surgery* 2012;255(6):1048–59.

82. Jusoh AC, Ammori BJ. Laparoscopic versus open distal pancreatectomy: a systematic review of comparative studies. *Surgical Endoscopy* 2012;26(4):904–13.

83. Lee SY, Allen PJ, Sadot E, D'Angelica MI, DeMatteo RP, Fong Y, et al. Distal pancreatectomy: A single institution's experience in open, laparoscopic, and robotic approaches. *Journal of the American College of Surgeons* 2015;220(1):18–27.

84. Schoellhammer HF, Fong Y, Gagandeep S. Techniques for prevention of pancreatic leak after pancreatectomy. *Hepatobiliary Surgery and Nutrition* 2014;3(5):276–87.

85. McMillan MT, Vollmer CM Jr. Predictive factors for pancreatic fistula following pancreatectomy. *Langenbeck's Archives of Surgery* 2014;399(7):811–24.

86. Bassi C, Dervenis C, Butturini G, Fingerhut A, Yeo C, Izbicki J, et al. Postoperative pancreatic fistula: an international study group (ISGPF) definition. *Surgery* 2005;138(1):8–13.

87. Lee CW, Pitt HA, Riall TS, Ronnekleiv-Kelly SS, Israel JS, Leverson GE, et al. Low drain fluid amylase predicts absence of pancreatic fistula following pancreatectomy. *Journal of Gastrointestinal Surgery* 2014;18(11):1902–10.

88. Bassi C, Molinari E, Malleo G, Crippa S, Butturini G, Salvia R, et al. Early versus late drain removal after standard pancreatic resections: results of a prospective randomized trial. *Annals of Surgery* 2010;252(2):207–14.

89. Kawai M, Kondo S, Yamaue H, Wada K, Sano K, Motoi F, et al. Predictive risk factors for clinically relevant pancreatic fistula analyzed in 1,239 patients with pancreaticoduodenectomy: multicenter data collection as a project study of pancreatic surgery by the Japanese Society of Hepato-Biliary-Pancreatic Surgery. *Journal of Hepato-Biliary-Pancreatic Sciences* 2011;18(4):601–8.

90. Bilimoria MM, Cormier JN, Mun Y, Lee JE, Evans DB, Pisters PW. Pancreatic leak after left pancreatectomy is reduced following main pancreatic duct ligation. *British Journal of Surgery* 2003;90(2):190–6.

91. Diener MK, Seiler CM, Rossion I, Kleeff J, Glanemann M, Butturini G, et al. Efficacy of stapler versus hand-sewn closure after distal pancreatectomy (DISPACT): a randomised, controlled multicentre trial. *Lancet* 2011;377(9776):1514–22.

92. Zhang H, Zhu F, Shen M, Tian R, Shi CJ, Wang X, et al. Systematic review and meta-analysis comparing three techniques for pancreatic remnant closure following distal pancreatectomy. *British Journal of Surgery* 2015;102(1):4–15.

93. Frozanpor F, Lundell L, Segersvard R, Arnelo U. The effect of prophylactic transpapillary pancreatic stent insertion on clinically significant leak rate following distal pancreatectomy: results of a prospective controlled clinical trial. *Annals of Surgery* 2012;255(6):1032–6.

94. Fujino Y, Sendo H, Oshikiri T, Sugimoto T, Tominaga M. A novel surgical technique to prevent pancreatic fistula in distal pancreatectomy using a patch of the falciform ligament. *Surgery Today* 2015;45(1):44–9.

95. Zhou Y, Zhang Z, Liu Y, Li B, Xu D. Pancreatectomy combined with superior mesenteric vein-portal vein resection for pancreatic cancer: a meta-analysis. *World Journal of Surgery* 2012;36(4):884–91.

96. Bockhorn M, Uzunoglu FG, Adham M, Imrie C, Milicevic M, Sandberg AA, et al. Borderline resectable pancreatic cancer: a consensus statement by the International Study Group of Pancreatic Surgery (ISGPS). *Surgery* 2014;155(6):977–88.

97. Almond M, Roberts KJ, Hodson J, Sutcliffe R, Marudanayagam R, Isaac J, et al. Changing indications for a total pancreatectomy: perspectives over a quarter of a century. *HPB* 2015;17(5):416–21.

98. Crippa S, Tamburrino D, Partelli S, Salvia R, Germenia S, Bassi C, et al. Total pancreatectomy: indications, different timing, and perioperative and long-term outcomes. *Surgery* 2011;149(1):79–86.

99. Hartwig W, Vollmer CM, Fingerhut A, Yeo CJ, Neoptolemos JP, Adham M, et al. Extended pancreatectomy in pancreatic ductal adenocarcinoma: definition and consensus of the International Study Group for Pancreatic Surgery (ISGPS). *Surgery* 2014;156(1):1–14.

100. Lassen K, Coolsen MM, Slim K, Carli F, de Aguilar-Nascimento JE, Schafer M, et al. Guidelines for perioperative care for pancreaticoduodenectomy: Enhanced Recovery After Surgery (ERAS®) Society recommendations. *Clinical Nutrition* 2012;31(6):817–30.

101. Balzano G, Bissolati M, Boggi U, Bassi C, Zerbi A, Falconi M, et al. A multicenter survey on distal pancreatectomy in Italy: results of minimally invasive technique and variability of perioperative pathways. *Updates in Surgery* 2014;66(4):253–63.

102. Braga M, Pecorelli N, Ariotti R, Capretti G, Greco M, Balzano G, et al. Enhanced recovery after surgery pathway in patients undergoing pancreaticoduodenectomy. *World Journal of Surgery* 2014;38(11):2960–6.

103. Coolsen MM, van Dam RM, van der Wilt AA, Slim K, Lassen K, Dejong CH. Systematic review and meta-analysis of enhanced recovery after pancreatic surgery with particular emphasis on pancreaticoduodenectomies. *World Journal of Surgery* 2013;37(8):1909–18.

104. Greenhalf W, Ghaneh P, Neoptolemos JP, Palmer DH, Cox TF, Lamb RF, et al. Pancreatic cancer hENT1 expression and survival from gemcitabine in patients from the ESPAC-3 trial. *Journal of the National Cancer Institute* 2014;106(1):djt347.

105. Neoptolemos JP, Stocken DD, Tudur Smith C, Bassi C, Ghaneh P, Owen E, et al. Adjuvant 5-fluorouracil and folinic acid vs observation for pancreatic cancer: composite data from the ESPAC-1 and -3(v1) trials. *British Journal of Cancer* 2009;100(2):246–50.

106. Jones OP, Melling JD, Ghaneh P. Adjuvant therapy in pancreatic cancer. *World Journal of Gastroenterology* 2014;20(40):14733–46.

107. Oettle H, Neuhaus P, Hochhaus A, Hartmann JT, Gellert K, Ridwelski K, et al. Adjuvant chemotherapy with gemcitabine and long-term outcomes among patients with resected pancreatic cancer: the CONKO-001 randomized trial. *JAMA* 2013;310(14):1473–81.

108. Murakami Y, Uemura K, Sudo T, Hashimoto Y, Nakashima A, Kondo N, et al. Long-term results of adjuvant gemcitabine plus S-1 chemotherapy after surgical resection for pancreatic carcinoma. *Journal of Surgical Oncology* 2012;106(2):174–80.

109. Sudo K, Nakamura K, Yamaguchi T. S-1 in the treatment of pancreatic cancer. *World Journal of Gastroenterology* 2014;20(41):15110–8.

110. Neoptolemos JP, Stocken DD, Bassi C, Ghaneh P, Cunningham D, Goldstein D, et al. Adjuvant chemotherapy with fluorouracil plus folinic acid vs gemcitabine following pancreatic cancer resection: a randomized controlled trial. *JAMA* 2010;304(10):1073–81.

111. Valle JW, Palmer D, Jackson R, Cox T, Neoptolemos JP, Ghaneh P, et al. Optimal duration and timing of adjuvant chemotherapy after definitive surgery for ductal adenocarcinoma of the pancreas: ongoing lessons from the ESPAC-3 study. *Journal of Clinical Oncology* 2014;32(6):504–12.

112. Robert PE, Leux C, Ouaissi M, Miguet M, Paye F, Merdrignac A, et al. Predictors of long-term survival following resection for ampullary carcinoma: a large retrospective French multicentric study. *Pancreas* 2014;43(5):692–7.

113. Neoptolemos JP, Moore MJ, Cox TF, Valle JW, Palmer DH, McDonald AC, et al. Effect of adjuvant chemotherapy with fluorouracil plus folinic acid or gemcitabine vs observation on survival in patients with resected periampullary adenocarcinoma: the ESPAC-3 periampullary cancer randomized trial. *JAMA* 2012;308(2):147–56.

114. Neoptolemos JP, Stocken DD, Friess H, Bassi C, Dunn JA, Hickey H, et al. A randomized trial of chemoradiotherapy and chemotherapy after resection of pancreatic cancer. *New England Journal of Medicine* 2004;350(12):1200–10.

115. Regine WF, Winter KA, Abrams RA, Safran H, Hoffman JP, Konski A, et al. Fluorouracil vs gemcitabine chemotherapy before and after fluorouracil-based chemoradiation following resection of pancreatic adenocarcinoma: a randomized controlled trial. *JAMA* 2008;299(9):1019–26.

116. Gillen S, Schuster T, Meyer Zum Buschenfelde C, Friess H, Kleeff J. Preoperative/neoadjuvant therapy in pancreatic cancer: a systematic review and meta-analysis of response and resection percentages. *PLoS Medicine* 2010;7(4):e1000267.

117. Chuong MD, Boggs DH, Patel KN, Regine WF. Adjuvant chemoradiation for pancreatic cancer: what does the evidence tell us? *Journal of Gastrointestinal Oncology* 2014;5(3):166–77.

118. Goodman KA, Regine WF, Dawson LA, Ben-Josef E, Haustermans K, Bosch WR, et al. Radiation Therapy Oncology Group consensus panel guidelines for the delineation of the clinical target volume in the postoperative treatment of pancreatic head cancer. *International Journal of Radiation Oncology, Biology, Physics* 2012;83(3):901–8.

119. Van Laethem JL, Verslype C, Iovanna JL, Michl P, Conroy T, Louvet C, et al. New strategies and designs in pancreatic cancer research: consensus guidelines report from a European expert panel. *Annals of Oncology* 2012;23(3):570–6.

120. Miura JT, Jayakrishnan TT, Amini A, Johnston FM, Tsai S, Erickson B, et al. Defining the role of adjuvant external beam radiotherapy on resected adenocarcinoma of the ampulla of Vater. *Journal of Gastrointestinal Surgery* 2014;18(11):2003–8.

121. Palta M, Patel P, Broadwater G, Willett C, Pepek J, Tyler D, et al. Carcinoma of the ampulla of Vater: patterns of failure following resection and benefit of chemoradiotherapy. *Annals of Surgical Oncology* 2012;19(5):1535–40.

122. Narang AK, Miller RC, Hsu CC, Bhatia S, Pawlik TM, Laheru D, et al. Evaluation of adjuvant chemoradiation therapy for ampullary adenocarcinoma: the Johns Hopkins Hospital–Mayo Clinic collaborative study. *Radiation Oncology* 2011;6:126.

123. Zhong J, Palta M, Willett CG, McCall SJ, McSherry F, Tyler DS, et al. Patterns of failure for stage I ampulla of Vater adenocarcinoma: a single institutional experience. *Journal of Gastrointestinal Oncology* 2014;5(6):421–7.

124. Alamo JM, Marin LM, Suarez G, Bernal C, Serrano J, Barrera L, et al. Improving outcomes in pancreatic cancer: key points in perioperative management. *World Journal of Gastroenterology* 2014;20(39):14237–45.

125. Christians KK, Evans DB. Additional support for neoadjuvant therapy in the management of pancreatic cancer. *Annals of Surgical Oncology* 2015;22(6):1755–8.

126. Delpero JR, Boher JM, Sauvanet A, Le Treut YP, Sa-Cunha A, Mabrut JY, et al. Pancreatic adenocarcinoma with venous involvement: is up-front synchronous portal-superior mesenteric vein resection still justified? A survey of the Association Francaise de Chirurgie. *Annals of Surgical Oncology* 2015;22(6):1874–83.

127. Barbier L, Turrini O, Gregoire E, Viret F, Le Treut YP, Delpero JR. Pancreatic head resectable adenocarcinoma: preoperative chemoradiation improves local control but does not affect survival. *HPB* 2011;13(1):64–9.

128. Laurence JM, Tran PD, Morarji K, Eslick GD, Lam VW, Sandroussi C. A systematic review and meta-analysis of survival and surgical outcomes following neoadjuvant chemoradiotherapy for pancreatic cancer. *Journal of Gastrointestinal Surgery* 2011;15(11):2059–69.

129. Festa V, Andriulli A, Valvano MR, Uomo G, Perri F, Andriulli N, et al. Neoadjuvant chemo-radiotherapy for patients with borderline resectable pancreatic cancer: a meta-analytical evaluation of prospective studies. *JOP: Journal of the Pancreas* 2013;14(6):618–25.

130. Golcher H, Brunner TB, Witzigmann H, Marti L, Bechstein W, Bruns C, et al. Neoadjuvant chemoradiation therapy with gemcitabine/cisplatin and surgery versus immediate surgery in resectable pancreatic cancer: results of the first prospective randomized phase II trial. *Strahlentherapie und Onkologie* 2015;191(1):7–16.

131. Moss AC, Morris E, Mac Mathuna P. Palliative biliary stents for obstructing pancreatic carcinoma. *Cochrane Database of Systematic Reviews* 2006;2:CD004200.

132. Ueda J, Kayashima T, Mori Y, Ohtsuka T, Takahata S, Nakamura M, et al. Hepaticocholecystojejunostomy as effective palliative biliary bypass for unresectable pancreatic cancer. *Hepato-gastroenterology* 2014;61(129):197–202.

133. Kahaleh M, Talreja JP, Loren DE, Kowalski TE, Poneros JM, Degaetani M, et al. Evaluation of a fully covered self-expanding metal stent with flared ends in malignant biliary obstruction: a multicenter study. *Journal of Clinical Gastroenterology* 2013;47(10):e96–100.

134. Petersen BT, Kahaleh M, Kozarek RA, Loren D, Gupta K, Kowalski T, et al. A multicenter, prospective study of a new fully covered expandable metal biliary stent for the palliative treatment of malignant bile duct obstruction. *Gastroenterology Research and Practice* 2013;2013:642428.

135. Saleem A, Leggett CL, Murad MH, Baron TH. Meta-analysis of randomized trials comparing the patency of covered and uncovered self-expandable metal stents for palliation of distal malignant bile duct obstruction. *Gastrointestinal Endoscopy* 2011;74(2):321–7, e1–3.

136. Maire F, Sauvanet A. Palliation of biliary and duodenal obstruction in patients with unresectable pancreatic cancer: endoscopy or surgery? *Journal of Visceral Surgery* 2013;150(3 Suppl.):S27–31.

137. Ly J, O'Grady G, Mittal A, Plank L, Windsor JA. A systematic review of methods to palliate malignant gastric outlet obstruction. *Surgical Endoscopy* 2010;24(2):290–7.

138. Siddiqui A, Spechler SJ, Huerta S. Surgical bypass versus endoscopic stenting for malignant gastroduodenal obstruction: a decision analysis. *Digestive Diseases and Sciences* 2007;52(1):276–81.

139. Bartlett EK, Wachtel H, Fraker DL, Vollmer CM, Drebin JA, Kelz RR, et al. Surgical palliation for pancreatic malignancy: practice patterns and predictors of morbidity and mortality. *Journal of Gastrointestinal Surgery* 2014;18(7):1292–8.

140. Morak MJ, Richel DJ, van Eijck CH, Nuyttens JJ, van der Gaast A, Vervenne WL, et al. Phase II trial of uracil/tegafur plus leucovorin and celecoxib combined with radiotherapy in locally advanced pancreatic cancer. *Radiotherapy and Oncology* 2011;98(2):261–4.

141. Sultana A, Tudur Smith C, Cunningham D, Starling N, Tait D, Neoptolemos JP, et al. Systematic review, including meta-analyses, on the management of locally advanced pancreatic cancer using radiation/combined modality therapy. *British Journal of Cancer* 2007;96(8):1183–90.

142. Faris JE, Wo JY. The controversial role of chemoradiation for patients with locally advanced pancreatic cancer. *Oncologist* 2013;18(9):981–5.

143. Cunningham D, Chau I, Stocken DD, Valle JW, Smith D, Steward W, et al. Phase III randomized comparison of gemcitabine versus gemcitabine plus capecitabine in patients with advanced pancreatic cancer. *Journal of Clinical Oncology* 2009;27(33):5513–8.

144. Petrioli R, Roviello G, Fiaschi AI, Laera L, Marrelli D, Roviello F, et al. Gemcitabine, oxaliplatin, and capecitabine (GEMOXEL) compared with gemcitabine alone in metastatic pancreatic cancer: a randomized phase II study. *Cancer Chemotherapy and Pharmacology* 2015;75(4):683–90.

145. Li Y, Sun J, Jiang Z, Zhang L, Liu G. Gemcitabine and S-1 combination chemotherapy versus gemcitabine alone for locally advanced and metastatic pancreatic cancer: a meta-analysis of randomized controlled trials in Asia. *Journal of Chemotherapy* 2015;27(4):227–34.

146. Gresham GK, Wells GA, Gill S, Cameron C, Jonker DJ. Chemotherapy regimens for advanced pancreatic cancer: a systematic review and network meta-analysis. *BMC Cancer* 2014;14:471.

147. Al-Hajeili M, Azmi AS, Choi M. Nab-paclitaxel: potential for the treatment of advanced pancreatic cancer. *OncoTargets and Therapy* 2014;7:187–92.

148. Conroy T, Desseigne F, Ychou M, Bouche O, Guimbaud R, Becouarn Y, et al. FOLFIRINOX versus gemcitabine for metastatic pancreatic cancer. *New England Journal of Medicine* 2011;364(19):1817–25.

149. Faris JE, Blaszkowsky LS, McDermott S, Guimaraes AR, Szymonifka J, Huynh MA, et al. FOLFIRINOX in locally advanced pancreatic cancer: the Massachusetts General Hospital Cancer Center experience. *Oncologist* 2013;18(5):543–8.

150. Von Hoff DD, Ervin T, Arena FP, Chiorean EG, Infante J, Moore M, et al. Increased survival in pancreatic cancer with nab-paclitaxel plus gemcitabine. *New England Journal of Medicine* 2013;369(18):1691–703.

151. Goldstein D, El-Maraghi RH, Hammel P, Heinemann V, Kunzmann V, Sastre J, et al. Nab-paclitaxel plus gemcitabine for metastatic pancreatic cancer: long-term survival from a phase III trial. *Journal of the National Cancer Institute* 2015;107(2).

152. Brower V. New approaches tackle rising pancreatic cancer rates. *Journal of the National Cancer Institute* 2014;106(12).

153. Aad G, Abajyan T, Abbott B, Abdallah J, Abdel Khalek S, Abdelalim AA, et al. Search for magnetic monopoles in sqrt[s]=7 TeV pp collisions with the ATLAS detector. *Physical Review Letters* 2012;109(26):261803.

32

Hepatocellular carcinoma

ROBERT P JONES, DANIEL H PALMER AND HASSAN Z MALIK

INCIDENCE AND AETIOLOGY

Liver cancer is the third most common cause of cancer death worldwide, with more than 745,000 deaths annually [1]. Hepatocellular carcinoma (HCC) comprises the overwhelming majority of primary liver cancers, with a steadily rising global burden [2]. There is wide variation in the geographic incidence of HCC, with >80% of cases occurring in Asia and sub-Saharan Africa with an incidence of 99 per 100,000. By contrast, incidence in Europe is considerably lower (approximately 5 per 100,000) [3]. In most populations, the incidence is higher in males than in females, with the greatest variation between genders seen in low-risk populations of Europe [4]. These wide variations in distribution reflect the varying incidence of aetiologic factors known to be integral to the development of hepatocellular carcinogenesis.

RISK FACTORS FOR HCC

Hepatitis B

Chronic hepatitis B virus (HBV) infection accounts for >50% of cases of HCC worldwide. HBV DNA has been shown to integrate into the genome of hepatocytes prior to the development of HCC and is thought to lead to a chromosomal instability subtype, promoting tumourigenesis [5].

HBV as a risk factor for HCC is supported by strong evidence that HBV vaccination programs have led to falls in the incidence of HCC in high-risk areas [6].

Hepatitis C

Hepatitis C virus (HCV) increases HCC by promoting end-stage liver disease, with the risk of HCC 17 times higher among patients with HCV than those without [7]. The exact mechanism by which HCC promotes carcinogenesis remains unclear, but the overwhelming majority of HCV positive patients with HCC have cirrhosis. It has been suggested that oxidative stress triggered by HCV infection leads to focal necrosis and compensatory cell division and turnover [8]. This necrosis can lead to the recruitment of Kupffer cells and hepatic stellate cells, leading to the accumulation of extracellular matrix protein and progression to cirrhosis, where high cellular turnover leads to HCC.

Alcohol

Numerous studies have implicated alcohol in the development of HCC, with clear evidence that lifetime alcohol exposure correlates with the incidence of HCC [9]. Hepatic metabolism of alcohol is thought to lead to the production of free radicals, causing intracellular oxidative stress eventually leading to a chronic inflammatory state [10].

Metabolic conditions

Because of the critical role of the liver in glucose metabolism, it is not surprising that obesity and diabetes mellitus (both of which involve impaired glucose handling) are significant independent risk factors for the development of HCC [11]. The global rise in obesity and diabetes is likely to lead to a significant increase in HCC developing on a background of hepatic non-alcoholic fatty liver disease (NAFLD) [12]. These patients often develop hepatic steatosis, with cellular adaptions to this environment increasing hepatocyte vulnerability to a 'second hit' [13]. Despite differences in underlying aetiology and pathogenesis, HCC developing in NAFLD is thought to behave in a fashion similar to that of HCC in HBV and HCV patients [14].

Other causes

Haemochromatosis is an autosomal recessive genetic disorder of iron metabolism that causes deposition of iron within the liver, leading to hepatic injury and hepatocarcinogenesis [15]. Aflatoxins are toxic fungal metabolites produced by *Aspergillus flavus* and *Aspergillus parasiticus*. These metabolites are converted to potent hepatotoxins by the cytochrome p450 system within the liver [16], with a clear correlation between aflatoxin-contaminated diets and HCC development [17].

Cohort studies have suggested that 60% of patients with HCC die of cancer-related causes, with the remaining 40% succumbing to their underlying parenchymal liver disease [18]. It is therefore critical that treatments for patients with HCC are considered in the context of both the cancer and the underlying parenchymal disease.

PATHOLOGY AND STAGING OF HEPATOCELLULAR CARCINOMA

Staging systems aim to stratify patients into groups with similar prognoses, and for HCC, they can be divided into clinical and pathological staging systems. Clinical staging systems are often designed to guide choice of therapy, the most commonly used being the Barcelona Clinic Liver Cancer (BCLC) Group staging system. Pathological staging systems are used after resection or transplantation and guide prognosis, the most commonly used being the American Joint Committee on Cancer–International Union Against Cancer (AJCC/UICC) system.

Barcelona Clinic Liver Cancer staging system

The BCLC system was initially designed to define both prognosis and optimal treatment for patients with HCC. As patients with HCC usually have underlying liver disease, the BCLC system was designed to reflect underlying liver function and patient performance status, as well as characteristics of the tumour (Figure 32.1) [27]. Underlying liver function is assessed using the Child–Pugh system

(Table 32.1) [28]. The score employs five clinical measures of parenchymal liver disease, with each measure scored between 1 and 3. A summative score is then used to categorize patients as Child A, B or C.

The BCLC system focuses on prognosis for patients with early disease who are most likely to benefit from aggressive therapy and has been demonstrated as an accurate predictor of long-term outcome [29]. However, the BCLC system has also been criticized as being too conservative with respect to surgical resection.

AJCC/UICC staging system

The AJCC/UICC staging system [32] is based on a retrospective central histology review of 557 surgically resected patients performed by the International Cooperative Study Group on Hepatocellular Carcinoma [33]. The group correlated histopathological findings with long-term outcome and identified tumour multimodality, size (only for multifocal disease) and the presence or absence of micro- or macrovascular invasion as prognostically important information. Consistent with historical studies [34], vascular invasion was identified as the most powerful histopathological prognostic indicator. The updated seventh edition of the AJCC/UICC staging manual reflects the importance of macroscopic vascular invasion by including a subdivision based on major vessel involvement to reflect the markedly varying prognosis for these patients (Table 32.2). Although the system was developed using a cohort of resected patients who had hepatitis C–related HCC, it has also been validated in patients with hepatitis B [35] and performed well in patients who have undergone liver transplantation as opposed to surgical resection [36]. However, its applicability to non-surgically treated patients remains unclear [37].

SURVEILLANCE FOR HCC IN HIGH-RISK POPULATIONS

As patients with underlying hepatic disease are known to be at significantly higher risk of developing HCC, surveillance programs to detect early lesions have been proposed. Although the evidence surrounding surveillance of high-risk groups remains limited [19], both US and European guidelines recommend surveillance for these patients. The British Society for Gastroenterology (BSG) [20], European Association for Study of the Liver (EASL) [21] and American Association for the Study of Liver Diseases (AASLD) [22] recommend routine ultrasound scanning in combination with serum α-fetoprotein (AFP) measurements in high-risk patients in an effort to detect earlier and therefore less advanced lesions, where more effective treatment can be offered. There is currently no clear evidence to identify an optimal surveillance interval. Tumour modelling has suggested it takes at least 5 months for even the fastest-growing HCC to reach a diameter of 3 cm [18]. Because treatments for HCC are markedly more effective for lesions <3 cm, an

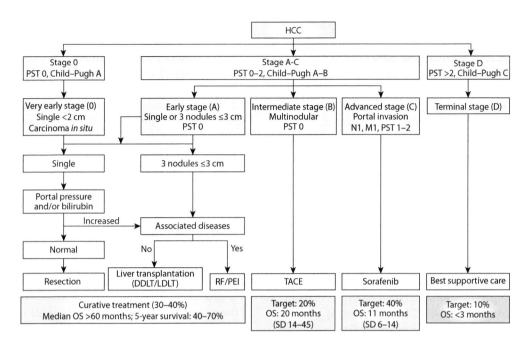

Figure 32.1 BCLC staging system. Patients with asymptomatic early tumours (stage 0–A) are candidates for curative therapies (resection, transplantation or local ablation). Asymptomatic patients with multinodular HCC (stage B) are suitable for transarterial chemoembolization (TACE), whereas patients with advanced symptomatic tumours or an invasive tumoural pattern (stage C), or both, are candidates for sorafenib. End-stage disease (stage D) includes patients with a very poor prognosis who should be treated by best supportive care. DDLT, deceased donor liver transplantation; LDLT, living donor liver transplantation; PEI, percutaneous ethanol injection; RF, radiofrequency ablation; OS, overall survival; PST, ECOG performance status. (Reproduced from Villanueva A, et al., *Nat Rev Gastroenterol Hepatol* 2013;10(1):34–42. With permission.)

Table 32.1 Child–Pugh classification

Measure	1 point	2 points	3 points
Bilirubin (μmol/L)	<34	34–50	>50
Albumin (g/dl)	>3.5	2.8–3.5	<2.8
INR[a]	<1.7	1.7–2.3	>2.3
Presence of ascites	None	Mild	Moderate/severe
Hepatic encephalopathy	None	Grade I–II	Grade III+

Note: The summative point score gives a Child–Pugh classification of A (5–6 points), B (7–9 points) or C (>10 points).

[a] International normalised ratio

Table 32.2 AJCC/UICC HCC staging system

AJCC stage	T classification	Description
Stage I	T1	Solitary tumour, no vascular invasion
Stage II	T2	Solitary tumour with vascular invasion *or* multifocal tumour ≤5 cm
Stage IIIA	T3a	Multiple tumours >5 cm
Stage IIIB	T3b	Single or multiple tumours of any size involving a major branch of the portal or hepatic vein
Stage IIIC	T4	Invasion of adjacent organs *or* perforation of visceral peritoneum
Stage IVA	Any stage with nodal disease	
Stage IVB	Any stage with distant metastases	

Source: With kind permission from Springer Science+Business Media: *AJCC Cancer Staging Manual*, 7th ed, 2010, 103–15, Edge SB, Byrd DR, Compton CC.

interval of 6 months is therefore commonly adopted. The endemic patient cohort often limits the effectiveness of surveillance programs, with around 50% of patients with alcoholic cirrhosis dropping out of surveillance follow-up within 5 years [18].

Serum AFP is commonly increased in patients with HCC, and serum levels >400 ng/ml are considered almost definitively diagnostic. However, AFP is limited as a tumour marker as levels may rise in active hepatitis without any evidence of HCC. In addition, small tumours (the detection of which is the primary objective of surveillance) may not produce sufficient AFP to allow the diagnosis. These inherent limitations are reflected in the widely varying sensitivity (39–65%) and specificity (76–94%) of AFP in detecting HCC [23].

Ultrasound scanning remains the most commonly used modality for identifying potential HCCs, and despite limitations in identifying lesions in nodular cirrhotic livers (with a reported sensitivity of 35–84% [24]), it remains appealing because of its low cost and lack of ionizing radiation.

Despite global recommendations supporting surveillance, empirical evidence is lacking. A large randomized controlled trial (RCT) comparing 6-monthly ultrasonography and serum AFP measurements with no surveillance demonstrated a significant survival advantage to surveillance (survival of screened participants was 66% vs. 31% at 1 year, 53% vs. 7% at 3 years, and 46% vs. 0% at 5 years) despite suboptimal adherence to the surveillance protocol (<60% of scheduled events were completed) [19].

Although the overwhelming majority of HCCs are detected during routine surveillance, emergency presentation because of spontaneous rupture may occur in up to 15% of patients [25]. Transarterial embolization remains the best method for haemostatic control. In patients with good underlying liver function, rupture should not be considered a contraindication to curative intent surgical resection [26].

Diagnosis and preoperative imaging for HCC

Imaging is a critical part of the pre-treatment assessment of HCC. Accurate tumour staging and anatomical assessment are essential to determine both technical and oncological resectability, as well as to exclude distant metastatic spread. Triple-phase CT of the chest, abdomen and pelvis and MRI of the liver are considered standard of care in most units. However, both MRI and CT have limited sensitivity and specificity for detection of lesions <1 cm, although this has improved with the use of liver-specific contrast agents [50]. There is also growing interest in the assessment of background liver fibrosis and cirrhosis with functional imaging techniques that use hepato-specific contrast medium [51]. The use of fluorodeoxyglucose–positron emission tomography (FDG-PET) to exclude extrahepatic involvement has been investigated, but it remains unclear whether this offers any benefit over standard CT of the chest, abdomen and pelvis [52].

SURGICAL RESECTION FOR HCC

Only 20–40% of patients with HCC are considered candidates for surgical resection [38]. However, with improved imaging and better perioperative management, surgical resection is increasingly considered the mainstay of treatment for patients with preserved hepatic function.

There remains considerable controversy over which patients should be considered surgical candidates. Although tumour size, vascular invasion and multifocal disease are recognized as poor prognostic indicators, none should be considered absolute contraindications to surgical intervention. For example, increasing tumour size is associated with increasing risk of microvascular invasion. However, a large tumour without microvascular invasion carries a prognosis similar to that of a small tumour with microvascular invasion [30].

Unlike microvascular invasion, macrovascular invasion of the major branches of the hepatic veins or the first- and second-order branches of the portal vein can be detected on preoperative imaging. Although technically difficult, surgical resection may be justified in selected patients; a series of 102 patients with macrovascular involvement of the hepatic or portal veins undergoing resection had a 5-year survival rate of 23%, with a median survival superior to that of non-surgically treated patients with comparable disease [39].

Multinodular lesions also present another management challenge. These may represent multiple discrete lesions occurring independently against a background of pro-carcinogenic parenchymal damage or may represent aggressive tumour biology with intrahepatic metastases. The BCLC system suggests that patients with >3 nodules or 2–3 nodules with one >3 cm should not be resected. However, recent reports have suggested 5-year survival of 39% in patients with this pattern of disease undergoing resection [40].

The BCLC staging system also suggests that resection should only be offered to patients with single lesions or three lesions <3 cm with good synthetic liver function, but this has been criticized as unduly cautious. A more pragmatic approach has been suggested by Zorzi et al., who defined the MD Anderson criteria for resection in chronic liver disease (Table 32.3) [41].

In general, oncological contraindications to resection are now taken to include (1) extrahepatic metastasis, (2) multiple and bilobar tumours, (3) involvement of the main bile duct and (4) presence of portal thrombus in the main portal vein or vena cava [42]. However, reasonable long-term outcomes from highly selected patients outside these contraindications have also been reported.

Preoperative evaluation of patients with HCC

Ensuring a good outcome for patients undergoing surgical resection for HCC relies on an accurate assessment of tumour stage, patient fitness and underlying liver function. This is particularly important when considering patients for

Table 32.3 MD Anderson Cancer Centre criteria for resection in patients with chronic liver disease

	Criteria
Minor resection	Child–Pugh A
	Bilirubin <110 µmol l^{-1}
	Absence of ascites
	Platelets >100 10^9 L^{-1}
Major resection	Criteria for minor resection plus
	Bilirubin <55 µmol L^{-1}
	Absence of portal hypertension
	Portal vein embolization for future liver remnant <40%

Source: Adapted from Zorzi D, et al., in *Hepatocellular Carcinoma*, New York: Springer, 2011, pp. 109–34.

larger resections, where the function of the future liver remnant (FLR) becomes critical.

ASSESSMENT OF UNDERLYING LIVER FUNCTION

Postoperative morbidity and mortality is known to increase with higher Child–Pugh score, and major liver resection is generally only considered feasible in patients with Child–Pugh A disease. Minor liver resection may be considered in Child–Pugh B, but remains a high-risk procedure. Child–Pugh classification has been criticized for underestimating surgical risk, as portal hypertension is not directly assessed as part of the scoring system. A clear correlation between portal hypertension and acute postoperative hepatic decompensation has been identified [43]. Portal hypertension can be assessed either by direct intravenous measurement or by radiological assessment of signs of hypertension (including splenomegaly and gastro-oesophageal varices). Some units also advocate the use of indocyanine green (ICG) clearance to directly assess liver function in higher-risk patients [44].

ASSESSMENT OF FUTURE LIVER REMNANT

Although Child–Pugh classification and ICG clearance assess overall liver function, they fail to provide specific information regarding the function of the liver parenchyma that will remain after resection (the FLR). There is a strong relationship between remnant liver volume and post-resection hepatic failure [45], and for patients considered for major hepatic resection assessment of volume of parenchyma left *in situ* as well as the underlying synthetic function is crucial. For patients with normal liver function, an FLR of 20% of total liver volume (TLV) is generally required, whereas 40% FLR may be necessary in patients with impaired hepatocyte function [46]. For some patients, inadequate FLR may be the only contraindication to surgical resection. For this group, preoperative radiological portal vein embolization (PVE) can be performed to induce hypertrophy in the proposed remnant liver increasing the FLR [47]. FLR hypertrophy after embolization is also a surrogate marker of underlying hepatic function, as well as a predictor of reduced perioperative morbidity, hepatic

decompensation and length of hospital stay [48]. Combination of TACE with lipiodol and an active chemotherapeutic agent followed by PVE is now recommended in patients with chronic liver disease being considered for major resection because of the increased hypertrophy and higher tumour responses than with PVE alone [49].

Surgical principles

The objectives of surgical resection for HCC can appear contradictory: (1) resection of all malignant and as much preoplastic tissue as possible, while (2) preserving enough functional hepatic parenchyma to reduce the risk of postoperative liver failure. HCC spreads within the liver by direct invasion of both the portal and hepatic venous system, and anatomical resection that includes removal of the entire venous drainage of an HCC is considered the optimal approach to increase the removal of occult micrometastases. There is a clear long-term survival advantage to anatomical versus non-anatomical resection [53,54], and this approach is now considered standard of care where underlying liver function allows. However, where a non-anatomical resection is considered (because of impaired hepatic function), resections with wide margins (1–2 cm) are associated with improved long-term survival [55,56]. Intraoperative blood loss remains the single strongest predictor of postoperative mortality, and low CVP anaesthesia is an essential technique to minimize bleeding during parenchymal transection [57]. Other techniques to minimize intraoperative blood loss include intermittent vascular exclusion (Pringle's manoeuver) or total vascular exclusion. Caution must be exercised in patients with borderline hepatic function who may not tolerate prolonged ischaemia well. However, intermittent occlusion with 15 minutes of clamping and 5 minutes of perfusion appears well tolerated, even in patients with cirrhosis [58]. In addition, an anterior surgical approach with reduced retraction and mobilization of the liver may also improve hepatic perfusion [59]. Although reports are limited, laparoscopic resection appears technically feasible with no impact on oncologic outcomes [60,61], with some groups suggesting lower postoperative morbidity and mortality [62].

These improvements in surgical technique have led to a reduction in mortality, with 30-day postoperative death consistently quoted as <5%, including patients with underlying cirrhosis [42].

Impact of disease features on long-term outcome after resection

Patients with solitary lesions without any evidence of micro- or macrovascular invasion (T1 disease) have a similar survival (approximately 55% at 5 years) irrespective of lesion size (Table 32.2; Figure 32.2). Patients with multiple lesions, none >5 cm, or patients with a solitary lesion with microvascular invasion were found to have a similar prognosis and are considered to have T2 disease, with a 5-year post-resection survival rate of 35%. Patients with multiple lesions, any of which is >5 cm, and those with major vascular invasion are considered to be T3, with a 5-year survival of 15% among those coming to resection [33].

Tumour size remains an important predictor of microvascular invasion, but it is important to recognize that large tumours without microvascular invasion carry a long-term outlook similar to that of small lesions with microvascular invasion. As microvascular invasion remains a histopathological diagnosis, resection remains the treatment of choice for these patients.

Disease recurrence after resection

Intrahepatic recurrence occurs in around 80% of cases within 5 years of resection [63–65]. There are no effective neoadjuvant or adjuvant treatment options to reduce risk of recurrence after resection. The STORM randomized controlled study assessed the impact of adjuvant sorafenib after curative surgical resection or ablation. Patients were treated with 400 mg sorafenib (n = 556) or placebo (n = 558), but no improvement in recurrence-free survival was demonstrated [66]. Interferon therapy has shown some promise in reducing recurrence, but is not currently used in routine clinical practice [67].

A recent randomized controlled study also suggested that antiviral therapies after resection might also reduce recurrence and improve overall survival. Huang et al. [68] randomized patients undergoing resection for HBV-related HCC to placebo or antiviral therapy (adefovir). The 1-, 3- and 5-year recurrence-free survival rates for the antiviral group and the control group were 84.0% vs. 85.0%, 37.9% vs. 50.3% and 27.1% vs. 46.1%, respectively. The corresponding overall survival rates for the two groups were 94.0% vs. 96.0%, 67.4% vs. 77.6% and 41.5% vs. 63.1%.

Intrahepatic recurrence after surgery is thought to consist of two discrete groups: patients who had missed micrometastases at initial staging and those who developed *de novo* lesions in diseased background liver [69]. The most effective approach to reducing intrahepatic recurrence of HCC is to remove both of these possibilities by performing liver transplantation.

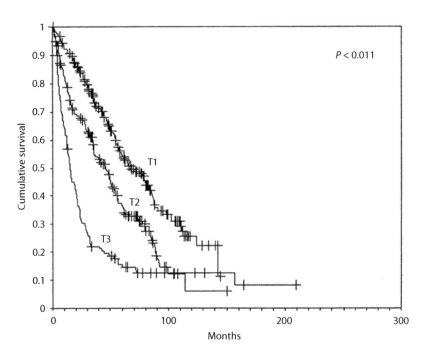

Figure 32.2 Survival of patients with resected HCC according to AJCC/UICC T stage. (Adapted from Vauthey JN, et al., *J Clin Oncol* 2002;20(6):1527–36.)

LIVER TRANSPLANTATION

Liver transplantation for HCC offers the advantage of not only definitively treating the tumour but also removing the diseased hepatic parenchyma, so reducing the potential for intrahepatic recurrence. The concept of organ transplantation for primary liver cancer was first described by Mazzaferro et al. in 1996 [70], who performed liver transplantation for patients with one hepatocellular carcinoma of ≤5 cm, or up to three nodules of ≤3 cm, and reported a 4-year overall survival of 75% and recurrence-free survival of 83%. Other groups have since replicated these results, and these inclusion criteria (Milan criteria) are now considered the benchmark indications for transplantation for HCC [21,71–73]. Patients outside these criteria can also be successfully downstaged using locoregional therapies (such as ablation), and following a period of observation with adequate disease control may be considered suitable candidates for transplantation [74].

A global shortage of organ donors inevitably leads to delays in transplantation, during which disease progression can occur. In some cases, disease can progress beyond transplantation criteria, with patients subsequently losing their opportunity for curative therapy [75]. Tumour progression has been reported in 15–33% of patients on waiting lists. This progression and dropout from the waiting list has a significant impact on the outcomes of transplantation for HCC when considered on an intention-to-treat basis: 2-year survival rate is 84% for patients with 62 days of waiting time, compared to 54% for patients with 162 days of waiting time [76]. In order to reduce the dropout rate because of disease progression, bridging therapies have been proposed. In addition to reducing dropout, treatment prior to resection may also improve disease-free survival (DFS) after transplantation [77,78]. Commonly utilized bridging therapies include radiofrequency ablation (RFA), TACE and liver resection. TACE and RFA are favoured because of their low morbidity and mortality [79,80]. Resection has also been proposed and may be justified where it delays or avoids the need for transplantation [74].

Despite the shortage of liver donors, several researchers have proposed expansion of current criteria for transplantation and have generated promising results, with the San Francisco group reporting that patients undergoing transplant for solitary tumours ≤6.5 cm, or ≤3 nodules with the largest lesion ≤4.5 cm and total tumour diameter ≤8 cm, had survival rates of 90% and 75.2% at 1 and 5 years [81]. However, it is clear that expanding criteria for transplantation does come at the cost of increased rates of recurrence. The balance between appropriately allocating scarce grafts to patients with the best long-term prognosis while maximizing the opportunity for cure for patients with limited other options remains a contentious topic.

Whether liver resection or liver transplantation is the optimal initial treatment for patients with good liver function and a tumour within the Milan criteria also remains

controversial [82,83]. Nathan and colleagues [84] performed a web-based assessment of choice of therapy (resection vs. transplantation vs. ablation) for early HCC by hepatobiliary surgeons and perhaps unsurprisingly found that surgical specialty (transplant hepatobiliary surgeons vs. non-transplant hepatobiliary surgeons) had a significant impact on management approach.

In view of the discrepancy between organ supply and demand, and the problems associated with liver transplantation, such as graft rejection, recurrent viral hepatitis, immunosuppression-related opportunistic infections and long-term medical complications, the potential value of liver resection followed by 'salvage' transplantation for tumour recurrence or deterioration of the hepatic function has also been proposed.

ABLATIVE THERAPIES FOR HCC

Ablation involves the introduction of heat energy to a tumour leading to cellular destruction. Radiofrequency ablation involves the application of high-frequency AC current (300–1000 kHz), causing tissue friction, heat generation and coagulation necrosis. The size of the ablation zone produced by existing RFA generators is 3–5 cm. Because of the potential for microvascular invasion and undetectable microsatellite nodules, an ablation margin of 0.5–1 cm is also recommended [85].

Although the size of the ablation zone produced by RFA can reach 5 cm, better outcomes are reported after ablation of small lesions [86]. Whether this is as a result of the less aggressive biology seen in smaller lesions or the destruction of surrounding tissue remains unclear. Indeed, the 2012 BCLC guideline update recommends RFA as first-line treatment for lesions <2 cm where transplantation is not considered an option [67]. Ablation for lesions >2 cm should be considered on a case-by-case basis. Most units adopt the Milan criteria (single HCC <5 cm, or <3 lesions all <3 cm) as inclusion criteria for RFA [87]. However, other factors such as operator's technical skill and general patient comorbidity should also be considered. For patients with borderline hepatic function, patients should also be able to tolerate the loss of hepatic parenchyma caused by the ablation.

Reports of local tumour progression after RFA vary. For lesions <5 cm, recurrence rates have been reported as 4.8–8.1%, 4.8–14.5% and 11.8–14.5% at 1-, 3- and 5-year follow-up, respectively (88,89). However, the wide heterogeneity in reporting makes accurate interpretation difficult. As previously described, anatomical resection is superior to non-anatomical resection in terms of reducing recurrence. It is therefore unsurprising that distant recurrence occurs more frequently after RFA than resection [87].

As a result of the excellent outcomes associated with RFA in small lesions, it has been suggested that RFA should replace resection as first-line treatment for small lesions. Meta-analysis of non-randomized retrospective studies has suggested better long-term outcome after resection [90], but only three prospective RCTs have been reported. Chen and colleagues [91] and Feng and colleagues [92] reported no difference in overall or DFS. By contrast, Huang et al. [93] reported significantly improved overall and DFS after resection, although loss to follow-up was much higher in the surgical resection group.

TRANSARTERIAL EMBOLIZATION AND CHEMOEMBOLIZATION

HCC is a vascular tumour, with the majority of its blood supply derived from the hepatic artery. Selective administration of intra-arterial agents is therefore a logical approach for treatment. Introduction of embolic agents can lead to the obstruction of blood vessels causing ischaemic tumour necrosis (transarterial embolization [TAE]), while combination with chemotherapy can also deliver high levels of local therapy by targeting supplying vessels and reducing tumour washout (TACE). A high-quality meta-analysis comparing TAE or TACE with best supportive care demonstrated a significant improvement in 2-year survival after TAE or TACE, ranging from 20% to 60% [94].

European guidelines now recommend TACE for patients with intermediate stage HCC (according to the BCLC classification) as standard of care (see Figure 32.1) [95]. However, this group comprises a wide spectrum in terms of liver function and tumour burden. Widely varying outcomes have been reported after TACE, with low albumin, high bilirubin or AFP and large tumour size now all recognized as predictors of long-term outcome after treatment (96). Radioembolization with yttrium-90 (Yt^{90})–labelled spheres has also shown potential in early clinical studies, with patients being downstaged or bridged with the intention of transplant [97].

SYSTEMIC CHEMOTHERAPY

Sorafenib is an oral multikinase inhibitor that blocks Raf signaling, vascular endothelial growth factor (VEGF), platelet-derived growth factor (PDGF) and c-Kit. It is both antiproliferative and antiangiogenic and remains the only agent to demonstrate proven survival benefit in advanced HCC. In a large phase 3 RCT, 602 patients with advanced HCC were treated with sorafenib or placebo. Median overall survival in the sorafenib group was 10.7 months (95% CI 9.4–13.3) vs. 7.9 months (95% CI 6.8–9.1) in the placebo group (hazard ratio 0.69, 95% CI 0.55–0.87; $p = 0.0001$) [98]. A similar benefit was demonstrated in a sister trial performed in an Asian population [99]. However, radiological response rate (by RECIST criteria) was less than 2%, suggesting that although sorafenib may improve overall survival, it is likely to have limited benefit in a neoadjuvant setting, where the goal may be to reduce tumour burden and convert patients to resectability. These results have established sorafenib as the standard of care for advanced hepatocellular carcinoma.

CONCLUSIONS

HCC remains a global health issue. Although the burden of hepatitis will decrease as a result of increasingly effective treatments, this will be counterbalanced by a rise in obesity and diabetes leading to an increase in NAFLD. Effective surveillance programs in these high-risk groups will hopefully increase the early detection of lesions, which can be more effectively treated. Liver transplantation is a highly effective therapy for early disease and offers the advantage of removing the protocarcinogenic diseased liver, reducing postoperative recurrence. However, transplantation is limited by donor shortage. Surgery remains the optimal therapy for patients with technically resectable disease and adequate underlying liver function and is no longer only offered for very early stage disease. For patients unsuitable for surgery, ablation offers an acceptable treatment option with good long-term results – especially for small lesions.

Although a number of important prognostic factors after surgical resection have been identified, traditional contraindications (such as large size or number of lesions) are increasingly being challenged by impressive long-term outcomes seen in these higher-risk groups. As the boundaries of surgical resection are pushed, optimal preoperative staging and assessment are critical to guide appropriate therapy. In addition, specialist perioperative care is essential to optimize outcome. For example, PVE may provide a quantitative assessment of actual hepatic regenerative capacity as well as increasing the safety of subsequent surgery.

Improved survival with HCC is likely to come from not only improved treatments but also earlier diagnosis and increasingly accurate staging and risk stratification. The multidisciplinary approach to HCC highlights the critical importance of managing these patients in an effective specialist multidisciplinary team.

REFERENCES

1. Ferlay J, Soerjomataram I, Dikshit R, Eser S, Mathers C, Rebelo M, et al. Cancer incidence and mortality worldwide: sources, methods and major patterns in GLOBOCAN 2012. *Int J Cancer* 2015;136(5):E359–86.
2. Altekruse SF, McGlynn KA, Reichman ME. Hepatocellular carcinoma incidence, mortality, and survival trends in the United States from 1975 to 2005. *J Clin Oncol* 2009;27(9):1485–91.
3. McGlynn KA, London WT. Epidemiology and natural history of hepatocellular carcinoma. *Best Pract Res Clin Gastroenterol* 2005;19(1):3–23.
4. El-Serag HB, Rudolph KL. Hepatocellular carcinoma: epidemiology and molecular carcinogenesis. *Gastroenterology* 2007;132(7):2557–76.
5. Brechot C, Pourcel C, Louise A, Rain B, Tiollais P. Presence of integrated hepatitis B virus DNA sequences in cellular DNA of human hepatocellular carcinoma. *Nature* 1980;286(5772):533–5.

6. Romanò L, Paladini S, Van Damme P, Zanetti AR. The worldwide impact of vaccination on the control and protection of viral hepatitis B. *Dig Liver Dis* 2011;43(Suppl. 1):S2–7.

7. Donato F, Boffetta P, Puoti M. A meta-analysis of epidemiological studies on the combined effect of hepatitis B and C virus infections in causing hepatocellular carcinoma. *Int J Cancer* 1998;75(3):347–54.

8. Cerutti PA. Oxy-radicals and cancer. *Lancet* 1994;344(8926):862–3.

9. Donato F, Tagger A, Gelatti U, Parrinello G, Boffetta P, Albertini A, et al. Alcohol and hepatocellular carcinoma: the effect of lifetime intake and hepatitis virus infections in men and women. *Am J Epidemiol* 2002;155(4):323–31.

10. Stewart S, Jones D, Day CP. Alcoholic liver disease: new insights into mechanisms and preventative strategies. *Trends Mol Med* 2001;7(9):408–13.

11. El-Serag HB, Hampel H, Javadi F. The association between diabetes and hepatocellular carcinoma: a systematic review of epidemiologic evidence. *Clin Gastroenterol Hepatol* 2006;4(3):369–80.

12. Jiang CM, Pu CW, Hou YH, Chen Z, Alanazy M, Hebbard L. Non alcoholic steatohepatitis a precursor for hepatocellular carcinoma development. *World J Gastroenterol* 2014;20(44):16464–73.

13. Browning JD, Horton JD. Molecular mediators of hepatic steatosis and liver injury. *J Clin Invest* 2004;114(2):147–52.

14. Kikuchi L, Oliveira CP, Alvares-da-Silva MR, Tani CM, Diniz MA, Stefano JT, et al. Hepatocellular carcinoma management in nonalcoholic fatty liver disease patients: applicability of the BCLC staging system. *Am J Clin Oncol* 2014; doi: 10.1097/COC.0000000000000134.

15. Bullen JJ, Ward CG, Rogers HJ. The critical role of iron in some clinical infections. *Eur J Clin Microbiol Infect Dis* 1991;10(8):613–7.

16. Guengerich FP, Shimada T. Oxidation of toxic and carcinogenic chemicals by human cytochrome P-450 enzymes. *Chem Res Toxicol* 1991;4(4):391–407.

17. Yeh FS, Yu MC, Mo CC, Luo S, Tong MJ, Henderson BE. Hepatitis B virus, aflatoxins, and hepatocellular carcinoma in southern Guangxi, China. *Cancer Res* 1989;49(9):2506–9.

18. Primary malignant tumours of the liver. In Garden OJ, Parks RW, eds., *Hepatobiliary & Pancreatic Surgery: A Companion to Specialist Practice*. Edinburgh: Saunders Elsevier, 2014, pp. 80–108.

19. Zhang BH, Yang BH, Tang ZY. Randomized controlled trial of screening for hepatocellular carcinoma. *J Cancer Res Clin Oncol* 2004;130(7):417–22.

20. Ryder SD, British Society of Gastroenterology. Guidelines for the diagnosis and treatment of hepatocellular carcinoma (HCC) in adults. *Gut* 2003;52(Suppl. 3):iii1–8.

21. Bruix J, Sherman M, Llovet JM, Beaugrand M, Lencioni R, Burroughs AK, et al. Clinical management of hepatocellular carcinoma. Conclusions of the Barcelona-2000 EASL Conference. European Association for the Study of the Liver. *J Hepatol* 2001;35(3):421–30.

22. Bruix J, Sherman M, Practice Guidelines Committee, American Association for the Study of Liver Diseases. Management of hepatocellular carcinoma. *Hepatology* 2005;42(5):1208–36.

23. Zhao YJ, Ju Q, Li GC. Tumor markers for hepatocellular carcinoma. *Mol Clin Oncol* 2013;1(4):593–8.

24. Peterson MS, Baron RL. Radiologic diagnosis of hepatocellular carcinoma. *Clin Liver Dis* 2001;5(1):123–44.

25. Marini P, Vilgrain V, Belghiti J. Management of spontaneous rupture of liver tumours. *Dig Surg* 2002;19(2):109–13.

26. Yeh CN, Lee WC, Jeng LB, Chen MF, Yu MC. Spontaneous tumour rupture and prognosis in patients with hepatocellular carcinoma. *Br J Surg* 2002;89(9):1125–9.

27. Bruix J, Llovet JM. Prognostic prediction and treatment strategy in hepatocellular carcinoma. *Hepatology* 2002;35(3):519–24.

28. Pugh RN, Murray-Lyon IM, Dawson JL, Pietroni MC, Williams R. Transection of the oesophagus for bleeding oesophageal varices. *Br J Surg* 1973;60(8):646–9.

29. Marrero JA, Fontana RJ, Barrat A, Askari F, Conjeevaram HS, Su GL, Lok AS. Prognosis of hepatocellular carcinoma: comparison of 7 staging systems in an American cohort. *Hepatology* 2005;41(4):707–16.

30. Pawlik TM, Poon RT, Abdalla EK, Zorzi D, Ikai I, Curley SA, et al. Critical appraisal of the clinical and pathologic predictors of survival after resection of large hepatocellular carcinoma. *Arch Surg* 2005;140(5):450–7; discussion 457–8.

31. Villanueva A, Hernandez-Gea V, Llovet JM. Medical therapies for hepatocellular carcinoma: a critical view of the evidence. *Nat Rev Gastroenterol Hepatol* 2013;10(1):34–42.

32. Edge SB, Byrd DR, Compton CC, et al. *AJCC Cancer Staging Manual*, 7th ed. New York: Springer Verlag, 2010.

33. Vauthey JN, Lauwers GY, Esnaola NF, Do KA, Belghiti J, Mirza N, et al. Simplified staging for hepatocellular carcinoma. *J Clin Oncol* 2002;20(6):1527–36.

34. Tsai TJ, Chau GY, Lui WY, Tsay SH, King KL, Loong CC, et al. Clinical significance of microscopic tumor venous invasion in patients with resectable hepatocellular carcinoma. *Surgery* 2000;127(6):603–8.

35. Poon RT, Fan ST. Evaluation of the new AJCC/UICC staging system for hepatocellular carcinoma after hepatic resection in Chinese patients. *Surg Oncol Clin N Am* 2003;12(1):35–50, viii.

36. Vauthey JN, Ribero D, Abdalla EK, Jonas S, Bharat A, Schumacher G, et al. Outcomes of liver transplantation in 490 patients with hepatocellular carcinoma: validation of a uniform staging after surgical treatment. *J Am Coll Surg* 2007;204(5):1016–27; discussion 1027–8.

37. Guglielmi A, Ruzzenente A, Pachera S, Valdegamberi A, Sandri M, D'Onofrio M, Iacono C. Comparison of seven staging systems in cirrhotic patients with hepatocellular carcinoma in a cohort of patients who underwent radiofrequency ablation with complete response. *Am J Gastroenterol* 2008;103(3):597–604.

38. Fong Y, Sun RL, Jarnagin W, Blumgart LH. An analysis of 412 cases of hepatocellular carcinoma at a Western center. *Ann Surg* 1999;229(6):790–9; discussion 799–800.

39. Pawlik TM, Poon RT, Abdalla EK, Ikai I, Nagorney DM, Belghiti J, et al. Hepatectomy for hepatocellular carcinoma with major portal or hepatic vein invasion: results of a multicenter study. *Surgery* 2005;137(4):403–10.

40. Ng KK, Vauthey JN, Pawlik TM, Lauwers GY, Regimbeau JM, Belghiti J, et al. Is hepatic resection for large or multinodular hepatocellular carcinoma justified? Results from a multi-institutional database. *Ann Surg Oncol* 2005;12(5):364–73.

41. Zorzi D, Vauthey J-N, Abdalla EK. Liver resection for hepatocellular carcinoma. In *Hepatocellular Carcinoma*. New York: Springer, 2011, pp. 109–34.

42. Belghiti J, Kianmanesh R. Surgical treatment of hepatocellular carcinoma. *HPB (Oxford)* 2005;7(1):42–9.

43. Bruix J, Castells A, Bosch J, Feu F, Fuster J, Garcia-Pagan JC, et al. Surgical resection of hepatocellular carcinoma in cirrhotic patients: prognostic value of preoperative portal pressure. *Gastroenterology* 1996;111(4):1018–22.

44. Torzilli G, Makuuchi M, Inoue K, Takayama T, Sakamoto Y, Sugawara Y, et al. No-mortality liver resection for hepatocellular carcinoma in cirrhotic and noncirrhotic patients: is there a way? A prospective analysis of our approach. *Arch Surg* 1999;134(9):984–92.

45. Shirabe K, Shimada M, Gion T, Hasegawa H, Takenaka K, Utsunomiya T, Sugimachi K. Postoperative liver failure after major hepatic resection for hepatocellular carcinoma in the modern era with special reference to remnant liver volume. *J Am Coll Surg* 1999;188(3):304–9.

46. Kubota K, Makuuchi M, Kusaka K, Kobayashi T, Miki K, Hasegawa K, et al. Measurement of liver volume and hepatic functional reserve as a guide to decision-making in resectional surgery for hepatic tumors. *Hepatology* 1997;26(5):1176–81.

47. Abdalla EK, Hicks ME, Vauthey JN. Portal vein embolization: rationale, technique and future prospects. *Br J Surg* 2001;88(2):165–75.

48. Vauthey JN, Chaoui A, Do KA, Bilimoria MM, Fenstermacher MJ, Charnsangavej C, et al. Standardized measurement of the future liver remnant prior to extended liver resection: methodology and clinical associations. *Surgery* 2000;127(5):512–9.

49. Aoki T, Imamura H, Hasegawa K, Matsukura A, Sano K, Sugawara Y, et al. Sequential preoperative arterial and portal venous embolizations in patients with hepatocellular carcinoma. *Arch Surg* 2004;139(7):766–74.

50. Ronot M, Vilgrain V. Hepatocellular carcinoma: diagnostic criteria by imaging techniques. *Best Pract Res Clin Gastroenterol* 2014;28(5):795–812.

51. Vauthey JN, Dixon E, Abdalla EK, Helton WS, Pawlik TM, Taouli B, et al. Pretreatment assessment of hepatocellular carcinoma: expert consensus statement. *HPB (Oxford)* 2010;12(5):289–99.

52. Wolfort RM, Papillion PW, Turnage RH, Lillien DL, Ramaswamy MR, Zibari GB. Role of FDG-PET in the evaluation and staging of hepatocellular carcinoma with comparison of tumor size, AFP level, and histologic grade. *Int Surg* 2010;95(1):67–75.

53. Hasegawa K, Kokudo N, Imamura H, Matsuyama Y, Aoki T, Minagawa M, et al. Prognostic impact of anatomic resection for hepatocellular carcinoma. *Ann Surg* 2005;242(2):252–9.

54. Regimbeau JM, Kianmanesh R, Farges O, Dondero F, Sauvanet A, Belghiti J. Extent of liver resection influences the outcome in patients with cirrhosis and small hepatocellular carcinoma. *Surgery* 2002;131(3):311–7.

55. Shi M, Guo RP, Lin XJ, Zhang YQ, Chen MS, Zhang CQ, et al. Partial hepatectomy with wide versus narrow resection margin for solitary hepatocellular carcinoma: a prospective randomized trial. *Ann Surg* 2007;245(1):36–43.

56. Poon RT, Fan ST, Ng IO, Wong J. Significance of resection margin in hepatectomy for hepatocellular carcinoma: a critical reappraisal. *Ann Surg* 2000;231(4):544–51.

57. Johnson M, Mannar R, Wu AV. Correlation between blood loss and inferior vena caval pressure during liver resection. *Br J Surg* 1998;85(2):188–90.

58. Imamura H, Seyama Y, Kokudo N, Maema A, Sugawara Y, Sano K, et al. One thousand fifty-six hepatectomies without mortality in 8 years. *Arch Surg* 2003;138(11):1198–206; discussion 1206.

59. Liu CL, Fan ST, Lo CM, Tung-Ping Poon R, Wong J. Anterior approach for major right hepatic resection for large hepatocellular carcinoma. *Ann Surg* 2000;232(1):25–31.

60. Croce E, Azzola M, Russo R, Golia M, Angelini S, Olmi S. Laparoscopic liver tumour resection with the argon beam. *Endosc Surg Allied Technol* 1994;2(3–4):186–8.

61. Vigano L, Laurent A, Tayar C, Tomatis M, Ponti A, Cherqui D. The learning curve in laparoscopic liver resection: improved feasibility and reproducibility. *Ann Surg* 2009;250(5):772–82.

62. Siniscalchi A, Ercolani G, Tarozzi G, Gamberini L, Cipolat L, Pinna AD, Faenza S. Laparoscopic versus open liver resection: differences in intraoperative and early postoperative outcome among cirrhotic patients with hepatocellular carcinoma – a retrospective observational study. *HPB Surg* 2014;2014:871251.

63. Regimbeau JM, Abdalla EK, Vauthey JN, Lauwers GY, Durand F, Nagorney DM, et al. Risk factors for early death due to recurrence after liver resection for hepatocellular carcinoma: results of a multicenter study. *J Surg Oncol* 2004;85(1):36–41.

64. Poon RT, Fan ST, Lo CM, Liu CL, Wong J. Long-term survival and pattern of recurrence after resection of small hepatocellular carcinoma in patients with preserved liver function: implications for a strategy of salvage transplantation. *Ann Surg* 2002;235(3):373–82.

65. Imamura H, Matsuyama Y, Tanaka E, Ohkubo T, Hasegawa K, Miyagawa S, et al. Risk factors contributing to early and late phase intrahepatic recurrence of hepatocellular carcinoma after hepatectomy. *J Hepatol* 2003;38(2):200–7.

66. Bruix J, Takayama T, Mazzaferro V, Chau GY, Yang J, Kudo M. STORM: a phase III randomized, double-blind, placebo-controlled trial of adjuvant sorafenib after resection or ablation to prevent recurrence of hepatocellular carcinoma (HCC). *J Clin Oncol* 2014;32(5s).

67. Forner A, Llovet JM, Bruix J. Hepatocellular carcinoma. *Lancet* 2012;379(9822):1245–55.

68. Huang G, Lau WY, Wang ZG, Pan ZY, Yuan SX, Shen F, et al. Antiviral therapy improves postoperative survival in patients with hepatocellular carcinoma: a randomized controlled trial. *Ann Surg* 2015; 261(1):56–66.

69. Llovet JM, Schwartz M, Mazzaferro V. Resection and liver transplantation for hepatocellular carcinoma. *Semin Liver Dis* 2005;25(2):181–200.

70. Mazzaferro V, Regalia E, Doci R, Andreola S, Pulvirenti A, Bozzetti F, et al. Liver transplantation for the treatment of small hepatocellular carcinomas in patients with cirrhosis. *N Engl J Med* 1996;334(11):693–9.

71. Bismuth H, Chiche L, Adam R, Castaing D, Diamond T, Dennison A. Liver resection versus transplantation for hepatocellular carcinoma in cirrhotic patients. *Ann Surg* 1993;218(2):145–51.

72. Jonas S, Bechstein WO, Steinmüller T, Herrmann M, Radke C, Berg T, et al. Vascular invasion and histopathologic grading determine outcome after liver transplantation for hepatocellular carcinoma in cirrhosis. *Hepatology* 2001;33(5):1080–6.

73. Clavien PA, Lesurtel M, Bossuyt PM, Gores GJ, Langer B, Perrier A, OLT for HCC Consensus Group. Recommendations for liver transplantation for hepatocellular carcinoma: an international consensus conference report. *Lancet Oncol* 2012;13(1):e11–22.

74. Jarnagin W, Chapman WC, Curley S, D'Angelica M, Rosen C, Dixon E, et al. Surgical treatment of hepatocellular carcinoma: expert consensus statement. *HPB (Oxford)* 2010;12(5):302–10.

75. Freeman RB, Edwards EB, Harper AM. Waiting list removal rates among patients with chronic and malignant liver diseases. *Am J Transplant* 2006;6(6):1416–21.

76. Llovet JM, Fuster J, Bruix J. Intention-to-treat analysis of surgical treatment for early hepatocellular carcinoma: resection versus transplantation. *Hepatology* 1999;30(6):1434–40.

77. Bharat A, Brown DB, Crippin JS, Gould JE, Lowell JA, Shenoy S, et al. Pre-liver transplantation locoregional adjuvant therapy for hepatocellular carcinoma as a strategy to improve longterm survival. *J Am Coll Surg* 2006;203(4):411–20.

78. Yao FY, Kinkhabwala M, LaBerge JM, Bass NM, Brown R, Kerlan R, et al. The impact of preoperative loco-regional therapy on outcome after liver transplantation for hepatocellular carcinoma. *Am J Transplant* 2005;5(4 Pt. 1):795–804.

79. Chapman WC, Majella Doyle MB, Stuart JE, Vachharajani N, Crippin JS, Anderson CD, et al. Outcomes of neoadjuvant transarterial chemoembolization to downstage hepatocellular carcinoma before liver transplantation. *Ann Surg* 2008;248(4):617–25.

80. Mazzaferro V, Battiston C, Perrone S, Pulvirenti A, Regalia E, Romito R, et al. Radiofrequency ablation of small hepatocellular carcinoma in cirrhotic patients awaiting liver transplantation: a prospective study. *Ann Surg* 2004;240(5):900–9.

81. Yao FY, Ferrell L, Bass NM, Watson JJ, Bacchetti P, Venook A, et al. Liver transplantation for hepatocellular carcinoma: expansion of the tumor size limits does not adversely impact survival. *Hepatology* 2001;33(6):1394–403.

82. Adam R, Azoulay D, Castaing D, Eshkenazy R, Pascal G, Hashizume K, et al. Liver resection as a bridge to transplantation for hepatocellular carcinoma on cirrhosis: a reasonable strategy? *Ann Surg* 2003;238(4):508–18; discussion 518–9.

83. Belghiti J, Cortes A, Abdalla EK, Régimbeau JM, Prakash K, Durand F, et al. Resection prior to liver transplantation for hepatocellular carcinoma. *Ann Surg* 2003;238(6):885–92; discussion 892–3.

84. Nathan H, Bridges JF, Schulick RD, Cameron AM, Hirose K, Edil BH, et al. Understanding surgical decision making in early hepatocellular carcinoma. *J Clin Oncol* 2011;29(6):619–25.

85. Rhim H, Goldberg SN, Dodd GD, Solbiati L, Lim HK, Tonolini M, Cho OK. Essential techniques for successful radio-frequency thermal ablation of malignant hepatic tumors. *Radiographics* 2001;21(Spec. no.):S17–35); discussion S36–9.

86. Livraghi T. Single HCC smaller than 2 cm: surgery or ablation: interventional oncologist's perspective. *J Hepatobiliary Pancreat Sci* 2010;17(4):425–9.

87. Kim YS, Lim HK, Rhim H, Lee MW. Ablation of hepatocellular carcinoma. *Best Pract Res Clin Gastroenterol* 2014;28(5):897–908.

88. Choi D, Lim HK, Rhim H, Kim YS, Lee WJ, Paik SW, et al. Percutaneous radiofrequency ablation for early-stage hepatocellular carcinoma as a first-line treatment: long-term results and prognostic factors in a large single-institution series. *Eur Radiol* 2007;17(3):684–92.

89. Waki K, Aikata H, Katamura Y, Kawaoka T, Takaki S, Hiramatsu A, et al. Percutaneous radiofrequency ablation as first-line treatment for small hepatocellular carcinoma: results and prognostic factors on long-term follow up. *J Gastroenterol Hepatol* 2010;25(3):597–604.

90. Duan C, Liu M, Zhang Z, Ma K, Bie P. Radiofrequency ablation versus hepatic resection for the treatment of early-stage hepatocellular carcinoma meeting Milan criteria: a systematic review and meta-analysis. *World J Surg Oncol* 2013;11(1):190.

91. Chen MS, Li JQ, Zheng Y, Guo RP, Liang HH, Zhang YQ, et al. A prospective randomized trial comparing percutaneous local ablative therapy and partial hepatectomy for small hepatocellular carcinoma. *Ann Surg* 2006;243(3):321–8.

92. Feng K, Yan J, Li X, Xia F, Ma K, Wang S, et al. A randomized controlled trial of radiofrequency ablation and surgical resection in the treatment of small hepatocellular carcinoma. *J Hepatol* 2012;57(4):794–802.

93. Huang J, Yan L, Cheng Z, Wu H, Du L, Wang J, et al. A randomized trial comparing radiofrequency ablation and surgical resection for HCC conforming to the Milan criteria. *Ann Surg* 2010;252(6):903–12.

94. Llovet JM, Real MI, Montaña X, Planas R, Coll S, Aponte J, et al. Arterial embolisation or chemoembolisation versus symptomatic treatment in patients with unresectable hepatocellular carcinoma: a randomised controlled trial. *Lancet* 2002;359(9319):1734–9.

95. European Organisation for Research and Treatment of Cancer. EASL-EORTC clinical practice guidelines: management of hepatocellular carcinoma. *J Hepatol* 2012;56(4):908–43.

96. Kadalayil L, Benini R, Pallan L, O'Beirne J, Marelli L, Yu D, et al. A simple prognostic scoring system for patients receiving transarterial embolisation for hepatocellular cancer. *Ann Oncol* 2013;24(10):2565–70.

97. Sangro B, Carpanese L, Cianni R, Golfieri R, Gasparini D, Ezziddin S, et al. Survival after yttrium-90 resin microsphere radioembolization of hepatocellular carcinoma across Barcelona Clinic Liver Cancer stages: a European evaluation. *Hepatology* 2011;54(3):868–78.

98. Llovet JM, Ricci S, Mazzaferro V, Hilgard P, Gane E, Blanc J-F, et al. Sorafenib in advanced hepatocellular carcinoma. *N Engl J Med* 2008;359(4):378–90.

99. Cheng AL, Kang YK, Chen Z, Tsao CJ, Qin S, Kim JS, et al. Efficacy and safety of sorafenib in patients in the Asia-Pacific region with advanced hepatocellular carcinoma: a phase III randomised, double-blind, placebo-controlled trial. *Lancet Oncol* 2009;10(1):25–34.

33

Carcinoma of the biliary tree and gallbladder

THOMAS GRUENBERGER, WOLFGANG SCHIMA, KOERT F D KUHLMANN
AND BIRGIT GRUENBERGER

INCIDENCE AND AETIOLOGY

Cancer of the biliary tree and gallbladder are considered rare in the Western world, with an overall incidence of about 5 per 100,000. About 12,000 new patients are diagnosed yearly in the United States [1].

Gallbladder cancer is the most common cancer of the biliary tract and accounts for 80–95% of cases [2]. Its incidence is highly dependent on geographic regions and ethnicities. Worldwide, the highest incidence rates are found in indigenous areas in Latin America and Asia. In female Mapuche Indians in Chile the incidence peaks at 27 per 100,000 each year [3]. The basis of these high incidence rates likely resides in the exposure to environmental factors, the high incidence of cholelithiasis and intrinsic genetic predisposition to carcinogenesis. Advancing age and obesity are general risk factors. Women are affected three to six times more often than men, possibly due to the higher incidence of cholelithiasis [4].

Irritation and chronic inflammation of the gallbladder mucosa are linked to malignant transformation and are therefore important factors in the development of gallbladder carcinoma. The main causative factor is cholelithiasis. The risk of developing gallbladder cancer in gallstone disease is dependent on stone size and type; cholesterol stones and a size >3 cm carry a significantly increased risk. Chronic cholecystitis can give rise to calcium deposits in the gallbladder wall. A gallbladder with extensive calcium deposits is defined as a porcelain gallbladder and malignancy is found in approximately 7% of cases [5].

Primary sclerosing cholangitis (PSC), a chronic fibro-inflammatory syndrome of the biliary tree, causes chronic inflammation of the biliary tree and leads to a high risk of developing gallbladder cancer, cholangiocarcinoma and hepatocellular carcinoma [6]. Chronic bacterial infections have also been described as risk factors for gallbladder and cholangiocarcinoma in multiple small studies. In particular, *Salmonella Typhi* and *Paratyphi* and *Helicobacter* cause a 12-fold risk increase [7].

Although most gallbladder polyps are non-neoplastic, approximately 5% of polyps progress to invasive carcinoma. Features that predict transformation to malignancy are polyp size above 10 mm, a solitary or sessile polyp and rapid polyp growth [4].

Another mechanism that is related to gallbladder cancer is an anomalous junction of the pancreaticobiliary duct. This is a congenital malformation in which the pancreatic duct drains into the biliary tract outside the duodenal wall. This anomaly allows pancreatic secretions to regurgitate into the bile ducts and gallbladder, which potentially leads to (pre)malignant changes in the mucosa [8].

Most cases of cholangiocarcinoma arise *de novo*. However, as in gallbladder cancer, inflammation and the link to malignant transformation play an important role. Patients with PSC have an annual risk of developing cholangiocarcinoma of 1.5% [9]. Parasitic infections such as *Clinorchis sinensis* and *Opisthorchis viverrini* (liver flukes) are closely related to an increased risk of developing cholangiocarcinoma, especially in southeast Asia where these infections are endemic [10]. Furthermore, chronic liver disease, especially hepatitis B and C, is recognized as a risk factor for cholangiocarcinoma with an odds ratio of 5 [11]. Due to biliary stasis, chronic reflux and subsequent chronic irritation of the biliary tree, patients with bile duct cystic disorders, including Caroli's disease, have a high risk of developing cholangiocarcinoma. The lifetime incidence ranges between 6% and 30% [12].

PATHOLOGY AND STAGING

In the most recent seventh edition of the American Joint Committee on Cancer (AJCC) staging system, biliary and gallbladder cancer is staged in four separate subtypes [13]: three cholangiocarcinoma subtypes (distal, perihilar and intrahepatic cholangiocarcinoma) and gallbladder carcinoma, which includes malignancies of the cystic duct.

Distal cholangiocarcinoma [13]

T-Stage

Tis	Carcinoma in situ
T1	Tumor confined to the bile duct
T2	Tumor invades beyond the wall of the bile duct
T3	Tumor invades the gallbladder, liver, pancreas, duodenum or other adjacent organs
T4	Tumor involves the coeliac axis or the superior mesenteric artery

Note: Distal cholangiocarcinoma arises from the common bile duct, between the confluence of the cystic duct with the common hepatic duct, and the ampulla of Vater.

N-Stage

N0	No regional lymph node metastases
N1	Regional lymph node metastases

Note: Regional lymph nodes are along the common bile duct, common hepatic artery, back toward the coeliac trunk, posterior and anterior pancreaticoduodenal nodes, and along the superior mesenteric vein and the right lateral wall of the superior mesenteric artery. Histological examination of a regional lymphadenectomy specimen will ordinarily include 12 or more lymph nodes. If the regional lymph nodes are negative, but the number ordinarily examined is not met, classify as pN0.

M-Stage

M0	No distant metastases
M1	Distant metastases

Staging groups for distal cholangiocarcinoma

Stage			
0	Tis	N0	M0
1a	T1	N0	M0
1b	T2	N0	M0
2a	T3	N0	M0
2b	T1–3	N1	M0
3	T4	Any N	M0
4	Any T	Any N	M1

Perihilar cholangiocarcinoma [13]

T-Stage

Tis	Carcinoma in situ
T1	Tumor confined to the bile duct, with extension up to the muscle layer or fibrous tissue
T2a	Tumor invades beyond the wall of the bile duct to surrounding adipose tissue
T2b	Tumor invades adjacent hepatic parenchyma
T3	Tumor invades unilateral branches of the portal vein or hepatic artery
T4	Tumor invades the main portal vein or its branches bilaterally, or the common hepatic artery, or the second-order biliary radicals bilaterally, or the unilateral second-order biliary radicals with contralateral portal vein or hepatic artery involvement

Note: Perihilar cholangiocarcinomas are tumors located in the extrahepatic biliary tree proximal to the origin of the cystic duct.

N-Stage

N0	No regional lymph node metastases
N1	Regional lymph node metastasis, including nodes along the cystic duct, common bile duct, hepatic artery and portal vein
N2	Metastasis to periaortic, pericaval, superior mesenteric artery and/or coeliac artery lymph nodes

M-Stage

M0	No distant metastases
M1	Distant metastases

Staging groups for perihilar cholangiocarcinoma

Stage			
0	Tis	N0	M0
1	T1	N0	M0

Continued

Stage			
2	T2a–b	N0	M0
3a	T3	N0	M0
3b	T1–3	N1	M0
4a	T4	Any N	M0
4b	Any T	N2	M0
	Any T	Any N	M1

Intrahepatic cholangiocarcinoma [13]

T-Stage

Tis	Carcinoma in situ
T1	Solitary tumor without vascular invasion
T2a	Solitary tumor with vascular invasion
T2b	Multiple tumors, with or without vascular invasion
T3	Tumor(s) perforating the visceral peritoneum or involving the local extrahepatic structures by direct invasion
T4	Tumor with periductal invasion

Note: Intrahepatic cholangiocarcinoma is a tumor within the liver, arising from the bile ducts proximal to the second-order bile ducts.

N-Stage*

N0	No regional lymph node metastases
N1	Regional lymph node metastases

* Right-liver intrahepatic cholangiocarcinoma regional lymph nodes include the hilar (common bile duct, hepatic arteries, portal vein and cystic duct), periduodenal and peripancreatic lymph nodes. Left-liver intrahepatic cholangiocarcinoma regional lymph nodes include the hilar and gastrohepatic lymph nodes.

Histological examination of a regional lymphadenectomy specimen will ordinarily include three or more lymph nodes. If the regional lymph nodes are negative, but the number ordinarily examined is not met, classify as pN0.

M-Stage*

M0	No distant metastases
M1	Distant metastases

* Spread to the coeliac or periaortic and caval lymph nodes is distant metastasis.

Staging groups for intrahepatic cholangiocarcinoma

Stage			
0	Tis	N0	M0
1	T1	N0	M0
2	T2	N0	M0

Continued

Stage			
3	T3	N0	M0
4a	T4	N0	M0
	Any T	N1	M0
4b	Any T	Any N	M1

Gallbladder cancer [13]

T-Stage

Tis	Carcinoma in situ
T1	Tumor invades lamina propria (T1a) or muscular layer (T1b)
T2	Tumor invades perimuscular connective tissue; no extension beyond serosa or into liver
T3	Tumor perforates the serosa (visceral peritoneum) and/or directly invades the liver and/or one other adjacent organ or structure, such as the stomach, duodenum, colon, pancreas, omentum or extrahepatic bile ducts
T4	Tumor invades main portal vein or hepatic artery or invades at least two extrahepatic organs or structures

N-Stage

N0	No regional lymph node metastasis
N1	Metastases to nodes along the cystic duct, common bile duct, hepatic artery and/or portal vein
N2	Metastases to periaortic, pericaval, superior mesenteric artery and/or coeliac artery lymph nodes

Note: Histological examination of a regional lymphadenectomy specimen will ordinarily include three or more lymph nodes. If the regional lymph nodes are negative, but the number ordinarily examined is not met, classify as pN0.

M-Stage

M0	No distant metastases
M1	Distant metastases

Staging groups for gallbladder cancer

Stage			
0	Tis	N0	M0
1a	T1	N0	M0
2	T2	N0	M0
3a	T3	N0	M0
3b	T1–3	N1	M0
4a	T4	Any N	M0
4b	Any T	N2	M0
	Any T	Any N	M1

DIAGNOSIS AND PREOPERATIVE STAGING

In general, contrast-enhanced multidetector CT (MDCT) or magnetresonance-cholangiopancreaticography (MRCP) with contrast-enhanced MRI is used for detection and staging of cancer of the biliary ducts or the gallbladder. MRCP has a high accuracy (98%) in the diagnosis of benign and malignant biliary diseases. For assessment of malignant disease MRCP has been shown to be superior to CT and ultrasound, with an accuracy of 96% vs 92% (CT) and 79% (US) [14]. State-of-the-art imaging techniques are vital for accurate assessment of resectability and, thus, for treatment planning. Contrast-enhanced MDCT (or MRI) should be performed in the arterial and the venous phases to allow assessment of the hepatic arterial and the portal venous system. MRCP offers superior soft tissue contrast for gallbladder lesions and extent of biliary tumor encasement. Diffusion-weighted MRI now plays an important role in the detection of hepatic metastases, enlarged regional lymph nodes and peritoneal carcinomatosis [15] and should be included in the routine MRI protocol.

The Liver Cancer Study Group of Japan distinguishes three macroscopic growth types of intrahepatic cholangiocarcinoma [16]: mass-forming, periductal-infiltrating, and intraductal growth types, with the mass-forming type being most common. Different imaging modalities may be used to detect and characterize the tumor, but in clinical practice both contrast-enhanced MDCT and MRI are generally used. At CT and MRI intrahepatic cholangiocarcinoma presents as a hypovascular mass with peripheral rim enhancement (Figure 33.1). The central, more fibrotic

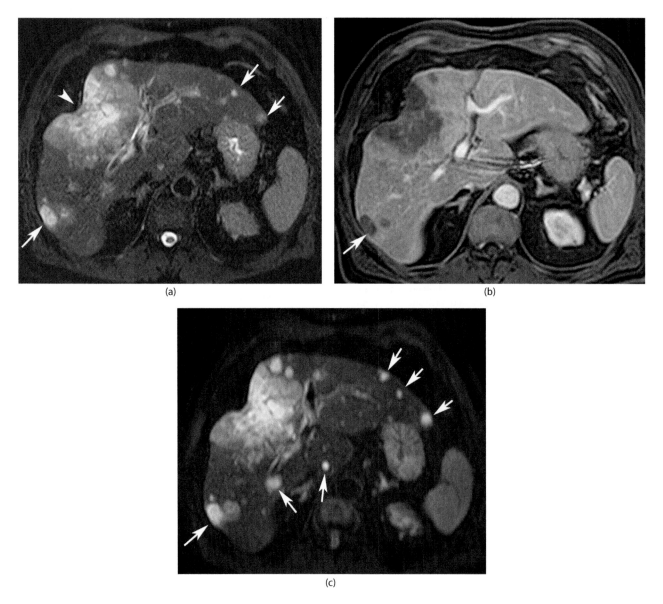

(a)

(b)

(c)

Figure 33.1 MRI of intrahepatic cholangiocarcinoma. (a) The T2-weighted pulse sequence demonstrates a large mass with capsular retraction (arrowhead) and metastatic lesions in both lobes (arrows). (b) The contrast-enhanced MR sequence shows the hypovascular lesion and two metastases in the right lobe (arrow). There is no encasement of the portal vein. (c) The diffusion-weighted pulse sequence not only shows the primary tumor, but also multiple metastases in both lobes (arrows).

part of the tumor is typically enhanced on delayed images obtained approximately 5 min after contrast injection. Capsule retraction is often seen, although it is not pathognomonic for cholangiocarcinoma. For tumor staging, contrast-enhanced images are important to demonstrate vascular invasion, satellite nodules and peritoneal spreading [17,18]. Diffusion-weighted MRI has been found to be very useful for the detection of small intrahepatic nodules, increasing the sensitivity of MRI (Figure 33.1).

MRCP with contrast-enhanced MRI has gained favour in assessment of hilar cholangiocarcinoma. MRCP allows delineation of proximal and distal extension of the tumor, which generally appears hypovascular at contrast-enhanced MRI. Dynamic contrast-enhanced series are valuable in the determination of hepatic arterial or portal venous infiltration (Figure 33.2). Park et al. showed that MRI with MCRP is equivalent to MDCT in combination with direct (invasive) cholangiography for assessment of biliary duct involvement (accuracy, 91% vs 85%) [19].

However, bi-phasic contrast-enhanced MDCT with short acquisition time may be superior to MRI for vascular infiltration in patients with poor health status because of the lower likelihood of breathing-related motion artefacts. In a larger series on surgically proven hilar cholangiocellular carcinoma (CCC), Lee et al. [20] could show CT has an accuracy of 85.5–92.7% for portal venous and arterial invasion and a positive predictive value for resectability of 71.4%. MRCP is the modality of choice to plan (temporary or palliative) biliary drainage. Biliary stents (plastic as well as metal) induce artefacts, which will impair visualization of adjacent small tumors (Figure 33.3). Moreover, biliary decompression induces biliary inflammation, which can severely interfere with the delineation of the longitudinal tumor extent into the biliary system. Thus, it is of utmost importance to perform cross-sectional imaging for staging of cholangiocarcinoma before obtaining biliary drainage.

In distal bile duct tumors, differentiation from pancreatic head cancer or periampullary tumors is difficult or

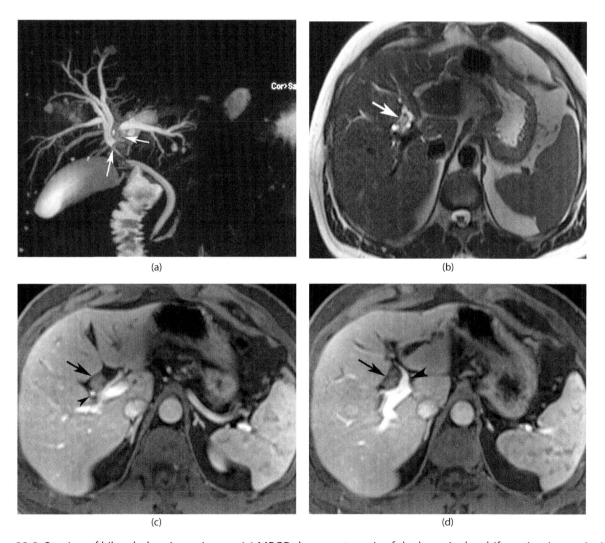

(a)

(b)

(c)

(d)

Figure 33.2 Staging of hilar cholangiocarcinoma. (a) MRCP shows a stenosis of the hepatic duct bifurcation (arrows) with intrahepatic bile duct dilatation. The segmental ducts are not affected by the stenosis. (b) The T2-weighted MR image in the axial plane shows the predominantly intraductal tumor growth (arrow). (c, d) Contrast-enhanced MR images show the tumor (arrow) in close proximity to the right hepatic artery (small arrowhead) and the portal vein bifurcation (large arrowhead), but without signs of infiltration.

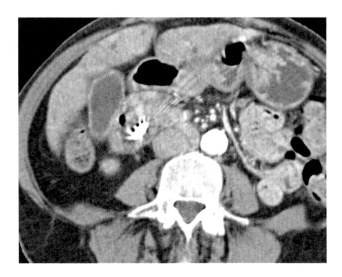

Figure 33.3 Artefacts induced by plastic stent application prior to imaging. In this patient with a small distal cholangiocarcinoma, stent-induced artefacts impair visualization of the tumor.

sometimes even impossible by imaging. Lack of pancreatic duct dilatation may favour the diagnosis of distal CCC, although this feature is not pathognomonic. Contrast-enhanced MDCT or MRI is used to determine biliary extent and possible vascular invasion.

Early gallbladder cancer may present as an incidental finding during ultrasound work-up for abdominal complaints, with non-specific findings such as a small polypoid lesion or wall thickening. On the other hand, a variety of benign gallbladder diseases may mimic gallbladder cancer. Especially focal wall thickening due to fundal type of adenomyomatosis or mass-forming xanthogranulomatous cholecystitis may be difficult to differentiate by imaging [21]. For detection and staging, either contrast-enhanced multidetector CT or MRI with MRCP should be performed. Typical imaging features include a discrete mass or focal wall thickening or, less commonly, diffuse wall thickening [22]. Use of liver-specific MR contrast agents improves assessment of the presence of liver invasion and the T-stage in general (accuracy, 86% vs 80%) (Figure 33.4) [23].

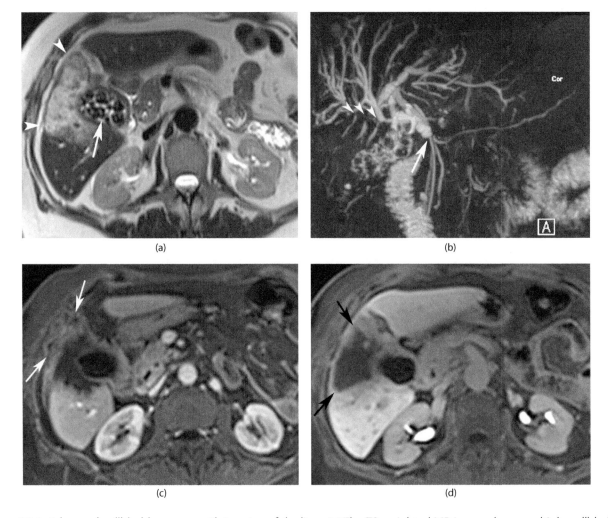

(a)　　　　　　　　　　　　　(b)

(c)　　　　　　　　　　　　　(d)

Figure 33.4 Advanced gallbladder cancer with invasion of the liver. (a) The T2-weighted MR image shows multiple gallbladder stones (arrow) and a mass invading the liver parenchyma (arrowheads). (b) MRCP demonstrates stenoses of the common hepatic duct (arrow) and of several segmental ducts in the right lobe (arrowheads), indicating advanced stage. (c, d) Enhanced MRI with liver-specific contrast material in the early phase (c) shows irregular peritoneal enhancement, suggestive of peritoneal carcinomatosis (arrows). In the hepato-biliary phase (d) extensive tumor infiltration into the liver is depicted (arrows).

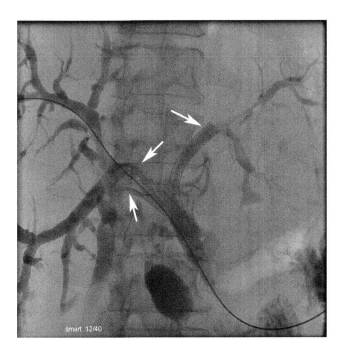

Figure 33.5 Palliative percutaneous drainage in unresectable hilar CCC: there are three stents (arrows) in place to achieve adequate bilateral biliary drainage.

A recent meta-analysis revealed a very high sensitivity (99%) of CT for assessment of gallbladder cancer resectability with a limited specificity of 76% [24]. This is caused by the limitations of contrast-enhanced CT to detect subtle signs of peritoneal carcinomatosis, invasion into the hilum, or distant metastases precluding radical surgery. The addition of preoperative PET to contrast-enhanced CT or MRI has only modest impact on the management of patients with gallbladder cancer [25].

Palliative drainage of hilar cholangiocarcinoma is necessary in the majority of patients, who are diagnosed at a stage when surgical resection is not an option. In general, self-expanding metal stents are superior to plastic biliary stents because of longer median patency times [26]. Percutaneous biliary drainage is more invasive than endoscopic procedures and has its role, when endoscopic drainage is not feasible (Figure 33.5). However, local expertise often guides the treatment approach in these patients and multimodality treatment is often required.

SURGERY FOR BILIARY AND PRIMARY GALLBLADDER CANCER

Surgical principles for the treatment of cholangiocellular carcinomas (CCCs) are usually defined by the existence of a multidisciplinary team (MDT) to correctly diagnose, outline a treatment plan, evaluate the patient's fitness for a major procedure and delineate the place for a neoadjuvant or perioperative medical oncology or radiation oncology therapy. As long as the patient is fit for major surgery and demonstrates with potential resectable disease radical resection is the cornerstone of CCC therapy. Prior to

resection, cardiac and respiratory function should be evaluated and volume measurement of the future remnant liver performed; the required percentage of remaining liver after resection is dependent on its function, which is usually impaired by fatty infiltration (therefore preoperative body mass index measurement essential) or fibrotic or cirrhotic transformation (unusual in CCCs) and especially after long-lasting biliary obstruction. If one of the above is present preservable volume should be kept above 40% of the total liver volume; otherwise 30% is accepted. Major hepatectomy has to be done with an anaesthesiology team that is aware of low-volume anaesthesia, intraoperative use of vasopressors to maintain minimum arterial blood pressure (around 100 mmHg) during liver transection and the specific postoperative volume management after intraoperative volume depletion. Postoperative alertness does not imperatively require ICU care but has to fulfil 4- to 6-hourly measurement of acid–base status, serum lactate, haemoglobin and glucose levels for the immediate 24 postoperative hours. Liver enzymes should be measured at least once within 6 h postoperatively. Watch out for early liver function parameters as bilirubin, prothrombin time (PTZ), albumin and thrombocytes. The liver resection technique itself is dependent on local expertise and even when studied in multiple settings, there was no technique found to be advantageous over another with regard to blood loss or perioperative morbidity and mortality. Liver resection including biliary duct resection and reconstruction should include postoperative local anastomotic drainage to detect potential leakage at an early stage. The essential requirement for the performance of safe major hepatectomy is the centre demonstration of a yearly mortality rate below 5% and a major morbidity rate below 30% (Dindo III–V) [27].

Although cholangiocarcinoma is a specific entity originating from small to large bile ducts, the required surgical procedures to perform a R0 resection are totally different depending on the exact location of the tumor and certainly the tumor's staging.

Intrahepatic cholangiocellular carcinoma

The intrahepatic cholangiocellular carcinoma (ICC) usually originates in normal underlying liver parenchyma and its radiological appearance is mostly typical as a mass-forming arterially enhancing tumor (see 'Diagnosis and Preoperative Staging' section above). Radical surgical removal with clear margins is the only accepted curative therapy. There are well-known prognostic parameters that should be taken into account when discussing prognosis, one of them being the lymph node spread, which led to the recommendation of routine lymphadenectomy at the level of the hepatoduodenal ligament during surgery [28]. Several other factors including size and number of tumors, the existence of satellite tumors, grading, and vascular and perineural invasion should be analyzed by the pathologist to guide decision for or against adjuvant chemotherapy (Figure 33.6). The evidence for the application of chemotherapy after surgery is

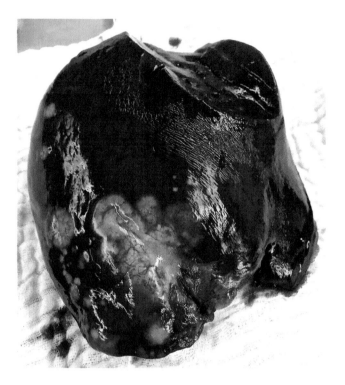

Figure 33.6 Intrahepatic cholangiocarcinoma with multiple satellites.

unfortunately still not prospectively studied [29]. ICCs are mostly diagnosed at advanced size requiring major hepatectomies. As long as minimum remaining liver volume is guaranteed with adequate in- and outflow, liver dysfunction is seldom a problem due to normal regenerating remnant liver [30].

Perihilar cholangiocellular carcinoma: Klatskin tumor

Diagnosis of perihilar cholangiocellular carcinoma (phCCC), or Klatskin tumor, and its allocation to a potential resectable candidate or a palliative case according to Bismuth's classification [31] are in a considerable number of patients only determinable with surgical exploration. Patients usually present with jaundice and require initial radiological staging before an endoscopic retrograde cholangiopancreatography (ERCP) or percutaneous transhepatic cholangiography (PTC) is performed, because the inserted drains or stents obscure the diagnosis and the determination of the extent of disease. The necessity of a biliary drainage prior to resection or immediate surgery demonstrated controversial results and has to be decided on by the treating team [32]. The anatomically longer left hepatic duct prior to segmental distribution implies more often an extended right hemihepatectomy in curative intent and requires in many cases a portal vein embolization (including the segment IV branches) to induce a hypertrophy of preservable segments II and III [33]. Segment I which is draining into the ductal bifurcation,

where the cancer lies, has to be removed in any potential curative procedure. Vascular resections at the hilum are possible and recommended by some groups, but their invasion affects immediate (postoperative morbidity and mortality) and long-term prognosis. Lymphadenectomy should be a standard procedure as in every CCC surgery. Liver transplantation (LT) in locally unresectable cases was tested in a multidisciplinary approach including pre-LT radiochemotherapy with interesting results but has not become standard of care due to unreproducible results and unusual inclusion and exclusion criteria (e.g. local lymph node involvement as a contraindication) [34].

Distal cholangiocellular carcinoma

Different to the other forms of CCC, distal cholangiocellular carcinoma (dCCC) requires the removal of the pancreatic head usually as partial duodenopancreatectomy (PDP) with extended bile duct removal up to the hilum. PDP is a standard procedure that includes relevant lymph node dissection and reconstruction of the stomach and the remaining pancreas in various ways to achieve macroscopic cure. Similar to the gallbladder cancer the involvement of ligamentary vascular structures often determines potential local radical surgery and can often only be explored intraoperatively. Interestingly the prognosis of dCCC is better than that of pancreas head adenocarcinoma and should therefore be separated from the latter [35].

Gallbladder cancer

Gallbladder cancer (GBC) has two typical presentations: diagnosed either incidentally in the histological work-up of a simple cholecystectomy or as symptomatic right upper quadrant tumor in an advanced stage. The former finding requires a staging CT and an exact histopathologic analysis of the following parameters prior to a decision of a re-resection: T-stage, cystic duct margin, involvement of resected lymph nodes, grading, perineural invasion and vascular invasion. Every T-stage above T1a and positivity of any mentioned parameters requires a reoperation where a segment IVb/V liver resection together with a ligamentary lymphadenectomy should be performed. The cystic duct should be re-excised, but the common bile duct should be kept in place as long as not microscopically involved, as its routine resection has not proven long-term benefit but increases postoperative morbidity [36,37]. If the gallbladder was not removed with a bag during laparoscopic resection or the gallbladder perforated (a bad prognostic factor) the port sides should be re-excised during a second procedure.

If a GBC is diagnosed during imaging or when patients present jaundiced evaluation of potential resectability is the key factor. Advanced T-stage including T4 tumors is not a contraindication for resectability as long as the tumor is located in the fundus; these tumors require major liver resection with potential resection of the transverse colon.

The achievement of a curative resection of an advanced tumor located at the infundibulum is much more difficult because it requires the resection of the bile duct, at least the bulbus duodeni and potentially the pancreatic head, together with a major hepatectomy, especially if right-sided vessels (right hepatic artery, right portal vein) are involved. The combination of a hepatectomy and a pancreatic head resection is only justified in young fit patients and should only be performed in recognized centres because the procedure's morbidity and mortality are higher than the usual compulsory numbers [38].

The prognosis of a GBC, if not diagnosed at a very early stage, is inferior to that for all other types of CCC, and evaluable data of adjuvant therapies are even more lacking.

Summary

CCCs, due to their rise in incidence, are becoming more and more relevant in MDT meetings, where they should be primarily discussed to decide therapeutic strategy because they require individual surgical approaches, based on different types.

NEOADJUVANT AND ADJUVANT THERAPIES

Complete surgical resection is the only potentially curative treatment in patients with biliary tract cancer. Nevertheless, the general outcome is disappointing. The 5-year survival rate after curative resection ranges from 5% to 10% in gallbladder cancer and 10% to 40% for cholangiocarcinoma. This high recurrence rate emphasizes the need for an adjuvant treatment. Unfortunately, most of the data reported are uncontrolled institutional series and retrospective analyses. Until now, there has been only one published randomized study [39]. In this trial, patients with pancreatic cancer, gallbladder cancer, biliary tract cancer and cancer of the ampulla Vateri were included to receive either mitomycin C (MMC) plus 5-fluorouracil (5-FU) or surgery alone. In the intent-to-treat analysis there was no statistically significant difference with regard to the median overall survival. Only patients with gallbladder cancer, who were not curatively resected, benefitted from postoperative chemotherapy: 8.9% 5-year survival in the chemotherapy group vs 0% in the control arm ($p = 0.0226$).

A systemic review and meta-analysis of adjuvant treatment of biliary tract cancer was published in 2012 [40]. Twenty studies, in which 6712 patients were included, were analyzed: one randomized trial of chemotherapy alone, two registry analyses and 17 institutional series. Patients were treated with chemotherapy, radiation or both modalities. There was a non-significant improvement in overall survival with any adjuvant treatment compared with surgery alone ($p = 0.06$). The greatest benefit for an adjuvant treatment was perceived in patients with positive resection margin or involved lymph nodes.

In a recently published paper, a nomogram was designed in which a possible benefit of an adjuvant radiochemotherapy in patients with resected gallbladder cancer was shown [41]. This model demonstrates a possible survival benefit in patients with at least T2 or N1 tumor.

Further clinical prospective randomized trials are urgently needed to define a standard approach after surgery. These trials should use recently developed treatment modalities including chemotherapy, radiotherapy and targeted therapies.

According to ESMO guidelines, adjuvant loco-regional treatment should be considered. According to the National Comprehensive Cancer Network (NCCN) guidelines, patients with R0 resection should be considered for observation, participation in a clinical trial or adjuvant chemotherapy (5-FU or gemcitabine based).

LOCALLY ADVANCED AND METASTATIC DISEASE

Most patients with biliary tract cancer are diagnosed with an advanced unresectable tumor. The prognosis of those is poor with a median survival of a few months and a 5-year survival rate of <5%.

In this palliative setting chemotherapy is the gold standard worldwide. Patients have to be in a good performance status without severe comorbidities, and it is necessary that a sufficient biliary decompression was performed before starting palliative chemotherapy in jaundiced patients. The goal of the palliative chemotherapy is not only to prolong survival but also improve quality of life.

The problem of nearly all published studies is the heterogeneity of the study population as well as the small sample size. In most of the studies patients with intrahepatic, extrahepatic, gallbladder cancer, cancer of the ampulla Vateri and even pancreatic cancer are included. Furthermore, most of the studies are retrospective.

In 1996, Glimelius et al. first described a significant prolongation of median survival in patients treated with 5-FU/LV vs best supportive care [42]. In addition, the treatment group also demonstrated improvement in quality of life.

Valle et al. published the prospective randomized phase III ABC-02 trial, in which gemcitabine was compared to gemcitabine–cisplatin [43]. There were 410 patients with locally advanced cholangiocarcinoma, gallbladder cancer or cancer of the ampulla Vateri included who were randomized to gemcitabine 1000 mg/m^2 on days 1, 8 and 15 every 4 weeks for six cycles or cisplatin 25 mg/m^2 followed by gemcitabine 1000 mg/m^2 on days 1 and 8 every 3 weeks for eight cycles. The primary endpoint, median overall survival, was met: 11.7 months in the combination group vs 8.1 months in the monotherapy group ($p = 0.001$) without added clinically significant toxicity. Additionally progression-free survival (PFS) was significantly prolonged: 8.0 vs 5.0 months in the gemcitabine–cisplatin vs gemcitabine alone group ($p < 0.001$). Based on these results, the combination chemotherapy of gemcitabine plus cisplatin is considered the standard of care as first-line chemotherapy for biliary tract cancer treatment.

If cisplatin is not applicable or if there is a contraindication for cisplatin, oxaliplatin can be used instead. Several phase II studies have shown antitumor activity and a good toxicity profile in patients with advanced or metastatic biliary tract cancer. For patients with a borderline performance status or a contraindication for a combination chemotherapy, 5-FU/LV, capecitabine or gemcitabine monotherapy is a reasonable option.

Targeted therapies, in combination with chemotherapy or alone, have improved response rates and progression-free and overall survival in various tumor entities. There are several trials published which investigate the role of molecular targeted therapies in biliary tract cancer patients. Tyrosine kinase inhibitors (TKIs) as single agents like erlotinib, lapatinib, sorafenib, sunitinib or selumetinib did not meet the primary endpoints and they have unfortunately not warranted further investigation. The combination of the two TKIs, sorafenib and erlotinib, also failed to meet the primary endpoint in the first-line treatment.

However, targeted therapies in combination with an effective chemotherapy backbone are generally more active. Combinations of gemcitabine and platinum-based drugs with targeted therapies like bevacizumab, cetuximab or erlotinib have shown more encouraging results. The only randomized phase III trial, with 268 patients receiving GEMOX plus erlotinib versus GEMOX alone, failed to show PFS benefit in the experimental arm [44]. Nevertheless, this trial demonstrated a significant improvement of the objective response rate (30% vs. 16%, $p = 0.005$). A phase II study of GEMOX and bevacizumab reported some antitumor activity with a tolerable safety profile [45]. In the BINGO trial, the addition of cetuximab to the combination chemotherapy GEMOX did not enhance activity among the 150 patients enrolled [46]. In contrast, a small study including 30 patients with advanced or metastatic biliary tract cancer showed encouraging results with three patients experiencing a complete radiological response, and a total of nine patients (33%) underwent surgical resection with curative intent after sufficient response to this combination therapy [47].

Recently a pooled analysis of clinical trials of chemotherapy and targeted therapy in advanced biliary tract cancer showed an excellent overview on published data: a total of 161 published trials comprising 6337 patients were analyzed [48]. The pooled results of the standard chemotherapy combination of gemcitabine with a platinum were median response rate 25.9%, tumor control rate 63.5%, time to tumor progression 5.3 months and overall survival 9.5 months, respectively. Triplets including gemcitabine, 5-FU and a platinum, as well as gemcitabine-based chemotherapy plus targeted therapy, were significantly superior to gemcitabine–platinum concerning tumor control and overall survival with no difference in response rates.

Although these data are encouraging, further efforts and additional data with randomized trials are needed to improve first-line treatment options for patients with advanced or metastatic biliary tract cancer.

A systematic review of second-line chemotherapy in advanced biliary tract cancer was published recently by Lamarca et al [49]. Twenty-five studies were eligible: 14 phase II clinical trials, 9 retrospective analyses and 2 case reports. Regimens used were, among others, docetaxel–erlotinib, gemcitabine, gemcitabine–cisplatin, iFAM, S1, irinotecan, FOLFOX and bortezomib. The mean OS was 7.2 months, and the mean progression-free survival, response rate and disease control rate were 3.2 months, 7.7% and 49.5%, respectively. Further prospective randomized studies are needed to evaluate the relative value of a second-line chemotherapy in this setting.

In patients with liver-limited disease loco-regional therapies can be considered. In a study by Vogl et al. 115 patients with non-resectable biliary tract cancer were treated with trans-arterial chemoembolization [50]. Agents used were gemcitabine, MMC or both as well as the combination of gemcitabine, MMC and cisplatin. The response rate was 8.7%; in 57.4% of the patients a stabilization was achieved. The median overall survival was 13 months. Radioembolization using yttrium-90 is the second loco-regional treatment modality evaluated. Al-Adra et al. performed a review of currently available data of 12 studies and demonstrated that the median OS was 15.5 months and a response rate of 28% and stabilization rate of 54% were achieved [51].

Photodynamic therapy (PDT) is a treatment option for intraluminal tumors and has been demonstrated to provide a survival benefit over simple biliary decompression in two prospective randomized studies. In the study by Ortner et al. the median overall survival was 498 days in the combination of PDT with Photofrin® and 98 days ($p < 0.0001$) with a biliary drainage without PDT [52]. In the second study the photosensitizer Photosan® was used [53]: the median overall survival was 630 days in the combination of biliary drainage and PTD vs 210 days with drainage alone. The most common side effects are cholangitis and phototoxicity of the skin.

REFERENCES

1. American Cancer Society. Cancer Facts and Figures 2014. New York: American Cancer Society, 2014. Available from http://www.cancer.org/research/cancerfactsstatistics/cancerfactsfigures2014/index.

2. Hundal R, Shaffer EA. Gallbladder cancer: epidemiology and outcome. *Clin Epidemiol* 2014; 6: 99–109.

3. Surveillance, Epidemiology and End Results Program (SEER). The four most common cancers for different ethnic populations 2013. Bethesda, MD: National Cancer Institute, 2013.

4. Randi G, Franceschi S, La Vecchia C. Gallbladder cancer worldwide: geographical distribution and risk factors. *Int J Cancer* 2006 118: 1591–1602.

5. Stephen AE, Berger DL. Carcinoma in the porcelain gallbladder: a relationship revisited. *Surgery* 2001; 129: 699–703.

6. Razumilava N, Gores GJ, Lindor KD. Cancer surveillance in patients with primary sclerosing cholangitis. *Hepatology* 2011; 54: 1842–1852.

7. Kumar S, Kumar S, Kumar S. Infection as a risk factor for gallbladder cancer. *J Surg Oncol* 2006; 93: 633–639.

8. Nomura T, Shirai Y, Sandoh N, Nagakura S, Hatakeyama K. Cholangiographic criteria for anomalous union of the pancreatic and biliary ducts. *Gastrointest Endosc* 2002; 55: 204–208.

9. Farrant JM, Hayllar KM, Wilkinson ML, et al. Natural history and prognostic variables in primary sclerosing cholangitis. *Gastroenterology* 1991; 100: 1710–1717.

10. Sithithaworn P, Yongvanit P, Duenngai K, Kiatsopit N, Pairojkul C. Roles of liver fluke infection as risk factor for cholangiocarcinoma. *J Hepatobiliary Pancreat Sci* 2014; 21: 301–308.

11. Palmer WC, Patel T. Are common factors involved in the pathogenesis of primary liver cancers? A meta-analysis of risk factors for intrahepatic cholangiocarcinoma. *J Hepatol* 2012; 57: 69–76.

12. Søreide K, Körner H, Havnen J, Søreide JA. Bile duct cysts in adults. *Br J Surg* 2004; 91: 1538–1548.

13. Edge SB, Byrd DR, Compton CC, et al., eds. *AJCC Cancer Staging Manual*, 7th ed. New York: Springer, 2010, pp. 211–217.

14. Singh A, Mann HS, Thukral CL, Singh NR. Diagnostic accuracy of MRCP as compared to ultrasound/CT in patients with obstructive jaundice. *J Clin Diagn Res* 2014; 8: 103–7.

15. Park MJ, Kim YK, Lim S, Rhim H, Lee WJ. Hilar cholangiocarcinoma: value of adding DW imaging to gadoxetic acid-enhanced MR imaging with MR cholangiopancreatography for preoperative evaluation. *Radiology* 2014; 270: 768–76.

16. Yamasaki S. Intrahepatic cholangiocarcinoma: macroscopic type and stage classification. *J Hepatobiliary Pancreat Surg* 2003; 10: 288–91.

17. Sainani NI, Catalano OA, Holalkere NS, Zhu AX, Hahn PF, Sahani DV. Cholangiocarcinoma: current and novel imaging techniques. *Radiographics* 2008; 28: 1263–87.

18. Ayuso JR, Pagés M, Darnell A. Imaging bile duct tumors: staging. *Abdom Imaging* 2013; 38: 1071–81.

19. Park HS, Lee JM, Choi JY, et al. Preoperative evaluation of bile duct cancer: MRI combined with MR cholangiopancreatography versus MDCT with direct cholangiography. *AJR Am J Roentgenol* 2008; 190: 396–405.

20. Lee HY, Kim SH, Lee JM, et al. Preoperative assessment of resectability of hepatic hilar cholangiocarcinoma: combined CT and cholangiography with revised criteria. *Radiology* 2006; 239: 113–21.

21. Deshmukh SD, Johnson PT, Sheth S, Hruban R, Fishman EK. CT of gallbladder cancer and its mimics: a pattern-based approach. *Abdom Imaging* 2013; 38: 527–36.

22. Mitchell CH, Johnson PT, Fishman EK, Hruban RH, Raman SP. Features suggestive of gallbladder malignancy: analysis of T1, T2, and T3 tumors on cross-sectional imaging. *J Comput Assist Tomogr* 2014; 38: 235–41.

23. Hwang J, Kim YK, Choi D, et al. Gadoxetic acid-enhanced MRI for T-staging of gallbladder carcinoma: emphasis on liver invasion. *Br J Radiol* 2014; 87: 20130608.

24. Li B, Xu XX, Du Y, et al. Computed tomography for assessing resectability of gallbladder carcinoma: a systematic review and meta-analysis. *Clin Imaging* 2013; 37: 327–33.

25. Leung U, Pandit-Taskar N, Corvera CU, et al. Impact of pre-operative positron emission tomography in gallbladder cancer. *HPB (Oxford)* 2014; 11: 1023–30.

26. Goenka MK, Goenka U. Palliation: hilar cholangiocarcinoma. *World J Hepatol* 2014; 6: 559–69.

27. Dindo D, Demartines N, Clavien PA. Classification of surgical complications: a new proposal with evaluation in a cohort of 6336 patients and results of a survey. *Annals of Surgery* 2004; 240: 205–213.

28. de Jong MC, Nathan H, Sotiropoulos GC, et al. Intrahepatic cholangiocarcinoma: an international multi-institutional analysis of prognostic factors and lymph node assessment. *Journal of Clinical Oncology* 2011; 29: 3140–3145.

29. Bridgewater J, Galle PR, Khan SA, et al. Guidelines for the diagnosis and management of intrahepatic cholangiocarcinoma. *Journal of Hepatology* 2014; 60: 1268–1289.

30. Mavros MN, Economopoulos KP, Alexiou VG, Pawlik TM. Treatment and prognosis for patients with intrahepatic cholangiocarcinoma: systematic review and meta-analysis. *JAMA Surgery* 2014; 149: 565–574.

31. Bismuth H, Nakache R, Diamond T. Management strategies in resection for hilar cholangiocarcinoma. *Annals of Surgery* 1992; 215: 31–38.

32. Iacono C, Ruzzenente A, Campagnaro T, et al. Role of preoperative biliary drainage in jaundiced patients who are candidates for pancreatoduodenectomy or hepatic resection: highlights and drawbacks. *Annals of Surgery* 2013; 257: 191–204.

33. Nagino M, Kamiya J, Nishio H, et al. Two hundred forty consecutive portal vein embolizations before extended hepatectomy for biliary cancer: surgical outcome and long-term follow-up. *Annals of Surgery* 2006; 243: 364–372.

34. Kelley RK, Hirose R, Venook AP. Can we cure cholangiocarcinoma with neoadjuvant chemoradiation and liver transplantation? Time for a multicenter trial. *Liver Transplantation* 2012; 18: 509–513.

35. Dickson PV, Behrman SW. Distal cholangiocarcinoma. *Surgical Clinics of North America* 2014; 94: 325–342.

36. Zhu AX, Hong TS, Hezel AF, Kooby DA. Current management of gallbladder carcinoma. *Oncologist* 2010; 15: 168–181.

37. Fuks D, Regimbeau J, Le Treut Y-P, et al. Incidental gallbladder cancer by the AFC-GBC-2009 Study Group. *World Journal of Surgery* 2011; 35: 1887–1897.

38. Lim C-S, Jang J-Y, Lee S, et al. Reappraisal of hepatopancreatoduodenectomy as a treatment modality for bile duct and gallbladder cancer. *Journal of Gastrointestinal Surgery* 2012; 16: 1012–1018.

39. Takada T, Hodaka A, Yasuda H, et al. Is postoperative adjuvant chemotherapy useful for gallbladder carcinoma? *Cancer* 2002; 95: 1685–1695.

40. Horgan AM, Amir E, Walter T, Knox JJ. Adjuvant therapy in the treatment of biliary tract cancer: a systematic review and meta-analysis. *Journal of Clinical Oncology* 2012; 30: 1934–1940.

41. Wang SJ, Lemieux A, Kalpathy-Cramer J, et al. Nomogram for predicting the benefit of adjuvant chemoradiotherapy for resected gallbladder cancer. *Journal of Clinical Oncology* 2011; 29: 4627–4632.

42. Glimelius B, Hoffman K, Sjödén P-O, et al. Chemotherapy improves survival and quality of life in advanced pancreatic and biliary cancer. *Annals of Oncology* 1996; 7: 593–600.

43. Valle J, Wasan H, Palmer DH, et al. Cisplatin plus gemcitabine versus gemcitabine for biliary tract cancer. *New England Journal of Medicine* 2010; 362: 1273–1281.

44. Lee J, Park SH, Chang H-M, et al. Gemcitabine and oxaliplatin with or without erlotinib in advanced biliary-tract cancer: a multicentre, open-label, randomised, phase 3 study. *Lancet Oncology* 2012; 13: 181–188.

45. Zhu AX, Meyerhardt JA, Blaszkowsky LS, et al. Efficacy and safety of gemcitabine, oxaliplatin, and bevacizumab in advanced biliary-tract cancers and correlation of changes in 18-fluorodeoxyglucose PET with clinical outcome: a phase 2 study. *Lancet Oncology* 2010; 11: 48–54.

46. Malka D, Cervera P, Foulon S, et al. Gemcitabine and oxaliplatin with or without cetuximab in advanced biliary-tract cancer (BINGO): a randomised, open-label, non-comparative phase 2 trial. *Lancet Oncology* 2014; 15: 819–828.

47. Gruenberger B, Schueller J, Heubrandtner U, et al. Cetuximab, gemcitabine, and oxaliplatin in patients with unresectable advanced or metastatic biliary tract cancer: a phase 2 study. *Lancet Oncology* 2010; 11: 1142–1148.

48. Eckel F, Schmid RM. Chemotherapy and targeted therapy in advanced biliary tract carcinoma: a pooled analysis of clinical trials. *Chemotherapy* 2014; 60: 13–23.

49. Lamarca A, Hubner RA, David Ryder W, Valle JW. Second-line chemotherapy in advanced biliary cancer: a systematic review. *Annals of Oncology* 2014; 25: 2328–2338.

50. Vogl TJ, Naguib NNN, Nour-Eldin N-EA, et al. Transarterial chemoembolization in the treatment of patients with unresectable cholangiocarcinoma: results and prognostic factors governing treatment success. *International Journal of Cancer* 2012; 131: 733–740.

51. Al-Adra DP, Gill RS, Axford SJ, et al. Treatment of unresectable intrahepatic cholangiocarcinoma with yttrium-90 radioembolization: a systematic review and pooled analysis. *European Journal of Surgical Oncology* 2015; 41: 120–127.

52. Ortner MEJ, Caca K, Berr F, et al. Successful photodynamic therapy for nonresectable cholangiocarcinoma: a randomized prospective study. *Gastroenterology* 2003; 125: 1355–1363.

53. Zoepf T, Jakobs R, Arnold JC, et al. Palliation of nonresectable bile duct cancer: improved survival after photodynamic therapy. *American Journal of Gastroenterology* 2005; 100: 2426–2430.

34

Liver metastases

MICHEL RIVOIRE, SERGE EVRARD AND THEO J M RUERS

INTRODUCTION

The liver is a common site for the development of metastases from primary tumors of various histologies. The site of the primary tumor is the main determinant of the management of patients. In general, we recognize liver metastases (LMs) from colorectal cancer, from neuroendocrine tumors and from non-colorectal non-neuroendocrine primary tumors. This chapter deals with the management of patients with LMs of colorectal origin and LMs from non-colorectal non-neuroendocrine origin. Management of LM from neuroendocrine tumors is discussed in the chapter on neuroendocrine tumors (Chapter 45).

LIVER METASTASES FROM COLORECTAL CANCER

Incidence

Colorectal cancer (CRC) is a major cause of morbidity and mortality throughout the world. It accounts for more

than 9% of all cancers. It is the third most common cancer worldwide and the fourth most common cause of death [1]. The cumulative lifetime risk is approximately 5%, and the incidence rate in the Western world is 45–50/100,000. It accounts for 12.2% of all cancer-related deaths in Europe [2]. LMs form the main cause of death in patients with CRC. At the time of diagnosis, 25% of patients have stage IV CRC (synchronous liver metastases) and ~50% of patients overall will develop LMs. For patients with isolated LMs the treatment strategy should be directed toward resection: unfortunately only a minority of patients (15–20%) with LMs are considered as candidates for surgery. The majority have unresectable disease and for these patients systemic chemotherapy is the standard of care. Without any treatment the median survival after detection of LM is approximately 9 months, depending on the extent of the disease at the time of diagnosis. Generally, colorectal LMs (CRLMs) do not cause any signs or symptoms. Only in advanced stages may patients suffer from cachexia, fatigue, icterus or sometimes pain due to stretching of the liver capsule. Recent efforts to optimize multidisciplinary management of patients with stage IV CRC have improved outcomes significantly by defining the indications for neoadjuvant chemotherapy to improve or permit surgical resection and to enhance surgical techniques for resectable metastases.

Surveillance and follow-up of patients with CRC

Given that ~30–50% of patients undergoing a curative CRC resection will ultimately develop recurrent disease, optimizing the surveillance strategy is paramount [3]. To detect LM at an early, potentially curable stage, patients with primary CRC should be actively screened for the presence of LMs at the time of diagnosis of the primary tumor as well as during follow-up after curative resection of the primary. Ideal pre- or postoperative protocol to follow CRC patients and to detect LMs at an early stage should include the following: (1) wide availability, (2) high sensitivity to detect small metastases or recurrence, (3) high specificity to ensure that those patients without disease are correctly labelled and (4) cost-efficiency. Currently, there is wide variation in follow-up after resection of the colorectal primary. Some authors have postulated that intensive follow-up would lead to early detection of metachronous tumors and thus improved survival, while others have questioned the need for follow-up at all. Numerous randomized controlled trials, meta-analyses and a Cochrane review [4] have been completed in the last decade to assess the impact of an intensive versus standard surveillance strategy on outcomes for post-resection CRC patients. In the Cochrane review, although the absolute numbers of recurrences were similar, intensive follow-up was associated with a significant survival benefit at 5 years compared to standard surveillance (OR 0.73, 95% CI 0.59–0.91). In addition, the time to recurrence was significantly reduced by –6.75 (95% CI –11.06 to –2.44), suggesting an earlier detection of recurrence in the high-intensity surveillance cohort. According to the National Comprehensive Cancer Network (NCCN) 2013 guidelines, patients who are fit enough to undergo liver surgery should undergo regular physical exam and carcinoembryonic antigen (CEA) measurements (every 3 months for 2 years and then every 6 months for 3 years) as well as annual computed tomography of the chest and abdomen for 5 years after surgery in high-risk patients (i.e. tumor with lymphatic or vascular invasion or poor differentiation) (Figure 34.1).

PATIENT SELECTION

Contemporary series have demonstrated that surgical therapy for CRLM is associated with 5- and 10-year survivals ranging from 25% to 74% (median 38%) and 9% to 50% (median 26%), respectively, depending on the study period and the underlying patient population. Survival following resection of CRLM varies and is dependent on clinical, tumor and molecular factors [5].

Clinical exam	Every 3 months during 3 years Then every 6 months during 2 years
Colonoscopy	At 1 or 2 years and then every 5 years
Abdomino-thoracic CT scan	Every year during 5 years
CEA	Every 3 months during 3 years Then every 6 months during 2 years

Figure 34.1 Surveillance and follow-up of patients with CRC.

Clinical preoperative factors

Historically, prognosis after resection has been largely based on preoperative patient and tumor-specific factors that have been mixed in scoring systems [6]. Results from studies have been heterogeneous and correlation with survival is poor. Factors that are related to survival after resection are the original staging of the primary tumor, a high preoperative CEA level (with a threshold of 200 ng/ml), the number of metastases (with a threshold of 4) and the size of the largest metastasis (with a threshold of 50 mm). For this latter factor, modern era chemotherapy regimens which are frequently used prior to surgery are able to downsize metastases. In this context, it is not clear if tumor size continues to hold important prognostic information. Response to chemotherapy – as evidenced by tumor size reduction – may be a more important and relevant prognostic marker than initial CRLM tumor size. While an association between synchronous LM as well as short disease-free interval and a worse prognosis have been noted, there is still no consensus on their impact on survival. One explanation for this controversy may be the impact of effective adjuvant (or neoadjuvant) chemotherapy.

Traditionally, the presence of extrahepatic disease (EHD) has been considered a contraindication to resection. With improvements in perioperative cross-sectional imaging, patient selection for resection, safety of surgical techniques and chemotherapy, improved survival following surgery for patients with EHD has been reported. EHD as a contraindication to surgery is now being challenged [7]. Nevertheless, it has been noted that the number of LMs as well as adverse locations of EHD is associated with prognosis: pulmonary metastases have the best prognosis and retroperitoneal lymph node metastases the worst.

Tumor factors

Microscopically negative surgical margins (R0) have traditionally been considered an important prognostic factor. What constitutes a 'truly' microscopically negative margin remains controversial and a margin width of more than 1 mm does not seem to be associated with a higher recurrence rate. It has been argued that it is biology, not millimetres, that dictates prognosis following resection. Some authors [8] did not find a difference in overall survival (OS) among patients undergoing an R0 versus R1 resection. These data may suggest that, in an era of more effective chemotherapies, leaving microscopic disease behind may result in increased local failure but not necessarily a worse OS. The impact of margin status on outcomes may therefore be influenced by patient and tumor factors, as well as the utilization of chemotherapy. Recently, attention has turned to the use of biological and molecular markers as a more accurate means to predict long-term outcomes. Patient and tumor-specific markers may provide more accurate predictions of survival after hepatic resection for colorectal metastases. Preoperative chemotherapy is being increasingly used, to allow previously unresectable patients to become resectable as well to increase the chance of cure of truly resectable patients. The use of preoperative systemic chemotherapy provides the opportunity to assess response. Response to chemotherapy assessed by standard cross-sectional imaging using the Response Evaluation Criteria in Solid Tumors (RECIST) has been shown to improve 5-year overall as well as disease-free survival (DFS) [9]. In addition to assessment on preoperative imaging, tumor response can be assessed on pathological examination after liver resection. Using a semi-quantitative scale of the number of residual cancer cells may allow classification of patients according to complete response (no residual cancer cells), major response (1–49% of residual cancer cells) or minor response (≥50% residual cancer cells), respectively. Such classification shows strong correlation with 5-year survival [10].

Molecular factors

The clinical behaviour of CRC is complex [11]. The emergence of biologic and molecular markers may allow for a more individualized approach to prognosis. Factors such as RAS, BRAF, thymidylate synthase, telomerase component hTERT and Ki-67, as well as circulating tumor cells and circulating tumor DNA, may help predict long-term prognosis following treatment of CRLM and lead to patient-specific prognostic information and treatments.

IMAGING TECHNIQUES AND RESULTS IN CRLM

Staging of patients with CRLM should concentrate on the accurate imaging of the number, size and location of the metastases within the liver as well as on the detection of possible EHD. Options available for hepatic imaging include ultrasound (US), computed tomography (CT), magnetic resonance imaging (MRI) and fluorodeoxyglucose–positron emission tomography (FDG-PET) [12].

US and contrast-enhanced US

Transabdominal US is operator dependent and plays a limited role in the diagnosis of CRLM, given its limited sensitivity of 50–75%. The addition of intravenous contrast improves sensitivity by about 20%, with results similar to those seen with multi-detector CT (MDCT). Intraoperative US (IOUS) combined with surgical exploration remains the standard for the detection of liver metastases. It alters the preoperative surgical plan in 20% of cases when compared to MDCT.

MDCT

MDCT is routinely used for the detection of CRLM and lung metastases. For the liver, contrast enhancement of the arterial and portal phases is required. CRLMs appear hypovascular (more evident during the portal venous phase) and hypodense compared to normal liver parenchyma. There is rim enhancement that subsequently washes out on later phases. The main limitations of MDCT are patient exposure to ionizing radiation, the potential for reactions to iodinated contrast and its inability to adequately characterize sub-centimetre lesions.

MRI

MRI is currently the most accurate imaging technique for the detection and characterization of CRLM, due to the recent technological advances and development of new contrast agents. It offers higher contrast resolution and the possibility of performing multi-parametric imaging, combining T1, T2 and diffusion-weighted imaging (DWI) with dynamic multiphasic contrast imaging. Several intravenous contrast agents are available to improve detection and characterization of liver lesions. They include gadolinium chelates (gadopentetate dimeglumine [Gd-DTPA]) routinely used as vascular contrast, or agents taken up by normal liver parenchyma, but excluded from metastatic lesions such as hepatobiliary agents (gadobenate dimeglumine [Gd-BOPTA] or gadoxetate disodium [Gd-EOB-DTPA]) used to improve characterization of small liver lesions. A combination of DWI and Gd-EOB-DTPA-enhanced imaging holds the best results for detection and characterization. The main limitations of MRI are costs, contraindications and access to radiological expertise (Figure 34.2).

PET and PET-CT

Optimal PET imaging is performed with a concurrent CT, providing a metabolic map of glucose uptake throughout the entire body. PET demonstrates high sensitivity and specificity for detection of CRLM, with the superiority of better detection of EHD over MDCT and MRI. However, the main limitations of PET are poor sensitivity, particularly for small lung nodules and in patients having recently received chemotherapy. Access to scanning may also be limited in some centres.

Comparison between imaging modalities

Each imaging modality has specific advantages and disadvantages, related to cost, speed of acquisition, use of ionizing radiation, risk of contrast reaction and local availability

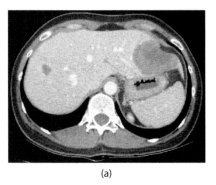
(a)

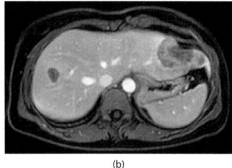
(b)

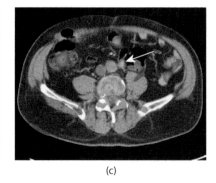
(c)

Figure 34.2 CRC liver metastases: (a) contrast-enhanced CT scan, (b) contrast-enhanced MRI and (c) FDG-PET showing retroperitoneal lymph node (white arrow).

and expertise. Recent meta-analyses support the use of MRI for the detection of CRLM and show that sensitivity and specificity on a per-patient basis for US, CT, MRI and FDG-PET are 63.0% and 97.6%, 74.8% and 95.6%, 81.1% and 97.2% and 93.8% and 98.7%, respectively [13]. On a per-lesion basis, sensitivity is 86.3%, 82.6%, 86.3% and 86.0%, respectively. MRI shows a better sensitivity than MDCT in per-patient and per-lesion analysis. In per-lesion analysis, the difference is higher when liver-specific contrast agents are administered and for lesions smaller than 10 mm. Data about FDG PET/CT are too limited for comparisons with other modalities.

RESECTION

Resection is the gold standard for the surgical treatment of CRLM [6]. It should be considered in all patients with metastatic disease confined to the liver, irrespective of the size, number or multilobar localization of the lesions, as long as all lesions can be removed adequately while leaving enough functional liver reserve.

Operative procedure

At laparotomy the abdomen is carefully inspected for EHD. Intraoperative US is performed in order to determine the number of metastases and to assess their localization in relation to the vascular structures and main bile ducts. Detailed knowledge of the segmental structure of the liver is essential for a safe surgical procedure. A large variety of resections can be undertaken, following the distribution of the metastases. There is a trend to avoid extensive resections when not absolutely indicated to obtain adequate margins. A liver-sparing approach offers significant better opportunities for secondary liver surgery and facilitates postoperative recovery. Surface-oriented metastases can be excised by non-anatomic wedge resections, whereas deeper solitary lesions can be treated by segmentectomy or bisegmentectomy. Large or multiple metastases are treated by right or left hepatectomy or multiple segmentectomies in case of bilobar disease. Several methods of vascular clamping can be applied to control intraoperative hemorrhage,

such as non-selective intermittent clamping of the portal triad (Pringle maneuver); complete vascular exclusion of the liver, including clamping of the hepatic pedicle and infra- and suprahepatic vena cava; and selective vascular occlusion or ligation of the hepatic artery, portal vein and hepatic vein of the depending site of the parenchymal resection. The venous pressure within the inferior vena cava should be maintained at a low level (<5 mmHg) to minimize blood loss during parenchymal dissection, especially in those cases where hepatic veins are not controlled. Parenchymal division can be performed in several ways. The easiest way is to crush small portions of liver tissue with small forceps. Smaller vessels that are encountered are coagulated, while larger vessels and biliary structures are ligated. Several instruments are available on the market to facilitate parenchymal dissection such as ultrasonic dissectors and water-jet dissectors. More recently, coagulation equipment has been developed to transect the liver tissue, by sealing the vascular structures or by coagulation of liver tissue with the help of radiofrequency energy. The choice of transection method is mainly based on the preference and expertise of the surgeon [14].

Perioperative mortality and morbidity

Although the mortality rate after hepatic resection has declined to less than 5%, in most major centres over the past 20 years, as a result of advances in operative techniques and perioperative care, it has been shown that actual population-based mortality rates for liver resection are higher than those reported in the literature from high-volume centres. Furthermore, most studies have quoted in-hospital or 30-day mortality, which may be as little as half the 90-day mortality rate that has now become the standard metric. In a recent population-based study from France, the in-hospital and 90-day mortality rates were 3.4% and 5.8%, respectively [15]. It has also recently been emphasized that the risk of death following hepatic surgery is lower at high-volume hospitals and patients treated at low-volume hospitals who have a complication are 40% more likely to die than patients with a complication in a high-volume hospital [16].

The morbidity rate after liver resection for CRLM still ranges from 23% to 56%, with a reoperation rate related to postoperative complications of around 5.2%. Furthermore, the recent development of effective chemotherapy regimens such as neoadjuvant or conversion strategies may be responsible for increased morbidity following hepatic resection for CRLM. Sepsis, wound infection, urinary tract infection and organ space infection are the most common complications. Male gender, previous cardiac operation, American Society of Anesthesiologists class 3 or higher score and disseminated cancer are significantly associated with higher complication rates [17]. In a recent meta-analysis of 2280 patients, 35% of patients experienced at least one postoperative complication. The occurrence of complications was associated with altered long-term oncological results [18]. Whether this association is the result of a direct cause–effect relationship or the consequence of a more extensive surgery for a higher tumor burden is still under debate. Nevertheless, in order to reduce complication rates, efforts should be made to reduce preoperative chemotherapy duration to a maximum of eight cycles (4 months), to avoid combined major liver and primary resections in case of synchronous metastases, to avoid major resections and consider two-stage procedures for bilateral metastases, to use portal vein embolization to reduce the risk of liver failure, and to favor non-anatomic resections or ablation rather than sacrificing a huge volume of healthy parenchyma, in patients presenting with multiple metastases [19].

Assessment of resectability

Over the past decade, the surgical approach to metastatic CRC has undergone a paradigm shift, as understanding of what can and should be resected grows. The border between clearly resectable and clearly unresectable disease is hazy and constantly evolving as large registries show good outcomes in subsets of patients whose tumors would previously not have been considered resectable. There have also been major developments in the use of chemotherapy for metastatic CRC, with the recognition that tumors in a subgroup of patients who present with unresectable disease can become resectable following systemic chemotherapy. Attempting to convert unresectable into resectable disease is a worthwhile aim, with 5-year survival rates for patients with tumors chemo-converted to resectability being similar to those of patients who underwent resection at presentation [20]. Response to chemotherapy is known to correlate with resection rate [21]. As a result, it is recommended that patients with unresectable liver-only disease should be treated with the most aggressive regimen possible. In a recent population-based study [22], the rate of hepatic resection following CRLM showed significant variation in its application across cancer networks and hospitals that was independent of case mix. These variations may reflect inequitable access to multimodal care, a lack of consensus regarding what constitutes resectable disease, and major differences in the use of downsizing

chemotherapy or use of different thresholds to determine which patients should be considered for resection [23]. Systematic referral to highly specialized multidisciplinary teams including both specialized surgeons and oncologists would reduce inequities in the use of resection for CRLM. It has been demonstrated that almost two-thirds of patients with CRLMs deemed unresectable by non-specialists are considered potentially resectable by specialist liver surgeons [24]. This highlights the need for ongoing education of non-specialists and the fact that *all* cases should be reviewed by a specialized MDT.

Repeat hepatectomy

Repeat curative intent hepatectomy for recurrence is being increasingly performed with associated survival rates identical to those of the first hepatectomy. The rationale behind repeat hepatectomy for recurrent disease is supported in part by a belief that the liver is often the sole site of recurrent metastases. The overall pattern of recurrence remains similar with regard to intrahepatic versus extrahepatic versus intra- plus extrahepatic disease. More importantly, the recurrence-free benefit of repeat curative intent surgery is similar regardless of the number of times previous surgery has been performed. The possibility of repeat hepatectomy with complete resection of all metastases should therefore always be considered in patients with recurrent disease. Owing to the high recurrence rate of CRLM, initial hepatectomies should be performed as efficiently as possible, integrating the possibility of repeat hepatectomy. Non-anatomical resections should therefore be preferred, saving the maximum amount of normal liver parenchyma, provided that safe tumor margins can be achieved [25].

ADJUVANT TREATMENT

The efficacy of adjuvant and palliative chemotherapy for primary and metastatic colon carcinoma has led to the development of studies integrating neoadjuvant or adjuvant chemotherapy in patients with resectable or resected liver metastases. The results are still uncertain as many variables interfere with the interpretation of these studies, such as variations in the timing (adjuvant or neoadjuvant), route (IV or regional infusion) and regimens used (e.g. fluoropyrimidine with or without oxaliplatin or irinotecan, targeted therapies).

Regional liver chemotherapy infusion

Regional liver chemotherapy infusion is a logical approach since the liver represents the main site of relapse after resection of hepatic metastases. This approach allows the delivery of high doses of chemotherapy to potential micrometastases remaining in the liver, while sparing extrahepatic organs. Combined hepatic artery infusion (HAI) plus systemic fluoropyrimidine-based adjuvant therapy significantly increases relapse-free survival [26]. A Cochrane meta-analysis shows that OS is not improved by HAI. The lack of survival benefit may be in part related to the morbidity of HAI and technical limitations [27]. Based on these results, and the availability of newer, active systemic agents and regimens, the value of HAI chemotherapy after resection of CRLM has to be questioned. In the future, it will be interesting to better evaluate locoregional chemotherapy regimens containing oxaliplatin or irinotecan.

Adjuvant chemotherapy

Adjuvant chemotherapy is simple, limits the risk of including patients with EHD and ensures that all of the enrolled patients have had complete macroscopic clearance of metastases. The usefulness of postoperative therapy by bolus 5-FU–leucovorin (5-FU–LV) has been assessed in two randomized studies comparing 6 months of postoperative chemotherapy to surgery alone, but both studies were closed prematurely as a result of slow accrual. A non-significant trend toward improvement of relapse-free and OS was observed. A pooled analysis of these studies has been reported [28]. The median DFS was 27.9 months in the chemotherapy arm and 18.8 months in the control arm. In the multivariate analysis, patients in the adjuvant chemotherapy group had a significantly reduced risk of relapse (HR 1.39, $p = 0.026$). The median OS was 62.2 months in the chemotherapy arm and 47.3 months in the control arm, but despite a strong trend, the difference was not statistically significant. Furthermore, a phase III study comparing 5-FU–LV versus 5-FU–LV–irinotecan (FOLFIRI) following R0 resection of CRLM reported 2-year DFS of 51% and 46%, respectively (HR 0.89, 95% CI 0.66–1.19, $p = 0.43$), similar to that reported for series of resection alone [29]. The evidence for adjuvant systemic chemotherapy after liver resection may therefore be considered marginal.

Preoperative chemotherapy

In cases of resectable CRLM, the postulated benefits of *preoperative chemotherapy* include (1) early treatment of micro-metastatic disease; (2) reduction of tumor volume, which allows 'easier' and more radical liver surgery; and (3) identification and exclusion from surgery of patients who have rapid disease progression during chemotherapy, which indicates aggressive tumor biology. However, preoperative chemotherapy can cause liver damage, which may increase the risk of postoperative complications. In addition, preoperative chemotherapy may also lead to the disappearance of metastases on radiological imaging, which might result in more difficult curative surgery. The EORTC group reported a randomized phase III trial comparing the administration of 12 perioperative FOLFOX-4 courses (6 preoperative and 6 postoperative) to surgery alone [30]. The resection rate was similar in both arms (83.5% vs. 83.0%). Postoperative complications were slightly higher in the chemotherapy group, but chemotherapy-related toxicity was low. The primary endpoint was the 3-year DFS, which was 7.2% higher in the

chemotherapy arm in the intent-to-treat analysis, 8.1% better if only eligible patients were retained and 9.2% better if only patients who underwent a liver resection were selected.

The long-term results at a median follow-up of 8.5 years showed that the addition of perioperative chemotherapy to surgery led to a non-significant 4% OS improvement in the chemotherapy arm after 5 years (HR 0.87, 95% CI 0.66–1.14, $p = 0.303$) [31]. The overall benefit in this study was modest, however, and the superiority of the FOLFOX-4 regimen was in the same range as that observed in the above-mentioned studies assessing adjuvant bolus 5-FU–leucovorin. Additionally, in the intent-to-treat analysis, the difference between the two arms was not statistically significant, probably as a result of a lack of power. Nevertheless, perioperative chemotherapy in patients with resectable LMs is now considered by most specialists to be a standard.

The situation is in fact more complex in clinical practice; for many multidisciplinary teams, chemotherapy is proposed after surgery in the case of metachronous metastases and is begun before surgery in the case of synchronous metastases or if at least two poor prognosis factors are present (more than one metastasis, tumor of more than 5 cm, nodal involvement of the primary, high CEA level). For the future, several questions remain unanswered. Is FOLFOX superior to LV–5-FU2? Is it possible to shorten the chemotherapy duration by using intensive regimens such as FOLFIRINOX? Is there a place for targeted therapies? Moreover, it is now likely that future trials will be carried out on selected subgroups of patients with a high risk of recurrence.

Risk of chemotherapy-induced liver damage

The major cause for concern when chemotherapy is used in resectable CRLM is its potential effects on the hepatic parenchyma and the subsequent implications this may have on surgical morbidity and mortality [32]. In the EORTC perioperative chemotherapy study, the incidence of postoperative complications was significantly increased in the FOLFOX arm compared to the surgery alone arm (25% vs. 16%, $p = 0.04$), although there was no difference in mortality. From a histological perspective, preoperative irinotecan is more likely to induce chemotherapy-associated steatohepatitis (CASH) or steatosis, while oxaliplatin is significantly associated with a sinusoidal dilatation. Patients with steatohepatitis may have an increased postoperative 90-day mortality rates (14.7% vs. 1.6%) [33]. These results suggest using only short-duration preoperative chemotherapy (3–4 months) and not waiting for the best tumor response. This is sufficient to provide chemosensitivity and tolerance data, facilitating use of the same chemotherapy regimen after surgery.

What to do in the case of complete response after chemotherapy

Modern chemotherapy regimens including oxaliplatin or irinotecan are associated with an objective response rate of 40–60% and a complete response rate of 5–10%.

Additionally, in a significant proportion of patients in whom a partial response is obtained, some of the metastases may be rendered undetectable on imaging. In these cases, it may be difficult for the surgeon to subsequently detect and remove all the initial metastases. At pathological analysis, metastatic sites which had apparently undergone a complete response on imaging criteria (RECIST) after neoadjuvant chemotherapy still had viable tumor in more than 80% of sites [34]. This may be a major problem for patients with resectable CRLM. These patients should be referred to the surgeon by the medical oncologist before the radiological disappearance of metastases.

MULTIDISCIPLINARY STRATEGIES TO IMPROVE RESECTABILITY

Conversion chemotherapy

Advances made by chemotherapy have been the major determinant of new therapeutic approaches concerning primarily unresectable patients. Bismuth and colleagues published the first large series of resections of initially unresectable CRLMs after induction chemotherapy. The 5-year OS rate after resection was 40%, which is comparable to that of liver resection for primarily resectable CRLMs [35]. It has been shown that in patients with unresectable CRLMs the response rate correlates with the rate of secondary resection [21]. This direct relationship between tumor response and resectability supports the strategy of using the most active regimens, particularly in patients with liver-limited metastases. In a recent systematic review, the response rate to chemotherapy in patients with unresectable CRLM was in the range of 43–79%, leading to an R0 resection rate of 23% in patients with initially unresectable disease [36]. This high secondary resectability rate was likely related to the high rate of patients with unresectable liver-only disease. These results were consistent with those of modern chemotherapy using a combination of irinotecan and oxaliplatin-based regimens, with or without cetuximab or bevacizumab. First-line chemotherapy regimens that include oxaliplatin or irinotecan in prospective randomized controlled trials have yielded response rates of 36–66% [37,38]. The addition of newly targeted molecular therapies (cetuximab, panitumumab or bevacizumab) has led to further improvements in response rates. Cetuximab added to oxaliplatin or irinotecan regimens appears to increase the response rate to 68% in randomized controlled trials [23,39]. The addition of bevacizumab to combined oxaliplatin and irinotecan regimens also increased the response rate to 65% in one phase III study [38].

Tumor ablation

In many patients with isolated CRLMs, resection of the metastases cannot result in adequate clearance of all tumor tissue from the liver. This may be the case because of either the number or location of metastases. Examples are patients with diffuse bilobar disease or with unresectable recurrence after previous liver surgery. In order to increase treatment options for patients with truly unresectable CRLMs, there is growing interest in ablative technologies, such as radiofrequency ablation (RFA) for localized tumor destruction. However, there remains a lack of clarity surrounding the role of ablation in the management of metastatic CRC. The main clinical issues are the efficacy of surgical hepatic resection versus RFA for resectable tumors, RFA approaches (open, laparoscopic or percutaneous) and the utility of RFA for unresectable tumors.

From a technical point of view, ablation should be performed during the course of a surgical procedure and limited to CRLMs of less than 30 mm, located at distance from the main bile duct. A recent report comparing two independent randomized controlled trials from the EORTC showed that the local recurrence rate per lesion, in patients treated with RFA or resection, did not appear to be different (6.2% vs. 5.5%) [40]. Local recurrences of lesions treated by RFA were more frequent when metastasis size exceeded 3 cm (21.4%). Percutaneous RFA procedures showed a much higher local recurrence rate, even in smaller metastases (16% for metastases ≤3 cm and 60% for metastases >5 cm). However, these results should be interpreted with caution since they were obtained with percutaneous conventional ultrasound-guided RFA which is inferior to CT-guided or magnetic resonance imaging–guided RFA (Figure 34.3).

The current consensus is that ablation should not be used as an alternative to resection but rather combined with it, in order to increase the chances of complete tumor clearance. Intraoperative ablation (whatever the source of energy used) is a real surgical procedure which must be performed by the surgeon who should have a good expertise in the use of intraoperative ultrasound and should know the technique for good needle placement under US guidance. Indeed, intraoperative ablation is a pragmatic non-anatomical concept, with a high propensity to spare healthy parenchyma. Combined ablation and resection (CARe) [41] is an option for patients in whom complete surgical resection is not possible. Taking advantage of the ability of liver-sparing ablations to destroy small metastases, and to best use resections for removal of large metastases, this is a rational de-escalating approach compared to more extensive hepatectomy. Furthermore, the positive impact of RFA on long-term outcomes has been independently demonstrated by two high-quality prospective studies. The EORTC CLOCC study compared systemic chemotherapy versus systemic chemotherapy plus RFA for patients with technically unresectable liver-limited disease [42]. Three-year DFS was improved in the combined RFA and chemotherapy arm (27.6% vs. 10%, $p = 0.025$) with a trend toward improved OS (median 45.3 months vs. 40.5, $p = 0.22$). In the French ARF 2003 single-arm phase II study, 52 patients with unresectable liver-limited disease were treated with a combined RFA and resection strategy [43]. One-year local DFS was 46% (95% CI 32–59) while 5-year OS was 43% (95% CI 21–64), demonstrating that RFA and resection can lead to good long-term survival.

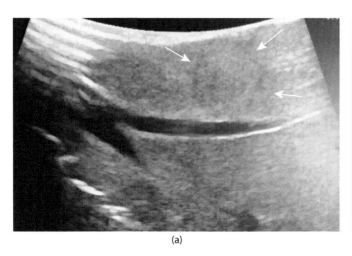
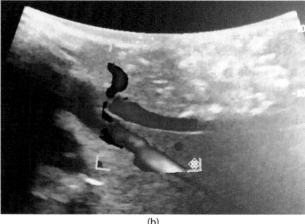

(a)   (b)

Figure 34.3 **(a)** A 2 cm colorectal metastasis, segment 7, beside the right hepatic vein. **(b)** After ablation (200 W), the metastasis appears to be hyperechoic. The coloured Doppler shows a persistent flow in the hepatic vein.

Portal vein embolization and staged resection

Resection of CRLM may lead to severe postoperative liver failure if the functional reserve of the future remnant liver (FRL) is too small. Two-stage hepatectomy (TSH) has been described to achieve curative resection in a selected group of patients with multiple bilobar CRLMs in whom complete resection could not have been achieved with a single procedure [44]. The current approach combines portal vein embolization (PVE) and tumor clearance of the FRL, followed by major resection when the FRL has achieved sufficient size. Tumor clearance of the non-embolized hemi-liver is undertaken before the application of PVE to avoid the risk of stimulating tumor growth [45]. PVE of one side of the liver leads to atrophy of the ipsilateral liver lobe and to compensatory hypertrophy of the contralateral liver lobe. It is indicated when the percentage of FRL is between 25% and 40% depending on its functional capacity and the duration of preoperative chemotherapy. The mean hypertrophy rate of the FRL is around 38%, in 2 to 4 weeks.

Contraindication of surgery directly related to PVE is rare (3.9%); insufficiency of the hypertrophic response, a technically unsuccessful procedure or complications leading to unresectability account for 2.8%, 0.7% and 0.4%, respectively [46]. In a recent systematic review of TSH in patients with initially unresectable CRLMs [47] postoperative morbidity and mortality after the first stage of TSH were 17% and 0.5%, respectively. PVE was used in 76% of patients. Ultimately, 352 of the initial 459 (77%) patients underwent the second stage of TSH. Major liver resection was undertaken in 84% of patients; the negative margin (R0) resection rate was 75%. Postoperative morbidity and mortality after the second stage of TSH were 40% and 3%, respectively. Median OS was 37 months in patients who completed both stages of TSH. The 3-year DFS rate was 20%. In patients who did not complete both stages of TSH, median survival was 16 months. These results have been confirmed by a recent

randomized controlled trial assessing prevention of perihepatic adhesions in patients with unresectable CRLM treated with TSH [48]. Further prospective controlled studies are required to better define criteria for the selection of patients for TSH and the exact roles of preoperative and interval chemotherapy and PVE.

Recently, associating liver partition and portal vein ligation for staged hepatectomy (ALPPS) has been increasingly used for extended right hepatectomy with marginal FRL. It is a two-stage procedure, for which a right portal vein ligation and a parenchymal transection are undertaken during the first stage. It induces more hypertrophy of the FRL (median 74%) in less time (median 9 days) than PVE [49]. The feasibility of the technique has been demonstrated, but the 90-day mortality remains as high as 11% and grade IIIa or higher complications occur in 44% of patients. Furthermore, data on oncologic long-term outcomes are missing [50]. This technique is still under investigation; analysis of registry data but also a randomized controlled trial of ALPPS versus TSH for CRLM should be undertaken.

SURGICAL MANAGEMENT OF SYNCHRONOUS CRLMs

The management of CRC with synchronous metastases is multimodal, including chemotherapy, radiotherapy for rectal primaries, local tumor ablation such as RFA and surgery. The use of systemic chemotherapy as the initial step allows immediate treatment of the liver disease, which is recognized as the most likely cause of patient death. The high response rates reported after first-line chemotherapy [36] support the concept of withholding surgery and selecting a biological cohort likely to benefit from surgery, avoiding aggressive treatment in patients most likely to benefit from palliative management only. The surgical strategy may be somewhat more difficult and there is still no consensus on the ideal management sequence. The need for surgical management of the two different tumor sites renders the combination of these modalities particularly complex regarding sequencing. Three approaches have been shaped regarding appropriate timing of surgical resection of primary and metastatic tumors.

In the 'classical' (or 'primary' first) approach, the primary is resected first and LM in a second operation [51]. The rationale is that the primary neoplasm should be managed first because it is the source of both further metastases and potential complications, including intestinal obstruction, perforation or bleeding. Its main drawback is the risk that CRLM may become unresectable during treatment of the primary tumor, especially if postoperative complications are encountered. In the 'simultaneous' approach, both resections are done in the same procedure. Its potential benefits include a single operation with an overall reduction in the total hospital length of stay [52]. In contrast to the classical approach, this approach may increase the complexity of the surgical procedure and the length of the operation, raising concern on safety and the long-term outcomes. In the 'liver-first' (or 'reverse') approach resection of LM precedes that of the primary tumor [53]. The aim of this approach is to avoid the possible risks of a combined procedure, at the same time avoiding the risks of delayed liver resection.

A recent systematic review suggested that none of the three surgical strategies (classical primary first, liver first or simultaneous resection) is inferior to the others [54]. All should be considered for patients with synchronous CRLM, with the exception of those with symptomatic primaries, in whom the liver-first approach is not suitable. None of the approaches has demonstrated better short- or long-term outcomes, and no subgroups of patients who would clearly benefit from a particular approach have been recognized.

RESULTS

Survival

It is estimated that 20% to 30% of patients with CRLMs are potential candidates for resection. Resection of isolated LM may substantially improve long-term outcomes [55]. Furthermore, recent published phase III chemotherapy trials in patients with previously untreated metastatic CRC have demonstrated substantial improvements in overall survival, with median OS times now ranging between 25 and 30 months with combination regimens [38,39]. As a result, the definition of resectable LM has changed over time, now focusing on the resection of all visible LMs while preserving at least a 20% to 25% liver remnant with adequate vascular supply and biliary drainage, with the expectation that such a resection would render the patient free of radiologically evident disease [56].

Despite the lack of randomized trial evidence, retrospective large-scale or population-based studies in patients who undergo complete surgical resection demonstrated the long-term survival benefit of hepatectomy for patients with resectable disease compared with those not undergoing liver surgery. Overall, the survival of patients who had LM resected is between 45% and 50% at 5 years and comparable to that of patients with stage III tumors [22,55].

Disease-free survival and tumor recurrence

The goal of hepatic surgery for CRLM should be to resect or completely ablate all LMs to provide the patient with the best chance at long-term cure. However, as the criteria for resection expand and more extensive surgeries are being performed, the incidence and pattern of recurrence following liver surgery may be altered. More than one-half of resected patients develop recurrence within 2 years. The patterns of failure are distributed relatively equally among intrahepatic, extrahepatic and intra- plus extrahepatic sites. In a recent cohort, DFS was 69.2% at 1 year and 30.0% at 5 years following curative intent surgery, the median DFS being 23.0 months [57]. The combination of modern chemotherapy with advances in surgical techniques has resulted in improvements in OS, but the actual overall rate of recurrence following curative intent surgery remains high (60% to 70%). Rather than decreasing recurrence rates, modern era multimodality curative intent therapy for CRLM appears to simply prolong the time to recurrence. Factors associated with a shorter DFS include rectum as the primary tumor site, primary tumor lymph node metastases, and synchronous presentation of primary tumor with hepatic metastases. The cumulative 5-year risk of intrahepatic recurrence is 50% to 55%. It appears to be highest over the first 3 years following surgery and subsequently reaches a plateau. It is influenced by margin status (R0 vs. R1 resection) as well as use of radiofrequency ablation, but not by the size and number of liver metastases. The cumulative 5-year risk of extrahepatic recurrence is 60% and continues to increase over time. It is influenced by more aggressive biologic factors such as primary tumor lymph node metastases, number of hepatic metastases greater than four and hepatic metastasis tumor size more than 5 cm.

LIVER METASTASES FROM NON-COLORECTAL AND NON-NEUROENDOCRINE PRIMARY TUMORS

The benefit of resection for non-colorectal, non-neuroendocrine (NCNN) LM remains unproven. Numerous studies, particularly in the last 15 years, have suggested that highly selected patients can have long-term survival after liver resection. However, in patients with technically resectable liver metastases, selection of patients for operation is difficult, complex and remains imperfect. Furthermore, the specific survival benefit of liver resection for NCNN metastases is difficult to differentiate from that of medical therapy, or from the natural history of the disease. Consideration must be given to the location of the primary tumor, biologic behaviour of the tumor (disease-free interval, tumor burden), presence of EHD (and whether it is resectable) and response of the tumor to systemic therapy. It is important to emphasize that, in general, liver resection in this setting is not curative, but instead may be life prolonging. Series that describe a collection of all types of NCNN LMs report a 3-year survival rate after resection between 30% and 45%, and a 5-year survival between 10% and 37% [58,59]. The most common primary tumor sites across these series are breast (25%), genitourinary (25%; testicular, ovarian, uterine, renal, adrenal and bladder), digestive tract (18%, including gastric, esophageal, duodenal, pancreatic and small bowel) and melanoma (9%; cutaneous and ocular). The remaining primary tumors (23%) include sarcoma (including gastrointestinal stromal tumors), head and neck, lung and LM from unknown primary tumor. The location of the primary tumor appears prognostically important. In a series of 1452 patients resected for NCNN liver metastases, patients were separated into three prognostic groups according to their primary tumor location [60]. Group 1 had a 5-year survival of more than 30% and comprised primaries of the breast and genitourinary system, as well as small bowel and ampullary tumors. Group 2 had 5-year survival between 15% and 30%, and included other foregut tumors (gastric, duodenal and exocrine pancreatic) and melanoma (cutaneous and uveal). Group 3 had a 5-year survival of less than 15% and comprised pulmonary, esophageal and head and neck tumors.

Data on individual histologic subtypes frequently come from small case series. Therefore, defining benefits of liver resection for individual patients is difficult. The best results have been achieved with LMs from genitourinary tumors, in particular from testicular germ-cell tumors where hepatic resection is performed to remove residual disease after induction chemotherapy [61]. For breast cancer, although LMs are frequent, resection is rarely indicated because it generally reflects disseminated disease. Several small series, however, report results of resection of these metastases in a highly selected group of patients with 5-year OS rates of over 25% [62]. A long interval between the primary tumor and liver recurrence as well as a negative lymph node status at the time of the primary tumor, hormone receptor positivity and response to preoperative chemotherapy are related to long-term survival. It should be emphasized that the available literature is scarce and the results concern a very small percentage of the total amount of metastatic breast cancer patients. For these reasons a conservative approach still seems most appropriate.

A recent case-controlled study found no difference between observation and resection for patients with NCNN gastrointestinal primaries [63]. This is consistent with most series that report poor long-term survival after resection for NCNN gastrointestinal LM. For gastric cancer, several Japanese series report more favorable results. In a selected group of patients with LMs from gastric cancer, 3-year survival after resection of LMs was close to 30%. Patients with a primary tumor not involving the serosa, and solitary and metachronous metastases of less than 5 cm, showed the best survival [64].

For sarcoma LMs, 5-year survival rates after resection vary between 15% and 20%. Even in patients with EHD at the time of liver resection, surgery may be considered, provided that complete removal of both liver and extrahepatic tumor is judged possible [65].

In melanoma patients, LMs are usually a marker of systemic disseminated disease and long-term survival after resection is rare [66]. Ocular melanoma often selectively metastasizes to the liver. Solitary liver lesions in ocular melanoma are, however, rare. A solitary liver lesion diagnosed in a patient with ocular melanoma often appears to be a precursor of more widespread liver disease in the near future, but resection may be possible in highly selected cases [67].

In conclusion, NCNN LMs generally indicate disseminated disease. Only in a highly selected group of patients may surgery be indicated and improve survival.

REFERENCES

1. Haggar FA, Boushey RP. Colorectal cancer epidemiology: incidence, mortality, survival, and risk factors. *Clin Colon Rectal Surg* 2009;22:191–197.
2. Hackl C, Neumann P, Gerken M, Loss M, Klinkhammer-Schalke M, Schlitt HJ. Treatment of colorectal liver metastases in Germany: a ten-year population-based analysis of 5772 cases of primary colorectal adenocarcinoma. *BMC Cancer* 2014;14:810.
3. Young PE, Womeldorph CM, Johnson EK, et al. Early detection of colorectal cancer recurrence in patients undergoing surgery with curative intent: current status and challenges. *J Cancer* 2014;5:262–271.
4. Jeffery M, Hickey BE, Hider PN. Follow-up strategies for patients treated for non-metastatic colorectal cancer. *Cochrane Database Syst Rev* 2007;CD002200.
5. Spolverato G, Ejaz A, Azad N, Pawlik TM. Surgery for colorectal liver metastases: the evolution of determining prognosis. *World J Gastrointest Oncol* 2013;5:207–221.
6. Fong Y, Fortner J, Sun RL, Brennan MF, Blumgart LH. Clinical score for predicting recurrence after hepatic resection for metastatic colorectal cancer: analysis of 1001 consecutive cases. *Ann Surg* 1999;230:309–318.
7. Hwang M, Jayakrishnan TT, Green DE, et al. Systematic review of outcomes of patients undergoing resection for colorectal liver metastases in the setting of extra hepatic disease. *Eur J Cancer* 2014;50:1747–1757.
8. de Haas RJ, Wicherts DA, Flores E, Azoulay D, Castaing D, Adam R. R1 resection by necessity for colorectal liver metastases: is it still a contraindication to surgery? *Ann Surg* 2008;248:626–637.
9. Adam R, Pascal G, Castaing D, et al. Tumor progression while on chemotherapy: a contraindication to liver resection for multiple colorectal metastases? *Ann Surg* 2004;240:1052–1061.

10. Blazer DG III, Kishi Y, Maru DM, et al. Pathologic response to preoperative chemotherapy: a new outcome end point after resection of hepatic colorectal metastases. *J Clin Oncol* 2008;26:5344–5351.

11. Neal CP, Garcea G, Doucas H, et al. Molecular prognostic markers in resectable colorectal liver metastases: a systematic review. *Eur J Cancer* 2006;42:1728–1743.

12. Adams RB, Aloia TA, Loyer E, Pawlik TM, Taouli B, Vauthey JN. Selection for hepatic resection of colorectal liver metastases: expert consensus statement. *HPB (Oxford)* 2013;15:91–103.

13. Floriani I, Torri V, Rulli E, et al. Performance of imaging modalities in diagnosis of liver metastases from colorectal cancer: a systematic review and meta-analysis. *J Magn Reson Imaging* 2010;31:19–31.

14. Lesurtel M, Selzner M, Petrowsky H, McCormack L, Clavien PA. How should transection of the liver be performed? A prospective randomized study in 100 consecutive patients: comparing four different transection strategies. *Ann Surg* 2005;242:814–22, discussion.

15. Farges O, Goutte N, Bendersky N, Falissard B. Incidence and risks of liver resection: an all-inclusive French nationwide study. *Ann Surg* 2012;256:697–704.

16. Spolverato G, Ejaz A, Hyder O, Kim Y, Pawlik TM. Failure to rescue as a source of variation in hospital mortality after hepatic surgery. *Br J Surg* 2014;101:836–846.

17. Virani S, Michaelson JS, Hutter MM, et al. Morbidity and mortality after liver resection: results of the patient safety in surgery study. *J Am Coll Surg* 2007;204:1284–1292.

18. Matsuda A, Matsumoto S, Seya T, et al. Does postoperative complication have a negative impact on long-term outcomes following hepatic resection for colorectal liver metastasis? A meta-analysis. *Ann Surg Oncol* 2013;20:2485–2492.

19. Tzeng CW, Vauthey JN. Postoperative complications and oncologic outcomes after resection of colorectal liver metastases: the importance of staying on track. *Ann Surg Oncol* 2013;20:2457–2459.

20. Adam R, Delvart V, Pascal G, et al. Rescue surgery for unresectable colorectal liver metastases downstaged by chemotherapy: a model to predict long-term survival. *Ann Surg* 2004;240:644–657.

21. Folprecht G, Grothey A, Alberts S, Raab HR, Kohne CH. Neoadjuvant treatment of unresectable colorectal liver metastases: correlation between tumour response and resection rates. *Ann Oncol* 2005;16:1311–1319.

22. Morris EJ, Forman D, Thomas JD, et al. Surgical management and outcomes of colorectal cancer liver metastases. *Br J Surg* 2010;97:1110–1118.

23. Folprecht G, Gruenberger T, Bechstein WO, et al. Tumour response and secondary resectability of colorectal liver metastases following neoadjuvant chemotherapy with cetuximab: the CELIM randomised phase 2 trial. *Lancet Oncol* 2010;11:38–47.

24. Jones RP, Vauthey JN, Adam R, et al. Effect of specialist decision-making on treatment strategies for colorectal liver metastases. *Br J Surg* 2012;99:1263–1269.

25. Wicherts DA, de Haas RJ, Salloum C, et al. Repeat hepatectomy for recurrent colorectal metastases. *Br J Surg* 2013;100:808–818.

26. Kemeny N, Huang Y, Cohen AM, et al. Hepatic arterial infusion of chemotherapy after resection of hepatic metastases from colorectal cancer. *N Engl J Med* 1999;341:2039–2048.

27. Nelson R, Freels S. Hepatic artery adjuvant chemotherapy for patients having resection or ablation of colorectal cancer metastatic to the liver. *Cochrane Database Syst Rev* 2006;CD003770.

28. Mitry E, Fields AL, Bleiberg H, et al. Adjuvant chemotherapy after potentially curative resection of metastases from colorectal cancer: a pooled analysis of two randomized trials. *J Clin Oncol* 2008;26:4906–4911.

29. Ychou M, Hohenberger W, Thezenas S, et al. A randomized phase III study comparing adjuvant 5-fluorouracil/folinic acid with FOLFIRI in patients following complete resection of liver metastases from colorectal cancer. *Ann Oncol* 2009;20:1964–1970.

30. Nordlinger B, Sorbye H, Glimelius B, et al. Perioperative chemotherapy with FOLFOX4 and surgery versus surgery alone for resectable liver metastases from colorectal cancer (EORTC Intergroup trial 40983): a randomised controlled trial. *Lancet* 2008;371:1007–1016.

31. Nordlinger B, Sorbye H, Glimelius B, et al. Perioperative FOLFOX4 chemotherapy and surgery versus surgery alone for resectable liver metastases from colorectal cancer (EORTC 40983): long-term results of a randomised, controlled, phase 3 trial. *Lancet Oncol* 2013;14:1208–1215.

32. Robinson SM, Wilson CH, Burt AD, Manas DM, White SA. Chemotherapy-associated liver injury in patients with colorectal liver metastases: a systematic review and meta-analysis. *Ann Surg Oncol* 2012;19:4287–4299.

33. Morris-Stiff G, Tan YM, Vauthey JN. Hepatic complications following preoperative chemotherapy with oxaliplatin or irinotecan for hepatic colorectal metastases. *Eur J Surg Oncol* 2008;34:609–614.

34. Benoist S, Brouquet A, Penna C, et al. Complete response of colorectal liver metastases after chemotherapy: does it mean cure? *J Clin Oncol* 2006;24:3939–3945.

35. Bismuth H, Adam R, Levi F, et al. Resection of nonresectable liver metastases from colorectal cancer after neoadjuvant chemotherapy. *Ann Surg* 1996;224:509–520.

36. Lam VW, Spiro C, Laurence JM, et al. A systematic review of clinical response and survival outcomes of downsizing systemic chemotherapy and rescue liver surgery in patients with initially unresectable colorectal liver metastases. *Ann Surg Oncol* 2012;19:1292–1301.

37. Ychou M, Rivoire M, Thezenas S, et al. A randomized phase II trial of three intensified chemotherapy regimens in first-line treatment of colorectal cancer patients with initially unresectable or not optimally resectable liver metastases. The METHEP trial. *Ann Surg Oncol* 2013;20:4289–4297.

38. Loupakis F, Cremolini C, Masi G, et al. Initial therapy with FOLFOXIRI and bevacizumab for metastatic colorectal cancer. *N Engl J Med* 2014;371:1609–1618.

39. Heinemann V, von Weikersthal LF, Decker T, et al. FOLFIRI plus cetuximab versus FOLFIRI plus bevacizumab as first-line treatment for patients with metastatic colorectal cancer (FIRE-3): a randomised, open-label, phase 3 trial. *Lancet Oncol* 2014;15:1065–1075.

40. Tanis E, Nordlinger B, Mauer M, et al. Local recurrence rates after radiofrequency ablation or resection of colorectal liver metastases. Analysis of the European Organisation for Research and Treatment of Cancer #40004 and #40983. *Eur J Cancer* 2014;50:912–919.

41. Evrard S, Poston G, Kissmeyer-Nielsen P, et al. Combined ablation and resection (CARe) as an effective parenchymal sparing treatment for extensive colorectal liver metastases. *PLoS One* 2014;9:e114404.

42. Ruers T, Punt C, van CF, et al. Radiofrequency ablation combined with systemic treatment versus systemic treatment alone in patients with non-resectable colorectal liver metastases: a randomized EORTC Intergroup phase II study (EORTC 40004). *Ann Oncol* 2012;23:2619–2626.

43. Evrard S, Rivoire M, Arnaud J, et al. Unresectable colorectal cancer liver metastases treated by intra-operative radiofrequency ablation with or without resection. *Br J Surg* 2012;99:558–565.

44. Wicherts DA, Miller R, de Haas RJ, et al. Long-term results of two-stage hepatectomy for irresectable colorectal cancer liver metastases. *Ann Surg* 2008;248:994–1005.

45. Narita M, Oussoultzoglou E, Jaeck D, et al. Two-stage hepatectomy for multiple bilobar colorectal liver metastases. *Br J Surg* 2011;98:1463–1475.

46. van Lienden KP, van den Esschert JW, de Graaf W, et al. Portal vein embolization before liver resection: a systematic review. *Cardiovasc Intervent Radiol* 2013;36:25–34.

47. Lam VW, Laurence JM, Johnston E, Hollands MJ, Pleass HC, Richardson AJ. A systematic review of two-stage hepatectomy in patients with initially unresectable colorectal liver metastases. *HPB (Oxford)* 2013;15:483–491.

48. Dupre A, Lefranc A, Buc E, et al. Use of bioresorbable membranes to reduce abdominal and perihepatic adhesions in 2-stage hepatectomy of liver metastases from colorectal cancer: results of a prospective, randomized controlled phase II trial. *Ann Surg* 2013;258:30–36.

49. Schnitzbauer AA, Lang SA, Goessmann H, et al. Right portal vein ligation combined with in situ splitting induces rapid left lateral liver lobe hypertrophy enabling 2-staged extended right hepatic resection in small-for-size settings. *Ann Surg* 2012;255:405–414.

50. Schadde E, Schnitzbauer AA, Tschuor C, Raptis DA, Bechstein WO, Clavien PA. Systematic review and meta-analysis of feasibility, safety, and efficacy of a novel procedure: associating liver partition and portal vein ligation for staged hepatectomy. *Ann Surg Oncol* 2015;22:3109–3120.

51. Chua HK, Sondenaa K, Tsiotos GG, Larson DR, Wolff BG, Nagorney DM. Concurrent vs. staged colectomy and hepatectomy for primary colorectal cancer with synchronous hepatic metastases. *Dis Colon Rectum* 2004;47:1310–1316.

52. Moug SJ, Smith D, Leen E, Roxburgh C, Horgan PG. Evidence for a synchronous operative approach in the treatment of colorectal cancer with hepatic metastases: a case matched study. *Eur J Surg Oncol* 2010;36:365–370.

53. Mentha G, Majno PE, Andres A, Rubbia-Brandt L, Morel P, Roth AD. Neoadjuvant chemotherapy and resection of advanced synchronous liver metastases before treatment of the colorectal primary. *Br J Surg* 2006;93:872–878.

54. Lykoudis PM, O'Reilly D, Nastos K, Fusai G. Systematic review of surgical management of synchronous colorectal liver metastases. *Br J Surg* 2014;101:605–612.

55. Kopetz S, Chang GJ, Overman MJ, et al. Improved survival in metastatic colorectal cancer is associated with adoption of hepatic resection and improved chemotherapy. *J Clin Oncol* 2009;27:3677–3683.

56. Abdalla EK, Adam R, Bilchik AJ, Jaeck D, Vauthey JN, Mahvi D. Improving resectability of hepatic colorectal metastases: expert consensus statement. *Ann Surg Oncol* 2006;13:1271–1280.

57. De Jong MC, Pulitano C, Ribero D, et al. Rates and patterns of recurrence following curative intent surgery for colorectal liver metastasis: an international multi-institutional analysis of 1669 patients. *Ann Surg* 2009;250:440–448.

58. Tan MC, Jarnagin WR. Surgical management of non-colorectal hepatic metastasis. *J Surg Oncol* 2014;109:8–13.

59. Fitzgerald TL, Brinkley J, Banks S, Vohra N, Englert ZP, Zervos EE. The benefits of liver resection for non-colorectal, non-neuroendocrine liver metastases: a systematic review. *Langenbecks Arch Surg* 2014;399:989–1000.

60. Adam R, Chiche L, Aloia T, et al. Hepatic resection for noncolorectal nonendocrine liver metastases: analysis of 1,452 patients and development of a prognostic model. *Ann Surg* 2006;244:524–535.

61. Rivoire M, Elias D, De CF, Kaemmerlen P, Theodore C, Droz JP. Multimodality treatment of patients with liver metastases from germ cell tumors: the role of surgery. *Cancer* 2001;92:578–587.

62. Adam R, Aloia T, Krissat J, et al. Is liver resection justified for patients with hepatic metastases from breast cancer? *Ann Surg* 2006;244:897–907.

63. Slotta JE, Schuld J, Distler S, Richter S, Schilling MK, Kollmar O. Hepatic resection of non-colorectal and non-neuroendocrine liver metastases – survival benefit for patients with non-gastrointestinal primary cancers – a case-controlled study. *Int J Surg* 2014;12:163–168.

64. Takemura N, Saiura A, Koga R, et al. Long-term outcomes after surgical resection for gastric cancer liver metastasis: an analysis of 64 macroscopically complete resections. *Langenbecks Arch Surg* 2012;397:951–957.

65. DeMatteo RP, Shah A, Fong Y, Jarnagin WR, Blumgart LH, Brennan MF. Results of hepatic resection for sarcoma metastatic to liver. *Ann Surg* 2001;234:540–547.

66. Aubin JM, Rekman J, Vandenbroucke-Menu F, et al. Systematic review and meta-analysis of liver resection for metastatic melanoma. *Br J Surg* 2013;100:1138–1147.

67. Rivoire M, Kodjikian L, Baldo S, Kaemmerlen P, Negrier S, Grange JD. Treatment of liver metastases from uveal melanoma. *Ann Surg Oncol* 2005;12:422–428.

35

Renal cell carcinoma

ROGIER K VAN DER VIJGH AND THEO M DE REIJKE

INCIDENCE AND AETIOLOGY

Renal cell carcinoma (RCC) represents 2–3% of all cancers [1]. Over the last two decades there has been an annual increase in global and European incidence of about 2%. This is due to the increased detection of incidental tumours by imaging techniques such as ultrasound (US) and computed tomography (CT) and probably also due to an increase in population risk factors such as obesity [2]. Tumours diagnosed incidentally are often smaller and of lower stage and are associated with higher rates of disease-free and overall survival than symptomatic cancers [3,4]. In 2012, there were approximately 84,400 new cases of RCC and 34,700 kidney cancer-related deaths within the European Union [5]. Mortality rates for renal cell cancer have remained stable in recent decades despite the increased incidence of the disease, with much of the increase probably being due to early stage disease picked up incidentally and hence having little impact on mortality.

RCC is the most common solid lesion within the kidney and accounts for approximately 90% of all kidney malignancies. There is a 1.5–1.8:1 predominance in men over women, with a peak incidence occurring between 60 and 70 years of age [5–7].

Lifestyle factors such as tobacco use, obesity and dietary factors are the most consistently identified risk factors for RCC, accounting for about 20% and 30% of cases, respectively [8,9]. Hypertension, medication use and genetic factors have also been demonstrated to increase the risk of RCC development. One-third of patients have two or more comorbidities [7]. Family history is associated with an increased risk for RCC development, with inherited forms of RCC accounting for approximately 2–4% of cases [5,6].

In addition to the already-mentioned predisposing factors, genetic factors clearly influence the risk of RCC. The von Hippel–Lindau syndrome is the most well-known hereditary form of RCC. In patients with a first- or second-degree relative with RCC a relative risk of 2.9 to 4.8 was reported [10]. Other forms of RCC that arise from germline mutations include type 1 papillary RCC (mutated c-Met gene), chromophobe RCC (mutated Birt–Hogg–Dubé gene) and type 2 papillary carcinoma (mutated fumarate hydratase gene).

There is no role for screening, except in cases of hereditary forms of renal cell cancer and patients who have been on prolonged hemodialysis.

DIAGNOSIS AND PREOPERATIVE IMAGING

The majority of patients present asymptomatically with incidentally diagnosed cancers. The classic triad of flank pain, gross haematuria and a palpable mass is now rare accounting for only 6–10% of cases. Flank pain is most often due to haemorrhage or ureteral obstruction, but can also result from locally advanced or invasive growth. In such symptomatic cases more advanced tumour stage is usually found [11]. Increasingly renal masses are found incidentally on imaging for other reasons, which may account for up to 67% of cases [7,12]. These tumours are more likely to be organ confined and are associated with a better prognosis [5,6].

In 20–30% of cases the presenting features are those of the paraneoplastic syndrome (e.g. anaemia, fever, polycythaemia and hypertension, hypercalcaemia, liver function disturbances) which, on investigation, lead to the diagnosis of RCC. Although physical examination has a limited role in diagnosing RCC the following findings may be signs of advanced disease: palpable abdominal mass, lymphadenopathy, non-reducing varicocele and bilateral lower extremity edema.

Preoperative imaging

The role of imaging in primary treatment planning is to determine the anatomical characteristics of the tumour including its size, location and relationship with the renal pelvis and collecting system, the presence of grossly enlarged lymph nodes and also the presence of distant metastases [12]. The differential diagnosis of a renal mass includes RCC renal adenoma, oncocytoma, angiomyolipoma, urothelial carcinoma, metastatic tumour, abscess, infarct, vascular malformation or pseudotumour. In particular, oncocytomas and angiomyolipomas can mimic RCC in preoperative imaging [5,12]. Renal masses can be classified as solid or cystic. With solid masses the most important criterion to differentiate a benign from a malignant mass is radiological enhancement. To determine whether there is enhancement of a renal mass both CT and magnetic resonance imaging (MRI) can be used. Contrast-enhanced US (CEUS) can be helpful in specific cases only, especially in patients with chronic renal failure with a relative contraindication to iodinated or gadolinium contrast media [5,12]. For cystic masses the Bosniak classification is widely adopted which determines the risk of malignancy by dividing renal cysts into five categories based on their CT image appearance [13]. Based on cyst appearances (e.g. wall thickening, presence of septa) and enhancement following contrast administration the risk of a cyst being a renal cancer can be discussed with the patient to plan further management.

For staging of a renal mass routine imaging of the chest must be performed. CT is the most accurate investigation for chest staging. However, at the very least, a plain chest X-ray should be performed. A bone scan or imaging of the brain is only indicated when there are specific clinical symptoms. Bone metastases from RCC are predominantly osteolytic and therefore MRI and CT are more sensitive investigations.

In the assessment of RCC 18F-FDG PET does not appear to be superior to conventional diagnostic modalities, such as CT or MRI. However, PET may provide additional value in the detection of distant metastases, because it typically images the entire body and therefore maps regions not routinely covered by conventional diagnostic imaging in the absence of organ-specific symptoms. 18F-FDG PET also appears to be superior to conventional skeletal scintigraphy for the diagnosis of bone metastases that have an osteolytic pattern of growth, as is the case in patients with RCC [14].

Tumour biopsy

Because of the high diagnostic accuracy of CT and MRI, renal tumour biopsy is not necessary before surgery in fit patients with a long predicted life expectancy and a clearly contrast-enhancing mass. The aim of a biopsy may be to distinguish between the benign or malignant nature of a renal tumour. In addition, it may be desirable to gain more precise information about the tissue diagnosis (grade, subtype) by means of a biopsy in order to decide on further treatment (selection of systemic treatment depending on the tumour type). The manner in which the biopsy is performed (cytological or histological) is determined by the clinical question. Core needle tumour biopsy is increasingly being used, especially to obtain histology before ablative treatment, to select patients for surveillance approaches and in cases where imaging is inconclusive. Another area where biopsies are increasingly being performed is in patients with metastatic or unresectable disease where systemic treatment depends on the histological type of the tumour.

In experienced hands biopsies of solid tumours show a high diagnostic yield (78–97%), high specificity (98–100%) and sensitivity (86–100%) for the diagnosis of malignancy. Fuhrman nuclear grading on the core biopsy specimen is not very reliable, however (43–75%). For cystic masses biopsies show low diagnostic yields and should therefore not be recommended. The incidence of symptomatic complications is low, with spontaneous resolving perinephric or subcapsular haematoma and haematuria as the most frequent complication. Only a small proportion of complications (<2%) require any form of intervention [5]. Also, needle tract seeding appears to be very rare [6].

Histological subtypes

Three major subtypes of RCC are important in clinical practice: clear cell, papillary (type 1 and 2) and chromophobe (Table 35.1).

Clear-cell RCC accounts for 80–90% of all RCCs and holds the worst prognosis compared to chromophobe and papillary subtype [15]. Five-year cancer-specific survival (CSS) rates are about 71% (69–73) in surgically treated patients. CSS varies with TNM stage, with 5-year CSS in T1 of 91% and in T4 of only 32%.

Papillary RCC accounts for 6–15% of all RCCs. It shows trisomies of chromosomes 7 and 17 and the loss of chromosome Y. There are two different subtypes based on histopathological criteria: the basophil phenotype (subtype 1)

Table 35.1 WHO classification 2004 for renal cell carcinomas

Subtype	Relative frequency (%)
Clear-cell RCC (synonym: common or conventional RCC)	80 (50–85)
Multilocular cystic clear-cell RCC	5
Papillary RCC	11
Chromophobe RCC	4
Collecting duct carcinoma (Bellini)	0.5
Renal medullary carcinoma	Rare
Tubulocystic carcinoma	Rare
Mucinous tubular and spindle cell carcinoma	Rare
Follicular RCC	Rare
RCC, unclassified	1.4
Translocation-linked RCC	Rare
Neuroblastoma-associated RCC	Rare

Table 35.2 Fuhrman grading system

Grade	Frequency (%)	Definition
1	10–15	Round, uniform nuclei, diameter ~10 mm, with small or absent nucleoli
2	35–55	Few irregular nuclear contours, diameter ~15 mm, nucleoli visible at 400×
3	25–35	Moderate to severely irregular nuclear contours, diameter ~20 mm, with large nucleoli visible at 100×
4	5–15	Similar to grade 3 with multilobular or bizarre polymorphic nuclei with irregular chromatin

has a better prognosis than the eosinophil phenotype (subtype 2). Exophytic growth, pseudonecrotic changes and pseudocapsule are typical signs of papillary RCC subtype 1. Ten-year survival rates of 80% versus 59% have been reported for subtypes 1 and 2, respectively, but a multivariate analysis has suggested that the difference was primarily a result of a higher tumour stage and nuclear grade in the subtype 2 group [16].

Chromophobe RCC accounts for 2–5% of all RCCs. It typically shows loss of chromosomes 2, 10, 13, 17 and 21. It has a relatively good prognosis with 5-year CSS rates of 93%, and 10-year CSS rates of 88.9% [5].

A relatively poor prognosis was found for patients who had unclassified RCC (5-year survival 24%), a sarcomatoid component (5-year survival 14.5–35%) or collecting duct carcinoma [17]. The presence of a focal sarcomatoid component appears to be an independent negative prognostic factor, independent of histopathological subtype, stage and grade, although a correlation with higher stage and grade has been reported. The presence of rhabdoid features is associated with a higher tumour stage and grade as well as an unfavourable prognosis, although it is not associated with a specific subtype of RCC.

Tumour grading

There is a clear relationship between grade and prognosis; the 5-year survival rates for Fuhrman grades G1, G2, G3, and G4 (see Table 35.2) were 94%, 86%, 59% and 31%, respectively [18].

Tumour staging

The prognostic value of the latest TNM edition for staging of RCC (see Table 35.3) has been confirmed in both single- and multi-institution studies [5].

For determination of prognosis anatomical, histological and clinical factors are considered. The anatomical factors (tumour size, venous invasion, renal capsular invasion, adrenal involvement, lymph node and distant metastasis) are embedded in the TNM classification. Higher stage correlates with worse survival rates [5]. Besides the TNM classification RENAL and PADUA criteria are additional methods to describe the anatomy of RCC in more detail [5,19,20].

Clinical factors include patient performance status, localized symptoms, cachexia, anaemia and platelet count [5].

SURGERY FOR PRIMARY OPERABLE CANCER

The current evidence suggests that localized (T1) renal tumours can best be managed by nephron-sparing surgery (NSS), irrespective of the surgical approach. Radical nephrectomy is associated with increased mortality from any cause and is an independent risk factor for new-onset chronic kidney disease, whereas CSS rates are comparable between partial and radical nephrectomy [5,6]. In deciding which tumour is suitable for a partial nephrectomy, radiological scoring systems, like RENAL and PADUA scores, can be helpful [19,20]. For T2 tumours and localized renal masses not suitable for NSS, laparoscopic radical nephrectomy is preferred over open radical nephrectomy. Laparoscopic radical nephrectomy is associated with a lower morbidity than open surgery, as oncological outcomes are equivalent [5].

Lymph node dissection and adrenalectomy

The role of lymph node dissection (LND) in RCC is still controversial. Blom and colleagues performed the only prospective randomized phase III trial to evaluate the potential benefit of extensive lymphadenectomy in patients with N0

Table 35.3 TNM classification (2010) of renal cell carcinoma

T: Primary tumour

TX	Primary tumour cannot be assessed
T0	No evidence of primary tumour
T1	Tumour 7 cm or less in greatest dimension, limited to the kidney
T1a	Tumour 4 cm or less
T1b	Tumour more than 4 cm but not more than 7 cm
T2	Tumour more than 7 cm in greatest dimension, limited to the kidney
T2a	Tumour more than 7 cm but not more than 10 cm
T2b	Tumour more than 10 cm, limited to the kidney
T3	Tumour extends into major veins or perinephric tissues but not into the ipsilateral adrenal gland and not beyond Gerota fascia
T3a	Tumour grossly extends into the renal vein or its segmental (muscle-containing) branches, or tumour invades perirenal or renal sinus fat (peripelvic) but not beyond Gerota fascia
T3b	Tumour grossly extends into vena cava below diaphragm
T3c	Tumour grossly extends into vena cava above the diaphragm or invades the wall of the vena cava
T4	Tumour invades beyond Gerota fascia (including contiguous extension into the ipsilateral adrenal gland)

N: Regional lymph nodes

NX	Regional lymph nodes cannot be assessed
N0	No regional lymph node metastasis
N1	Metastasis in a single regional lymph node
N2	Metastasis in more than one regional lymph node

M: Distant

M0	No distant metastasis
M1	Distant metastasis

and M0 disease [21]. After a median follow-up of 5 years, only 17% of patients developed progressive disease or died; rates of progression and survival were similar in both treatment groups. The long-term data showed no difference in survival between patients with or without extensive lymphadenectomy [22]. In patients with localized disease without clinical evidence of lymph node metastases, no survival advantage of an LND in conjunction with a radical nephrectomy was demonstrated. If there are clinical signs of enlarged lymph nodes, in patients with localized disease, the survival benefit of an LND is unclear. An LND for staging purposes can be considered in these cases.

Ipsilateral adrenalectomy during radical or partial nephrectomy does not provide a survival advantage [23]. Therefore, adrenalectomy should only be performed when there are intra-operative or radiological signs of adrenal involvement or in the case of upper pole renal tumours.

Patients who undergo adrenalectomy for adrenal metastases typically have a very poor prognosis, as most of these patients already have distant metastases [24].

Tumour thrombus

A tumour thrombus in the inferior vena cava (IVC) which in some cases may even extend into the right atrium (4–10% of cases) is a significant adverse prognostic factor. In non-metastatic disease, low-quality data suggest that the tumour thrombus should be excised if the performance status of the patient allows it. The 5-year survival rate for patients with RCC and a tumour thrombus in the IVC is 47–72% for non-metastatic patients and 0–20% for metastatic patients [25]. There is no evidence to support one surgical approach over another. Neither is there any high-level evidence that adjunctive preoperative procedures, like tumour embolization or placement of an IVC filter, offer any benefits. Evidently, these patients should be treated in specialized centres with cardiopulmonary surgery support.

Alternatives to surgery

Alternatives to surgery include active surveillance (AS) and ablative techniques (e.g. cryoablation and radiofrequency ablation [RFA]). In those cases where a small tumour is detected, there is a considerable chance (up to >25%) that the tumour is benign [26]. Active surveillance is defined as the initial monitoring of tumour size by serial abdominal imaging (US, CT or MRI) with delayed intervention reserved for those tumours that show clinical progression during follow-up. Elderly and comorbid patients with incidentally detected small renal masses have relatively low RCC-specific mortality and a significant competing other cause mortality. Furthermore, AS cohorts show that the growth rate of small renal masses is low and progression to metastatic disease is rare (1–2%) [5,6]. It has to be noted that there are no validated AS protocols yet and not all patients undergo tumour biopsy before inclusion in AS studies. Therefore, AS data are likely to be biased by observing benign tumours as well. As a result of the above-mentioned reasons AS should be discussed with elderly or comorbid patients with a limited life expectancy.

Only low quality of evidence is available about the oncological outcomes and morbidity of RFA and cryoablation treatment. Both techniques can be performed percutaneously or laparoscopically with probably similar results. When compared to partial nephrectomy low-quality data show a tendency toward a higher local recurrence rate for minimal invasive therapies [5,6]. Cryoablation and RFA treatment can be discussed with elderly and comorbid patients with small renal masses (<4 cm) and a limited life expectancy.

Embolization

If a patient has an inoperable or metatstatic renal tumour transarterial embolization can be performed to palliate serious haematuria. Seldomly, preoperative embolization is indicated in order to reduce vascularization of the kidney, because a hilar tumour could jeopardize early arterial ligation. The benefit is, however, not proven and controversial, because it has never clearly been proven that subsequent radical nephrectomy is easier. About 43% of patients experience a post-infarct or post-embolization syndrome, which is characterized by fever, local pain and malaise; these symptoms resolve spontaneously after approximately 36–48 h.

NEOADJUVANT AND ADJUVANT THERAPIES

Several adverse prognostic factors have been identified following radical nephrectomy based on the TNM system, clinical factors and also molecular markers. Based on three randomized trials, there is, however, no evidence that adjuvant therapy improves survival after nephrectomy, using different treatment strategies of immunotherapeutic approaches, e.g. interferon-alpha (IFN-α), interleukin-2 (IL-2), a combination of the two and tumour vaccines [27–30]. Several phase III randomized controlled trial (RCTs) of adjuvant treatment with tyrosine kinase inhibitors (e.g. sunitinib, sorafenib, pazopanib, axitinib and everolimus) are ongoing, but results are still awaited. It remains questionable if these will show any advantage in adjuvant treatment in resectable renal tumours.

Adjuvant radiotherapy following nephrectomy has also not been shown to provide any advantage in terms of local disease control or survival [31].

Follow-up

Follow-up for RCC is done to detect recurrent or metastatic disease (predominantly lung, liver and bone) at an early stage, because surgical resection is still the best treatment option if feasible. Check-ups are based on initial tumour characteristics and depend on type of treatment (e.g. AS, ablative treatment and surgical resection, either partial or complete resection). Follow-up investigations include local imaging to check the operated kidney if a partial nephrectomy was performed, and chest CT or conventional X-ray should exclude the presence of distant metastases. Metastases can present at very unusual locations and patients should be instructed to report unusual manifestations. Besides investigating for tumour recurrence also laboratory checks (creatinine, liver function tests, alkaline phosphatase and calcium) and blood pressure measurement should be performed regularly. The schedule for follow-up is individualized based on initial tumour characteristics, age and comorbidity. The usual follow-up lasts 5 to 10 years.

METASTATIC DISEASE

Cytoreductive nephrectomy

In locally advanced or metastatic disease curative treatment is only possible if surgery can excise all tumour deposits. Data suggest that this can even be achieved in patients with single- or oligo-metastatic resectable disease. For most patients though, cytoreductive nephrectomy is palliative, and systemic treatment is necessary. Two trials investigated if there was a benefit of cytoreductive surgery. The SWOG 8949 and EORTC-GU 30947 randomized metastatic patients to IFN-α treatment only and radical tumour nephrectomy followed by IFN-α. Overall survival was 3 months longer in patients who received combination therapy (average survival 11 months vs. 8 months) [32,33]. Data suggest that there is an increased long-time survival for patients treated with IFN-α and cytoreductive nephrectomy compared to IFN-α treatment alone. There are no data available yet about cytoreductive nephrectomy combined with tyrosine kinase inhibitors, but two trials are underway investigating the combination with sunitinib.

In the case of metastatic disease, compressing the spinal cord, or in the case of an osteolytic defect, direct surgical decompression and stabilization is the preferred treatment followed by radiation.

Brain metastases are resected if technically feasible, but in the case of multiple lesions irradiation of the whole brain or stereotactic radiation is advised.

Systemic therapy

RCC is resistant to most forms of chemotherapy (except the very aggressive Bellini duct carcinoma) because of high levels of the multi-drug resistance protein P-glycoprotein. At this moment no effective chemotherapeutic agents are available.

Systemic treatment options for RCC include immunotherapy, drugs that target vascular endothelial growth factor (VEGF) and mammalian target of rapamycin (mTOR). To decide which drug, or combination of drugs, is the appropriate first-line treatment tumours should be categorized in high, intermediate or low risk by the Memorial Sloan Kettering Cancer Center criteria (MSKCC), also called the Motzer criteria [34]. Variables prior to treatment that were shown to be associated with short survival in a multivariate analysis were:

- Karnofsky performance score of <80
- Serum LDH of >1.5 times the upper limit of normal
- Low haemoglobin
- Hypercalcaemia corrected for albumin
- Not having undergone a nephrectomy (this was later modified in 'interval between nephrectomy and the occurrence of metastases of 1 year or shorter')

Patients can be classified in three prognostic categories by means of these five variables. Patients with none of these factors (the group with a favourable prognosis, approximately 25% of all patients) have a median life expectancy of 20 months. Patients with one to two factors (the group with intermediate prognosis, 53% of all patients) have a median life expectancy of 10 months, while patients with three to five factors (the group with poor prognosis, 22% of

Table 35.4 Systemic treatment mRCC

RCC type	MSKCC risk group	First-line therapy[a]	Second-line therapy	Third-line therapy
Clear cell	Good or intermediate	Sunitinib IFN-α + bevacizumab pazopanib	Everolimus after prior TKI	Everolimus after prior TKI
			Sorafenib after prior cytokine therapy	
			Pazopanib after prior cytokine therapy	
	Poor	Temsirolimus		
Non-clear cell	Good	No standard		
	Intermediate	No standard		
	Poor	No standard		
Remaining non-clear cell		No standard		

Source: Escudier B, et al., *J Clin Oncol* 2009; 27: 3312–8; Hudes G, et al., *New Engl J Med* 2007; 356: 2271–81; Motzer RJ, et al., *J Clin Oncol* 2009; 27: 3584–90; Reprinted from *The Lancet*, 370, Escudier B, Pluzanska A, Koralewski P, et al., Bevacizumab plus interferon alfa-2a for treatment of metastatic renal cell carcinoma: a randomised, double-blind phase III trial, pp. 2103–11, Copyright (2007), with permission from Elsevier; Reprinted from *The Lancet*, 372, Motzer RJ, Escudier B, Oudard S, et al., Efficacy of everolimus in advanced renal cell carcinoma: a double-blind, randomised, placebo-controlled phase III trial, pp. 449–56, Copyright (2008), with permission from Elsevier; Sternberg CN, et al., *J Clin Oncol* 2010; 28: 1061–8 [35–40].

all patients) have a median life expectancy of approximately 4 months. It is important to note that reliable data about systemic treatment are available only for clear-cell RCC.

Several treatment modalities have entered into clinical practice; however, the best moment to start is still not known, because the progression of metastatic disease can vary.

Immunotherapy

Immunotherapy consists of treatment with IFN-α or IL-2.

IFN-α showed response rates of 6–15%. It improves survival with 3 to 5 months and reduces the risk of tumour progression with approximately 25%. These rates though seem only applicable to some patient subgroups including patients with clear-cell histology, good risk criteria as defined by the Motzer criteria and metastases only in the lung. When IFN-α is combined with either bevacizumab, sunitinib or pazopanib better response rates are reported as well as increased progression-free survival rates.

IL-2 has been used for decades in the treatment of metastatic RCC with response rates ranging from 7% to 27%. Although the optimal regimen is not yet known, long-term complete responses have been shown with high-dose bolus IL-2. Compared to IFN-α, the toxicity of IL-2 is much greater.

Drugs that target VEGF

VEGF overexpression promotes neoangiogenesis; this contributes to RCC development and progression. Multiple drugs that affect VEGF have been approved for treating metastatic RCC: sorafenib, sunitinib, bevacizumab and pazopanib. Studies established combination therapy with

IFN-α and sunitinib, bevacizumab or pazopanib as first-line treatment in patients with treatment-naïve metastatic clear-cell RCC with good- to intermediate-risk scores according to Motzer criteria (Table 35.4).

Patients with a good or intermediate prognosis after nephrectomy for metastatic clear-cell RCC should be treated with sunitinib or bevacizumab and IFN-α. An alternative is pazopanib. Given there is a difference in side effects and administration, this decision should be made on an individual basis.

Drugs that target mTOR

Everolimus and temsirolimus are the two approved drugs that inhibit mammalian target of rapamycin (mTOR). Temsirolimus showed favourable results in median overall survival (10.9 vs. 7.3 months) compared to IFN-α monotherapy as first-line treatment in high-risk metastatic RCC, according to the Motzer criteria. A combination of IFN-α and temsirolimus showed no benefit in overall survival compared to temsirolimus alone.

Everolimus is established in the treatment of VEGF-refractory disease. In this selected group median progression-free survival under everolimus treatment was 4 months compared to 1.9 months in the placebo control group.

CONCLUSION

In conclusion, first-line systemic therapy for low- to intermediate-risk metastatic RCC is IFN-α combined with either sunitinib, pazopanib or bevacuzimab. Temsirolimus showed the most favourable results in high-risk RCC patients.

REFERENCES

1. Parkin DM, Pisani P, Ferlay J. Estimates of the worldwide incidence of eighteen major cancers in 1985. *Int J Cancer* 1993; 54: 594–606.

2. Lightfoot N, Conlon M, Kreiger N, Bissett R, Desai M, Warde P, Prichard HM. Impact of noninvasive imaging on increased incidental detection of renal cell carcinoma. *Eur Urol* 2000; 37: 521–7.

3, Beisland C, Medby PC, Beisland HO. Renal cell carcinoma: gender difference in incidental detection and cancer-specific survival. *Scand J Urol* 2002; 36: 414–8.

4. Dinney CP, Awad SA, Gajewski JB, Belitsky P, Lannon SG, Mack FG, Millard OH. Analysis of imaging modalities, staging systems, and prognostic indicators for renal cell carcinoma. *Urology* 1992; 39: 122–9.

5. Ljungberg B, Bensalah K, Bex A, et al. EAU guidelines on renal cell carcinoma. *Eur Urol* 2015; 67: 913–24.

6. Novick AC, Campbell SC, Belldegrun A, et al. AUA guideline for management of the clinical stage 1 renal mass. Linthicum, MD: American Urological Association. http://www.auanet.org/common/pdf/education/clinical-guidance/Renal-Mass.pdf.

7. Laguna MP, Algaba F, Cadeddu J, et al. Current patterns of presentation and treatment of renal masses: a Clinical Research Office of the Endourological Society prospective study. *J Endourol Endourol Soc* 2014; 28: 861–70.

8. Bergstrom A, Hsieh CC, Lindblad P, Lu CM, Cook NR, Wolk A. Obesity and renal cell cancer – a quantitative review. *Br J Cancer* 2002; 85: 984–990.

9. Mellemgaard A, Engholm G, McLaughlin JK, Olsen JH. Risk factors for renal cell carcinoma in Denmark. I. Role of socioeconomic status, tobacco use, beverages, and family history. *Cancer Causes Control* 1994; 5: 105–13.

10. Gago-Dominguez M, Yuan JM, Castelao JE, Ross RK, Yu MC. Family history and risk of renal cell carcinoma. *Cancer Epidemiol Biomarkers Prev* 2001; 10: 1001–4.

11. Lee CT, Katz J, Fearn PA, Russo P. Mode of presentation of renal cell carcinoma provides prognostic information. *Urol Oncol* 2002; 7: 135–40.

12. Wagstaff PGK, Zondervan PJ, de La Rosette JJMCH, Laguna MP. The role of imaging in the active surveillance of small renal mass. *Current Urol Rep* 2014; 15: 386.

13. Israel GM, Bosniak MA. 2005. An update of the Bosniak renal cyst classification system. *Urology* 2005; 66: 484–88.

14. Aide N, Cappele O, Bottet P, et al. Efficiency of [(18) F]FDG PET in characterising renal cancer and detecting distant metastases: a comparison with CT-SCAN. *Eur J Nucl Med Mol Imaging* 2003; 30: 1236–45.

15. Cheville JC, Lohse CM, Zincke H, Weaver AL, Blute ML. Comparisons of outcome and prognostic features among histologic subtypes of renal cell carcinoma. *Am J Surg Pathol* 2003; 27: 612–24.

16. Mejean A, Hopirtean V, Bazin JP, et al. Prognostic factors for the survival of patients with papillary renal cell carcinoma: meaning of histological typing and multifocality. *J Urol* 2003; 170; 764–7.

17. Amin MB, Amin MB, Tamboli P, et al. Prognostic impact of histologic subtyping of adult renal epithelial neoplasms: an experience of 405 cases. *Am J Surg Pathol* 2002; 26: 281–91.

18. Ficarra V, Righetti R, Pilloni S, D'amico A, Maffei N, Novella G, et al. Prognostic factors in patients with renal cell carcinoma: retrospective analysis of 675 cases. *Eur Urol* 2002; 41: 190–8.

19. Ficarra V, Novara G, Secco S, et al. Preoperative aspects and dimensions used for an anatomical (PADUA) classification of renal tumours in patients who are candidates for nephron-sparing surgery. *Eur Urol* 2009; 56: 786–93.

20. Parsons RB, Canter D, Kutikov A, Uzzo RG. RENAL nephrometry scoring system: the radiologist's perspective. *Am J Roentgenol* 2012; 199: W355–59.

21. Blom JH, Van Poppel H, Marechal JM, Jacqmin D, Sylvester R. Schroder FH, De Prijck L. Radical nephrectomy with and without lymph node dissection; preliminary results of the EORTC randomized phase III protocol 30881. *Eur Urol* 1999; 36: 570–75.

22. Blom JH, van Poppel H, Maréchal JM, Jacqmin D, Schröder FH, de Prijck L, Sylvester R, EORTC Genitourinary Tract Cancer Group. Radical nephrectomy with and without lymph-node dissection: final results of European Organization for Research and Treatment of Cancer (EORTC) randomized phase 3 trial 30881. *Eur Urol* 2009; 55: 28–34.

23. Leibovitch I, Raviv G, Mor Y, Nativ O, Goldwasser B. Reconsidering the necessity of ipsilateral adrenalectomy during radical nephrectomy for renal cell carcinoma. *Urology* 1995; 46: 316–20.

24. Paul R, Mordhorst J, Busch R, Leyh H, Hartung R. Adrenal sparing surgery during radical nephrectomy in patients with renal cell carcinoma: a new algorithm. *J Urol* 2001; 166: 59–62.

25. Zisman A, Wieder JA, Pantuck AJ, et al. Renal cell carcinoma with tumor thrombus extension: biology, role of nephrectomy and response to immunotherapy. *J Urol* 2003; 169: 909–16.

26. Richard PO, Jewett MA, Bhatt JR, et al. Renal tumor biopsy for small renal masses: a single-center 13-year experience. *Eur Urol* 2015; 68: 1007–13.

27. Pizzocaro G, Piva L, Colavita M, et al. Interferon adjuvant to radical nephrectomy in Robson stages II and III renal cell carcinoma: a multicentric randomized study. *J Clin Oncol* 2001; 19: 425–31.

28. Messing EM, Manola J, Wilding G, et al. Phase III study of interferon alfa-NL as adjuvant treatment for resectable renal cell carcinoma: an Eastern Cooperative Oncology Group/Intergroup trial. *J Clin Oncol* 2003; 21: 1214–22.

29. Atzpodien J, Schmitt E, Gertenbach U, et al. Adjuvant treatment with interleukin-2- and interferon-alpha2a-based chemoimmunotherapy in renal cell carcinoma post tumour nephrectomy: results of a prospectively randomised trial of the German Cooperative Renal Carcinoma Chemoimmunotherapy Group (DGCIN). *Br J Cancer* 2005; 92: 843–6.

30. Jocham D, Richter A, Hoffmann L, et al. Adjuvant autologous renal tumour cell vaccine and risk of tumour progression in patients with renal-cell carcinoma after radical nephrectomy: phase III, randomised controlled trial. *Lancet* 2004; 363: 594–9.

31. Kjaer M, Frederiksen PL, Engelholm SA. Postoperative radiotherapy in stage II and III renal adenocarcinoma. A randomized trial by the Copenhagen Renal Cancer Study Group. *Int J Radiat Oncol Biol Phys* 1987; 13: 665–72.

32. Mickisch GH, Garin A, van Poppel H, de Prijck L, Sylvester R, European Organisation for Research and Treatment of Cancer (EORTC) Genitourinary Group. Radical nephrectomy plus interferon-alfa-based immunotherapy compared with interferon alfa alone in metastatic renal-cell carcinoma: a randomised trial. *Lancet* 2001; 358: 966–70.

33. Flanigan RC, Mickisch G, Sylvester R, Tangen C, Van Poppel H, Crawford ED. Cytoreductive nephrectomy in patients with metastatic renal cancer: a combined analysis. *J Urol* 2004; 171: 1071–6.

34. Motzer RJ, Bander NH, Nanus DM. Renal cell carcinoma. *New Engl J Med* 1996; 335: 865–75.

35. Motzer RJ, Hutson TE, Tomczak P, et al. Overall survival and updated results for sunitinib compared with interferon alfa in patients with metastatic renal cell carcinoma. *J Clin Oncol* 2009; 27: 3584–90.

36. Escudier B, Pluzanska A, Koralewski P, et al. Bevacizumab plus interferon alfa-2a for treatment of metastatic renal cell carcinoma: a randomised, double-blind phase III trial. *Lancet* 2007; 370: 2103–11.

37. Sternberg CN, Davis ID, Mardiak J, et al. Pazopanib in locally advanced or metastatic renal cell carcinoma: results of a randomized phase III trial. *J Clin Oncol* 2010; 28: 1061–8.

38. Hudes G, Carducci M, Tomczak P, et al. Temsirolimus, interferon alfa, or both for advanced renal-cell carcinoma. *New Engl J Med* 2007; 356: 2271–81.

39. Escudier B, Eisen T, Stadler WM, et al. Sorafenib for treatment of renal cell carcinoma: final efficacy and safety results of the phase III treatment approaches in renal cancer global evaluation trial. *J Clin Oncol* 2009; 27: 3312–8.

40. Motzer RJ, Escudier B, Oudard S, et al. Efficacy of everolimus in advanced renal cell carcinoma: a double-blind, randomised, placebo-controlled phase III trial. *Lancet* 2008; 372: 449–56.

36

Urothelial carcinoma of the bladder and upper tract

ANNEKE C M KUSTERS AND THEO M DE REIJKE

INTRODUCTION

Urothelial carcinoma (UC) can affect any portion of the urinary tract, which includes the renal pelvis, the ureter, the bladder and the prostatic and penile urethra. The normal urothelial is composed of several different cell subtypes and is usually three to seven layers thick. Basal cells attach to the lamina propria basement membrane; a few intermediate cell layers separate the basal cells from apical cells known as umbrella cells. Umbrella cells project into the lumen of the urinary tract and serve a key role in providing a barrier against solutes and waste products in the urine.

The exact etiology of urothelial carcinoma is unknown, but clearly it is multifactorial. Certain genetic predispositions and exposure of urothelium to chemical carcinogens or other irritating stimuli (infection, inflammation and radiation) probably lead to alterations in DNA, which cause the normal cell cycle to go awry, promoting the development of a malignancy. Not surprisingly, UC is often a field change disease with the entire urothelium susceptible to malignancy.

Although the most common, urothelial carcinoma is not the only primary malignancy affecting the urinary tract. Pure squamous cell carcinoma accounts for around 3–5% of all bladder tumors in Western countries [1]. Primary adenocarcinoma is the third most common epithelial tumor of the bladder; it represents 1–2% of all bladder tumors. Other rare primary bladder tumors include micropapillary subtype, sarcomas, carcinosarcomas, small-cell carcinomas, pheochromocytomas, lymphomas and melanomas. Similarly, squamous cell carcinomas, adenocarcinoma, sarcomas and small-cell carcinomas can involve the upper urinary tract. Of upper tract tumors 1–7% are squamous cell carcinomas. The focus of this chapter is on urothelial carcinomas, and distinctions are made between those tumors arising primarily within the bladder and those of the upper tracts.

INCIDENCE AND ETIOLOGY

Bladder cancer (BC) accounts for 90–95% and upper tract urothelial carcinomas (UTUCs) only for 5–10% of the urothelial carcinomas (UCs) [2]. Urothelial tumors are three times more common in men than women and upper tract tumors occur three to four times more commonly in the renal pelvis than in the ureter. The incidence of urothelial cancer increases with age and is most common in the fifth to seventh decade [3,4]. The age-standardized (world) mortality rates are 2–10 per 100,000 males and 0.5–4 per 100,000 females [5]. At the initial diagnosis of bladder cancer, 70% of cases are non-muscle invasive bladder cancer (NMIBC) and approximately 30% muscle-invasive bladder cancer (MIBC). Approximately one-third of patients diagnosed with MIBC have undetected metastases at the time of treatment for the primary tumor [2,3]. The association of BC and UTUCs is well documented but poorly understood. In primary bladder cancer, UTUCs occur in 2–4%, but of patients who have UTUCs, 30–75% subsequently can develop bladder cancer [4,6]. The incidence of UTUCs is significantly increased if carcinoma in situ (CIS) is found in the bladder. UTUCs are often multifocal and recurrent and whatever the etiology, recurrences are mostly seen in the ipsilateral upper tract; the incidence of contralateral UTUCs is only 2–6% [2,4]. With the presence of CIS the incidence of bilateral disease increases up to 30%. The natural history of UTUCs differs from that of bladder cancer: 60% of UTUCs are invasive at diagnosis compared with only 30% of bladder tumors [2].

The incidence of UC has decreased, possibly reflecting a dropping impact of causative agents, mainly smoking and occupational exposure. Tobacco smoking is the most important risk factor for UC, accounting for 30–50% of cases [2,5]. People who ever smoked have two to four times the risk of UC, and this risk tends to grow with both longer duration and more intense smoking. Stopping diminishes the risk immediately, 30% after 1–4 years and 60% after 25 years [5]. Occupational exposure to aromatic amines, polycyclic aromatic hydrocarbons and chlorinated hydrocarbons is the second most important risk factor for UC, accounting for 20% of UC [2,5]. Such occupational exposure occurs mainly in industrial branches processing paint, dye, metal and petroleum products. Another risk factor is exposure to ionizing radiation, and chemotherapy is also connected with increased risk of bladder cancer. Risk factors for particularly invasive squamous cell carcinoma are bladder schistosomiasis, chronic urinary tract infection, radiation, stones and a permanent catheter [2,5]. High consumption of fluids, vegetables and fruits has been associated with a decrease in the risk of bladder cancer, although studies are inconsistent [5]. Familial bladder cancer is a fairly rare phenomenon; nevertheless numerous striking case reports described familial clustering, usually with early age at onset [5]. There are familial and hereditary cases of UTUCs, manifested as Lynch's syndrome. This condition is predominantly associated with hereditary colonic and endometrial tumors but also with UTUCs if there is an MSH2 mutation present [4]. A more recent cause of UTUCs is the Chinese herb nephropathy. Slimming pills containing the herb *Aristolochia fangchi*, a potent carcinogen, cause this progressive form of fibrosing nephropathy. Other etiological factors include excessive coffee drinking and Balkan nephropathy, a condition characterized by the development of low-grade, multiple and often bilateral UTUCs in small populations in specific geographical clusters [4].

PATHOLOGY AND STAGING

The 2002 tumor, node, metastasis (TNM) classification approved by the Union Internationale Contre le Cancer (UICC) has been widely accepted for bladder cancer and UTUCs. It was updated in 2009, but it has no changes for bladder tumors (Table 36.1).

Until 2004, the most common classification used for grading urothelial cancers was the World Health Organization (WHO) classification of 1973, which distinguished only three grades: low, intermediate and high. A new classification system was developed in 2004 better reflecting the potential growth of these tumors, which

Table 36.1 Urothelial carcinoma of the bladder staging

Primary tumor (T)

TX	Primary tumor cannot be assessed
T0	No evidence of primary tumor
Ta	Non-invasive papillary carcinoma
Tis	Carcinoma in situ: 'flat tumor'
T1	Tumor invades subepithelial connective tissue
T2	Tumor invades muscle
T2a	Tumor invades superficial muscle (inner half)
T2b	Tumor invades deep muscle (outer half)
T3	Tumor invades perivesical tissue
T3a	Microscopically
T3b	Macroscopically (extravesical mass)
T4	Tumor invades any of the following: prostate, uterus, vagina, pelvic wall, abdominal wall
T4a	Tumor invades prostate, uterus, vagina
T4b	Tumor invades pelvic wall, abdominal wall

Regional lymph nodes (N)

NX	Regional lymph nodes cannot be assessed
N0	No regional lymph node metastasis
N1	Metastasis in a single lymph node, ≥2 cm in greatest dimension
N2	Metastasis in a single lymph node, >2 cm but ≤5 cm in greatest dimension, or multiple lymph nodes, none >5 cm in greatest dimension
N3	Metastasis in a lymph node, >5 cm in greatest dimension

Distant metastasis (M)

MX	Distant metastasis cannot be assessed
M0	No distant metastasis
M1	Distant metastasis

Table 36.2 WHO grading system

Urothelial papilloma
Papillary urothelial neoplasm of low malignant potential (PUNLMP)
Low-grade papillary urothelial carcinoma
High-grade papillary urothelial carcinoma

should also diminish inter- and intra-observer variability. Based on detailed specific cytological and architectural criteria, urothelial lesions are now divided into four grades: papilloma, papillary urothelial neoplasia of low malignant potential (PUNLMP), low grade (LGUC) and high grade (HGUC) (Table 36.2) [2,7]. Tumors should be graded using both the 1973 and 2004 WHO classifications, because most clinical trials published so far on bladder tumors have been performed using the 1973 WHO classification.

Primary pure adenocarcinomas of the bladder are rare, representing approximately 2% of all malignant bladder neoplasms. Adenocarcinomas can arise from cystitis cystica et glandularis or surface glandular metaplasia, most commonly in the region of the trigone and posterior wall. The other 20–35% of bladder adenocarcinomas arise within urachal remnants in the bladder dome [7]. Microscopically the tumor is most often composed of colonic-type glandular epithelium and often contains abundant extracellular mucin. In the differential diagnosis one must consider the possibility of adenocarcinoma involving the bladder by either metastasis or direct invasion from other sites [7].

DIAGNOSIS AND PREOPERATIVE IMAGING

The mean age at presentation of upper tract urothelial cancers is 65 years and is slightly older than for bladder tumors [8]. On initial presentation, approximately 70–80% of patients with bladder cancer have disease that does not invade the muscle, which has historically been referred to as superficial bladder cancer, nowadays non-muscle invasive bladder cancer (NMIBC). Among these patients, approximately 20–40% may progress to muscle invasion, underscoring the need for effective treatment of the initial and recurrent disease. The remaining 20–30% will present with *de novo* muscle-invasive bladder cancer, and if left untreated, only about 15% will survive 2 years [9,10]. Thus, 80% of patients with muscle-invasive disease harbor this potentially lethal tumor at the time of initial diagnosis. Unlike bladder tumors, 50–60% of urothelial tumors of the renal pelvis are invasive at presentation [8].

The classical presentation of bladder carcinoma is hematuria (75%), which is typically intermittent, gross, painless and present throughout micturition. Pain (33%) associated with bladder cancer is usually the result of CIS and advanced (T2–4) tumors. The combination of dysuria, frequency and urgency is suggestive for CIS [2,4]. The diagnosis of UTUC may be fortuitous. The symptoms are generally non-specific. The most common symptom of UTUC is gross or microscopic hematuria (70–80%). Flank pain occurs in 20–40% of the cases, and a lumbar mass is present in 10–20% of the cases [2].

Although often unremarkable, a complete physical examination should be performed in patients with (suspicion of) bladder cancer, including digital rectal examination and bimanual examination of the vagina in women. Abnormalities can be found: solid pelvic mass, induration of the prostate gland and inguinal adenopathy.

Computed tomography (CT) consisting of a four-phase urography is the imaging technique with the highest diagnostic accuracy for UTUC. Indications of a pyelum or ureter tumor are filling defects in the calyces, renal pelvis and ureters; hydronephrosis; and wall thickening of the pelvis or ureter. Magnetic resonance (MR) urography is indicated in patients who cannot undergo CT urography usually when radiation or iodinated contrast media are contraindicated [2]. Both CT and MRI may be used for assessment of local invasion of BC, but they are unable to diagnose accurately microscopic invasion of perivesical fat (T3a). The principal aim of CT and MRI is therefore to detect T3b disease or higher and lesions in the upper urinary tract. The assessment

of metastases to lymph nodes based simply on size is limited by the inability of both CT and MRI to identify metastases in normal-sized or minimally enlarged nodes. The sensitivity for detection of lymph node metastases is as low as 48–87% [2]. CT and MRI are the diagnostic techniques of choice to detect metastases to lung and liver. Metastases to bones or brain at the presentation of invasive bladder cancer are rare. A bone scan and additional brain imaging are therefore not routinely indicated unless the patient has specific symptoms or signs suggestive for bone or brain metastases. MRI is more sensitive and specific for diagnosing bone metastases than bone scintigraphy [2]. Currently, there is no evidence supporting the routine use of positron emission tomography–computed tomography (PET-CT) in the nodal staging of bladder cancer.

Urinary cytology of voided urine or bladder wash cytology has a median sensitivity of only 35% and median specificity of 94% [3]. In the presence of high-grade cancers it has a high sensitivity and therefore cytology is mainly used for the follow-up of high-risk tumors. Cytological interpretation is investigator dependent. Evaluation can be hampered by low cellular yield, presence of urinary tract infections, stones or intravesical instillations [2–4]. Cytology should be performed on fresh urine with adequate fixation. Morning urine is not suitable.

On suspicion of BC, the initial investigation is a flexible white-light cystoscopy in the outpatient department to confirm the presence, number, location and type of the tumor(s). White-light cystoscopy might be reliable for papillary tumors; flat carcinomas (particularly CIS), multifocal growth and microscopic lesions are more difficult to detect. Photodynamic diagnosis (PDD) uses a photoactive substance, 5-aminolaevulinic acid (ALA) or hexaminolevulinic acid (HAL). It accumulates 20 times more in neoplastic areas than normal tissue and enhances the visual difference between normal and neoplastic tissue after illumination with light of the appropriate wavelength [2,3] (Figure 36.1).

Tumor detection rates increased by 20–90% with similar specificity [3]. Another endoscopic technique is narrow-band imaging (NBI), which depends on sequential green and blue illumination by two optical filters with wavelengths of 415 and 540 nm that correspond to the absorption spectrum of

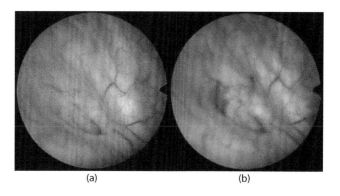

(a)   (b)

Figure 36.1 (a) White light cystosocopy showing no suspicious areas, (b) PDD positive lesion which showed carcinoma in situ.

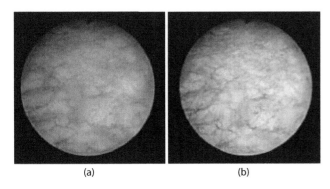

(a)   (b)

Figure 36. 2 (a) White light cystoscopy showing possible lesion, (b) NBI enhanced vascularized areas which showed papillary tumour (TaG2).

haemoglobin. It can be used for detailed visualization of the mucosal surface and tissue microvasculature [3] (Figure 36.2).

PDD and NBI could be considered, especially if a T1 high-grade tumor is present, to demonstrate associated CIS. The advantage of NBI is that no instillation is used and it can be done immediately in the outpatient setting.

Transurethral resection of bladder tumor (TURBT) in combination with bimanual examination is the surgical procedure used to diagnose, stage and treat primary and recurrent NMIBC, so TURBT is both a diagnostic and a therapeutic operation. The initial TURBT has three main goals: (1) to obtain pathological material for histological typing and grading; (2) to determine the presence, depth and type of tumor invasion; and (3) to remove if possible all visible lesions [2,11].

In the case of suspicion of a tumor in the upper tract, diagnostic semirigid or flexible ureterorenoscopy is used to visualize the entire upper urinary tract and biopsy possible lesions in the ureter, renal pelvis and collecting system. Ureterorenoscopy facilitates selective ureteral sampling for cytology and ureteroscopic biopsies can determine tumor grade in approximately 90% of cases with a low false-negative rate [2,4]. Combining ureterorenoscopic biopsy grade, diagnostic imaging findings and urinary cytology may help decision making on radical nephroureterectomy versus endoscopic treatment.

SURGERY FOR PRIMARY OPERABLE CANCER

TURBT

The initial treatment of NMIBC is complete transurethral resection of [all visible] bladder tumor (TURBT), which is usually carried out at the time of diagnosis. Before TURBT bimanual palpation should be performed, and if a palpable lesion is present before the resection it should be repeated after TURBT. Complete and correct TURBT, including detrusor muscle, is essential for optimal staging and decision making to achieve a good prognosis [2,11]. When abnormal areas of urothelium are seen, it is advised to take cold-cup biopsies or biopsies with a resection loop. Biopsies from normal-looking

mucosa including the prostatic urethra should be performed in patients with positive urinary cytology and absence of visual tumor. These so-called random biopsies are not routinely recommended with TaT1 tumors, as the likelihood of detecting CIS in low-risk tumors is extremely low (<2%) [2]. Incomplete resection and understaging of bladder tumors is well known. Because the treatment of muscle-invasive tumors is completely different, a second TURBT is recommended (1) after incomplete initial TUR, (2) if there is no muscle in the specimen after initial TUR (with exception of Ta G1 tumors and CIS), (3) in all T1 tumors and (4) in all G3 tumors [2,11]. Muscle invasion has been found on re-resection in up to 50% of cases when initially no muscularis propria was present at initial TURBT, and in up to 14% of cases when muscle was present in an original T1 tumor [12]. TURBT is associated with a low (5%) overall complication rate [13]. The most common complication is bleeding [2]. The most serious complication is a bladder perforation occurring in 1.3–3.5% of the cases [14,15]. This can happen when the tumor is located on the lateral bladder wall, because the obturator nerve can then be triggered, resulting in an unexpected adduction of the leg. Although tumor seeding is a concern when the bladder is perforated, documented cases of extravesical pelvic disease are rare.

An estimated 40–80% of NMIBC recur within 6–12 months if managed with a radical TURBT without additional therapy, and 10–25% will develop into progressive disease including muscle invasion, regional or metastatic disease. The most important prognostic factors for progression are histologic stage and grade. Other factors include the presence of multifocal disease, the frequency of recurrence, the tumor size and the presence or absence of concomitant CIS [2,16]. Risk assessment is needed for defining an appropriate individual treatment strategy. The European Association of Urology (EAU) guidelines recommend a simple risk stratification scheme with low risk including patients with solitary Ta G1 first occurrence, intermediate risk as multifocal or recurrent Ta T1 G1–2, and high risk as any high-grade Ta or T1 or CIS [2]. Low-grade tumors have a high probability of recurrence, an estimated 60–80%, but are unlikely to progress to high-grade or invasive cancer. High-grade tumors have a similar recurrence probability but a much higher risk of progression into muscle invasion cancer [2,16].

BLADDER INSTILLATIONS

To prevent the chance of recurrence low-risk patients are treated with a single dose of immediate postoperative intravesical chemotherapy (most commonly mitomycin C) within 24 h and cystoscopic surveillance. In low-risk patients cystoscopy is performed after 3 months and if no recurrence is observed, the next cystoscopic check is done 9 months later and then yearly up to approximately 5 years. Bacillus Calmette–Guèrin (BCG) is never given immediately post TURBT, because of the risk of disseminating the tuberculous bacilli. Intermediate-risk patients are treated with either chemotherapy (e.g. mitomycin C weekly × 6 followed by monthly instillations) or BCG (induction phase weekly × 6, followed by maintenance instillations at months 3, 6, 12, 18, 24, 30 and 36), while patients with high-risk disease should be treated with induction and maintenance BCG instillations [2]. BCG maintenance instillations last at least 1 year, but can be extended up to 3 years if tolerated. Serious side effects occur in <5% of all patients undergoing BCG treatment. BCG toxicity can be divided into local, systemic and allergic side effects. Local toxicities are generally more common and less severe than systemic toxicity, but they are more often the cause of treatment interruption [17]. Local side effects include frequency, pain (57–71%), hematuria (20%) and bladder contracture (3%) [18]. Systemic side effects generally occur in the first 6 months of treatment and can be divided into infectious (bacterial cystitis, epididymitis, prostatitis, urethral infections and systemic infections) and non-infectious (arthralgia, skin reactions and anaphylaxis) types. BCG-itis occurs at a rate of 2–6% of the serious side effects [19]. It must be considered when patients have high fever during more than 48 h after instillation. It is a severe systemic BCG infection that can cause, e.g. bronchopulmonary lesions and granulomatous hepatitis. It should be treated with rifampicin, isoniazid and prednisone.

Patients with intermediate- and high-risk NMIBC should have a more rigorous follow-up with 3-monthly cystoscopy in the first year and also upper tract imaging, and follow-up should at least be 10 years and perhaps lifelong in the high-risk group.

RADICAL CYSTECTOMY

Radical cystectomy with pelvic lymph node dissection (PLND) is recommended for patients with MIBC T2–4 N0–x M0. Other indications include high-risk and recurrent NMIBC, BCG-resistant CIS, T1 G3 as well as extensive papillary disease that cannot be controlled with TURBT and intravesical therapy alone [2]. In men, the prostate is traditionally removed with the cystectomy specimen, as it can be involved with the urothelial tumor or harbor a secondary malignancy. The incidence of prostatic involvement varies with individual tumor characteristics as well as the technique used to assess the prostate specimen. Incidental adenocarcinoma of the prostate can be detected in about half of the specimens. However, select patients can be considered for sparing of the prostate, and in properly selected patients the oncological safety and functional outcomes have been demonstrated [20]. If the urethra is involved with urothelial cancer, urethrectomy is generally performed at the time of cystectomy.

Classically the standard of treatment for MIBC in women has been anterior exenteration, which included removal of the bladder, urethra, uterus, ovaries, fallopian tubes and a portion of the anterior vaginal wall. With the refinement of surgical techniques and careful patient selection, certain gynecological organs, urethra and the anterior vaginal wall can be spared [21]. In fact, there is a low incidence of secondary gynecological malignancies incidentally found at cystectomy, and direct extension of urothelial tumors into adjacent organs, if present, is usually suspected preoperatively or determined intraoperatively [22].

The open procedure has been the mainstay of treatment for decades. Laparoscopic radical cystectomy (LRC) offers patients the potential of less morbidity and earlier convalescence, while maintaining oncological efficacy. Early experience with (robot-assisted) LRC has shown that there is a longer learning curve. The laparoscopic removal of the bladder and prostate is rather straightforward for experienced pelvic laparoscopic surgeons, but the accompanying intracorporeal construction of the urinary diversion had posed the main technical challenge. Likewise, extending the limits of the laparoscopic PLND to include the presacral, proximal common iliac and retroperitoneal lymph nodes has presented technical challenges. The oncological equivalence or non-inferiority of (robot-assisted) LRC has yet to be confirmed [23].

A recent randomized trial, performed by experienced surgeons at a single high-volume center, showed similar rates of perioperative complications and lengths of hospital stay among patients who underwent robot-assisted surgery and those who underwent open surgery [24]. In selected centers (robot-assisted) LRC can be performed [24]. PLND is an essential component of the surgical procedure: (1) some patients with lymph node involvement might be cured if these nodes are removed, (2) staging is more accurate and (3) a far more anatomic RC is possible after a thorough PLND and allows safer dissection. A prospective study showed a significantly lower 5-year survival rate for patients with no LND or only dissection of the obturator lymph nodes compared to those who underwent a standard LND. But the presence of gross lymph node metastases has been viewed as evidence of systemic disease, and despite a meticulous LND, long survival among such patients is rare [25]. Prognosis following radical cystectomy depends on pathological stage and extent of lymph node involvement. The 5- and 10-year overall survival rates for extravesical, lymph node–negative disease were 47% and 27%, respectively [26]. Complications related to radical cystectomy may be directly related to pre-existing patient comorbidities as well as the surgical procedure itself, the bowel anastomosis or the urinary diversion. Risk factors for complications are advanced age, prior abdominal surgery, extravesical disease and prior radiotherapy. Radical cystectomy with urinary diversion is associated with an overall complication rate of up to 56% and an almost 10% 30-day mortality rate in patients aged >80 years [19].

URINARY DIVERSION

Urinary tract reconstruction attempts to provide an acceptable alternative to the native bladder by creating adequate storage and continence or an acceptable conduit. In exceptional cases an internal diversion can be created connecting the ureters to the sigmoid. In these cases the patient should have demonstrated adequate anal sphincter control; otherwise urinary leakage will develop that is impossible to handle. In older patients (>80 years) a direct bilateral ureterocutaneostomy can be created in order to avoid intestinal anastomosis, because this has been demonstrated to increase postoperative morbidity. An incontinent urinary diversion is still the most common type of reconstruction of the lower urinary tract performed in conjunction with radical cystectomy, the uretero-ileal cutaneostomy (Bricker) being the most widespread technique. Simplicity and good functional outcome are two features that make this conduit an attractive approach [2,26].

The overall incidence of complications associated with ileal conduits is substantial, partly because many are elderly patients with comorbidities. Complication rates of 20–56% have been reported at <30 days and 28–81% at >30 days [26]. Early complications are anastomotic leak, enteric fistula, bowel obstruction, prolonged ileus and necrosis of the conduit. The most common long-term complications are stomal or peristomal problems, parastomal hernia, conduit stenosis, stenosis in the uretero-enteric anastomosis, urinary tract infections, stone formation and upper tract deterioration. With intestinal urinary diversion there is the possibility of hyperchloraemic metabolic acidosis due to a net absorption of ammonium from the urine.

Patients should be under lifelong surveillance and the follow-up should comprise measures to detect cancer recurrence, deterioration of renal function, stoma problems, infections and metabolic conditions (e.g. bicarbonate, vitamin B12) [2,26]. Urologists have presumed that the development of continent diversions would replicate the normal voiding pattern and provide improved quality of life (QoL) over the incontinent diversions, but a real improvement has been difficult to demonstrate. Both continent and incontinent diversions have high-perceived overall satisfaction at 1 year [27]. Continent diversions require a high-volume, low-pressure reservoir. Important is good counseling of the patients preoperatively, because an orthotopic bladder substitution is not a normal bladder and the patient has to strain to empty the bladder and sometimes has to perform clean intermittent self-catheterization and mucus can sometimes block the urethra.

Different bowel segments have been used, i.e. ileocoecum, colon (ascendens, transverse, descending) and ileum [28]. Conventional wisdom suggests the need for an anti-reflux mechanism (nipple valve, split-cuff ureteric nipple, LeDuc technique) to prevent deterioration in renal function, as reflux nephropathy can develop with high pressure in the reservoir [28,29]. However, reflux prevention in a low-pressure detubularized reservoir might not be as beneficial as anticipated and has a higher stricture rate of 4–29% against 1.5–5% with the direct ureterointestinal implantation technique [29]. Two kinds of continent reservoirs can be created: (1) the cutaneous diversion (appendix stoma, intussuscepted ileal nipple) and (2) the orthotopic bladder substitution (reservoir connected to the urethra). Clean intermittent catheterization (CIC) is necessary with a continent cutaneous diversion, but also if an orthotopic bladder substitution was created CIC is

reported in up to 50% of cases [28]. Contraindications for a continent diversion are impaired renal function (creatinine > 150 µmol/L); severely impaired liver function; severe intestinal disease; inadequate intellectual capacity, dexterity or mobility; incompliant patients for active postoperative re-education and regular follow-up; and specifically for the orthotopic bladder substitution urinary stress incontinence, damaged rhabdomyosphincter or incompetent urethra and tumor infiltration of the distal prostatic urethra in men or bladder neck in women [28,29]. Continent diversions are prone to stone formation. Risk factors are foreign body material, residual urine, bacteriuria, hypercalciuria and hypocitraturia [28]. They are also prone to incontinence and stenosis of the appendix or ileal nipple or the bladder neck [28,29]. Furthermore, complications are more or less the same as with an incontinent urinary deviation and lifelong follow-up is required.

BLADDER-PRESERVING THERAPY

Radical cystectomy comes with considerable morbidity such as erectile dysfunction, urinary leakage, urinary tract infection and most important, loss of normal bladder function. Bladder-preserving therapy may then offer an alternative to radical cystectomy with possible reduction of side effects [30]. Radiation monotherapy results in an unacceptable low likelihood of local disease control of ≈40% with 5-year survival rates of 38–59% for T2 disease and 14–39% for T3–T4 disease [2,31]. Combined modality therapy for bladder preservation can be an alternative in selected patients, leading to similar local control and survival rates, with the QoL advantage of retaining a functional bladder. In quality of life studies 85% of patients reported no or only mild bladder symptoms, 22% had mild to moderate bowel symptoms and half of men reported normal erectile function [30,32].

Two of the bladder-preserving therapies are brachytherapy in combination with external beam radiotherapy (EBRT) and partial cystectomy. A recent systematic review showed a survival similar to that of radical cystectomy for muscle-invasive bladder cancer, but it must be mentioned that patients with ≤T2 tumors represent the largest group and it comprises a highly selected group of patients with solitary tumors. A common late effect of brachytherapy is the development of ulceration at the implantation site. This late effect occurs in about 10% of the patients at 6 months post-therapy, usually asymptomatic and self-limiting. It is important to recognize this late effect and avoid unnecessary biopsies. Fistula formation is very rare in 2–5% of cases [30].

There will be cystoscopic and cytological assessment of the treatment response and prompt salvage cystectomy for non-responders [31]. Currently it is more or less standard to combine EBRT with chemotherapy in order to improve outcome. Five- and ten-year overall survival rates are 52% and 35%, respectively [30]. There is no significant difference with radical cystectomy [30,33]. However, there are negative effects of cisplatin-based chemotherapy, such as ototoxicity and renal function impairment. And more importantly, a high dose of external beam radiotherapy to the intestine leads to gastrointestinal complication rates of 6.5–10%. Moreover, 2.3% of all patients needed surgical treatment for bowel strictures following radical radiotherapy [30,33]. Over the past 20–25 years, accumulated data show that bladder-preserving treatments provide a safe and effective alternative to radical cystectomy [31]. Careful selection of patients is, however, needed. The best candidates for bladder-preserving therapy have MIBC with a solitary lesion, with no carcinoma in situ and without hydronephrosis, have sufficient renal function to tolerate platinum-based chemotherapy and have had radical TURBT [31].

RADICAL NEPHROURETERECTOMY

The management of UTUCs is constantly being driven to include minimally invasive technology. Radical nephroureterectomy (RNU) with a bladder cuff remains the 'reference standard' treatment of UTUCs and is recommended for all patients with high-grade or invasive UTUC. Laparoscopic RNU has become the standard of care at many centers but the open approach to the distal ureter remains superior to modern laparoscopic techniques [2,4]. Extended LND might be of benefit during RNU for high-stage disease. Lymph node metastasis generally occurs in 13–44% of patients, depending on tumor stage and extent of LND. Recent evidence suggests significant survival benefit in patients with pT3 disease and higher that underwent LND compared with no LND [4]. Segmental ureterectomy or distal ureterectomy with a psoas hitch or a Boari flap can be performed in the case of a local ureteral tumor [2,4]. Ureteroscopic ablation of UTUCs is best reserved for patients with small, low-grade tumors that have no evidence of invasion or local metastasis, and in whom the risk of subsequent renal failure after definitive surgical resection outweighs that of tumor progression. The tumor is biopsied for pathological analysis and then ablated with electrocautery or preferably laser (Holmium:Yag) [2,4].

NEOADJUVANT AND ADJUVANT THERAPIES

The management of MIBC requires a multimodal approach, including the integration of perioperative chemotherapy. Cisplatin-based chemotherapy represents the cornerstone of the management of patients with advanced urothelial bladder cancer [2,27]. Methotrexate, vinblastine, doxorubicin and cisplatin (MVAC) are recommended for patients with T2–4a cN0 M0 bladder cancer with performance status 0–1 and a normal renal function. The regimen gemcitabine and cisplatin (GC) is less toxic and achieves a response and survival similar to that of MVAC, but remains untested in a prospective trial in the neoadjuvant setting. Carboplatin may be considered in patients with an impaired renal function [27].

There are several potential benefits to the use of chemotherapy in the neoadjuvant rather than the adjuvant setting.

First, administration of chemotherapy before surgery avoids the potential for postoperative recovery and complications that might affect the ability to administer adjuvant chemotherapy. Second, the use of neoadjuvant chemotherapy allows for *in vivo* drug sensitivity testing, which might also provide important prognostic information. Third, chemotherapy might lead to tumor downstaging and allows for less morbid surgery or potentially converts unresectable to resectable disease. Finally, the ability to monitor the primary tumor during treatment allows for discontinuation of ineffective chemotherapy if there is evidence of disease progression [2,27].

For patients who respond to neoadjuvant chemotherapy, known as responders, and especially those who show a complete response (pT0 N0), neoadjuvant chemotherapy has a major impact on overall survival. From randomized studies and a systematic review, a 5–8% improvement in overall survival can be expected with neoadjuvant cisplatin-containing chemotherapy [34–37]. A disadvantage of neoadjuvant chemotherapy is that clinical staging using CT or MRI may often results in over- and understaging and has a staging accuracy of only 70%. Overtreatment is the possible negative consequence. Another disadvantage is that delayed cystectomy might compromise the outcome in patients not sensitive to chemotherapy. This is avoided with adjuvant chemotherapy [2,26]. Although adjuvant studies have been problematic and underpowered to detect a survival advantage, in all they suggest a benefit for the use of adjuvant cisplatin-based chemotherapy in patients with T3, T4 or node-positive disease. Several ongoing trials are attempting to further address the use of adjuvant chemotherapy.

LOCALLY ADVANCED AND METASTATIC DISEASE

Salvage chemotherapy for advanced UC with conventional chemotherapeutic agents (MVAC, GC) yields suboptimal response rates of ≈20% and a median survival of 6–9 months. Renal dysfunction, poor performance status and advanced age are relatively common and preclude cisplatin chemotherapy. Carboplatin-based combined regimens are feasible in such patients, but appear to be suboptimal [2,38]. Ongoing randomized trials are now evaluating anti-PD1 and anti-PDL1 regimens in this population.

REFERENCES

1. Bostwick DG and JN Eble. *Urologic Surgical Pathology*. St. Louis: Mosby-Year Book, 1997.
2. Babjuk M, M Burger, R Zigeuner, et al. EAU guidelines on non-muscle-invasive urothelial carcinoma of the bladder: update 2013. *Eur Urol* 2013(64): 639-53
3. Lee CSD, CY Yoon, and JA Witjes. The Past, Present and Future of Cystoscopy: The Fusion of Cystoscopy and Novel Imaging Technology. *BJU International* 2008(102): 1228-33.

4. Maddineni SB, NW Clarke, DE Sutherland, and TW Jarrett. Aetiology, Diagnosis and Management of Urothelial Tumours of the Renal Pelvis and Ureter. *BJU International* 2008(102): 302–6.

5. Wu X, MM Ros, J Gu, and L Kiemeney. Epidemiology and Genetic Susceptibility to Bladder Cancer. *BJU International* 2008(102): 1207–15.

6. Huben RP, AM Mounzer, and GP Murphy. Tumor Grade and Stage as Prognostic Variables in Upper Tract Urothelial Tumors. *Cancer* 1988(62): 2016–20.

7. Tavora F and JI Epstein. Bladder Cancer, Pathological Classification and Staging. *BJU International* 2008(102): 1216–20.

8. Campbell MF, PC Walsh, and AB Retik. *Campbell's Urology*, 8th ed. Philadelphia: Saunders, 2002: 2732–84.

9. Prout GR and VF Marshall. The Prognosis with Untreated Bladder Tumors. *Cancer* 1956(9): 551–8.

10. Stein JP, G Lieskovsky, R Cote, et al. Radical Cystectomy in the Treatment of Invasive Bladder Cancer: Long-Term Results in 1,054 Patients. *Journal of Clinical Oncology* 2001(19): 666–75.

11. Herr HW and S Machele Donat. Quality Control in Transurethral Resection of Bladder Tumours. *BJU International* 2008(102): 1242–46.

12. Jakse G, F Algaba, PU Malmström, and W Oosterlinck. A Second-Look TUR in T1 Transitional Cell Carcinoma: Why? *European Urology* 2004(45): 539–46.

13. Collado A, GE Chéchile, J Salvador, and J Vicente. Early Complications of Endoscopic Treatment for Superficial Bladder Tumors. *Journal of Urology* 2000(164): 1529–32.

14. Balbay MD, E Cimentepe, A Unsal, O Bayrak, A Koç, and Z Akbulut. The Actual Incidence of Bladder Perforation Following Transurethral Bladder Surgery. *Journal of Urology* 2005(174): 2260–62. Discussion 2262–63.

15. Desgrandchamps F, M Teren, L Dal Cortivo, JP Marolleau, P Bertheau, JM Villette, A Cortesse, P Teillac, A Le Duc, and FC Hamdy. The Effects of Transurethral Resection and Cystoprostatectomy on Dissemination of Epithelial Cells in the Circulation of Patients with Bladder Cancer. *British Journal of Cancer* 1999(5): 832–34.

16. Braasch MR, A Böhle, and MA O'Donnell. Risk-Adapted Use of Intravesical Immunotherapy. *BJU International* 2008(102): 1254–64.

17. Van der Meijden APM, RJ Sylvester, W Oosterlinck, W Hoeltl, and AV Bono. Maintenance Bacillus Calmette-Guerin for Ta T1 Bladder Tumors Is Not Associated with Increased Toxicity: Results from a European Organisation for Research and Treatment of Cancer Genito-Urinary Group Phase III Trial. *European Urology* 2003(4): 429–34.

18. Hall MC, SS Chang, G Dalbagni, RS Pruthi, JD Seigne, EC Skinner, J Stuart Wolf, and PF Schellhammer. Guideline for the Management of Nonmuscle Invasive Bladder Cancer (Stages Ta, T1, and Tis): 2007 Update. *Journal of Urology* 2007(6): 2314–30.

19. Lerner SP and JLS Au. Risk-Adapted Use of Intravesical Chemotherapy. *BJU International* 2008(102): 1247–53.

20. Nieuwenhuijzen JA, W Meinhardt, and S Horenblas. Clinical Outcomes after Sexuality Preserving Cystectomy and Neobladder (Prostate Sparing Cystectomie) in 44 Patients. *Journal of Urology* 2005(173): 1314–7.

21. Ali-el-Dein B, M Abdel-Latif, A Ahammallah, et al. Local Urethral Recurrence after Radical Cystectomy and Orthotopic Bladder Substitution in Women: A Prospective Study. *Journal of Urology* 2004(171): 275–8.

22. Chang SS, E Cole, JA Smith Jr, et al. Pathological Findings of Gynecologic Organs Obtained at Female Radical Cystectomy. *Journal of Urology* 2002(168): 147–9.

23. Stephenson AJ and IS Gill. Laparoscopic Radical Cystectomy for Muscle-Invasive Bladder Cancer: Pathological and Oncological Outcomes. *BJU International* 2008(102): 1296–301.

24. Bochner BH. A Randomized Trial of Robot-Assisted Laparoscopic Radical Cystectomy. *New England Journal of Medicine* 2014(4): 398–90.

25. Thalmann GN and JP Stein. Outcomes of Radical Cystectomy. *BJU International* 2008(102): 1279–88.

26. Gudjónsson S, T Davidsson, and W Månsson. Incontinent Urinary Diversion. *BJU International* 2008(102): 1320–25.

27. Milowsky MI, WM Stadler, and DF Bajorin. Integration of Neoadjuvant and Adjuvant Chemotherapy and Cystectomy in the Treatment of Muscle-Invasive Bladder Cancer. *BJU International* 2008(102): 1339–44.

28. Fisch M and JW Thüroff. Continent Cutaneous Diversion. *BJU International* 2008(102): 1314–19.

29. Thurairaja R, FC Burkhard, and UE Studer. The Orthotopic Neobladder. *BJU International* 2008(102): 1307–13.

30. Bos MK, RO Marmolejo, RNR Coen, and BR Pieters. Bladder Preservation with Brachytherapy Compared to Cystectomy for T1-T3 Muscle-Invasive Bladder Cancer: A Systematic Review. *Journal of Contemporary Brachytherapy* 2014(2): 191–99.

31. Mak RH, AL Zietman, NM Heney, DS Kaufman, and WU Shipley. Bladder Preservation: Optimizing Radiotherapy and Integrated Treatment Strategies. *BJU International* 2008(102): 1345–53.

32. Rodel C. Combined-Modality Treatment and Selective Organ Preservation in Invasive Bladder Cancer: Long-Term Results. *Journal of Clinical Oncology* 2002(14): 3061–71.

33. James ND, SA Hussain, E Hall, et al. Radiotherapy with or without Chemotherapy in Muscle-Invasive Bladder Cancer. *New England Journal of Medicine* 2012(16): 1477–88.

34. Sherif A, L Holmberg, E Rintala, O Mestad, J Nilsson, S Nilsson, and PU Malmström. Neoadjuvant Cisplatinum Based Combination Chemotherapy in Patients with Invasive Bladder Cancer: A Combined Analysis of Two Nordic Studies. *European Urology* 2004(3): 297–303.

35. Grossman HB, RB Natale, CM Tangen, et al. Neoadjuvant Chemotherapy Plus Cystectomy Compared with Cystectomy Alone for Locally Advanced Bladder Cancer. *New England Journal of Medicine* 2003(9): 859–66.

36. Australian Bladder Cancer Study, Norwegian Bladder, Club Urologico, and Espanol De Tratamiento. Chemotherapy for Muscle-Invasive Bladder Cancer: A Randomised Controlled Trial. http://www.ncbi.nlm.nih.gov/pubmed/10470696

37. International Collaboration of Trialists on Behalf of the Medical Research Council Advanced Bladder Cancer Working Party. Neoadjuvant Cisplatin, Methotrexate, and Vinblastine Chemotherapy for Muscle-Invasive Bladder Cancer: A Randomised Controlled Trial. *Lancet* 1999(345): 533–40.

38. Sonpavde G and CN Sternberg. Treatment of Metastatic Urothelial Cancer: Opportunities for Drug Discovery and Development. *BJU International* 2008(102): 1354–60.

37

Prostate cancer

LONA VYAS AND DEREK J ROSARIO

EPIDEMIOLOGY

In 2012, prostate cancer accounted for 15% of all cancers diagnosed worldwide with an estimated total of 1.1 million new cases. Two-thirds of these were in the developed world. The highest incidence rates were found in Australasia and North America (Figure 37.1) and the incidence appears to be rising on all continents.

Although prostate-specific antigen (PSA) testing and biopsy protocols may be contributing to this with identification of early non-clinically significant disease (lead time bias), other factors such as changing demographics with an ageing population, increasing obesity, hypogonadism and changes in dietary patterns may be implicated in a true increased incidence of the disease.

Prostate cancer is a disease of elderly men. Post-mortem studies (Table 37.1) have demonstrated histological evidence of prostate cancer in around 10% of men in their third decade, rising with increasing age with a similar prevalence worldwide. Actual clinical presentation of prostate cancer is rare below the age of 40 years and rises with age (Figure 37.2). Epidemiological data suggest the environment and possibly diet have a direct effect on progression from an indolent state to a more aggressive clinical meaningful disease. For instance, Japanese and Asian Americans have a 20-fold increased risk of developing clinical prostate cancer compared to Japanese men living in Japan. Men of African and Afro-Caribbean origin have the highest risk of dying of the disease, followed by Caucasian men and finally Asians, who have the lowest risk.

It is estimated that the lifetime risk of being diagnosed with prostate cancer in the developed world is currently around 1 in 8 (12%) and rising; the risk of dying from prostate cancer is around 3% and remaining static. Thus prostate cancer poses a rather unusual paradigm among cancers – it is the fifth highest cause of cancer deaths among men worldwide, yet the incidence far outweighs its mortality, particularly in high-income countries with well-developed healthcare systems. In low-income nations with less developed healthcare systems, the statistics are somewhat different, with rising incidence and mortality. There is less variation worldwide in mortality rates than in incidence rates, likely reflecting earlier diagnosis and more effective treatment in developed healthcare systems. Nevertheless,

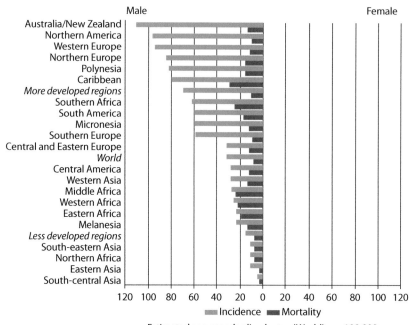

Figure 37.1 Age-standardized global incidence and mortality rates of clinical prostate cancer with highest incidence in Australasia, 2012. (Reprinted with permission of Globocan, World Health Organization, Available at http://globocan.iarc.fr/old/bar_sex_site.asp?selection=24191&title=Prostate&statistic=2&populations=6&window=1&grid=1&color1=5&color1e=&color2=4&color2e=&submit=%C2%A0Execute.)

Table 37.1 Post-mortem prevalence rates of prostate cancer worldwide (%)

Age	US white	US black	Japan	Spain	Greece	Hungary
21–30	8	8	0	4	0	0
31–40	31	31	20	9	0	27
41–50	37	43	13	14	3	20
51–60	44	46	22	24	5	28
61–70	65	70	35	32	14	44
71–80	83	81	41	33	31	58
81–90			48		40	73

Source: After Delongchamps NB, et al., Cancer Control 2006; 13(3): 158–168.

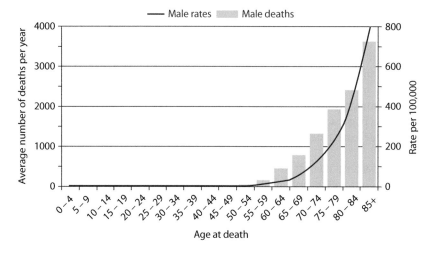

Figure 37.2 Average number of deaths per year and age-specific mortality rates, males, UK, 2010–2012. (Reprinted with permission of Cancer Research UK, Available at http://www.cancerresearchuk.org/health-professional/cancer-statistics/statistics-by-cancer-type/prostate-cancer/mortality#heading-One.)

the increasing incidence and treatment rates have major implications for health resource management, particularly given the ageing population worldwide.

RISK FACTORS

Age and ethnicity form the main risk factors for development of prostate cancer, but other risk factors that have been identified include the following.

Anthropometry

A recent analysis of the literature suggested an increased risk of prostate cancer in obese men, mainly for advanced disease, and an increased risk with increasing height. Obese men often have lower PSA but higher risk of disease at initial presentation, extracapsular spread, recurrence post-treatment, metastasis and death.

Family history

Inherited prostate cancer is found in approximately 5% of cases. It tends to occur in younger men (usually under 60 years of age) and is associated with a number of gene mutations including 1q (HPC1 locus), Xp and Y, and 8p (MSR-1 locus). It is also associated with the BRCA2 gene on 13q. If a man has one first-degree relative affected by prostate cancer, his risk of developing the disease is double that of the general population. If two or more first-degree relatives are affected this increases up to 11-fold (Table 37.2).

Diet and growth factors

High saturated fat has also been found to increase prostate cancer cell growth together with high dairy protein and calcium. High fat consumption can lead to increased production of insulin and insulin-like growth factors (IGFs), which might explain the link with obesity. Inhibitory factors include vitamin D, polyphenols and lycopenes.

Sedentary lifestyle

There is evidence that men who lead a more active life have a lower mortality from prostate cancer. It is estimated

Table 37.2 Influence of family history of prostate cancer on lifetime risk of developing the disease

Family history	Lifetime risk (%)
No history	8
Father with prostate cancer at ≥60 years	12
1 brother affected at ≥60 years	15
Father affected before age 60 years	20
1 brother affected before age 60 years	25
2 male relatives with prostate cancer[a]	30
3 or more affected male relatives	35–45

Source: After Bratt O, et al., *J Urol* 2002; 168(3): 906.
[a] First-degree relatives.

that >3 h/week of exercise is associated with better outcomes possibly by reducing IGF-1 levels.

DIAGNOSIS AND STAGING

Prostate-specific antigen

Prostate-specific antigen (PSA) is a 34 kDa glycoprotein kallikrein produced exclusively by the prostate by both benign and malignant cells. It is found in large quantities in ejaculated semen where its main function appears to be liquefaction of seminal coagulum. Far smaller quantities are found in the serum, mostly complexed with circulating protease inhibitors such as alpha-1-chymotrypsin and alpha-2-macroglobulin. The half-life of circulating PSA is approximately 2.2 days.

As PSA is an organ-specific protease, and not a cancer-specific marker, it lacks specificity for detection of prostate cancer; PSA levels are elevated in benign prostatic hyperplasia, prostatitis, urinary tract infections and following blunt or iatrogenic trauma to the lower urinary tract (e.g. cystoscopy, catheterization). However, the overall level of PSA and changes in PSA level with time remain the best independent variables in the prediction of prostate cancer, far better than digital rectal examination (DRE), imaging (transrectal ultrasound) or any other marker described to date.

PSA has revolutionized the diagnosis of prostate cancer and its management. Prior to widespread PSA testing, the majority of cases of prostate cancer presented with evidence of advanced disease. Since the advent of PSA testing, the age at presentation has come down, with the majority of cases now presenting as localized (and therefore potentially curable) disease, which has often led to the question of population screening. The European randomized study of screening for prostate cancer with PSA testing, a trial involving more than 160,000 men, showed an absolute reduction in prostate cancer mortality of approximately 20% to 30% at 13 years. Conversely, the US randomized screening trial of the prostate, lung, colorectal and ovarian cancer (PLCO study) concluded there was no evidence of mortality benefit at 13 years using annual PSA and DRE compared to opportunistic screening; however, significant concerns remain about the conduct of the study and the level of contamination by PSA testing in the control arm. Nevertheless, the risk of overdiagnosing non-significant disease along with the potential harms associated with unnecessary treatment mean that the overall benefit has been judged insufficient to justify population-based PSA screening. Both the UK cancer screening council and the US Preventive Services Task Force (USPSTF) have recommended against PSA-based screening for prostate cancer. However, testing of asymptomatic men as well as men with unrelated lower urinary tract symptoms remains widespread and no doubt is contributing to the increasing incidence seen.

Table 37.3 Predictive value of PSA and DRE for TRUS biopsy prostate cancer diagnosis

PSA ng/ml	0.1–1.0	1.1–2.5	2.6–4.0	4–10	>10
DRE normal	10%	17%	23%	26%	>50%
DRE abnormal	15%	30%	40%	50%	75%

Source: Reynard J, et al., *Oxford Handbook of Urology*, 3rd ed., Oxford: Oxford University Press, 2013.

There are a number of areas where PSA testing has established clinical utility:

- Monitoring of response to treatment of advanced prostate cancer
- Detection of recurrent disease, e.g. after radical prostatectomy
- Risk prediction for complications of benign prostatic obstruction

PSA is a useful risk indicator, in conjunction with DRE, for the presence of prostate cancer on biopsy. Table 37.3 outlines the risk of finding prostate cancer on biopsy at any given level of PSA.

PSA counselling

Given the controversy surrounding the value of PSA in diagnosing asymptomatic disease, PSA counselling is mandatory before offering a PSA and DRE to asymptomatic men. An explanation of the potential disadvantages of an abnormal result must be given. The potential harm must be weighed against the potential benefit of finding a clinically significant prostate cancer diagnosed at an earlier stage with these assessments. When counselling asymptomatic men one should include the following points:

- Prostatic biopsy carries with it morbidity (bleeding, sepsis, discomfort and retention) and may miss the cancer.
- Sensitivity of PSA (usually applied as a specific cut-off or age-related cut-off) is around 80% so a false negative result is possible.
- Specificity is low, a false positive result is possible; indeed the majority of men with an elevated PSA will not have prostate cancer.
- Prostate cancer will be identified in around 1 in 20 men undergoing opportunistic PSA testing.
- Treatment may not be necessary or curative.
- Treatment-related morbidity might diminish quality of life and affect insurance.

The prostate cancer risk management programme has produced a useful tool for counselling the patient for PSA screening.

Prostate biopsy

The diagnosis of prostate cancer is most commonly based on transrectal needle biopsy of the prostate gland carried out under local anaesthesia with antibiotic cover in an ambulatory setting. There is a risk of severe post-biopsy sepsis (approximately 1%) with some authors suggesting an increased rate in recent years due to the development of quinolone-resistant bacterial strains. More recently, given the potential risk of infection, transperineal biopsy has become more acceptable, but usually requires sedation or regional anaesthesia. Biopsies have traditionally been carried out systematically, with most protocols recommending 10–12 cores for a first-time biopsy and more where re-biopsy is indicated following a negative initial biopsy.

The role of pre-biopsy MRI in directing targeted biopsies is showing some promise, with a number of studies indicating that the use of MRI improves localization of disease and reduces the number of negative biopsies. The most common complications after prostate biopsies are haematuria, haematochezia, haemoejaculate and acute retention requiring a catheter. Extensive perineal bruising and sexual dysfunction seem to be more associated with transperineal prostate mapping than the traditional transrectal route.

Imaging

There is growing interest in the use of pre-biopsy multiparametric prostate MRI (mpMRI) as a means of reducing biopsy-associated morbidity and the detection of low-risk disease. mpMRI appears to have reasonable sensitivity for detecting cancers (Figure 37.3), with increasing detection rates with larger tumour sizes and higher Gleason scores, but the problem of verification bias remains, with little prospective evidence in biopsy-naive men as to the true sensitivity, specificity and positive and negative predictive values of the investigation. Additionally questions remain around variability in interpretation and cost-effectiveness of mpMRI as suitable for triage test before biopsy. The Prostate Imaging Reporting and Data System (PI-RADS) has been developed to address inter- and intra-observer reproducibility.

Studies such as the multicentre UK-based prostate MRI study (PROMIS), which is soon to report, will provide prospective documentation of the sensitivity, specificity, PPV and NPV of multiparametric MRI of the prostate, as well as providing information on the relative merits of transperineal and transrectal biopsy. MRI is currently used as an adjunct to allow localization of a target for biopsy, rather than an isolated test for diagnosis. mpMRI enables targeted biopsies, especially in anterior tumours, which can be missed by DRE and systematic biopsies, and re-biopsies in clinically suspicious patients.

Once diagnosed, imaging is important in the staging of prostate cancer, particularly in high-risk disease (*vide infra*). Routine staging investigations are considered unnecessary in low-risk disease, with nomograms usually providing sufficient information to aid management. Both MRI and CT can be used to detect nodal disease, prior to radical treatment. For detection of distant metastases, the traditional investigation of choice has been Tc-labelled

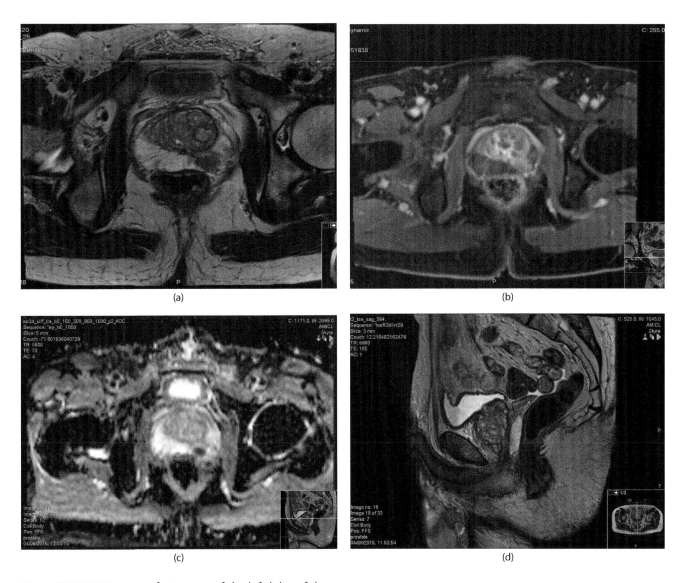

Figure 37.3 MRI images of a tumour of the left lobe of the prostate.

dynamic bone scintigraphy, although whole body MRI has better sensitivity than bone scans or CT.

STAGING, GRADING AND RISK CLASSIFICATION

There are two widely used classification systems for prostate cancer: the TNM system and the Jewitt–Whitmore classifications systems (Figure 37.4). Nomograms exist (e.g. Partin's nomogram) that allow prediction of the overall stage of disease based on the clinical T stage, serum PSA and biopsy Gleason grade.

TNM classification system

T stage is assessed as a clinical stage by findings on DRE, a radiological stage on imaging (TRUS, MRI) or a histological examination of the prostate specimen after radical prostatectomy (RP). Clinical staging is prefixed with *c* and pathological staging with *p*.

Nodal stage is most commonly assessed by CT or MRI. MRI can be used to detect nodes >8 mm in maximal diameter; however, given that size criteria do not reliably identify affected nodes (sensitivity ranges from 0% to 70% with a positive predictive value of 50%), bilateral extended pelvic lymphadenectomy is the gold standard assessment of N staging. This is most commonly carried out in conjunction with radical prostatectomy.

For the *M stage*, in the presence of a serum PSA >100 ng/ml the risk of metastases is virtually 100% and often a biochemical M stage is determined by a very high PSA level.

Jewitt–Whitmore classification

The tumour is classified as stages A to D.

Stage A: This is asymptomatic localized disease detected on pathological assessment of the tissue (e.g. from transurethral resection of the prostate [TURP]); the tumour cells are limited to the prostate.

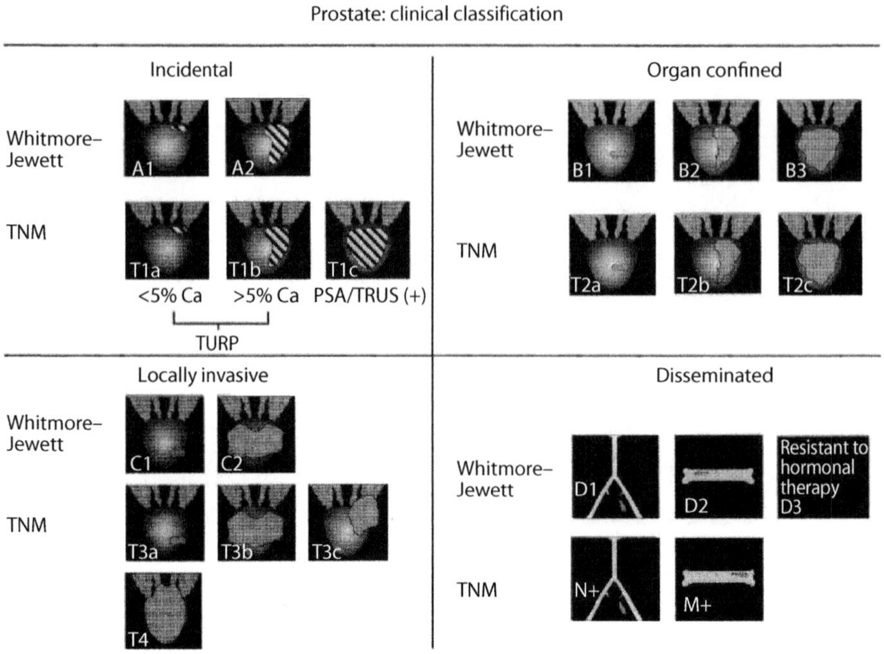

Prostate: clinical classification

Figure 37.4 Comparison of TNM and Whitmore–Jewett clinical classification. (From Garnick MB and Fair WR, *Ann Intern Med* 1996; 125: 118–125.)

Stage B: The tumour is limited to the prostate but palpable (detectable in a rectal examination) or detectable by an elevated PSA.

- B0 limited to the prostate, not detectable; high PSA
- B1 a single tumour nodule in a prostate lobe
- B2 diffuse, involves one or both lobes of the prostate

Stage C: The tumour cells are found outside the extension limited to surrounding tissues or seminal vesicles.

Stage D: This includes metastasis to the regional lymph glands, or at a distance from the bones, organs (liver, lungs) or other tissues.

Figure 37.4 shows a comparison between the classification systems.

Grading of prostate cancer

Prostate cancer is an adenocarcinoma of the ductal or acinar epithelium (>95%). Transitional cell carcinoma can occur in the prostatic urethra, ducts or stroma. Both prostatic sarcoma and secondary metastases to the prostate are rare. Macroscopically, these cancers are hard and white, although a soft mucin-producing variety does exist. Microscopically the basal cell layer is absent and the basement membrane is breached by malignant cells invading the prostatic fibromuscular stroma.

Most adenocarcinomas are located in the peripheral zone and they are predominantly multifocal. A proportion of cancers arise from the anterior zone, which are difficult to reach with transrectal ultrasound (TRUS)–guided prostate biopsy. The grading system for adenocarcinoma of the prostate is called the Gleason system, named after the Minneapolis pathologist who first described it in 1966. This system is a tissue grading system, unlike the more common cell grading seen in most cancers.

The system uses low-power microscopy to grade the adenocarcinoma from 1–5 according to the resemblance the malignant tissue bears to normal gland-forming differentiation. Under the original description, the most prevalent pattern (dominant pattern) and the next most prevalent (secondary pattern) are each awarded a grade between 1 and 5. The two are then simply added together to give the total Gleason score of between 2 and 10 (Figure 37.5). In practice, patterns 1 and 2 are almost unheard of, particularly on needle biopsy; thus the lowest score commonly seen is 6, which is responsible for around 80% of cancers diagnosed on needle biopsy.

Gleason score correlates well with prognosis and remains one of the most important prognostic indicators: the higher the score, the worse the prognosis associated with the disease. Cancers of the same prognostic score have a worse prognosis if the predominant Gleason score is higher, i.e. 4 + 3 = 7 is generally worse than 3 + 4 = 7. Furthermore, small areas of higher-grade disease seen on biopsy which do not get reported as the primary or secondary grade may have a significant impact on prognosis. It should be remembered that treatment to the prostate, including radiotherapy and androgen deprivation, has an effect on Gleason scoring and therefore cautious interpretation is necessary in patients having biopsies while already on or after treatment.

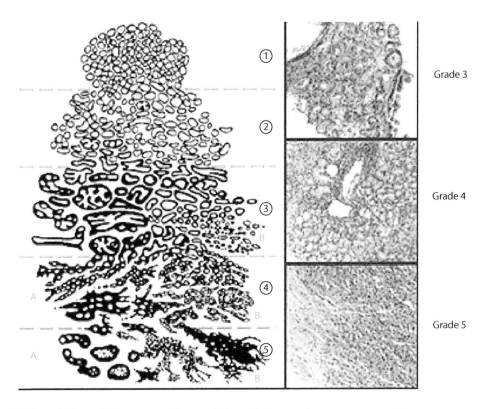

Figure 37.5 Original description of Gleason grading on left, with the modern common patterns seen on needle biopsy on the right. Available at http://www.curcuminjournal.com/gleason-scores.html.

		Low risk	Intermediate risk	High risk	
Definition		PSA <10 ng/mL and GS <7 and cT1-2a	PSA 10–20 ng/mL or GS 7 or cT2b	PSA >20 ng/mL or GS >7 or cT2c	Any PSA Any GS cT3-4 or cN+
			Localized		Locally advanced

Figure 37.6 EAU guidelines for definitions of localized and locally advanced prostate cancer. (From EAU guidelines, 2015. Available at http://uroweb.org/wp-content/uploads/09-Prostate-Cancer_LR.pdf)

Clinical presentation and risk stratification

From a clinical perspective, it is most convenient to divide prostate cancer into localized, locally advanced and metastatic disease.

LOCALIZED DISEASE

Prostate cancer tends to be a slow-growing cancer and as such localized disease is associated with relatively few specific symptoms. Most men are diagnosed on prostate biopsy, based on an elevated PSA test. Where symptoms are present (lower urinary tract symptoms, voiding discomfort, haematoejaculate or haematuria) these are usually caused by coexisting benign prostatic hyperplasia. Indeed, all other things being equal, prostate cancer on biopsy is more likely in a man without LUTS than in one with LUTS, at a similar elevation of PSA. The PSA level in localized disease is rarely in excess of 20 ng/ml: levels significantly above this generally indicate locally advanced or indeed metastatic disease and should initiate further staging investigations.

There exist a number of guidelines and nomograms to help classify localized prostate cancer to aid management plans. The most commonly used are based on the D'Amico risk criteria, which originally described the outcomes in treated cohorts of men with prostate cancer (Figure 37.6).

LOCALLY ADVANCED DISEASE

Locally advanced disease may present with progressive LUTS, with a time frame over months (rather than several years as is the case in BPH). Haematuria as a presenting symptom is unusual (approximately 1% of all cases of haematuria).

METASTATIC DISEASE

Metastatic prostate cancer most commonly presents with non-specific constitutional symptoms (anorexia, cachexia, lethargy, malaise). The classical presentation of an elderly man with progressive lower urinary tract symptoms and backache is rarely seen in the developed world these days, but is far more common in under-resourced nations.

Occasionally men present with obstructive uropathy (renal failure due to ureteric obstruction or chronic retention) or genital or lower limb lymphoedema. Bone pain, pathological fractures, cauda equina syndrome, spinal cord compression and haematological abnormalities such as anaemia and coagulopathies are similarly unusual but with catastrophic consequences where the underlying diagnosis is missed.

MANAGEMENT OF PROSTATE CANCER

Prostate cancer is often an indolent cancer, progressing slowly over many years. Previous studies have shown that mortality from localized prostate cancer is predominantly age related, with a 75% cancer-specific survival with untreated prostate cancer. The prognosis of higher-grade (Gleason 8–10) disease is less favourable; nevertheless survival exceeding 10 to 15 years without treatment is not unheard of. This aspect of the natural history of prostate cancer has led to the statement that more men die with prostate cancer rather than of prostate cancer, which still has some truth; however as outlined in the introduction, prostate cancer remains one of the most common causes of cancer death. Balancing the adverse events associated with treatment versus the relative indolence of the disease means that when considering the optimal treatment option for any man, an individualized approach should be followed taking into account comorbidities, quality of life and patient choice. The therapies offered could include monitoring of the disease, surgery, radiation therapy, either as brachytherapy or external beam, and focal therapies. Decisions regarding prostate cancer management should be made after all treatments have been discussed at a multidisciplinary forum (including urologists, uropathologists, oncologists, nurse specialists and uro-radiologists). Figure 37.7 outlines the general options for treatment according to disease stage.

Active monitoring

In the majority of men with clinically localized disease, radical treatment is unlikely to affect overall survival and indeed carries adverse effects that affect quality of life.

The treatment of a man with localized prostate cancer, whose cancer may never have progressed in his lifetime to significant disease has been termed 'overtreatment'. It is important to bear in mind that there is no reliable marker of overtreatment in any individual, although younger age (<70 years), with a predicted life expectancy (>10–15 years), higher Gleason grade, tumour volume and PSA level are all considered markers of significant progression to clinically symptomatic prostate cancer if left untreated. Where monitoring of clinically localized prostate cancer is being carried out with the express intention of deferring radical curative treatment for progressive disease, monitoring is termed 'active surveillance' (AS). AS protocols have been developed to reduce overtreatment of low-risk localized prostate cancer, with a number of approaches described (Table 37.4). All of these include regular DRE, PSA measurement, prostate imaging and possible repeated biopsies, but the exact combination varies and optimal timing is unclear. AS is most suitable for men with D'Amico very low or low-risk disease, but even in the most mature AS protocols, progression to locally advanced or indeed metastatic disease can occur without an obvious trigger.

Radical prostatectomy

RP is an established procedure that is generally well tolerated. Potential risks include prolonged hospitalization, lymphocele formation (particularly with extended pelvic lymphadenectomy), perioperative cardiovascular complications and rarely death (0.25%). Longer-term complications include urinary incontinence (1–10%), sexual dysfunction (25–90%), rectal injury (<1%), bladder neck stenosis, urethral stricture and bowel dysfunction. To date radical retropubic prostatectomy is the only radical treatment option for localized prostate cancer demonstrated to be associated with better survival than active monitoring; the Scandinavian study (SPCG-4) initiated in 1989 found a survival benefit for RP compared to watchful waiting, including improved overall and disease-specific mortality with an estimated number needed to treat (NNT) of 8 to save one life. This was most evident in younger men (under 65 years), although there was a

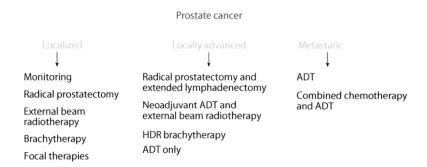

Figure 37.7 First-line treatment options for prostate cancer.

Table 37.4 Comparison of different published AS protocols

Institution	PSA testing	DRE	Repeat biopsy	Imaging (MRI)	Progression protocol
PRIAS	3 monthly years 1–2 6 monthly years 3–10 Annually year 10 onward	3 monthly years 1–2 6 monthly years 3–10 Annually year 10 onward		No	PSA-DT <3 years PSA-DT 3–10 repeat biopsy ≥3 positive biopsies GS >6 After 1 year of F/U
Klotz	3 monthly years 1–2 6 monthly years 3 onward	3 monthly years 1–2 6 monthly years 3 onward	Repeat biopsy within year 1 Year 4 Year 7 3–4 yearly until aged 80 years	Yes	PSA-DT <3 years (after 2009) PSA-DT triggered repeat biopsy or mpMRI Palpable nodule
Johns Hopkins	6 monthly	6 monthly	Annual biopsy	Yes	PSA-DT >0.15 ng/ml GS ≥7 >2 cores positive >50% cancer involvement
Royal Marsden	3 monthly years 1–2 6 monthly 3 years onward	3 monthly years 1–2 6 monthly 3 years onward	Repeat biopsy 2–4 yearly	Yes	PSA velocity >1 ng/ml/year Clinical progression on DRE GS >4 + 3 on repeat biopsy Patient choice
ProTecT	3 monthly year 1 6 monthly year 2 onward	3 monthly year 1 6 monthly year 2 onward	None	No	If PSA rise >50% in 1 year repeat PSA 6–9 weeks and review for possible repeat biopsy

Note: mpMRI = multiparametric MRI; PSA velocity = absolute annual increase in serum PSA (ng/ml/year); PSA-DT = PSA density.

reduced risk of metastatic disease spread and the requirement for androgen deprivation therapy (ADT) in men of all ages. The findings of the more recent PIVOT study carried out during the era of widespread PSA testing in the US suggested surgery carried no benefit; however, it has to be borne in mind that the average age of men in this study was 67 with 15% of the recruits in very poor general health and a 50% non-cancer mortality within 10 years of randomization.

Thus it appears that surgery remains the gold standard for the treatment of localized prostate cancer for men with an estimated life expectancy of 10 years or more. Salvage radical prostatectomy can be offered after radiotherapy but the complication rate appears to be higher than that for the primary procedure (e.g. up to 40% urinary incontinence).

The situation regarding locally advanced prostate cancer is more controversial. Multiple series have demonstrated significant overall survival and cancer-specific survival in this group of men (Table 37.5). However, there are no current direct comparative data with radiotherapy, which in conjunction with ADT remains the radical treatment of choice in most cases of locally advanced disease.

The main arguments for radical prostatectomy in locally advanced disease are:

1. Clinical overstaging and grading occurs in around 25% of men for whom surgery alone would be a viable option.
2. The situation following radical treatment with regard to disease recurrence is clear-cut; any detectable PSA indicates failure of treatment with an early option for adjuvant treatment.
3. The Swedish observational study of outcomes in more than 34,000 men at 15 years following surgery or radiotherapy suggests an advantage of surgery over radiotherapy as primary treatment.
4. Avoidance of ADT with its attendant adverse events and potential cardiovascular risk.

The role of extended pelvic lymphadenectomy in high-risk localized disease and locally advanced disease is even more controversial. Although there are no published results to date documenting long-term survival benefit, the benefit of removing lymph nodes harbouring micrometastases provides improved prognostic information and potentially delays the addition of systemic therapies such as ADT or chemotherapy.

Table 37.5 Radical prostatectomy for higher clinical stage (T3) in contemporary series

| Author (year) | No. patients | Adjuvant treatment | Overall survival | | Cancer-specific survival | |
			5 years	10 years (15 years)	5 years	10 years (15 years)
Ward et al. (2005)	842	62%	90%	76% (53%)	95%	90% (79%)
Carver et al. (2006)	176	36%[a]	88%	75% (69%)	94%	85% (76%)
Loeb et al. (2007)	288	15%	91%°	74%	92%[§]	88%
Freedland et al. (2007)	56	0%	—	—	98%	91% (84%)
Xylinas et al. (2009)	100	25%	85%	—	90%	—

Source: Alan JW, Louis RK, Alan WP, Craig AP, Campbell-Walsh Urology, 10th ed., Saunders: Campbell's Walsh Urology, 2011.

SURGICAL TECHNIQUE

With RP the entire prostate and seminal vesicles are removed en bloc with or without an extended pelvic lymphadenectomy. The bladder neck is reconstructed and is anastomosed with the remaining urethral sphincter. The procedure can be accomplished via an open retropubic approach, a perineal approach or a laparoscopic approach, with or without robotic assistance. The minimally invasive approach is associated with less blood loss and quicker recovery than open surgery. Robotic-assisted laparoscopic radical prostatectomy (RALP) has rapidly become the most popular approach, although no strong data exist demonstrating clear benefits in terms of cancer clearance, continence and potency rates over other approaches. Surgeon experience and volume together with careful patient selection are likely the most common factors influencing outcome rather than the approach per se; however RALP has a shorter learning curve, more consistent early results and is a better training platform for the procedure. Nerve-sparing surgery should be attempted in preoperatively potent patients with low risk for extracapsular disease.

The main goals are to excise the gland completely to obtain negative margins, to gain favourable oncological outcomes while not impinging on quality of life, namely urinary continence and sexual function. This is commonly referred to as the surgical pentafecta, which includes lack of postoperative complications, negative surgical margins, continence, potency and biochemical recurrence-free survival.

COMPLICATIONS OF RADICAL PROSTATECTOMY

Bleeding

Since the classical description by Walsh of the dorsal venous complex (Santorini's plexus) significant blood loss during RP has become a rare event. There is an avascular plane present between this venous complex and prostate, which is a landmark to gain dorsal venous plexus (DVC) control.

Urinary incontinence

The apex is intimately related to the distal sphincter mechanism. The puboprostatic ligaments insert onto the distal third of the posterior surface of the pubic bone, just adjacent and anterior to the urethral sphincter. These play an important role in preserving continence, and careful dissection at the apex preserving the ligaments and urethral length will minimize the risk of damage to the sphincter.

Sexual dysfunction

The neurovascular bundles arise from the hypogastric plexus bilaterally, course around the seminal vesicles and lie adjacent to the posterolateral margins of the prostate, providing vascular and autonomic supply for erectile function. Sparing these during the course of prostatectomy allows preservation of sexual function in most, but not all, cases.

Rectal injury (<1%)

The posterior aspect of the prostate is intimately related to the anterior aspect of the rectum separated only by Denonvilliers' fascia, which should be taken en bloc with the specimen. The rectum is at risk particularly when operating on locally advanced disease or as a salvage procedure, for example, following brachytherapy.

Post-prostatectomy biochemical failure and adjuvant therapy

Six weeks after RP, a serum PSA level of 0.05 ng/ml is generally considered an important cut-off. Biochemical failure is usually defined as a PSA level above 0.05 ng/ml at any point of follow-up beyond this time frame. At such low levels, the dilemma lies in determining whether the recurrence is local, thereby amenable to adjuvant external beam radiotherapy or systemic (metastatic). Prediction of the benefit of adjuvant local treatment is rendered easier if the results of an extended lymphadenectomy are available. Metastatic disease is usually indicated by high PSA kinetics (PSA doubling time <6 months or a PSA velocity >0.5 ng/ml/month) or lymph node positivity. In the absence of detectable PSA postoperatively, adjuvant external radiotherapy can also be offered as a treatment following RP in men with positive surgical margins to improve the biochemical and clinical disease-free survival.

The true benefit of this approach, as well as the matter of ideal patient selection, is currently being addressed by the international RADICALS trial.

Other surgical options for management of prostate cancer

FOCAL AND PARTIAL THERAPIES

Given the documented adverse event profile of the standard radical options for the treatment of localized prostate cancer, there is considerable interest in partial prostatic or focal therapies. The aim here is to obliterate the cancer while minimizing the collateral damage to normal tissues and hence adverse events such as urinary incontinence and sexual dysfunction. Patient selection remains of critical importance as around 80–85% of men with prostate cancer have multifocal disease. Approaches such as sequencing treatment to one lobe of the prostate and then to the other are currently being explored. A number of technologies have been described with varying evidence of efficacy and duration of follow-up. An added benefit of these technologies is they might be of benefit in local disease control following failure of external beam radiation.

CRYOTHERAPY

This is a day-case procedure performed under general anaesthetic. Ultrasound-guided cryoprobes are placed transperineally. These deliver argon or liquid nitrogen at –20°C to –40°C. Cell necrosis occurs after two freeze–thaw cycles. The urethra, external sphincter and rectum are protected. The PSA nadir is usually achieved around 3 months after treatment and 96% of men achieve a PSA <0.2 ng/ml. Possible complications include erectile dysfunction, incontinence, lower urinary tract symptoms and pelvic pain.

HIGH-INTENSITY FOCUSED ULTRASOUND

High-intensity focused ultrasound (HIFU) utilizes focused ultrasound to cause selective destruction of tissues at up to 4 cm depth without damaging adjacent tissues such as the rectum. Tissue is heated to >85°C leading to coagulative necrosis. Through use of a transrectal ultrasound probe to transmit high-energy ultrasound waves, 77% of men achieve a PSA nadir of <0.5 ng/ml within 4 months. In a small study two-thirds remained disease free at 2 years. Possible complications include erectile dysfunction, urinary retention, urethral stricture, stress incontinence and rectourethral fistula.

VASCULAR-TARGETED PHOTODYNAMIC THERAPY

Vascular-targeted photodynamic (VTP) therapy involves the use of a photosensitizing agent (TOOKAD®) in association with a low-power near-infrared laser (753 nm) light to destroy targeted tissues. The laser fibres are inserted into the prostate under ultrasound guidance via a perineal template under general anaesthesia. The photosensitizer is then infused intravenously while only the targeted areas of the prostate are laser illuminated. The procedure induces irreversible damage to the local vascular endothelium causing thrombosis, stasis and vascular occlusion, leading to tumour necrosis. Optimal results are obtained in prostates with a volume of between 25 and 70 cc. The procedure has an excellent safety record, but minimal long-term data of efficacy. Possible complications include erectile dysfunction, urinary retention, urethral stricture, stress urinary incontinence and rectourethral fistula.

TRANSURETHRAL RESECTION OF THE PROSTATE

Lower urinary tract symptoms in association with localized prostate cancer are commonly caused by benign prostatic obstruction. Under these circumstances, a limited transurethral resection of the prostate (TURP) can relieve symptoms and reduce the risk of retention or worsening symptoms in men due to undergo brachytherapy or external beam radiotherapy. In locally advanced disease, outflow obstruction can occur from tumour growth. Alternatives for symptomatic improvement in such cases include ADT alone or TURP. Judicious resection to prevent urinary incontinence is indicated, particularly in a repeat procedure where local tumour infiltration or scarring might result in obliteration of the usual surgical landmarks.

NON-SURGICAL OPTIONS

Radiotherapy

In localized prostate cancer, three-dimensional conformal radiotherapy (3D-CRT) with or without intensity-modulated radiotherapy (IMRT) is thought to be a curative treatment option, in the absence of comparative evidence with active monitoring or surgery. For high-risk patients, long-term androgen deprivation therapy before and during radiotherapy is recommended, because of demonstrable superiority in overall survival at 10 years. In fit patients with locally advanced prostate cancer, the recommended treatment is external beam radiotherapy (EBRT) plus long-term ADT (*vide infra*). It is however becoming increasingly apparent that despite the oncological benefits associated with such an approach, long-term ADT might be associated with an increased risk of cardiovascular mortality in men with pre-existing cardiovascular disease.

In low-risk patients with a prostate volume of <50 ml transperineal brachytherapy (implantation of radioactive seeds) can be an alternative with or without an external radiation boost.

Biochemical failure after radiation therapy is more difficult to define than following radical prostatectomy. The current consensus is to consider a rising PSA level to more than 2 ng/ml above the nadir PSA (lowest PSA level after treatment) as indicative of biochemical failure. This may take some time to manifest itself, particularly in the setting of neoadjuvant ADT. In patients with BCF who are candidates for local salvage therapy, prostate mpMRI can guide biopsy. Selected men with localized prostate cancer at initial diagnosis and with histologically proven recurrence in the absence of metastatic disease can be treated with salvage RP (SRP), but this is usually only offered in high-volume centres.

Systemic therapy

ANDROGEN DEPRIVATION THERAPY

The dependence of prostate cancer on androgenic stimulation places androgen deprivation therapy (ADT) on the main stage of treatment in several circumstances, including as sole primary treatment for advanced or metastatic disease, as neoadjuvant with radiation therapy (DXT), as adjuvant therapy after surgery and for progression of disease following radical primary therapy. ADT in metastatic disease results in palliation of symptoms and can delay complications such as spinal cord compression; nevertheless randomized trials provide evidence for improved overall survival when ADT is combined with radiation for intermediate- and high-risk localized disease as well as locally advanced and node positive disease after radical radiotherapy or prostatectomy. More recent studies have confirmed significant survival benefit for men with advanced disease given both ADT and taxane-based chemotherapy in combination (chemohormonal therapy). Although ADT in isolation is not curative, many patients experience long-term remissions in cases of advanced or metastatic disease.

ADT can be achieved by surgical or medical castration. The perceived psychological effects of surgical orchidectomy mean that chemical castration is most commonly utilized in clinical practice, although in men with high-volume metastatic disease or impending spinal cord compression, bilateral orchidectomy might still have a role to play. Luteinizing hormone-releasing hormone (LHRH) agonists have been available for several years. These cause an initial rise in LH and therefore testosterone levels and thus require concomitant therapy with a peripheral androgen receptor antagonist to avoid an initial tumour volume increase termed 'clinical flare'. This can lead to increased bone pain, acute bladder outlet obstruction, obstructive renal failure, spinal cord compression and fatal cardiovascular events. Anti-androgen therapy needs to be continued for around 4 weeks after initiation of LHRH agonist therapy at which point LH and associated testosterone levels will reach castrate levels. In recent years, LHRH antagonists such as degarelix have become available. Degarelix results in rapid LH and testosterone suppression, similar to that seen with surgical castration.

The benefits of ADT must be weighed against the expected adverse effects which include fatigue, cognitive changes, depression and decrease in libido and sexual function. Hot flushes can occur with severe flushes affecting approximately 30% of men. Reduction in bone density can occur in up to 3–4% of men at 12 months of commencing ADT. The risk of osteoporosis increases with duration of therapy with almost 81% of men having osteoporosis at 10 years. As well as vitamin D and calcium supplements, zolendronic acid and denosumab can be used in severe cases. More recently, concerns regarding increased risk of adverse cardiovascular events, particularly in association with the LHRH agonists, have arisen. Although cause and effect remains unproven, it is recommended that routine evaluation of cardiovascular risk status is carried out in men on ADT with periodic checking of blood pressure, lipid profile and glucose levels. Supervised exercise programmes have been shown to reduce many of the adverse events associated with ADT with concomitant improvement in disease-specific quality of life. The wider role of lifestyle interventions, including reduction of cardiovascular risk and improvement in survival, is currently being studied in international studies such as the STAMINA and the GAP4 programmes.

CASTRATION-RESISTANT PROSTATE CANCER

Circulating androgens play a critical role in the development and progression of prostate cancer: ever since the initial description of orchiectomy for symptomatic metastatic prostate cancer by Huggins and Hodges, endocrine therapy in the form of ADT has formed the cornerstone of primary treatment for advanced prostate cancer. ADT can be achieved through surgical castration by bilateral orchiectomy or medical castration by gonadotropin-releasing hormone (GnRH) analogues, either agonists or antagonists. Response to ADT occurs in around 80% of primary cases of prostate cancer, with demonstrable clinical, radiological and biochemical improvement, often lasting several years (but typically 2–2½ years for men presenting with metastatic disease), a fact that signifies the pivotal role of the androgen receptor in most cases of prostate cancer. Despite the initial response to ADT in the remainder, progression to castrate-resistant prostate cancer (CRPC) is inevitable, should the man not succumb to other disease processes. Metastatic castrate-resistant prostate cancer (mCRPC) is the lethal form of prostate cancer; although there are a variety of treatment options available to ameliorate disease progression (Table 37.6), mCRPC remains incurable.

It was previously thought that mCRPC development represented loss of androgen responsiveness. However, what seems most likely is that expression and functionality of the androgen receptor is almost never lost in mCRPC: androgen receptor sensitivity is retained with stimulation and growth occurring at extremely low levels of circulating androgens through a number of mechanisms including stem cell involvement, overexpression, coactivator upregulation, gene amplification, androgen receptor splice-variant expression or mutation (Figure 37.8). As such, novel inhibitors of androgen synthesis and second-generation anti-androgens have been identified, with better pharmacokinetic targeting, providing new hope for men with mCRPC. It is clear

Table 37.6 Newer generation agents used in the treatment of castration-resistant prostate cancer

Therapeutic agent	Mechanism of action	Clinical trial status	Therapeutic efficacy
Docetaxel	Stabilization of tubulin, induction of cell cycle arrest and inhibition of cell proliferation	FDA approved	Overall survival benefit and palliation of cancer-associated symptoms
Cabazitaxel	Stabilization of tubulin, induction of cell cycle arrest and inhibition of cell proliferation	FDA approved for men after failure of docetaxel	Overall survival benefit and palliation of cancer-associated symptoms
Sipuleucel-T (Provenge)	Enhancement of men's autologous antigen-presenting cells to induce cytotoxic response against prostate cancer cells	FDA approved	Increase in overall survival but not progression-free survival
Abiraterone acetate	Irreversible inhibition of CYP17 and subsequent androgen synthesis	FDA approved in the pre- and post-docetaxel settings	Increase in overall survival (almost 4 months), radiographic progression-free survival, time to PSA progression and palliation of cancer-associated symptoms
MDV3100 (enzalutamide)	AR antagonist preventing nuclear translocation and binding to chromatin	FDA approved in the post-docetaxel setting Phase III clinical trial in comparison with placebo in chemotherapy-naive men	Increase of overall survival (4.8 months), radiographic progression-free survival and time to PSA progression; similar benefits reported
BEZ235	Inhibition of PI3K	Phase I or II clinical trials in combination with abiraterone acetate (NCT01717898)	Results pending
RAD001 (everolimus)	Inhibition of mTOR	Phase II clinical trial in combination with bicalutamide (NCT00630344)	Failure to show increase in time to progression
Alpharadin (radium-223)	An alpha emitter which selectively targets bone metastases with alpha particles	Phase III clinical trial in men who had received, were not eligible to receive or declined docetaxel	Increase of overall survival (median 14.0 months vs. 11.2 months [placebo]; hazard ratio 0.70)
Dovitinib (TK1258)	Inhibition of FGFR	Phase II clinical trial in men after failure of docetaxel-based chemotherapy (NCT01741116)	Results pending
Cabozatinib (XL184)	Inhibition of c-MET	Phase II clinical trial in men with mCR prostate cancer (NCT01428219) Phase III clinical trial in comparison with prednisone in men previously treated with docetaxel and abiraterone or MDV3100 (COMET-1, NCT01605227) Phase III clinical trial in comparison with mitoxantrone and prednisone (COMET-2, NCT01522443)	Reduction of soft tissue lesions, resolution of bone scans, increase of progression-free survival, results pending in phase III trials

Source: Adapted from Karantanos T, et al., Oncogene 2013; 32(49): 5501.

however that in most cases of mCRPC, a dynamic situation exists which poses an ongoing challenge to the development of truly effective disease-modifying treatments. Although many of the newer treatments for mCRPC continue to target the androgen axis, resistance to the agent with subsequent disease progression remains the norm. Anti-androgens in the form of flutamide and bicalutamide have been available for many years, with some evidence for providing additive benefit to ADT in terms of reduction in PSA levels (so-called complete androgen blockade) but little

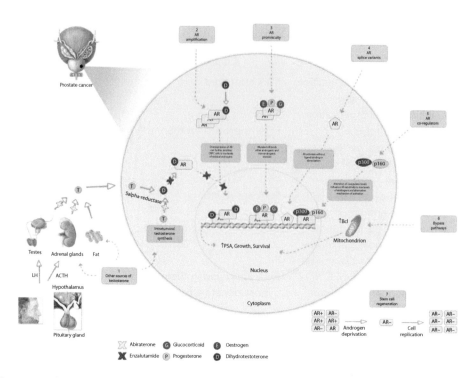

Figure 37.8 Mechanisms of ongoing androgen responsiveness in castrate-resistant prostate cancer. (Adapted with permission from Greasley R, et al., *Cancer Manag Res* 2015; 7: 153–164.)

evidence of improved survival. Several phenomena such as the development of resistance to the initial agent and the anti-androgen withdrawal response (AAWR) demonstrate that adaptive changes such as coactivator upregulation with subsequent paradoxical agonist effects of the anti-androgen occur. Additionally, *in vitro* and *in vivo* studies have demonstrated the ability of anti-androgens to induce AR mutations, again resulting in paradoxical stimulation of tumour progression. Cross-resistance to agents with different mechanisms of action, such as abiraterone and enzalutamide, has been suggested by the results of smaller clinical trials, but the true benefits of simultaneous use and drug sequencing have yet to be demonstrated clinically. Finally, truly androgen-independent tumour progression via cross talk with MAP-kinase pathways (EGF and IGF-1) occurs, with some evidence to suggest that anti-androgens such as flutamide act directly on these pathways. Multiple mechanisms with resistance to novel anti-androgens exist and have been recently reviewed (Yuan et al. 2014). One of the major mechanisms that have been postulated to be responsible for an overall resistance to conventional and next-generation ADT is the synthesis of androgen receptor splice variants (AR-V). Overexpression of AR-V at mRNA and protein levels in prostate cancer tissue is associated with disease progression and poor prognosis.

1. Extragonadal production. Androgens from other sources such as adrenal glands, adipose tissue and intratumoral production bind and activate the androgen receptor despite absence of gonadal-derived androgens.

2. Amplification. Prostate cancer cells become sensitized to low levels of circulating androgens post-castration by increasing the production of androgen receptor via gene amplification.

3. Promiscuity. Mutations (mostly mis-sense) of the ligand binding domain (LBD) of the androgen receptor expand the binding specificity, allowing non-androgenic steroids such as oestrogen (E), progesterone (P) and glucocorticoid (G) to bind and activate the androgen receptor.

4. Splice variants. Constitutively active splice variants result in ligand-independent receptor activation allowing protein translocation without the need for ligand binding or dimerization. Some splice variants promote castration resistance and anchorage-independent growth through coupling to the full-length mRNA production.

5. Coregulator alteration. Alteration of the levels of coactivators and corepressors, signalling intermediates between the AR and transcriptional machinery, affects activation by sensitizing to lower levels of androgen and alternative activation mechanisms.

6. Bypass pathway. Prostate cancer cells develop the ability to evade apoptosis and survive when exposed to low levels of androgen via upregulation of the molecule Bcl-2, a regulator of programmed cell death.

7. Stem cell regeneration. Possible source of continual supply of androgen-independent population of prostate cancer cells after ADT.

FURTHER READING

Books

EAU guidelines
Campbell–Walsh Urology, Volume 3.

Papers

Andriole G, et al. Prostate cancer screening in the Randomized Prostate, Lung, Colorectal and Ovarian Cancer Screening Trial: mortality results after 13 years of follow up. *J Natl Cancer Inst* 2012; 104(2): 125–132.

Bill-Axelson A, Holmberg L. Radical prostatectomy or watchful waiting in early prostate cancer. *N Engl J Med* 2014; 370(10): 932–942.

Bill-Axelson A, Holmberg L, Ruutu M, et al. Radical prostatectomy versus watchful waiting in early prostate cancer. *N Engl J Med* 2005; 352(19): 1977–1984.

Bratt O, et al. Hereditary prostate cancer: clinical aspects. *J Urol* 2002; 168(3): 906.

Bul M, et al. Active surveillance for low risk prostate cancer worldwide: the PRIAS study. *Eur Urol* 2013; 63(4) 507–603.

D'Amico A, Kantoff P. Longterm follow up of a randomized trial of radiation with or without androgen deprivation therapy for localized prostate cancer. *JAMA* 2015; 314(12): 1291–1293.

Delongchamps NB, et al. The role of prevalence in the diagnosis of prostate cancer. *Cancer Control* 2006; 13(3): 158–168.

Garnick M, Fair W. Prostate cancer: emerging concepts part 1. *Ann Intern Med* 1996; 125(2): 118–125.

Gnanapragasam V, Neal D. The role of surgery in high risk localised prostate cancer. *BJU Int* 2012; 109(5): 648–658.

Greasley R, Khabazhaitajer M, Rosario DJ. A profile of enzalutamide for the treatment of advanced castration resistant prostate cancer. *Cancer Manag Res* 2015; 7: 153–164.

Huggins C, Hodges CV. Studies on prostatic cancer. I. The effect of castration, of estrogen and androgen injection on serum phosphatases in metastatic carcinoma of the prostate. *CA Cancer J Clin* 1972; 22(4): 232–240.

James N, Sydes M. Survival with newly diagnosed metastatic prostate cancer in the "docetaxel era": data from 917 patients in the control arm of the STAMPEDE Trial. *Eur Urol* 2015; 67(6); 1028–1038.

Karantanos T, Corn PG, Thompson TC. Prostate cancer progression after androgen deprivation therapy: mechanisms of castrate resistance and novel therapeutic approaches. *Oncogene* 2013; 32(49): 5501.

Klotz L, et al. Long-term follow-up of a large active surveillance cohort of patients with prostate cancer. *J Clin Oncol* 2015; 33(3): 272–277.

Maughan B, Antonarakis E. Optimal sequencing of docetaxel and abiraterone in men with metastatic castration-resistant prostate cancer. *Prostate* 2015; 75(15): 1814–1820.

McCain J. Drugs that offer a survival advantage for men with bone metastases resulting from castration resistant prostate cancer. *Pharm Therapeut* 2014; 39(2): 130–137.

Schroder F, et al. Screening and prostate cancer mortality: results of the European Randomised Study of Screening for Prostate Cancer (ERSPC) at 13 years of follow up. *Lancet* 2014; 384(9959): 2027–2035.

Sooriakumaran P, et al. Comparative effectiveness of radical prostatectomy and radiotherapy in prostate cancer: observational study of mortality outcomes. *BMJ* 2014; 348: g1502.

Studer U, Collette L. Morbidity from pelvic lymphadenectomy in men undergoing radical prostatectomy. *Eur Urol* 2006; 50(5): 887–889.

Sweeney C, Chamberlain D. Insights into E3805: the CHAARTED trial. *Future Oncol* 2015; 11(6): 897–898.

Walsh P, Lepor H. The role of radical prostatectomy in the management of prostatic carcinoma. *Cancer* 1987; 60(3 Suppl.): 526–537.

Wilt T, Wheeler T. Radical prostatectomy versus observation for localised prostate cancer. *N Engl J Med* 2012; 367(3): 203–213.

Yuan X, Cai C, Chen S, Yu Z, Balk SP. Androgen receptor functions in castration-resistant prostate cancer and mechanisms of resistance to new agents targeting the androgen axis. *Oncogene* 2014; 33(22): 2815–2825.

WEBSITES

https://www.gov.uk/government/publications/prostate-specific-antigen-testing-evidence-document

http://www.uspreventiveservicestaskforce.org/Page/Document/RecommendationStatementFinal/prostate-cancer-screening

TRIAL WEBSITES

http://www.radicals-trial.org

http://www.stampedetrial.org

http://www.ctu.mrc.ac.uk/our_research/research_areas/cancer/studies/promis

38

Testicular tumours

CELINE P E ASSELBERGS AND THEO M DE REIJKE

INCIDENCE AND ETIOLOGY

Testicular tumours represent a relatively rare malignancy accounting for approximately 1% to 1.5% of all malignancies in men and 5% of urological tumours in general. Nevertheless, testicular cancer is the most common solid malignancy in men between the ages of 15 and 40. The incidence in industrialized countries is about 3 to 10 new cases per 100,000 males per year and increases worldwide. The peak incidence for non-seminoma germ cell tumour (NSGCT) is in the third decade, and for seminoma in the fourth decade [1]. The remaining 5% of non–germ cell tumours comprise mainly lymphoma presenting in adult men (age range 50–70 years); other tumours include sex cord tumours (Sertoli cell tumours, Leydig cell tumours) in adults and paratesticular tumours (rhabdomyosarcoma in infants and leiomyosarcoma in adults).

Several etiological risk factors are known: prior history of germ cell tumour (GCT), the presence of a contralateral tumour or intratubular germ cell neoplasia (testicular intraepithelial neoplasia [TIN]), Klinefelter's syndrome, positive family history of testicular tumours among first-grade relatives, cryptorchidism, hypotrophic testicle and infertility [1].

When the developed follow-up and treatment algorithms are strictly followed, the cure rate of testicular tumours is excellent [1–4]. Prognosis is most favourable in low-volume disease with a 99% 5-year survival rate for all stage I tumours but less favourable rates (~60%) for the rarer cases of advanced tumours with visceral metastases.

PATHOLOGICAL CLASSIFICATION

Testicular tumours can be subdivided according to a recommended pathological classification system as introduced by the World Health Organization (WHO) (Table 38.1) [5]. Ninety-five percent of malignant testicular tumours are GCT, classified as either seminoma or NSGCT [3,4]. Occasionally GCTs occur in extragonadal primary sites, usually found in mid-line anatomic locations, e.g. retroperitoneum, mediastinum or cerebrum. Their management is the same as for testicular GCT [2,3].

CLINICAL PRESENTATION

Patients usually present with a unilateral, painless testicular swelling. There might be testicular discomfort or swelling that mimics an epididymitis or orchitis, with subsequent

Table 38.1 Pathological classification of germ cell tumours

- Intratubular germ cell neoplasia, unclassified type (IGCNU)
- Seminoma (including cases with syncytiotrophoblastic cells)
- Spermatocytic seminoma (mention if there is sarcomatous component)
- Embryonal carcinoma
- Yolk sac tumour
- Choriocarcinoma
- Teratoma (mature, immature, with malignant component)
- Tumours with more than one histological type (specify percentage of individual components)

Source: Data from European Association of Urology, Guidelines on testicular cancer, 2011, http://www.uroweb.org.

delay of diagnosis. A recent trauma to the scrotal region can also reveal the presence of a testicular mass. Some patients present with symptoms attributable to metastatic disease. Many men carry out self-examination as a result of increased public awareness about testicular cancer, and many such cases reveal epididymal cysts, a hydrocele or normal anatomy. The important step in clinical examination is to establish whether the mass is intratesticular, indicating a high risk that it is a malignant growth.

The examination of the testis may be restricted by the presence of a hydrocele that can develop secondary to a testicular tumour or by the presence of incidental epididymal cysts.

A thorough physical examination of the affected and contralateral testis is necessary. The abdomen should be palpated for evidence of nodal disease or visceral involvement. Inguinal or supraclavicular lymphadenopathy, gynaecomastia or thoracic involvement must also be assessed [1–4].

DIAGNOSTICS AND INITIAL MANAGEMENT

If there is suspicion of a testicular tumour immediate diagnostics should be performed and there is general consensus that the treatment should be performed within 5 days.

An ultrasound (US) examination of both testes should always be performed and has a sensitivity to detect a testicular mass of almost 100% [1–4]. Besides imaging the affected testis, the contralateral testis should also be investigated to exclude microcalcifications.

The next essential step is to determine the serum tumour markers. Although not uniquely specific for GCT, they provide important information when present about tumour burden, tumour type and response to treatment and possible relapse. If they are elevated then sequential postoperative measurements will indicate whether they fall

to normal, indicating a stage I tumour that has been completely removed, or they remain elevated indicating metastatic disease even if further imaging is normal. Lactate dehydrogenase (LDH), alpha-fetoprotein (AFP) and β–human chorionic gonadotrophin (β-HCG) have established roles in diagnosis and staging, determining prognosis and assessment of treatment outcome. They should be determined before, during and after treatment and are used in the follow-up.

LDH is a less specific marker than AFP and β-HCG. Its concentration is proportional to tumour volume. AFP is produced by non-seminomatous cells and has a half-life of approximately 5 to 7 days. If AFP is elevated and histology does not identify non-seminomatous areas the tumour should still be treated as such. β-HCG, with a half-life of 1 to 3 days, can be found in either type of testicular GCT. Negative tumour markers do not exclude a testicular cancer [1–4].

Cryopreservation and hormonal analyses

Every patient of fertile age should be offered sperm banking prior to undergoing any therapeutic intervention that may compromise fertility, preferably before orchiectomy, but in any case before adjuvant chemotherapy or radiotherapy [1–4].

The EAU guideline gives a grade B recommendation concerning fertility investigations: total testosterone, LH, FSH and semen analysis [1].

Biopsy of the contralateral testis

There is no reason for a standard contralateral biopsy, unless when dealing with high-risk patients for contralateral TIN (testicular volume <12 ml, history of cryptorchidism and age <40 years). Without these risk factors, testicular microlithiasis is not an indication for biopsy or further US screening [1–4].

The treatment of TIN (with a healthy contralateral testis) consists of either orchiectomy or active surveillance, with a risk of 50% within 5 years to develop a testicular cancer. In patients diagnosed with TIN and a solitary testis, local radiotherapy is the standard treatment [1].

Inguinal orchidectomy

All patients with suspected testicular mass should undergo radical inguinal orchidectomy with division of the spermatic cord at the level of the internal inguinal ring. Scrotal violation should be avoided [1–4]. There is no need for testicular biopsy to confirm the diagnosis.

Organ-sparing surgery may be considered for synchronous bilateral tumours <2 cm or in a tumour in a mono-testis with sufficient preoperative testosterone levels [1,2,4].

In patients presenting with life-threatening advanced disease, chemotherapy can be started immediately and orchiectomy may be delayed until clinical stabilization has occurred [1,2].

Histological types

SEMINOMA

The majority of seminoma (~85%) are 'classical' in their appearance with approximately 10% demonstrating anaplastic features. A small number are described as spermatocytic seminomas which are recognized as benign tumours and not GCT.

NON-SEMINOMA

These tumours are characterized by exhibiting cellular elements from all three primitive developmental layers, endoderm, mesoderm and ectoderm. Cellular elements may include glandular tissue, respiratory or gastrointestinal morphology, neurological tissue and bone, or cartilaginous or skin structures. In addition embryological tissues such as trophoblastic cells, yolk cell elements and choriocarcinoma may be seen. The American classification lists each element, whereas the UK classification subdivides into four main categories:

- Teratoma differentiated (TD) containing both mature and immature elements
- Malignant teratoma intermediate (MTI) containing teratoma with malignant transformation and can include embryonal carcinoma
- Malignant teratoma undifferentiated (MTU) describing embryonal carcinoma
- Malignant teratoma trophoblastic describing choriocarcinoma which may contain other malignant elements

STAGING

Imaging

Computed tomography (CT) scanning of the abdomen and pelvis is required in determining the state of retroperitoneal lymph nodes and lung or liver metastases [1–4]. Although the NCCN guideline on testicular cancer advises chest X-ray, in Europe chest CT is recommended to evaluate the thorax and mediastinal lymph nodes [1,3]. Up to 10% of patients can present with small subpleural nodes, not visible on X-ray. If an extensive tumour burden is found a brain CT may be indicated to exclude cerebral metastatic disease. Magnetic resonance imaging (MRI) shows higher sensitivity and specificity than US scanning of the testis for diagnosing testicular tumours and is comparable to CT scanning to detect retroperitoneal lymph nodes. However, MRI is less cost-effective and therefore not standard investigation in the diagnosis and staging of testicular cancer. Nevertheless, it can be used when US and abdominopelvic CT scans are not conclusive or the patient has a contrast allergy or a contraindication for CT scanning. At staging, there is no need for a bone scan unless metastases are suspected [1]. Primary retroperitoneal lymph node dissection in the case of negative imaging is generally not performed in Europe unless there is a high-risk tumour, e.g. lymphovascular invasion.

Serum tumour markers

As mentioned earlier, serum markers are important for staging, prognosis and follow-up. Post-orchidectomy, markers must be evaluated repeatedly to assess decline according to their half-life [1–4].

Prognostic classification

Prognosis and management of GCT are based on the clinical stage of disease. The recommended staging system is the 2009, 7th edition, tumour node metastasis (TNM) classification of the American Joint Committee on Cancer (AJCC) and the International Union Against Cancer (UICC) (Table 38.2).

Combined with serum tumour marker levels, stage groups have been defined (Table 38.3) [5].

In 1997, the International Germ Cell Cancer Consensus Group (IGCCCG) developed a prognostic factor-based staging system which reflects the extent of the disease based on identification of clinically independent factors: primary tumour location, elevation of tumour marker levels and presence of non-pulmonary visceral metastasis (Table 38.4) [6].

Progression-free survival

For stage I disease, different prognostic risk factors have been suggested, based on histopathological features in the primary tumour. For seminoma, both tumour size ≥4 cm and invasion of tumour in the rete testis have been identified as predictors in recurrence. The most valid predictors for occult metastatic disease in NSGCT are vascular invasion of the primary tumour, as well as proliferation rate (>70%) and presence of embryonal carcinoma (>50%) [1,2,4].

When both seminoma and NSGCT elements are present in the primary tumour, treatment is according to the NSGCT algorithms as an NSGCT is the clinically more aggressive tumour [1–4].

TREATMENT OF SEMINOMA AFTER ORCHIECTOMY

Stage I

The disease-specific survival in patients with stage I seminoma is approximately 100%, regardless of the treatment strategy (surveillance, radiotherapy to the abdominal lymph nodes or one course of chemotherapy with carboplatin) chosen after initial orchidectomy [7]. Currently, the preferred treatment option in informed and compliant patients with stage I disease is surveillance.

The risk of relapse after orchiectomy alone is approximately 15% to 20% within 5 years, due to subclinical metastatic disease occurring mostly in infra-diaphragmatic lymph nodes. In low-risk patients (tumour size ≤4 cm, no

Table 38.2 TNM classification of testicular cancer

pT: Primary tumour

pTX: Primary tumour cannot be assessed

pT0: No evidence of primary tumour (e.g. histological scar in testis)

pTis: Intratubular germ cell neoplasia (testicular intraepithelial neoplasia)

pT1: Tumour limited to testis and epididymis without vascular/lymphatic invasion; tumour may invade tunica albuginea but not tunica vaginalis

pT2: Tumour limited to testis and epididymis with vascular/lymphatic invasion, or tumour extending through tunica albuginea with involvement of tunica vaginalis

pT3: Tumour invades spermatic cord with or without vascular/lymphatic invasion

pT4: Tumour invades scrotum with or without vascular/lymphatic invasion

cN: Regional lymph nodes

NX: Regional lymph nodes cannot be assessed

N0: No regional lymph node metastasis

N1: Metastasis with a lymph node mass 2 cm or less in greatest dimension or multiple lymph nodes, none more than 2 cm in greatest dimension

N2: Metastasis with a lymph node mass more than 2 cm but not more than 5 cm in greatest dimension, or multiple lymph nodes, any one mass more than 2 cm but not more than 5 cm in greatest dimension

N3: Metastasis with a lymph node mass more than 5 cm in greatest dimension

pN: Pathological

pNX: Regional lymph nodes cannot be assessed

pN0: No regional lymph node metastasis

pN1: Metastasis with a lymph node mass 2 cm or less in greatest dimension and 5 or fewer positive nodes, none more than 2 cm in greatest dimension

pN2: Metastasis with a lymph node mass more than 2 cm but not more than 5 cm in greatest dimension, or more than 5 nodes positive, none more than 5 cm, or evidence or extranodal extension of tumour

pN3: Metastasis with a lymph node mass more than 5 cm in greatest dimension

cM: Distant metastasis

MX: Distant metastasis cannot be assessed

M0: No distant metastasis

M1: Distant metastasis

M1a: Non-regional lymph node(s) or lung

M1b: Other sites

S: Serum tumour markers

Sx: Serum marker studies not available or not performed

S0: Serum marker study levels within normal limits

S1: LDH $< 1.5 \times$ N U/l *and* β-HCG < 5.000 mIU/ml *and* AFP < 1.000 ng/ml

S2: LDH $1.5–10 \times$ N U/l *or* β-HCG $< 5.000–50.000$ mIU/ml *or* AFP $1.000–10.000$ ng/ml

S3: LDH $> 10 \times$ N U/l *or* β-HCG > 50.000 mIU/ml *or* AFP > 10.000 ng/ml

Source: Data from European Association of Urology, Guidelines on testicular cancer, 2011, http://www.uroweb.org; Edge S, et al., *AJCC Cancer Staging Manual*, 7th ed., New York: Springer Verlag, 2010.

rete testis invasion) the recurrence under surveillance is as low as 6% at 5 years; therefore, adjuvant treatment is not recommended in these cases. For some patients, surveillance will not be applicable. Also, the prognostic risk factors might indicate treatment with one or two courses of single-agent carboplatin (AUC 7). Carboplatin results in similar recurrence rates and survival as adjuvant radiotherapy, is well tolerated and is associated with less morbidity. Radiotherapy (10 × 2 Gy to a para-aortic field) is recommended only to those patients not suitable for surveillance or chemotherapy [1].

Stage IIA

As in stage I, the overall survival rate is almost 100%, with a relapse-free survival of 92%. The mainstay of treatment is radiotherapy (30 Gy directed to a 'hockey stick field'; e.g. the para-aortal region and the ipsilateral iliac lymph nodes) [1].

Table 38.3 Stage grouping of testicular cancer

Stage	T	N	M	S
Stage 0	pTis	N0	M0	S0, SX
Stage I	pT1–T4	N0	M0	SX
Stage IA	pT1	N0	M0	S0
Stage IB	pT2–pT4	N0	M0	S0
Stage IS	Any patient/TX	N0	M0	S1–S3
Stage II	Any patient/TX	N1–N3	M0	SX
Stage IIA	Any patient/TX	N1	M0	S0, S1
Stage IIB	Any patient/TX	N2	M0	S0, S1
Stage IIC	Any patient/TX	N3	M0	S0, S1
Stage III	Any patient/TX	Any N	M1a	SX
Stage IIIA	Any patient/TX	Any N	M1a	S0, S1
Stage IIIB	Any patient/TX	N1–N3	M0	S2
	Any patient/TX	Any N	M1a	S2
Stage IIIC	Any patient/TX	N1–N3	M0	S3
	Any patient/TX	Any N	M1a	S3
	Any patient/TX	Any N	M1b	Any S

Source: Data from European Association of Urology, Guidelines on testicular cancer, 2011, http://www.uroweb.org; Edge S, et al., *AJCC Cancer Staging Manual*, 7th ed., New York: Springer Verlag, 2010.

Table 38.4 Prognostic-based staging system for metastatic GCT

Good prognosis group

Seminoma
(90% of cases)
5-year PFS 82%
5-year survival 86%

All of the following criteria:
- Any primary site
- No non-pulmonary visceral metastases
- Normal AFP
- Any HCG
- Any LDH

NSGCT (56% of cases)
5-year PFS 89%
5-year survival 92%

All of the following criteria:
- Testis/retroperitoneal primary
- No non-pulmonary visceral metastases
- AFP < 1.000 ng/ml
- HCG < 5.000 IU/L
- LDH < 1.5 × N

Intermediate prognosis group

Seminoma
(10% of cases)
5-year PFS 67%
5-year survival 72%

All of the following criteria:
- Any primary site
- Non-pulmonary visceral metastases
- Normal AFP
- Any HCG
- Any LDH

(Continued)

Table 38.4 *(Continued)* Prognostic-based staging system for metastatic GCT

Intermediate prognosis group

NSGCT (28% of cases)
5-year PFS 75%
5-year survival 80%

The following criteria:
- Testis/retroperitoneal primary
- No non-pulmonary visceral metastases
- AFP 1.000–10.000 ng/ml or
- HCG 5.000–50.000 IU/L or
- LDH 1.5–10 × N

Poor prognosis group

Seminoma
No patients classified as poor prognosis

NSGCT (16% of cases)
5-year PFS 41%
5-year survival 48%

Any of the following criteria:
- Mediastinal primary
- Non-pulmonary visceral metastases
- AFP > 10.000 ng/ml or
- HCG > 50.000 IU/L or
- LDH > 10 × N

Source: Data from European Association of Urology, Guidelines on testicular cancer, 2011, http://www.uroweb.org; International Germ Cell Cancer Collaborative Group, *J Clin Oncol* 1997; 15: 594–603.

Stage IIB

Combination cisplatin-based chemotherapy (four courses of etoposide and cisplatin [EP] or three courses of bleomycin, etoposide and cisplatin [BEP]) is an alternative to radiotherapy as mentioned for stage IIA. After radiotherapy (36 Gy), overall survival is again around 100%, with a relapse-free survival of 90%. Chemotherapy achieves a similar level of disease control, but is more toxic in the short term [1].

Stages IIC and III

Cisplatin-based chemotherapy is used for both groups of patients. According to the IGCCCG risk classification, in patients with good prognosis, three cycles of BEP are recommended. In the intermediate prognosis risk group, four cycles of BEP are standard treatment with a 5-year survival rate of approximately 80% [1].

TREATMENT OF NSGCT AFTER ORCHIECTOMY

Stage I

In general, three different treatment options are available for stage I NSGCT: surveillance, adjuvant chemotherapy and nerve-sparing retroperitoneal lymph node dissection (NS-RPLND), which can be performed laparo-scopically. Nearly 30% of patients have subclinical metasta-ses and will relapse within 12 months if surveillance alone is offered.

As mentioned earlier, vascular invasion is the most important risk factor for presumed risk of relapse. Using this risk-stratifying approach, pT1 tumours without vascular invasion are considered low risk and pT2–T4 tumours with vascular invasion high risk. Correlating this to the recom-mended treatment options, long-term survival approaches 100% with all available treatment options. Patients with low-risk tumours should be advised to undergo long-term (at least 5 years) surveillance. This means that the patient should be motivated to have a stringent follow-up sched-ule, and compliance to this scheme is essential. If this is not feasible, adjuvant chemotherapy (two cycles of BEP) or NS-RPLND is a treatment option. Patients with high-risk tumours preferably undergo adjuvant chemotherapy (two cycles of BEP), although surveillance and NS-RPLND remain options for those not willing to undergo adjuvant chemotherapy. Positive lymph nodes in both risk groups warrant chemotherapy (two cycles of BEP) [1].

Stages IIA and IIB

MARKER POSITIVE

Low-volume NSGCT with elevated markers should be treated like good or intermediate prognosis risk groups, with three or four cycles of BEP. Also, a patient might opt for NS-RPLND, as primary chemotherapy and primary NS-RPLND have comparable outcomes (cure rates approach 98%), although side effects and toxicity differ [1].

MARKER NEGATIVE

Treatment options in marker negative stages IIA and IIB are either primary NS-RPLND or surveillance to clarify stage, as an alternative to primary chemotherapy. If NS-RPLND is cho-sen and vital GCT diagnosed, two adjuvant cycles of BEP are advisable. A NS-RPLND without vital tumour warrants sur-veillance. Small lymph nodes on imaging might not represent metastases, thus implying the risk of over-treatment. This may be avoided by repeated staging after 6 weeks of surveillance. Regression of a lesion leads to observation only. In unchanged and progressive lesions, a NS-RPLND must be performed because of suspected teratoma or undifferentiated malignant tumour. Progressive disease which became marker positive should be treated with BEP chemotherapy according to the IGCCCG recommendations. An alternative to the surveil-lance strategy with suspicion of an undifferentiated malignant tumour is a (CT-guided) biopsy, if technically possible [1].

Stage III

In advanced metastatic NSGCT, chemotherapy is advised in the same regimen as in stage IIC and III seminoma. The poor prognosis risk group has a 5-year progression-free

survival rate between 45% and 50% and receives, as the intermediate group, four cycles of BEP [1].

MANAGEMENT OF GCT AFTER ADJUVANT THERAPY: RESIDUAL DISEASE

Restaging by means of imaging and re-evaluation of the tumour markers is the cornerstone of management after adjuvant therapy for GCT.

Seminoma

In patients with normal markers and without residual lesion or a residual lesion ≤3 cm on imaging, surveillance is rec-ommended. If there is evidence of a residual mass of >3 cm after first-line adjuvant therapy (even with normal tumour markers), a fluorodeoxyglucose–positron emission tomog-raphy (FDG-PET) for determination of viability of this lesion should be performed 2 months after chemotherapy in order to decide whether surveillance or active treatment should be performed.

Salvage chemotherapy, surgery or radiotherapy is indi-cated if there is progression of the seminoma. If β-HCG is elevated, the preferred treatment after first-line chemo-therapy is salvage chemotherapy. Radiotherapy can be considered in localized lesions. In patients with progres-sive seminoma without β-HCG progression, a histological biopsy or surgery of the lesion should confirm the diagnosis, before salvage chemotherapy is given [1].

NSGCT

Even if there is marker normalization after primary adjuvant treatment, any visible residual lesion, especially >1 cm, should be surgically resected within 4–6 weeks of comple-tion of chemotherapy to rule out residual cancer or teratoma. Residual masses after BEP induction chemotherapy contain viable cancer in 10%, mature teratoma in 50% and necrotic-fibrotic tissue in 40% of the patients. To date, it is not pos-sible to distinguish between these histological findings on imaging, which makes residual tumour resection mandatory. In lesions <1 cm, observation is accepted. If pathology of a completely resected residual lesion shows necrosis, mature or immature teratoma or vital tumour in <10% of total volume, follow-up is justified. When there is incomplete resection of vital tumour, poor prognosis patients should be treated with adjuvant cisplatin-based chemotherapy [1].

MANAGEMENT OF GCT AFTER ADJUVANT THERAPY: RELAPSE OR REFRACTORY DISEASE

Relapsed disease is diagnosed by an increase in serum tumour markers or evidence of disease on imaging.

Relapses after initial chemotherapy generally require addi-tional cisplatin-based combination salvage chemotherapy (four cycles of etoposide, ifosfamide and cisplatin [PEI/VIP], four cycles of paclitaxel, ifosfamide and cisplatin [TIP] or four cycles of vinblastine, ifosfamide and cisplatin [VeIP]). This results in long-term remissions in approximately 50% of patients.

If there is relapse after salvage chemotherapy, salvage surgery should be considered (if technically feasible). Approximately 25% of long-term survival may be achieved.

All patients with late relapses (≥2 years after end of chemotherapy for metastatic NSGCT) should undergo immediate radical surgery of all lesions in order to completely resect undifferentiated GCT, mature teratoma or secondary non-GCT. If these lesions are not (completely) resectable, induction salvage chemotherapy before surgical resection is advised after histological assessment with biopsy. Also, when β-HCG marker levels rise rapidly, salvage chemotherapy is advised prior to resection. Radiotherapy can be considered in localized, not surgically resectable relapses [1].

FOLLOW-UP OF PATIENTS WITH TESTICULAR TUMOURS

According to the existing literature and guidelines, different follow-up schedules have been proposed. The primary objective of ideal follow-up should be early detection of relapse and monitoring of the contralateral testis. According to the time of maximal risk of recurrence, the interval between examinations and duration of follow-up should be determined. One should be aware of an increased long-term risk of development of secondary malignancies after chemotherapy and radiotherapy. Also, tests must be accurate and should be directed at the most likely sites of recurrence [1–4]. Table 38.5 shows the recommended minimum follow-up schedule according to the latest EAU guidelines [1].

Minimal annually abdominal CT in cases of retroperitoneal teratoma.

In seminoma, FGD-PET/CT 2 (and 4) months post-chemotherapy where there is any mass >3 cm.

Indications for a chest CT are abnormalities detected on chest X-ray or after pulmonary resection. Indications for a brain CT are headache, focal neurological findings or any central nervous system symptoms.

During treatment and follow-up special attention should be given to the side effects that can be caused by the different treatments. Patients with advanced disease have been shown to have better outcomes when treated in centers with experience treating patients with testis cancer [8].

The cisplatin is nephrotoxic and adequate baseline renal function is needed for safe administration, with the dose based on the patient's weight and height. The drug is given intravenously with a crystalloid infusion to maintain good renal perfusion. It can induce significant nausea and vomiting. In addition cisplatin is neurotoxic and can result in both peripheral neuropathy affecting the fingers and toes and ototoxicity causing loss of high-frequency hearing. Although often reversible, the recovery process can take up to 2 years.

Bleomycin has the rare but fatal complication of progressive pulmonary fibrosis causing irreversible damage to the lung resulting in progressive and ultimately fatal hypoxia. Etoposide can induce bone marrow suppression resulting in

Table 38.5a Proposed follow-up schedule for post-orchiectomy surveillance, radiotherapy or chemotherapy: seminoma stage I

Procedure	Year			
	1	2	3–4	5–10
Physical examination	3 times	3 times	Once every year	Once every year
Tumour markers	3 times	3 times	Once every year	Once every year
Chest X-ray	2 times	2 times		
Abdominopelvic CT	2 times	2 times		

Source: Data from European Association of Urology, Guidelines on testicular cancer, 2011, http://www.uroweb.org.

Table 38.5b Proposed follow-up schedule for post-orchiectomy surveillance: NSGCT stage I

Procedure	Year			
	1	2	3–5	6–10
Physical examination	4 times	4 times	Once every year	Once every year
Tumour markers	4 times	4 times	Once every year	Once every year
Chest X-ray	2 times	2 times		
Abdominopelvic CT	2 times (at 3 and 12 months)			

Source: Data from European Association of Urology, Guidelines on testicular cancer, 2011, http://www.uroweb.org.

Table 38.5c Proposed follow-up schedule for post-orchiectomy NS-RPLND or chemotherapy: NSGCT stage I

	Year			
Procedure	1	2	3–5	6–10
Physical examination	4 times	4 times	Once every year	Once every year
Tumour markers	4 times	4 times	Once every year	Once every year
Chest X-ray	2 times	2 times		
Abdominopelvic CT	Once	Once		

Source: Data from European Association of Urology, Guidelines on testicular cancer, 2011, http://www.uroweb.org.

Table 38.5d Proposed follow-up schedule for advanced GCT

	Year			
Procedure	1	2	3–5	Thereafter
Physical examination	4 times	4 times	Twice every year	Once every year
Tumour markers	4 times	4 times	Twice every year	Once every year
Chest X-ray	4 times	4 times	Twice every year	Once every year
Abdominopelvic CT	2 times	2 times	As indicated	As indicated
Chest CT	As indicated	As indicated	As indicated	As indicated
Brain CT	As indicated	As indicated	As indicated	As indicated

Source: Data from European Association of Urology, Guidelines on testicular cancer, 2011, http://www.uroweb.org.

a reduction in the number of white blood cells and platelets. Cases of secondary leukemia have been described. Any sign of infection or abnormal bruising requires prompt attendance at the hospital. Hair loss (alopecia) is usual.

Of particular importance is the effect of the chemotherapeutic agents on the germinal epithelium of the remaining testis. Spermatogenesis is eradicated by the chemotherapy, but generally returns to normal after about 12 months. For this reason all patients are offered sperm banking before starting chemotherapy. If for some reason spermatogenesis does not return, *in vitro* fertilization would be an option for the couple. There is no evidence to suggest that a pregnancy may be abnormal if it occurs while spermatogenesis is undergoing recovery, and so contraception is not required.

Long-term late complications remain an area of investigation, but secondary malignancies and cardiovascular disease have both been associated with GCT chemotherapy [9–11].

REFERENCES

1. European Association of Urology. Guidelines on testicular cancer. 2011. http://www.uroweb.org.
2. Oldenburg J, Fosså S, Nuver J, et al. Testicular seminoma and non-seminoma: ESMO clinical practice guidelines for diagnosis, treatment and follow-up. *Ann Oncol* 2013; 24(Suppl. 6): vi125–vi132.
3. National Comprehensive Cancer Network. Clinical practice guidelines in oncology. Testicular cancer. 2014. http://nccn.org.
4. Swedish and Norwegian Testicular Cancer Group SWENOTECA. http://www.swenoteca.org.
5. Edge S, Byrd D, Compton C, Fritz A, Greene F, Trotti A. *AJCC Cancer Staging Manual*, 7th ed. New York: Springer Verlag, 2010.
6. International Germ Cell Cancer Collaborative Group. International germ cell consensus classification: a prognostic factor-based staging system for metastatic germ cell cancers. *J Clin Oncol* 1997; 15: 594–603.
7. Oliver RT, Mason MD, Mead GM, et al. Radiotherapy versus single-dose carboplatin in adjuvant treatment of stage I seminoma: a randomised trial. *Lancet* 200; 366: 293–300.
8. Collette L, Sylvester RJ, Stenning SP, et al. Impact of the treating institution on survival of patients with "poor-prognosis" metastatic nonseminoma. European Organization for Research and Treatment of Cancer Genito-Urinary Tract Cancer Collaborative Group and the Medical Research Council Testicular Cancer Working Party. *J Natl Cancer Inst* 1999; 91: 839–46.
9. Huddart RA, Norman A, Shahidi M, et al. Cardiovascular disease as a long-term complication of treatment for testicular cancer. *J Clin Oncol* 2003; 21: 1513–23.
10. Zagars GK, Ballo MT, Lee AK, Strom SS. Mortality after cure of testicular seminoma. *J Clin Oncol* 2004; 22: 640–7.
11. van den Belt-Dusebout AW, de Wit R, Gietema JA, et al. Treatment-specific risks of second malignancies and cardiovascular disease in 5-year survivors of testicular cancer. *J Clin Oncol* 2007; 25: 4370–8.

39

Gynaecological oncology

GABRIELLA FERRANDINA AND GIOVANNI SCAMBIA

CERVICAL CANCER

Incidence and aetiology

Cervical cancer is the fourth most frequently diagnosed malignancy in women, accounting for an estimated 528,000 new cases in 2012 worldwide [1]. The incidence varies widely between countries with 13 cases/100,000 women/year in the US, 34 cases/100,000 women/year in the European Union and up to 40 cases/100,000 women/year in some African countries.

Human papilloma virus (HPV) plays a critical role in cervical carcinogenesis and is identifiable in almost all cervical tumor tissues [2]. HPV infection increases with the number of sexual partners and is linked to the early start of sexual activity. Moreover, smoking, sexually transmitted disease, use of oral contraceptives and immunosuppressive conditions may act as co-factors.

HPV sub-types 16, 18, 31, 51, 52 and 58 are the most commonly detected. Viral infection occurs at the basal layer of the cervical mucosa and is followed by HPV DNA replication; in the presence of co-factors, immune-mediated

HPV clearance, which normally occurs in 90% of cases, is impaired, thus favouring persistent infection. Infection from high-risk HPV sub-types increases the risk of developing epithelial lesions with progressive severity (low-grade intraepithelial lesions [LSILs] to high-grade intraepithelial lesions [HSILs]) and reduces the chance of remission. Indeed, progression from LSIL to HSIL is characterized by HPV DNA integration into the cellular genome and initiation of carcinogenesis through the upregulation of E6/E7 viral oncogenes and blocking of tumor suppressor genes [2]. It has been suggested that these lesions could take up to 10–20 years to evolve toward invasive carcinoma.

Pathology and tumor spread

Squamous cell carcinoma is documented in 70–80% of malignant cervical tumors, while adenocarcinomas account for only 5–20%. Cervical cancer spreads via local invasion with extension to the vagina, and the parametria up to the pelvic side wall, ureters, bladder and rectum. Lymphatic invasion takes place through external iliac, obturator, internal iliac and common iliac lymph nodes up to the aortic lymph nodes. Hematogeneous spread mainly involves bone, liver and lung.

Diagnosis and staging

Early cervical cancer may be asymptomatic; if present, symptoms are predominantly intermittent or post-coital vaginal bleeding. Diagnostic suspicion of cervical cancer is usually suggested by an abnormal finding on cytological smear and confirmed by cervical biopsy. In more advanced disease, symptoms can include pelvic pain, lower limb lymphedema and venous thromboembolism. Urinary or ano-rectal fistula is a less common presenting feature.

Staging is performed according to the International Federation of Gynaecology and Obstetrics (FIGO) staging system (Table 39.1) and includes gynaecologic examination under anaesthesia, colposcopy, endocervical curettage, hysteroscopy, cystoscopy or proctoscopy in cases where there is a suspicion of rectal or bladder invasion [3].

Imaging techniques such as CT, PET/CT scan (considered optional in FIGO stage ≤IB1) or MRI are also helpful in treatment planning. Surgical staging (often by means of laparoscopic lymphadenectomy) can be adopted for stage IB2 up to stage IVA disease [4].

Screening and prevention

The main method of screening is cervical cytology (Papanicolaou smear), which has a 60–70% sensitivity and a 95–98% specificity. More recent liquid-based methods of collection of cervical cytology have been shown not to be superior to conventional cytology [5]. HPV DNA tests are incorporated into cervical cytology in women aged 30–65 years, since they result in a more accurate prediction of risk of developing HSIL and adenocarcinoma [5]. Moreover, the cobas® HPV DNA test, which tests for the HPV 16 and 18 sub-types, and pooled results for additional 12 high-risk HPV DNA sub-types have been approved by the FDA as primary screening in women >25 years old and is increasingly also used in Europe.

Screening should be done from the age of between 21 and 25 years until 30 years, with cervical cytology; women aged 30–65 years should undergo cytology and HPV testing every 5 years, or cytology alone every 3 years. After 65 years, screening may be interrupted in the absence of risk factors.

Bivalent vaccines against HPV 16 and 18, and quadrivalent vaccines (against HPV 6, 11, 16 and 18) have been shown to reduce by up to 98% the incidence of adenocarcinoma in situ and HSIL [6]. The nonavalent vaccine (for HPV 6, 11, 16, 18, 31, 33, 45, 52 and 58) has been recently approved by the FDA in females (9–26 years old) and males (9–15 years old). Secondary prevention through the Pap test is still needed, especially in less developed countries.

Treatment

Early stage cervical carcinomas (FIGO stages IA and IB1) are mostly managed by a surgical approach, although radiotherapy can be adopted in selected situations.

Table 39.1 FIGO staging: cervical cancer

FIGO stage			Definition
I			Tumor confined to the cervix
	IA		Disease involves ≤5 mm of the cervical stroma and ≤7 mm in greatest diameter lateral dimension
		IA1	Disease involves ≤3 mm of the cervical stroma and ≤7 mm in greatest diameter lateral dimension
		IA2	Disease involves >3–5 mm of the cervical stroma and ≤7 mm in greatest diameter lateral dimension
	IB		Clinically visible disease limited to the cervix or preclinical cancers greater than stage IA
		IB1	Lesions ≤4 cm
		IB2	Lesions >4 cm
II			Tumor invades beyond the uterus, but not to the pelvic side wall or the lower third of the vagina
	IIA		No obvious parametrial involvement
		IIA1	Tumor size ≤4 cm
		IIA2	Tumor size >4 cm
	IIB		Unilateral or bilateral parametrial involvement
III			Tumor involves the lower third of the vagina and/or to the pelvic side wall and/or causes hydronephrosis or a non-functioning kidney
		IIIA	Tumor involves the lower third of the vagina with no extension to the pelvic side wall
		IIIB	Tumor extends to the pelvic side wall and/or hydronephrosis or non-functioning kidney
IV			Tumor spreads beyond the true pelvis or involves (biopsy proven) the mucosa of the bladder or rectum; a bullous edema does not allow a case to be allocated to stage IV
		IVA	Tumor spreads to adjacent organs
		IVB	Tumor spreads to distant organs

STAGE IA1

If fertility preservation is required, patients can be managed by cervical conization (preferably cold-knife conization); in case of negative margins and in the absence of lympho-vascular space invasion (LVSI), pelvic lymphadenectomy is omitted since the risk of lymph node involvement is less than 1%. If margins are positive, a second conization (or trachelectomy) can be performed. If LVSI is positive, pelvic lymphadenectomy is recommended. If fertility preservation is not required, simple hysterectomy [7,8] (Tables 39.2 and 39.3) can be performed, and lymphadenectomy is recommended if LVSI is positive.

STAGE IA2

If fertility preservation is required, patients can be treated with conization only if LVSI is negative; if LVSI is positive, radical trachelectomy (removal of cervix and proximal parametrial tissues and a 1–2 cm vaginal cuff) plus pelvic lymphadenectomy is performed.

If fertility preservation is not required, simple hysterectomy or modified radical hysterectomy (Tables 39.2 and 39.3) can be performed according to LVSI status. In patients considered unfit for surgery radiotherapy can be employed.

For stage IA1 with positive LVSI and stage IA2, sentinel lymph node mapping can also be considered, since it represents a valid method for lymph node assessment especially in the group of patients with a less than 2 cm tumor size, and in women with a stage of disease less than IB2 [9].

STAGES IB1–IIA1

In this group of patients, surgical and radiotherapeutic approaches have been shown to provide equivalent results in terms of clinical outcomes [10]: 5-year survival was 83% for radical hysterectomy plus pelvic lymphadenectomy versus 74% in patients treated with external beam radiotherapy plus brachytherapy.

Adjuvant treatment is required in the presence of pathological high-risk factors (positive surgical margins, positive lymph nodes or microscopic parametrial involvement); these patients would obtain a greater benefit in survival when given adjuvant chemoradiation versus radiation only (4-year survival, 81% vs. 71%, respectively) [11]. When preservation of fertility is required trachelectomy or cold-knife conization can be performed in selected cases of stage IB1 with a tumor size less than 2 cm, without lymph node involvement.

Neo-adjuvant platinum-based chemotherapy before trachelectomy or conization has also been employed in selected patients bearing squamous tumors between 2 and 4 cm with the exception of more aggressive histological sub-types.

Table 39.2 Hysterectomy: Piver classification

I	II	III	IV	V
Extrafascial hysterectomy	**Modified radical hysterectomy**	**Classical radical hysterectomy**		
Identification of ureters, rolling them outside the field without dissection	Ureters are dissected in the para-cervical region but not resected from the pubovesical ligaments	Ureters are dissected and resected from the pubovesical ligaments except for a small part where the umbilical bladder artery is situated to the level of penetration into the bladder	Ureters are completely dissected from the pubovesical ligaments and umbilical bladder artery is sacrificed	Excision of part of the ureter or bladder and reimplantation of the ureter
Uterine artery is dissected lateral to the ureters	Uterine artery is dissected besides and medial to the ureters	Uterine arteries are cut off at the origin of hypogastric region	Uterine arteries are cut off at the origin of hypogastric region	
Utero-sacral and cardinal ligaments are not removed	Utero-sacral and cardinal ligaments are excised midway from their sacral insertion	Utero-sacral ligaments are excised at their sacred insertion	Utero-sacral ligaments are excised at their sacred insertion	
No excision of part of vagina	Resection of the cardinal ligaments up to their medial half	Cardinal ligaments are resected as close to the pelvic wall as possible	Cardinal ligaments are resected as close to the pelvic wall as possible	
		Half vagina is removed	3/4 of vagina is removed	

Source: Piver MS, et al., *Obstet Gynecol* 1974;44(2):265–72.

Table 39.3 Hysterectomy: Querleu and Morrow classification

Type						
	B		C		D	
A	B1	B2	C1	C2	D1	D2
Extrafascial hysterectomy	Ureters are deperitonized and rolled to the lateral side		Ureters are fully mobilized		Full resection of the para-cervical tissue up to the wall of pelvic bone together with the hypogastric vessels, exposing the sciatic routes	
Palpation of the ureters without dissection of the ureteral layer	Partial resection of the utero-sacral and vesico-uterine ligaments		Section of utero-sacral ligaments at the level of the rectum		Ureter fully ambulant	
	Section of para-cervical tissue at ureteral tunnel level		Section of vesico-uterine ligaments at the level of the bladder			Resection of muscle and adjacent fascia
	≥10 mm vagina from the cervix or the tumor		Complete resection of para-cervical tissues			
	No removal of lateral para-cervical lymph nodes	Removal of lateral para-cervical lymph nodes	15–20 mm from the vagina resected toward the cervix or tumor and correspondent paracolpos			
			Preservation of the autonomous nerves	No preservation of the autonomous nerves		

Source: Querleu D, Morrow CP, Lancet Oncol 2008;9(3):297–303.

STAGES IB2–IVA

In locally advanced cervical cancer patients the current standard of care is represented by chemoradiotherapy only [12], usually with a cisplatin-based chemotherapy regime plus external beam radiation and brachytherapy. According to the longest follow-up study of such regimes, the 5-year survival rate was significantly higher for chemoradiation than for radiation only (73% vs. 52%, respectively) [13].

Neo-adjuvant chemotherapy followed by radical surgery has been proposed as another way to manage locally advanced disease. Indeed, this approach has been shown to provide a reduction of 35% of the risk of death from disease compared to radiation only [14].

Pelvic exenteration (removal of uterus together with the bladder or ano-rectum or both) can be considered in very selected cases affected by stage IVA disease complicated by urogenital or anorectal fistula.

FIGO STAGE IVB AND RECURRENT DISEASE

In the metastatic setting, and in patients with recurrent disease, platinum-based treatment is employed with a palliative intent [15]. Indeed, the clinical outcome of these patients remains dismal with a median survival of around a year. Advanced cervical cancer patients receiving cisplatin–paclitaxel plus bevacizumab experienced a 3.7-month increase of median survival compared with cisplatin–paclitaxel only (median survival, 17.5 vs. 14.3 months, respectively) [16].

In cases of local recurrence after primary surgery only, salvage chemoradiation may represent a valid option. Conversely, if primary treatment consisted of chemoradiation, the loco-regional recurrence may be managed by pelvic exenteration or laterally extended endopelvic resection plus intra-operative radiotherapy.

Prognosis

Prognosis of cervical cancer patients is mainly influenced by the stage of disease and lymph node status: in stage I disease, 5-year survival is around 90%, while in patients affected by stage IB2–II cervical cancer it remains around 70–75%. The prognosis of stage III–IV disease remains disappointing (5-year survival around 60%), while it remains dismal for metastatic disease (5-year survival around 10%).

ENDOMETRIAL CANCER

Incidence and aetiology

Endometrial carcinoma represents the most common of all gynaecologic malignancies with an incidence of 20–25 new cases/100,000/year [17]. Only 5–10% of patients are <40 years old, while the incidence rises up to 90/100,000/year in the age cohort between 60 and 69 years.

Two different types of endometrial carcinoma are recognized: type I tumors (almost 90% of cases) show an endometrioid histological sub-type and are associated with endometrial hyperplasia. Exposure to unopposed oestrogens plays a major role in pathogenesis; indeed, in postmenopausal women, oestrogen production taking place in adipose tissue represents a relevant risk factor, supporting the relationship between obesity and the risk of disease development. Other risk factors include chronic anovulation, polycystic ovarian syndrome, oestrogen replacement therapy and use of tamoxifen for breast cancer. A small proportion of endometrial cancer (almost 2%) is associated with the hereditary non-polyposis colorectal carcinoma (HNPCC) syndrome, a condition characterized by mutations of the *mismatch repair gene* system. Women with HNPCC have up to an 80% lifetime risk of developing colorectal cancer, but also ovarian (10%) and endometrial (almost 60%) cancer [18]. Type I endometrial carcinomas express variable levels of oestrogen receptor (ER) and progesterone receptor (PR) expression, as well as mutation of the pTEN and β-catenin genes: the presence of microsatellite instability is a distinctive feature of endometrial adenocarcinomas associated with Lynch syndrome. Endometrioid tumors are often diagnosed at an early stage and usually have an indolent disease course (Figure 39.1).

In contrast, type II tumors (about 10% of cases) are usually either a serous or clear cell histological sub-type, and are associated with atrophic endometrium and adjacent endometrial intraepithelial carcinoma. These tumors are characterized by loss of ER and PR expression and mutation of the p53 gene; they are frequently diagnosed at an advanced stage and follow an aggressive clinical course (Figure 39.1).

Tumor spread

Endometrial cancer spreads via direct invasion of the myometrium, extension to the endocervical canal and vagina, and involvement of the ovaries and fallopian tubes. Lymphatic infiltration may occur through lymphatic vessels of the round ligament up to the inguinal lymph nodes, or through lymphatic vessels of the broad ligaments, thus reaching pelvic lymph nodes; aortic lymph node stations are involved when tumor cells are drained through vessels of the ovarian pedicle. Hematogeneous spread mainly involves the bone, liver, lung and brain.

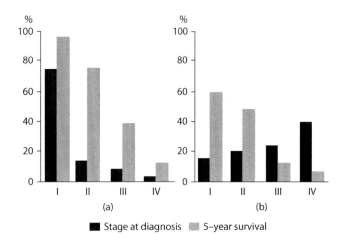

■ Stage at diagnosis   ■ 5–year survival

Figure 39.1 Distribution by stage, and 5-year survival rate in endometrioid (a) and serous (b) endometrial cancer.

Diagnosis and staging

The most common symptom of endometrial cancer is abnormal uterine bleeding; this occurs very early, thus leading to a prompt diagnosis in almost 70% of cases. Usually, the first diagnostic step in postmenopausal women complaining of vaginal bleeding is a gynaecologic examination, and transvaginal ultrasound (TV/US) examination. Hysteroscopy-guided endometrial biopsy is the standard for diagnosis with a sensitivity of up to 92% [19]. Staging procedures include a gynaecologic examination, chest X-ray and imaging to evaluate myometrial invasion, cervical involvement and extra-uterine disease: TV/US is equivalent to pelvic MRI for the detection of myometrial invasion and cervical involvement, and represents the investigation of choice since it is easily available, cheap and quick. Diagnostic CT scan and MRI are equivalent for the identification of lymph node involvement. The revised FIGO staging system has provided more detailed sub-staging of stage I and II disease, as well as stage IIIC disease (Table 39.4). In particular, the dismal clinical outcome of cases with aortic rather than pelvic lymph node involvement has been emphasized [3].

Treatment: Surgery for primary operable cancer

In apparent early stage disease, a surgical approach represents standard treatment, with the exception of patients considered unfit for surgery because of severe co-morbidities, who are usually triaged to radiation or hormonal therapies.

Equivalent disease-specific survival rates combined with more favourable perioperative outcome have been reported in patients managed by laparoscopic approaches [20,21]; therefore, minimally invasive techniques (totally laparoscopic, laparoscopic-assisted vaginal hysterectomy and robotic surgery) have currently replaced the open laparotomy approach. Staging procedures include peritoneal washings, inspection

Table 39.4 FIGO staging: carcinoma of the corpus uteri

I			Tumor confined to the corpus uteri
	IA		No or <50% myometrial invasion
	IB		≥50% myometrial invasion
II			Cervical stroma involvement, but tumor does not extend beyond the uterus[a]
III			Local and/or regional spread of the tumors
	IIIA		Uterine serosa and/or adnexae[b]
	IIIB		Vaginal and/or parametrial involvement
	IIIC		Metastases to pelvic and/or aortic lymph nodes
		IIIC1	Positive pelvic lymph nodes
		IIIC2	Positive aortic lymph nodes with or without pelvic lymph node involvement
IV			Tumor invasion of bladder and/or bowel mucosa
	IVA		Bladder and/or bowel mucosa involvement
	IVB		Distant metastases including intra-abdominal and/or inguinal lymph nodes

[a] Isolated endocervical glandular involvement should be considered stage I.
[b] Positive cytology should be reported separately without changing the stage.

of the abdominal cavity, biopsies of suspicious lesions, total hysterectomy and bilateral salpingo-oophorectomy.

The decision about whether to perform pelvic lymphadenectomy is based on risk factors partly based on frozen section analysis: in cases where the extent of myometrial invasion is *less than* 50% and the grade only 1 or 2, the risk of pelvic lymph node involvement is very low (2–4%), and lymphadenectomy can be omitted.

A recent meta-analysis indicated that pelvic lymphadenectomy has a very limited impact on the survival of patients with early stage disease [22]; however, controversy still exists about the role of lymphadenectomy in patients with high-risk factors. Therefore, in cases where the extent of myometrial invasion is less than 50%, but the disease is grade 3, or more than 50% and any grade of differentiation, pelvic lymphadenectomy is recommended. Results about the performance of a sentinel lymph node procedure in this clinical setting are promising but need to be consolidated [23].

In cases of apparent stage II disease, optimal surgery is generally considered to be by modified radical hysterectomy (Tables 39.2 and 39.3), bilateral salpingo-oophorectomy and pelvic lymphadenectomy. Aortic lymphadenectomy is performed in cases of pelvic lymph node involvement or intra-operative identification of lymphadenopathy, since aortic lymph node involvement in the absence of pelvic lymph node metastasis is very rare (about 1%).

In cases of tumors clinically extending outside of the uterus (stage III–IVA disease), cytoreduction represents the clinical goal of surgery, although a multimodal approach taking advantage of radiotherapy and chemotherapy is often required. In stage IVA disease pelvic exenteration can be considered. In the metastatic setting, surgery or radiation may be carried out with a palliative intent.

Adjuvant therapy

The administration of adjuvant treatment (and the precise type) is determined by the extent of myometrial invasion, grade of differentiation and lymph node status; however, tumor size of greater than 2 cm, age and LVSI status also have to be considered. Therefore, in stage I disease, patients with low-risk endometrial cancer (myometrial invasion ≤50%, grade 1 or 2), which account for almost 55% of cases, are treated with observation only.

Results from the PORTEC2 trial showed that in patients with myometrial invasion of ≤50% plus grade 3 disease or myometrial invasion of greater than 50% with grade 1 or 2 disease, brachytherapy provides survival outcomes equivalent to those obtained with pelvic radiotherapy, which was associated with a less favourable toxicity profile and worse quality of life than brachytherapy [24]. These intermediate- and high-risk patients may be triaged to vaginal brachytherapy, or pelvic radiation in the presence of adverse risk factors.

In cases with myometrial invasion of greater than 50% and grade 3 disease, the risk of distant recurrence is quite high, indicating that systemic treatment may be advantageous. Attempts to combine chemotherapy and radiotherapy in high-risk patients have been made: in particular, chemotherapy followed by radiotherapy has proven more effective than radiation alone.

The phase III randomized PORTEC trial (still ongoing) has been designed to compare concomitant chemoradiation followed by chemotherapy versus pelvic radiation only, in cases with myometrial invasion of less than 50% plus grade 3 disease and positive LVSI, and myometrial invasion of greater than 50% plus grade 3, stage II or IIIA, or stage IIIC or IIIB if parametrial invasion only, or stage IA (with invasion), IB, II or III with serous or clear cell histology.

Salvage therapy

For metastatic patients, multi-agent regimens incorporating platinum and paclitaxel are used and achieve up to a 50–60% response; however, survival still remains dismal with a 5-year rate of around 10%. In patients with slowly progressing and asymptomatic disease, progestins may be utilized.

Encouraging outcome data have come from the combination of bevacizumab (an antibody against vascular endothelial growth factors [VEGFs]) and conventional platinum–paclitaxel, which has been shown to provide a survival advantage over chemotherapy alone [25]. Moreover, several lines of evidence emphasize the clinical role of mTOR inhibitors [26].

Fertility preservation

The selection of patients who can be offered conservative treatment is very important: stage IA (no myometrial invasion) grade 1 patients are considered the best candidates. Oral progestins (megestrol acetate 160–320 mg/day or medroxyprogesterone acetate 400–600 mg/day, for 6 months) or use of a levonorgestrel-releasing intra-uterine device represents the most common option [27].

The rate of pathological complete response to treatment is 70–75%. In unresponsive patients, hysterectomy has to be planned. In case of recurrence, a re-challenge with progestins can still be offered with a high chance of success. Up to 30% of such patients will achieve a subsequent live birth with a higher frequency when assisted reproduction techniques are employed.

EPITHELIAL OVARIAN CARCINOMA

Epidemiology and risk factors

Epithelial ovarian carcinomas originate from ovarian surface epithelium and account for almost 90% of malignant ovarian tumors. This neoplasia represents the second most common gynaecologic tumor; 9–15 new cases/100,000 women/year are diagnosed in developed countries, while 2–5 new cases/100,000 women/year are documented in Africa and Asia [17].

Diagnosis is rare before age 40, while incidence shows a progressive increase with age, up to 40–45 cases/100,000/women/year in women over the age of 70. Other risk factors include early age at menarche, late age at menopause, infertility and nulliparity. Pregnancies, tubal ligation or more than 1 year of oral contraceptive use seem to play a protective role [28]. Recent data seem to confirm that the use of fertility drugs is safe [29].

Different clinical manifestations of hereditary ovarian cancer have been described including hereditary ovarian cancer syndrome, hereditary breast and ovarian cancer (HBOC) syndrome and HNPCC. Up to 10% of all ovarian cancers are hereditary and are associated with a dominant autosomal genetic predisposition with a high penetrance: of these, 90% are linked to BRCA gene mutations. BRCA proteins are involved in the homologous recombination-based mechanisms of DNA repair; therefore, when a deleterious mutation occurs, inactivation of BRCA protein results in inadequate repair of DNA strand breaks and a higher susceptibility to DNA damage.

The lifetime risk of developing ovarian cancer is 1.4–1.8% in the general population, while it rises up to 40–60% in case of BRCA1 mutation and 10–25% in cases of BRCA2 mutation [30].

Pathogenesis and histopathology

Besides the theory of incessant ovulation, which postulates that chronic trauma at each ovulation may lead to malignant transformation of the surface epithelium of the ovary, a new model sustains that tubal cells are the precursor of serous ovarian cancer. The demonstration of serous tubal intraepithelial carcinoma (STIC) in the absence of any ovarian lesions in BRCA positive women undergoing prophylactic salpingo-oophorectomy suggests that malignant cells of the distal fallopian tube may exfoliate and implant in the ovary where they could be exposed to sex hormones and pro-inflammatory cytokines able to promote progression. Conversely, endometrioid carcinomas may originate from transformation of endometriotic implants, while mucinous and Brenner tumors may result from metaplastic peritoneal elements. A dualistic model of ovarian carcinoma has acknowledged the relevance of molecular characterization and has proposed the classification of ovarian cancer into type I tumors (low-grade serous, mucinous, endometrioid, clear cell and Brenner carcinomas) and type II tumors (high-grade serous and endometrioid carcinoma, undifferentiated tumors and carcinosarcomas) (Figure 39.2).

Screening

Despite the efforts made to set up a screening strategy combining TV/US together with different schedules of CA-125 assessments, none of the studies has proved the efficacy of routine screening in terms of reduction of ovarian cancer mortality in the general population [31].

On the other hand, in high-risk women (i.e. women carriers of a BRCA mutation or reporting a family history for breast or ovarian carcinoma), screening is recommended and should be started at the age of 35 years, since BRCA-mutated ovarian carcinomas are generally diagnosed earlier than sporadic ones. However, since there is no clear evidence that this approach translates into a survival benefit, these women are advised to proceed to prophylactic salpingo-oophorectomy as soon as childbearing is accomplished.

In recent years, based on the theory of the tubal origin of ovarian cancer, salpingectomy or fimbriectomy has been advocated as a temporary risk-reducing strategy for selected young women.

Signs and symptoms and diagnosis

Ovarian cancer is very often asymptomatic in its early stages and can be detected at routine TV/US. In advanced stages,

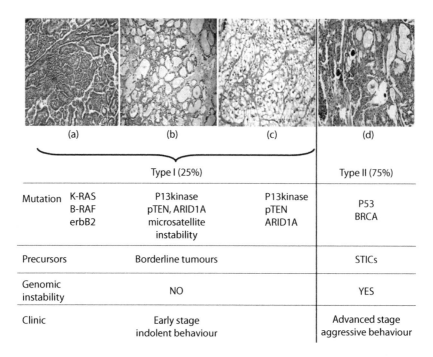

		Type I (25%)		Type II (75%)
	(a)	(b)	(c)	(d)
Mutation	K-RAS B-RAF erbB2	P13kinase pTEN, ARID1A microsatellite instability	P13kinase pTEN ARID1A	P53 BRCA
Precursors		Borderline tumours		STICs
Genomic instability		NO		YES
Clinic		Early stage indolent behaviour		Advanced stage aggressive behaviour

Figure 39.2 Main distinctive morphological, molecular and clinical differences in type I and type II tumors. (a) Low-grade serous ovarian carcinoma. (b) Low-grade endometrioid carcinoma. (c) Clear cell carcinoma. (d) High-grade serous carcinoma.

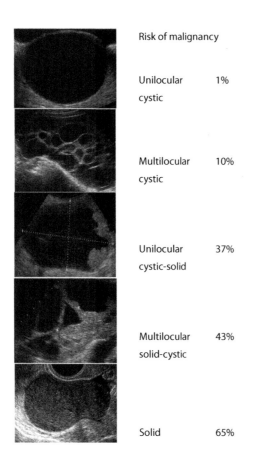

Risk of malignancy	
Unilocular cystic	1%
Multilocular cystic	10%
Unilocular cystic-solid	37%
Multilocular solid-cystic	43%
Solid	65%

Figure 39.3 Transvaginal ultrasound evaluation of adnexal masses: morphologic features and risk of malignancy.

symptoms include nausea, constipation, abdominal pain, asthenia and dyspnoea in cases of pleural effusion. Due to the presence of non-specific symptoms, ovarian malignancy is often not suspected in a timely manner and the patient is treated for benign gastrointestinal conditions such as irritable bowel for months. Gynaecologic examination may indicate the presence of pelvic or abdominal masses; TV/US plays a key role in the characterization of adnexal mass morphology, echogenicity and vascularization (Figure 39.3). These findings together with serum CA-125 levels, as well as age, and menopausal status contribute to the calculation of the risk of malignancy. Abdomino-pelvic CT scan represents a useful tool to estimate the extent and sites of disease, and more accurately plan the type of surgical procedures.

Routes of spread and staging

Ovarian cancer spreads within the pelvis and abdominal cavity in the vast majority of cases: peritoneal disease in the diaphragm, liver and spleen is often documented as well as involvement of the omentum, small and large bowel, mesentery and upper abdominal structures (porta hepatis, lesser omentum, celiac trunk lymph nodes) (Figure 39.4). Hematogeneous diffusion to the spleen, liver and extra-abdominal organs can also occur. Isolated involvement of the retroperitoneum is documented in about 10% of cases.

Ovarian cancer is surgically staged according to the FIGO staging system, which has recently been revised [32] (Table 39.5).

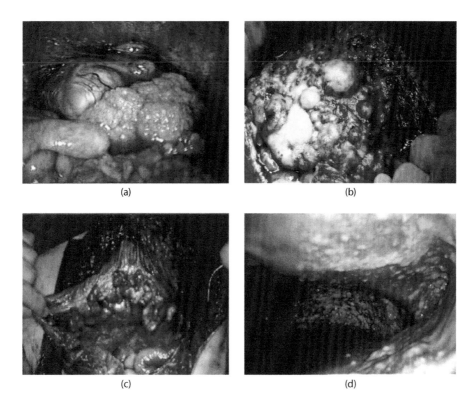

Figure 39.4 Representative sites of disease in advanced ovarian cancer. (a) Presence of a left ovarian mass with exophytic tumor nodules. (b) Omentum appears completely replaced by large tumor nodules ('omental cake'). (c) Several tiny nodules involve serosa of mesentery and bowel. (d) Diffuse carcinomatosis of right hemidiaphragm: tiny tumor seedings appear confluent.

Table 39.5 FIGO staging: ovarian cancer

FIGO stage			Definition
I			Tumor confined to ovaries
	IA		Tumor limited to one ovary, capsule intact, no tumor on surface, negative washing
	IB		Tumor involves both ovaries; otherwise like IA
	IC		Tumor limited to one or both ovaries
		IC1	Surgical spill
		IC2	Capsule rupture before surgery or tumor on ovarian surface
		IC3	Malignant cells in the ascites or peritoneal washing
II			Tumor involves one or both ovaries with pelvic extension (below the pelvic brim) or primary peritoneal cancer
	IIA		Extension and/or implant on uterus and/or fallopian tubes
	IIB		Extension to other pelvic intraperitoneal tissues
III			Tumor involves one or both ovaries with cytologically or histologically confirmed spread to the peritoneum outside the pelvis and/or metastasis to the retroperitoneal lymph nodes
	IIIA		Positive retroperitoneal lymph nodes and/or microscopic metastasis beyond the pelvis
		IIIA1	Only retroperitoneal lymph nodes
			IIIA1 (i) Metastasis ≤10 mm
			IIIA1 (ii) Metastasis >10 mm
		IIIA2	Microscopic, extrapelvic peritoneal metastasis ± positive retroperitoneal lymph nodes
	IIIB		Macroscopic, extrapelvic, peritoneal metastasis ≤2 cm ± positive retroperitoneal lymph nodes Includes extension to capsule of liver/spleen
	IIIC		Macroscopic, extrapelvic, peritoneal metastasis >2 cm ± positive retroperitoneal lymph nodes Includes extension to capsule of liver/spleen
IV			Distant metastasis excluding peritoneal metastasis
	IVA		Pleural effusion with positive cytology
	IVB		Hepatic and/or splenic parenchymal metastasis, metastasis to extra-abdominal organs (including inguinal lymph nodes and lymph nodes outside of the abdominal cavity

Primary treatment

EARLY STAGE DISEASE

Surgery plays a crucial role in the management of ovarian carcinoma and should be carried out by trained gynaecologic oncology surgeons in the context of a tertiary referral center. In early stage disease (almost 20% of cases), surgery permits accurate staging and complete removal of disease: peritoneal washing, random peritoneal biopsies and biopsies of any suspicious lesion, total hysterectomy, bilateral salpingo-oophorectomy, omentectomy and pelvic and aortic lymphadenectomy are performed more and more frequently through laparoscopy. Correct application of all procedures translates into a rate of upstaging of between 10% and 30%.

The FIGO classification recommends selective assessment of pelvic and aortic lymph nodes, while some studies suggest that surgeons should perform systematic pelvic (≥20 lymph nodes) and aortic (≥15 lymph nodes) lymphadenectomy even in stage IA disease: the rate of lymph node involvement is dictated by the presence of bilateral ovarian lesions, ascites, positive cytology, sub-stage, serous histological type and grade [33]. Nonetheless the therapeutic benefit of lymphadenectomy remains to be established. Fertility preservation may be considered in stage IA G1–G2, providing that all staging procedures are accomplished; careful evaluation of the endometrium is required in the case of endometrioid histological sub-type.

The efficacy of adjuvant chemotherapy has been demonstrated by two randomized phase III studies [34]. Long-term evaluation of ICON1 results showed that adjuvant chemotherapy provided the highest benefit in high-risk patients (stages IB–IC, grade 2 and all stages, grade 3), with a survival improvement of 18% [35].

ADVANCED STAGE DISEASE

Almost 70–80% of ovarian cancer is diagnosed at an advanced stage; surgical exploration is aimed at evaluating disease extension and achieving removal of all macroscopic lesions. Indeed, maximal cytoreductive surgery and achievement of complete cytoreduction (i.e. no macroscopic residual tumor) have been shown to provide better survival figures with a median survival prolongation of 2.3 months for each 10% increase in the rate of complete cytoreduction [36]. Given the presence of widespread abdominal disease, aggressive surgical procedures may include radical pelvic surgery, bowel resection and removal of upper abdominal disease foci (resection of diaphragm, splenectomy, etc.), although this is associated with an increased rate of severe complications (around 22–24%) and death (around 4%) [37].

Neo-adjuvant chemotherapy (NACT) with delayed surgery (i.e. interval debulking surgery [IDS]) has been demonstrated to increase rates of optimal debulking and reduce surgery-related complications. Despite the fact that two randomized phase III trials have reported non-inferiority of NACT compared to primary surgery in terms of clinical outcome in the face of more favourable perioperative results, [38,39] this approach is usually considered for patients considered unfit for surgery, and in the case of unresectable disease. The major reasons precluding the achievement of complete cytoreduction include the presence of multiple parenchymal liver metastases, infiltration of multiple sites in the pancreas or duodenum, infiltration of the porta hepatis or truncus celiacus, deep infiltration of the radix mesenterii, involvement of the superior mesenteric artery, diffuse and confluent carcinomatosis of the stomach or small bowel, not completely resectable extra-abdominal disease with the exception of resectable inguinal lymph nodes, and solitary para-cardiac and retrocrural lymph nodes. Laparoscopy may be useful to assess the chance of optimal cytoreduction through specific predictive scores of the extent of intra-abdominal disease [40].

Combined chemotherapy with carboplatin and paclitaxel has been the gold standard since 1996 based on several phase III randomized studies [41]. None of the efforts made to improve the efficacy of this first-line chemotherapy regime through the use of novel doublets, the incorporation of a third drug and maintenance therapy have proved to be superior to the standard. In this scenario, the adoption of a weekly schedule of carboplatin (AUC = 2) and paclitaxel (80 mg/m^2) has resulted in a large improvement of survival in a Japanese phase III randomized study [42]. However, these results did not modify the standard regimen since the study was limited to Asiatic patients.

In 2005, the NCI released an alert supporting the use of intraperitoneal chemotherapy in stage III ovarian cancer patients submitted to optimal cytoreduction; this was based on the results of the GOG272 randomized study which reported a prolongation of median survival of 15.9 months in favour of intraperitoneal chemotherapy versus the standard [43]; however, due to significant toxicity, intraperitoneal chemotherapy was deliverable in only 42% of patients, thus limiting the routine use of this approach. Recently, based on the favourable results obtained by the incorporation of bevacizumab to first-line chemotherapy and as maintenance therapy, this drug has been approved in the adjuvant treatment of stage IIIB–IV ovarian cancer patients [44,45].

Salvage treatment

Recurrence or progression of disease is documented in about 20–30% of early stage patients and in 70–80% of advanced stage disease. The time interval from completion of platinum-based chemotherapy and recurrence (defined as platinum-free interval [PFI]) represents a critical parameter for prognostic characterization and choice of treatment; if PFI is ≤6 months, patients are considered platinum resistant and are triaged to non-platinum drugs. Recent evidence from the AURELIA trial has proved the benefit of adding bevacizumab to standard drugs in terms of higher response rates and even prolongation of survival compared to the standard [46]. In patients defined as platinum sensitive (PFI > 6 months), secondary cytoreduction can be considered, especially in cases of isolated recurrence; otherwise, these patients may be treated with platinum-based combinations according to their performance status, residual neurotoxicity, refusal of alopecia and so on. This approach has been modified by the results of the OCEANS study which showed the superiority of using bevacizumab with platinum–gemcitabine compared to the standard [47].

Finally, encouraging results have been reported for olaparib, a PARP inhibitor with selective activity in ovarian cancer associated with a BRCA mutation: a phase II randomized study has shown that olaparib administered as maintenance therapy in platinum-sensitive recurrent ovarian cancer has reduced the risk of disease progression by 65% compared to placebo [48], thus leading to approval for this subset of patients at the end of 2014.

Novel perspectives for the exploitation of PARP inhibitors come from the demonstration that several epigenetic alterations may alter BRCA function (so-called *BRCAness*), thus possibly expanding the number of patients who might benefit from this class of drugs.

Overall, 5-year survival is around 80% in stage I disease and 50–60% for stage II patients. In advanced stage disease these figures drop down to 30% for stage II and 10% for stage IV patients.

NON-EPITHELIAL OVARIAN CARCINOMA

Ovarian germ cell tumors

These tumors are rare (incidence = 0.4/100,000/year), and almost 70% of cases are diagnosed in women under 20 years of age, thus raising fertility preservation issues. The most frequent ovarian germ cell tumors are dysgerminoma (about 50%) and yolk sac tumor (about 10%) [49]. Staging systems and procedures are the same as for early ovarian carcinoma, with the exception of lymphadenectomy, the role of which is still controversial [50]. When fertility preservation is required, staging has to be carried out preserving the contralateral ovary and uterus.

Adjuvant chemotherapy is usually administered in patients with anything greater than stage IA dysgerminoma. In immature teratoma, adjuvant chemotherapy is administered in stage IA G2–G3 and in patients with >stage IA. The most common regimen is the combination bleomycin, etoposide and cisplatin (BEP). Clinical outcome is excellent with a cure rate of more than 90% in early stage disease.

Sex cord–stromal cell ovarian tumors

These tumors have an incidence of approximately 0.2/100,000/year; they include heterogeneous types of tumors originating from cells of the sex cords and ovarian stroma. Granulosa cell tumors are the most common; they include an adult form (almost 95% of cases) and a juvenile form (5% of cases). Granulosa cell tumors are

hormonally active and can result in abnormal vaginal bleeding when occurring during postmenopause or menstrual abnormalities or precocious pseudo-puberty when diagnosed in pre-menarche age [51]. They are diagnosed at stage I in 80–90% of cases and show an indolent behaviour with recurrence of disease after even 30 years since diagnosis. Staging systems and surgical procedures are the same as for germ cell tumors; in particular, when fertility preservation is required, careful evaluation of the endometrium is needed in order to exclude hyperplastic or neoplastic lesions. Adjuvant chemotherapy is required in stage IIA–IV. BEP represents the most commonly utilized regimen.

Sertoli–Leydig tumors contain cells reminiscent of testicular development and are able to produce androgen hormones and cause signs of virilization in 70–80% of cases. Sometimes, they show the presence of heterologous elements, a characteristic associated with a more aggressive outcome. Adjuvant treatment is administered in stage IA Sertoli–Leydig tumors in case of poor grade of differentiation or heterologous elements, and in >stage IA tumors. Besides BEP, carboplatin–paclitaxel has been shown to provide equivalent efficacy and a more favourable toxicity profile [51].

VULVAR CANCER, VAGINAL CANCER, UTERINE SARCOMA AND GESTATIONAL TROPHOBLASTIC DISEASE

Vulvar cancer

Vulvar carcinoma is the fourth most frequent gynaecological malignancy, accounting for about 5% of cases [17]. It includes two distinct entities: the first type is very rare and usually diagnosed in younger women. This type of disease is strongly associated with vulvar intraepithelial neoplasia (VIN) associated with HPV infection; additional factors (sexually transmitted disease, smoking and low socio-economic status) can contribute to the pathogenesis of this disease [52]. The second type of vulvar carcinoma is usually diagnosed in older patients (mean age = 65 years) who frequently complain of a long history of vulvar pruritus and who may have a previous diagnosis of dystrophic or atrophic disease. Documentation of HPV infection is very rare. Squamous cell carcinoma is the most common histological type (95% of cases); vulvar melanoma is the second most common vulvar malignancy.

The vast majority of patients present with a vulvar mass which appears fleshy, bleeds easily or is ulcerated. Classical routes of vulvar cancer spread include extension to contiguous organs, lymphatic spread to the groin and iliac lymph nodes up to the aortic lymph nodes, and hematogeneous dissemination.

Frequent symptoms include itching, burning, discharge and pain according to the site and extent of disease. A diagnosis of vulvar carcinoma is usually made by vulvar biopsy. In cases with apparently multifocal disease, or

Table 39.6 FIGO staging: vulvar carcinoma

FIGO stage		Definition
IA		Size ≤2 cm, confined to vulva or perineum
		Stromal invasion ≤1 mm, no metastatic lymph node involvement
IB		Size ≥2 cm, confined to vulva or perineum
		Any size with stromal invasion ≥1 mm
II		Any size, extension to lower 1/3 urethra, lower 1/3 vagina, anal involvement, no metastatic lymph node involvement
III		Any size, with or without extension to upper 2/3 urethra, upper 2/3 vagina, anal involvement
	IIIA	1 lymph node metastasis (≥5 mm)
		1–2 lymph node metastases (≤5 mm)
	IIIB	≥2 lymph node metastases (≥5 mm)
		≥3 lymph node metastases (≤5 mm)
	IIIC	Metastatic lymph nodes with extra-capsular spread
IVA		Involves 2/3 urethra and/or vagina, bladder and/or rectal mucosa or fixed to pelvic bones
		Fixed/ulcerated inguinal lymph nodes

very extensive disease, mapping of lesions and evaluation of disease-free margins should be performed. Exclusion of multifocal squamous lesions should be carried out through Pap smear, colposcopy and careful evaluation of the vagina.

Staging of vulvar carcinoma (Table 39.6) is based on pathological evaluation of tumor size and invasion, disease extension and eventual metastatic involvement of lymph nodes [3]. However, CT scan or PET/CT should also to be taken into account. Additional examinations (cystoscopy, proctoscopy, etc.) are performed if needed.

Early stage vulvar carcinoma is managed mostly by radical local excision (RLE) with inguinal lymphadenectomy (unilateral or bilateral on the basis of tumor location), unless patients are considered unfit for surgery, and then triaged to radiotherapy with or without chemotherapy. A minimum tumor-free tissue margin of 1 cm should be achieved. Stage IA tumors can be safely managed by RLE only regardless of tumor location, since the rate of lymph node involvement is minimal. In case of stage IB ≤2 cm diameter, localized on one vulvar side, ipsilateral groin lymphadenectomy should be performed. Conversely, if the primary lesion is located centrally, inguinal lymphadenectomy should be bilateral [53].

Stage II patients should be considered individually, based on the site of the tumor, and extension to the clitoris, urethra or rectal mucosa. When possible, sparing of the clitoris and urethra should considered; also, for lesions very close to the anus, preoperative chemoradiation could be considered. Bilateral inguinal lymphadenectomy is required.

Since only 30% of early stage patients bear inguino-femoral metastases, the issue of sparing postoperative complications associated with lymphadenectomy is of clinical relevance. A sentinel lymph node biopsy provides high sensitivity and negative predictive values of 92% and 97%, respectively, thus leading many to consider this technique

an accurate approach in staging vulvar squamous cell carcinoma stage IB/II <4 cm [54].

Adjuvant treatment is required in cases of metastatic inguinal lymph nodes; in particular, cases with any lymph node macrometastasis (≥5 mm) as well as patients with ≥2 micrometastatic (<5 mm) lymph nodes or extra-capsular spread are treated with inguinal and pelvic irradiation.

Stage III–IVA disease (Figure 39.5) can be amenable to radical surgery in selected cases; pelvic exenteration can be offered in cases of ano-rectal or bladder fistula. In order to reduce the extent of surgery and consequent complications, preoperative chemoradiation can be utilized; otherwise, exclusive chemoradiation can also be performed [55]. As far as lymph node management is concerned, bilateral inguinal lymphadenectomy is carried out in cases of negative imaging. In cases with bulky lymphadenopathy, surgery can be performed unless infiltration of vascular structures or bone is documented.

In stage IVB disease, chemotherapy has to be employed and usually includes cisplatin-based regimens similar to those used in uterine cervical cancer patients [56].

Five-year survival is almost 90% in early stage patients without lymph node involvement, while it drops down to 50–60% in cases with metastatic lymph nodes. Stage IV patients have a poor clinical outcome with median progression-free survival ranging from 3 to 10 months.

Vaginal cancer

Vaginal carcinoma accounts for only 2–3% of gynaecological malignancies with an incidence of approximately 0.6 cases/100,000 women/year and a mortality rate of 30% [17]. It usually affects postmenopausal women, who often have a history of vaginal intraepithelial neoplasia, prior pelvic radiation and previous hysterectomy. Sexual promiscuity, smoking and previous ano-genital tumors are additional risk factors [57].

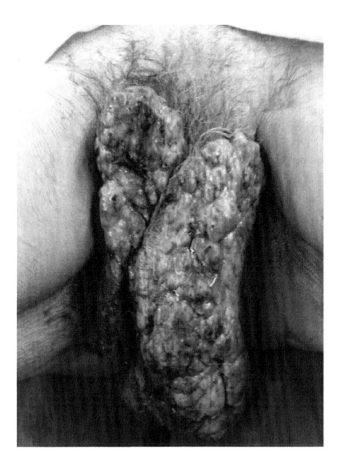

Figure 39.5 Voluminous, fleshy, easily bleeding mass originating from the left hemivulva, involving anterior and posterior perineum, urethra and distal portion of vagina. Inguino-femoral lymph nodes were palpable bilaterally. The patient was triaged to total pelvic exenteration, Bricker pouch, definitive colostomy inguino-femoral lymphadenectomy and reconstructive surgery.

In the vast majority of cases (80%) vaginal carcinoma presents a squamous histology, while adenocarcinoma is less frequently diagnosed.

The main routes of vaginal cancer spread include direct extension to paravaginal tissues, parametria and vulva, or to contiguous organs such as the bladder and ano-rectum. Lymphatic infiltration is indicated by the site of the primary tumor: vaginal carcinoma of the upper vagina is drained by lymphatic vessels following the uterine vessels, thus involving pelvic lymph nodes; lymphatic drainage of the distal vagina follows the vulvar lymphatic network and involves primarily the groin lymph nodes. In cases of tumor located in the mid-vagina, both routes of lymphatic diffusion may be involved [57]. Hematogeneous spread may occur and involves lung and bone.

The most frequent symptoms are vaginal bleeding or watery, malodorous vaginal discharge. Urinary or ano-rectal symptoms can be associated with bladder or anal involvement. Diagnosis of vaginal carcinoma is made by vaginal biopsy, and disease should be clinically staged according to the FIGO staging system [3] (Table 39.7).

Table 39.7 FIGO staging: vaginal cancer

FIGO stage	Definition
I	Limited to vaginal wall
II	Involving paravaginal tissues
III	Involves pelvic wall[a]
IVA	Involves bladder and/or rectal and/or direct extension beyond the true pelvis
IVB	Spread to distant organs

[a] Pelvic wall refers to muscle, fascia, neurovascular structures and skeletal portions of the bony pelvis.

Careful examination of the vaginal walls should be performed, if needed, under anaesthesia, and possible origin from the uterine cervix or vulva should be excluded. Other investigations including chest X-rays, cystoscopy and proctoscopy are performed in cases with suspicion of involvement of the bladder or ano-rectum. CT scan, PET/CT scan or MRI and pelvic US can be useful, but should not modify the initial stage.

The mainstay of treatment for squamous cell carcinomas of the vagina is radiotherapy (external beam radiation with or without brachytherapy) or brachytherapy only. Several factors, including extent and site of disease, thickness and morphology, should be considered when deciding treatment. The whole vagina is commonly included in the radiation field as well as paravaginal tissues up to the pelvic wall and pelvic lymph nodes, unless the tumor is located in the distal vagina, thus requiring irradiation of the groin lymph nodes. However, in the case of small lesions, brachytherapy can be employed [58,59]. The efficacy of concomitant chemoradiation has been investigated; however, the therapeutic role of this multimodal treatment has to be further evaluated.

The role of surgery seems limited to patients with stage I disease involving only the proximal vagina which can be managed through upper colpectomy, radical hysterectomy and pelvic lymphadenectomy; pelvic exenteration can be considered in stage IV tumor associated with vesico-vaginal or recto-vaginal fistula, or in cases of central recurrence after radiotherapy.

In metastatic or recurrent disease, systemic therapy utilizes drugs and combinations similar to those used in cervical cancer patients [57].

Five-year overall survival is around 95% for stage I and 75% for stage II disease; patients bearing stage III or IVA disease present worse outcomes, with 5-year overall survival around 70% and 53%, respectively [59].

Uterine sarcoma

The incidence of uterine sarcomas is low with 1.6–3 new cases/100,000 women/year. They include leiomyosarcomas which originate from smooth muscles cells, and endometrial stromal tumors (including endometrial stromal sarcoma and undifferentiated endometrial sarcoma) arising from endometrial stromal cells [60].

Leiomyosarcomas seem to be associated with previous pelvic radiation and have a very poor prognosis. Endometrial stromal sarcomas are associated with obesity and diabetes, show ER and PR expression in a high percentage of cases and exhibit indolent behaviour. Conversely, undifferentiated endometrial sarcomas represent a completely different entity, since they exhibit divergent chromosomal alterations, low expression of ER and PR and a worse clinical outcome [61].

Early symptoms and signs of uterine sarcomas include abnormal vaginal bleeding, discharge or pelvic pain, and a rapidly growing pelvic mass can often be documented. However, diagnosis can be made incidentally after surgery for asymptomatic uterine myomas (0.1–0.3%) [61]. In the case of a histologic diagnosis of uterine sarcoma after uterine curettage or hysteroscopic biopsy, staging work-up includes chest X-rays, abdomino-pelvic CT scan or MRI and TV/US; FIGO staging classification is based on pathologic examination (Table 39.8).

When disease is clinically limited to the uterus, standard treatment is surgery and includes hysterectomy, bilateral salpingo-oophorectomy and removal of all suspicious lesions [60]. In April 2014, the FDA released an alert discouraging laparoscopic morcellation during hysterectomy or myomectomy for myomas based on the increased risk of intra-abdominal spread of unexpected uterine sarcoma and worse survival.

Preservation of the ovaries can be considered in selected young women, since salpingo-oophorectomy seems not to affect prognosis. Ovarian preservation can also be considered in patients affected by early stage endometrial stromal sarcomas [62]. Lymphadenectomy is not required given the rate of retroperitoneal involvement is very rare and should be carried out only if there is pre- or intra-operative documentation of lymphadenopathy.

For stage II–IV disease, the goal is complete cytoreduction and procedures will be conditioned by intra-operative findings. Adjuvant treatment of stage I leiomyosarcoma and undifferentiated endometrial sarcoma is not clearly defined; chemotherapy is usually administered because of the high risk of systemic recurrence, despite the lack of pertinent randomized studies.

For stage II–IVA disease chemotherapy is the standard approach, and radiation may be employed for palliation of symptoms. The combination of gemcitabine–docetaxel is usually employed in the adjuvant treatment of leiomyosarcomas, but other regimens can be administered [59]. In stage I endometrial stromal sarcoma, hormone therapy including progestins or aromatase inhibitors can be administered, while it is recommended in more advanced stages. Radiotherapy may be employed for symptom palliation.

The prognosis of leiomyosarcoma and undifferentiated endometrial sarcoma is poor with 5-year survival rates of 50–60% in stage I and 5–10% in more advanced disease.

For endometrial stromal sarcoma, 10-year survival is 95–98% in stage I disease and 60–70% in more advanced cases.

Gestational trophoblastic disease

Gestational trophoblastic disease (GTD) arises from placental tissue and includes benign conditions (complete or partial mole, placental site nodule) and malignant conditions (gestational trophoblastic neoplasia [GTN]) which include invasive mole, choriocarcinoma, placental site trophoblastic tumor and epithelioid trophoblastic tumor.

Molar pregnancy occurs in 0.5–1 cases/1000 pregnancies in developed countries, while incidence rises up to 12/1000 pregnancies in Asiatic areas [63].

Complete mole is characterized by transparent vesicles corresponding to hydropic villi; no structured villi or fetal

Table 39.8 FIGO staging: leiomyosarcoma, undifferentiated endometrial sarcoma and endometrial stroma sarcoma

FIGO stage		Definition
I		Tumor limited to uterus
	IA	≤5 cm in greatest dimension
	IB	>5 cm in greatest dimension
II		Tumor extends beyond the uterus, but within the pelvis
	IIA	Involves adnexa
	IIB	Involves other pelvic tissues
III		Tumor infiltrates abdominal tissues
	IIIA	1 site
	IIIB	>1 site
	IIIC	Regional lymph node metastasis
IVA		Invades bladder or rectum
IVB		Distant metastasis (including intra-abdominal or inguinal lymph nodes; excluding adnexa, pelvic and abdominal tissues)

Table 39.9 Gestational trophoblastic neoplasia: WHO prognostic scoring system

Risk factor	Score			
	0	1	2	4
Age, years	<40	≥40	—	—
Antecedent pregnancy	Mole	Abortion	Term	—
Interval from index pregnancy (months)	<4	4–6	7–12	>12
Pretreatment hCG (IU/L)	<1,000	1,000–10,000	10,000 to <100,000	≥100,000
Largest tumor size (cm)	<3	3–4	≥5	—
Site of metastases	Lung	Spleen, kidney	Gastrointestinal tract	Brain, liver
No. of metastases identified	—	1–4	5–8	>8
Previous failed chemotherapy	—	—	Single drug	≥2 drugs

parts are present. Conversely, partial mole shows variable villous size, focal edema and hyperplasia, and sometimes fetal remnants. Usually, pathologically the diagnosis of GTD is made by curettage of the uterine cavity; although hysterectomy can be performed in cases where childbearing is no longer desired, it is rarely offered to patients. After evacuation, serial assessment of human chorionic gonadotropin (hCG) is carried out, and oral contraceptives are recommended.

Evolution to GTN is often heralded by hCG elevation: invasive mole is a morphologically benign tumor with high invasiveness and metastatic potential (15% of cases). Diagnosis is often not histological but is based on persistent elevation of hCG.

Choriocarcinoma usually presents as a friable, hemorrhagic mass composed of only cytotrophoblasts and syncitiotrophoblasts, with absence of villi (otherwise, diagnosis of an invasive mole). This neoplasia has a high propensity for hematogeneous spread. Staging work-up includes hCG, chest X-ray, CT scan, TV/US examination or MRI.

FIGO stage I corresponds to disease confined to the uterus, stage II refers to disease limited to genital structures (adnexa, vagina, broad ligament), stage III refers to lung involvement and stage IV corresponds to other metastatic sites. The risk factor scoring system is used for prognostic and therapeutic determination (Table 39.9).

Patients with stage I disease and patients with stage II–III and a low-risk score (<7) achieve 90–100% survival, with single agent chemotherapy [64]. In cases of resistant disease (10% of cases), or in stage IV patients and stage II–III with a high-risk score (≥7), treatment requires a multi-agent regimen. Surgery can play a role in cases of sanctuary localization of disease showing resistance to chemotherapy, or in palliative cases.

Placental trophoblastic tumor and epithelioid trophoblastic tumors show low levels of hCG and a slow growth rate. Given the poor response to chemotherapy, surgery is the cornerstone of treatment. Adjuvant chemotherapy is recommended in stage ≥II and in metastatic disease and consists of platinum-containing regimens. Prognosis is excellent (survival almost 100%) in non-metastatic patients, but drops down to 50–60% survival in metastatic patients.

REFERENCES

1. International Agency for Research on Cancer. Cervical cancer estimated incidence, mortality, and prevalence worldwide in 2012. Geneva: World Health Organization, 2012. Available at http://globocan.iarc.fr/old/FactSheets/cancers/cervix-new.asp.
2. Asiaf A, Ahmad ST, Mohammad SO, Zargar MA. Review of the current knowledge on the epidemiology, pathogenesis, and prevention of human papillomavirus infection. *Eur J Cancer Prev* 2014;23(3):206–24.
3. Mutch D. The new FIGO staging system for cancers of the vulva, cervix, endometrium and sarcomas. *Gynecol Oncol* 2009;115(3):325–28.
4. Siegel CL, Andreotti RF, Cardenes HR, et al. American College of Radiology. ACR Appropriateness Criteria® pretreatment planning of invasive cancer of the cervix. *J Am Coll Radiol* 2012;9(6):395–402.
5. Schlichte MJ, Guidry J. Current cervical carcinoma screening guidelines. *J Clin Med* 2015;4(5):918–32.
6. Schiller JT, Castellsagué X, Garland SM. A review of clinical trials of human papillomavirus prophylactic vaccines. *Vaccine* 2012;30(Suppl. 5):F123–38.
7. Piver MS, Rutledge F, Smith JP. Five classes of extended hysterectomy for women with cervical cancer. *Obstet Gynecol* 1974;44(2):265–72.
8. Querleu D, Morrow CP. Classification of radical hysterectomy. *Lancet Oncol* 2008;9(3):297–303.
9. Kadkhodayan S, Hasanzadeh M, Treglia G, et al. Sentinel node biopsy for lymph nodal staging of uterine cervix cancer: a systematic review and meta-analysis of the pertinent literature. *Eur J Surg Oncol* 2015;41(1):1–20.
10. Landoni F, Maneo A, Colombo A, et al. Randomised study of radical surgery versus radiotherapy for stage Ib-IIa cervical cancer. *Lancet* 1997;350(9077):535–40.
11. Peters WA 3rd, Liu PY, Barrett RJ 2nd, et al. Concurrent chemotherapy and pelvic radiation therapy compared with pelvic radiation therapy alone as adjuvant therapy after radical surgery in high-risk early-stage cancer of the cervix. *J Clin Oncol* 2000;18:1606–13.

12. Chemoradiotherapy for Cervical Cancer Meta-Analysis Collaboration (CCCMAC). Reducing uncertainties about the effects of chemoradiotherapy for cervical cancer: individual patient data meta-analysis. *Cochrane Database Syst Rev* 2010;(1):CD008285.

13. Eifel PJ, Winter K, Morris M, et al. Pelvic irradiation with concurrent chemotherapy versus pelvic and para-aortic irradiation for high-risk cervical cancer: an update of radiation therapy oncology group trial (RTOG) 90-01. *J Clin Oncol* 2004;22(5):872–80.

14. Neoadjuvant Chemotherapy for Locally Advanced Cervical Cancer Meta-Analysis Collaboration. Neoadjuvant chemotherapy for locally advanced cervical cancer: a systematic review and meta-analysis of individual patient data from 21 randomised trials. *Eur J Cancer* 2003;39(17):2470–86.

15. Chao A, Cheng-Tao Chao A, Lin CT, Lai CH. Updates in systemic treatment for metastatic cervical cancer. *Curr Treat Options Oncol* 2014;15(1):1–13.

16. Tewari KS, Sill MW, Long HJ 3rd, et al. Improved survival with bevacizumab in advanced cervical cancer. *N Engl J Med* 2014;370(8):734–43.

17. Siegel R, Ma J, Zou Z, Jemal A. Cancer statistics, 2014. *CA Cancer J Clin* 2014;64(1):9–29.

18. Tzortzatos G, Andersson E, Soller M, Askmalm MS, et al. The gynecological surveillance of women with Lynch syndrome in Sweden. *Gynecol Oncol* 2015;138(3):717–22.

19. Gkrozou F, Dimakopoulos G, Vrekoussis T, et al. Hysteroscopy in women with abnormal uterine bleeding: a meta-analysis on four major endometrial pathologies. *Arch Gynecol Obstet* 2015;291(6):1347–54.

20. Obermair A, Janda M, Baker J, et al. Improved surgical safety after laparoscopic compared to open surgery for apparent early stage endometrial cancer: results from a randomised controlled trial. *Eur J Cancer* 2012;48(8):1147–53.

21. Walker JL, Piedmonte MR, Spirtos NM, et al. Laparoscopy compared with laparotomy for comprehensive surgical staging of uterine cancer: Gynecologic Oncology Group Study LAP2. *J Clin Oncol* 2009;27(32):5331–6.

22. Kim HS, Suh DH, Kim MK, et al. Systematic lymphadenectomy for survival in patients with endometrial cancer: a meta-analysis. *Jpn J Clin Oncol* 2012;42(5):405–12.

23. Kang S, Yoo HJ, Hwang JH, et al. Sentinel lymph node biopsy in endometrial cancer: meta-analysis of 26 studies. *Gynecol Oncol* 2011;123(3):522–7.

24. Nout RA, Smit VT, Putter H, et al. PORTEC Study Group. Vaginal brachytherapy versus pelvic external beam radiotherapy for patients with endometrial cancer of high-intermediate risk (PORTEC-2): an open-label, non-inferiority, randomised trial. *Lancet* 2010;375(9717):816–23.

25. Lorusso D, Ferrandina G, Colombo N, et al. Randomized phase II trial of carboplatin-paclitaxel (CP) compared to carboplatin-paclitaxel-bevacizumab (CP-B) in advanced (stage III-IV) or recurrent endometrial cancer: The MITO END-2 trial. 2015 ASCO Annual Meeting. *J Clin Oncol* 2015;33(Suppl.):abstr. 5502.

26. Amadio G, Masciullo V, Ferrandina MG, Scambia G. Emerging drugs for endometrial cancer. *Expert Opin Emerg Drugs* 2014;19(4):497–509.

27. Rodolakis A, Biliatis I, Morice P, et al. Society of Gynecological Oncology Task Force for Fertility Preservation: clinical recommendations for fertility-sparing management in young endometrial cancer patients. *Int J Gynecol Cancer* 2015;25(7):1258–65.

28. American College of Obstetricians and Gynecologists. ACOG practice bulletin. Management of adnexal masses. *Obstet Gynecol* 2007;110(1):201–14.

29. Diergaarde B, Kurta ML. Use of fertility drugs and risk of ovarian cancer. *Curr Opin Obstet Gynecol* 2014;26(3):125–9.

30. Mavaddat N, Peock S, Frost D, et al. Cancer risks for BRCA1 and BRCA2 mutation carriers: results from prospective analysis of EMBRACE. *J Natl Cancer Inst* 2013;105(11):812–22.

31. Clarke-Pearson DL. Clinical practice. Screening for ovarian cancer. *N Engl J Med* 2009;361(2):170–7.

32. Prat J. FIGO Committee on Gynecologic Oncology. Staging classification for cancer of the ovary, fallopian tube, and peritoneum. *Int J Gynecol Obstet* 2014;124:1–5.

33. Powless CA, Aletti GD, Bakkum-Gamez JN, Cliby WA. Risk factors for lymph node metastasis in apparent early-stage epithelial ovarian cancer: implications for surgical staging. *Gynecol Oncol* 2011;122(3):536–40.

34. Trimbos JB, Parmar M, Vergote I, et al. International Collaborative Ovarian Neoplasm trial 1 and Adjuvant ChemoTherapy In Ovarian Neoplasm trial: two parallel randomized phase III trials of adjuvant chemotherapy in patients with early-stage ovarian carcinoma. *J Natl Cancer Inst* 2003;95(2):105–12.

35. Collinson F, Qian W Fossati R, et al. Optimal treatment of early stage ovarian cancer. *Ann Oncol* 2014;25:1165–71.

36. Bristow RE, Tomacruz RS, Armstrong DK, Trimble EL, Montz FJ. Survival effect of maximal cytoreductive surgery for advanced ovarian carcinoma during the platinum era: a meta-analysis. *J Clin Oncol* 2002;20(5):1248–59.

37. Chi DS, Zivanovic O, Levinson KL, et al. The incidence of major complications after the performance of extensive upper abdominal surgical procedures during primary cytoreduction of advanced ovarian, tubal, and peritoneal carcinomas. *Gynecol Oncol* 2010;119(1):38–42.

38. Vergote I, Trope CG, Amant F, et al. Neoadjuvant chemotherapy or primary surgery in stage IIIC or IV ovarian cancer. *N Engl J Med* 2010;363:943–53.

39. Kehoe S, Hook J, Nankivell M, et al. Primary chemotherapy versus primary surgery for newly diagnosed advanced ovarian cancer (CHORUS): an open-label, randomised, controlled, non-inferiority trial. *Lancet* 2015;386:249–57.

40. Fagotti A, Vizzielli G, De Iaco P, et al. A multicentric trial (Olympia-MITO 13) on the accuracy of laparoscopy to assess peritoneal spread in ovarian cancer. *Am J Obstet Gynecol* 2013;209(5):462.e1–11.

41. Vasey PA. Ovarian cancer: front-line standard treatment in 2008. *Ann Oncol* 2008;19(Suppl. 7):vii61–6.

42. N Katsumata, M Yasuda, F Takahashi, et al. Dose-dense paclitaxel once a week in combination with carboplatin every 3 weeks for advanced ovarian cancer: a phase 3, open-label, randomised controlled trial. *Lancet* 2009;374:1331–8.

43. Armstrong DK, Bundy B, Wenzel L, et al. Intraperitoneal cisplatin and paclitaxel in ovarian cancer. *N Engl J Med* 2006;354:34–43.

44. Burger RA, Brady MF, Bookman MA, et al. Incorporation of bevacizumab in the primary treatment of ovarian cancer. *N Engl J Med* 2011;365:2473–83.

45. Perren TJ, Swart AM, Pfisterer J, et al. A phase 3 trial of bevacizumab in ovarian cancer. *N Engl J Med* 2011;365:2484–96.

46. Pujade-Lauraine E, Hilpert F, Weber B, et al. Bevacizumab combined with chemotherapy for platinum-resistant recurrent ovarian cancer: the AURELIA open-label randomized phase III trial. *J Clin Oncol* 2014;32(13):1302–8.

47. Aghajanian C, Blank SV, Goff BA, et al. OCEANS: a randomized, double-blind, placebo-controlled phase III trial of chemotherapy with or without bevacizumab in patients with platinum-sensitive recurrent epithelial ovarian, primary peritoneal, or fallopian tube cancer. *J Clin Oncol* 2012;30:2039–45.

48. Ledermann J, Harter P, Gourley C, et al. Olaparib maintenance therapy in platinum-sensitive relapsed ovarian cancer. *N Engl J Med* 2012;366:1382–1392.

49. Colombo N, Peiretti M, Garbi A, et al. Non-epithelial ovarian cancer: ESMO clinical practice guidelines for diagnosis, treatment and follow-up. *Ann Oncol* 2012;23(Suppl. 7):vii20–26.

50. Kleppe M, Amkreutz LCM, van Gorp T, et al. Lymph node metastasis in stage I and II sex cord stromal and malignant germ cell tumors: a systematic review. *Gynecol Oncol* 2014;133:124–7.

51. Ray-Coquard I, Brown J, Provencher DM, et al. Gynecologic Cancer Intergroup (GCIG) consensus review for ovarian sex cord-stromal tumors. *Int J Gynaecol Cancer* 2014;24:S42–7.

52. Medeiros F, Nascimento AF, Crum CP. Early vulvar squamous neoplasia: advances in classification, diagnosis, and differential diagnosis. *Adv Anat Pathol* 2005;12(1):20–26.

53. Saito T, Kato K. Management of lymph nodes in the treatment of vulvar cancer. *Int J Clin Oncol* 2007;12(3):187–91.

54. Hassanzade M, Attaran M, Treglia G, et al. Lymphatic mapping and sentinel node biopsy in squamous cell carcinoma of the vulva: systematic review and meta-analysis of the literature. *Gynecol Oncol* 2013;130(1):237–45.

55. Shylasree TS, Bryant A, Howell RE. Chemoradiation for advanced primary vulval cancer. *Cochrane Database Syst Rev* 2011;(4):CD003752.

56. Reade CJ, Eiriksson LR, Mackay H. Systemic therapy in squamous cell carcinoma of the vulva: current status and future directions. *Gynecol Oncol* 2014;132:780–8.

57. Gadducci A, Fabrini MG, Lanfredini N, Sergiampietri C. Squamous cell carcinoma of the vagina: natural history, treatment modalities and prognostic factors. *Crit Rev Oncol Hematol* 2015;93(3):211–24.

58. Hiniker SM, Roux A, Murphy JD, et al. Primary squamous cell carcinoma of the vagina: prognostic factors, treatment pattern, and outcomes. *Gynecol Oncol* 2013;131:380–385.

59. Chyle V, Zagars CK, Wheeler JA, et al. Definitive radiotherapy for carcinoma of the vagina: outcome and prognostic factors. *Int J Radiat Oncol Biol Phys* 1996;35:891–905.

60. Amant F, Floquet A, Friedlander M, et al. Gynecologic Cancer Intergroup (GCIG) Consensus review for endometrial stromal sarcoma. *Int J Gynecol Cancer* 2014;24:S67–72.

61. El-Khalfaoui K, du Bois A, Heitz F, et al. Current and future options in the management and treatment of uterine sarcoma. *Ther Adv Med Oncol* 2014;6(1):21–28.

62. Jin Y, Deng CY, Tian QJ, et al. Fertility sparing treatment of low grade endometrial stromal sarcoma. *Int J Clin Exp Med* 2015;8(4):5818–21.

63. Lurain JR. Gestational trophoblastic disease I: epidemiology, pathology, clinical presentation and diagnosis of gestational trophoblastic disease, and management of hydatidiform mole. *Am J Obstet Gynecol* 2010, 203(6):531–9.

64. Mangili G, Lorusso D, Brown J, et al. Trophoblastic disease review for diagnosis and management. *Int J Gynecol Cancer* 2014;24(S3):S109–16.

40

Skin cancer: Squamous cell carcinoma and basal cell carcinoma

IBRAHIM EDHEMOVIĆ

INCIDENCE AND AETIOLOGY

There are two major types of skin cancers: melanoma and non-melanoma. The vast majority of non-melanoma skin cancers (NMSCs) (Figure 40.1) comprise squamous cell carcinoma (SCC) and basal cell carcinoma (BCC), and both together are the most common human cancers [1]. BCC is more common than SCC, accounting for about 74% of NMSCs, while SCC accounts for approximately 23% [2]. The term *NMSC* is mostly used to define both BCC and SCC; however, there are also much less common types, such as Merkel cell carcinoma and skin adnexal carcinomas, Kaposi sarcoma and other types of sarcomas and lymphomas. All these less common types account for approximately 1–3% of all NMSCs.

It is not easy to obtain detailed and correct data about the incidence of NMSC because some cancer registries do not register all NMSCs [2] or they do not register BCC and SCC separately [3]. The worldwide incidence varies considerably which probably reflects not only different exposure to risk factors in different countries but also different methodology and completeness of data. The highest incidence of BCC is in Australia (>1000) and the lowest is in Africa (1) per 100,000 person-years. The incidence of SCC in Europe in 1997 varied from less than 10 in Nordic countries to 28.9

in Switzerland per 100,000 person-years [4,5]. In Slovenia, in the period from 2007 to 2011, the average incidence of SCC and BCC was 18.1 and 78.7 per 100,000 person-years, respectively [6]. In all countries, the incidence of NMSC is increasing over time; however, in the countries with a low incidence, it is rising at a much slower rate than in the countries with a high incidence [5].

Predisposing factors

ULTRAVIOLET RADIATION

For both BCC and SCC, exposure to ultraviolet radiation (sunlight, tanning beds and occupational exposure) is the most important risk factor. These tumours may arise anywhere on the skin. The most commonly affected areas are those exposed to the sun. In a study on 145 cases of SCC in Australia [7], 73% cases were localized on the head and neck and dorsal aspects of the hands and forearms, while the remaining 27% cases were distributed on other parts of the body. The pattern and type of exposure differ among different types of skin cancer [8,9]. The main mechanism is UV-induced cumulative DNA damage, usually to the TP53 tumour suppressor gene. Failure to repair these mutations results in tumour development. A severe bout of sunburn

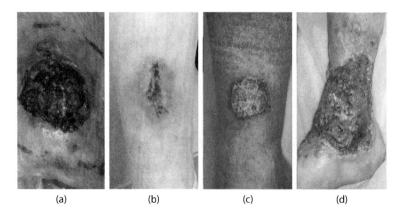

(a)   (b)   (c)   (d)

Figure 40.1 Examples of BCC and SCC: BCC on the forehead (a) and on the lower leg (b). SCC on the lower leg (c) and on the ankle (d). (Courtesy of Boris Jancar, MD, MSc, Institute of Oncology Ljubljana, Slovenia.)

may not be more mutagenic and carcinogenic than a mild sunburn [10]. Ultraviolet radiation with wavelengths between 310 and 320 nm may contribute more to mutation formation [10].

IMMUNOSUPPRESSION

Immunosuppressed renal transplant recipients are at an elevated risk of developing NMSC, particularly SCC. It has been shown [11,12] that in these patients, compared to the healthy population, the probability of developing more aggressive SCC and BCC is up to 250 times and 10 times higher, respectively. Also, 47% of lung transplant recipients developed new NMSC after 10 years [13]. In HIV-positive patients compared to HIV-negative patients, the incidence rate of BCC and SCC is 2.1- and 2.6-fold higher, respectively [14]. It seems that an altered immune response caused by transplantation immunosuppressive drugs and HIV plays an important role [15] in increasing the risk of developing NMSC.

HUMAN PAPILLOMA VIRUS

There is an association between human papilloma virus (HPV) and SCC. HPV is not found in all SCCs; however, it is found more often in immunosuppressed than in immunocompetent patients with SCC [16]. HPV is also found in 60% of immunosuppressed and in 36% of immunocompetent patients with BCC [17]. The role of HPV and the mechanisms involved in these associations are still not clear.

IONIZING RADIATION

Exposure to ionizing radiation elevates risk of skin cancer. In the study of 80,158 atomic bomb survivors in Japan [18], the authors noted a significant excess of relative risk for BCC and Bowen disease. A study on childhood cancer survivors [19] showed that radiation therapy was associated with a 6.3-fold increase in risk of skin cancer compared to those who were not irradiated.

Other known risk factors include chronic arsenic exposure, naevoid basal cell nevus syndrome (Gorlin syndrome), psoralen therapy, smoking, aging and chemical carcinogens.

PATHOLOGY AND STAGING

Pathology

The skin consists of three main layers: the epidermis (outermost superficial layer), the dermis (middle layer) and the subcutis (the deepest layer). The epidermis consists of five layers: stratum basale, stratum spinosum (these two layers form stratum germinativum), stratum granulosum, stratum lucidum and stratum corneum (the most superficial layer). Basal cell carcinoma arises from the stratum basale and SCC arises from the stratum spinosum (Figure 40.2). Both BCC and SCC arise from keratinocytes and histologically resemble epidermal keratinocytes [20], and both are referred to as NMSC; however, there are significant histopathological as well as clinical differences between them.

Examples of BCC and SCC are shown in Figures 40.1 and 40.3. BCC can appear in different clinical forms. The most frequent form is a white-pink nodule with telangiectasia, thickened borders and central ulceration. In a review of 1039 consecutive cases of basal cell carcinoma [21], Sexton and colleagues identified five major histological patterns: nodular (21%), superficial (17%), micronodular (15%), infiltrative (7%) and morpheic (1%). A mixed pattern (two or more major histologic patterns) was present in 38.5% of cases. Basosquamous type is considered a high-risk feature [22].

The clinical appearance of SCC is highly variable. It appears mostly in the form of a solid or dense, skin-coloured plaque or papule, mostly with ulceration, hyperkeratosis and raised borders. Histologically, there are numerous subtypes [23], such as acantholytic SCC, spindle cell SCC and verrucous carcinoma.

Premalignant lesions

ACTINIC KERATOSIS

Actinic keratosis (AK) is a precursor lesion of cutaneous SCC. Usually, they appear as multiple hyperkeratotic or scaly lesions. Some of them will progress to SCC. There is

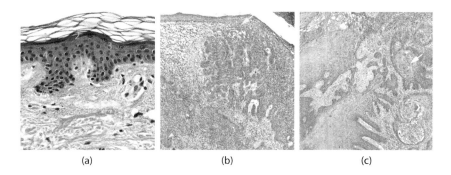

Figure 40.2 (a) Layers of the epidermis in normal skin: stratum basale (1), stratum spinosum (2), stratum granulosum (3), stratum lucidum (4) and stratum corneum (5). (b) BCC arising from stratum basale (yellow arrow). (c) SCC arising from stratum spinosum and infiltrating into the dermis (green arrow) with tumour islands showing keratinization (white arrow). (Courtesy of Barbara Gazic, MD, PhD, Institute of Oncology Ljubljana, Slovenia.)

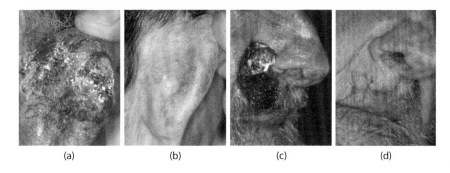

Figure 40.3 Good cosmetic results after radiation therapy: SCC on the posterior aspect of auricle – before (a) and after (b) the treatment. BCC at the base of the nose – before (c) and after (d) the treatment. (Courtesy of Boris Jancar, MD, MSc, Institute of Oncology Ljubljana, Slovenia.)

a huge variability in estimated lifetime risk for one single AK to progress to SCC (from 0.1% to 10.2% [24]). Keeping in mind the multiplicity of such lesions, a more significant lifetime risk of progression is estimated to be between 6% and 10% [25,26]. Another study showed that people with more than 10 AKs had a cumulative probability of 14% of developing an SCC within 5 years [27]. SCC and AK share the same risk factors: excessive exposure to UV radiation, immunosuppression, the presence of HPV infection and already presented AK or SCC [26]. AK can be considered as an early form of carcinoma in situ [28]. It is best treated with cryotherapy or topically with imiquimod [29]. Other treatment options may also be used (curettage, shave excision, photodynamic therapy, carbon dioxide laser). AKs that have an atypical appearance or do not respond to appropriate therapy should be biopsied [30].

BOWEN'S DISEASE

The term *Bowen's disease* refers to *in situ* SCC of the skin. Bowen's disease and SCC share the same risk factors as AK (see above). There are genital subtypes which include erythroplasia of Queyrat, bowenoid papulosis and vulval intraepithelial neoplasia. Most studies suggest that the risk of invasive carcinoma is about 3% [31], whereas the risk of malignant transformation associated with erythroplasia of Queyrat is estimated to be around 10% [32]. Treatment

options include cryotherapy, imiquimod, 5-fluorouracil (5-FU) topically, curettage or excision.

Staging

The most recent staging system, proposed by the International Union Against Cancer (UICC), is published in the seventh edition of the TNM classification [33] (Table 40.1) and is almost identical to that published by the American Joint Committee on Cancer (AJCC) [34]. Staging of the tumours located on the eyelid, vulva and penis is classified separately from other skin locations.

Primary SCC may also be classified as high-risk or low-risk SCC, depending on additional characteristics. Some of these characteristics have already been recognized in the seventh edition of TNM classification under high-risk features (Table 40.1). In addition to these tumour-related high-risk features, National Comprehensive Cancer Network (NCCN) guidelines [30] also recognize patient-related high-risk features: size ≥6, 10 or 20 mm (depending on location – face, forehead and scalp or trunk and extremities, respectively), poorly defined borders, recurrent tumour, immunosuppression, site of previous radiation therapy or chronic ulceration, rapid tumour growth and neurologic symptoms. Furthermore, other authors [35] recognize additional patient-related high-risk features: coexisting chronic

Table 40.1 TNM clinical classification primary tumour (T)[a]

TX	Primary tumour cannot be assessed
T0	No evidence of primary tumour
Tis	Carcinoma in situ
T1	Tumour 2 cm or less in greatest dimension
T2	Tumour more than 2 cm in greatest dimension
T3	Tumour with invasion of deep structures, e.g. muscle, bone, cartilage, jaws, and orbit
T4	Tumour with direct or perineural invasion of skull base or axial skeleton

Regional lymph nodes (N)

NX	Regional lymph nodes cannot be assessed
N0	No regional lymph node metastasis
N1	Metastasis in a single lymph node, 3 cm or less in greatest dimension
N2	Metastasis in a single lymph node, more than 3 cm but not more than 6 cm in greatest dimension, or in multiple lymph nodes, none more than 6 cm in greatest dimension
N3	Metastasis in a lymph node, more than 6 cm in greatest dimension

Distant metastasis (M)

M0	No distant metastasis
M1	Distant metastasis

pTNM pathological classification

pT	Corresponds to T category
pN	Corresponds to N category
pN0	Histological examination of a regional lymphadenectomy specimen will ordinarily include 6 or more lymph nodes; if the lymph nodes are negative, but the number ordinarily examined is not met, classify as pN0
pM1	If microscopically confirmed

High-risk features

Depth/invasion	>4 mm thickness
	Clark level IV
	Perineural invasion
	Lymphovascular invasion
Anatomic location	Primary site ear
	Primary site non-glabrous lip
Differentiation	Poorly differentiated or undifferentiated

Histopathological grading (G)

GX	Grade cannot be assessed
G1	Well differentiated
G2	Moderately differentiated
G3	Poorly differentiated
G4	Undifferentiated

Stage grouping

Stage 0	Tis	N0	M0
Stage I	T1	N0	M0
Stage II	T2	N0	M0
Stage III	T3	N0	M0
	T1, T2, T3	N1	M0
Stage IV	T1, T2, T3	N2, N3	M0
	T4	N any	M0
	T any	N any	M1

Source: Sobin LH, Gospodarowicz MK, Wittekind C, *UICC TNM Classification of Malignant Tumours*, 7th ed., Oxford: Blackwell Publishing, 2010. Copyright © Blackwell Publishing Ltd. Reproduced with permission of Blackwell Publishing Ltd.

Note: In the case of multiple simultaneous tumours, the tumour with the highest T category is classified and the number of separate tumours is indicated in parentheses, e.g., T2(5).

[a] AJCC considers stage I tumours with more than one high-risk feature as stage II.

lymphocytic leukemia, organ transplantation and positive margins after excision. The presence of any of these tumour- or patient-related features implies a high-risk tumour.

DIAGNOSIS AND PREOPERATIVE IMAGING

Diagnosis

Many NMSCs have a typical clinical appearance; however, definitive diagnosis can be achieved only by biopsy and histological confirmation. Three typical biopsy techniques are shave, punch and excision. All three techniques can be performed under local anaesthesia in outpatient settings. Shave biopsy is performed using a scalpel positioned parallel to the skin; unfortunately, using this technique, the full skin thickness specimen is almost never possible to obtain. Punch biopsy is performed using a specially designed knife (trephine) to cut out a cylindrically shaped piece of skin. The punch biopsy skin specimen contains the full skin thickness. Excisional biopsy, in the case of small tumours, implies the removal of the tumour with clinically uninvolved margins. In the case of a favourable histological diagnosis, excisional biopsy can be considered a definitive treatment. In the case of a larger tumour, only a part of the tumour is removed (incisional biopsy).

Another useful tool for diagnosis is cytological assessment. In the majority of cases, it enables safe and quick diagnosis for a fraction of the price. The skin lesions are best sampled by scraping or by fine-needle aspiration biopsy without anaesthesia. In experienced hands, the accuracy is high. The study by Daskalopoulou et al [36]. showed only one false-positive and six false-negative diagnoses in 513 cases. Another study from Özden et al [37]. showed that cytodiagnosis of BCC was concordant with the histopathology results in 80% of cases of BCC.

Preoperative imaging

BCC metastasizes very rarely, so there is no need for any imaging for detecting distant metastasis, though this type of tumour can be locally very aggressive. If clinically suspicious (fixed, large tumours), the extent of tumour invasion in the affected area is best assessed by CT or MRI scan.

SCC has more potential to metastasize than BCC, especially in immunosuppressed patients with high-risk tumour features. These patients have a significantly higher probability of developing metastases in regional lymph nodes [38] as well as distant metastases [39]. In addition to regional lymph nodes, the most common sites for distant metastases are the in-transit sites, lung and bone [39]. In the case of high-risk patients, ultrasound examination of the regional lymph node basins with ultrasound-guided fine-needle aspiration biopsy of suspicious nodes should be performed. Additionally, chest CT scan, bone scintigraphy and other appropriate imaging investigations should be carried out in the case of clinical suspicion of distant metastases.

TREATMENT OPTIONS FOR LOCALIZED DISEASE

The goal of treatment is to cure the disease, while preserving functionality and cosmesis as much as possible. In most cases, the disease will be localized. In such cases, local treatment only will be sufficient to effect cure.

Surgical excision

Surgical excision is the most widely used treatment approach. There is no clear evidence to indicate how wide surgical margins should be; however, for the low-risk SCC 4 mm is recommended. For high-risk tumours 6 mm should be sufficient [40].

The advantages of surgical excision are the possibility of histological analysis, no need for repeated procedures, no serious side effects in the majority of cases and a relatively short treatment spell.

BCCs metastasize to the regional lymph nodes extremely rarely (0.0028–0.5%) [41,42]. In contrast, SCC will develop nodal metastases in 3–6% of patients with low-risk tumour characteristics and in up to 40% [38] of patients with high-risk tumour characteristics. In a study published by the American Joint Committee on Cancer (AJCC) [43], the authors showed that 11.2% of T2 tumours and 60% of T4 tumours had a positive sentinel lymph node biopsy (SLNB). The authors of this study proposed an alternative T-staging system based on the presence of four high-risk features (poor differentiation, perineural invasion, tumour diameter ≥2 cm, invasion beyond the subcutaneous fat). This alternative staging system could more accurately identify a group of patients eligible for SLNB. These high-risk patients may benefit from SLNB, though no guidelines on the routine use of sentinel lymph node biopsy in such patients are currently available [44].

Mohs micrographic surgery

Developed by Dr Frederick Mohs in 1938 and improved over the past decades, Mohs micrographic surgery evolved into an effective method for excising NMSC. Mohs technique differs from conventional excision techniques in that the thin layers of skin are serially excised and histologically evaluated using frozen sections. Mohs technique ensures clear margins and allows maximal preservation of the healthy skin avoiding the need to estimate where excision margins should be.

Radiation therapy

The radiation therapy is the treatment of choice if NMSCs are large or localized to areas where extensive mutilation with or without reconstruction is required to obtain clear margins (e.g. lip, ears or nose). Patients may also elect to have radiotherapy instead of surgery if preferred. Radiotherapy results in a high rate of local control with a low rate of serious side effects [45]. Cosmetic results are good (Figure 40.3). With radiation therapy, there is no need for reconstruction or skin grafting; however, the treatment can take weeks. Its biggest disadvantage is the lack of histological analysis.

Thermal ablative methods

Curettage down to the base of the tumour followed by electrodesiccation is an ablative therapy for the management of superficial NMSC. It is a fast method for destroying the tumour; however, margins cannot be assessed. It is also possible to combine curettage and cryosurgery instead of electrodesiccation to avoid more extensive connective tissue damage associated with the electrodestruction without affecting recurrence rate [46]. Cryotherapy alone is also one of the ablative methods used for the treatment of superficial NMSC. Freezing the tissue down to −60°C causes, among other effects, ice crystal formation, cell membrane damage, blood flow stasis and finally cell death. The major drawback of ablative methods is the lack of margin assessment.

Non-thermal ablative methods

Electrochemotherapy (ECT) with bleomycin and cisplatin combines reversible electroporation and cytotoxic drugs. It has been shown that ECT is an effective treatment option for both SCC and BCC on the head and neck with complete response rates varying from 41% to 100% [47,48]. Unlike the thermal ablative methods, ECT does not cause thermal tissue injury and has a minimal impact on the healthy skin surrounding the tumour.

Topical treatment

The most widely known topical agents for the treatment of superficial NMSC are imiquimod (IQ) and 5-fluorouracil (5-FU). IQ, through cytokine induction, locally enhances immune pathways, resulting in immunomodulating, antiviral and antitumour effects [49]. IQ 5% cream is used for the treatment of T1 NMSC [50] and Bowen's disease. 5-FU is a cytotoxic agent which may also be used in the form of a topically applied cream. The reported efficacy of both agents varies from 42% to 100% [51].

Photodynamic therapy

Photodynamic therapy (PDT) combines drugs and light of a specific wavelength [52]. A topically applied inactive prodrug (5-aminolaevulinic acid or methyl aminolevulinate) is intracellularly converted into a photoactivated metabolite (protoporphyrin IX) which causes cellular damage when exposed to light [53]. It is used for BCC, but not for SCC.

TREATMENT OPTIONS FOR LOCALLY ADVANCED AND METASTATIC DISEASE

While the vast majority of NMSC can be successfully treated with excision or other local treatment modalities, there is a subset of locally advanced lesions which are more aggressive and metastasize, resulting in severe morbidity and mortality. These lesions require a much more complex treatment; however, there is little reliable information regarding the management of locally advanced disease. The presence of high-risk features does not mean that the tumour is locally advanced. Actually, there is no widely recognized definition of locally advanced disease. The definition of locally advanced disease appeared in literature in 2004 [54] in a study conducted by Kwan et al [55]. as an inclusion criterion. The authors considered an NMSC to be locally advanced disease if it fulfilled one of the following criteria: T2 or above (>2 cm) according to UICC TNM classification or node-positive disease [55].

The probability of a BCC metastasizing is extremely low. Therefore, the treatment strategy in these patients is focused only on local control. In the case of resectability without severe mutilation, surgery would be the first option [22]. Radiotherapy also provides a high rate of local control [56]. In the case of non-resectability, radiotherapy should be considered the definitive treatment [22].

In cases where a patient with a BCC is unsuitable for either surgery or radiotherapy, a new drug may provide an alternative. This is vismodegib, a small-molecule inhibitor of the hedgehog pathway [57] with a 30% objective response rate in locally advanced BCC [22].

Primary therapy for resectable locally advanced SCC is surgery. In cases of non-resectable tumours or if severe mutilation may result from such surgery, primary chemoradiation should be considered.

In the case of proven nodal disease (by fine-needle aspiration biopsy or open biopsy), regional lymphadenectomy should be performed. In the case of more positive lymph nodes, adjuvant radiotherapy should be considered [30]. Radiation or chemoradiation therapy without surgery can also be used for the treatment of metastatic regional lymph nodes; however, there are insufficient data to support either primary radiation therapy or surgery alone. In cases where very extensive surgery would be necessary, radiotherapy may be the treatment of choice.

Patients with locally advanced but not metastatic SCC, who are not amenable for local treatment, may be treated with systemic therapy (targeted agents, biological response modifiers and chemotherapy). Meta-analysis from Behshad and colleagues [58] showed that systemic treatment was effective, with an overall systemic response of 72% and duration of response of 42 weeks. This treatment approach applies also for metastatic disease. There are no data supporting a surgical approach in patients with distant metastases.

NEOADJUVANT AND ADJUVANT THERAPIES

There are very few data collected from small, non-randomized trials showing good response rates to neo-adjuvant systemic therapy [59] in patients with NMSC. Currently, neoadjuvant systemic therapy is not included in the treatment guidelines [30]. There is also a lack of data supporting the use of adjuvant chemotherapy. A phase III study by Brewster and colleagues [60] did not now show any benefit for patients with advanced SCC receiving 13-cis-retinoic acid plus interferon-alpha compared to patients receiving no adjuvant therapy.

Adjuvant radiotherapy, alone or in combination with chemotherapy, is utilized to reduce the rate of recurrence in high-risk NMSC patients in whom the probability of residual disease is high. It is indicated in cases of positive margins, perineural invasion, multiple recurrences and invasion of bone or nerves [61]. Adjuvant radiotherapy may also be indicated in cases of large tumour size, rapid growth, recurrent disease and neurological compromise at presentation [44]. To date there are no data quantifying the benefit of adjuvant radiation therapy.

PROGNOSIS

The prognosis of low-risk BCC is most favourable. After completing local treatment, the probability of recurrence is less than 0.5%; however, in the presence of perineural invasion, it may rise to 7.7% even after Mohs micrographic surgery [62]. If left untreated it may result in significant morbidity.

SCC is a more aggressive disease. The prognosis depends on the presence or absence of high-risk features. A study by Clayman and colleagues [63] showed that 3-year disease-specific survival was 100% for patients with no risk factors compared to 70% for patients with at least one high-risk factor. The probability of local recurrence and metastases also depends on the number and type of high-risk features, ranging from 3.1% to 53.6% [64] and up to 40%, respectively [38].

ACKNOWLEDGEMENTS

The author thanks Barbara Gazic, MD, PhD; Boris Jancar, MD, MSc; Katja Jarm, MD, PhD; and Ziva Pohar Marinsek, MD, PhD – all from the Institute of Oncology Ljubljana, Slovenia, for their help in preparing the manuscript.

REFERENCES

1. Diepgen TL, Mahler V. The epidemiology of skin cancer. *Br J Dermatol* 2002; 146 (Suppl. 61): 1–6.
2. National Cancer Intelligence Network. Non-melanoma skin cancer in England, Scotland, Northern Ireland, and Ireland. 2013. http://www.ncin.org.uk/view?rid=2178 (assessed 23 December 2014).
3. Bonenkamp JJ. Squamous cell carcinoma and basal cell carcinoma of the skin. In Poston JG, Beauchamp RD, Ruers JMT, ed., *Textbook of Surgical Oncology*, 1st ed. Boca Raton, FL: Taylor & Francis, 2007, pp. 304–9.
4. Levi F, Franceschi S, Te VC, Randimbison L, La Vecchia C. Trends of skin cancer in the Canton of Vaud, 1976–92. *Br J Cancer* 1995; 72(4): 1047–53.
5. Lomas A, Leonardi-Bee J, Bath-Hextall F. A systematic review of worldwide incidence of nonmelanoma skin cancer. *Br J Dermatol* 2012; 166(5): 1069–80.
6. Cancer Registry of Slovenia. 2014. http://www.onko-i.si/eng/crs/ (assessed 11 December 2014).
7. English DR, Armstrong BK, Kricker A, Winter MG, Heenan PJ, Randell PL. Demographic characteristics, pigmentary and cutaneous risk factors for squamous cell carcinoma of the skin: a case-control study. *Int J Cancer* 1998; 76(5): 628–34.
8. National Cancer Institute at the National Institutes of Health. Skin cancer treatment (PDQ®). 2013. http://www.cancer.gov/cancertopics/pdq/treatment/skin/HealthProfessional/page1#section_1.1 (assessed 1 October 2014).
9. Moan J, Grigalavicius M, Baturaite Z, Dahlback A, Juzeniene A. The relationship between UV exposure and incidence of skin cancer. *Photodermatol Photoimmunol Photomed* 2015; 31: 26–35.
10. Runger TM. Much remains to be learned about how UVR induces mutations. *J Invest Dermatol* 2013; 133(7): 1717–9.
11. Hartevelt MM, Bavinck JN, Kootte AM, Vermeer BJ, Vandenbroucke JP. Incidence of skin cancer after renal transplantation in the Netherlands. *Transplantation* 1990; 49(3): 506–9.
12. Moloney FJ, Comber H, O'Lorcain P, O'Kelly P, Conlon PJ, Murphy GM. A population-based study of skin cancer incidence and prevalence in renal transplant recipients. *Br J Dermatol* 2006; 154(3): 498–504.
13. Rashtak S, Dierkhising RA, Kremers WK, Peters SG, Cassivi SD, Otley CC. Incidence and risk factors for skin cancer following lung transplantation. *J Am Acad Dermatol* 2015; 72(1): 92–8.
14. Silverberg MJ, Leyden W, Warton EM, Quesenberry CP Jr, Engels EA, Asgari MM. HIV infection status, immunodeficiency, and the incidence of non-melanoma skin cancer. *J Natl Cancer Inst* 2013; 105(5): 350–60.
15. Muehleisen B, Jiang SB, Gladsjo JA, Gerber M, Hata T, Gallo RL. Distinct innate immune gene expression profiles in non-melanoma skin cancer of immunocompetent and immunosuppressed patients. *PLoS One* 2012; 7(7): e40754.
16. Wang J, Aldabagh B, Yu J, Arron ST. Role of human papillomavirus in cutaneous squamous cell carcinoma: a meta-analysis. *J Am Acad Dermatol* 2014; 70(4): 621–9.
17. Shamanin V, Hausen Hz, Lavergne D, Proby CM, Leigh IM, Neumann C, et al. Human papillomavirus infections in nonmelanoma skin cancers from renal transplant recipients and nonimmunosuppressed patients. *J Natl Cancer Inst* 1996; 88(12): 802–11.
18. Sugiyama H, Misumi M, Kishikawa M, Iseki M, Yonehara S, Hayashi T, et al. Skin cancer incidence among atomic bomb survivors from 1958 to 1996. *Radiat Res* 2014; 181(5): 531–9.
19. Perkins JL, Liu Y, Mitby PA, Neglia JP, Hammond S, Stovall M, et al. Nonmelanoma skin cancer in survivors of childhood and adolescent cancer: a report from the Childhood Cancer Survivor Study. *J Clin Oncol* 2005; 23(16): 3733–41.
20. Karimkhani C, Boyers LN, Dellavalle RP, Weinstock MA. It's time for "keratinocyte carcinoma" to replace the term "nonmelanoma skin cancer". *J Am Acad Dermatol* 2015; 72(1): 186–7.
21. Sexton M, Jones DB, Maloney ME. Histologic pattern analysis of basal cell carcinoma. Study of a series of 1039 consecutive neoplasms. *J Am Acad Dermatol* 1990; 23(6 Pt. 1): 1118–26.
22. National Comprehensive Cancer Network. 2014. Basal cell skin cancers. http://www.nccn.org/professionals/physician_gls/pdf/nmsc.pdf (assessed 20 December 2014).
23. Rinker MH, Fenske NA, Scalf LA, Glass LF. Histologic variants of squamous cell carcinoma of the skin. *Cancer Control* 2001; 8(4): 354–63.
24. Marks R, Rennie G, Selwood TS. Malignant transformation of solar keratoses to squamous cell carcinoma. *Lancet* 1988; 1(8589): 795–7.
25. Dodson JM, DeSpain J, Hewett JE, Clark DP. Malignant potential of actinic keratoses and the controversy over treatment. A patient-oriented perspective. *Arch Dermatol* 1991; 127(7): 1029–31.
26. Salasche SJ. Epidemiology of actinic keratoses and squamous cell carcinoma. *J Am Acad Dermatol* 2000; 42(1 Pt. 2): 4–7.

27. Moon TE, Levine N, Cartmel B, Bangert JL, Rodney S, Dong Q, et al. Effect of retinol in preventing squamous cell skin cancer in moderate-risk subjects: a randomized, double-blind, controlled trial. Southwest Skin Cancer Prevention Study Group. *Cancer Epidemiol Biomarkers Prev* 1997; 6(11): 949–56.

28. Guenthner ST, Hurwitz RM, Buckel LJ, Gray HR. Cutaneous squamous cell carcinomas consistently show histologic evidence of in situ changes: a clinicopathologic correlation. *J Am Acad Dermatol* 1999; 41(3): 443–8.

29. Sligh JE Jr. New therapeutic options for actinic keratosis and basal cell carcinoma. *Semin Cutan Med Surg* 2014; 33(4 Suppl.): S76–80.

30. National Comprehensive Cancer Network. 2014. Squamous cell skin cancers. http://www.nccn.org/professionals/physician_gls/pdf/squamous.pdf (assessed 20 December 2014).

31. Cox NH, Eedy DJ, Morton CA, on behalf of the British Association of Dermatologists Therapy Guidelines and Audit Subcommittee. Guidelines for management of Bowen's disease: 2006 update. *Br J Dermatol* 2007; 156(1): 11–21.

32. Cox NH, Eedy DJ, Morton CA. Guidelines for management of Bowen's disease. *Br J Dermatol* 1999; 141(4): 633–41.

33. International Union Against Cancer (UICC). Carcinoma of skin. In Sobin LH, Gospodarowicz MK, Wittekind C, eds., *TNM Classification of Malignant Tumours*, 7th ed. Oxford: Wiley-Blackwell, 2010, pp. 165–8.

34. Edge SB, Byrd DR, Carducci MA, Compton CC, Fritz AG, Greene FL, et al., eds. *Cancer Staging Manual*, 7th ed. New York: Springer, 2009.

35. Cranmer LD, Engelhardt C, Morgan SS. Treatment of unresectable and metastatic cutaneous squamous cell carcinoma. *Oncologist* 2010; 15(12): 1320–8.

36. Daskalopoulou D, Gourgiotou K, Thodou E, Vaida S, Markidou S. Rapid cytological diagnosis of primary skin tumours and tumour-like conditions. *Acta Derm Venereol* 1997; 77(4): 292–5.

37. Özden MG, Maier T, Bek Y, Ruzicka T, Berking C. Cytodiagnosis of erosive melanoma and basal cell carcinoma of the skin using cutaneous tissue smear. *Clin Exp Dermatol* 2013; 38(3): 251–61.

38. Krediet JT, Beyer M, Lenz K, Ulrich C, Lange-Asschenfeldt B, Stockfleth E, et al. Sentinel lymph node and risk factors for predicting metastasis in cutaneous squamous cell carcinoma. *Br J Dermatol* 2015; 172: 1029–36.

39. Martinez J, Otley CC, Stasko T. Defining the clinical course of metastatic skin cancer in organ transplant recipients: a multicenter collaborative study. *Arch Dermatol* 2003; 139(3): 301–6.

40. Brodland DG, Zitelli JA. Surgical margins for excision of primary cutaneous squamous cell carcinoma. *J Am Acad Dermatol* 1992; 27(2 Pt. 1): 241–8.

41. Mohan SV, Chang AL. Advanced basal cell carcinoma: epidemiology and therapeutic innovations. *Curr Dermatol Rep* 2014; 3(1): 40–5.

42. Moser S, Borm J, Mihic-Probst D, Jacobsen C, Kruse Gujer AL. Metastatic basal cell carcinoma: report of a case and review of the literature. *Oral Surg Oral Med Oral Pathol Oral Radiol* 2014; 117(2): e79–82.

43. Schmitt AR, Brewer JD, Bordeaux JS, Baum CL. Staging for cutaneous squamous cell carcinoma as a predictor of sentinel lymph node biopsy results: meta-analysis of American Joint Committee on Cancer criteria and a proposed alternative system. *JAMA Dermatol* 2014; 150(1): 19–24.

44. Palyca P, Koshenkov VP, Mehnert JM. Developments in the treatment of locally advanced and metastatic squamous cell carcinoma of the skin: a rising unmet need. *Am Soc Clin Oncol Educ Book* 2014; e397–404.

45. Cho M, Gordon L, Rembielak A, Woo TCS. Utility of radiotherapy for treatment of basal cell carcinoma: a review. *Br J Dermatol* 2014; 171(5): 968–73.

46. Peikert JM. Prospective trial of curettage and cryosurgery in the management of non-facial, superficial, and minimally invasive basal and squamous cell carcinoma. *Int J Dermatol* 2011; 50(9): 1135–8.

47. Campana LG, Mali B, Sersa G, Valpione S, Giorgi CA, Strojan P, et al. Electrochemotherapy in non-melanoma head and neck cancers: a retrospective analysis of the treated cases. *Br J Oral Maxillofac Surg* 2014; 52(10): 957–64.

48. Mali B, Jarm T, Snoj M, Sersa G, Miklavcic D. Antitumor effectiveness of electrochemotherapy: a systematic review and meta-analysis. *Eur J Surg Oncol* 2013; 39(1): 4–16.

49. Lacarrubba F, Potenza MC, Gurgone S, Micali G. Successful treatment and management of large superficial basal cell carcinomas with topical imiquimod 5% cream: a case series and review. *J Dermatolog Treat* 2011; 22(6): 353–8.

50. Firnhaber JM. Diagnosis and treatment of basal cell and squamous cell carcinoma. *Am Fam Physician* 2012; 86(2): 161–8.

51. Chitwood K, Etzkorn J, Cohen G. Topical and intralesional treatment of nonmelanoma skin cancer: efficacy and cost comparisons. *Dermatol Surg* 2013; 39(9).

52. Samarasinghe V, Madan V. Nonmelanoma skin cancer. *J Cutan Aesthet Surg* 2012; 5(1): 3–10.

53. Morton CA, McKenna KE, Rhodes LE, on behalf of the British Association of Dermatologists Therapy Guidelines and Audit Subcommittee and the British Photodermatology Group. Guidelines for topical photodynamic therapy: update. *Br J Dermatol* 2008; 159(6): 1245–66.

54. Maly TJ, Sligh JE. Defining locally advanced basal cell carcinoma. *J Drugs Dermatol* 2014; 13(5): 528–9.

55. Kwan W, Wilson D, Moravan V. Radiotherapy for locally advanced basal cell and squamous cell carcinomas of the skin. *Int J Radiat Oncol Biol Phys* 2004; 60(2): 406–11.

56. Cho M, Gordon L, Rembielak A, Woo TC. Utility of radiotherapy for treatment of basal cell carcinoma: a review. *Br J Dermatol* 2014; 171(5): 968–73.

57. Sandhiya S, Melvin G, Kumar SS, Dkhar SA. The dawn of hedgehog inhibitors: vismodegib. *J Pharmacol Pharmacother* 2013; 4(1): 4–7.

58. Behshad R, Garcia-Zuazaga J, Bordeaux JS. Systemic treatment of locally advanced nonmetastatic cutaneous squamous cell carcinoma: a review of the literature. *Br J Dermatol* 2011; 165(6): 1169–77.

59. Denic S. Preoperative treatment of advanced skin carcinoma with cisplatin and bleomycin. *Am J Clin Oncol* 1999; 22(1): 32–4.

60. Brewster AM, Lee JJ, Clayman GL, Clifford JL, Reyes MJ, Zhou X, et al. Randomized trial of adjuvant 13-cis-retinoic acid and interferon alfa for patients with aggressive skin squamous cell carcinoma. *J Clin Oncol* 2007; 25(15): 1974–8.

61. Mendenhall WM, Amdur RJ, Hinerman RW, Cognetta AB, Mendenhall NP. Radiotherapy for cutaneous squamous and basal cell carcinomas of the head and neck. *Laryngoscope* 2009; 119(10): 1994–9.

62. Leibovitch I, Huilgol SC, Selva D, Richards S, Paver R. Basal cell carcinoma treated with Mohs surgery in Australia III. Perineural invasion. *J Am Acad Dermatol* 2005;53(3): 458–63.

63. Clayman GL, Lee JJ, Holsinger FC, Zhou X, Duvic M, El-Naggar AK, et al. Mortality risk from squamous cell skin cancer. *J Clin Oncol* 2005; 23(4): 759–65.

64. Rowe DE, Carroll RJ, Day CL Jr. Prognostic factors for local recurrence, metastasis, and survival rates in squamous cell carcinoma of the skin, ear, and lip. Implications for treatment modality selection. *J Am Acad Dermatol* 1992; 26(6): 976–90.

41

Skin: Melanoma

KONSTANTINOS LASITHIOTAKIS, ODYSSEAS ZORAS AND CHARLES BALCH

INCIDENCE AND MORTALITY

Globally, melanoma is a rare tumour that accounts for less than 2% of incident cancer cases in males and females. However, the incidence of melanoma varies considerably throughout the world and in fair-skinned populations of Australia, Northern America and Europe it may reach 30–40 per 100,000 persons-years. In the European Union, melanoma is the seventh most common cancer with 83,000 new cases diagnosed a year and 15,000 deaths [1]. Melanoma incidence rates have increased significantly for the last five decades and they keep increasing in several medium- to high-incidence regions causing doubling of the rates every 10–20 years. Increasing melanoma rates have been attributed to a progressive change from occupational to predominantly recreational sun exposure patterns mainly in populations of European origin along with a change of dressing habits. Notably, the highest increases of melanoma incidence in women after the 1950s occurred for melanomas of the leg when the length of skirts was decreasing. In men, the highest increases in melanoma rates were reported for the trunk. At the same time, skin cancer awareness was increasing due to improvement in living standard and several educational campaigns in industrialized countries [2].

Most melanomas accounting for the increased incidence are thin tumours (<1 mm) which are generally curable with adequate surgery. Consequently, mortality from melanoma has increased at a considerably slower pace than incidence. Contemporary data show that death rates continue to climb particularly among elderly patients, particularly males.

This is an important high-risk group among melanoma patients. It is associated with dismal prognostic factors, such as tumour thickness, histological ulceration and nodular type. Older patients have lower skin cancer awareness and lower rates of self-examination and participation in screening programs [3]. Deteriorating vision, loss of a partner as well as poor access to health care contribute to late diagnosis and the dismal outcome of melanomas in the elderly. Therefore, targeting this group by preventative campaigns could be beneficial.

RISK FACTORS AND GENETIC PREDISPOSITION

Most melanomas develop in individuals with fair skin pigmentation. Therefore, traits such as red hair, blue eyes, white skin prone to sunburn and unable to tan and freckles are associated with an increased risk of melanoma. It is rare in non-white populations where it occurs mainly on sun-protected sites such as the palms, soles and mucosal surfaces. The most consistent risk factor for melanoma is the presence of a high number of benign moles (common melanocytic nevi) and the presence of atypical nevi. The latter are benign moles exhibiting some of the 'ABCD' characteristics of early melanoma. Patients with atypical mole syndrome (>100 common nevi >2 mm and two or more atypical nevi) are at a particularly high risk of developing cutaneous melanoma. Indices of solar damage of the skin such as solar elastosis, solar lentigines and solar keratoses are linked to melanoma risk. Solar keratoses and non-melanoma skin cancer are risk factors in older patients who may develop melanoma in chronically sun exposed sites (i.e. face, ears and lentigo maligna) [4]. A history of previous melanoma increases the risk approximately 10-fold for developing a second primary most commonly within 2 years after the diagnosis of the first primary lesion. A family history of melanoma is also a significant risk factor [5].

Ultraviolet radiation exposure is the predominant environmental risk factor. Case-control studies have repeatedly identified recreational intermittent sun exposure, such as on sunny holidays, as well as a history of sunburn as the key behavioural factors for melanoma [6]. Ultraviolet (UV) irradiation is the human carcinogen present in sunlight. It is subcategorized as UVA (l = 320–400 nm), UVB (l = 280–320 nm) and UVC (l = 200–280 nm). UVC is biologically irrelevant since it is absorbed by oxygen and ozone and does not reach the surface of the earth. UVA and UVB radiations both exert a carcinogenic effect on the skin. UVA constitutes 98.7% of UV radiation that reaches the earth's surface and can indirectly cause DNA damage through the formation of reactive oxygen radicals. This accounts for approximately 90% of skin melanomas. UVB causes direct DNA damage and sunburn through the formation of pyrimidine dimers [7]. Sunbeds and sunlamps used for artificial tanning emit in the range of UVA and increase the risk of melanoma particularly when used at a young age. Psoralen UVA radiation therapy (PUVA) is a common and effective treatment of psoriasis and other dermatological conditions which increases significantly the risk for skin melanoma several years after exposure. Individualized melanoma risk assessment tools based on data from large case-control studies are available* [8,9].

Approximately 5–10% of melanoma is hereditary and 40% of that is caused by mutations in the cyclin-dependent kinase inhibitor 2A gene (CDKN2A p16) which is a tumour suppressor gene. The familial atypical multiple mole and melanoma (FAMMM) syndrome characterizes melanoma in the setting of a positive family history, a high number of melanocytic nevi and the presence of atypical nevi. In these families the CDKN2A mutation is associated with melanoma occurrence in up to 90% of patients as well as with pancreatic cancer [10]. A much rarer syndrome due to mutation in the cyclin-dependent kinase 4 (CDK4) gene has also been described in melanoma families that render it insensitive to p16 inhibition, thereby promoting oncogenesis. Xeroderma pigmentosum (XP) is a rare autosomal recessive disorder of XP genes that repair DNA damage caused by UV radiation. It is characterized by extreme sun sensitivity and development of BCC, SCC and melanomas early in childhood. Loss of function polymorphisms in the melanocortin-1 receptor (MC1R) have been associated with red–blonde hair, photosensitive skin and high risk for melanoma [11].

* The NCI risk tool is available at http://www.cancer.gov/melanomarisktool/ and the Victorian Melanoma Service risk calculator available at http://www.victorianmelanomaservice.org/calculator/

PREVENTION AND SCREENING

Primary prevention of melanoma should aim to reduce strong sun exposure. Complete sun avoidance is impossible; thus a reasonable message to the patients should be 'don't burn, don't tan'. Practical messages of sun protection have been included in several campaigns such as the 'Slip, Slop, Slap, Seek, Slide' (slip on sun-protective clothing, slop on sunscreen, slap on a broad-brimmed hat, seek shade, slide on sunglasses). Sunscreens should protect against UVA and UVB with an SPF of ≥30. They should be applied 20 minutes before exposure and re-applied after water exposure or after 2 h. Sun-protective clothing, broad-brimmed hats and UV-protective sunglasses are also very effective against UV exposure. The use of sunbeds and sunlamps should be strongly discouraged. With regard to secondary prevention, there is recent evidence showing improved outcomes associated with both clinician and patient screening. Population-based and work-based screening in Australia and the United States has been associated with a decrease in the incidence of thick melanomas and overall melanoma mortality [12–14]. SCREEN, a 1-year-long statewide screening program in Germany, has resulted in 50% reduction in melanoma mortality 5 years after the end of the screening program [8,9]. These promising findings led to a nationwide expansion of the program since 2008 aiming at individuals older than 35 years. However, due to the lack of evidence from randomized studies and the high associated costs, current guidelines do not suggest physician screening for melanoma. Periodic skin self-examination is encouraged by national and international organizations and it should be coupled with public awareness campaigns as well as with educational activities of involved professions such as primary care physicians, medical students, nursing staff and non-clinicians such as hair-professionals, physiotherapists and chiropractors. Finally, it may be more meaningful to target screening patients at high risk for melanoma (i.e. older age and high numbers of moles) [3,8,9].

PATHOLOGY AND STAGING

Most melanomas develop initially confined to the epidermis for several years, during a horizontal or 'radial' growth phase during which they are curable with adequate surgery. Later, with the accumulation of genetic abnormalities they expand beyond the basal membrane to the dermis, in a 'vertical' growth phase, where they acquire metastatic potential. Melanoma in situ is a form of radial growth phase melanoma. Superficial spreading melanoma is the most common subtype accounting for three-quarters of the total number of melanomas, and it can arise *de novo* (in previously healthy skin) or in association with pre-existent nevus in up to one-third of cases (Figure 41.1a). Nodular melanomas lack a radial growth phase, develop rapidly and are associated with a worse prognosis (Figure 41.1b). Lentigo maligna melanoma

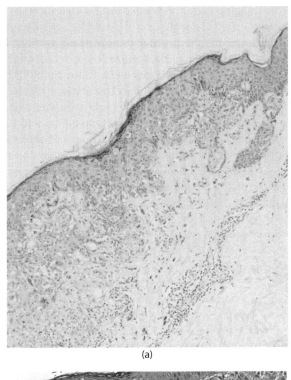

(a)

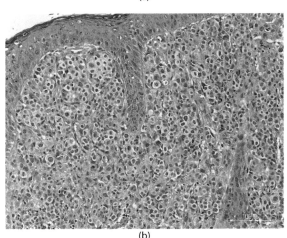

(b)

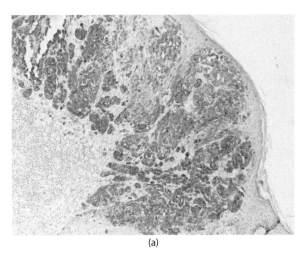

(a)

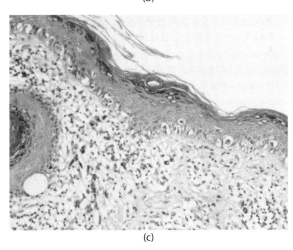

(c)

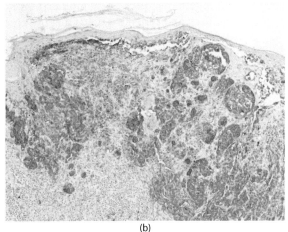

(b)

is characterized by melanocytic proliferation along the dermo-epidermal junction in the radial phase and signs of heavy sun damage such as epidermal atrophy and solar elastosis (Figure 41.1c). Acral lentiginous melanoma (ALM) is the least common histological subtype but it is the most common type of melanoma among Asian and dark-skinned individuals. Immunohistochemistry can be helpful in ambiguous cases or in lesions lacking pigment (amelanotic). Commonly used markers are S-100, melanoma antigen recognized by T-cells/melanocyte antigen (MART-1/Melan-A), human melanoma black-45 (HMB-45), micropthalmia-associated transcription factor (MITF), MIB-1 (Ki-67 or mindbomb E3 ubiquitin protein ligase 1 protein) and tyrosinase (Figure 41.2). Histologically uncertain cases should be reviewed by experienced skin pathologists. In such cases, comparative genomic hybridization (CGH) or fluorescence *in situ* hybridization (FISH) to detect chromosomal aberrations can be helpful [15].

Essential elements of the histology report and significant prognostic factors for primary melanoma with implications

Figure 41.1 (a) Superficially spreading melanoma. (b) Nodular melanoma. (c) Lentigo maligna melanoma. (Courtesy of Maria Tzardi, Professor of Pathology, University of Crete, Medical School.)

Figure 41.2 Immunohistochemistry for melanoma. (a) Melanoma antigen recognized by T-cells/melanocyte antigen (MART-1/Melan-A). (b) Human melanoma black-45 (HMB-45). *(Continued)*

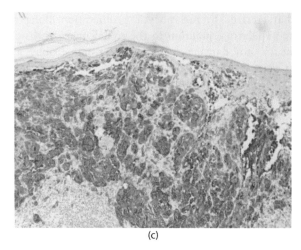

(c)

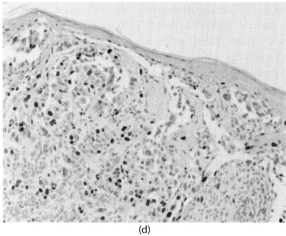

(d)

Figure 41.2 (Continued) Immunohistochemistry for melanoma. (c) Protein S-100. (d) Ki-67 (or MIB-1, mind-bomb E3 ubiquitin protein ligase 1 protein). (Courtesy of Maria Tzardi, Professor of Pathology, University of Crete, Medical School.)

for the management of the patient are Breslow tumour thickness, ulceration, mitotic rate per square millimetre, Clark level of invasion, deep and peripheral status margins (positive or negative) and microscopic satellitosis. Additional factors include location, regression and the presence of tumour-infiltrating lymphocytes, growth phase, angiolymphatic invasion, neurotropism, desmoplacia and histological subtype [16]. TNM staging of melanoma incorporates pathological information from primary tumour and regional lymph nodes and is presented in Table 41.1. An online melanoma prediction tool based on the AJCC melanoma database predicts the clinical outcome for an individual patient with localized or regional melanoma.*

The initial work-up for patients with melanoma is controversial due to a lack of evidence. Its most important elements are a careful history, review of systems and physical examination. Most guidelines agree that for asymptomatic patients with stage I or II melanoma,

* Available at http://www.melanomaprognosis.org/

routine imaging is not warranted as the identification of metastatic disease is negligible, at around 1%, with a relatively high rate of false positive examinations. In stage III patients, the use of imaging upstages the disease in up to 30% and changes their management. Thus, body CT or PET/CT studies are worthwhile in this setting [17]. Stage IV patients require comprehensive evaluation with MR or CT of the brain, and CT of the chest, abdomen and pelvis, or PET/CT scan, because the likelihood of detecting additional lesions is higher. This is particularly important when curative surgery for distant metastasis is contemplated. Serum LDH should be measured in all stage IV patients as it has prognostic significance. Finally, symptomatic patients of any stage should be assessed with appropriate investigations [16].

DIAGNOSIS

A full medical history should systematically assess risk factors and symptoms of metastatic disease. The physical examination of the skin should be systematic including all skin surfaces, intertriginous areas, web spaces, palms, soles, unpolished nails and scalp. Genital, ocular and mucosal surfaces should be examined or preferentially recommended as part of routine gynaecological, ophthalmological and dental examinations. Most melanomas arise as pigmented skin lesions that change visibly over a period of months to years. Changes in pigmented lesions over the course of days are most likely benign resulting from trauma or inflammation [18]. The ABCDE rule has been developed to identify lesions that are suspicious for melanoma (Figure 41.3 and Table 41.2). No clear guidelines on how to use these criteria in the clinical setting exist. However, it is safe to refer patients who report at least one of the ABCDE features to specialist doctors. This is associated with 97% sensitivity and 37% specificity in identifying a new lesion as melanoma [19]. Itching, tenderness, ulceration and bleeding are also associated with melanoma, the latter two in advanced tumours. Superficially spreading melanoma is the most common melanoma type and it commonly has the typical ABCDE characteristics (Figure 41.4). The 'ugly duckling sign' is used to indicate a lesion that is distinctly different from surrounding skin lesions of the patient. The nodular type of melanoma lacks typical characteristics and presents as a small shiny lesion with striking colour (Figure 41.5). Lentigo maligna melanoma (LMM) arises as a pigmented macule on chronically sun-exposed skin and can be difficult to distinguish from benign solar lentigo (Figure 41.6). Acral lentiginous melanoma (ALM) is more common among dark-skinned individuals in palmo-plantar sites and nail beds (Figure 41.7). They develop as macular lesions masked by a thickened stratum corneum and are frequently confused with benign lesions such as common warts, callus, fungal infections, subungual haematomas, and ingrowing or infected toenails. 'Hutchinson's sign' is specific for subungual melanoma and it designates

Table 41.1 Seventh AJCC TNM staging of melanoma

Stage	Primary tumour variables		Regional lymph node variables		Ma	5-year survival %
0	Tis	*In situ*	N0		M0	
IA	T1a	<1.0 mm, U(–) or M(+)	N0		M0	97
IB	T1b	<1.0 mm, U(+) or (M+)	N0		M0	92
	T2a	1.01–2.0 mm, U(–)	N0		M0	
IIA	T2b	1.01–2.0 mm, U(+)	N0		M0	80
	T3a	2.01–4.0 mm, U(–)	N0		M0	
IIB	T3b	2.01–4.0 mm, U(+)	N0		M0	70
	T4a	>4.0 mm, U(–)	N0		M0	
IIC	T4b	>4.0 mm, U(+)	N0		M0	53
IIIA	T1–4a	Any thickness, U(–)	N1a	1 LN, micro	M0	78
	T1–4a	Any thickness, U(–)	N2a	2–3 LNs, micro	M0	
IIIB	T1–4b	Any thickness, U(+)	N1a	1 LN, micro	M0	59
	T1–4b	Any thickness, U(+)	N2a	2–3 LNs, micro	M0	
	T1–4a	Any thickness, U(–)	N1b	1 LN, macro	M0	
	T1–4a	Any thickness, U(–)	N2b	2–3 LNs, macro	M0	
	T1–4a	Any thickness, U(–)	N2c	In transit/satellite	M0	
IIIC	T1–4b	Any thickness, U(+)	N1b	1 LN, macro	M0	40
	T1–4b	Any thickness, U(+)	N2b	2–3 LNs, macro	M0	
	T1–4b	Any thickness, U(+)	N2c	In transit/satellite	M0	
	Any T	Any thickness	N3	>3 LNs or matted LNs, or in transit/satellite plus LNs	M0	
IV	Any T	Any thickness	Any N	Skin, subcutaneous, distant LNs, n.l. LDH	M1a	62[b]
				Lung, n.l. LDH	M1b	53[b]
				Other visceral or high LDH	M1c	33[b]

Source: Balch C, et al., *Melanoma Staging and Clinical Classification*, edited by C Balch, et al. 5th ed. St Louis, MO: Quality Medical Publishing, 2009.

Note: U(+)/U(–), with/without histological ulceration; M(+)/M(–), with/without mitoses >1 mm²; LNs, regional lymph nodes; n.l., within normal range; LDH, lactate dehydrogenase.

[a] Refers to distant metastasis (M stage).
[b] One-year overall survival.

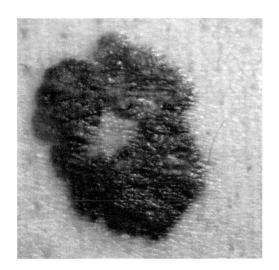

Figure 41.3 ABCD rule for the early detection of melanoma. For definitions of the letters refer to Table 41.1. (From Department of Surgical Oncology, University of Crete.)

Table 41.2 ABCDE characteristics of early melanoma

Asymmetry: If a lesion is bisected, one-half is not identical to the other half

Border irregularities: Uneven, scalloped or notched edges

Colour variegation

Diameter ≥6 mm

Evolving: A lesion that is changing in size, shape or colour, or a new lesion

extension of black pigmentation to the nail fold or hyponychium (Figure 41.8). Melanomas of any type can be amelanotic, lacking any apparent pigmentation, and thus can be confused with benign tumours [15].

Photography can be used to ensure accurate identification of the lesions referred for excision by the surgeon, to facilitate diagnosis of early melanoma in patients

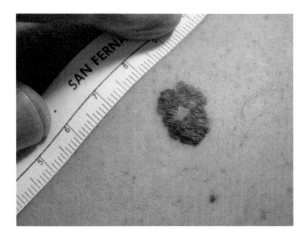

Figure 41.4 Superficially spreading melanoma (SSM). (From Department of Surgical Oncology, University of Crete.)

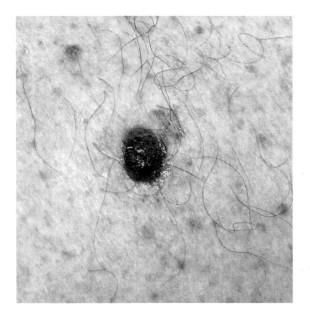

Figure 41.5 Nodular melanoma. (Courtesy of Dr George Evangelou, Consultant Dermatologist, University Hospital of Heraklion.)

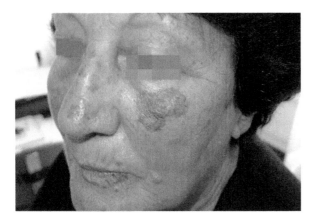

Figure 41.6 Lentigo maligna melanoma. (Courtesy of Dr George Evangelou, Consultant Dermatologist, University Hospital of Heraklion.)

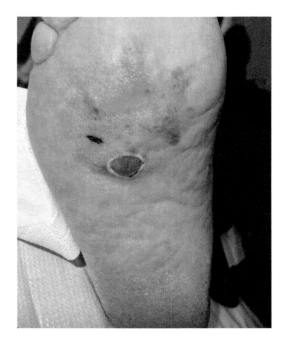

Figure 41.7 Acral lentiginous melanoma. (Courtesy of Dr George Evangelou, Consultant Dermatologist, University Hospital of Heraklion.)

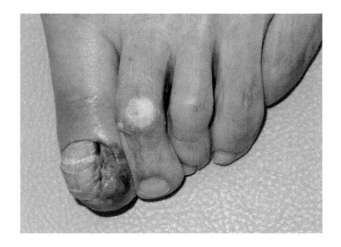

Figure 41.8 Subungual melanoma. (Courtesy of Dr George Evangelou, Consultant Dermatologist, University Hospital of Heraklion.)

with several atypical nevi (total body photography) and to monitor individual lesions for change (close-up photography). Dermatoscopy increases diagnostic sensitivity by up to 20% in the hands of experienced examiners [8,9] (Figure 41.9). All skin lesions that are suspicious for melanoma should be biopsied. An excisional biopsy of the entire lesion with a margin of 1–2 mm of normal skin and part of the subcutaneous fat is the technique of choice. Wider margins are not necessary and may compromise subsequent wide excision and sentinel node biopsy. Incisional biopsies should be avoided because of the risk of sampling error, but they may be occasionally acceptable

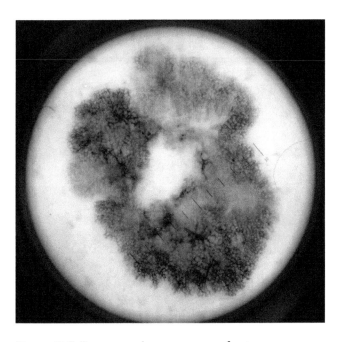

Figure 41.9 Dermoscopic appearance of cutaneous melanoma (macroscopically shown in Figure 41.3a). (From Department of Surgical Oncology, University of Crete.)

Table 41.3 Resection margins for primary cutaneous melanoma

Tumour thickness	Recommended margins[a] (cm)
In situ	0.5–1
≤1 mm	1
1.01–2.00 mm	1–2
>2.00 mm	2

[a] Taken at the time of surgery, *not* as taken by the pathologist.

Lymphatic mapping and sentinel node biopsy

Lymphatic mapping and sentinel node biopsy (SNB) are standard of care for patients with non-palpable regional lymph nodes who are at substantial risk of regional lymph node metastasis. These include the majority of patients with tumours ≥1.00 mm (T2, T3 and T4) and those less than 1.00 mm with secondary adverse features (ulceration, mitotic rate of ≥1/mm^2, level IV depth, lymphovascular invasion) and a tumour thickness of >0.7 mm [16,26]. Lymphatic mapping (lymphoscintigraphy) increases the accuracy of SNB by identifying the site but also the number of sentinel nodes at each location. It is particularly helpful in revealing nodal basins draining from primary sites located in areas of ambiguous or dual lymphatic drainage, unexpected lymphatic drainage pathways and nodes that lie between the tumour site and a recognized lymph node group (interval nodes) [27]. SNB is a valuable prognostic tool. It identifies patients who may benefit from adjuvant treatment and stratifies appropriately candidates for clinical trials. It offers more detailed staging information than an elective lymph node dissection because it allows more extensive histological and immunohistological examination of a limited number of nodes. It is a minimally invasive test with a low morbidity which reduces up to 80% the number of negative elective lymphadenectomies and their complications. When performed in experienced hands the false negative rate of SNB is well below 5%. SNB followed by completion lymphadenectomy if it is positive reduces significantly the rates of regional recurrences compared with observation alone. It also reduces the rates of deep groin resections which are associated with higher morbidity. Multicenter Selective Lymphadenectomy Trial-I (MSLT-I) showed that SNB-based management of the regional lymph nodes increases the recurrence-free and disease-specific survival of patients with intermediate thickness melanomas (1.2 to 3.5 mm) and has both staging and prognostic value for tumours thicker than 3.5 mm [28] (Figure 41.12).

Lymph node dissection

Completion lymphadenectomy is offered to patients with a positive SNB as well as in patients with palpable lymph nodes after pathological confirmation of the presence of melanoma metastases (Figure 41.10). Baseline imaging to

for very large lesions or for certain sites, including the face, palm or sole, ear, distal digit, or subungual lesions. Shave biopsies are not acceptable because only the superficial portion of the tumour is removed resulting in underestimation of tumour thickness, and even subsequent surgical excision is hampered by fibrosis and scarring at the base of the biopsy that make it impossible to assess its thickness accurately [16].

SURGICAL TREATMENT

Primary tumour

Wide local excision is the definitive treatment of primary cutaneous melanoma. It includes surgical resection of the biopsy site en bloc with the surrounding normal skin and the subcutaneous tissue down to the muscular fascia. The rationale for WLE is to remove all remaining microscopic satellite lesions and malignant cells in order to achieve durable local control of the disease and cure patients without metastasis. Margin width in melanoma is based on several prospective randomized trials [20–25]. For melanoma in situ margins of 0.5–1 cm are recommended. Tumours with thickness ≥1 mm are adequately resected with 1 cm margin and tumours with thickness 1.01–2.00 mm should be resected with 1–2 cm margins to accommodate individual anatomic and functional considerations. Tumours >2.00 mm are resected with 2 cm margins (Table 41.3). Mohs micrographic surgery and staged excision methods may be used in melanomas near sensitive anatomic structures in order to minimize resection margins without compromising local control.

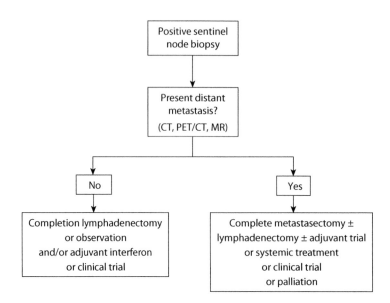

Figure 41.10 Treatment algorithm for patients with metastasis in the sentinel node.

rule out distant metastasis and pathological examination of the nodes with fine-needle aspiration (FNA) or core needle lymph node biopsy should be done prior to lymph node dissection (LND). LND offers long-term regional control of the disease in a subset of patients and prevents devastating bulky regional recurrence even in those who will develop and die of distant metastasis. Complete removal of all nodal tissue is recommended. Sampling or partial lymphadenectomy has no place in melanoma management. The level of dissection is controversial. Many surgeons advocate deep dissections in all cases which, however, is associated with higher morbidity. A less aggressive and still reasonable approach is to reserve ilio-obturator dissections for patients with multiple macroscopic positive femoral nodes or positive Cloquet's node and in patients with imaging evidence of ilio-obturator involvement [16,29]. Patients with clinically apparent iliac nodes are potentially curable and resectable. A proportion of these patients, reaching 40%, can still be cured [30]. Axillary dissection for melanoma should include levels I, II and III. Involvement of the axillary vein is not a contraindication for resection even when reconstruction of the vein is not to be performed. Complete removal of all macroscopic disease is necessary since postoperative radiation and systemic chemotherapy are rarely effective if macroscopic melanoma is left behind. Complications in the short term include infection, haemorrhage, skin edge necrosis, wound dehiscence and lymphocele. Long-term morbidity comprises paraesthesia and lymphoedema. The complication may occur in up to 50% of patients and is higher in the groin than in the axillary LNDs and in deep versus superficial dissections [31]. Melanomas of the head and neck with a positive SNB are treated with selective neck dissection (i.e. dissection of the draining basins) and superficial parotidectomy according to the anatomical site [32]. Selective neck dissection should be modified to include more basins on the basis of the lymphatic mapping [33]. Patients with palpable lymph nodes are at higher risk for recurrence and metastasis may be present in any level of the neck. Thus they require modified radical neck dissection of all five levels, with preservation of the sternocleidomastoid muscle, the spinal accessory nerve and the internal jugular vein unless directly involved with tumour. Additionally superficial parotidectomy should be performed [34].

ADJUVANT TREATMENT

Evidence from meta-analysis of randomized controlled trials supports the therapeutic efficacy of interferon-alpha-2b (IFN-α2b) in patients with high-risk melanoma in terms of disease-free survival and, to a lesser extent, overall survival [35] (Figures 41.11 and 41.12). These are patients with melanoma stages IIB and III. The optimal treatment schedule is controversial. Best available evidence suggests that options should include high-dose IFN-α2b with a planned duration of 1 year or pegylated interferon with a planned duration of up to 5 years [16,36]. Pegylated IFN-α2b is a long-acting analogue that can be administered weekly and for longer durations, allowing for adjustments of dosage in order to reduce discontinuation of treatment due to toxicity [37]. However, many experts do not advocate its extended use in high-risk patients because the evidence is not as solid as for IFN-α2b [38]. High-dose IFN-α is associated with serious adverse effects. Granulocytopenia and fatigue which can often be debilitating are reported by the majority of patients. Liver toxicity, thyroid dysfunction and depression are common. These adverse effects may require dose modification or cessation of treatment in a significant proportion of patients. Aggressive biochemotherapy may increase relapse-free survival compared with high-dose interferon, but at the cost of significantly higher toxicity [39]. Enrolment in clinical

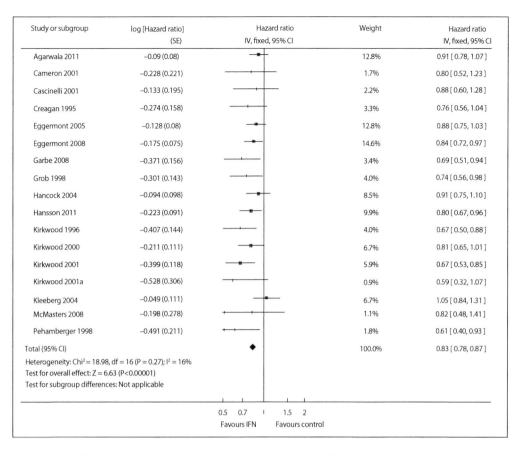

Figure 41.11 Meta-analysis of randomization of studies on the adjuvant use of interferon in high-risk melanoma patients. Effects on relapse-free survival. (Reproduced with permission from Mocellin S, et al., *Cochrane Database Syst Rev* 6:CD008955.)

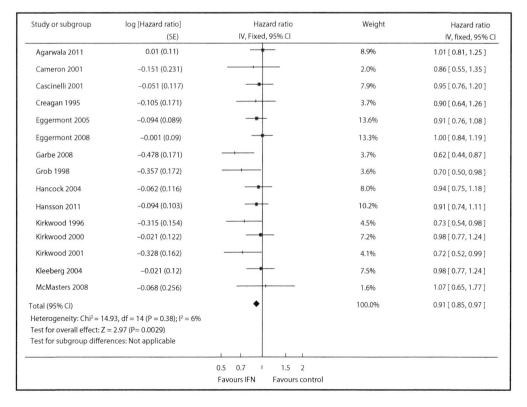

Figure 41.12 Effects on overall survival. (Reproduced with permission from Mocellin S, et al., *Cochrane Database Syst Rev* 6:CD008955.)

trials is strongly encouraged and several agents are under evaluation in the adjuvant setting. These include ipilimumab (anti-CTLA-4 [cytotoxic T-lymphocyte-associated protein 4]), anti-PD1 (programmed cell death protein 1), bevacizumab (anti-VEGF [vascular endothelial growth factor]), BRAF (b-rapidly accelerated fibrosarcoma) inhibitors, MEK (mitogen extracellular signal-regulated kinase) inhibitors, GM-CSF (granulocyte-macrophage colony-stimulating factor) and tumour vaccines.

TREATMENT OF LOCAL, SATELLITE AND IN-TRANSIT METASTASIS

Local metastasis is defined as recurrence of tumour within 2 cm from previous scar of definite resection of the primary tumour. Satellite and in-transit metastases represent disease within the regional and subdermal lymphatics located within 2 cm of the primary tumour and between 2 cm and the regional lymph nodes, respectively (Figures 41.13 and 41.14). These arbitrary definitions are included in the AJCC system for the purposes of clinical trials. In practice it is often impossible to differentiate local from in-transit metastasis and the classification

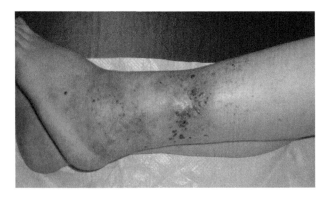

Figure 41.13 Unresectable local satellite metastasis from melanoma. (From Department of Surgical Oncology, University of Crete.)

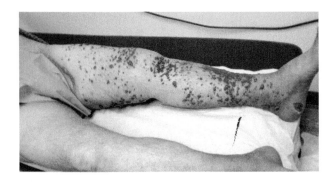

Figure 41.14 Bulky in-transit melanoma metastasis. Primary tumour excision scar is obvious on the heel. (From Department of Surgical Oncology, University of Crete.)

does not change the management of the patient [16]. Among patients with clinical stage I and II melanoma in-transit metastasis will appear in around 5% and it reaches 30% in stage III disease [40]. SNB and lymph node dissection does not increase the risk of local or in-transit recurrence, as previously thought [28]. Patients with local or in-transit recurrence should be carefully investigated with history, physical examination and imaging to rule out distant disease. Lymphatic mapping and SNB, even in cases who have undergone previous SNB and lymph node dissection, may still offer significant prognostic information, but its role remains to be defined [41].

Complete surgical resection of local or in-transit metastases with negative margins is the treatment of choice. Wide margins are not indicated. In the case of histologically positive margins the decision regarding re-resection should be balanced against expected morbidity. Resection of local or in-transit metastases should also be considered even in patients with distant disease to improve the quality of life by reducing associated bleeding or pain. For unresectable in-transit melanoma of the limbs, isolated limb perfusion (ILP) or infusion is the most effective treatment offering palliation and preservation of the limb to the majority of patients. ILP is a surgical procedure for delivering high doses of anticancer agents into the tumour-bearing limb avoiding systemic effects. Vascular isolation of the limb is performed at the level of the iliac or femoral vessels depending on the extent of disease in the limb (Figure 41.15). For the upper limb the level of axillary or subclavian vessels is chosen. Perfusion catheters are inserted via venotomy or arteriotomy and limb isolation is achieved by a tourniquet in the root of the limb. Consequently the limb is connected to an extracorporeal oxygenation circuit (Figure 41.16). Usually the procedure is done under mild

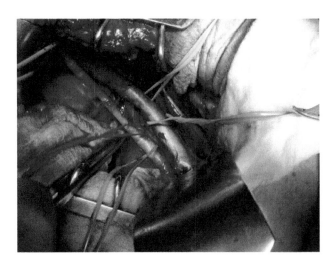

Figure 41.15 Dissected external iliac artery and vein during ilioinguinal lymphadenectomy and hyperthermic isolated limb perfusion (HILP) for melanoma in transit. (From Department of Surgical Oncology, University of Crete.)

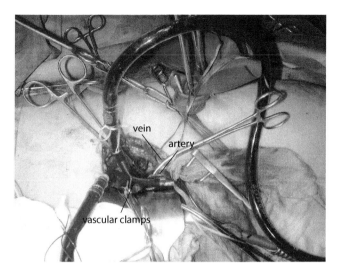

Figure 41.16 Hyperthermic isolated limb perfusion (HILP) for melanoma in transit. Extracorporeal circulation catheters in the external iliac artery and vein, vascular clamps placed proximally to both vessels and Esmarch's tourniquet in the root of the limb (#). (From Department of Surgical Oncology, University of Crete.)

hyperthermia (38.5–40°C) of the limb which improves tumour response. In this case air blankets are used to heat the limb and its temperature is monitored throughout the procedure with subcutaneous and muscle thermometers. The most common cytotoxic agent used is melfalan. The addition of tumour necrosis factor–alpha (TNF-α) may increase tumour response rates. However, because of the high toxicity of TNF-α continuous monitoring of leakage to the systemic circulation is mandatory. This is usually achieved with the use of radioisotopes. Leakage exceeding 10% is usually an indication for cessation of the procedure if it cannot be corrected with appropriate adjustments of the catheters and the circuit. At the end of the procedure the limb is flushed out with crystalloid solution, catheters are removed and vessels are repaired [42,43].

Contraindications for ILP are patients unfit to undergo a major surgical procedure and severe peripheral vascular disease. Local toxicity occurs in virtually all the patients and it is mainly mild erythema or oedema (Wieberdink II grade) which is considerable in around 15% (grade III). Serious toxicity involving extensive epidermolysis or evident damage to the deep tissues causing definite functional disturbances, threatening or manifesting compartment syndrome (grade IV) and a reaction that may mandate amputation (grade V) is described in less than 2% and 1%, respectively of patients undergoing ILP. Deep venous thrombosis may occur as well as persistent lymphoedema. Serious systemic toxicity (grades III and IV) in the form of myelosuppression and cardiovascular and gastrointestinal problems occurs in less than 10% of patients. Complete response rates of up to 70% with the use of TNF-α can be expected with overall response rates and limb salvage rates exceeding 90% [42].

Isolated limb infusion (ILI) is a less invasive form of regional chemotherapy which is performed with percutaneous catheterization of the vessels. It does not require a membrane oxygenator, it has a shorter duration and it is associated with lower systemic morbidity, making it very appealing for patients unfit to undergo ILP. Response rates are comparable to those of ILP [44]. Other treatment options for in-transit melanoma include LASER ablation, intralesional interleukin-2 injection, interferon or Bacille Calmette–Guérin, electrochemotherapy, radiotherapy and systemic therapy [45].

In the era of SNB, regional lymph node recurrence is expected in around 5% of patients undergoing prior lymph node dissection and is more common in patients with a high number of involved lymph nodes and extranodal involvement [28]. Redissection of the surgical node basin with curative intent after thorough work-up to rule out disseminated disease is the treatment of choice. Excision of the lesion with a clear margin is a less satisfactory alternative. For unresectable recurrence usually due to neurovascular involvement, radiotherapy or systemic therapy or inclusion in clinical trial should be considered [16].

TREATMENT OF DISTANT METASTASIS

The aims of medical treatment for stage IV melanoma are prolongation of overall survival and progression-free survival and improvement of quality of life. Currently there are three main categories of medical treatment for stage IV melanoma: immunotherapy, targeted therapies and chemotherapy.

Immunotherapy stimulates or reinforces the immune system against melanoma. High-dose interleukin-2 (IL-2) can increase overall survival and cure a small proportion of patients. Its use is hampered by severe cardiorespiratory and infectious toxicity and should be restricted to fit patients and in centres with experience in managing adverse effects [16]. Cytotoxic T-lymphocyte antigen 4 (CTLA-4) is a T-cell receptor which acts as an inhibitor of T-cell activation. Targeting this receptor with ipilimumab, a monoclonal antibody against CTLA-4, stimulates an immune response against the tumour. Phase III trials showed that ipilimumab alone or combined with DTIC increased overall survival in patients with stage IV melanoma. Hepatic and immune system–related toxicity (colitis, rash and hypophysitis) are the most common side effects. Programmed cell death-1 (anti PD1) is another key immune checkpoint receptor expressed by activated T-cells. Monoclonal antibodies against PD1 have produced significant prolongation of overall survival in metastatic melanoma and are under extensive evaluation in combination with chemotherapy and other agents [46]. Response patterns in patients on immunotherapy with the aforementioned agents differ considerably from those of conventional chemotherapy. First, patients may experience early worsening of the disease, responses take longer to become clinically apparent and patients without objective responses may experience long periods of stable disease. Thus, immune response criteria should be applied rather than Response Evaluation Criteria in Solid Tumors (RECIST) criteria to avoid early discontinuation of treatment in patients who may eventually benefit from these treatments [47].

Patients with metastatic melanoma should have their tumour tested for the BRAF V600 mutation which predicts response to targeted treatment with BRAF or a MEK inhibitor. This is present in more than half of patients with metastatic melanomas. Objective responses in more than 50% of patients can be expected with prolongation of overall survival; however, most patients will progress while on treatment. Serious toxicity includes the development of squamous cell carcinoma and keratoacanthomas of the skin in up to one-fourth of the patients that develop within weeks from the initiation of the treatment. These can be treated surgically and no discontinuation of treatment is necessary [48]. Tumours that do not harbour the BRAF V600 mutation should be tested for activating mutation of the c-kit gene. These mutations are more common in acrolentiginous and mucosal melanomas and predict response to imatinib, a tyrosine kinase inhibitor [49].

Cytotoxic chemotherapy has a limited role in the initial treatment of stage IV melanoma. It is used as second- or third-line treatment in patients not responding to immunotherapy or targeted treatments. Dacarbazine is the most active single agent with response rates up to 20% but does not have a proven survival benefit [50]. Temozolomide has comparable activity with its analogue dacarbazine, with the additional benefit of oral administration and penetration of the blood brain barrier [51]. Other agents used in melanoma treatment are carboplatin, paclitaxel and nitrosureas alone or in combination with regimens of biochemotherapy as salvage treatments. For the moment there is no evidence regarding the optimal sequence of treatment for stage IV disease. Therefore it is reasonable to consider immunotherapy, targeted agents or clinical trials as first-line treatment for stage IV disease. In patients with rapidly progressive, bulky metastases and high LDH levels, who have generally very short survival, the use of targeted therapies may be advantageous because it is associated with rapid responses as opposed to immunotherapy. Since cytotoxic chemotherapy does not produce a survival benefit, it should be reserved for patients not suitable or not responding to first-line treatment.

METASTASECTOMIES

In non-randomized studies, complete resection of oligometastatic disease has been associated with overall survival rates exceeding 30% at 4 years [52]. Retrospective analysis of data of the MSLT-1 trial showed that more than half of stage IV patients may be amenable to complete resection of their disease [53]. On the other hand, it is likely that the favourable outcome of patients undergoing complete resection of distant metastasis is biased on the selection of the fittest patients with biologically less

aggressive disease. In any case, stringent patient selection is crucial when surgery is contemplated for stage IV melanoma. Preoperative work-up should include extensive imaging with the use of brain MR and PET/CT is necessary to rule out occult metastatic disease not amenable to surgery. Patients with M1a disease (i.e. skin, distant nodes and soft tissues) have relatively longer survival, making an aggressive surgical approach defensible. In these cases, surgery should be performed early before lesions become bulky and symptomatic requiring extensive resections with a high morbidity [54]. Wide excisions are preferable to the degree this is anatomically possible. In distant node metastasis, complete clearance of the respective nodal basin is recommended. There is no limit on the number or sites of visceral metastasis that can be resected. Only complete resection of all metastatic disease should be considered and certainly patients most likely to experience long disease-free survival are those with oligometastatic disease to one organ, a long disease-free interval and good performance status. Palliative resection of metastases to GI tract causing bleeding or obstruction should be considered on an individualized basis. Resection of a second recurrence may be beneficial in selected patients [55]. The role of novel systemic treatments in the neoadjuvant or adjuvant setting for stage IV disease is not clear yet.

ROLE OF RADIATION TREATMENT

Radiation treatment is a useful option for patients with melanoma on an individualized basis. It should be considered in the treatment of lentigo maligna or lentigo maligna melanoma if surgery is not an option, in the case of a positive or close margin when re-excision is not an option, as adjuvant treatment in desmoplastic melanoma with neurotropism and in inoperable mucosal melanomas of the head and neck. It may reduce local relapse in patients undergoing lymph node dissection with high numbers of involved lymph nodes and extranodal extension [56]. In the palliative setting radiation treatment is used for local, in-transit or lymph node relapse when surgery or regional chemotherapy is not an option. It can offer symptom relief in patients with bone metastasis and spinal cord compression and, to a much lesser degree, in patients with lung, liver and abdomino-pelvic disease. Whole brain radiation treatment should be considered as an adjuvant to surgery and stereotactic radiotherapy for brain metastasis. Poor prognosis patients with brain metastases, low performance status and uncontrolled extracranial disease should be treated with whole brain radiation therapy [16].

FOLLOW-UP

The main value of follow-up visits in melanoma is to detect earlier potentially curable locoregional disease and second primaries. The frequency of surveillance and the use of imaging studies are controversial due to lack of high-level evidence. Two-thirds of the recurrences occur within the first 2 years and the majority within 4 years from primary diagnosis. Half of relapses are identified in the regional lymph nodes, 20% are local or regional and 30% are distant metastasis [57]. Most experts and guidelines agree that a stage-escalating approach is reasonable. Patients with melanoma stages I–IIA are at low risk for recurrence, and extensive imaging has low detection yields and unacceptably high false positive rates [58]. These patients are unlikely to benefit from imaging unless they become symptomatic and may well be followed up with clinical examinations every 6–12 months. Factors such as a personal or family history of melanoma, the presence of atypical moles and patient or doctor concern may modify this scheme [16]. Patients with stages IIB–IV are at higher risk for recurrence and more detailed surveillance may be justified. This may include history and physical examination with cross-sectional imaging of the chest, abdomen or pelvis with CT or PET/CT every 3–6 months for 2 years and then every 6–12 months for the following 3 years and then annually as clinically indicated. Annual brain MRI may also be considered. European guidelines (European Society of Medical Oncology, German Cancer Society, German Dermatologic Society and Swiss Melanoma Guidelines) advocate the use of lymph node ultrasound and measurement of serum $S100\beta$ every 3–12 months in patients with stage I–III melanoma. Most experts and guidelines agree that patients' education toward skin and node examination and alarming symptoms of recurrence, coupled with lifelong skin surveillance, is mandatory for all stages [59].

REFERENCES

1. Ferlay, J., I. Soerjomataram, M. Ervik, et al. 2013. GLOBOCAN 2012 v1.0, cancer incidence and mortality worldwide: IARC CancerBase No. 11. Lyon: International Agency for Research on Cancer. Available from http://globocan.iarc.fr (accessed 8 November 2014).
2. Lasithiotakis, K. G., U. Leiter, R. Gorkievicz, et al. 2006. The incidence and mortality of cutaneous melanoma in southern Germany: trends by anatomic site and pathologic characteristics, 1976 to 2003. *Cancer* 107 (6):1331–9.
3. Lasithiotakis, K. G., I. E. Petrakis, and C. Garbe. 2010. Cutaneous melanoma in the elderly: epidemiology, prognosis and treatment. *Melanoma Res* 20 (3):163–70.
4. Rigel, D. S. 2010. Epidemiology of melanoma. *Semin Cutan Med Surg* 29 (4):204–9.
5. Mann, G. J., and H. Tsao. 2009. Clinical genetics and risk assessment of melanoma. In *Cutaneous Melanoma*, edited by C. Balch, A. N. Houghton, A. J. Sober, S. J. Soong, M. B. Atkins, and J. F. Thompson. St Louis, MO: Quality Medical Publishing.
6. Gandini, S., F. Sera, M. S. Cattaruzza, et al. 2005. Meta-analysis of risk factors for cutaneous melanoma: II. Sun exposure. *Eur J Cancer* 41 (1):45–60.
7. Volkovova, K., D. Bilanicova, A. Bartonova, S. Letasiova, and M. Dusinska. 2012. Associations between environmental factors and incidence of cutaneous melanoma. Review. *Environ Health* 11 (Suppl. 1):S12.
8. Mayer, J. E., S. M. Swetter, T. Fu, and A. C. Geller. 2014a. Screening, early detection, education, and trends for melanoma: current status (2007–2013) and future directions: part I. Epidemiology, high-risk groups, clinical strategies, and diagnostic technology. *J Am Acad Dermatol* 71 (4):599 e1–599 e12; quiz 610, 599 e12.
9. Mayer, J. E., S. M. Swetter, T. Fu, and A. C. Geller. 2014b. Screening, early detection, education, and trends for melanoma: current status (2007–2013) and future directions: part II. Screening, education, and future directions. *J Am Acad Dermatol* 71 (4):611 e1–611 e10; quiz 621–2.
10. Goldstein, A. M., M. Chan, M. Harland, et al. 2006. High-risk melanoma susceptibility genes and pancreatic cancer, neural system tumors, and uveal melanoma across GenoMEL. *Cancer Res* 66 (20):9818–28.
11. Williams, P. F., C. M. Olsen, N. K. Hayward, and D. C. Whiteman. 2011. Melanocortin 1 receptor and risk of cutaneous melanoma: a meta-analysis and estimates of population burden. *Int J Cancer* 129 (7):1730–40.
12. Schneider, J. S., D. H. Moore, M. L. Mendelsohn. 2008. Screening program reduced melanoma mortality at the Lawrence Livermore National Laboratory, 1984 to 1996. *J Am Acad Dermatol* 58:741–9.
13. Aitken, J. F., M. Elwood, P. D. Baade, P. Youl, and D. English. 2010. Clinical whole-body skin examination reduces the incidence of thick melanomas. *Int J Cancer* 126:450–8.
14. Swetter, S. M., R. A. Pollitt, T. M. Johnson, D. R. Brooks, and A. C. Geller. 2012. Behavioral determinants of successful early melanoma detection. *Cancer* 118:3725–34.
15. Pack, S. C., A. J. Sober, H. Tsao, M. Mihm, and T. M. Johnson. 2008. Cutaneous melanoma. In *Fitzpatrick's Dermatology in General Medicine*, edited by K. Wolf, L. A. Goldsmith, S. I. Katz, B. A. Gilchrest, A. S. Paller, and D. J. Leffel. New York: McGraw Hill, 2008.
16. NCCN [National Comprehensive Cancer Network]. 2014. Melanoma (Version 1.2015). Fort Washington, PA: NCCN, 2014. Available from http://www.nccn.org/professionals/physician_gls/f_guidelines.asp#melanoma (accessed 21 December 2014).
17. Bastiaannet, E., T. Wobbes, O. S. Hoekstra, et al. 2009. Prospective comparison of [18F]fluorodeoxyglucose positron emission tomography and

computed tomography in patients with melanoma with palpable lymph node metastases: diagnostic accuracy and impact on treatment. *J Clin Oncol* 27 (28):4774–80.

18. Halpern, A. C., A. A. Marghoob, A. J. Sober. 2009. *Clinical Characteristics of Melanoma*, edited by C. Balch, A. N. Houghton, A. J. Sober, S. J. Soong, M. B. Atkins, and J. F. Thompson. 5th ed. St Louis, MO: Quality Medical Publishing.

19. Thomas, L., P. Tranchand, F. Berard, T. Secchi, C. Colin, and G. Moulin. 1998. Semiological value of ABCDE criteria in the diagnosis of cutaneous pigmented tumors. *Dermatology* 197 (1):11–7.

20. Veronesi, U., N. Cascinelli, J. Adamus, et al. 1988. Thin stage I primary cutaneous malignant melanoma. Comparison of excision with margins of 1 or 3 cm. *N Engl J Med* 318 (18):1159–62.

21. Cohn-Cedermark, G., L. E. Rutqvist, R. Andersson, et al. 2000. Long term results of a randomized study by the Swedish Melanoma Study Group on 2-cm versus 5-cm resection margins for patients with cutaneous melanoma with a tumor thickness of 0.8–2.0 mm. *Cancer* 89 (7):1495–501.

22. Khayat, D., O. Rixe, G. Martin, et al. 2003. Surgical margins in cutaneous melanoma (2 cm versus 5 cm for lesions measuring less than 2.1-mm thick). *Cancer* 97 (8):1941–6.

23. Gillgren, P., K. T. Drzewiecki, M. Niin, et al. 2011. 2-cm versus 4-cm surgical excision margins for primary cutaneous melanoma thicker than 2 mm: a randomised, multicentre trial. *Lancet* 378 (9803):1635–42.

24. Balch, C. M., S. J. Soong, T. Smith, et al. 2001. Long-term results of a prospective surgical trial comparing 2 cm vs. 4 cm excision margins for 740 patients with 1–4 mm melanomas. *Ann Surg Oncol* 8 (2):101–8.

25. Thomas, J. M., J. Newton-Bishop, R. A'Hern, et al. 2004. Excision margins in high-risk malignant melanoma. *N Engl J Med* 350 (8):757–66.

26. Gershenwald, J. E., D. G. Coit, V. K. Sondak, and J. F. Thompson. 2012. The challenge of defining guidelines for sentinel lymph node biopsy in patients with thin primary cutaneous melanomas. *Ann Surg Oncol* 19 (11):3301–3.

27. Uren, R. F., R. B. Howman-Giles, D. Chung, and J. F. Thompson. 2005. Role of lymphoscintigraphy for selective sentinel lymphadenectomy. *Cancer Treat Res* 127:15–38.

28. Morton, D. L., J. F. Thompson, A. J. Cochran, et al. 2014. Final trial report of sentinel-node biopsy versus nodal observation in melanoma. *N Engl J Med* 370 (7):599–609.

29. Essner, R., R. Scheri, M. Kavanagh, H. Torisu-Itakura, L. A. Wanek, and D. L. Morton. 2006. Surgical management of the groin lymph nodes in melanoma in the era of sentinel lymph node dissection. *Arch Surg* 141 (9):877–82; discussion 882–4.

30. Badgwell, B., Y. Xing, J. E. Gershenwald, et al. 2007. Pelvic lymph node dissection is beneficial in subsets of patients with node-positive melanoma. *Ann Surg Oncol* 14 (10):2867–75.

31. Shaw, J. H., and E. M. Rumball. 1990. Complications and local recurrence following lymphadenectomy. *Br J Surg* 77 (7):760–4.

32. Pathak, I., C. J. O'Brien, K. Petersen-Schaeffer, et al. 2001. Do nodal metastases from cutaneous melanoma of the head and neck follow a clinically predictable pattern? *Head Neck* 23 (9):785–90.

33. Lin, D., B. L. Franc, M. Kashani-Sabet, and M. I. Singer. 2006. Lymphatic drainage patterns of head and neck cutaneous melanoma observed on lymphoscintigraphy and sentinel lymph node biopsy. *Head Neck* 28 (3):249–55.

34. Tufaro, A. P., S. K. Mithani, J. A. Califano III, and A. Shaha. 2009. Neck dissection and parotidectomy for melanoma. In *Cutaneous Melanoma*, edited by C. Balch, A. N. Houghton, A. J. Sober, S. J. Soong, M. B. Atkins, and J. F Thompson. St Louis, MO: Quality Medical Publishing.

35. Mocellin, S., M. B. Lens, S. Pasquali, P. Pilati, and V. Chiarion Sileni. 2013. Interferon alpha for the adjuvant treatment of cutaneous melanoma. *Cochrane Database Syst Rev* 6:CD008955.

36. Dummer, R., A. Hauschild, M. Guggenheim, L. Jost, G. Pentheroudakis, and Esmo Guidelines Working Group. 2010. Melanoma: ESMO Clinical Practice Guidelines for diagnosis, treatment and follow-up. *Ann Oncol* 21 (Suppl. 5):v194–7.

37. Eggermont, A. M., S. Suciu, A. Testori, et al. 2012. Long-term results of the randomized phase III trial EORTC 18991 of adjuvant therapy with pegylated interferon alfa-2b versus observation in resected stage III melanoma. *J Clin Oncol* 30 (31):3810–8.

38. Kaufman, H. L., J. M. Kirkwood, F. S. Hodi, et al. 2013. The Society for Immunotherapy of Cancer consensus statement on tumour immunotherapy for the treatment of cutaneous melanoma. *Nat Rev Clin Oncol* 10 (10):588–98.

39. Flaherty, L. E., M. Othus, M. B. Atkins, et al. 2014. Southwest Oncology Group S0008: a phase III trial of high-dose interferon Alfa-2b versus cisplatin, vinblastine, and dacarbazine, plus interleukin-2 and interferon in patients with high-risk melanoma – an intergroup study of cancer and leukemia group B, Children's Oncology Group, Eastern Cooperative Oncology Group, and Southwest Oncology Group. *J Clin Oncol* 32 (33):3771–8.

40. Mervic, L. 2012. Time course and pattern of metastasis of cutaneous melanoma differ between men and women. *PLoS One* 7 (3):e32955.

41. Beasley, G. M., P. Speicher, K. Sharma, et al. 2014. Efficacy of repeat sentinel lymph node biopsy in patients who develop recurrent melanoma. *J Am Coll Surg* 218 (4):686–92.

42. Moreno-Ramirez, D., L. de la Cruz-Merino, L. Ferrandiz, R. Villegas-Portero, and A. Nieto-Garcia. 2010. Isolated limb perfusion for malignant melanoma: systematic review on effectiveness and safety. *Oncologist* 15 (4):416–27.

43. Zoras, O., ed. 2007. *Isolated Limb Perfusion.* 1st ed. Athens: Pashalides Medical Publications.

44. Kroon, H. M., A. M. Huismans, P. C. Kam, and J. F. Thompson. 2014. Isolated limb infusion with melphalan and actinomycin D for melanoma: a systematic review. *J Surg Oncol* 109 (4):348–51.

45. Gabriel, E., and J. Skitzki. 2015. The role of regional therapies for in-transit melanoma in the era of improved systemic options. Cancers (Basel) 7 (3):1154–77.

46. Topalian, S. L., M. Sznol, D. F. McDermott, et al. 2014. Survival, durable tumor remission, and long-term safety in patients with advanced melanoma receiving nivolumab. *J Clin Oncol* 32 (10):1020–30.

47. Wolchok, J. D., A. Hoos, S. O'Day, et al. 2009. Guidelines for the evaluation of immune therapy activity in solid tumors: immune-related response criteria. *Clin Cancer Res* 15 (23):7412–20.

48. Flaherty, K. T., C. Robert, P. Hersey, et al. 2012. Improved survival with MEK inhibition in BRAF-mutated melanoma. *N Engl J Med* 367 (2):107–14.

49. Hodi, F. S., C. L. Corless, A. Giobbie-Hurder, et al. 2013. Imatinib for melanomas harboring mutationally activated or amplified KIT arising on mucosal, acral, and chronically sun-damaged skin. *J Clin Oncol* 31 (26):3182–90.

50. Eggermont, A. M., and J. M. Kirkwood. 2004. Re-evaluating the role of dacarbazine in metastatic melanoma: what have we learned in 30 years? *Eur J Cancer* 40 (12):1825–36.

51. Quirt, I., S. Verma, T. Petrella, K. Bak, and M. Charette. 2007. Temozolomide for the treatment of metastatic melanoma: a systematic review. *Oncologist* 12 (9):1114–23.

52. Sosman, J. A., J. Moon, R. J. Tuthill, et al. 2011. A phase 2 trial of complete resection for stage IV melanoma: results of Southwest Oncology Group Clinical Trial S9430. *Cancer* 117 (20):4740–6.

53. Howard, J. H., J. F. Thompson, N. Mozzillo, et al. 2012. Metastasectomy for distant metastatic melanoma: analysis of data from the first Multicenter Selective Lymphadenectomy Trial (MSLT-I). *Ann Surg Oncol* 19 (8):2547–55.

54. Leung, A. M., D. M. Hari, and D. L. Morton. 2012. Surgery for distant melanoma metastasis. *Cancer J* 18 (2):176–84.

55. Ollila, D. W., E. C. Hsueh, S. L. Stern, and D. L. Morton. 1999. Metastasectomy for recurrent stage IV melanoma. *J Surg Oncol* 71 (4):209–13.

56. Burmeister, B. H., M. A. Henderson, J. Ainslie, et al. 2012. Adjuvant radiotherapy versus observation alone for patients at risk of lymph-node field relapse after therapeutic lymphadenectomy for melanoma: a randomised trial. *Lancet Oncol* 13 (6):589–97.

57. Scally, C. P., and S. L. Wong. 2014. Intensity of follow-up after melanoma surgery. *Ann Surg Oncol* 21 (3):752–7.

58 Bastiaannet, E., W. J. Oyen, S. Meijer, et al. 2006. Impact of [18F]fluorodeoxyglucose positron emission tomography on surgical management of melanoma patients. *Br J Surg* 93 (2):243–9.

59. Trotter, S. C., N. Sroa, R. R. Winkelmann, T. Olencki, and M. Bechtel. 2013. A global review of melanoma follow-up guidelines. *J Clin Aesthet Dermatol* 6 (9):18–26.

42

Thyroid cancer

SAMIRA M SADOWSKI, XAVIER M KEUTGEN AND ELECTRON KEBEBEW

INCIDENCE AND AETIOLOGY

Thyroid cancer accounts for only 1% of all epithelial malignancies, but represents 95% of all endocrine malignancies. The incidence of thyroid cancer in the United States and Europe is about three cases per 100,000 population per year [1]. Its incidence has significantly increased worldwide [2] with the overall annual average percentage change in incidence of thyroid cancer of 6.2% for men and 7.3% for women from 1999 to 2008, largely due to increased detection of smaller tumors [3,4]. Given the increasing incidence of thyroid cancer, proper and cost-effective diagnosis and management of thyroid cancer is paramount.

Once a thyroid nodule has been detected, the basis of any evaluation consists of a complete history and physical examination. Important risk factors should be assessed, such as a history of thyroid cancer in a first-degree relative, a history of head and neck irradiation [5,6], a history of multiple endocrine neoplasia (MEN), rapid growth of a nodule or associated lymphadenopathy. Male patients and patients younger than 30 or older than 60 years have a higher risk of having a malignant tumor [7]. A recent study on the incidence and characteristics of radiation-associated thyroid cancer detected during a systematic screening program initiated for at-risk children and adolescents in Belarus showed that the risk of this cancer is age and dose related and that radiation may result in more aggressive disease [8].

Approximately 95% of thyroid cancers are of follicular cell origin, with papillary thyroid cancer (PTC) comprising 85% of these cases. Most non-medullary thyroid cancers (NMTCs) are sporadic; however, approximately 3–8% of NMTCs are familial [9,10]. Familial non-medullary thyroid cancer (FNMTC) can occur as a minor component of familial cancer syndromes (Gardner, Cowden and Werner syndromes and Carney complex) or as non-syndromic familial disease [11]. Population studies have shown that the risk of thyroid cancer increases ninefold in patients with a first-degree relative with thyroid cancer [12,13]. FNMTC is defined as when two or more first-degree relatives are affected [14]. When three or more first-degree relatives are affected, the probability that their cancer is FNMTC is greater than 95%, compared with 31–38% when only two first-degree relatives are affected [12].

Our understanding of the molecular events that lead to thyroid cancer initiation and progression has improved and some of these findings may have potential in improving diagnosis and prognostication. Most thyroid cancers of follicular cell origin have genetic alterations in the MAPK pathways (activating mutations in *RET, RAS* and *BRAF*) and PI3k/Akt pathway (inactivating *PTEN* mutations), and inactivating *TP53* and *TERT* mutations.

Fusion of genes encoding receptor tyrosine kinases with other genes is common in papillary thyroid cancer (PTC). They include RET and NTRK which when rearranged with other genes (*RET/PTC* and *NTRK* rearrangements) encode a protein with constitutive tyrosine kinase activity. The chimeric RET/PTC protein activates the RAS-RAF-MAPK pathway and induces cell proliferation and tumorigenesis. The *RET/PTC* rearrangement is frequent in radiation-associated PTC and occurs in 15–45% of sporadic papillary thyroid carcinoma [15], with the most common types being *RET/PTC1* and *RET/PTC3* [16]. *RET/PTC1* is frequent in classic PTC and has been associated with more favourable tumor behaviour. However, tumors harbouring *RET/PTC3* rearrangements have been associated with aggressive behaviour and advanced stage at diagnosis [17].

A mutation in RAS encodes a small G-protein that propagates the signal from the receptor tyrosine kinase to the MAPK and PI3K/Akt pathways. Mutations in *NRAS* are more frequent in follicular thyroid cancer (40–50%) than in PTC (0–16%; all of these are follicular variant) [18]. *RAS* mutations are more frequent in the encapsulated follicular variant of PTC.

BRAF is a serine-threonine kinase of the RAF family. The most common point mutation occurs in codon 600 and results in a valine-to-glutamine transversion (V600E), resulting in constitutive activation of the BRAF kinase. This results in phosphorylation of downstream MAPK targets such as MEK1/2 and ERK1/2, leading to increased cellular proliferation, de-differentiation, angiogenesis and thyroid cancer initiation [19]. This mutation is the most common alteration in PTC and has been associated with more aggressive disease, characterized by extra-thyroidal extension, lymph node metastasis, advanced TNM stage and higher recurrence rates [20].

The *PAX8/PPARγ* chromosomal rearrangement is a fusion of *PAX8*, a thyroid-specific transcription factor, with the peroxisome proliferator-activated receptor gamma gene (*PPARγ*) involved in cancer cell differentiation. The rearrangement has been identified in up to 50% of follicular thyroid cancers, some follicular adenomas, and also in the follicular variant of PTC [21]. *PAX8/PPARγ* has been associated with younger age at presentation and a higher rate of vascular invasion and distant metastases [22].

Most thyroid cancers arise from the follicular cells and are well-differentiated thyroid cancers (WDTCs). The most aggressive, but rare, type of thyroid cancer is anaplastic (undifferentiated) thyroid cancer (ATC). Differentiated thyroid cancers of follicular cell origin can be syndromic or non-syndromic. Patients with familial syndromes such as familial adenomatous polyposis (FAP), Cowden's syndrome, Werner syndrome and Peutz–Jeghers syndrome have a higher risk of developing thyroid cancer. About 1–2% of patients with FAP develop PTC, and up to 10% of patients with Cowden's syndrome will develop follicular thyroid cancer [23]. FAP is an inherited syndrome characterized by the development of hundreds to thousands of adenomatous polyps in the colon and has an incidence of approximately 1 per 10,000 births. FAP is caused by a mutation in the adenomatous polyposis coli (*APC*) gene, which is inherited in an autosomal dominant manner. Because colorectal polyps are not always symptomatic, the first manifestation of FAP or clue to its diagnosis may be colorectal cancer or an extra-intestinal manifestation, such as thyroid cancer. Cowden's syndrome is an intestinal polyposis syndrome characterized by the development of hamartomatous polyps and is inherited in an autosomal dominant manner. It is caused by inactivating mutations in the phosphatase and tensin homolog (*PTEN*) gene. Differentiated thyroid cancer,

predominantly follicular thyroid cancer, is the second most frequent cancer, after breast cancer, found in patients with Cowden's syndrome.

Medullary thyroid cancer (MTC) arises from the parafollicular cells that secrete calcitonin and accounts for 5–7% of all thyroid cancer cases. The parafollicular cells are of neural crest origin, account for 1% of thyroid cells and are most numerous at the junction of the upper third and lower two-thirds of the thyroid lobes. In all MTCs, there is positive immunohistochemical staining for calcitonin and carcinoembryonic antigen (CEA), and the serum levels for both of these are elevated in subjects with MTC. Lymph node metastases are found in 20–30% of patients with a tumor of less than 1 cm and in up to 90% of patients with a tumor larger than 4 cm [24]. Metastases may arise in the liver, lungs and bones.

MTC may be hereditary (familial) in about 20–25% of cases [25]. Sporadic MTC can occur at any age, but its incidence peaks between the fourth and sixth decades of life. It usually presents with a palpable nodule located in the upper third of a thyroid lobe, and may be associated with diarrhea and hot flushes in patients with advanced and metastatic disease.

Inherited MTC syndromes (part of MEN2) affect approximately 1 in 30,000 individuals [26] and consist of three distinct familial MTC syndromes: MEN2A (Sipple's syndrome), familial MTC (FMTC) and MEN2B. MEN2 is an autosomal dominant hereditary cancer syndrome that imparts a 50% risk of transmitting the disorder to the offspring of a carrier. It is caused by missense mutations in the *RET* protooncogene that result in gain of function [27]. All three clinical subtypes of MEN2 are characterized by the presence of MTC. Affected individuals initially develop C-cell hyperplasia that progresses to MTC. The most common clinical subtype of MEN2 is type 2A. The typical age of onset of this condition is the third or fourth decade of life and it is characterized by a triad of features: MTC, pheochromocytoma and primary hyperparathyroidism. Nearly 90% of these gene carriers will develop MTC, and their risk of developing unilateral or bilateral pheochromocytoma is as high as 57%. In addition, 15–30% of these gene carriers will develop primary hyperparathyroidism. MEN2B is characterized by the presence of MTC, marfanoid habitus, medullated corneal nerve fibres, ganglioneuromatosis of the gut and oral mucosa and pheochromocytoma [28]. FMTC is a clinical variant of MEN2A in which MTC is the only manifestation. To prove that a particular kin has FMTC, it is necessary to demonstrate the absence of pheochromocytoma or primary hyperparathyroidism in two or more generations within a family or to have a *RET* mutation identified only in kindred with FMTC [28].

All patients with a personal medical history of primary C-cell hyperplasia, MTC or MEN2 or a family history should be offered germline *RET* mutation testing. For MEN2B, this should be done shortly after birth. For MEN2A and FMTC, this should be done before 5 years of age [28].

PATHOLOGY AND STAGING

Most thyroid cancers arise from the follicular thyroid cells and histologically are classified into PTC (including histologic variants), follicular thyroid cancer, Hürthle cell carcinoma, poorly differentiated thyroid cancer and ATC. MTC comprises about 5–7% of all thyroid cancers. Patients with WDTC usually have a good prognosis, with a 10-year survival rate of approximately 90%. Nevertheless, about 20% of patients experience disease recurrence and WDTC-related deaths [29–31].

Thyroid cancer is classified according to the TNM staging system (Table 42.1), where patient's age at diagnosis plays an important part. For example, any tumor size, with or without extra-thyroidal extension (T1–4), or any N lesion in a patient 45 years or younger is considered stage I disease. However, in patients older than 45 years of age, the stage depends on tumor size, lymph node involvement and the presence or absence of distant metastases [32]. In addition to the TNM staging, several prognostic classification systems have been used (e.g. AGES, AMES, MACIS), all of which accurately predict prognosis (Table 42.2) [33]. Both the European Thyroid Association and the American Thyroid Association (ATA) have proposed practical guidelines to estimate the risk of recurrence, in which the TNM parameters are integrated with additional clinical features, such as histological variants, results of post-ablative whole body scans and serum thyroglobulin (Tg) levels [30,34].

Serum calcitonin plays an important role in diagnosing and predicting the prognosis of MTC. Data suggest that routine serum calcitonin screening may detect C-cell hyperplasia and MTC at an earlier stage, allowing for prophylactic thyroidectomy and improved overall survival [34]. Some centres rely on pentagastrin stimulation testing to increase diagnostic specificity.

DIAGNOSIS AND PREOPERATIVE IMAGING

Patients with thyroid cancer present in various ways, including self-identification (40.1%), health care provider identification (29.8%) and incidental detection (30.1%) [35]. Patients may have symptoms and signs of hyper- or hypothyroidism, but the vast majority of patients are euthyroid. Some patients may have local symptoms from their tumor, which include dysphagia and hoarseness.

Thyroid function tests should include measurement of serum thyrotropin (TSH) levels to determine the functional status of the thyroid gland. If the TSH level is abnormal, free T3 and T4 should be checked. Some studies have reported that high TSH levels (hypothyroidism) in patients with a thyroid nodule are associated with a higher risk of thyroid cancer [36].

A diagnostic thyroid ultrasound (US) should be performed in all patients with a suspected thyroid nodule, goiter with a

Table 42.1 TNM classification system for differentiated thyroid cancer

	Definition
T1	Tumor diameter 2 cm or smaller
T2	Primary tumor diameter >2 to 4 cm
T3	Primary tumor diameter >4 cm limited to the thyroid or with minimal extra-thyroidal extension
T4a	Tumor of any size extending beyond the thyroid capsule to invade subcutaneous soft tissues, larynx, trachea, esophagus or recurrent laryngeal nerve
T4b	Tumor invades prevertebral fascia or encases carotid artery or mediastinal vessels
TX	Primary tumor size unknown, but without extra-thyroidal invasion
N0	No metastatic nodes
N1a	Metastases to level VI (pretracheal, paratracheal and prelaryngeal = Delphian lymph nodes)
N1b	Metastases to unilateral, bilateral, contralateral cervical or superior mediastinal nodes
NX	Nodes not assessed at surgery
M0	No distant metastases
M1	Distant metastases
MX	Distant metastases not assessed

Stage	Patient age <45 years	Patient age 45 years or older
I	Any T, any N, M0	T1, N0, M0
II	Any T, any N, M1	T2, N0, M0
III		T3, N0, M0
		T1, N1a, M0
		T2, N1a, M0
		T3, N1a, M0
IVA		T4a, N0, M0
		T4a, N1a, M0
		T1, N1b, M0
		T2, N1b, M0
		T3, N1b, N0
		T4a, N1b, M0
IVB		T4b, any N, M0
IVC		Any T, any N, M1

Source: Adapted Edge S, et al., AJCC Cancer Staging Manual, 7th ed., New York: Springer, 2010.

dominant nodule or incidentally discovered thyroid nodules on imaging (via computed tomography [CT], magnetic resonance imaging [MRI] or ^{18}F-fluorodeoxyglucose–positron emission tomography [^{18}FDG-PET]) [34]. Thyroid US is useful for assessing whether the nodule has features suspicious for cancer, for detecting additional thyroid nodules, for

Table 42.2 Staging system and method of tumor risk calculation

Staging system	Calculation method
AGES (age, grade, extent, size)	Total score = 0.05 × age in years (if aged ≥40) or + 0 (if aged <40) + 1 (if tumor grade 2) or + 3 (if tumor grade 3 or 4) + 1 (if extra-thyroidal invasion) + 3 (if distant spread) + 0.2 × tumor size (maximum diameter in cm) Four risk groups: Group 1 = score <4.00 Group 2 = score 4.01–4.99 Group 3 = score 5.00–5.99 Group 4 = score ≥6
AMES (age, metastases, extent, size)	Low-risk group: 1. All younger patients without distant metastases (men <41 years, women <51 years) 2. All older patients with: a. Intrathyroidal papillary cancer or minor tumor capsular involvement follicular carcinoma and b. Tumor size <5 cm and c. No distant metastases High-risk group: 1. All patients with distant metastases 2. All older patients with: a. Major capsular involvement papillary cancer or major capsular involvement follicular carcinoma and b. Tumor size ≥5 cm
MACIS (metastases, age, complete resection, invasion, size)	Total score = 3.1 (if aged ≤39 years) or 0.08 × age (if aged ≥40 years) + 0.3 × tumor size in cm + 1 (if not completely resected) + 1 (if locally invasive) + 3 (if distant metastases) Four risk groups: Group 1 = <6.0 Group 2 = 6.0–6.99 Group 3 = 7.0–7.99 Group 4 = >8.0

Source: Adapted from Lang BH, et al., *Annals of Surgery* 2007;245(3):366–78.

determining the presence of cervical lymph node metastasis and for facilitating fine-needle aspiration (FNA) biopsies of the suspicious nodules and lymph nodes. Therefore, US is the best initial imaging modality, as it allows for diagnosis and treatment planning [5].

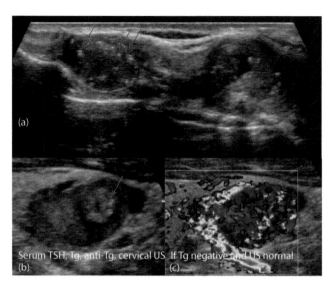

Serum TSH, Tg, anti-Tg, cervical US If Tg negative and US normal

Figure 42.1 Ultrasound features suspicious for malignancy. A 53-year-old man, with bilateral thyroid nodules on ultrasound. (a) The right thyroid lobe shows several masses, with the largest 1.7 × 1.2 cm in size and microcalcifications (red arrows). (b) An echopenic and heterogeneous mass is shown in the left thyroid. The mass is approximately 2.1 × 1.1 cm, partially calcified (red arrow), and its vascularity is imaged via colour-flow Doppler study (c) Pathology of nodules confirms classic PTC.

Features suspicious for malignancy detectable by US are thyroid nodules with microcalcifications, hypoechogenicity, irregular margins, absence of a halo, solid composition and intranodular vascularity or a taller-than-wide nodule (Figure 42.1) [37].

Other imaging modalities have been used to characterize thyroid nodules, such as CT, MRI and ¹⁸FDG-PET. They are not routinely used unless there is suspicion of a locally invasive tumor or distant metastases [34]. Recent CT studies on malignant thyroid nodules showed more frequent nodular or rim calcifications, a taller-than-wide ratio greater than 1 and a higher mean attenuation. An FNA biopsy was recommended based on these features [38]. MRI studies revealed a delayed washout pattern associated with thyroid cancer [39], and in ¹⁸FDG-PET studies, an SUV cut-off value of 4.2 allowed differentiation between benign and malignant nodules. These nodules should then be biopsied using FNA [40].

The most accurate and cost-effective initial diagnostic test to evaluate patients with thyroid nodules, and exclude a thyroid cancer diagnosis, is a thyroid FNA biopsy and cytologic examination [34]. Several guidelines have been established to determine which thyroid nodule features should dictate a thyroid FNA biopsy, as outlined in Table 42.3. The Bethesda system (Table 42.4) for reporting thyroid cytopathology has been implemented at most medical centres and provides uniform criteria for classifying cytologic diagnoses and a risk estimate of thyroid cancer for each of these cytopathologic categories [41,42]. The risk of malignancy varies for each of these categories. In a majority of cases, thyroid FNA biopsies distinguish between benign

Table 42.3 Sonographic and clinical features of thyroid nodules and recommendation for FNA

Nodule sonographic or clinical features	Recommended nodule threshold size for FNA
High-risk history[a]	
Nodule *with* suspicious sonographic features[b]	>5 mm
Nodule *without* suspicious sonographic features[b]	>5 mm
Abnormal cervical lymph nodes	All[c]
Microcalcifications present in nodule	≥1 cm
Solid nodule	
and hypoechoic	>1 cm
and iso- or hyperechoic	≥1–1.5 cm
Mixed cystic–solid nodule	
with any suspicious ultrasound features[b]	≥1.5–2 cm
without suspicious ultrasound features	≥2 cm
Spongiform nodule	≥2 cm[d]
Purely cystic nodule	FNA not indicated[e]

Source: Modified from Cooper DS, et al., *Thyroid* 2009;19(11): 1167–214.

[a] High-risk history: History of thyroid cancer in one or more first-degree relatives; history of external beam radiation as a child; exposure to ionizing radiation in childhood or adolescence; prior hemithyroidectomy with discovery of thyroid cancer, [18]FDG avidity on PET scanning; MEN2/FMTC-associated RET protooncogene mutation, calcitonin >100 pg/ml.

[b] Suspicious features: Microcalcifications, hypoechoic, increased nodular vascularity, infiltrative margins, taller than wide on transverse view.

[c] FNA cytology may be obtained from the abnormal lymph node in lieu of the thyroid nodule.

[d] Sonographic monitoring without biopsy may be an acceptable alternative.

[e] Unless indicated as therapeutic modality.

and malignant nodules. However, a significant number of FNA diagnoses are inconclusive, falling into one of three Bethesda categories: follicular lesion of undetermined significance (FLUS) or atypia of undetermined significance (AUS), follicular neoplasm (FN), and suspicious for malignancy, often collectively referred to as indeterminate diagnoses. Between 5% and 42% of thyroid FNA diagnoses reported belong in this category [41]. A similar classification proposed by the Royal College of Pathologists in the UK is used in many centres and its categories corresponding to the Bethesda system are shown in Table 42.4.

According to the ATA guidelines [34], genetic mutation analysis for molecular markers might be considered for patients with indeterminate cytology, as determined by FNA biopsy analysis, to help guide management. In this context, the BRAF[V600E] mutation, the most prevalent genetic alteration observed in 29–87% of PTCs, and considered an early

genetic event in thyroid cancer progression, has been shown to be a possible new prognostic marker in PTC [43,44]. Several reports have described the association of this mutation with factors related to a poor prognosis, such as the presence of extra-thyroidal extension, lymph node metastasis, advanced tumor stage and reduced disease-free interval and patient survival. Molecular testing of thyroid FNA biopsies to identify a panel of mutations, including BRAF[V600E], *RAS*, *RET/PTC* and *PAX8/PPARγ*, has been shown to help decide the appropriate therapeutic approach when indeterminate FNA results are obtained [45].

However, additional markers are needed to reliably diagnose malignancy, especially when the mutation detection tests are negative and the FNA biopsy results are indeterminate. A commercially available gene expression classifier panel (142 genes) using genome-wide gene expression profiling based on the expression pattern of mRNA extracted from FNA needle passes has shown some potential. This approach was initially shown to distinguish benign from malignant thyroid nodules, with a sensitivity of 92% and specificity of 52% [46]. Unfortunately it was most accurate only in the AUS category of thyroid FNA biopsy results, and a follow-up independent study showed higher false-negative results than initially reported [47].

SURGICAL TREATMENT OF THYROID CANCER

Surgical removal of the thyroid and involved cervical lymph nodes is the main pillar of thyroid cancer therapy. Additional therapeutic options include radioactive iodine (RAI) treatment and TSH suppression and occasionally chemotherapy and external beam radiotherapy (XRT).

Well-differentiated thyroid cancer

Total thyroidectomy is defined as the complete removal of both lobes of the thyroid. Near-total thyroidectomy is defined as the removal of both thyroid lobes except for a small amount of thyroid tissue (≤1 g on one side, to protect the recurrent laryngeal nerve or parathyroid glands). Hemithyroidectomy is defined as the removal of a thyroid lobe, including the thyroid isthmus. Because the survival rate of WDTC is very high, independent of disease stage, there are no large randomized trials comparing the extent of thyroidectomy for those patients, since it would take an excessively large number of patients to show a small potential difference.

We recommend that patients with a diagnosis of PTC ≥1 cm undergo a total or near-total thyroidectomy. The appropriate extent of a thyroidectomy for PTC smaller than 1 cm is controversial, as it is unclear whether a hemithyroidectomy results in the same rate of recurrent disease and mortality. Most surgeons will agree that a well-differentiated, unifocal PTC <1 cm, in a young patient with no history of neck radiation, without extra-thyroidal extension or positive cervical nodes, is at

Table 42.4 Risk stratification for indeterminate thyroid nodules on FNA, according to National Cancer Institute classification

Classification Bethesda (UK-RCP)	Terminology	Approximate cancer risk (%)	Treatment
Bethesda I (Thy 1)	Non-diagnostic	5–18	Repeat biopsy
Bethesda II (Thy 2)	Benign	0–5	None
Bethesda III (Thy 3a)	Follicular lesion of indeterminate significance (FLUS), atypia	5–10	Repeat biopsy or perform hemithyroidectomy
Bethesda IV (Thy 3f)	Follicular or Hürthle cell neoplasm (FN)	20–30	Hemithyroidectomy
Bethesda V (Thy 4)	Suspicious for cancer	50–75	Total or hemithyroidectomy
Bethesda VI (Thy 5)	Cancer	92–100	Total thyroidectomy[a]

Note: UK-RCP = United Kingdom Royal College of Pathologists.
[a] Hemithyroidectomy could be considered for low-risk well-differentiated thyroid cancer (i.e. papillary thyroid cancer 1 cm or less).

low risk of recurrence and can therefore be treated with a hemithyroidectomy [34,48].

Regardless of the extent of thyroidectomy, the goal of surgery should be complete resection of the tumor, including any disease extension beyond the thyroid capsule, as well as removal of affected cervical lymph nodes since residual micro- or macroscopic disease in lymph nodes may be the source of disease recurrence [49–51].

If postoperative RAI ablation and Tg surveillance is planned, care must be taken to remove all macroscopically visible tumor and normal thyroid tissue, during the initial operation. This will maximize the efficacy of postoperative adjuvant treatment [52,53].

Although some groups selectively use observation instead of surgical therapy for small WDTC, this strategy remains controversial [54,55]. Since our group has recently demonstrated that up to 12% of thyroid cancer–related deaths occur in patients with PTC ≤2 cm, active surveillance for PTC less than 1 cm and no risk factor [56].

Surgical management of indeterminate thyroid nodules

Patients with indeterminate lesions on preoperative FNA should be informed of the likelihood of malignancy, which is dependent on the cytopathological classification (Table 42.4). Bethesda III lesions in most cases can be observed and re-biopsied due to their low likelihood of malignancy. Bethesda IV and V lesions should be surgically removed. Most surgeons recommend a diagnostic hemithyroidectomy in these cases. Intraoperative frozen section analysis for indeterminate thyroid nodules is of limited use since pathologists rely on the presence of capsular or vascular invasion to distinguish follicular or Hürthle cancer from adenomas, which cannot be accurately analyzed in frozen sections. Moreover, sampling errors predispose this test to false-negative results since some thyroid cancers may only have focal extra-thyroidal invasion. Lastly, artefacts related

to the process of freezing can mimic invasion and therefore lead to false-positive results [57,58].

Completion thyroidectomy should be offered to patients for whom a total thyroidectomy would have been recommended if the diagnosis had been definitive before surgery. A direct or indirect laryngoscopy for evaluation of vocal cord function should be performed even in patients without symptoms such as hoarseness, dysphagia or aspiration.

Mutation analysis, which detects mutations in the *BRAF*, *RAS*, *RET/PTC* and *PAX-8-PPARy* genes, can potentially be helpful in determining the malignancy status and extent of thyroidectomy necessary in some patients with cytologically indeterminate thyroid nodules [59]. Since mutation-positive indeterminate nodules are malignant in the vast majority of cases, patients with mutation-positive nodules >1 cm should undergo total thyroidectomy during the initial operation. However, due to the low prevalence of mutations in indeterminate lesions, the need for diagnostic thyroidectomy in mutation-negative nodules, and the high costs associated with routine mutation testing at this time, most clinicians refrain from using mutation analysis routinely [60].

Lymph node dissection and sentinel lymph node biopsy

It is estimated that 60–90% of patients with PTC will have lymph node metastasis, most of which will be microscopic [48]. Since most lymph node metastases occur in the central neck compartment (level VI), some surgeons advocate a routine prophylactic ipsilateral central neck dissection (pCND) during the initial thyroidectomy. Proponents of routine pCND argue that (1) dissection of the level VI compartment reduces the risk of persistent or recurrent PTC and therefore the need for reoperation in the recurrent laryngeal nerve region, (2) level VI dissection can be done safely by experienced surgeons and (3) more reliable staging may change postoperative treatment decisions.

Opponents of routine pCND argue that (1) there is added potential risk of damage to the recurrent laryngeal nerve and of postoperative hypoparathyroidism; (2) even with the known 60–90% frequency of microscopic level VI lymph node metastases, disease-free survival remains excellent and lymph node metastasis relapse remains infrequent; and (3) as long as RAI treatment is planned, dissection of non-palpable involved lymph nodes is probably not essential. Although there have been multiple retrospective studies evaluating outcomes for patients who did and did not undergo pCND, no prospective randomized studies have been performed. This would require a prohibitively large number of patients with long-term follow-up to determine a difference in clinical recurrence [61].

Sentinel lymph node biopsy (SLNB) has been studied in thyroid cancer with the aim of identifying those patients with central node involvement who would benefit from a central node dissection during their initial thyroidectomy. However, recent studies have found that the costs associated with implementation of SLNB may outweigh any potential benefit of reduction in morbidity attributable to central compartment dissection [62].

For patients with clinical evidence of lymph node metastases, removal of the level VI and VII (upper mediastinum) lymph node compartments and, if the ipsilateral lateral nodes are involved, a functional modified radical neck dissection (MRND) should be undertaken (Figure 42.2). An MRND includes dissection of the level II, III and IV compartments. The sternocleidomastoid muscle, the internal jugular veins (IJVs) and the spinal accessory nerve are usually spared during this dissection. However, if an IJV is involved with the tumor, it can be resected. If both IJVs are involved, a staged operation should be performed (one side first, followed by the other side 2–6 weeks later). Some surgeons believe that a more selective approach to dissection

of levels I and V compartments can be undertaken and that those levels should be included only if they are clinically or radiographically involved [63]. Isolated removal of macroscopically involved lymph nodes during the thyroidectomy, also referred to as 'berry picking', is not recommended.

Complications of thyroid surgery

The common complications of thyroidectomy include hypoparathyroidism and recurrent or superior laryngeal nerve injury, transient or permanent. Other complications include hemorrhage (0.5%) and surgical site infection (0.5%). It is crucial that one be familiar with the anatomy of both recurrent and superior laryngeal nerves in order to avoid injury.

The external branch of the superior laryngeal nerve innervates the cricothyroid muscle and courses 1–2 cm upward of the superior thyroid pole in most cases. Special care must be taken not to injure it while ligating and dividing the superior thyroid pole vessels. The recurrent laryngeal nerve takes an oblique course from lateral to medial after wrapping around the innominate artery on the right side, and a course parallel to the trachea in the trachea-esophageal groove after wrapping around the aortic arch on the left side. The recurrent laryngeal nerve is non-recurrent in less than 1% of patients, usually on the right side. This may be predicted preoperatively on a CT scan by recognizing the origin of the right subclavian artery directly from the aortic arch. It is our practice to identify and trace the recurrent laryngeal nerve during the thyroidectomy, in order to avoid inadvertent injury. The recurrent laryngeal nerve can usually be found at one of three locations: (1) inferiorly, at the level of the inferior thyroid artery, which it crosses posterior to the inferior parathyroid gland; (2) further cephalad, at the tubercle of Zuckerkandl (often referred to as the arrow that points to the nerve); and (3) superiorly, at its insertion at the level of the cricoid cartilage.

We routinely use intraoperative nerve monitoring (IONM) for all thyroid cases. While IONM has not been shown to decrease nerve injury rates, it can be useful in confirming nerve function and is therefore of value, especially in reoperations [64].

In order to avoid postoperative hypoparathyroidism, special attention needs to be given to avoiding disruption of the blood supply to the parathyroid glands, which originates from the inferior thyroid artery and courses from lateral to medial. The thyroidectomy specimen should always be inspected for inadvertent removal of one or more parathyroid glands. Suspicion of parathyroid gland removal may be confirmed via frozen section examination and, if confirmed, the gland should be re-implanted in the ipsilateral sternocleidomastoid muscle and the site marked with a clip.

Locally advanced thyroid cancer

When aggressive or invasive thyroid cancer is suspected, a direct or indirect laryngoscopy should be performed

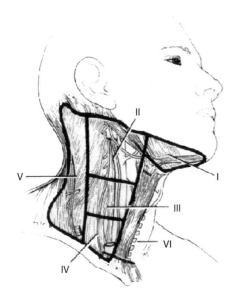

Figure 42.2 Anatomical neck compartments.

to evaluate vocal cord function. If the ipsilateral nerve is paralyzed, an R0 resection should be attempted, including resection of the recurrent laryngeal nerve, if necessary. If, however, both vocal cords are functioning, the nerve should be preserved, if possible, even if this results in an R1 resection. It is reasonable to resect the outer muscle wall of the esophagus or to shave the tumor off the trachea if those structures are involved. However, when there is full-thickness invasion of the trachea, a wedge resection (not involving more than one-third the circumference) or a segmental resection may be necessary, though this is rarely done.

Patients with metastatic WDTC should undergo resection of their primary tumor. If the distant metastatic sites are stable, become non-iodine avid or threaten to cause local symptoms (e.g. brain), a palliative resection or ablative treatment of the metastasis may be considered [34].

ATC warrants special consideration, since almost half of all patients will present with locally invasive or distant disease, and the tumor doubling time can be very short. Moreover, it accounts for approximately one-third of all thyroid cancer–related deaths [56]. Best management practices for ATC include rapid airway assessment and tumor staging, diagnosis based on FNA or core needle biopsy and cytologic examination. If possible, expeditious surgical resection with grossly negative margins should be performed. Alternatively, chemo-radiotherapy may help in reducing the size of the primary tumor before surgery is attempted.

Prophylactic and therapeutic thyroidectomy for medullary thyroid cancer

Recommendations for prophylactic thyroidectomy in familial MTC and MEN2A are dependent on the codon mutation in the *RET* protooncogene. Patients with codon mutations 768, 790, 791, 804 and 891 in *RET* are at lower risk of developing early-onset MTC. Prophylactic thyroidectomy (including level VI neck compartment if there is clinical evidence of disease) should therefore be performed between the 5th and 10th years of life. Patients with *RET* codon mutations 609, 611, 618, 620, 630 and 634 are part of the intermediate risk group and should undergo prophylactic thyroidectomy (including level VI neck compartment if there is clinical evidence of disease) by age 5. Patients with MEN2B and *RET* codon mutations 883, 918 and 922 have the most aggressive disease and should undergo prophylactic total thyroidectomy (including level VI neck compartment if there is clinical evidence of disease) by age 1.

Therapeutic total thyroidectomy for sporadic MTC should include bilateral central neck dissection (level VI). Ipsilateral or bilateral lateral neck dissection is done if US imaging shows evidence of metastatic lymph nodes or if calcitonin levels are high, the primary tumor is larger than 1 cm and there is no evidence of distant metastases. Patients with familial MTC should also routinely undergo therapeutic total thyroidectomy with bilateral level VI dissection.

Here again, unilateral or bilateral lateral neck dissection is warranted only if US imaging reveals positive lymph nodes. Exceptions to this rule include MEN2B patients diagnosed with MTC later in life and patients with high calcitonin levels without evidence of distant metastatic disease [65].

Postoperative surveillance and recurrence management

Follow-up of patients with WDTC should include annual physical exams and measurements of Tg and Tg antibodies in all patients who have had a total or near-total thyroidectomy, with or without RAI therapy. In many centres, neck US and RAI or PET scans are also performed. Figure 42.3 shows our protocol at the time of initial follow-up. Tg antibodies can interfere with measurement of Tg levels and therefore should be assessed every time Tg levels are measured.

Patients with MTC should undergo calcitonin and CEA level measurements, as well as US imaging, annually. Up to 50% of patients with MTC will have persistently elevated postoperative calcitonin levels. Management of these patients is particularly challenging, since there is often no recognizable evidence of macroscopic disease [65].

Patients with suspicion of local recurrence should undergo an FNA biopsy to confirm the diagnosis. Therapeutic re-do compartmental neck dissection should follow if this is a first recurrence without evidence of distant disease by imaging studies and calcitonin levels.

ADJUVANT AND NEOADJUVANT THERAPIES

Using RAI as an adjuvant treatment has two distinctive benefits in thyroid cancer management. First, it enables the ablation of any residual microscopic disease after surgery. Second, it makes the use of serum Tg more sensitive as a postoperative tumor marker for persistent or recurrent WDTC. There are several ways to prepare a patient for adjuvant RAI treatment: levothyroxine withdrawal for at least 4 weeks; liothyronine treatment for 2–4 weeks, followed by withdrawal for 2 weeks; or recombinant TSH administration. All options should lead to an increase in TSH levels, to >30 mIU/L, which allows for an increased uptake of iodine by the remaining thyroid tissues [34]. Patients typically receive low-dose RAI as a screening and calibration dose, followed by a calculated therapeutic dose based on dosimetry data. The goal of dosimetry is to deliver an appropriate dose of I^{131}, thereby decreasing the risk of bone marrow suppression, fibrosis and secondary malignancies. Other more common side effects of RAI therapy include destruction of the salivary glands and subsequent xerostomia [66]. Contraindications to RAI treatment include pregnancy and lactation.

Postoperative RAI therapy is recommended for PTC when distant metastases, tumors >4 cm, gross extra-thyroidal extension, aggressive tumor histology (e.g. tall cell variant) and intrathyroidal vascular invasion are detected.

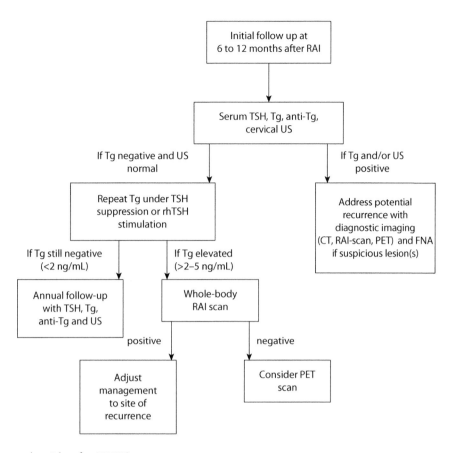

Figure 42.3 Follow-up algorithm for WDTC.

Patients with PTC 1 to 4 cm in size should undergo RAI treatment if they have positive lymph nodes, any of the other high-risk features mentioned above, if their baseline non-stimulated thyroglobulin level is >2 ng/ml, or if their stimulated Tg level is >10 ng/ml [34]. Follicular thyroid cancer and Hürthle cell carcinoma are relatively more aggressive and therefore RAI treatment is indicated in all these tumors >1 cm. However, less than 10% of Hürthle cell carcinomas are iodine avid, and therefore RAI therapy is of limited use in treating those lesions [67]. Patients with minimally invasive follicular thyroid cancer also may not need RAI therapy as the risk of recurrent or persistent disease is low and these patients have near-normal life expectancies [68–70].

Postoperative TSH suppression has been shown to improve outcomes in thyroid cancer. Thyroid hormone treatment with a target TSH level of <0.1 mIU/L is recommended for aggressive thyroid cancers, while a TSH slightly below the normal level (0.1–0.5 mIU/L) is considered adequate for low-risk WDTCs [34]. Adverse side effects of TSH suppression therapy may include subclinical thyrotoxicosis, increased risk of ischemic heart disease and atrial fibrillation in elderly patients, and osteoporosis in post-menopausal women. Neoadjuvant or adjuvant XRT, with or without chemotherapy, can be added to improve resectability or symptoms for locally advanced

thyroid cancer [71]. Recently, tyrosine kinase inhibitors (TKIs) have been evaluated in WDTC, ATC and MTC. TKIs, such as vandetanib and cabozantinib, have been approved for treating advanced MTC and their use results in improved progression-free survival. Sorafenib has also been used to treat late-stage WDTC and its use results in improved progression-free survival in RAI-negative thyroid cancer of follicular cell origin [72,73]. Phase III studies demonstrated significantly prolonged progression-free survival in patients treated with these agents [74].

REFERENCES

1. Schlumberger M. [Papillary and follicular thyroid carcinoma] [in French]. *Annales d'endocrinologie* 2007;68(2–3):120–8.
2. McLeod DS, Sawka AM, Cooper DS. Controversies in primary treatment of low-risk papillary thyroid cancer. *Lancet* 2013;381(9871):1046–57.
3. Simard EP, Ward EM, Siegel R, Jemal A. Cancers with increasing incidence trends in the United States: 1999 through 2008. *CA: A Cancer Journal for Clinicians* 2012;62(2):118–28.
4. Zevallos JP, Hartman CM, Kramer JR, Sturgis EM, Chiao EY. Increased thyroid cancer incidence corresponds to increased use of thyroid

ultrasound and fine-needle aspiration: a study of the Veterans Affairs health care system. *Cancer* 2015;121(5):741–46.

5. Rosen JE, Stone MD. Contemporary diagnostic approach to the thyroid nodule. *Journal of Surgical Oncology* 2006;94(8):649–61.

6. Yip L, Carty SE. Systematic screening after Chernobyl: insights on radiation-induced thyroid cancer. *Cancer* 2015;121(3):339–40.

7. Krikorian A, Kikano G. Thyroid nodules: when is an aggressive evaluation warranted? *Journal of Family Practice* 2012;61(4):205–8.

8. Zablotska LB, Nadyrov EA, Rozhko AV, Gong Z, Polyanskaya ON, McConnell RJ, et al. Analysis of thyroid malignant pathologic findings identified during 3 rounds of screening (1997–2008) of a cohort of children and adolescents from Belarus exposed to radioiodines after the Chernobyl accident. *Cancer* 2015;121(3):457–66.

9. Moses W, Weng J, Kebebew E. Prevalence, clinico-pathologic features, and somatic genetic mutation profile in familial versus sporadic nonmedullary thyroid cancer. *Thyroid* 2011;21(4):367–71.

10. Vriens MR, Suh I, Moses W, Kebebew E. Clinical features and genetic predisposition to hereditary nonmedullary thyroid cancer. *Thyroid* 2009;19(12):1343–9.

11. Kebebew E. Hereditary non-medullary thyroid cancer. *World Journal of Surgery* 2008;32(5):678–82.

12. Charkes ND. On the prevalence of familial nonmedullary thyroid cancer in multiply affected kindreds. *Thyroid* 2006;16(2):181–6.

13. Hemminki K, Eng C, Chen B. Familial risks for nonmedullary thyroid cancer. *Journal of Clinical Endocrinology and Metabolism* 2005;90(10):5747–53.

14. Malchoff CD, Malchoff DM. Familial nonmedullary thyroid carcinoma. *Cancer Control* 2006;13(2):106–10.

15. Nikiforova MN, Nikiforov YE. Molecular diagnostics and predictors in thyroid cancer. *Thyroid* 2009;19(12):1351–61.

16. Santoro M, Dathan NA, Berlingieri MT, Bongarzone I, Paulin C, Grieco M, et al. Molecular characterization of RET/PTC3: a novel rearranged version of the RET proto-oncogene in a human thyroid papillary carcinoma. *Oncogene* 1994;9(2):509–16.

17. Sugg SL, Ezzat S, Zheng L, Freeman JL, Rosen IB, Asa SL. Oncogene profile of papillary thyroid carcinoma. *Surgery* 1999;125(1):46–52.

18. Zhu Z, Gandhi M, Nikiforova MN, Fischer AH, Nikiforov YE. Molecular profile and clinical-pathologic features of the follicular variant of papillary thyroid carcinoma. An unusually high prevalence of ras mutations. *American Journal of Clinical Pathology* 2003;120(1):71–7.

19. Vasko V, Espinosa AV, Scouten W, He H, Auer H, Liyanarachchi S, et al. Gene expression and functional evidence of epithelial-to-mesenchymal transition in papillary thyroid carcinoma invasion. *Proceedings of the National Academy of Sciences of the United States of America* 2007;104(8):2803–8.

20. Xing M, Westra WH, Tufano RP, Cohen Y, Rosenbaum E, Rhoden KJ, et al. BRAF mutation predicts a poorer clinical prognosis for papillary thyroid cancer. *Journal of Clinical Endocrinology and Metabolism* 2005;90(12):6373–9.

21. Marques AR, Espadinha C, Catarino AL, Moniz S, Pereira T, Sobrinho LG, et al. Expression of PAX8-PPAR gamma 1 rearrangements in both follicular thyroid carcinomas and adenomas. *Journal of Clinical Endocrinology and Metabolism* 2002;87(8):3947–52.

22. Nikiforova MN, Lynch RA, Biddinger PW, Alexander EK, Dorn GW 2nd, Tallini G, et al. RAS point mutations and PAX8-PPAR gamma rearrangement in thyroid tumors: evidence for distinct molecular pathways in thyroid follicular carcinoma. *Journal of Clinical Endocrinology and Metabolism* 2003;88(5):2318–26.

23. Harb WJ, Sturgis EM. Differentiated thyroid cancer associated with intestinal polyposis syndromes: a review. *Head & Neck* 2009;31(11):1511–9.

24. Scollo C, Baudin E, Travagli JP, Caillou B, Bellon N, Leboulleux S, et al. Rationale for central and bilateral lymph node dissection in sporadic and hereditary medullary thyroid cancer. *Journal of Clinical Endocrinology and Metabolism* 2003;88(5):2070–5.

25. Lodish M. Multiple endocrine neoplasia type 2. *Frontiers of Hormone Research* 2013;41:16–29.

26. Mulligan LM, Kwok JB, Healey CS, Elsdon MJ, Eng C, Gardner E, et al. Germ-line mutations of the RET proto-oncogene in multiple endocrine neoplasia type 2A. *Nature* 1993;363(6428):458–60.

27. Hansford JR, Mulligan LM. Multiple endocrine neoplasia type 2 and RET: from neoplasia to neurogenesis. *Journal of Medical Genetics* 2000;37(11):817–27.

28. Kloos RT, Eng C, Evans DB, Francis GL, Gagel RF, Gharib H, et al. Medullary thyroid cancer: management guidelines of the American Thyroid Association. *Thyroid* 2009;19(6):565–612.

29. Jemal A, Siegel R, Ward E, Hao Y, Xu J, Thun MJ. Cancer statistics, 2009. *CA: A Cancer Journal for Clinicians* 2009;59(4):225–49.

30. Pacini F, Schlumberger M, Dralle H, Elisei R, Smit JW, Wiersinga W. European consensus for the management of patients with differentiated thyroid carcinoma of the follicular epithelium. *European Journal of Endocrinology* 2006;154(6):787–803.

31. Eustatia-Rutten CF, Corssmit EP, Biermasz NR, Pereira AM, Romijn JA, Smit JW. Survival and death causes in differentiated thyroid carcinoma. *Journal of Clinical Endocrinology and Metabolism* 2006;91(1):313–9.

32. Edge S, Labow D, Carduci M. *AJCC Cancer Staging Manual*. 7th ed. New York: Springer, 2010.

33. Lang BH, Lo CY, Chan WF, Lam KY, Wan KY. Staging systems for papillary thyroid carcinoma: a review and comparison. *Annals of Surgery* 2007;245(3):366–78.

34. Cooper DS, Doherty GM, Haugen BR, Kloos RT, Lee SL, Mandel SJ, et al. Revised American Thyroid Association management guidelines for patients with thyroid nodules and differentiated thyroid cancer. *Thyroid* 2009;19(11):1167–214.

35. Mevawalla N, McMullen T, Sidhu S, Sywak M, Robinson B, Delbridge L. Presentation of clinically solitary thyroid nodules in surgical patients. *Thyroid* 2011;21(1):55–9.

36. Kim HK, Yoon JH, Kim SJ, Cho JS, Kweon SS, Kang HC. Higher TSH level is a risk factor for differentiated thyroid cancer. *Clinical Endocrinology* 2013;78(3):472–7.

37. Moon WJ, Jung SL, Lee JH, Na DG, Baek JH, Lee YH, et al. Benign and malignant thyroid nodules: US differentiation – multicenter retrospective study. *Radiology* 2008;247(3):762–70.

38. Yoon DY, Chang SK, Choi CS, Yun EJ, Seo YL, Nam ES, et al. The prevalence and significance of incidental thyroid nodules identified on computed tomography. *Journal of Computer Assisted Tomography* 2008;32(5):810–5.

39. Tezelman S, Giles Y, Tunca F, Gok K, Poyanli A, Salmaslioglu A, et al. Diagnostic value of dynamic contrast medium enhanced magnetic resonance imaging in preoperative detection of thyroid carcinoma. *Archives of Surgery* 2007;142(11):1036–41.

40. Boeckmann J, Bartel T, Siegel E, Bodenner D, Stack BC Jr. Can the pathology of a thyroid nodule be determined by positron emission tomography uptake? *Otolaryngology – Head and Neck Surgery* 2012;146(6):906–12.

41. Bose S, Walts AE. Thyroid fine needle aspirate: a post-Bethesda update. *Advances in Anatomic Pathology* 2012;19(3):160–9.

42. Cibas ES, Ali SZ. The Bethesda system for reporting thyroid cytopathology. *Thyroid* 2009;19(11):1159–65.

43. Zheng X, Wei S, Han Y, Li Y, Yu Y, Yun X, et al. Papillary microcarcinoma of the thyroid: clinical characteristics and BRAF(V600E) mutational status of 977 cases. *Annals of Surgical Oncology* 2013;20(7):2266–73.

44. Xing M. BRAF mutation in papillary thyroid cancer: pathogenic role, molecular bases, and clinical implications. *Endocrine Reviews* 2007;28(7):742–62.

45. Yip L, Wharry LI, Armstrong MJ, Silbermann A, McCoy KL, Stang MT, et al. A clinical algorithm for fine-needle aspiration molecular testing effectively guides the appropriate extent of initial thyroidectomy. *Annals of Surgery* 2014;260(1):163–8.

46. Alexander EK, Kennedy GC, Baloch ZW, Cibas ES, Chudova D, Diggans J, et al. Preoperative diagnosis of benign thyroid nodules with indeterminate cytology. *New England Journal of Medicine* 2012;367(8):705–15.

47. McIver B, Castro MR, Morris JC, Bernet V, Smallridge R, Henry M, et al. An independent study of a gene expression classifier (afirma) in the evaluation of cytologically indeterminate thyroid nodules. *Journal of Clinical Endocrinology and Metabolism* 2014;99(11):4069–77.

48. Grant CS. Papillary thyroid cancer: strategies for optimal individualized surgical management. *Clinical Therapeutics* 2014;36(7):1117–26.

49. Hay ID, Bergstralh EJ, Goellner JR, Ebersold JR, Grant CS. Predicting outcome in papillary thyroid carcinoma: development of a reliable prognostic scoring system in a cohort of 1779 patients surgically treated at one institution during 1940 through 1989. *Surgery* 1993;114(6):1050–7; discussion 7–8.

50. Shah MD, Hall FT, Eski SJ, Witterick IJ, Walfish PG, Freeman JL. Clinical course of thyroid carcinoma after neck dissection. *Laryngoscope* 2003;113(12):2102–7.

51. Wang TS, Dubner S, Sznyter LA, Heller KS. Incidence of metastatic well-differentiated thyroid cancer in cervical lymph nodes. *Archives of Otolaryngology – Head & Neck Surgery* 2004;130(1):110–3.

52. Lin JD, Chao TC, Huang MJ, Weng HF, Tzen KY. Use of radioactive iodine for thyroid remnant ablation in well-differentiated thyroid carcinoma to replace thyroid reoperation. *American Journal of Clinical Oncology* 1998;21(1):77–81.

53. Mazzaferri EL. An overview of the management of papillary and follicular thyroid carcinoma. *Thyroid* 1999;9(5):421–7.

54. Ito Y, Miyauchi A, Kihara M, Higashiyama T, Kobayashi K, Miya A. Patient age is significantly related to the progression of papillary microcarcinoma of the thyroid under observation. *Thyroid* 2014;24(1):27–34.

55. Ito Y, Uruno T, Nakano K, Takamura Y, Miya A, Kobayashi K, et al. An observation trial without surgical treatment in patients with papillary microcarcinoma of the thyroid. *Thyroid* 2003;13(4):381–7.

56. Nilubol N, Kebebew E. Should small papillary thyroid cancer be observed? A population-based study. *Cancer* 2015;121(7):1017–24.

57. Callcut RA, Selvaggi SM, Mack E, Ozgul O, Warner T, Chen H. The utility of frozen section evaluation for follicular thyroid lesions. *Annals of Surgical Oncology* 2004;11(1):94–8.

58. Udelsman R, Westra WH, Donovan PI, Sohn TA, Cameron JL. Randomized prospective evaluation of frozen-section analysis for follicular neoplasms of the thyroid. *Annals of Surgery* 2001;233(5):716–22.

59. Keutgen XM, Filicori F, Fahey TJ 3rd. Molecular diagnosis for indeterminate thyroid nodules on fine needle aspiration: advances and limitations. *Expert Review of Molecular Diagnostics* 2013;13(6):613–23.

60. Filicori F, Keutgen XM, Buitrago D, AlDailami H, Crowley M, Fahey TJ 3rd, et al. Risk stratification of indeterminate thyroid fine-needle aspiration biopsy specimens based on mutation analysis. *Surgery* 2011;150(6):1085–91.

61. Carling T, Carty SE, Ciarleglio MM, Cooper DS, Doherty G, Kim LT, et al. American Thyroid Association (ATA) – design and feasibility of a prospective randomized controlled trial of prophylactic central lymph node dissection for papillary thyroid carcinoma. *Thyroid* 2012;22(3):237–44.

62. Balasubramanian SP, Brignall J, Lin HY, Stephenson TJ, Wadsley J, Harrison BJ, et al. Sentinel node biopsy in papillary thyroid cancer – what is the potential? *Langenbeck's Archives of Surgery* 2014;399(2):245–51.

63. Lim YC, Choi EC, Yoon YH, Koo BS. Occult lymph node metastases in neck level V in papillary thyroid carcinoma. *Surgery* 2010;147(2):241–5.

64. Pisanu A, Porceddu G, Podda M, Cois A, Uccheddu A. Systematic review with meta-analysis of studies comparing intraoperative neuromonitoring of recurrent laryngeal nerves versus visualization alone during thyroidectomy. *Journal of Surgical Research* 2014;188(1):152–61.

65. American Thyroid Association Guidelines Task Force, Kloos RT, Eng C, Evans DB, Francis GL, Gagel RF, et al. Medullary thyroid cancer: management guidelines of the American Thyroid Association. *Thyroid* 2009;19(6):565–612.

66. Blumhardt R, Wolin EA, Phillips WT, Salman UA, Walker RC, Stack BC Jr, et al. Current controversies in the initial post-surgical radioactive iodine therapy for thyroid cancer: a narrative review. *Endocrine-Related Cancer* 2014;21(6):R473–84.

67. Kushchayeva Y, Duh QY, Kebebew E, Clark OH. Prognostic indications for Hurthle cell cancer. *World Journal of Surgery* 2004;28(12):1266–70.

68. D'Avanzo A, Treseler P, Ituarte PH, Wong M, Streja L, Greenspan FS, et al. Follicular thyroid carcinoma: histology and prognosis. *Cancer* 2004;100(6):1123–9.

69. Goffredo P, Cheung K, Roman SA, Sosa JA. Can minimally invasive follicular thyroid cancer be approached as a benign lesion? A population-level analysis of survival among 1,200 patients. *Annals of Surgical Oncology* 2013;20(3):767–72.

70. Sugino K, Kameyama K, Ito K, Nagahama M, Kitagawa W, Shibuya H, et al. Outcomes and prognostic factors of 251 patients with minimally invasive follicular thyroid carcinoma. *Thyroid* 2012;22(8):798–804.

71. Smallridge RC, Ain KB, Asa SL, Bible KC, Brierley JD, Burman KD, et al. American Thyroid Association guidelines for management of patients with anaplastic thyroid cancer. *Thyroid* 2012;22(11):1104–39.

72. Elisei R, Schlumberger MJ, Muller SP, Schoffski P, Brose MS, Shah MH, et al. Cabozantinib in progressive medullary thyroid cancer. *Journal of Clinical Oncology* 2013;31(29):3639–46.

73. Wells SA Jr, Robinson BG, Gagel RF, Dralle H, Fagin JA, Santoro M, et al. Vandetanib in patients with locally advanced or metastatic medullary thyroid cancer: a randomized, double-blind phase III trial. *Journal of Clinical Oncology* 2012;30(2):134–41.

74. Krajewska J, Jarzab B. Novel therapies for thyroid cancer. Expert opinion on pharmacotherapy. *Expert Opinion on Pharmacotherapy* 2014;15(28):1–12.

43

Adrenal tumours

ATUL BAGUL AND SABA BALASUBRAMANIAN

ANATOMY AND PHYSIOLOGY OF THE ADRENAL GLAND

The adrenal glands are situated within a compartment of the renal fascia in relation to the upper poles of the kidneys. The right is smaller and triangular, and the left larger and crescentic. The right adrenal gland is located partially behind the inferior vena cava and superior to the right kidney, whereas the left adrenal is anteromedial to the left kidney.

The arterial blood supply for both glands arises from the abdominal aorta, the inferior phrenic artery and the renal artery. The venous drainage is mostly via the main adrenal vein that drains into the inferior vena cava on the right and the renal vein on the left side. Histologically, the adrenal gland is comprised of an outer cortex derived from mesoderm and an inner medulla derived from the neural crest, i.e. the ectoderm. Table 43.1 shows the hormones secreted by the various layers of the adrenal gland and their key regulatory mechanisms.

This chapter focuses on adrenal malignancies with a brief mention of functioning adenomas and incidentalomas. The medical management of patients with functioning tumours, adrenal hyperplasia or paediatric adrenal tumours is beyond the scope of this chapter.

EPIDEMIOLOGY

Adrenal gland tumours arise from the cortex or the medulla and can be benign or malignant, the latter being either primary or secondary. Tumours may be functioning or non-functioning (Table 43.2). Functioning tumours secrete hormones which either may present as specific clinical syndromes or are diagnosed on biochemical testing (subclinical tumours). Hypofunction (adrenal insufficiency) may occasionally be the presenting feature of bilateral adrenal metastases.

Adrenal tumours are relatively rare in comparison with tumours in other organs. Incidentally detected tumours of the adrenal gland (incidentalomas) are on the increase with the increased use of cross-sectional imaging such as computed tomography (CT) and magnetic resonance imaging (MRI). Incidentalomas are present in approximately 2.1% of individuals from autopsy series and the incidence rises with age [1].

Cushing's syndrome (all causes) affects mainly adults aged 20–50 years with an incidence of 2.5 per million population per year [2]. The incidence of Conn's syndrome is around 0.8 per million per year [3], and the incidence of pheochromocytomas ranges from 1.55 to 1.9 per million per year [3,4].

Adrenocortical carcinoma (ACC) is a rare tumour with reported age-adjusted incidence rates of 0.72–2 persons per million population per year [5–7]. ACC typically has a bimodal age distribution in the first and fourth decades of life. At the time of diagnosis, only 30% of these malignancies are confined to the adrenal gland [8,9]. Adrenal tumours can be sporadic or familial. Although no environmental risk factors have been identified, genetic predisposition may

Table 43.1 Hormones secreted by the various layers of the adrenal gland and their principal regulatory mechanisms

Adrenal gland	Hormones	Regulation
Cortex		
Zona glomerulosa (15%)	Aldosterone	Renin–angiotensin system
Zona reticularis (70%)	Cortisol, sex steroids	ACTH (negative feedback mechanism)
Zona fasciculata (15%)	Sex steroids	ACTH (negative feedback mechanism)
Medulla		
	Catecholamines and metabolites	As part of the autonomic nervous system

Table 43.2 Adrenal tumours or tumour-like lesions

Adrenal cortex
Adenomas – functioning and non-functioning
Adrenocortical carcinoma – functioning and non-functioning

Adrenal medulla
Pheochromocytoma – benign and malignant
Ganglioneuroma, ganglioneuroblastoma and neuroblastoma

Miscellaneous
Adrenal metastases
Cysts
Hematomas
Myelolipomas
Other rare tumours

Table 43.3 Familial syndromes associated with adrenal lesions

Adrenal tumour	Syndrome	Chromosomal defect
Adrenocortical	Carney's syndrome	Defects in Ch 2p16 and PRKARIA gene in Ch 17q22
	Congenital adrenal hyperplasia	Defect in 21-hydroxylase gene on Ch 6p21.3
	Li–Fraumeni syndrome	Defect in TP53 gene in Ch 17q13
	McCune–Albright syndrome	Defect in GNAS1 gene in Ch 20q13
	MEN type I	Defect in Menin gene in Ch 11q13
	Beckwith–Wiedemann syndrome	Defects in Ch 11p15
Pheochromocytoma	von Hippel–Lindau type II	Defect in VHL gene in Ch 3p25–26
	MEN type II	Defect in RET gene in Ch 10q11.2
	Neurofibromatosis type I	Defect in NF1 gene in Ch 17q11.2
	Paraganglioma syndromes	Defects in mitochondrial genes SDHB (Ch 1p36.13) SDHD (Ch 11q23)

Note: Ch = chromosome.

underlie a significant proportion of them. Familial syndromes associated with an increased risk of cortical and medullary tumours are shown in Table 43.3. Most cancers occur in people with no family history.

PRESENTATION

Hormonal effects

Clinical effects of hormones secreted by the tumour include hyperaldosteronism, hypercortisolism, pheochromocytoma and virilizing or feminizing features. Around 80% of adrenocortical malignancies present with evidence of steroid hormone excess (Table 43.4) [10,11].

Primary hyperaldosteronism results from excess secretion of aldosterone from the adrenal cortex. This usually arises either from an adenoma (Conn's syndrome) or from bilateral adrenal hyperplasia. Rare causes include unilateral adrenal hyperplasia, ACC and glucocorticoid-suppressible hyperaldosteronism. In patients with hypertension, careful screening will demonstrate primary hyperaldosteronism in 5–13%, of which aldosterone-producing adenoma is the cause in about 28% [12]. The only specific clinical feature is hypertension. Biochemical findings include raised plasma aldosteronism, low plasma renin activity, hypokalemia, hypernatremia and alkalosis.

Hypercortisolism results from excess secretion of cortisol from the adrenal cortex. The excess secretion can be adrenocorticotropic hormone (ACTH) dependent (excess ACTH secretion from the pituitary [in 70%] when it is referred to as Cushing's disease) or ectopic sites (in 15%) or ACTH independent (in 15%). The latter are usually due to adrenal adenomas or carcinomas but can rarely be due to bilateral hyperplasia, primary pigmented nodular adrenal disease

Table 43.4 Symptoms attributable to hormone excess in functional adrenal tumours

Aldosterone excess
Excessive thirst
Frequent urination
High blood pressure
Muscle cramp
Weakness

Cortisol excess
Depression
Easy bruising
Fat behind neck and shoulders
Hair growth
Irregular periods
Weakness in legs
Weight gain around chest and abdomen
  (central obesity)

Estrogen excess
Gynecomastia
Early puberty in girls
Lack of sex drive and impotence

Testosterone excess
Deepening voice
Acne
Excessive growth of facial and body hair
Increased muscle mass
Irregular periods

(Carney's complex) or McCune–Albright syndrome [13]. Clinical features include abnormal fat deposition, myopathy, fragile skin with easy bruising and poor healing, osteopenia, hypertension, diabetes, psychological symptoms, reduced libido, menstrual irregularities and hirsutism in women and growth retardation in children.

Pheochromocytoma arises from the adrenal medulla or extra-adrenal chromaffin tissue resulting in the hypersecretion of catecholamines and their metabolites. They may be asymptomatic or present as cardiovascular syndromes (such as myocardial infarction, arrhythmias and uncontrolled hypertension), cerebrovascular events, panic attacks, anxiety and occasionally hyperglycemia. Previously undiagnosed pheochromocytoma may be incidentally detected at abdominal surgery. No attempt should be made to excise the pheochromocytoma in a pharmacologically unprepared patient. Pheochromocytoma is rarely encountered in pregnancy or labour when it may be confused with other hypertensive syndromes related to pregnancy. Delayed diagnosis can adversely affect both mother and fetus [14].

Virilizing and feminizing tumours of the adrenal gland are extremely uncommon and often associated with raised levels of other hormones such as cortisol. They are almost always symptomatic and malignant.

Local symptoms

The vast majority of adrenal tumours are not associated with any local or abdominal symptoms. Some malignant tumours can infiltrate the retroperitoneum and adjacent organs and present with haemorrhage, local pressure symptoms such as pain or organ-specific symptoms from metastases.

Incidental lesions

Adrenal lesions (Table 43.2) are often detected as an incidental finding during investigation of other abdominal pathology (incidentalomas). The prevalence of such lesions ranges from 0.1% during general health screening with ultrasound to 4.3% in cancer patients. These lesions become increasingly common with age, with a prevalence of 7% in patients aged 70 and above [1]. The reported incidence of functioning tumours in adrenal incidentalomas varies widely due to variation in the extent of biochemical screening. A prospective study of patients from 33 hospitals in Sweden showed that 5% of lesions in 381 patients were hormonally active [15].

SCREENING AND DIAGNOSTIC STRATEGIES

Screening

The rarity of adrenal malignancies and the relative abundance of incidental benign lesions make adrenal cancer and pheochromocytoma unsuitable diseases for general population screening. Screening by abdominal CT and biochemical testing may be appropriate for those proven to be gene carriers of familial syndromes described in Table 43.3.

Diagnosis

Biochemical testing is mandatory in the evaluation of all adrenal masses. This will confirm a suspected clinical diagnosis, detect subclinical hormonal syndromes, obtain baseline hormonal levels in patients with functioning tumours and help confirm biochemical cure after surgery and detect recurrence.

1. **Cushing's syndrome:** Biochemical tests for the confirmation of hypercortisolism include measurement of urinary-free cortisol, midnight plasma or late-night salivary cortisol and low-dose (overnight and 48-h) dexamethasone suppression test. The cause of hypercortisolism is determined by measuring plasma ACTH, a corticotropin-releasing hormone (CRH) test and sometimes a high-dose dexamethasone suppression test [12].

2. **Pheochromocytoma:** Urine and plasma catecholamines (epinephrine and norepinephrine) and their metabolites (metanephrine, normetanephrine and vanillylmandelic acid) are commonly measured. Plasma-free metanephrines have been shown to be a highly accurate test for the diagnosis of pheochromocytoma [16].

3. **Conn's syndrome:** In patients with hypertension, serum potassium, plasma aldosterone levels and renin activity are measured to diagnose hyperaldosteronism. A raised ratio of plasma aldosterone concentration to plasma renin activity is a sensitive test for autonomous aldosterone production [10].

4. **Sex hormone-secreting tumours:** Serum levels of dehydroepiandrosterone (DHEA), 17-OH-progesterone, androstenedione, testosterone and 17-OH-estradiol are measured in patients with feminizing or virilizing syndromes.

Many of these tests have a normal range, a borderline range and a clearly abnormal range. The tests have differing sensitivities and specificities depending on the threshold level chosen. Performing more than one test for a suspected hormonal excess or insufficiency may often help in securing a biochemical diagnosis. It is important to keep in mind that several variables such as drugs and dietary factors influence the results of these tests and that repeat measurements are often of value in borderline scenarios. Interested readers are referred to other sources for detailed information on these and additional tests [1,12,13,16–18].

Cross-sectional imaging is essential to confirm the adrenal abnormality, laterality and size, to identify obvious malignant features, and to monitor for recurrence after initial treatment in those with cancer. In patients with an incidentaloma, adrenal cancer accounts for 2% of tumours that are 4 cm or less, 6% of tumours 4.1–6 cm and 25% of tumours >6 cm. CT scan is the currently preferred modality for the diagnosis and characterization of adrenal tumours (Figure 43.1). Density measurements on non-contrast CT and enhancement patterns on contrast and delayed washout images are all important in the characterization of adrenal

tumours. MRI is as effective as CT scan and can be used to evaluate lesions that are indeterminate on CT.

Findings suggestive of malignancy include invasion into adjacent structures, associated lymphadenopathy, the presence of metastases, irregular tumour margins, heterogeneity and more than 10 Hounsfield units on CT scan. MRI features of malignancy also include reduced fat content, isointensity to the liver on T1-weighted images, intermediate to moderate intensity on T2-weighted images, and enhancement after gadolinium contrast with slow washout [10].

Functional imaging using iodine-123 metaiodobenzylguanidine (MIBG) scanning is useful in the detection of pheochromocytomas (Figure 43.2) with a reported sensitivity and specificity of 91% and 100%, respectively [19]. It is strongly recommended in those at high risk of extraadrenal disease. This includes those with a family history of pheochromocytoma, suggestive of familial syndromes associated with pheochromocytoma and a large adrenal tumour (>5 cm) [18].

Localization tests such as selective venous catheterization of the adrenal veins for differential determination of the aldosterone–cortisol ratio can help in differentiating between

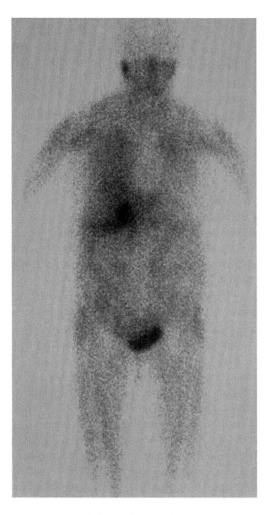

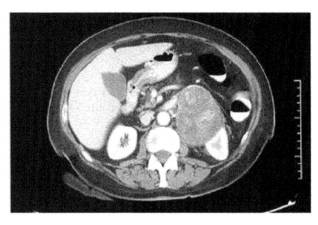

Figure 43.1 A cross-sectional CT image showing a heterogeneous adrenal tumour on the left side. Histology confirmed adrenocortical cancer.

Figure 43.2 Metaiodobenzyl-guanidine (MIBG) scan showing increased uptake on the right side in a patient with right adrenal pheochromocytoma.

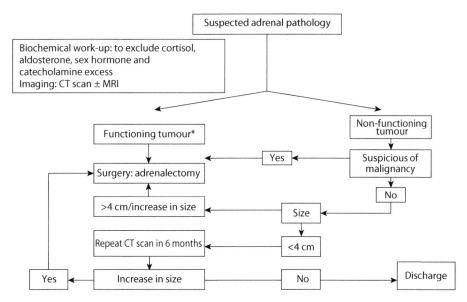

*The management of subclinical Cushing's syndrome and medically treated Conn's adenomas is controversial. Some of these patients may need further studies such as adrenal venous sampling to differentiate between single-gland and bilateral disease.

Figure 43.3 A suggested approach for diagnosis and treatment of adrenal gland tumours without evidence of extra-adrenal disease.

unilateral and bilateral Conn's disease. This is useful in patients with a high probability of an aldosterone-producing adenoma but with equivocal findings of unilateral disease on CT scan [12].

Biopsy of adrenal tumours is rarely indicated in the management of adrenal tumours and should never be undertaken on retroperitoneal lesions in the region of the adrenal gland without ruling out a pheochromocytoma by biochemical testing. Comprehensive biochemical and imaging evaluation gives sufficient information for appropriate management in the vast majority of cases. Functioning tumours and those with a high risk of malignancy (>4 cm) need surgical excision and small non-functioning tumours can be observed safely. Relative indications for percutaneous biopsy, however, include large retroperitoneal tumours of uncertain origin, a non-functioning adrenal mass in a patient previously treated for cancer, and therapeutic aspiration of cysts [20].

A pragmatic algorithm for the initial investigation and treatment of the adrenal mass in patients without evidence of extra-adrenal disease is shown in Figure 43.3. This algorithm is only a guide that needs to be tailored to local facilities and expertise. Interpretation of the results of diagnostic tests and planning appropriate treatment require multidisciplinary input from a team comprising surgeons, endocrinologists, biochemists and radiologists.

SURGERY

Indications

Adrenalectomy is indicated for masses with biochemical or radiological features suggestive of malignancy, in masses of more than 4 cm in diameter and in functioning tumours [21–23]. Long-term cost benefits over medical

therapy have also been demonstrated for patients with Conn's syndrome [24], where the main objective is control of blood pressure and avoidance of side effects of medication. The indications for surgery are less certain in patients with subclinical Cushing's syndrome with small tumours and Conn's syndrome with well-controlled blood pressure. Small non-functioning lesions, asymptomatic adrenal cysts and myelolipomas may be managed conservatively.

Perioperative management

Perioperative medical management of these patients in collaboration with medical endocrinologists and anaesthetists is essential for a good outcome. Table 43.5 outlines the issues for consideration for any patient undergoing adrenalectomy. Informed written consent prior to surgery should include the risk of conversion to open surgery, injury to adjacent intra-abdominal viscera, the risk of residual and recurrent disease, major bleeding, wound and intra-abdominal infection, and general complications associated with major surgery such as chest infection, cardio-respiratory problems, venous thromboembolism and the occasional need for management in a high dependency or intensive care unit.

Laparoscopic versus open adrenalectomy

Various surgical approaches are available for adrenalectomy (Table 43.6). The choice of operation depends on whether the disease is unilateral or bilateral, the size of tumour, risk of malignancy, other abdominal disease or previous surgery, body habitus and most importantly the surgeon's expertise. Several observational studies have demonstrated the safety and efficacy of the laparoscopic approach. Immediate benefits include reduction in postoperative pain, blood loss, and

Table 43.5 Issues to consider in patients undergoing adrenal surgery

General considerations

Perioperative thromboprophylaxis (especially in those with hypercortisolism)

Critical care facilities in the early postoperative period (especially in phaeochromocytoma)

Availability of cross-matched blood

Appropriate postoperative tests to confirm biochemical cure

Phaeochromocytoma

Gradual increase of alpha-blockers to ensure maximum preoperative alpha-blockade

Beta-blockers (if needed) only after adequate prior alpha-blockade

Adequate preoperative hydration to prevent postoperative hypotension

Intensive intra- and postoperative monitoring of blood pressure

Monitoring and treatment of postoperative hypoglycemia

Cushing's syndrome

Perioperative steroid supplementation to prevent relative adrenal insufficiency

Ensure adequate function by the other adrenal gland (by basal cortisol or synacthen test) before stopping steroids postoperatively

Conn's syndrome

Stop aldosterone antagonists postoperatively and withdrawal of other anti-hypertensive agents in accordance with local protocols

Table 43.6 Surgical approaches to the adrenal gland

Laparoscopic approach

Transperitoneal
    Anterior
    Lateral
Retroperitoneal
    Lateral
    Posterior

Open approach

Anterior
Posterior
Thoracoabdominal

wound infection, reduced hospitalization, and early return to normal activity. The laparoscopic approach is now the preferred approach for all benign adrenal tumours [17] and can be considered suitable for tumours up to 7–8 cm in size. For tumours with a high likelihood of being malignant, the open approach is recommended due to oncological concerns regarding clearance and the risk of tumour seeding due to capsular rupture and tumour spillage during laparoscopy, increasing the risk of local recurrence [25].

A hand-assisted laparoscopic approach enables direct handling and excision of larger tumours, preserving some of the benefits of laparoscopy for these lesions. A thoracoabdominal approach may sometimes be required for excision of very large lesions [8].

Transperitoneal and retroperitoneal approaches

The transperitoneal approach may be anterior or lateral; the retroperitoneal approach may be posterior or lateral. The transperitoneal approach with the patient in lateral position is most commonly used [24] and has advantages of a larger working space and easily identifiable landmarks. The retroperitoneal approach, however, is said to be associated with shorter hospital stay and earlier recovery. This is especially true when the procedure is performed by experienced surgeons in large-volume centres [25,26]. Two randomized controlled trials comparing the retroperitoneal and transperitoneal laparoscopic approaches did not find any significant difference in important clinical outcomes [27,28]. The retroperitoneal approach is, however, useful in those with previous intra-abdominal surgery (avoids adhesions and reopening scarred planes) and those undergoing bilateral adrenalectomy (avoids need for repositioning).

The key steps in laparoscopic adrenalectomy include correct positioning of the patient and port placement. In the transperitoneal approach, careful mobilization of the liver on the right side and the spleen with the tail of the pancreas on the left side is important. In the retroperitoneal approach, high insufflation pressures (20 to 28 mmHg) are considered crucial not only to improve exposure but also to minimize bleeding from small vessels [25]. Meticulous dissection along avascular planes and early identification and division of major feeding vessels facilitate safe mobilization of the gland. During the operation, it is important to avoid grasping the tumour or adrenal gland and leaving behind remnants of adrenal tissue to reduce the risk of persistent or recurrent disease.

MALIGNANT TUMOURS OF THE ADRENAL GLAND

Adrenocortical cancer

Most patients with ACC (~80%) present with clinical or biochemical evidence of hormonal excess [28], often mixed. Non-functioning cancers may present with abdominal or back pain, with or without systemic symptoms of fever, weight loss and anorexia.

The diagnosis of ACC is sometimes suspected preoperatively on the basis of imaging findings, but is usually confirmed by histology following an adrenalectomy. The distinction between benign and malignant adrenal tumours on histology may be difficult. Malignant potential is indicated by the presence of three or more [29,30] of nine histological features (Table 43.7). Broad fibrous bands are also a characteristic feature of malignant adrenocortical tumours [10].

STAGING

For adrenocortical cancers, the Macfarlane staging system, initially proposed in 1958 and later modified by Sullivan and

Table 43.7 Histological criteria of malignancy in adrenocortical lesions

High nuclear grade
High mitotic rate (>5/50 high power fields)
Atypical mitoses
Clear cells comprising ≤25% of the tumour
Diffuse architecture (≥33% of tumour)
Microscopic necrosis
Venous invasion
Sinusoidal invasion
Capsular invasion

Table 43.8 TNM system

Tumour (T)
T1	Tumour ≤5 cm in size, invasion absent
T2	Tumour >5 cm in size, invasion absent
T3	Tumour locally invasive not involving adjacent organs
T4	Tumour invading adjacent organs

Nodes (N)
N0	No nodal involvement
N1	Involvement of regional lymph nodes

Metastases (M)
M0	No metastases
M1	Metastases present

Table 43.9 Comparison of the TNM and Macfarlane stagings for adrenocortical cancer

Macfarlane staging	Description of the Macfarlane staging	TNM
I	<5 cm, confined to the adrenal gland	T1N0M0
II	>5 cm, confined to the adrenal gland	T2N0M0
III	Involvement of lymph nodes or tumour extending beyond the adrenal gland but without metastases	T1N1M0 T2N1M0 T3N0M0
IV	Tumour extending beyond the adrenal gland with lymph node involvement or distant metastases	T3N1M0 T4N1M0 Any T Any N, M1

colleagues [31] along with a proposed TNM system [28], is generally used (Table 43.8). Table 43.9 compares the two systems.

TREATMENT

Adrenalectomy is the recommended treatment for stage I and II tumours. For patients with a clear preoperative diagnosis of malignancy, open surgery with en bloc resection of the adrenal gland and any enlarged lymph nodes offers the best chance of achieving R0 resection and thereby cure. Concomitant lymphadenectomy, nephrectomy and rarely liver resection may sometimes be necessary (Figure 43.4).

Rupture of the tumour capsule during surgery is associated with a high rate of local recurrence. Extension of tumour into the inferior vena cava (Figure 43.5) is not considered a metastatic disease and complete removal should be attempted [32]. The value of surgical treatment in stage III or IV disease remains controversial [8]. R0 resection in stage III patients may confer some survival benefit; however,

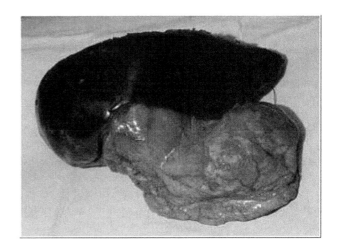

Figure 43.4 En bloc resection of the adrenal gland, kidney and segments 5, 6 and 7 of the liver for locally advanced adrenocortical cancer on the right side.

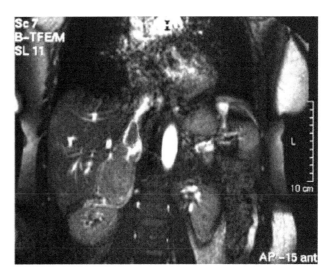

Figure 43.5 MRI (coronal section) showing right adrenocortical cancer invading into the inferior vena cava.

debulking or palliative resection does not influence survival [33,34].

For patients with local recurrence, there is evidence that repeat resection (if complete) may improve survival [34]. Resection of solitary metastasis may be indicated in the absence of diffuse metastatic disease or major vessel involvement [35]. Adrenocortical tumours are generally considered resistant to radiotherapy. Radiotherapy, however, can result in an objective reduction in tumour bulk in unresectable disease, and is effective in the palliation of symptoms [8]. Adjuvant radiotherapy in patients with stage III or high-risk stage II patients has been shown in small case series to improve local control [10,36].

The only organ-specific chemotherapeutic drug in adrenocortical cancer is mitotane (o,p′-DDD), which suppresses adrenal steroid secretion and causes necrosis of adrenal tissue. Although mitotane controls excess tumoural hormone secretion in the majority of patients, reduction in tumour bulk occurs in only 25% [37]. Optimal response occurs at blood mitotane concentrations above 14 mg/ml [38], but this is tempered by significant gastrointestinal (nausea, vomiting, anorexia and diarrhea) and neurological side effects (lethargy, depression and somnolence).

Supraphysiological doses of glucocorticoid replacement are necessary as mitotane induces steroid insufficiency and increases metabolic clearance of exogenous steroids [10]. Although mitotane is often used in metastatic disease in an attempt to control the syndrome of hormone excess [37] and to prolong survival [39], its efficacy as an adjuvant agent is doubtful, although a recent retrospective review of 177 patients suggested an improvement in recurrence-free survival [40]. The use of single agents (cisplatin, suramin and gossypol) and combined chemotherapy regimens with or without mitotane has been reported in small case series.

Phase II studies of two combination regimens (etoposide, doxorubicin, cisplatin and mitotane in one and streptozocin and mitotane in another) in unresectable adrenocortical cancer showed measurable reduction in tumour bulk in 48.6% [41] and 36% [42], respectively. Patients with advanced disease under consideration for chemotherapy should be enrolled in clinical trials for objective assessment of response and effectiveness.

A multinational phase III randomized control trial (FIRM-ACT: First International Randomized Trial in Locally Advanced and Metastatic Adrenocortical Carcinoma Treatment) compared mitotane, doxorubicin, etoposide and cisplatin (EDP-M) in one arm to mitotane and streptozotocin (Sz-M) in the other [43]. The trial included a total of 304 patients and compared these regimes, as both first- and second-line treatments. Although overall survival was not significantly different (14.8 and 12 months, respectively), objective response rate and progression-free survival clearly favoured the EDP-M arm. Given these data and the comparable rates of serious adverse events and quality of life in these groups, most experts now advocate EDP-M as first-line therapy for patients requiring cytotoxic treatment [44]. Adrenostatic drugs such as ketoconazole, metyrapone or etomidate are occasionally used in patients symptomatic from hormone excess uncontrolled by mitotane treatment alone [10].

Interested readers are referred to a detailed review on this topic for further information [44].

OUTCOMES

For adrenocortical cancer, large series have quoted overall 5-year survival rates of between 22 and 23% [45,46] in the late 1980s, and 37–38% more recently [47,48]. Although the exact reason for this improvement is unclear, this may be due to the increasing use of mitotane or the increasing proportion of smaller tumours in the more recent series. The role of adjuvant treatments in improving outcomes in this cohort is unclear [49,50]. The international randomized ADIUVO trial (www.adiuvo-trial.org) comparing mitotane with a strategy of watchful waiting in patients who have had a complete resection is currently ongoing.

PROGNOSTIC FACTORS

Early stage and curative resection of adrenocortical cancer is a key determinant of survival [5]. However, at the time of diagnosis, only 35% of ACC are confined to the adrenal. Metastases commonly occur in the liver, lungs, bone and retroperitoneal lymph nodes. Most patients with metastases at diagnosis die within 1 year [8]. Tumour size and age are other prognostic factors; smaller tumours [51] and young age [8] favour a better outcome. A short duration between onset of symptoms and diagnosis [8] and a low mitotic rate [45] are also associated with a good prognosis.

Malignant pheochromocytoma

Malignancy in pheochromocytoma ranges from 11.6 to 23% [52–54] in large series. As with adrenocortical cancer, there are no absolute histological criteria to differentiate between benign and malignant pheochromocytomas. Malignancy is diagnosed when there is clear evidence of local invasion into periadrenal tissues or metastatic spread in non-chromaffin tissue. The common sites of metastases include bone, lung, liver and lymph nodes. Clinical features associated with an increased risk of malignancy are abdominal pain, a short history, large (>5 cm) tumours, extra-adrenal location, patients with succinate dehydrogenase complex subunit B (SDHB) mutations, persistent postoperative hypertension, and raised plasma and urinary dopamine and dihydroxyphenylalanine [16,52,53].

Histological features associated with malignancy include confluent tumour necrosis, presence of vascular invasion, intracytoplasmic hyaline globules [55] and S100 positive sustentacular cells [56]. It is important to note that local capsular or vascular invasion does not in isolation predict malignant behaviour. All patients with pheochromocytomas require lifelong surveillance due to the difficulty in differentiating between benign and malignant tumours. There are no staging classifications for malignant pheochromocytomas.

TREATMENT AND OUTCOMES

Radical surgery is the mainstay of treatment and due to the rarity of the condition, there are few large studies on other forms of treatment. Alpha-blockers can be used for symptomatic relief. In a review of 116 patients with malignant pheochromocytomas treated in 24 different centres, treatment with iodine-131-MIBG was found to result in symptomatic improvement in 76% of patients and objective reduction in tumour bulk in 30%.

A survival benefit was seen in responders [57]. Combination chemotherapy with cyclophosphamide, vincristine and dacarbazine is associated with response rates of 57% [58] but the benefit on survival is unclear. The 5-year survival rate for malignant pheochromocytomas after surgery was 20% in a small series of 10 patients [52].

Adrenal metastases

In a series of 1000 consecutive autopsies in patients with cancer, adrenal metastases were demonstrated present in 27% of cases [59]. Clinical presentation occurs usually in three different ways: during staging investigations for cancer, incidentalomas and local pressure effects. The latter group is rare and only accounted for 4% in a series of 464 patients [60]. In a series of patients who underwent surgery for incidentalomas, a past history of cancer increases the likelihood of the lesion being metastatic to 52% [61]. The most common primary cancers that metastasize to the adrenal gland are lung cancer, followed by stomach, esophagus and liver or bile ducts cancers [60,62]. Usually, the primary site is apparent and the disease is widespread. Retrospective observational data suggest that adrenalectomy may benefit some patients with an isolated metastasis [63,64].

REFERENCES

1. Grumbach MM, Biller BM, Braunstein GD, et al. Management of the clinically inapparent adrenal mass ("incidentaloma"). *Ann Intern Med* 2003; 138: 424–9.
2. Lindholm J, Juul S, Jorgensen JO, et al. Incidence and late prognosis of Cushing's syndrome: a population-based study. *J Clin Endocrinol Metab* 2001; 86: 117–23.
3. Andersen GS, Toftdahl DB, Lund JO, et al. The incidence rate of phaeochromocytoma and Conn's syndrome in Denmark, 1977–1981. *J Hum Hypertens* 1988; 2: 187–9.
4. Hartley L, Perry-Keene D. Phaeochromocytoma in Queensland – 1970–83. *Aust N Z J Surg* 1985; 55: 471–5.
5. Soreide JA, Brabrand K, Thoresen SO. Adrenal cortical carcinoma in Norway, 1970–1984. *World J Surg* 1992; 16: 663–7.
6. Bilimoria KY, Shen WT, Elaraj D, et al. Adrenocortical carcinoma in the United States: treatment utilization and prognostic factors. *Cancer* 2008; 113(11): 3130–6.
7. Kerkhofs TM, Verhoeven RH, Van der Zwan JM, et al. Adrenocortical carcinoma: a population-based study on incidence and survival in the Netherlands since 1993. *Eur J Cancer* 2013; 49: 2579–86.
8. Wajchenberg BL, Albergaria Pereira MA, Medonca BB, et al. Adrenocortical carcinoma: clinical and laboratory observations. *Cancer* 2000; 88: 711–36.
9. Fassnacht M, Allolio B. Epidemiology of adrenocortical carcinoma. In Hammer GD, Else T, eds., *Adrenocortical Carcinoma: Basic Science and Clinical Concepts.* New York: Springer, 2010: 23–29.
10. Allolio B, Fassnacht M. Adrenocorticl carcinoma: clinical update. *J Clin Endocrinol Metab* 2006; 91: 2027–37.
11. Allolio B, Fassnacht M. Clinical presentation and initial diagnosis In Hammer GD, Else T, eds., *Adrenocortical Carcinoma: Basic Science and Clinical Concepts.* New York: Springer, 2010: 31–47.
12. Young WF Jr. Minireview: primary aldosteronism changing concepts in diagnosis and treatment. *Endocrinology* 2003; 144: 2208–13.
13. Newell-Price J, Bertagna X, Grossman AB, Nieman LK. Cushing's syndrome. *Lancet* 2006; 367: 1605–17.
14. Potts JM, Larrimer J. Pheochromocytoma in a pregnant patient. *J Fam Pract* 1994; 38: 289–93.
15. Bulow B, Ahren B. Adrenal incidentaloma – experience of a standardized diagnostic programme in the Swedish prospective study. *J Intern Med* 2002; 252: 239–46.
16. Lenders JW, Pacak K, Walther MM, et al. Biochemical diagnosis of pheochromocytoma: which test is best? *JAMA* 2002; 287: 1427–34.
17. Nieman LK, Ilias I. Evaluation and treatment of Cushing's syndrome. *Am J Med* 2005; 118: 1340–6.
18. Lenders JW, Eisenhofer G, Mannelli M, Pacak K. Phaeochromocytoma. *Lancet* 2005; 366: 665–75.
19. Lumachi F, Tregnagh A, Zucchetta P, et al. Sensitivity and positive predictive value of CT, MRI and 123I-MIBG scintigraphy in localizing pheochromocytomas: a prospective study. *Nucl Med Commun* 2006; 27: 583–7.
20. Neri LM, Nance FC. Management of adrenal cysts. *Am Surg* 1999; 65: 151–63.
21. Sywak M, Pasieka JL. Long-term follow-up and cost benefit of adrenalectomy in patients with primary hyperaldosteronism. *Br J Surg* 2002; 89: 1587–93.
22. Shen WT, Sturgeon C, Duh QY. From incidentaloma to adrenocortical carcinoma: the surgical management of adrenal tumours. *J Surg Oncol* 2005; 89: 186–92.
23. Gonzalez RJ, Shapiro S, Sarlis N, et al. Laparoscopic resection of adrenal cortical carcinoma: a cautionary note. *Surgery* 2005; 138: 1078–85.
24. Assalia A, Gagner M. Laparoscopic adrenalectomy. *Br J Surg* 2004; 91: 1259–74.

25. Walz MK, Alesina PF, Wenger FA, et al. Posterior retroperitoneoscopic adrenalectomy result of 560 procedures in 520 patients. *Surgery* 2000; 140(6): 943–8; discussion 948–50.

26. Fernandez-Cruz L, Saenz A, Benarroch G, et al. Laparoscopic unilateral and bilateral adrenalectomy for Cushing's syndrome. Transperitoneal and retroperitoneal approaches. *Ann Surg* 1996; 224: 727–34.

27. Rubinstein M, Gill TS, Aron M, et al. Prospective, randomized comparison of transperitoneal versus retroperitoneal laparoscopic adrenalectomy. *J Urol* 2005; 174: 442–5.

28. Norton JA. Adrenal tumours. In DeVita VTJ, Hellman S, Rosenberg SA, eds., *Cancer: Principles and Practice of Oncology*, 7th ed. Philadelphia: Lippincott Williams and Wilkins, 2005: 1528–39.

29. Weiss LM. Comparative histologic study of 43 metastasizing and nonmetastasizing adrenocortical tumours. *Am J Surg Pathol* 1984; 8: 163–9.

30. Medeiros LJ, Weiss LM. New developments in the pathologic diagnosis of adrenal cortical neoplasms. A review. *Am J Clin Pathol* 1992; 97: 73–83.

31. Sullivan M, Boileau M, Hodges CV. Adrenal cortical carcinoma. *J Urol* 1978; 120: 660–5.

32. Chiche L, Dousset B, Kieffer E, Chapuis Y. Adrenocortical carcinoma extending into the inferior vena cava: presentation of a 15-patient series and review of the literature. *Surgery* 2006; 139: 15–27.

33. Henley DJ, van Heerden JA, Grant CS, et al. Adrenal cortical carcinoma – a continuing challenge. *Surgery* 1983; 94: 926–31.

34. Causeret S, Monneuse O, Mabrut JY, et al. [Adrenocortical carcinoma: prognostic factors for local recurrence and indications for reoperation. A report on a series of 22 patients] [in French]. *Ann Chir* 2002; 127: 370–7.

35. Schulick RD, Brennan MF. Long-term survival after complete resection and repeat resection in patients with adrenocortical carcinoma. *Ann Surg Oncol* 1999; 6: 719–26.

36. Markoe AM, Serber W, Micaily B, et al. Radiation therapy for adjunctive treatment of adrenal cortical carcinoma. *Am J Clin Oncol* 1991; 14: 170–4.

37. Hahner S, Fassnacht M. Mitotane for adrenocortical carcinoma treatment. *Curr Opin Investig Drug* 2005; 6: 386–94.

38. Haak HR, Hermans J, van de Velde CJ, et al. Optimal treatment of adrenocortical carcinoma with mitotane: results in a consecutive series of 96 patients. *Br J Cancer* 1994; 69: 947–51.

39. Ilias I, Alevizaki M, Philippou G, et al. Sustained remission of metastatic adrenal carcinoma during long-term administration of low-dose mitotane. *J Endocrinol Invest* 2001; 24: 532–5.

40. Terzolo M, Angeli A, Fassnacht M, et al. Adjuvant mitotane treatment for adrenocortical carcinoma. *N Engl J Med* 2007; 356: 2372–80.

41. Berruti A, Terzolo M, Sperone P, et al. Etoposide, doxorubicin and cisplatin plus mitotane in the treatment of advanced adrenocortical carcinoma: a large prospective phase II trial. *Endocr Relat Cancer* 2005; 12: 657–66.

42. Khan TS, Imam H, Juhlin C, et al. Streptozocin and o,p'DDD in the treatment of adrenocortical cancer patients: long-term survival in its adjuvant use. *Ann Oncol* 2000; 11: 1281–7.

43. First International Randomized Trial in Locally Advanced and Metastatic Adrenocortical Carcinoma Treatment. www.firm-act.org/, June 2007.

44. Fassnacht M, Kroiss M, Allolio B. Update in adrenocortical carcinoma. *J Clin Endocrinol Metab* 2013; 98(12): 4551–64.

45. Venkatesh S, Hickey RC, Selin RV, et al. Adrenal cortical carcinoma. *Cancer* 1989; 64: 765–9.

46. Luton JP, Cerdas S, Billaud L, et al. Clinical features of adrenocortical carcinoma, prognostic factors, and the effect of mitotane therapy. *N Engl J Med* 1990; 322: 1195–201.

47. Icard P, Goudet P, Charpenay C, et al. Adrenocortical carcinomas: surgical trends and results of a 253-patient series from the French Association of Endocrine Surgeons Study Group. *World J Surg* 2001; 25: 891–7.

48. Abiven G, Coste J, Groussin L, et al. Clinical and biological features in the prognosis of adrenocortical cancer: poor outcome of cortisol-secreting tumours in a series of 202 consecutive patients. *J Clin Endocrinol Metab* 2006; 91: 2650–5.

49. Stojadinovic A, Ghossein RA, Hoos A, et al. Adrenocortical carcinoma: clinical, morphologic, and molecular characterization. *J Clin Oncol* 2002; 20: 941–50.

50. Fassnacht M, Johanssen S, Fenske W, et al. Improved survival in patients with stage II adrenocortical carcinoma followed up prospectively by specialized centers. *J Clin Endocrinol Metab* 2010; 95: 4925–4932.

51. Harrison LE, Gaudin PB, Brennan MF. Pathologic features of prognostic significance for adrenocortical carcinoma after curative resection. *Arch Surg* 1999; 134: 181–5.

52. John H, Ziegler WH, Hauri D, Jaeger P. Pheochromocytomas: can malignant potential be predicted? *Urology* 1999; 53: 679–83.

53. Glodny B, Winde G, Herwig R, et al. Clinical differences between benign and malignant pheochromocytomas. *Endocr J* 2001; 48: 151–9.

54. Goldstein RE, O'Neill JA, Holcomb GW, et al. Clinical experience over 48 years with pheochromocytoma. *Ann Surg* 1999; 229: 755–64.

55. Linnoila RI, Keiser HR, Steinberg SM, Lack EE. Histopathology of benign versus malignant sympathoadrenal paragangliomas: clinicopathologic study of 120 cases including unusual histologic features. *Hum Pathol* 1990; 21: 1168–80.

56. Unger P, Hoffman K, Pertsemlidis D, et al. S100 protein-positive sustentacular cells in malignant and locally aggressive adrenal pheochromocytomas. *Arch Pathol Lab Med* 1991; 115: 484–7.

57. Loh KC, Fitzgerald PA, Matthay KK, et al. The treatment of malignant pheochromocytoma with iodine-131 metaiodobenzyl-guanidine (131I-MIBG): a comprehensive review of 116 reported patients. *J Endocrinol Invest* 1997; 20: 648–58.

58. Averbuch SD, Steakley CS, Young RC, et al. Malignant pheochromocytoma: effective treatment with a combination of cyclophosphamide, vincristine, and dacarbazine. *Ann Intern Med* 1988; 109: 267–73.

59. Abrams HL, Spiro R, Goldstein N. Metastases in carcinoma; analysis of 1000 autopsied cases. *Cancer* 1950; 3: 74–85.

60. Lam KY, Lo CY. Metastatic tumours of the adrenal glands: a 30 year experience in a teaching hospital. *Clin Endocrinol (Oxf)* 2002; 56: 95–101.

61. Lenert JT, Barnett CC, Kudelka AP, et al. Evaluation and surgical resection of adrenal masses in patients with a history of extraadrenal malignancy. *Surgery* 2001; 130: 1060–7.

62. Hess KR, Varadhachary GR, Taylor SH, et al. Metastatic patterns in adenocarcinoma. *Cancer* 2006; 106: 1624–33.

63. Sarela AI, Murphy I, Coit DG, Conlon KC. Metastasis to the adrenal gland: the emerging role of laparoscopic surgery. *Ann Surg Oncol* 2003; 10: 1191–6.

64. Sebag F, Calzolari F, Harding J, et al. Isolated adrenal metastasis: the role of laparoscopic surgery. *World J Surg* 2006; 30: 888–92.

44

Parathyroid cancer

SHEILA FRASER AND STAN SIDHU

INTRODUCTION

There are two pairs of parathyroid glands, a superior and an inferior gland, on each side of the neck. The locations of the parathyroid glands are typically symmetrical. Although the majority of individuals have four glands, a small percentage of people will have supernumerary glands.

The glands develop during 5–6 weeks of gestation. The superior glands arise from the dorsal aspect of the fourth pharyngeal pouch and descend with the thyroid. They are usually found outside the thyroid's fibrous capsule at the upper pole of the thyroid, in a postero-lateral position. Most commonly they are located just above the junction of the RLN and the inferior thyroid artery. Occasionally, in 1% of the population, the superior glands can be found in a retro-pharyngeal or retro-oesophageal location.

The inferior glands arise from the dorsal aspect of the third pharyngeal pouch while the thymus develops from the ventral aspect. The inferior parathyroids descend caudally and anteriorly with the thymus and have a longer descent. Due to this they have a more variable location and can lie near the lower pole of the thyroid, within the thymus or even in the upper mediastinum. The embryology of the parathyroid glands is important, as its understanding provides insight into the variable and sometimes ectopic locations of parathyroid tumours, including cancers.

The chief cells of the parathyroid glands secrete parathyroid hormone (PTH) and regulate calcium homeostasis.

Small drops in serum calcium levels activate calcium-sensing receptors on the chief cells, instigating the synthesis and release of PTH. Serum calcium levels are raised by increased renal tubular calcium reabsorption and osteoclast-driven bone resorption. PTH stimulates the 1-alpha hydroxylase enzyme in the kidney to convert 25-hydroxyvitamin D to its active metabolite 1,25-dihydroxyvitamin D, stimulating calcium and phosphate absorption by the gastrointestinal tract.

INCIDENCE AND AETIOLOGY

Primary hyperparathyroidism is common, with an annual incidence of 1–4 per 1000 people in the general population [1,2]. Primary hyperparathyroidism is the third most common endocrine disorder. The prevalence of primary hyperparathyroidism increases with age and is most common in post-menopausal women, with a 3–4:1 ratio of women to men [3].

Primary hyperparathyroidism is due to autonomous and excessive PTH secretion by one or more of the parathyroid glands, causing hypercalcaemia. Over the past few decades this has changed from a condition that presented symptomatically to one that is often asymptomatic and discovered on routine blood tests.

The most common cause of primary hyperparathyroidism, in 87–90% patients, is a benign single-gland adenoma. In 3% patients, there is more than one adenoma, and in a further 10% four-gland hyperplasia occurs. Parathyroid cancer is extremely rare and accounts for less than 1% of cases of primary hyperparathyroidism. The prevalence of parathyroid cancer in the general population is only 0.005%.

In contrast to primary hyperparathyroidism caused by benign parathyroid adenomas or hyperplasia, parathyroid cancer has an equal incidence between men and women. Patients are on average almost a decade younger than those diagnosed with benign disease.

The aetiology of parathyroid cancer is unknown, although implicated risk factors include exposure to external ionizing radiation and end-stage renal dialysis. Parathyroid cancer is associated with rare genetic syndromes including hyperparathyroidism–jaw tumour syndrome (HPT-JT) and familial isolated primary hyperparathyroidism. HPT-JT is an autosomal dominant disorder with mutations in the CDC73 (also called HRPT2) gene. It is characterized by parathyroid tumours (of which 10–15% are parathyroid carcinomas) and fibro-osseous tumours of the jawbone. HPT-JT patients are also prone to renal abnormalities, including Wilms' tumours, hamartomas and polycystic disease [4].

Familial isolated primary HPT is an autosomal dominant condition considered to represent an early stage of either multiple endocrine neoplasia type 1 (MEN1) or HPT-JT syndromes. Patients have mutations in the MEN1 or HRPT2 genes and are prone to primary hyperparathyroidism and an increased risk of parathyroid carcinoma in the latter category. Occasional cases of parathyroid cancer have been reported in patients with multiple endocrine neoplasia type 1 (MEN1) and 2A (MEN2A) syndromes.

Sporadic cases of parathyroid cancer normally demonstrate mutations in the HRPT2 gene. This is a tumour suppressor gene that codes for the protein parafibromin, loss of expression of which is associated with parathyroid cancer. However, HRPT2 mutations can be occasionally seen in benign parathyroid adenomas.

PATHOLOGY AND STAGING

Due to the rare occurrence of parathyroid cancer, it is not currently staged by the American Joint Committee on Cancer [5].

The distinction between parathyroid adenoma and carcinoma is often not easy, even on histopathological examination. In certain cases, the diagnosis is clear, as specified in the histopathological criteria for parathyroid cancer by the World Health Organization (WHO). This includes vascular or peri-neural space invasion, capsular penetration and expansion into adjacent tissues or the presence of metastases. However, these characteristics are only seen in the minority of cases [6].

In 1973 Schantz and Castleman proposed a classic histological definition of parathyroid cancer with features of a trabecular pattern, mitotic figures, a thick fibrous band and capsular or vascular invasion. Again, these features are frequently absent. In addition, irregular fibrosis secondary to previous haemorrhage in a parathyroid adenoma can potentially result in a false positive diagnosis [7,8].

Immunohistochemistry can be helpful in the differentiation of benign parathyroid adenomas and carcinomas. Immunocytochemical markers, such as the proliferation marker Ki-67, can be positive in both benign and malignant tumours, but are more frequent in malignancy. Other promising markers include galectin-3 and human telomerase reverse transcriptase (hTERT) [7,9].

The HRPT2 gene is mutated in most sporadic parathyroid cancers. If an atypical adenoma or suspected parathyroid carcinoma is seen during histopathological examination, immunohistochemistry for parafibromin may be useful. Loss of parafibromin expression occurs in approximately 70% of parathyroid cancers and a small proportion of adenomas, resulting in high specificity but low sensitivity for parathyroid cancer. The positive expression of parafibromin does convincingly imply a benign adenoma [10,11].

The protein gene product 9.5 (PGP 9.5), encoded by *ubiquitin carboxyl-terminal esterase L1* (*UCHL1*), has been suggested as a supplementary marker to support the diagnosis of parathyroid cancer. Positive immunohistochemistry staining for PGP 9.5, together with negative parafibromin staining, confirms malignancy. PGP 9.5 also has been reported to have higher sensitivity, but similar specificity, than parafibromin [10].

The reported incidence of parathyroid cancer has increased recently, although it is not yet clear whether it is more frequent than previously thought, or whether better immunochemistry techniques have allowed for a more confident diagnosis [12].

DIAGNOSIS

Clinical features

The majority of parathyroid carcinomas (95%) are functional. Patients usually present with the clinical features of elevated serum calcium. Typically calcium and PTH levels are extremely high, with corrected calcium higher than 3.0 mmol/L and PTH five times greater than the upper limit of normal [13]. However, it should be borne in mind that most patients presenting with calcium levels higher than 3.0 mmol/L do not have parathyroid cancer, but primary hyperparathyroidism due to benign disease.

Due to the high calcium and PTH levels, patients are generally more symptomatic than those presenting with benign primary hyperparathyroidism. Symptoms include bone pain or fractures (90%), renal calculi or impairment (50–80%), fatigue, weakness, depression, confusion and constipation. It is rare in benign primary hyperparathyroidism to have coexistent bony and renal involvement, but this can be demonstrated in up to 40% patients with parathyroid carcinoma. Recurrent severe pancreatitis, anaemia and peptic ulcer disease can also occur.

A palpable parathyroid mass in the neck is virtually never associated with benign primary HPT (Figure 44.1).

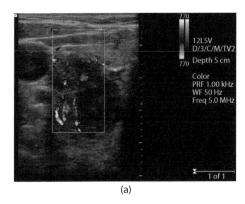 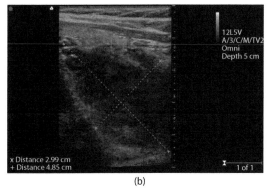

(a)　　　　　　　　　　　　　　　(b)

Figure 44.1 Mass demonstrated below the lower pole of the right thyroid lobe. It is irregular, large and has a disordered vascular pattern. (a) Transverse view; (b) longitudinal view.

However 30–76% patients with parathyroid cancer are reported to have a palpable mass and this should raise the suspicion of malignancy [14].

Very rarely, parathyroid cancer is non-functional and patients have normal calcium and PTH levels [15]. Patients typically present with a neck mass, dysphagia or hoarseness. The majority of these patients present late and have a poor prognosis.

Although hyperparathyroidism is a common cause of hypercalcaemia, other causes should be considered.

Investigations

It is often difficult to make the diagnosis of parathyroid cancer preoperatively. Initial investigations are those performed to establish a diagnosis of primary hyperparathyroidism. Biochemical tests include serum PTH, calcium, phosphate and albumin levels. A 24-h urinary calcium or fractional excretion of calcium is performed to exclude benign familial hypocalciuric hypercalcaemia (FHH), signified by a low urinary calcium excretion compared to primary hyperparathyroidism. Hypophosphataemia is frequently seen in primary hyperparathyroidism due to the increased renal excretion of phosphate.

In primary hyperparathyroidism, surgery has moved away from the traditional four-gland exploration to minimally invasive surgery. Most patients will therefore undergo imaging preoperatively to identify patients with single-gland disease and facilitate minimally invasive surgery.

The most common imaging studies performed in primary hyperparathyroidism are ultrasonography and technetium 99m-sestamibi scintigraphy. Neck ultrasound can provide valuable general information about an enlarged parathyroid. However, it is operator dependent and cannot access the mediastinum or retro-oesophageal areas. It also has reduced sensitivity in patients with multinodular thyroid disease [16]. Ultrasound features of parathyroid cancer are not always present, but characteristically include heterogeneity, hypoechogenicity and irregular borders [17].

Sestamibi scanning is currently the most common nuclear imaging study used in primary hyperparathyroidism.

Parathyroid adenomas have a high concentration of oxyphilic cells, with a large number of mitochondria. Sestamibi concentrates in the mitochondria and so adenomas have an increased sestamibi uptake. Although thyroid tissue also concentrates sestamibi, the lesser number of mitochondria results in relatively rapid washout of the isotope. A persistent uptake of sestamibi demonstrated on delayed imaging is typical of parathyroid adenomas. The sensitivity of sestamibi is greater than 80%, but rises with increasing gland weight [18]. Although small tumours may not be easy to find on sestamibi, this is not usually a problem with parathyroid cancer.

Single-photon emission computed tomography/computed tomography (SPECT/CT) can be used in combination with sestamibi scanning for improved anatomical localization of parathyroid adenomas and has been reported to slightly increase the sensitivity (Figure 44.2).

More recently 4D CT (with images in the axial, coronal and sagittal planes plus the fourth dimension derived from contrast phases) has been used to detect parathyroid adenomas not identified on traditional imaging. It provides both functional and anatomical information and increases the sensitivity of preoperative localization. However, the larger radiation doses required prevent its routine use [19].

If parathyroid cancer is suspected preoperatively on the basis of clinical and biochemical features (severity of end organ damage, a palpable gland or very high serum calcium and PTH levels), further imaging may be useful. Both CT and MRI provide additional information on the anatomical location of the lesion, the possibility of local invasion and cervical lymph node involvement. MRI with gadolinium and fat suppression is better at visualizing the soft tissues in the neck and is superior in patients with recurrent cancer, where surgical clips can cause artefacts on CT scanning [5].

Fluorodeoxyglucose (FDG) PET-CT scanning is not routinely used in parathyroid cancer, but can be a sensitive tool in the detection of persistent or recurrent disease. However, small lesions may not be demonstrated on FDG PET-CT and postoperative inflammation may give a false positive result.

Fine-needle aspiration (FNA) of a suspected parathyroid cancer is not recommended prior to the initial surgery. Not only can it be difficult to differentiate between benign and

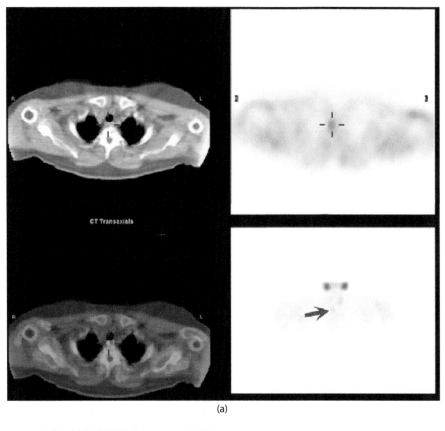

(a)

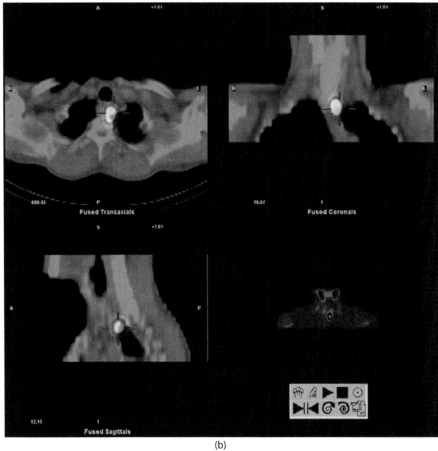

(b)

Figure 44.2 (a) SPECT/CT imaging for parathyroid localization. (b) SPECT/CT imaging for parathyroid localization.

malignant disease on cytology, but there is a risk of causing tumour rupture and seeding along the FNA tract [20].

Selective venous sampling is an invasive procedure that is rarely used as it is expensive, time-consuming and has potentially serious complications. It may provide extra information in patients with negative or equivocal non-invasive scans and is generally reserved for patients who have had previously unsuccessful neck surgery or where ectopic glands are suspected. The left and right thymic veins, inferior thyroid veins and large veins of the neck and chest are sampled and the result considered positive if there is a twofold gradient between the sampled vein and a peripheral vein [21].

MANAGEMENT

Surgery in primary hyperparathyroidism

The standard operation for primary hyperparathyroidism has traditionally been a bilateral neck exploration, with cure rates of more than 95% when performed by an experienced surgeon. During this operation, all four glands are identified and examined and the enlarged glands are removed. More recently, there has been a shift toward minimally invasive surgery, as the majority of patients have single-gland disease causing primary hyperparathyroidism. This approach reduces the risk of postoperative hypoparathyroidism as

only one side of the neck is explored and allows for a better cosmetic result. The imaging studies described above have allowed for this focused approach.

Many surgeons use techniques such as intra-operative PTH assay to confirm removal of the correct parathyroid gland and to ensure further exploration is not necessary (Figure 44.3). However, the effectiveness of these techniques remains unclear. If there are doubts regarding whether resection of parathyroid tissue or a lymph node has occurred, tissue can be sent for frozen section to check the histology.

Intra-operative PTH (IOPTH) monitoring works on the premise that PTH has a very short half-life of only 3–5 minutes. An operation is considered successful if there is more than a 50% drop in intra-operative PTH levels between the baseline value and 10–15 minutes after parathyroid removal.

Radioguided minimally invasive parathyroid surgery uses the principles of sestamibi scanning in an operative setting. The patient is injected with radioactive technetium 99m-sestamibi 2 h prior to an operation. By the time the operation takes place the sestamibi has washed out of the thyroid and concentrated in the parathyroid lesion. A gamma ray detection probe is placed on the neck and the incision made over the point of maximal radioactivity. The sterile probe can be used within the surgical wound to further localize the lesion [22].

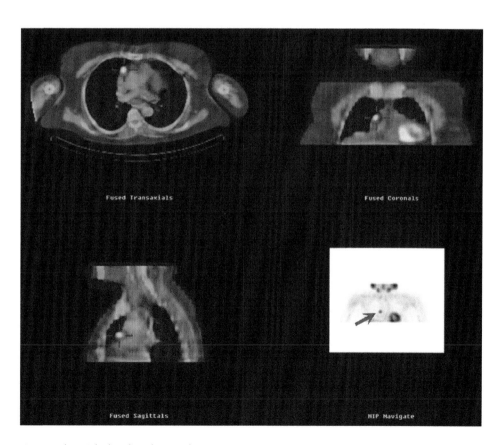

Figure 44.3 Ectopic parathyroid gland in the mediastinum.

Surgery for parathyroid cancer

As for benign disease, surgery remains the primary management of parathyroid cancer. The best chance of cure is complete surgical resection at the initial operation with microscopically negative margins [23].

Often the diagnosis of parathyroid cancer is suspected intra-operatively. Parathyroid cancer appears as a firm mass, surrounded by a whitish grey capsule. It is usually significantly larger than a benign adenoma and is adherent to the adjacent thyroid or cervical tissues [24]. Parathyroid cancers typically weigh between 2 and 10 g, with a mean weight of 7 g and a median size of 3.3 cm. If an initial minimally invasive approach has been undertaken, the surgical wound should be extended to adequately visualize the tumour and adjacent structures. En bloc resection of the tumour and adjacent structures is recommended. The minimum recommended operation is a parathyroidectomy and ipsilateral hemithyroidectomy to obtain clear margins.

There remains controversy regarding the need for and extent of central neck lymph node dissection at the initial operation. The cervical lymph nodes are involved in 15–30% of cases [25]. Many authors advise an ipsilateral central lymph node dissection performed en bloc along with a hemithyroidectomy and parathyroidectomy. Others would advocate a formal central lymph node dissection if the tumour invades any local structure, but would otherwise only resect adjoining or suspicious trachea–oesophageal lymph nodes. If there are any doubts, a frozen section of concerning lymph nodes can be performed intra-operatively [26,27]. A lateral neck dissection is not necessary, unless there is preoperative evidence of abnormally enlarged lateral neck lymph nodes.

Any adherent adjacent tissue should be resected along with the surgical specimen. If the recurrent laryngeal nerve is involved, then this should be sacrificed. The trachea or oesophagus can be affected and consideration should be given to surgical resection of the tracheal wall or muscular layer of the oesophagus [20,28]. This can be undertaken at the primary operation, if suspected prior to surgery, or as a staged procedure.

It is important to keep the tumour capsule intact. Breach of the capsule intra-operatively has been shown to correlate with both local tumour recurrence and distant metastases [7,29].

Surgery for parathyroid cancer not recognized at the first operation

In around 25% of cases, parathyroid cancer is not recognized intra-operatively by the surgeon. Despite the recommendation for initial aggressive en bloc resection of the tumour, almost 85% of patients receive inadequate surgery at the primary surgery [30]. Of those patients who only undergo a routine parathyroidectomy, 50% will develop local recurrence. For this reason, a second operation consisting of a hemithyroidectomy, with removal of the ipsilateral central lymph nodes, is recommended.

Postoperative care and follow-up for parathyroid cancer

Surgical risks include recurrent laryngeal nerve injury and injury to the trachea or oesophagus.

If there is no evidence of distant metastases, the hypercalcaemia should settle within 24 h. Calcium levels should be monitored closely as patients often develop hungry bone syndrome with symptomatic hypocalcaemia and hypophosphataemia. In hungry bone syndrome, rapid bone remineralization occurs after the correction of severe hyperparathyroidism, causing a severe and protracted hypocalcaemia. It is difficult to maintain adequate calcium levels on oral calcium and vitamin D supplements alone. Patients frequently need temporary intravenous calcium gluconate therapy, in combination with oral calcium and active vitamin D supplementation. Magnesium levels ought to be checked and be replaced as necessary.

Patients with parathyroid cancer require long-term follow-up. Although the majority of parathyroid cancer recurrences occur 2 to 5 years following initial resection, late recurrence is well documented. Once calcium levels are stable in the postoperative period, it is advised to check calcium and PTH levels 3 monthly in the first year and then 6 monthly afterwards.

If there are any clinical or biochemical concerns, cross-sectional neck imaging (ultrasound, MRI or CT) should be arranged to assess for loco-regional recurrence. In addition whole body scanning, including PET-CT and bone scans, may be required to evaluate for the presence of distant metastases. Although FNA is not recommended for use in the primary diagnosis, it can be helpful to distinguish between recurrent disease and scar tissue if there are any doubts and further surgery is being considered [31].

Non-functional parathyroid cancer presents a challenge to follow-up. Along with clinical examination, ultrasound or MRI scanning at 6-monthly intervals for the first 2 years has been suggested; however, there are no recommended guidelines.

RECURRENT AND METASTATIC DISEASE

Parathyroid cancer runs an indolent course, but recurrence after surgical resection is high. Between 33% and 78% of patients have recurrent or metastatic disease causing persistent hyperparathyroidism [32]. The most frequent site for recurrence is loco-regional, commonly secondary to incomplete initial surgery.

In all patients with a local recurrence, further surgery should be considered, although there is an increased risk of surgical complications, especially recurrent laryngeal nerve damage. Re-explorations are typically not easy due to dense scar tissue and the loss of clear anatomical planes. Patients often require several operations for loco-regional disease, increasing their risk of surgical complications [20,33].

About 30% patients with parathyroid cancer have distant metastases at presentation. Parathyroid cancer metastasizes by both the lymphatic and haematogenous routes. The most frequent site of metastasis is the lung, followed by the liver, although bone, pleura and brain metastases have also been reported. Resection of distant metastases is recommended to reduce the associated symptomatic hypercalcaemia and potentially improve patient survival [25,31].

Although surgical resection of local recurrences and distant metastases is often not curative, it can relieve symptoms and reduce serum calcium levels with effects lasting months to years depending on the extent of disease. Multiple operations, even in the palliative setting, can be helpful.

ALTERNATIVE TREATMENT OPTIONS IN PARATHYROID CANCER

Radiotherapy

There is limited data on the effectiveness of radiotherapy in parathyroid cancer and it was previously thought not to be helpful. However more recently, there have been several reports of increased disease-free survival in high-risk patients who received adjuvant external beam radiotherapy [34,35]. It is difficult to perform large multi-centred randomized trials to assess the effectiveness of radiotherapy due to the rarity of the condition.

Chemotherapy

There is limited evidence for the use of chemotherapy in metastatic parathyroid cancer and there are no standard protocols for treatment. It is generally reserved for symptomatic patients with inoperable disease. There have been case reports of successful therapy, with varied chemotherapy agents including cyclophosphamide, 5-fluorouracil and dacarbazine [36,37]. Treatment should be considered on an individual basis.

Palliative treatment

The main aim of treatment in inoperable parathyroid cancer is to control the effects of PTH-driven hypercalcaemia. The majority of deaths are due to the metabolic complications of hypercalcaemia rather than metastatic disease.

Patients can present with a hypercalcaemic crisis, known as parathyrotoxicosis. Until this is controlled, surgical treatment is contraindicated. Clinically patients present as a medical emergency, with dehydration, drowsiness, confusion, cardiac arrhythmias and even coma.

The main aim of treatment in a hypercalcaemic crisis is to reduce the severity of hypercalcaemia by stimulating calcium excretion by the kidney, thereby preventing irreversible damage to the renal, cardiac and cerebral systems. Patients are rehydrated with intravenous 0.9% saline to increase the extracellular volume; usually 4–6 L of fluid is required over a 24-h period. Intravenous saline promotes natriuresis which in turn causes calciuresis (renal calcium excretion). Loop diuretics, such as furosemide, were previously used to increase the renal excretion of calcium but are now only recommended if fluid overload develops. Thiazide diuretics have the opposite effect, decreasing the renal excretion of calcium, and should be stopped in patients taking them regularly.

After rehydration, intravenous bisphosphonates are used to reduce osteoclast-mediated bone resorption and decrease serum calcium levels. Usually pamidronate (30 to 90 mg depending on severity of hypercalcaemia at 20 mg per hour) or zolendronate (4 mg over 15 minutes) is used. Bisphosphonates take 2 to 4 days to reach a maximal response and so calcium levels are measured regularly to ensure hypocalcaemia does not occur. Zolendronic acid has been reported to have a faster onset of action than pamidronate with a longer time to relapse. However, there are more reported side effects including osteonecrosis of the jaw, and gastrointestinal, cardiac and renal side effects. Hypercalcaemia is usually well controlled initially with bisphosphonates. However, patients become refractory to the effects over time and require further intervention [38].

The natural antagonist to PTH is calcitonin, which inhibits osteoclast-mediated bone resorption and increases renal calcium excretion. It is useful for the treatment of acute hypercalcaemia, especially in patients with a poor response to bisphosphonates. It has a synergistic effect in combination with glucocorticoids. It is not suitable for the long-term control of hypercalcaemia as it has a limited effect after a few days and there have been reports of anaphylaxis to calcitonin in patients allergic to salmon [31].

Cinacalcet is a calcimimetic agent that binds to the calcium-sensing receptor on the surface of parathyroid cells. It increases the receptor's sensitivity to extra-cellular calcium and reduces PTH secretion and subsequently serum calcium levels. An international multi-centre trial demonstrated that cinacalcet is effective in lowering serum calcium levels and maintaining these levels in patients with inoperable parathyroid cancer. Most patients tolerate cinacalcet well and doses range from 60 to 360 mg daily in divided doses. Cinacalcet is licensed for use in the UK for patients with parathyroid cancer and is an effective long-term palliative treatment [32,39].

A monoclonal antibody, denosumab, has recently been trialled in patients with parathyroid cancer and refractory hypercalcaemia, when conventional treatments have failed. It prevents osteoclast activity by inhibiting the activation of nuclear factor kB ligand at the receptor. It is currently licensed for treatment of post-menopausal osteoporosis and to reduce skeletal-related events in patients with bone metastases. Recent case reports have described successful and sustained treatment of resistant hypercalcaemia [40,41].

PROGNOSIS

Although parathyroid cancer is slow growing, it has a tendency for local recurrence and can metastasize by both lymphatic and haematogenous routes. The majority of deaths occur from the consequence of hypercalcaemia rather than the disease itself. Five-year survival rates range from 50% to 85% and 10-year survival rates are between 49% and 77%. Some of the improvement in survival in recent years reflects the recent advances in the medical treatment of hypercalcaemia for inoperable parathyroid cancer. However, surgery remains the mainstay of treatment and should be considered even in the palliative setting.

REFERENCES

1. Pallan S, Rahman MO, Khan AA. Diagnosis and management of primary hyperparathyroidism. *BMJ* 2012;344:e1013.
2. Yu N, Donnan PT, Murphy MJ, Leese GP. Epidemiology of primary hyperparathyroidism in Tayside, Scotland, UK. *Clin Endocrinol (Oxf)* 2009;71(4):485–93.
3. Fraser WD. Hyperparathyroidism. *Lancet* 2009;374(9684):145–58.
4. Cavaco BM, Barros L, Pannett AA, Ruas L, Carvalheiro M, Ruas MM, et al. The hyperparathyroidism-jaw tumour syndrome in a Portuguese kindred. *QJM* 2001;94(4):213–22.
5. Evangelista L, Sorgato N, Torresan F, Boschin IM, Pennelli G, Saladini G, et al. FDG-PET/CT and parathyroid carcinoma: review of literature and illustrative case series. *World J Clin Oncol* 2011;2(10):348–54.
6. Witteveen JE, Haak HR, Kievit J, Morreau H, Romijn JA, Hamdy NA. Challenges and pitfalls in the management of parathyroid carcinoma: 17-year follow-up of a case and review of the literature. *Horm Cancer* 2010;1(4):205–14.
7. Johnson SJ, Sheffield EA, McNicol AM. Best practice no 183. Examination of parathyroid gland specimens. *J Clin Pathol* 2005;58(4):338–42.
8. Schantz A, Castleman B. Parathyroid carcinoma. A study of 70 cases. *Cancer* 1973;31(3):600–5.
9. Osawa N, Onoda N, Kawajiri H, Tezuka K, Takashima T, Ishikawa T, et al. Diagnosis of parathyroid carcinoma using immunohistochemical staining against hTERT. *Int J Mol Med* 2009;24(6):733–41.
10. Howell VM, Gill A, Clarkson A, Nelson AE, Dunne R, Delbridge LW, et al. Accuracy of combined protein gene product 9.5 and parafibromin markers for immunohistochemical diagnosis of parathyroid carcinoma. *J Clin Endocrinol Metab* 2009;94(2):434–41.
11. Juhlin CC, Hoog A. Parafibromin as a diagnostic instrument for parathyroid carcinoma – lone ranger or part of the posse? *Int J Endocrinol* 2010:324964.
12. Brown S, O'Neill C, Suliburk J, Sidhu S, Sywak M, Gill A, et al. Parathyroid carcinoma: increasing incidence and changing presentation. *ANZ J Surg* 2011;81(7–8):528–32.
13. Digonnet A, Carlier A, Willemse E, Quiriny M, Dekeyser C, de Saint Aubain N, et al. Parathyroid carcinoma: a review with three illustrative cases. *J Cancer* 2011;2:532–7.
14. Shane E. Clinical review 122: parathyroid carcinoma. *J Clin Endocrinol Metab* 2001;86(2):485–93.
15. Wilkins BJ, Lewis JS Jr. Non-functional parathyroid carcinoma: a review of the literature and report of a case requiring extensive surgery. *Head Neck Pathol* 2009;3(2):140–9.
16. Noda S, Onoda N, Kashiwagi S, Kawajiri H, Takashima T, Ishikawa T, et al. Strategy of operative treatment of hyperparathyroidism using US scan and (99m)Tc-MIBI SPECT/CT. *Endocr J* 2014;61(3):225–30.
17. Sharretts JM, Kebebew E, Simonds WF. Parathyroid cancer. *Semin Oncol* 2010;37(6):580–90.
18. Norton KS, Johnson LW, Griffen FD, Burke J, Kennedy S, Aultman D, et al. The sestamibi scan as a preoperative screening tool. *Am Surg* 2002;68(9):812–5.
19. Brown SJ, Lee JC, Christie J, Maher R, Sidhu SB, Sywak MS, et al. Four-dimensional computed tomography for parathyroid localization: a new imaging modality. *ANZ J Surg* 2015;85(6):483–87.
20. Wei CH, Harari A. Parathyroid carcinoma: update and guidelines for management. *Curr Treat Options Oncol* 2012;13(1):11–23.
21. Ogilvie CM, Brown PL, Matson M, Dacie J, Reznek RH, Britton K, et al. Selective parathyroid venous sampling in patients with complicated hyperparathyroidism. *Eur J Endocrinol* 2006;155(6):813–21.
22. Goldstein RE, Blevins L, Delbeke D, Martin WH. Effect of minimally invasive radioguided parathyroidectomy on efficacy, length of stay, and costs in the management of primary hyperparathyroidism. *Ann Surg* 2000;231(5):732–42.
23. Schulte KM, Talat N, Galata G, Gilbert J, Miell J, Hofbauer LC, et al. Oncologic resection achieving r0 margins improves disease-free survival in parathyroid cancer. *Ann Surg Oncol* 2014;21(6):1891–7.
24. Sidhu PS, Talat N, Patel P, Mulholland NJ, Schulte KM. Ultrasound features of malignancy in the preoperative diagnosis of parathyroid cancer: a retrospective analysis of parathyroid tumours larger than 15 mm. *Eur Radiol* 2011;21(9):1865–73.
25. Artinyan A, Guzman E, Maghami E, Al-Sayed M, D'Apuzzo M, Wagman L, et al. Metastatic parathyroid carcinoma to the liver treated with radiofrequency ablation and transcatheter arterial embolization. *J Clin Oncol* 2008;26(24):4039–41.
26. Hsu KT, Sippel RS, Chen H, Schneider DF. Is central lymph node dissection necessary for parathyroid carcinoma? *Surgery* 2014;156(6):1336–41.

27. Ricci G, Assenza M, Barreca M, Liotta G, Paganelli L, Serao A, et al. Parathyroid carcinoma: the importance of high clinical suspicion for a correct management. *Int J Surg Oncol* 2012:649148.

28. Dotzenrath C, Goretzki PE, Sarbia M, Cupisti K, Feldkamp J, Roher HD. Parathyroid carcinoma: problems in diagnosis and the need for radical surgery even in recurrent disease. *Eur J Surg Oncol* 2001;27(4):383–9.

29. Wang CA, Gaz RD. Natural history of parathyroid carcinoma: diagnosis, treatment, and results. *Am J Surg* 1985;149(4):522–7.

30. Hundahl SA, Fleming ID, Fremgen AM, Menck HR. Two hundred eighty-six cases of parathyroid carcinoma treated in the U.S. between 1985–1995: a National Cancer Data Base Report. The American College of Surgeons Commission on Cancer and the American Cancer Society. *Cancer* 1999;86(3):538–44.

31. Al-Kurd A, Mekel M, Mazeh H. Parathyroid carcinoma. *Surg Oncol* 2014;23(2):107–14.

32. Silverberg SJ, Rubin MR, Faiman C, Peacock M, Shoback DM, Smallridge RC, et al. Cinacalcet hydrochloride reduces the serum calcium concentration in inoperable parathyroid carcinoma. *J Clin Endocrinol Metab* 2007;92(10):3803–8.

33. Schulte KM, Talat N. Diagnosis and management of parathyroid cancer. *Nat Rev Endocrinol* 2012;8(10):612–22.

34. Munson ND, Foote RL, Northcutt RC, Tiegs RD, Fitzpatrick LA, Grant CS, et al. Parathyroid carcinoma: is there a role for adjuvant radiation therapy? *Cancer* 20031;98(11):2378–84.

35. Rasmuson T, Kristoffersson A, Boquist L. Positive effect of radiotherapy and surgery on hormonally active pulmonary metastases of primary parathyroid carcinoma. *Eur J Endocrinol* 2000;143(6):749–54.

36. Bowyer SE, White AM, Ransom DT, Davidson JA. R esistant hypercalcaemia in metastatic parathyroid carcinoma. *Med J Aust* 2013;198(10):559–61.

37. Bukowski RM, Sheeler L, Cunningham J, Esselstyn C. Successful combination chemotherapy for metastatic parathyroid carcinoma. *Arch Intern Med* 1984;144(2):399–400.

38. Major PP, Coleman RE. Zoledronic acid in the treatment of hypercalcemia of malignancy: results of the international clinical development program. *Semin Oncol* 2001;28(2 Suppl. 6):17–24.

39. Block GA, Martin KJ, de Francisco AL, Turner SA, Avram MM, Suranyi MG, et al. Cinacalcet for secondary hyperparathyroidism in patients receiving hemodialysis. *N Engl J Med* 2004 Apr 8;350(15):1516–25.

40. Karuppiah D, Thanabalasingham G, Shine B, Wang LM, Sadler GP, Karavitaki N, et al. Refractory hypercalcaemia secondary to parathyroid carcinoma: response to high-dose denosumab. *Eur J Endocrinol* 2014;171(1):K1–5.

41. Vellanki P, Lange K, Elaraj D, Kopp PA, El Muayed M. Denosumab for management of parathyroid carcinoma-mediated hypercalcemia. *J Clin Endocrinol Metab* 2014;99(2):387–90.

45

Neuroendocrine tumours of the gastrointestinal tract

MENNO R VRIENS AND INNE H M BOREL RINKES

INTRODUCTION

In this chapter we concentrate on the following neuroendocrine tumours: carcinoid tumours and pancreatic endocrine tumours.

Carcinoid tumours, related to the gastrointestinal tract, can be found in the stomach, jejunum, ileum, appendix, ascending colon and colorectal. Carcinoid primary tumours occur in the appendix (38%), ileum (23%) and rectum (13%). Flushing is the most frequent symptom (94%), followed by diarrhoea (78%) and abdominal pain or cramping (51%). Other symptoms include endocardial fibrosis, wheezing, myopathy, arthritis, arthralgias and changes in mental state. Carcinoid syndrome occurs in fewer than 10% of patients with carcinoid tumours and has an incidence of about 3.2–5 cases per million of the population per year and results from excessive secretion of hormone products into the systemic circulation (e.g. adrenocorticotropic hormone [ACTH], gastrin, pancreatic polypeptide, insulin, tachykinins, vasoactive intestinal polypeptide [VIP], serotonin or 5-hydroxyindoleacetic acid [5-HIAA]).

Carcinoid syndrome does not usually develop until a tumour has metastasized, usually to the liver. The incidence of metastases in carcinoid tumours is less than 2% in tumours smaller than 1 cm and almost 100% in tumours greater than 2 cm. Surgical removal of the tumours is the primary therapeutic option; chemotherapy is less effective. Octreotide is the primary medical therapy for the management of certain symptoms associated with carcinoid syndrome.

Pancreatic endocrine tumours occur in 1 per 100,000 of the population. In this chapter we discuss the incidence, diagnostics, treatment and prognosis of gastrinomas, insulinomas, glucagonomas, VIP-secreting tumours (VIPomas), somatostatinomas, pancreatic polypeptide-secreting tumours (PPomas) and non-functioning islet cell tumours (Table 45.1).

Optimal imaging and staging of the disease are the most important factors in both medical and surgical treatment of neuroendocrine tumours. Localization of the primary tumour and exclusion of metastatic disease, before performing surgery, is best practice. When liver metastases have been identified and considered for resection, resectability of both solitary and multifocal lesions should be determined [1].

IMAGING

At present, gastrointestinal carcinoid tumours are often difficult to diagnose because of their small size and multiplicity. Endoscopy and endoscopic ultrasonography provide sensitive tools for visualizing gastric and duodenal carcinoids. Proctoscopy and colonoscopy together with ultrasonography can visualize rectal and sigmoid carcinoids. However, primary midgut tumours are difficult to diagnose. On occasion, they can be detected on barium enema, but usually lymph node and liver metastases (when at least 0.5–1 cm in diameter) are detected by computed tomography (CT) and magnetic resonance imaging (MRI) [2–4]. The current most sensitive diagnostic procedure for optimal management of patients with neuroendocrine tumours is

Table 45.1 Pancreatic endocrine tumours

Types	Incidence per million per year	Clinical features
Gastrinomas	0.5–4	Peptic ulcers, diarrhoea
Insulinomas	2–4	Hypoglycemia, neuroglycopenic
Glucagonomas, erythema	1	Necrolytic migratory
VIPomas	1	Watery diarrhoea syndrome
Somatostatinomas, neurofibromatosis	0.025	Non-specific
PPomas	<1	Jaundice due to compression
Non-functioning tumours	<1	Pain, jaundice

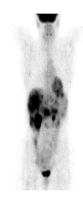

Figure 45.1 Galium-68 DOTATATE scintogram of a patient with metastatic small bowel carcinoid tumour showing activity at the site of the primary tumour, regional lymph node metastases and liver metastases.

somatostatin receptor scintigraphy (SRS) (Figure 45.1). The sensitivity of SRS for the detection of carcinoid tumours has been reported to lie between 80% and 100% in different studies. There is no significant difference between foregut, midgut and hindgut tumours. Scintigraphy also provides a more accurate staging of the disease by demonstrating tumour sites which are not shown by conventional imaging. It also indicates the number of somatostatin receptors which may indicate efficacy of treatment with octreotide [2]. In a recent study Dimitroulopoulos et al. evaluated the diagnostic sensitivity and accuracy and the cost-effectiveness of SRS in the detection of gastroenteropancreatic carcinoid tumours and their metastases in comparison with conventional imaging methods. They concluded that SRS imaging is a very sensitive method for the detection of gastroenteropancreatic carcinoids but is less sensitive than ultrasound and CT in the detection of liver metastases. Between several imaging combinations, the combination of chest X-ray–upper abdominal CT/SRS shows the highest sensitivity (89%) with a cost of more than $1000 [5].

Next to SRS, positron emission tomography (PET) is a non-invasive technique for measurement of regional tracer accumulation and quantification. PET has already provided much improved sensitivity in the localization of both primary and metastatic neuroendocrine tumours [6]. In the future, improved cameras and new tracers might further improve the sensitivity and specificity of SRS and PET, but already tumours as small as 2 mm can be visualized with the current PET technique [2].

Li and Beheshti state that in the case of metastatic disease no single imaging technique identifies all the metastatic sites of neuroendocrine tumours. The best results may be obtained with a combination of functional imaging such as PET and SRS and morphological imaging with CT and MRI. Many molecular imaging and therapy modalities for neuroendocrine tumours are under investigation or being developed. The usefulness of these

modalities, however, has to be evaluated by well-designed and multicentre studies [7].

BIOCHEMICAL MARKERS

The biochemical diagnosis of endocrine digestive tumours is based on general and specific markers. The best general markers are chromogranin A and pancreatic polypeptide (PP). Specific markers for endocrine tumours include insulin, gastrin, glucagon, VIP, somatostatin and the primary catabolic product of serotonin, 5-HIAA [8]. Chromogranin A is a glycoprotein which is widely expressed in neuroendocrine cells and constitutes one of the most abundant components of secretory granules. Chromogranin A immunohistochemistry is the main step in the diagnosis of neuroendocrine tumours. Increased levels of chromogranin A have been reported in 50–80% of pancreatic endocrine tumours. Serum pancreatic polypeptide alone shows a sensitivity of between 40% and 55%. Determination of plasma insulin and proinsulin concentrations by radioimmunoassay has simplified the diagnosis for insulinomas. For gastrinomas the combination of serum gastrin concentration and a basal acid output (BAO) and pentagastrin-stimulated acid output (MAO) is the most sensitive. The diagnosis of a glucagonoma is made on the basis of a raised fasting plasma glucagon concentration. Somatostatinomas are associated with excessive somatostatin secretion. VIPomas (Verner–Morrison syndrome) are associated with secretion of VIP. Carcinoid is usually diagnosed by increased 24-h urinary 5-HIAA levels.

CARCINOIDS

In general, radical surgical resection is considered to be the treatment of choice. However, in many instances carcinoids are found incidentally and are often not diagnosed until after surgery, when ileus or obstruction, ischemia or other abdominal disturbances occur. Whenever carcinoids are diagnosed preoperatively, e.g. following endoscopic biopsy, surgery has to be considered, along with perioperative measures to

Table 45.2 Risk of developing a gastric carcinoid in patients with ABG, MEN-1-associated type, or sporadic ZES

Background pathology	Risk of developing carcinoid (%)	Risk of developing metastases in the case of carcinoid
ABG (type I)	1	Exceptional
MEN-1/ZES (type II)	20–30	Up to 30%
Sporadic ZES (type III)	0–1	50–100%

prevent a carcinoid crisis during surgery (e.g. administration of octreotide). Surgical treatment is dominated by the location of the primary tumour [1].

Gastric carcinoids

Gastric endocrine tumours usually grow from enterochromaffin-like (ECL) cells. They are rare neoplasms occurring in one to two per million of the population per year. Three types of tumour may be distinguished on the basis of the background gastric pathology: type I, which develops in atrophic body gastritis (ABG), represents 70–80% of the cases; type II, which is associated with multiple endocrine neoplasia (MEN) and Zollinger–Ellison syndrome, represents 5% of gastric carcinoids; and the sporadic type III, which is not associated with any background pathology, represents the remaining 15–25% (Table 45.2). This classification plays a major role in determining the optimal approach to these diseases [9].

Due to their indolent course, an appropriate treatment for type I gastric carcinoids, localized in the gastric fundus or body, would be surveillance endoscopic follow-up based on gastroscopy with multiple gastric biopsy [10], and a conservative approach with endoscopic resection and eventually somatostatin analogues. Gastric carcinoids do not tend to metastasize. Type II carcinoids are often multiple and thus not suitable for complete endoscopic resection. They develop in the gastric fundus or body, and rarely in the antrum as well. Regional lymph node involvement has been described in 30% of patients. In these cases the somatostatin analogue octreotide has been demonstrated to be effective at reducing tumour growth [11]. Surgery is the treatment of choice for type III gastric carcinoid, which grows from the gastric fundus or body. This carcinoid has an aggressive tumour behaviour (liver and lymph node metastases are frequent) and a high risk of tumour-related death. There is no place for somatostatin analogues.

Carcinoids of jejunum, ileum and ascending colon

Carcinoids arising in the distal jejunum and ileum (Figure 45.2) have a worse prognosis than duodenal, gastric

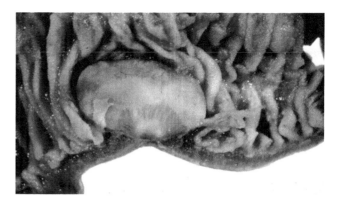

Figure 45.2 Typical small bowel 'carcinoid' tumour, which may have been present for many years before becoming symptomatic.

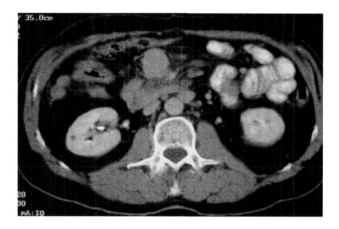

Figure 45.3 Abdominal CT scan showing typical large lymph node metastasis in the mesentery.

and rectal carcinoids, since they frequently lead to metastases to the adjacent lymph nodes (Figure 45.3), liver and other sites. The 10-year survival rate is approximately 43%, and this is more favourable if the primary tumour has been removed and liver metastases are absent. Therefore, in patients with small carcinoids in the ileum that have been discovered incidentally during endoscopy, a generous resection of ileum and distal jejunum is recommended. Aggressive palliative cytoreductive surgical treatment of the primary tumour, lymph node metastases and even liver metastases can ameliorate symptoms and improve survival in patients with advanced disease [12].

Appendiceal carcinoid

Carcinoids of the appendix are rare and are usually detected incidentally after appendectomy. Tumours less than 1 cm hardly ever metastasize and are treated by appendectomy. Tumours larger than 2 cm require a right-sided hemicolectomy because of a significant risk of metastatic spread, even when primary surgery (appendectomy) has been radical. Treatment for lesions 1–2 cm is controversial and needs further characterization of the tumour and careful patient risk evaluation [13]. Median survival is 5–8 years. For surgically resectable tumours 10-year survival rates of more than 60% have been reported.

Colorectal carcinoid

Small colorectal carcinoids may be treated by either polypectomy or transanal local excision, but for tumours larger than 2 cm in diameter an oncological resection is mandatory [1]. Carcinoid tumours are about twice as likely to occur in the rectum than in the colon. They grow slowly and have about a 1/300,000 chance of metastasizing. However, if carcinoid tumours do spread (to lymph nodes or liver) the survival rates mimic those of colorectal cancer.

ISLET CELL TUMOURS

Gastrinomas

Zollinger–Ellison syndrome (ZES) is characterized by peptic ulcers of the upper gastrointestinal tract failing to heal despite maximal medical therapy, diarrhoea and marked gastric acid hypersecretion associated with a gastrin-secreting tumour (gastrinoma). ZES might be associated with multiple endocrine neoplasia type 1 (MEN-1). To identify the localization of gastrinoma several imaging techniques have been proposed. Compared with ultrasound, CT and MRI, SRS is capable of locating the tumour in 80% of cases and of identifying it even in anatomic sites other than the pancreas and duodenum. A new technique called the selective arterial secretagogue injection (SASI) test is able to identify even small tumours with a high sensitivity and specificity (both 90%) [14]. The two main principal therapeutic strategies are to control both the gastric acid hypersecretion and the growth of the neoplasia. The best surgical treatment is excision of gastrinoma before metastatic spread has occurred. However, about 50% of patients have metastases at the time of operation. Somatostatin analogue can reduce both gastric acid hypersecretion and serum gastrin levels. Moreover, they have an antiproliferative effect. Chemotherapy, interferon and embolization are indicated in rapidly evolving tumours or in cases in which the tumoural symptoms cannot be treated by other approaches [15]. In a prospective study involving 123 patients with sporadic gastrinoma who had a surgical resection of tumour, Norton et al. showed cure rates of 40% at 5 years and 34% at 10 years [16].

In general, the progression of gastrinomas is relatively slow with a combined 5-year survival rate of 65% and 10-year survival rate of 51%. In patients with ZES and MEN-1 the most important predictor of survival is the development of liver metastases. Since patients with ZES and MEN-1 with tumours of 2 cm or more have an increased probability of developing liver metastases, surgical exploration is recommended in these patients.

Duodenotomy has improved both the tumour detection rate and the cure rate and should be routinely performed. Whipple pancreaticoduodenectomy results in the highest probability of cure in both sporadic and MEN-1 gastrinoma patients as it removes the entire gastrinoma triangle. However, the excellent long-term survival of these patients with fewer operations and the increased operative mortality and long-term morbidity of Whipple make its current role in the management of these patients unclear until studies are done to clarify these issues [17].

Insulinomas

Insulinomas are the most frequent of all islet cell tumours, with an incidence of two to four cases per million of the population per year. Insulinomas are characterized by fasting hypoglycemia and neuroglycopenic symptoms. The episodic nature of the hypoglycemic attacks is due to the intermittent insulin secretion by the tumour. The majority of insulinomas are intrapancreatic, benign and solitary. They are equally distributed between the head, body and tail of the pancreas. Approximately 85% of insulinomas occur singly, 6–13% are multiple and 4–6% are associated with MEN-1. The overall 5-year survival has been reported to approach 97% [18]. Surgical resection is the treatment of choice. A multimodal approach to detect primary tumours, which may include CT, SRS and endoscopic ultrasonography, is recommended. Preoperative imaging combined with intraoperative ultrasonography should enable accurate tumour localization in more than 95% of patients, and blind pancreatic resection in the absence of tumour detection is not recommended [19]. Nesidioblastosis has to be considered, if invasive localization studies do not reveal a tumour in the absence of MEN-1. This is a rare condition, which is treated by diazoxide or streptozotocin, or by surgery [1]. Laparoscopic surgery, especially for small insulinomas located in the body and tail, is feasible and safe [20]. Enucleation will suffice in most cases of solitary insulinoma, but the surgeon has to pay special attention to the location of the tumour in relation to the pancreatic duct. Splenic salvage with or without preservation of the splenic vessels is feasible. In case of splenectomy pneumococcal vaccination has to be given.

Other islet cell tumours

The estimated incidence of glucagonomas is one per million of the population per year. The glucagonoma syndrome reflects the catabolic action of excessively elevated glucagon levels. Necrolytic migratory erythema is a common presenting feature, found in 70% of all patients. Glucagonomas are occasionally part of MEN-1 and commonly occur in the tail of the pancreas. Extrapancreatic glucagonomas are extremely rare. Approximately 60–70% of glucagonomas are already metastatic at the time of diagnosis; these tumours tend to grow slowly and patients may survive for many years [1,18]. Glucagonomas are generally large at presentation (>5 cm diameter); visualization is usually easy. Diagnostic laparoscopy to determine the extent of spread of disease and a definitive operation strategy is recommended. Cytoreductive surgery in slowly progressing tumours like glucagonomas should always be considered. Following cytoreductive surgery in the presence of (liver) metastases and palliative chemotherapy, a 5-year survival rate of 50% may be achieved [21].

VIPomas are tumours which secrete VIP [22]. The incidence is one per million of the population per year. Of these tumours 50% are already malignant at the time of diagnosis and associated with the watery diarrhoea syndrome (Verner–Morrison syndrome). Due to severe symptoms, an aggressive surgical treatment is warranted. VIPomas in the corpus or tail of the pancreas require distal pancreatectomy; pancreaticoduodenectomy should be considered for tumours in the pancreatic head [1]. As symptoms are often so severe, blind distal pancreatectomy may be performed if a primary tumour cannot be found. Liver metastases should be resected if technically possible. Surgical treatment, as extensive as possible, in combination with somatostatin analogues or chemotherapy when necessary, may result in prolonged survival, even in patients with advanced disease.

The 5-year survival rate is 60% for patients with metastases and 94% for patients without metastases [18]. Somatostatinomas are rare tumours, large at presentation and often located in the head of the pancreas or duodenum, especially in patients with neurofibromatosis (von Recklinghausen's disease). Between 70% and 92% demonstrate metastatic spread at diagnosis. Pancreaticoduodenectomy should be performed in patients with a respectable lesion without liver metastases. The overall 5-year survival rate is 75%, or 60% when metastases are present [18]. PPomas are, like somatostatinomas, large at presentation (>5 cm) and located in the head of the pancreas. The foremost clinical feature is jaundice by compression of the bile duct [1]. Pancreaticoduodenectomy is the surgical procedure of choice.

Non-functioning islet cell tumours are usually advanced when diagnosed and therefore large in diameter (6–10 cm). The initial clinical presentation is pain (in 36% of patients) and jaundice (in 28% of patients). The malignancy rate, based on the findings of metastatic growth outside the pancreas, peri-neural or vascular invasion, varies from 62% to 92% [18].

SRS can be helpful in differentiating these tumours from exocrine pancreatic carcinomas. Aggressive resection is indicated, if distant metastases cannot be found. In 60% of cases, distant metastases are already encountered. Overall 5-year survival rates are estimated around 75% [23,24].

LIVER METASTASES OF NEUROENDOCRINE TUMOURS

Neuroendocrine tumours behave in a protracted and predictable way, which allows for multiple therapeutic options. Even in the presence of hepatic metastases, the standard treatment is surgery, either with curative intent or for more tumour cytoreduction, i.e. resection of 90% or more of the tumour volume [25]. Moreover, surgical clearance of the largest lesions should be considered prior to radionuclide treatment to increase the latter's efficacy in cases of extensive metastases, both intra- and extrahepatic [26].

Surgery for liver metastases is often impossible due to their diffuse spread; cure is only possible in 5–10%. In half of hepatic patients, resection is combined with resection of the primary tumour and adjacent lymph nodes. Vascular interventions such as embolization, chemoembolization or radioembolization, and other local ablative therapies like radiofrequency ablation, interstitial laser coagulation, alcohol injection and regional hyperthermia, can be used for the treatment of liver metastases. Surgical treatment appears to result in outstanding long-term survival and amelioration of symptoms. Furthermore, there is mounting evidence of the benefit of resecting symptomatic primary NETs in the presence of inoperable liver disease [26].

Non-surgical treatment options for liver metastases of neuroendocrine tumours include long-acting somatostatin receptor antagonists (LARs), interferon, chemotherapy and hepatic artery embolization with and without chemotherapy [27]. When patients with progressive metastatic disease are unresponsive to these options for treatment, total hepatectomy can be a final solution. However, liver transplantation is only rarely feasible [12]. Liver transplantation for patients with symptomatic liver metastases is associated with an overall 5-year survival of 65% and a median survival of 8 years, and immediate relief from hormone-related symptoms.

A promising treatment modality for patients with symptomatic liver metastases of neuroendocrine tumours is the peptide receptor radionuclide therapy with somatostatin analogue [1]. Most recently, two trials (PROMID [28] and CLARINET [29]) have demonstrated effective tumour static treatment of inoperable metastatic NETs using both commercially available long-acting somatostatin analogues. As yet neither has been tested in the adjuvant setting following apparently curative resection of either primary or metastatic NETs, but it is hoped that such studies should commence in the near future.

Last is the role of peptide receptor radionuclide therapy (PRRT) [30]. PRRT utilizes the high binding affinity of various analogues of somatostatin to the over-expressed somatostatin receptors found on most NETs (regardless of their functional activity). When labelled with either radioactive yttrium or lutetium significant uptake of radio-labelled somatostatin analogue by the NET cells leads to significant tumour death, with many authors reporting partial response by Response Evaluation Criteria in Solid Tumours (RECIST) criteria. These treatments can be repeated, but caution has to be advised because of bone marrow and renal toxicity [31].

REFERENCES

1. Van Lanschot J, Gouma D, Jansen P, et al. *Textbook of Integrated Medical and Surgical Gastroenterology.* Houten, Netherlands: Bohn Stafleu Van Loghum, 2004: 416–20.

2. Oberg K, Eriksson B. Nuclear medicine in the detection, staging and treatment of gastrointestinal carcinoid tumors. *Best Pract Res Clin Endocrinol Metab* 2005; 19: 265–7.

3. Oberg K. Neuroendocrine gastrointestinal tumors – a condensed overview of diagnosis and treatment. *Ann Oncol* 1999; 10 (Suppl. 2): S3–8.

4. Chaplin M, Buscombe J, Hilson A. Carcinoid tumors. *Lancet* 1998; 352: 799–805.

5. Dimitroulopoulos D, Xynopoulos D, Tsamakidis K, et al. Scintigraphic detection of carcinoid tumors with a cost effectiveness analysis. *World J Gastroenterol* 2004; 10: 3628–33.

6. Ganim R, Norton J. Recent advances in carcinoid pathogenesis, diagnosis and management. *Surg Oncol* 2000; 9: 173–9.

7. Li S, Beheshti M. The radionuclide molecular imaging and therapy of neuroendocrine tumors. *Curr Cancer Drug Targets* 2005; 5: 139–48.

8. Tomassetti P, Migliori M, Lalli S, et al. Epidemiology, clinical features and diagnosis of gastroentero-pancreatic endocrine tumors. *Ann Oncol* 2001; 12 (Suppl. 2): S95–9.

9. Delle Fave G, Capurso G, Milione M, et al. Endocrine tumors of the stomach. *Best Pract Res Clin Gastroenterol* 2005; 19: 659–73.

10. Annibale B, Azzoni C, Corleto V, et al. Atrophic body gastritis with enterochromaffin-like cell dysplasia are at increased risk for the development of type I gastric carcinoid. *Eur J Gastroenterol Hepatol* 2001; 13: 1449–56.

11. Tomassetti P, Migliori M, Caletti G, et al. Treatment of type II gastric carcinoid tumors with somatostatin analogues. *N Engl J Med* 2000; 343: 551–4.

12. Herder de W. Tumors of the midgut (jejunum, ileum and ascending colon, including carcinoid syndrome). *Best Pract Res Clin Gastroenterol* 2005; 19: 705–15.

13. Stinner B, Rothmund M. Neuroendocrine tumors (carcinoids) of the appendix. *Best Pract Res Clin Gastroenterol* 2005; 19: 729–38.

14. Imamura M, Komoto I, Ota S. Changing treatment strategy for gastrinoma in patients with Zollinger-Ellison syndrome. *World J Surg* 2006; 30: 1–11.

15. Pellicano R, De Angelis C, Resegotti A, et al. Zollinger-Ellison syndrome in 2006: concepts from a clinical point of view. *Panminerva Med* 2006; 48: 33–40.

16. Norton J, Fraker D, Alexander H, et al. Surgery to cure the Zollinger Ellison syndrome. *N Engl J Med* 1999; 341: 635–44.

17. Norton J. Surgical treatment and prognosis of gastrinoma. *Best Pract Res Clin Gastroenterol* 2005; 19: 799–805.

18. Oberg K, Eriksson B. Endocrine tumors of the pancreas. *Best Pract Res Clin Gastroenterol* 2005; 19: 753–81.

19. Tucker O, Crotty P, Conlon K. The management of insulinoma. A review. *Br J Surg* 2006; 93: 264–75.

20. Assalia A, Gagner M. Laparoscopic pancreatic surgery for islet cell tumors of the pancreas. *World J Surg* 2004; 28: 1239–47.

21. Chastain M. The glucagonoma syndrome; a review of its features and discussion of new perspectives. *Am J Med Sci* 2001; 321: 306–20.

22. Nikou GC, Toubanakis C, Nikolaou P, et al. VIPomas: an update in diagnosis and management in a series of 11 patients. *Hepatogastroenterology* 2005; 52: 1259–65.

23. Schwab M, Knoll MR, Jentschura D, Hagmuller E. Hormone inactive neuroendocrine tumors of the pancreas. *Chirurg* 1997; 68: 705–9.

24. Panzuto F, Nasoni S, Falconi M, et al. Prognostic factors and survival in endocrine tumor patients: comparison between gastrointestinal and pancreatic localization. *Endocr Relat Cancer* 2005; 12: 1083–92.

25. Atwell T, Charboneau J, Que F, et al. Treatment of neuroendocrine cancer metastasic to the liver: the role of ablative techniques. *Cardiovasc Intervent Radiol* 2005; 28: 409–21.

26. Ahmed A, Turner G, King B, et al. Midgut neuro-endocrine tumours with liver metastases. Results of the UKI NETS study. *Endocr Relat Cancer* 2009; 16: 885–94.

27. Norton J. Surgical treatment of neuroendocrine metastases. *Best Pract Res Clin Gastroenterol* 2005; 19; 577–83.

28. Rinke A, Müller HH, Schade-Brittinger C, et al. Placebo-controlled, double-blind, prospective, randomized study on the effect of octreotide LAR in the control of tumor growth in patients with meta-static neuroendocrine midgut tumors: a report from the PROMID Study Group. *J Clin Oncol* 2009; 27(28): 4656–63.

29. Caplin ME, Pavel M, Ćwikła JB, et al. Lanreotide in metastatic enteropancreatic neuroendocrine tumors. *N Engl J Med* 2014; 371(3): 224–33.

30. Vinjamuri S, Gilbert TM, Banks M, et al. Peptide receptor radionuclide therapy with 90Y-DOTATATE/90Y-DOTATOC in patients with progressive metastatic neuroendocrine tumours: assessment of response, survival and toxicity. *Br J Cancer* 2013; 108: 1440–8.

31. Ramage JK, Ahmed A, Ardill J, et al. Guidelines for the management of gastroenteropancreatic neuro-endocrine (including carcinoid) tumours (NETs). *Gut* 2012; 61: 6–32.

46

Bone sarcoma

ROBERT J GRIMER AND MICHAEL PARRY

INCIDENCE AND AETIOLOGY

Bone sarcomas arising from mesenchymal tissue are rare, accounting for only 0.2% of all new cancer diagnoses in the UK, an incidence of only 8.2 cases per million of the population [1]. The most common sarcomas arising from bone are osteosarcoma (OS), Ewing's sarcoma (EWS) and chondrosarcoma (CS). The first two of these demonstrate a high incidence in children and adolescents, representing approximately 4% of all malignancies in children under the age of 14 (Figure 46.1). The overall estimated incidence is 2.6 per million for OS, 1.9 per million for EWS and 2.9 per million for CS. There is, however, a wide variety of other less common primary bone tumours broadly included under the category of undifferentiated pleomorphic sarcomas (UPSs) or spindle cell sarcomas of the bone. These comprise a diagnostically heterogenous group of malignant tumours including fibrosarcoma, malignant fibrous histiocytoma, leiomyosarcoma and undifferentiated sarcoma. While the age distribution of these tumours is similar to that of chondrosarcoma, the distribution is more like that of osteosarcoma. They typically represent between 2% and 5% of all primary bone tumours. The management of these malignancies is similar to that of the more common primary bone tumours, with comparable outcomes [2]. The remaining primary malignancy of bone burden constitutes notochordal tumours (chordoma), malignancy in giant cell tumours, angiosarcoma and liposarcoma of the bone. Chordomas, which are derived from primitive notochordal remnants, can arise in the spine or base of the skull with an incidence of one per million per year.

For all sarcomas of the bone, the incidence is more common in males than females, excluding chondrosarcoma for which the incidence is equal. Most cases of primary bone sarcoma are sporadic, the aetiology remaining largely unknown. However, approximately 70% of osteosarcomas, for example, demonstrate mutations in tumour suppressor genes or in DNA helicases. There is an increased incidence of osteosarcoma in patients with the Li–Fraumeni syndrome, involving the tp53 tumour suppressor gene [3], and also those with retinoblastoma, involving the RB1 gene [4]. Rarer conditions involving mutations on the DNA helicases, responsible for the unwinding of DNA prior to replication, including the BLM gene, resulting in Bloom syndrome, and RECQL4 genes, resulting in Rothmund–Thomson syndrome, result in an increased preponderance for osteosarcoma. Secondary osteosarcoma has been associated with pre-existing Paget's disease, with sarcomatous degeneration occurring in 0.1–0.95% of patients with Paget's disease [5], and the incidence increasing with polyostotic Paget's disease [6]. Secondary osteosarcoma may also result in the field of previous therapeutic irradiation or following occupational exposure. It results from DNA damage and subsequent genomic instability in non-cancerous target cells within the previously irradiated field. These tumours are rare with an estimated risk of 0.03–0.08% in a previously irradiated bone [6–9] and a range of latency of onset between 3 and 50 years. Radiation-induced osteosarcomas are aggressive tumours, often arising in central locations which makes treatment difficult. Prognosis is related to the ability to resect the tumour with clear margins [10].

In the case of Ewing's sarcoma, more than 95% of tumours demonstrate EWS-ETS fusion gene rearrangements, most commonly the result of translocations between chromosome 22 and chromosome 11 (t22;11 [q24;q12 translocation]) or 21 (t21;22 [q22;q12]). The ETS transcription factor family is responsible for regulating cellular differentiation, the cell cycle, cell migration and apoptosis. Hence, mutations will

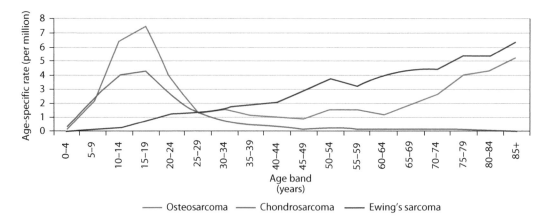

Figure 46.1 Age-specific incidence of the three most common bone tumours. (UK data from the National Cancer Intelligence Unit, http://www.ncin.org.uk/publications/data_briefings/bone_sarcomas_incidence_and_survival.)

result in deregulation of programmed cell death and disruption of cell cycle control.

Chondrosarcomas can be sub-classified as primary conventional chondrosarcomas, arising *de novo* in bone without a pre-existing lesion, and secondary chondrosarcomas, arising from a benign pre-existing chondroid lesion, most commonly an osteochondroma. Secondary chondrosarcomas represent a different entity from dedifferentiated chondrosarcomas which arise from a pre-existing chondroid lesion, but are characterized by a high-grade sarcoma, typically of a different histology (often osteosarcoma), adjacent to the low-grade cartilaginous tumour. Dedifferentiation does occur in secondary chondrosarcoma, but the rate is low, approximately 5% [11], compared to 15% in primary chondrosarcoma [12]. The majority (88%) of secondary chondrosarcomas arise from pre-existing osteochondromas, with solitary osteochondromas carrying a slightly higher risk than multiple osteochondromas [13–15]. In the case of hereditary multiple exostoses (HMEs), a rare familial disease characterized by multiple osteochondromas, mutations are seen in the EXT1, EXT2 and EXT3 genes, with variable phenotypic manifestations. The lifelong risk of malignant degeneration in HME is between 1% and 5%. Secondary chondrosarcoma is seen in patients with Ollier's disease (multiple enchondromas) and Maffucci syndrome (multiple enchondromas and soft tissue haemangiomas). Estimates of malignant transformation in Ollier's disease range from 10% to 40% [16–19] and in Maffucci syndrome from 15% to 20% [20,21], though this risk is increased in the pelvis, scapula and long flat bones [19]. Other benign cartilaginous lesions that have been reported to give rise to secondary chondrosarcoma include solitary enchondromas, synovial chondromatosis and chondromyxoid fibroma.

The most frequent site for bone tumours to arise is shown in Table 46.1. More than 60% of primary bone tumours will arise in the long bones of the lower limb, most commonly around the knee. The second most common site of origin is the pelvis, sacrum and coccyx, accounting for a further 18%, with an additional 13% of tumours arising from the upper limb and shoulder girdle [1].

PATHOLOGY

Primary bone tumours are classified on the basis of their principal cell type and have been defined by the World Health Organization (WHO) [22]. Tissue diagnosis is critical to the management of sarcomas of the bone and, due to their rare incidence, should be performed by experts in the management and diagnosis of bone sarcomas working in a multidisciplinary team. The handling and processing of material harvested at biopsy is critical to allow novel techniques, increasingly relied upon for diagnosis. Tissue imprints can be used to allow fluorescent in situ hybridization (FISH), cells can be cultured to allow further cytogenetic analysis, tissue should be processed for immunohistochemical analysis and samples should be banked for further research and analysis. These techniques have improved diagnosis and allowed targeted therapies, which previously were underutilized due to misdiagnosis. For example, Ewing's sarcoma is a small blue round cell tumour and shares many histological features with neuroblastoma. However, the diagnosis can be confirmed by identifying the characteristic translocation of chromosome 22 using immunohistochemistry.

The pathological diagnosis of chondrosarcoma can be very difficult due to the indistinct spectrum of disease represented by benign chondroid lesions and low-grade malignant lesions. Sarcomatous features are represented by the presence of malignant chondroid tissue which demonstrates hypercellularity, binucleate cells, multiple cells in lacunae, atypical nuclei and myxoid changes in the hyaline cartilage matrix. Some or many of these features may be present in osteochondroma, highlighting the difficulty in accurately diagnosing the malignant potential of the lesion. In such cases, correlation with radiographic and clinical features aids the diagnosis. A slow-growing lesion present for a number of years without significant change in size with a thin cartilage cap (as it is this component of the lesion that undergoes malignant transformation) is unlikely to represent a malignant chondroid lesion.

Table 46.1 Location of bone tumours split by the three most common diagnoses, with the others categorized as UPS

Site/diagnosis	Chondrosarcoma	Ewing's	Osteosarcoma	UPS	Grand total	% of total
Ankle and foot	36	46	59	19	160	4.1
Arm	81	29	41	17	168	4.3
Distal femur	108	79	733	158	1078	27.8
Fibula	8	61	72	10	151	3.9
Pelvis	264	190	134	89	677	17.5
Proximal femur	182	92	103	56	433	11.3
Proximal humerus	103	63	175	27	368	9.5
Proximal tibia	45	78	349	56	528	13.6
Shoulder girdle	52	31	23	12	118	3.0
Trunk	96	44	33	19	192	5.0
Grand total	975	713	1722	463	3873	

Source: Data from Royal Orthopaedic Hospital Oncology Service, Birmingham.

An accurate tissue diagnosis is imperative not only in guiding treatment but also in predicting the natural history of the tumour. Some tumours are rapidly growing with high metastatic potential (e.g. OS, EWS and dedifferentiated CS), while others are much slower growing with less metastatic potential (e.g. parosteal OS, low-grade CS, chordoma and adamantinoma).

DIAGNOSIS AND PREOPERATIVE IMAGING

Despite advances in clinician education and improvements in referral pathways for specialist investigation, the diagnosis of bone sarcomas is often delayed [23,24]. Primary care physicians, particularly when dealing with children and adolescents, must hold a low index of suspicion for malignancy. Symptoms vary but worrisome features from the history include pain, particularly night pain, pain not responding to simple analgesia and persistent pain following injury, as well as prior benign or malignant lesions, family history and previous radiotherapy. All too often, young patients are not referred for investigation, as the diagnosis is not considered. A recent injury does not rule out a malignant pathology and must not prevent investigation. The duration of symptoms prior to diagnosis is often measured in months and for slow-growing tumours such as chondrosarcoma or chordoma, in years. In an attempt to rectify these delays in diagnosis, the National Institute of Health and Care Excellence (NICE) in the UK issued guidelines for the improvement in care for patients presenting with sarcomas [25].

The biopsy of a suspected bone sarcoma must be performed in an institution specializing in the diagnosis and care of these tumours and must be performed according to strict guidelines aimed at minimizing potential morbidity and progression of disease stage as a result of biopsy. In the majority of cases, sufficient material can be retrieved through core needle biopsy often controlled by x-ray, ultrasound or computed tomography [26]. Where possible, biopsy should be undertaken after staging studies as this

will allow assessment of the true extent of the lesion and guide the location of the most representative area of the lesion for biopsy, taking into consideration future potential limb salvage surgery. If open biopsy is required, the incision should be performed in line with the expected incision for definitive resection and should not cross osseo-fascial compartments so as to minimize contamination. Material should be sent for frozen section to ensure a sufficient representative sample has been obtained, and a sample must always be sent for microbiological culture. In the case of malignant aggressive tumours of bone, the biopsy tract must be considered contaminated and should be placed to allow its excision at the time of definitive resection.

Staging involves the accurate assessment of the degree of local and systemic disease and must be completed for all patients with a new diagnosis of bone sarcoma, by a multidisciplinary team specializing in the treatment of such cancers. Local staging requires a minimum of plain radiography and MRI of the affected extremity. Systemic staging, identifying distant metastases and skip lesions must include a CT scan of the chest and traditionally a radionuclide bone scan with Tc-99m. Increasing evidence is appearing of the advantages of whole-body MRI, FDG-PET and PET/CT in the staging of sarcomas of the bone [27], and these will no doubt play an important role in the future. Evidence of metastatic disease is present at the time of diagnosis in approximately 15–22% of patients with osteosarcoma [28,29], 30% of patients with Ewing's sarcoma [30] and 15% with chondrosarcoma [31].

A number of staging systems have been proposed for sarcomas of the bone; perhaps the most commonly applied is the Enneking system [32,33]. According to this system, the majority of primary bone tumours are stage IIB or III at diagnosis. More recently, the TNM system, universally adopted for non-mesenchymal malignancies, has been applied to sarcomas. While this should allow greater ease of comparison between pathology, there are limitations when applied to sarcomas of the bone as, for example, in the case of Ewing's sarcoma, nodal metastases are an infrequent occurrence (Table 46.2).

Table 46.2 AJCC staging system

Stage	Bone sarcoma
Ia	Low grade, ≤8 cm
Ib	Low grade, >8 cm
IIa	High grade, ≤8 cm
IIb	High grade, >8 cm
III	Any tumour with skip metastases
IV	Any with distant metastases at diagnosis

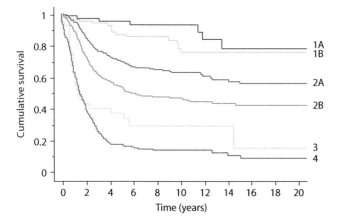

Figure 46.2 Kaplan–Meier survival curve showing the effect of stage on prognosis for all bone sarcomas. (From Royal Orthopaedic Hospital Oncology Service data.)

Regardless of the system adopted, the stage of disease has clinical significance to both the patient and clinician due to the association of poorer prognosis with advanced stage disease (Figure 46.2).

SURGERY FOR PRIMARY OPERABLE CANCER

The management of patients with bone sarcomas must be carried out by a multidisciplinary team including clinicians, pathologists, radiologists and oncologists together with appropriate expertise governed on a case-by-case basis, for example, vascular, general, urological, spinal, thoracic and plastic surgical specialists, as well as dedicated specialist nurses and rehabilitation experts.

The resection of all detectable tumour, including metastases, is the cornerstone of treatment of the majority of sarcomas of the bone. For primary operable tumours, the options are tumour excision with limb salvage or amputation. In the case of tumour resection, this should encompass resection with a clear margin including the pseudocapsule of the tumour and a cuff of normal tissue. The margin of resection will be governed by preoperative local staging imaging. The classic paper by Enneking defined margins as either intralesional (through the tumour), marginal (through the pseudocapsule), wide (through normal tissue) or radical (compartmentectomy, usually by amputation). There is no doubt that neoadjuvant chemotherapy can change the significance of the margin achieved, with a good chemotherapy response dramatically reducing the risk of local recurrence for the same margin achieved. The key factor affecting the width of the margin is usually the closest critical structure – commonly the neurovascular bundle.

The decision between carrying out limb salvage or amputation is governed by the expected postoperative limb function, potential for complications, psychological acceptance and oncological outcomes. Quality-of-life studies suggest that patients adapt equally well to amputation as limb salvage [34,35]. Most importantly, no significant difference exists between the survival rates for amputation and those for limb salvage surgery [36–38], but as survival is affected by the margins achieved at resection, limb salvage must not be favoured over amputation where the potential to compromise a complete resection exists. Limb salvage is possible for approximately 85% of appendicular tumours [36]. Local recurrence rates for amputation and limb salvage are similar and approximately 5% for osteosarcoma [38,39], 9% for Ewing's sarcoma [40] and 25% for chondrosarcoma [31].

Options for reconstruction in limb salvage include endoprosthetic replacement, allograft–prosthetic composite, allograft using donated bone or extracorporeal sterilization and reimplantation of the patient's own bone, and arthrodesis. Each option has its advantages and application is governed on a case-by-case basis. Endoprosthetic replacement offers mobilization and stability, though it incurs the risks of mechanical failure (18%) and infection (11%) [41]. Allograft–prosthetic composite affords the advantages of early stability with the potential biologic benefits of allograft bone. Allografts, particularly osteoarticular allografts, can be used to reconstruct complex structures including joints allowing reattachment of soft tissues. However, the complications are potentially high, including fracture, non-union and infection rates as high as 20% [42–45].

Limb salvage can be particularly challenging in the skeletally immature as reconstruction often requires excision or compromise of the physes, particularly those around the knee, with subsequent implications for limb length discrepancy. This can be counteracted with the use of an extendible endoprosthesis allowing interval lengthening comparable to that of the contralateral limb [46] (Figure 46.3). Lengthening can be achieved either minimally invasively, necessitating multiple surgical interventions and the concurrent increased risk of periprosthetic infection, or non-invasively through extracorporeal magnetic distraction of a motor within the implant.

For tumours involving the distal femur or proximal tibia in skeletally immature patients, intercalary resection and 180° rotation of the distal leg, recreating the knee joint with the prior ankle joint, is an option [36,47]. Following rotationplasty, a prosthesis is worn at the knee for ambulation, and gait analysis demonstrates improved kinematics when compared to above-knee amputation [48]. However, the procedure is technically challenging and some patients and families cannot tolerate the cosmetic disfigurement of the neo-knee joint.

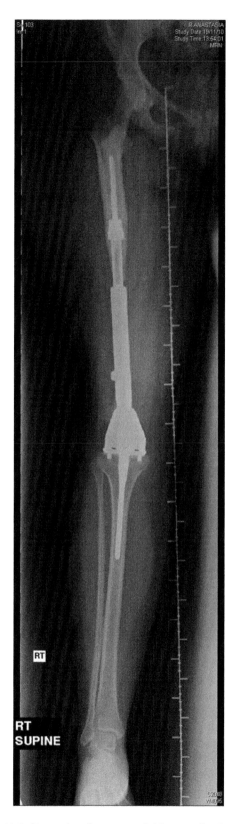

Figure 46.3 Example of an extendable prosthesis inserted in a 10-year-old child for an osteosarcoma of the distal femur. She is now 23 and walks normally. Her leg lengths are equal after undergoing 6 cm of lengthening of the femoral component. Note how the host bone of the femur has overgrown the proximal part of the prosthesis 'locking' it in place.

NEOADJUVANT AND ADJUVANT THERAPIES

Neoadjuvant chemotherapy has been used for most patients with osteosarcoma and Ewing's sarcoma for well over 35 years [49]. A series of trials has shown the value of multidrug regimens for both tumour types [50,51]. In osteosarcoma the principal drugs used are doxorubicin, cisplatin, ifosfamide and high-dose methotrexate, in various combinations to avoid chemoresistance and increase the rate of tumour necrosis [39,50,52,53]. The aim of this chemotherapy is to try to shrink the tumour while also treating the micrometastatic disease [36,54]. Patients without radiologically detectable metastases are considered to have micrometastases and so are treated with the same neoadjuvant regimen. Neoadjuvant chemotherapy allows the assessment of the tumour's sensitivity to chemotherapy following definitive surgical resection, itself a predictor of local recurrence and disease-free survival [39]. For those demonstrating a good response to neoadjuvant chemotherapy (defined as a tumour necrosis rate of $\geq 90\%$), the same adjuvant chemotherapy regimen is administered postoperatively. Patients with a poor response to neoadjuvant chemotherapy (defined as a tumour necrosis rate of $<90\%$) may still benefit from adjuvant chemotherapy [55]. However, despite variations in agents, duration and dose, such salvage attempts have not demonstrated an improvement in disease-free survival for patients with poorly responding tumours [39,56]. The role of radiation therapy in the treatment of osteosarcoma is limited to palliation as this tumour is largely radiation resistant.

In cases of Ewing's sarcoma, most patients with apparently localized disease will have subclinical micrometastases and so any treatment must include systemic therapy in combination with local control through radiotherapy or surgery. As Ewing's sarcoma is often sensitive to chemotherapy, most patients will receive neoadjuvant chemotherapy, regardless of the extent of the local disease [51]. A number of trials have evaluated the role of differing agents and differing durations in the neoadjuvant treatment of Ewing's sarcoma. Current regimens in the United States rely on vincristine, doxorubicin and cyclophosphamide, alternating with ifosfamide and etoposide [57,58]. A number of pan-European trials have investigated the role of neoadjuvant and adjuvant chemotherapy in Ewing's sarcoma. The European Ewing Sarcoma Study Group (EURO-Ewing-99) assessed the role of additional cyclophosphamide in good responders following conventional vincristine, ifosfamide, doxorubicin and etoposide (VIDE) and demonstrated no superior outcome when compared to conventional vincristine, actinomycin-D and ifosfamide [59,60], while the current EURO-Ewing-2008 trial is exploring the role of additional bisphosphonates. The Children's Oncology Group (COG) aimed to assess the effect of dose intensification (AEWS0031), while the Italian/Scandinavian ISG/SSG III trial investigated the role of additional busulfan–melphalan high-dose therapy with stem cell support for poor responders to neoadjuvant therapy chemotherapy [61,62].

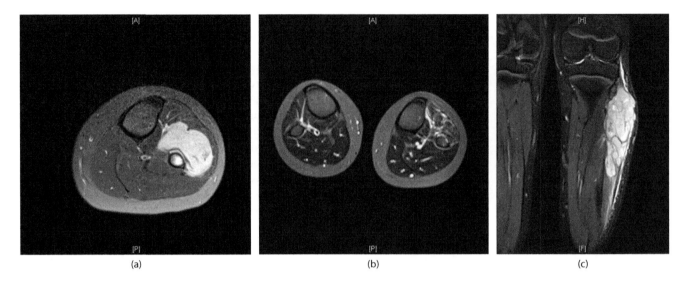

(a)   (b)   (c)

Figure 46.4 Cautionary tale about Ewing's sarcoma. A 13-year-old boy had a Ewing's sarcoma of the proximal fibula with significant soft tissue extension. (a) Following chemotherapy all of the soft tissue tumour resolved. (b) He underwent resection of the proximal fibula with a thin cuff of muscles around it, preserving the peroneal nerve. There was no viable tumour seen in the resected specimen. Within 1 year, however, he developed a large local recurrence in the soft tissues (c) and required above-knee amputation. Sterilizing the whole of the original tumour area is essential in all sarcoma surgery.

Multimodal neoadjuvant chemotherapy in Ewing's sarcoma will often produce a dramatic shrinkage of the tumour with a concurrent reduction in symptoms.

Local control is achieved by surgical resection whenever possible. The main principle is that all of the initially involved tissue must be sterilized by either surgical excision or radiotherapy, no matter how effective the chemotherapy, and the two are often used in combination (Figure 46.4). This will result in the lowest risk of recurrence. Radiotherapy alone is reserved for unresectable tumours, but does result in a higher rate of local recurrence which is associated with a very poor prognosis [63–66].

LOCALLY ADVANCED AND METASTATIC DISEASE

As recurrence and hence survival is significantly affected by attaining a clear margin at local control [67–69], amputation must be considered for tumours which are unresectable by any other means. Such tumours will often be extending out of the primary bone, violating a number of compartments, and will be encircling the neurovascular bundle as well as multiple muscles and often joints. While it is of course possible to resect all of these, the reconstruction options or the oncological margins that can be achieved may mean that amputation is the preferred option both for oncological reasons and for better function. Amputation is required in approximately 15% of patients with primary bone tumours. The need for amputation will depend on the location and extent of the tumour, the capabilities of the operating team and the wishes of the patient.

For tumours arising around the ankle and hindfoot, amputation may be considered for local control above limb salvage as reconstruction options are limited and function is often excellent following below-knee amputation [70]. For tumours around the knee, primary amputation may be considered if tumour involves not only the knee joint, but also surrounding soft tissues and encircles the neurovascular bundle. For tumours invading the knee, or knee involvement due to iatrogenic contamination or inappropriate biopsy technique, extra-articular resection may be considered [71,72]. However, it should be noted that despite, at worst, functional outcomes comparable to those of more conventional intra-articular resections, extra-articular resection carries a complication rate approximating 40% [73,74]. Careful assessment of patients and counselling of the potential for significant complications must be completed prior to undertaking an extra-articular resection. In children particularly, rotationplasty offers a more functional alternative.

The surgical treatment of pelvic tumours presents a unique set of challenges, due to the proximity of neurovascular and visceral structures and the complex anatomy of the pelvis. Achieving surgical margins in pelvic resection is often difficult [75]. With advances in imaging and non-surgical treatment modalities, the use of limb salvage as opposed to amputation has demonstrated reliable outcomes in the treatment of osseous pelvic sarcoma [41,76–80]. Several reconstruction options have been proposed including iliofemoral or ischiofemoral arthrodesis, massive allografts, endoprosthetic reconstruction and bone sterilization and reimplantation. However, for all these reconstruction options, significant rates of early and late complications have been reported (Figure 46.5). Early complications such as infection or instability may delay adjuvant chemotherapy with a subsequent impact on oncological outcomes. One of the simplest procedures is an internal hemipelvectomy without reconstruction which can lead to a surprisingly good level of function (Figure 46.6) [81]. For extensive tumours involving the pelvis, careful consideration must be given to balancing satisfactory surgical margins with function and patient preferences. There is still a role for hindquarter amputation for extensive tumours of the pelvis. This operation can offer a reasonable chance of survival, and although there is major functional loss, improvements in prosthetics are increasingly allowing patients to become mobile again, with many returning to work [82,83].

For tumours of the upper limb, limb salvage should be undertaken when at all possible, as all amputations in

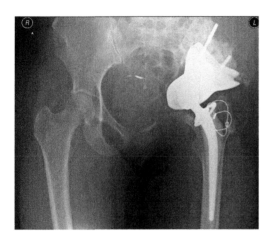

Figure 46.5 Example of a hemipelvectomy for a chondrosarcoma of the pelvis treated by excision and reconstruction with a custom made pelvic endoprosthetic replacement. The implant failed to integrate and migrated over a period of 5 years requiring removal of the prosthesis.

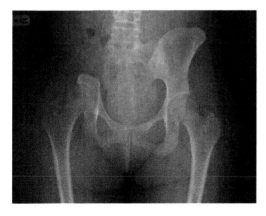

Figure 46.6 Example of an internal hemipelvectomy for a radiation-induced osteosarcoma of the ilium. No reconstruction was used and the patient walked without any need for walking aids.

the upper limb will result in significant loss of function. Fortunately, upper limb tumours tend to present at an earlier stage than those in the pelvis and lower limb. However, survival after upper limb amputation is often poor as it tends to be reserved for large or multifocal tumours, or for palliation [84–86]. Microsurgical, allograft and prosthetic options have advanced significantly [87–89] with amputation reserved for only unresectable tumours.

LOCAL RECURRENCE

Despite advances in adjuvant therapies, the prognosis for sarcomas of the bone is affected by the development of recurrent disease. In slow-growing tumours of the bone where wide margins are difficult to achieve, for example, chordoma of the sacrum, local recurrence is almost inevitable with rates ranging between 43% and 85% [90]. This should be contrasted with Ewing's sarcoma where the development of local recurrence has a catastrophic effect on survival which diminishes to <10% at 5 years with recurrent disease [91–93]. The treatment of local recurrence in Ewing's sarcoma depends on the site of the recurrence, previous treatment and individual patient considerations. Radiotherapy to isolated bone lesions may provide symptomatic relief while radical resection may improve outcome [94].

The prognosis for patients after local recurrence of osteosarcoma is generally poor, despite aggressive multimodal treatment [95,96]. The management of local recurrence in the case of osteosarcoma, particularly on the background of limb salvage surgery, remains controversial. Improved survival in the presence of osseous recurrence is seen with clear margins following resection of the recurrence (including amputation), and a time lag of >18 months between diagnosis and local recurrence [96–98]. The effect of resection margin on the treatment of local recurrence in osteosarcoma is significant with some advocating that amputation must be considered when a margin of >1 cm cannot be achieved with limb salvage [99]. The use of second-line chemotherapy remains uncertain if the recurrence has been completely surgically removed.

In recent years, a number of focused conventional radiotherapy strategies, including intensity-modulated radiotherapy (IMRT), and non-conventional particle therapies (carbon ion and proton therapy) have demonstrated promising results in the treatment of primary tumours particularly in unresectable regions (especially chordomas), but also in the management of local recurrence [100–102]. As these modalities become more freely available, evidence for their efficacy and applications will no doubt expand.

METASTATIC DISEASE

Sarcomas of the bone metastasize primarily to the lung. Pulmonary metastases occur in approximately 40% of patients with sarcomas of the bone. Pulmonary metastases lead to a significant deterioration in survival with only 20–40% of those with pulmonary metastases surviving 5 years. In the case of primary metastatic osteosarcoma, treatment intent is the same as that for non-metastatic osteosarcoma. In select patient subsets, a prognosis similar to that of non-metastatic groups is seen, albeit with the addition of surgical removal of all metastatic deposits. Approximately 30% of those with primary metastatic osteosarcoma and >40% of those who achieve a complete surgical remission become long-term survivors. In the case of recurrent metastases in osteosarcoma, surgical resection must be considered as unoperated metastatic disease is almost universally fatal, while more than 30% of those who achieve a second surgical remission survive >5 years. Even those with multiple pulmonary recurrences should be considered for repeated surgical resection. There are at present no accepted regimens for second-line chemotherapy in osteosarcoma, though combinations of ifosfamide, etoposide and carboplatin are often employed.

In the case of Ewing's sarcoma, patients with pulmonary metastases at diagnosis require special consideration, as those treated with the same regimens as non-metastatic disease have a worse prognosis. As previously discussed, several studies have assessed the efficacy of time-compressed, intensive high-dose chemotherapy together with autologous stem cell rescue for patients with metastatic disease. Patients with pulmonary metastases should be considered for whole lung irradiation [94] with surgical resection of residual disease. Ifosfamide and etoposide should be considered if not previously administered. Second-line agents including topotecan, irinotecan, busulfan, melphalan, thiotepa and temozolomide have demonstrated reasonable response in metastatic Ewing's sarcoma [51,103,104]. Given the poor outcomes associated with unresected metastatic Ewing's sarcoma, even aggressive myeloablative approaches should be considered [105].

REFERENCES

1. National Cancer Intelligence Network. Bone sarcoma: incidence and survival rates in England. Available from http://www.ncin.org.uk/publications/data_briefings/bone_sarcoma_incidence_and_survival_rates_in_england_october_2012.
2. Pakos EE, Grimer RJ, Peake D, Spooner D, Carter SR, Tillman RM, et al. The "other" bone sarcomas: prognostic factors and outcomes of spindle cell sarcomas of bone. *J Bone Joint Surg Br* 2011;93(9):1271–8.
3. Hayden JB, Hoang BH. Osteosarcoma: basic science and clinical implications. *Orthop Clin North Am* 2006;37(1):1–7.
4. Wang LL. Biology of osteogenic sarcoma. *Cancer J* 2005;11(4):294.
5. Mangham DC, Davie MW, Grimer RJ. Sarcoma arising in Paget's disease of bone: declining incidence and increasing age at presentation *Bone* 2009;44(3):431–6.
6. Huvos AG, Butler A, Bretsky SS. Osteogenic sarcoma associated with Paget's disease of bone. A clinicopathologic study of 65 patients. *Cancer* 1983;52(8):1489–95.
7. Mark RJ, Poen J, Tran LM, Fu YS, Selch MT, Parker RG. Postirradiation sarcomas. A single-institution study and review of the literature. *Cancer* 1994;73(10):2653–62.
8. Mavrogenis AF, Pala E, Guerra G, Ruggieri P. Post-radiation sarcomas. Clinical outcome of 52 patients. *J Surg Oncol* 2011;105(6):570–6.
9. Mavrogenis AF, Angelini A, Pala E, Calabro T, Bianchi G, Casadei R, et al. Radiation-induced sarcomas. *J Long Term Eff Med Implants* 2011;21(3):233–40.
10. Kalra S, Grimer RJ, Spooner D, Carter SR, Tillman RM, Abudu A. Radiation-induced sarcomas of bone: factors that affect outcome. *J Bone Joint Surg Br* 2007;89(6):808–13.
11. Staals EL, Bacchini P, Mercuri M, Bertoni F. Dedifferentiated chondrosarcomas arising in pre-existing osteochondromas. *J Bone Joint Surg Am* 2007;89(5):987.
12. Staals EL, Bacchini P, Bertoni F. Dedifferentiated central chondrosarcoma. *Cancer* 2006;106(12):2682–91.
13. Ahmed AR, Tan T-S, Unni KK, Collins MS, Wenger DE, Sim FH. Secondary chondrosarcoma in osteochondroma: report of 107 patients. *Clin Orthop Relat Res* 2003;411:193–206.
14. Altay M, Bayrakci K, Yildiz Y, Erekul S, Saglik Y. Secondary chondrosarcoma in cartilage bone tumors: report of 32 patients. *J Orthop Sci* 2007;12(5):415–23.
15. Garrison RC, Unni KK, McLeod RA, Pritchard DJ, Dahlin DC. Chondrosarcoma arising in osteochondroma. *Cancer* 2006;49(9):1890–7.
16. Liu J, Hudkins PG, Swee RG, Unni KK. Bone sarcomas associated with Ollier's disease. *Cancer* 1987;59(7):1376–85.
17. Schaison FF, Anract PP, Coste FF, De Pinieux GG, Forest MM, Tomeno BB. Chondrosarcoma secondary to multiple cartilage diseases. Study of 29 clinical cases and review of the literature. *Rev Chir Orthop Reparatrice Appar Mot* 1999;85(8):834–45.
18. Schwartz HS, Zimmerman NB, Simon MA, Wroble RR, Millar EA, Bonfiglio M. The malignant potential of enchondromatosis. *J Bone Joint Surg Am* 1987;69(2):269–74.
19. Verdegaal SHM, Bovée JVMG, Pansuriya TC, Grimer RJ, Ozger H, Jutte PC, et al. Incidence, predictive factors, and prognosis of chondrosarcoma in patients with Ollier disease and Maffucci syndrome: an international multicenter study of 161 patients. *Oncologist* 2011;16(12):1771–9.
20. Lewis RJ, Ketcham AS. Maffucci's syndrome: functional and neoplastic significance. Case report and review of the literature. *J Bone Joint Surg Am* 1973;55(7):1465–79.

21. Sun TC, Swee RG, Shives TC, Unni KK. Chondrosarcoma in Maffucci's syndrome. *J Bone Joint Surg Am* 1985;67(8):1214–9.

22. Fletcher CD, World Health Organization, International Agency for Research on Cancer. *WHO Classification of Tumours of Soft Tissue and Bone.* Lyon: IARC Press, 2013.

23. Goyal S, Roscoe J, Ryder WDJ, Gattamaneni HR, Eden TOB. Symptom interval in young people with bone cancer. *Eur J Cancer* 2004;40(15):2280–6.

24. Grimer RJ, Briggs TWR. Earlier diagnosis of bone and soft-tissue tumours. *J Bone Joint Surg Br* 2010;92(11):1489–92.

25. National Collaborating Centre for Cancer. *Guidance on Cancer Services: Improving Outcomes for Patients with Sarcoma.* London: National Institute for Health and Care Excellence Press, 2006.

26. Saifuddin A, Clarke A. Biopsy of bone and soft tissue sarcomas. In Bentley G, ed., *European Surgical Orthopaedics and Traumatology.* Berlin: Springer, 2014, pp. 3995–4016.

27. Ciliberto M, Maggi F, Treglia G, Padovano F, Calandriello L, Giordano A, et al. Comparison between whole-body MRI and fluorine-18-fluorodeoxyglucose PET or PET/CT in oncology: a systematic review. *Radiol Oncol* 2013;47(3):206–18.

28. Kaste SC, Pratt CB, Cain AM, Jones-Wallace DJ, Rao BN. Metastases detected at the time of diagnosis of primary pediatric extremity osteosarcoma at diagnosis: imaging features. *Cancer* 1999;86(8):1602–8.

29. Ozaki T, Flege S, Kevric M, Lindner N, Maas R, Delling G, et al. Osteosarcoma of the pelvis: experience of the Cooperative Osteosarcoma Study Group. *J Clin Oncol* 2003;21(2):334–41.

30. Rodríguez-Galindo C, Navid F, Liu T, Billups CA, Rao BN, Krasin MJ. Prognostic factors for local and distant control in Ewing sarcoma family of tumors. *Ann Oncol* 2008;19(4):814–20.

31. Fiorenza F, Abudu A, Grimer RJ, Carter SR, Tillman RM, Ayoub K, et al. Risk factors for survival and local control in chondrosarcoma of bone. *J Bone Joint Surg Br* 2002;84(1):93–9.

32. Enneking WF, Spanier SS, Goodman MA. A system for the surgical staging of musculoskeletal sarcoma. *Clin Orthop Relat Res* 1980;(153):106–20.

33. Enneking WF. A system of staging musculoskeletal neoplasms. *Clin Orthop Relat Res* 1986;(204):9–24.

34. Meyers PA, Gorlick R. Osteosarcoma. *Pediatr Clin North Am* 1997;44(4):973–89.

35. Rougraff BT, Simon MA, Kneisl JS, Greenberg DB, Mankin HJ. Limb salvage compared with amputation for osteosarcoma of the distal end of the femur. A long-term oncological, functional, and quality-of-life study. *J Bone Joint Surg Am* 1994;76(5):649–56.

36. Grimer RJ. Surgical options for children with osteosarcoma. *Lancet Oncol* 2005;6(2):85–92.

37. Simon MA, Aschliman MA, Thomas N, Mankin HJ. Limb-salvage treatment versus amputation for osteosarcoma of the distal end of the femur. *J Bone Joint Surg Am* 1986;68(9):1331–7.

38. Bacci G, Ferrari S, Lari S, Mercuri M, Donati D, Longhi A, et al. Osteosarcoma of the limb. *J Bone Joint Surg Br* 2002;84:88–92.

39. Ferrari S. Neoadjuvant chemotherapy with high-dose ifosfamide, high-dose methotrexate, cisplatin, and doxorubicin for patients with localized osteosarcoma of the extremity: a joint study by the Italian and Scandinavian sarcoma groups. *J Clin Oncol* 2005;23(34):8845–52.

40. Bacci G, Forni C, Longhi A, Ferrari S, Donati D, De Paolis M, et al. Long-term outcome for patients with non-metastatic Ewing's sarcoma treated with adjuvant and neoadjuvant chemotherapies. 402 patients treated at Rizzoli between 1972 and 1992. *Eur J Cancer* 2004;40(1):73–83.

41. Jeys LM, Kulkarni A, Grimer RJ, Carter SR, Tillman RM, Abudu A. Endoprosthetic reconstruction for the treatment of musculoskeletal tumors of the appendicular skeleton and pelvis. *J Bone Joint Surg Am* 2008;90(6):1265–71.

42. Grimer R. Excision and reconstruction around the knee. In Bentley G, ed., *European Surgical Orthopaedics and Traumatology.* Berlin: Springer, 2014, pp. 4223–40.

43. Ogilvie CM, Crawford EA, Hosalkar HS, King JJ, Lackman RD. Long-term results for limb salvage with osteoarticular allograft reconstruction. *Clin Orthop Relat Res* 2009;467(10):2685–90.

44. Mankin HJ, Hornicek FJ, Raskin KA. Infection in massive bone allografts. *Clin Orthop Relat Res* 2005;(432):210–6.

45. Sorger JI, Hornicek FJ, Zavatta M, Menzner JP, Gebhardt MC, Tomford WW, et al. Allograft fractures revisited. *Clin Orthop Relat Res* 2001;382:66.

46. Goulding KA, Gaston CL, Grimer RJ. Outcomes and options for prosthetic reconstruction after tumour resection about the knee. *Curr Surg Rep* 2014;2(2):42.

47. Nichter LS, Menendez LR. Reconstructive considerations for limb salvage surgery. *Orthop Clin North Am* 1993;24(3):511–21.

48. Fuchs B, Kotajarvi BR, Kaufman KR, Sim FH. Functional outcome of patients with rotationplasty about the knee. *Clin Orthop Relat Res* 2003;415:52–8.

49. Jaffe N, Paed D, Traggis D, Salian S, Cassady JR. Improved outlook for Ewing's sarcoma with combination chemotherapy (vincristine, actinomycin D and cyclophosphamide) and radiation therapy. *Cancer* 1976;38(5):1925–30.

50. Carrle D, Bielack SS. Current strategies of chemotherapy in osteosarcoma. *Int Orthop* 2006;30(6):445–51.

51. Ludwig JA. Ewing sarcoma: historical perspectives, current state-of-the-art, and opportunities for targeted therapy in the future. *Curr Opin Oncol* 2008;20(4):412–8.

52. Longhi A, Errani C, De Paolis M, Mercuri M, Bacci G. Primary bone osteosarcoma in the pediatric age: state of the art. *Cancer Treat Rev* 2006;32(6):423–36.

53. Meyers PA, Schwartz CL, Krailo MD, Healey JH, Bernstein ML, Betcher D, et al. Osteosarcoma: the addition of muramyl tripeptide to chemotherapy improves overall survival: a report from the Children's Oncology Group. *J Clin Oncol* 2008;26(4):633–8.

54. Hosalkar HS, Dormans JP. Limb sparing surgery for pediatric musculoskeletal tumors. *Pediatr Blood Cancer* 2004;42(4):295–310.

55. Meyers PA, Heller G, Healey J, Huvos A, Lane J, Marcove R, et al. Chemotherapy for nonmetastatic osteogenic sarcoma: the Memorial Sloan-Kettering experience. *J Clin Oncol* 1992;10(1):5–15.

56. Smeland S, Müller C, Alvegard TA, Wiklund T, Wiebe T, Björk O, et al. Scandinavian Sarcoma Group Osteosarcoma Study SSG VIII: prognostic factors for outcome and the role of replacement salvage chemotherapy for poor histological responders. *Eur J Cancer* 2003;39(4):488–94.

57. Grier HE, Krailo MD, Tarbell NJ, Link MP, Fryer CJH, Pritchard DJ, et al. Addition of ifosfamide and etoposide to standard chemotherapy for Ewing's sarcoma and primitive neuroectodermal tumor of bone. *N Engl J Med* 2003;348(8):694–701.

58. Grier HE, Krailo MD, Tarbell NJ, Link MP, Fryer CJH, Pritchard DJ, et al. Addition of ifosfamide and etoposide to standard chemotherapy for Ewing's sarcoma and primitive neuroectodermal tumor of bone. *N Engl J Med* 2003;348(8):694–701.

59. Juergens C, Weston C, Lewis I, Whelan J, Paulussen M, Oberlin O, et al. Safety assessment of intensive induction with vincristine, ifosfamide, doxorubicin, and etoposide (VIDE) in the treatment of Ewing tumors in the EURO-E.W.I.N.G. 99 clinical trial. *Pediatr Blood Cancer* 2006;47(1):22–9.

60. Ladenstein R, Potschger U, Le Deley MC, Whelan J, Paulussen M, Oberlin O, et al. Primary disseminated multifocal Ewing sarcoma: results of the Euro-Ewing 99 trial. *J Clin Oncol* 2010;28(20):3284–91.

61. Womer RB, West DC, Krailo MD, Dickman PS, Pawel BR, Grier HE, et al. Randomized controlled trial of interval-compressed chemotherapy for the treatment of localized Ewing sarcoma: a report from the Children's Oncology Group. *J Clin Oncol* 2012;30(33):4148–54.

62. Ferrari S, Sundby Hall K, Luksch R, Tienghi A, Wiebe T, Fagioli F, et al. Nonmetastatic Ewing family tumors: high-dose chemotherapy with stem cell rescue in poor responder patients. Results of the Italian Sarcoma Group/Scandinavian Sarcoma Group III protocol. *Ann Oncol* 2011;22(5):1221–7.

63. Dunst J, Schuck A. Role of radiotherapy in Ewing tumors. *Pediatr Blood Cancer* 2004;42(5):465–70.

64. Dunst J, Jurgens H, Sauer R, Pape H, Paulussen M, Winkelmann W, et al. Radiation therapy in Ewing's sarcoma: an update of the CESS 86 trial. *Int J Radiat Oncol Biol Phys* 1995;32(4):919–30.

65. Donaldson SS. Ewing sarcoma: radiation dose and target volume. *Pediatr Blood Cancer* 2004;42(5):471–6.

66. Bolek TW, Marcus RB, Mendenhall NP, Scarborough MT, Graham-Pole J. Local control and functional results after twice-daily radiotherapy for Ewing's sarcoma of the extremities. *Int J Radiat Oncol Biol Phys* 1996;35(4):687–92.

67. Gupta GR, Yasko AW, Lewis VO, Cannon CP, Raymond AK, Patel S, et al. Risk of local recurrence after deltoid-sparing resection for osteosarcoma of the proximal humerus. *Cancer* 2009;115(16):3767–73.

68. Davis AM, Kandel RA, Wunder JS, Unger R, Meer J, O'Sullivan B, et al. The impact of residual disease on local recurrence in patients treated by initial unplanned resection for soft tissue sarcoma of the extremity. *J Surg Oncol* 1997;66(2):81–7.

69. Blakely ML, Spurbeck WW, Pappo AS, Pratt CB, Rodriguez-Galindo C, Santana VM, et al. The impact of margin of resection on outcome in pediatric non-rhabdomyosarcoma soft tissue sarcoma. *J Pediatr Surg* 1999;34(5):672–5.

70. Refaat Y, Gunnoe J, Hornicek FJ, Mankin HJ. Comparison of quality of life after amputation or limb salvage. *Clin Orthop Relat Res* 2002;397:298.

71. Capanna R, Scoccianti G, Campanacci DA, Beltrami G, De Biase P. Surgical technique: extraarticular knee resection with prosthesis-proximal tibia-extensor apparatus allograft for tumors invading the knee. *Clin Orthop Relat Res* 2011;469(10):2905–14.

72. Zwolak P, Kühnel SP, Fuchs B. Extraarticular knee resection for sarcomas with preservation of the extensor mechanism: surgical technique and review of cases. *Clin Orthop Relat Res* 2010;469(1):251–6.

73. Ieguchi M, Hoshi M, Aono M, Takada J, Ohebisu N, Kudawara I, et al. Knee reconstruction with endoprosthesis after extra-articular and intra-articular resection of osteosarcoma. *Jap J Clin Oncol* 2014;44(9):812–7.

74. Hardes J, Henrichs MP, Gosheger G, Gebert C, Höll S, Dieckmann R, et al. Endoprosthetic replacement after extra-articular resection of bone and soft-tissue tumours around the knee. *Bone Joint J* 2013;95-B(10):1425–31.

75. Carter SR, Eastwood DM, Grimer RJ, Sneath RS. Hindquarter amputation for tumours of the musculoskeletal system. *J Bone Joint Surg Br* 1990;72(3):490–3.

76. Bell RS, Davis AM, Wunder JS, Buconjic T, McGoveran B, Gross AE. Allograft reconstruction of the acetabulum after resection of stage-IIB sarcoma. Intermediate-term results. *J Bone Joint Surg Am* 1997;79(11):1663–74.

77. Langlais F, Lambotte JC, Thomazeau H. Long-term results of hemipelvis reconstruction with allografts. *Clin Orthop Relat Res* 2001;388:178–86.

78. Ueda T, Kakunaga S, Takenaka S, Araki N, Yoshikawa H. Constrained total hip megaprosthesis for primary periacetabular tumors. *Clin Orthop Relat Res* 2013;471(3):741–9.

79. Fisher NE, Patton JT, Grimer RJ, Porter D, Jeys L, Tillman RM, et al. Ice-cream cone reconstruction of the pelvis: a new type of pelvic replacement: early results. *J Bone Joint Surg Br* 2011;93(5):684–8.

80. Campanacci D, Chacon S, Mondanelli N, Beltrami G, Scoccianti G, Caff G, et al. Pelvic massive allograft reconstruction after bone tumour resection. *Int Orthop* 2012;36(12):2529–36.

81. Gebert C, Gosheger G, Winkelmann W. Hip transposition as a universal surgical procedure for periacetabular tumors of the pelvis. *J Surg Oncol* 2009;99(3):169–72.

82. Grimer RJ, Chandrasekar CR, Carter SR, Abudu A, Tillman RM, Jeys L. Hindquarter amputation: is it still needed and what are the outcomes? *J Bone Joint Surg Br* 2013;95(1):127–31.

83. Houdek MT, Kralovec ME, Andrews KL. Hemipelvectomy: high-level amputation surgery and prosthetic rehabilitation. *Am J Phys Med Rehabil* 2014;93(7):600–8.

84. Bhagia SM, Elek EM, Grimer RJ, Carter SR, Tillman RM. Forequarter amputation for high-grade malignant tumours of the shoulder girdle. *J Bone Joint Surg Br* 1997;79(6):924–6.

85. Rickelt J, Hoekstra H, van Coevorden F, de Vreeze R, Verhoef C, van Geel AN. Forequarter amputation for malignancy. *Br J Surg* 2009;96(7):792–8.

86. Puhaindran ME, Chou J, Forsberg JA, Athanasian EA. Major upper-limb amputations for malignant tumors. *J Hand Surg Am* 2012;37(6):1235–41.

87. Athanasian EA, Healey JH. Resection replantation of the arm for sarcoma: an alternative to amputation. *Clin Orthop Relat Res* 2002;395:204–8.

88. Abdeen A, Hoang BH, Athanasian EA, Morris CD, Boland PJ, Healey JH. Allograft-prosthesis composite reconstruction of the proximal part of the humerus: functional outcome and survivorship. *J Bone Joint Surg Am* 2009;91(10):2406–15.

89. Windhager R, Millesi H, Kotz R. Resection-replantation for primary malignant tumours of the arm. An alternative to fore-quarter amputation. *J Bone Joint Surg Br* 1995;77(2):176–84.

90. Ruggieri P, Angelini A, Ussia G, Montalti M, Mercuri M. Surgical margins and local control in resection of sacral chordomas. *Clin Orthop Relat Res* 2010;468(11):2939–47.

91. Rodríguez-Galindo C, Navid F, Liu T, Billups CA, Rao BN, Krasin MJ. Prognostic factors for local and distant control in Ewing sarcoma family of tumors. *Ann Oncol* 2008;19(4):814–20.

92. Bacci G, Longhi A, Ferrari S, Mercuri M, Barbieri E, Bertoni F, et al. Pattern of relapse in 290 patients with nonmetastatic Ewing's sarcoma family tumors treated at a single institution with adjuvant and neoadjuvant chemotherapy between 1972 and 1999. *Eur J Surg Oncol* 2006;32(9):974–9.

93. Bacci G, Longhi A, Ferrari S, Mercuri M, Versari M, Bertoni F. Prognostic factors in non-metastatic Ewing's sarcoma tumor of bone: an analysis of 579 patients treated at a single institution with adjuvant or neoadjuvant chemotherapy between 1972 and 1998. *Acta Oncol* 2006;45(4):469–75.

94. Rodriguez-Galindo C, Billups CA, Kun LE, Rao BN, Pratt CB, Merchant TE, et al. Survival after recurrence of Ewing tumors. *Cancer* 2002;94(2):561–9.

95. Bacci G, Longhi A, Cesari M, Versari M, Bertoni F. Influence of local recurrence on survival in patients with extremity osteosarcoma treated with neoadjuvant chemotherapy: the experience of a single institution with 44 patients. *Cancer* 2006;106(12):2701–6.

96. Rodriguez-Galindo C, Shah N, McCarville MB, Billups CA, Neel MN, Rao BN, et al. Outcome after local recurrence of osteosarcoma. *Cancer* 2004;100(9):1928–35.

97. Franke M, Hardes J, Helmke K, Jundt G, Jürgens H, Kempf-Bielack B, et al. Solitary skeletal osteosarcoma recurrence. Findings from the Cooperative Osteosarcoma Study Group. *Pediatr Blood Cancer* 2011;56(5):771–6.

98. Takeuchi A, Lewis VO, Satcher RL, Moon BS, Lin PP. What are the factors that affect survival and relapse after local recurrence of osteosarcoma? *Clin Orthop Relat Res* 2014;472(10):3188–95.

99. Loh AHP, Navid F, Wang C, Bahrami A, Wu J, Neel MD, et al. Management of local recurrence of pediatric osteosarcoma following limb-sparing surgery. *Ann Surg Oncol* 2014;21(6):1948–55.

100. Tsujii H, Kamada T. A review of update clinical results of carbon ion radiotherapy. *Jpn J Clin Oncol* 2012;42(8):670–85.

101. Nikoghosyan AV, Rauch G, Münter MW, Jensen AD, Combs SE, Kieser M, et al. Randomised trial of proton vs. carbon ion radiation therapy in patients with low and intermediate grade chondrosarcoma of the skull base, clinical phase III study. *BMC Cancer* 2010;10:606–12.

102. McDonald MW, Linton OR, Shah MV. Proton therapy for reirradiation of progressive or recurrent chordoma. *Int J Radiat Oncol Biol Phys* 2013;87(5):1107–14.

103. McTiernan A, Driver D, Michelagnoli MP, Kilby AM, Whelan JS. High dose chemotherapy with bone marrow or peripheral stem cell rescue is an effective treatment option for patients with relapsed or progressive Ewing's sarcoma family of tumours. *Ann Oncol* 2006;17(8):1301–5.

104. Wagner LM, McAllister N, Goldsby RE, Rausen AR, McNall-Knapp RY, McCarville MB, et al. Temozolomide and intravenous irinotecan for treatment of advanced Ewing sarcoma. *Pediatr Blood Cancer* 2007;48(2):132–9.

105. Burdach S, van Kaick B, Laws HJ, Ahrens S, Haase R, Körholz D, et al. Allogeneic and autologous stem-cell transplantation in advanced Ewing tumors. *Ann Oncol* 2000;11:1451–62.

47

Extremity soft tissue sarcoma

NICHOLAS C EASTLEY, ANDREW J HAYES AND ROBERT U ASHFORD

INCIDENCE AND AETIOLOGY

Soft tissue sarcomas (STSs) are a diverse group of malignant tumours that originate from mesenchymal tissue. They account for just 1% of all cancers, and despite presenting in a bimodal distribution, they are still considerably more common in the elderly (85%). There are more than 50 different subtypes of STS subcategorized by their histological appearance, although overall the group remain relatively rare compared to their benign soft tissue tumour counterparts (100:1). Overall 13,100 new cases of STS are diagnosed annually in the European Union and approximately 8500 annually in the US [1,2].

The most common site for a STS is in the lower limb, but they can be found in almost any anatomical location (Table 47.1) [13]. Overall more than 50% of cases occur in either the upper or lower limb. The most common histological subtypes include liposarcomas, leiomyosarcomas and synovial sarcomas, but the majority of STSs found in children and young adults are rhabdomyosarcomas.

Most STSs are sporadic with an unknown aetiology. Several rare genetic syndromes predisposing to STSs have however been recognized, including hereditary retinoblastoma (involving a germline mutation of the retinoblastoma gene), Li–Fraumeni syndrome [3] (involving P53 mutations) and neurofibromatosis type 1 which is linked primarily with malignant peripheral nerve sheath tumours [4]. Some STSs are associated with viral infections including human herpes virus (Kaposi sarcoma) and Epstein–Barr virus (a subset of leiomyosarcomas). Others have been linked with environmental factors including the previous administration of radiotherapy [5]. The most common example of this is found in the breast when radiotherapy is the major predisposing factor for cutaneous angiosarcomas [6,7]. Certain chemicals have also been implicated in the development of STS including vinyl chloride (linked specifically with hepatic angiosarcoma) [8] and dioxins (linked with STSs generally) [9]. In rare cases lymphangiosarcoma can be found in cases of chronic lymphoedema (termed Stewart–Treves syndrome following a mastectomy [10]), and cutaneous angiosarcomas have also been linked with non-functioning arteriovenous fistulae in renal dialysis patients [11].

Genetically STSs can be broadly classified into one of two groups [12]. Around 20% of STSs have simple genetic mutations (usually balanced translocations or oncogene mutations) and a stable karyotype. The tumour-specific nature of some of these mutations makes their detection of diagnostic use, for example, the EWS mutation in Ewing's STS and the reciprocal translocation between chromosome 18 and the X chromosome in synovial sarcoma. The remaining 80% of STSs have less specific mutations that include non-balanced translocations, genetic deletions and amplifications. These mutations characteristically result in unbalanced karyotypes and significant genomic instability.

Table 47.1 Anatomical distribution of soft tissue sarcomas

Site	Incidence (%)
Lower limb and girdle	40
Upper limb and girdle	20
Retroperitoneum	15
Trunk	10
Head and neck	10
Other	5

Source: Adapted from Cormier JN, Pollock RE, *CA Cancer J Clin* 2004;54:94–109; Clark M, et al., *N Engl J Med* 2005;353(7):701–11.

PATHOLOGY AND STAGING

Pathology

Histologically STSs are classified according to the World Health Organization (WHO) classification based on their morphological appearance [14]. Although all STSs originate from mesenchymal tissue there is huge variation in the histopathological subtypes. Complicating matters further, certain STSs have the ability to dedifferentiate, occasionally into non-mesenchymal cells.

Inaccuracies in histological diagnoses should be avoided at all costs as different STSs behave entirely differently. To minimize the risk of this all potential STSs should be reviewed by specialist sarcoma pathologists, even if samples need to be transported to facilitate this. A specialist histopathological review will also enable other rare non-malignant soft tissue masses that have radiological appearances similar to those of STS (e.g. nodular fasciitis) to be diagnosed with greater accuracy.

Staging

Histopathological staging allows prognosis to be predicted based on a tumour's characteristics. The risk of recurrence and metastatic disease can also be predicted, and therefore also the role of any non-surgical oncologic treatments. The staging system most commonly used for STSs is the American Joint Committee on Cancer (AJCC) and International Union Against Cancer (UICC) system summarized in Table 47.2 [20,21]. In contrast to the TNM staging used for other cancers this system includes grade as an important prognostic indicator.

Grading

Grading allows a tumour's clinical behaviour to be predicted based on its histological variables. The most commonly used grading system in Europe for STSs is the three-tier Trojani system which scores tumours according to three characteristics – histological subtype or

differentiation, degree of tumour necrosis and mitotic count [15]. Grading is not possible for STSs previously treated with chemotherapy or radiotherapy, or cases of STS recurrence. Accuracy is key, as errors may result in incorrect staging and subsequent treatment. In North America a two- or four-tier grading system is more commonly used based on similar principles [16].

DIAGNOSIS AND PREOPERATIVE IMAGING

Presentation

STSs classically present as a slowly growing lump which may be painful. In rare cases a patient may complain of symptoms resulting from local neurovascular invasion. STSs are most frequently located deep to the deep fascia, although not always. All soft tissue lesions larger than 4 cm, deep to fascia, increasing in size or causing pain should be referred to units experienced in the management of soft tissue tumours. Recurrence of a previously benign lesion is also concerning and warrants investigation.

Unfortunately there is often a significant time delay between the initial presentation of many STSs in primary care and subsequent referral to an appropriate tertiary centre [17]. This should be avoided as larger STSs have a poorer prognosis and a higher chance of metastatic spread at presentation [18].

Imaging

DIAGNOSTIC

Diagnostic imaging is key to identifying potentially malignant characteristics in soft tissue lesions. All imaging should be reviewed by radiologists experienced in soft tissue tumours to maximize the accuracy of any diagnoses made, predictions made about a tumour's resectability and patient staging.

Ultrasonography (US) is often the first-line modality used to investigate soft tissue lesions due to its widespread availability and relatively low cost [19]. When undertaken by specialist musculoskeletal radiologists it can provide useful information, although it is a user-dependent investigation and may be less accurate in assessing deeper lesions [19].

Magnetic resonance imaging (MRI) is considered the gold standard investigation in soft tissue lesions. This is based on its accurate ability to characterize a tumour's pseudo-capsule and inflammatory zone, and quantify any local soft tissue or neurovascular infiltration. All potential STS cases should undergo an MRI prior to definitive management decisions being made. However, it is worth noting that even MRI has insufficient diagnostic accuracy to diagnose an STS, and all forms of imaging should be considered an adjunct to a diagnostic biopsy. Whole-body MRI (WB-MRI) scans are used in particular in myxoid liposarcoma to detect multi-focal disease.

Table 47.2 Tumour, grade, node and metastasis staging system of the AJCC for Soft-Tissue Sarcoma and the UICC

Tumour

TX	Primary tumour cannot be assessed
T0	No evidence of primary tumour
T1	Tumour ≤5 cm in greatest dimension
T1a	Superficial tumour
T1b	Deep tumour
T2	Tumour >5 cm in greatest dimension
T2a	Superficial tumour
T2b	Deep tumour

Grade

G1	Well differentiated
G2	Moderately differentiated
G3	Poorly differentiated
G4	Undifferentiated

Lymph Node Status

NX	Regional lymph nodes cannot be assessed
N0	No regional lymph node metastasis
N1	Regional lymph node metastasis[a]

Distant Metastasis

M0	No distant metastasis
M1	Distant metastasis

Stage	Tumour	Lymph node involvement	Metastatic spread	Grade	5-year survival[a]
1A	T1a	N0	M0	G1, GX	86%
	T1b	N0	M0	G1, GX	
1B	T2a	N0	M0	G1, GX	
	T2b	N0	M0	G1, GX	
2A	T1a	N0	M0	G2, G3	72%
	T1b	N0	M0	G2, G3	
2B	T2a	N0	M0	G2	
	T2b	N0	M0	G2	
3	T2a, T2b	N0	M0	G3	52%
	Any T	N1[a]	M0	Any G	
4	Any T	Any N	M1	Any G	10%

Source: Edge S, et al., in *AJCC Cancer Staging Manual*, Edge S, et al., eds., 7th ed., New York: Springer, 2010, pp. 291–6; Greene F, et al., *AJCC Cancer Staging Manual*, 6th ed., New York: Springer Verlag, 2002.
Note: Associated 5-year survival rates are also shown.
[a] Data include retroperitoneal and intra-thoracic tumours.

Computed tomography (CT) can be used in cases when MRI is contraindicated and where claustrophobia prohibits a patient's willingness to undergo MRI. Haematogenous spread to the lung is the most common mode of STS spread and unfortunately will be present at presentation in a significant proportion of cases. All confirmed cases of STS should therefore undergo a chest CT to facilitate early staging. Extending this CT to include the abdomen and pelvis should also be considered for all trunk and lower limb lesions. Dependent on STS subtype additional imaging may be required to facilitate staging (e.g. CNS imaging in angiosarcoma as per ESMO and European Sarcoma Network Working Group guidelines [22]).

Positron emission tomography–computed tomography (PET-CT) scans have a limited and evolving role in the management of STSs. Current indications include pre-ablative surgery and pre-metastasectomy to exclude occult metastases and in NF-1 to detect multi-focal malignant peripheral nerve sheath tumours. Indications are increasing and there is evidence that PET-CT is useful in both staging and grading of STSs [23].

FOLLOW-UP

There is no standardized follow-up protocol for STS patients following attempted curative treatment. The most common protocol includes clinical examination and chest radiographs performed 3 monthly for the first 2 years postoperatively, 6 monthly for the following 3 years and then annually until potential discharge 10 years post-resection. Any lung lesions of concern should be investigated further with a chest CT. If any clinical evidence of local recurrence is found during follow-up an MRI of the area of concern should be performed.

Biopsy

Any lesion with concerning radiological features should undergo a biopsy planned in conjunction with a soft tissue tumour multi-disciplinary team (MDT) or tumour board prior to definitive treatment. The aim of a biopsy is to confirm a histological diagnosis and facilitate tumour grading.

Standard principles should be adhered to when biopsying potentially malignant soft tissue lesions. The approach to biopsy should be determined by a surgeon experienced in the management of malignant soft tissue tumours. In most cases of percutaneous biopsy in the United Kingdom ultrasound (superficial and in some cases deep) or CT (deep) is used to guide clinicians to target lesions safely.

Compartmental barriers should not be breached unless absolutely unavoidable, and if curative resections are subsequently performed biopsy tracts should be removed en bloc with the specimen. During an incisional biopsy fastidious haemostasis should be ensured to minimize any potential tissue seeding by haematoma. Regardless of biopsy technique multiple (usually three or more) specimens should be taken, ideally from the periphery of the lesion to avoid any central necrotic tissue. An additional sample should also be taken for microbiological assessment to exclude infection.

Several techniques can be used to biopsy soft tissue lesions including core needle biopsy (CNB), fine-needle aspiration (FNA) and incisional (open) biopsy. CNB's low morbidity, diagnostic accuracy [24–26] and ability to facilitate STS grading in more than 86% of cases [27] make it the technique of choice at the majority of institutions.

The inabilities of FNA to provide information on tissue architecture or facilitate immunohistochemical analysis are significant disadvantages. However, the technique is still used widely in certain regions, including Scandinavia [28], and provides an attractive option to diagnose superficial metastatic disease when a primary lesion's histology is already established.

Generally the morbidity associated with incisional (open) biopsies means they are performed less commonly than the closed techniques. An open biopsy may still be adopted however when a CNB fails to provide adequate information to facilitate treatment planning, or alternatively when there is discordance between imaging and histopathology.

At open biopsy a frozen section to confirm diagnostic tissue is desirable [24].

SURGERY FOR PRIMARY OPERABLE CANCER

Technique

The most effective curative treatment for the majority of STSs is surgical resection. The aim of surgery is to widely excise the STS (achieving negative histological margins) leaving a functional limb. In the majority of cases surgery will be combined with either induction or adjuvant radiotherapy. In certain STSs, particularly those seen in the paediatric population (Ewing's, rhabdomyosarcoma), induction chemotherapy is also be used. After the resected specimen is removed en bloc it should be marked with skin sutures to orientate the pathology team in cases of unplanned positive margins and the need for a further surgical resection. Metallic clips should be used to mark the resected tumour's bed to guide any postoperative radiotherapy.

Surgical margins

Historically the descriptive system that has been used to describe STS resection margins was proposed by Enneking [29]. In this original classification margins are described as radical, wide, marginal or intra-lesional depending on the plane of resection's relationship to the tumour, the tumour's pseudo-capsule and reactive zone, and the anatomical compartment in which the tumour is found (Figure 47.1).

Enneking described a radical resection as the removal of the entire anatomical compartment containing the STS. A reliable characteristic of STSs is their relative inability to invade fascia or bone, and therefore anatomical boundaries are often respected. This characteristic means that a radical resection should ensure removal of all STS tissue (microscopic and macroscopic), but with obvious functional consequences.

A wide resection includes the tumour (with an intact pseudo-capsule) and the tumour's reactive zone. Although a cuff of surrounding normal tissue is excised in a wide resection it should be recognized that in high-grade STSs microscopic skip lesions may still be missed. In practical terms a wide resection would normally include the involved muscle and adjacent fascia or periosteum, but not any uninvolved neurovascular structures or muscles within the anatomical compartment.

A marginal resection includes the tumour (with an intact pseudo-capsule) but not the entire reactive zone of the tumour. A marginal excision is usually performed when a tumour's reactive zone includes adjacent or nearby neurovascular structures that if resected may leave a significant functional impairment. Marginal excisions leave a significant risk of residual microscopic disease for high-grade tumours or infiltrative low-grade tumours. Despite this for certain low-grade tumours (such as well-differentiated

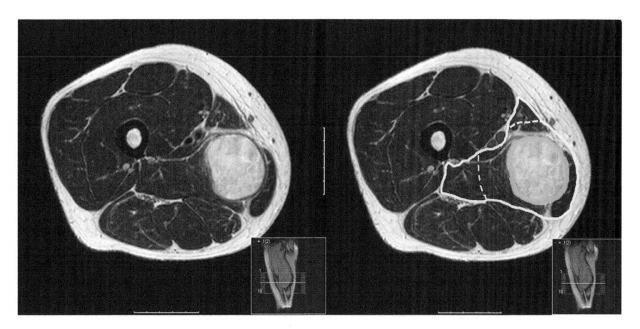

Figure 47.1 Two axial MRI scan images showing a large STS (green) in the adductor compartment of the right thigh. The image on the right highlights the femoral artery (red) and vein (blue) and the planes of dissection that would result in a radical (yellow line) or smaller wide (dashed yellow line adjustments) margin of resection.

liposarcomas) marginal resections may ensure local control [30] and offer the advantage of maintaining function over a wide resection.

An intra-lesional resection leaves macroscopic remnants of tumour. This can be either planned (e.g. curettage) or unplanned as an inadvertent excision (the so-called whoops procedure). A whoops procedure should be avoided due to the negative impact on long-term prognosis [31].

Limb conservation versus amputation

Limb STSs often arise adjacent to or invade key neurovascular structures (Figure 47.2). In this situation several surgical strategies can be adopted. The first decision to be made is whether to adopt a limb-sparing surgical approach or to perform an amputation. If a limb-conserving procedure is chosen a decision must then be made whether to perform a resection that will have a planned marginal or positive margin (to protect the involved neurovascular structures) or a more radical excision (accepting that the involved structures must be sacrificed.)

In most low-grade lesions microscopic infiltration of the reactive zone is unlikely, with the exception of myxofibrosarcomas (which are recognized by their high local recurrence rates [32]). As a result long-term local control may follow a planned marginal excision combined with adjuvant radiotherapy, making this approach wholly appropriate and amputation unnecessary for these lesions.

For higher-grade lesions the 'limb-sparing versus amputation' decision is less clear-cut. It has long been known that an unplanned intra-lesional or marginal resection of an intermediate or high-grade STS can compromise local control and cure, and historically it was this knowledge that

formed the basis for the higher rates of primary, proximal amputations performed. More recently however comparable outcomes in terms of disease-free and overall survival have been reported following less extensive, planned, limb-sparing surgeries combined with adjuvant radiotherapy [33]. Based on this, the current absolute indications for a primary amputation for a STS are now rare and continue to fall as the armoury of techniques available to reconstruct vascular and soft tissue defects continues to grow. Currently only around 9% of STS patients undergo an amputation with curative intent. Relative indications for a primary amputation include local recurrence, gross neurovascular involvement and fungating tumours. Decisions regarding the appropriate level for amputation should be decided preoperatively in an MDT setting with input from sarcoma radiologists, specialist sarcoma surgeons and reconstructive plastic surgeons. Multiple options are available including forequarter, above-elbow, below-elbow, hemipelvectomy, hip disarticulation, above-knee and below-knee amputations. Skin and soft tissues from the limbs can be utilized as pedicle flaps as required [34]. Regardless of the level chosen detailed preoperative counselling and postoperative access to limb prostheses and rehabilitation are essential.

If limb-sparing surgery is felt appropriate but significant neurovascular structures are found adjacent to a STS, a decision of whether to sacrifice these structures to gain wider histological margins must also be made. Although local recurrence rates of just 3.6% have been reported following planned, marginal STS excisions in this scenario in soft tissue tumour units [30], it should also be recognized that a major lower limb nerve resection does not necessarily lead to a non-functional outcome [35]. In reality therefore either approach can often be justified, and clearly this

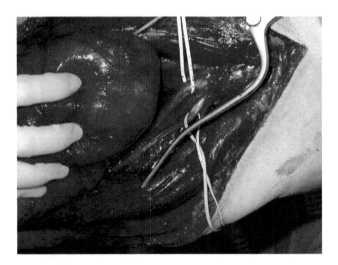

Figure 47.2 Large well-differentiated liposarcoma in hamstring compartment. As shown the tumour was intimately associated with the common peroneal and tibial nerves (shown in vascular slings) which had divided in the upper thigh, and so a planned marginal resection with nerve preservation was performed.

decision must be made in close conjunction with patients, with frank discussions held over the implications of any neurovascular structure's sacrifice.

Reconstructive surgery

In order to obtain wide margins in extensive superficial or fungating STSs skin removal en bloc with the tumour will be necessary. Although primary wound closure is possible without reconstructive surgery in the majority of STS resection surgeries, up to 38% of patients may require some form of soft tissue reconstruction [36]. Even after re-resections following unplanned incomplete resections soft tissue reconstruction is only required in around 17% of cases [37].

Surgical planning for potentially problematic (large) STSs should be done preoperatively with a reconstructive plastic surgeon. Simple skin grafting is not usually appropriate given the frequency that radiotherapy is utilized as skin grafts tolerate radiotherapy very poorly. As a consequence pedicled or free myocutaneous tissue transfers are often required. Reconstruction of the abdominal wall can be achieved relatively simply using prolene mesh, while reconstruction of the chest wall may be more complex and will require the input of a specialist thoracic surgeon.

NEOADJUVANT AND ADJUVANT THERAPIES

Radiotherapy

Radiotherapy is often administered for trunk, limb girdle and extremity STSs to improve local control in the United

Kingdom [38,39]. Specific indications include intermediate or high-grade tumours larger than 5 cm (regardless of excision margins) and any incompletely excised STS. Radiotherapy probably has little benefit in low-grade STSs or small (less than 5 cm) STSs which are completely excised. In these scenarios regardless of tumour grade the risk of local recurrence is already low [40,41]. Radiotherapy may prove a useful adjunct if recurrence does occur in these cases. Radiotherapy has no effect on metastatic disease-free survival or overall survival in STS.

Standard radiotherapy can be administered as external beam therapy or brachytherapy (when the radiation source is placed into or adjacent to the area being treated). Despite the increased dose delivery permitted with brachytherapy both techniques have comparable local control rates [39], and in the United Kingdom external beam therapy is usually performed due to its ease of delivery and availability.

Intensity-modulated radiation therapy (IMRT) is an emerging technique increasingly offered in STS centres which facilitates the administration of concave radiation dose distributions and gradients. This allows radiation to be directed more accurately than in standard external beam radiotherapy, and so spares any uninvolved, nearby anatomical structures (Figure 47.3). For this reason IMRT should be considered in STSs adjacent to particularly radiosensitive structures that would otherwise necessitate a reduction in radiation dose such as the spinal cord.

Proton therapy (proton beam therapy) is another external beam radiation therapy which is unique in its use of protons as the source of radiation delivered to the target tissue. Despite the high targeting accuracy that proton therapy allows, its extremely high costs mean that only a few centres in Europe currently offer the treatment. At present only STSs located in extremely critical locations (e.g. skull base or paraspinal spinal region) and paediatric rhabdomyosarcomas are considered for referral to one of these centres from the United Kingdom.

Neoadjuvant Versus Adjuvant Radiotherapy

Although traditionally adjuvant (postoperative) radiotherapy has been used in the United Kingdom there has been a recent paradigm shift to a preference for the use of neoadjuvant (preoperative) radiotherapy. Although both approaches result in comparable local control rates [42,43], both have advantages and disadvantages. Preoperative radiotherapy may induce tumour shrinkage, improving resectability of large tumours and also requiring a lower radiation dose than adjuvant therapy (typically 50 Gy compared with 66 Gy). Despite this preoperative therapy remains associated with a higher rate of postoperative wound complications and may also hamper the histopathological assessment of any resected specimens due to tissue destruction. Considering these issues it has been proposed that preoperative radiotherapy be

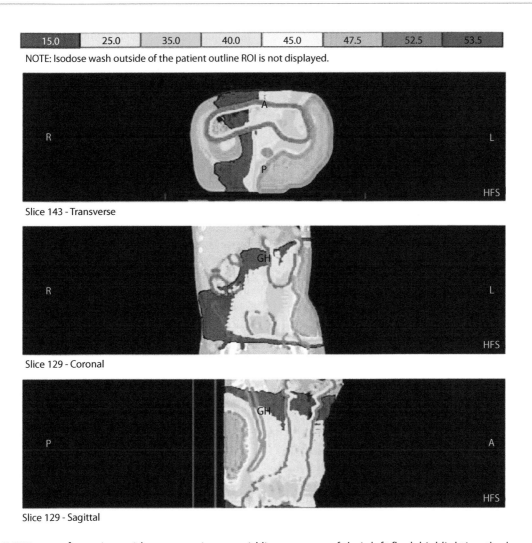

Figure 47.3 IMRT scan of a patient with an extensive myxoid liposarcoma of their left flank highlighting the large convex radiation treatment volumes that can be delivered accurately.

adopted for STSs adjacent to key radiosensitive structures, in regions associated with low postoperative complication rates, in particularly large STSs that will require a large radiation field, and for those STS subtypes that are particularly radiosensitive (such as myxoid liposarcomas) [43,44]. Despite the associations between wound complications and preoperative radiotherapy it may also be prudent to use preoperative radiotherapy in particularly difficult anatomical sites already prone to wound complications (e.g. the groin and popliteal fossae). This slightly counterintuitive approach means that even if a wound complication does occur, local oncological therapy need not be withheld to allow soft tissue healing or reconstruction. One relative contraindication to preoperative radiotherapy that should be recognized is the case of a rapidly growing, predominantly radioinsensitive STS subtype (such as an undifferentiated pleomorphic sarcoma) found close to a critical neurovascular structure. In this scenario if disease progression occurs throughout a course of radiotherapy (as occurs in about 30% of cases) an initially resectable tumour may become unresectable

due to the development of more extensive neurovascular involvement, and close monitoring is obviously therefore required during treatment.

COMPLICATIONS

Radiotherapy is associated with significant early and late complications. These include the risk of subsequent malignancies, localized lymphoedema, fibrosis, joint stiffness, pathological fractures and as discussed above, wound complications.

Chemotherapy

Neoadjuvant chemotherapy is generally not used for STSs in the United Kingdom other than in a few histological subtypes that consistently show a good response (e.g. rhabdomyosarcoma and soft tissue Ewing's sarcoma). Overall there is no clear evidence that preoperative chemotherapy improves survival. Approximately 13% of patients show a significant response (leading to higher local control rates [45] and improvements in disease-specific survival in the short to medium term [46]). A similar proportion appear to progress during treatment and so require more extensive surgery. Despite this it should be recognized that certain STS subtypes respond more consistently to chemotherapy [47]. Examples include angiosarcomas which have been reported as showing a significant response to taxanes (paclitaxel) in up to 89% of cases [48], and leiomyosarcomas of which up to 50% appear to respond to a combination of gemcitabine and docetaxel [49].

The role of adjuvant chemotherapy in STSs is also limited. A meta-analysis performed in 1999 of 14 small randomized trials assessing doxorubicin-based chemotherapy regimes in STSs showed no significant impact on relapse-free survival or overall survival [50]. Although an update including four newer trials resulted in some improvement in these outcomes [51], the toxicities of the regimes tested mean that adjuvant chemotherapy still has little place for non-metastatic STS in the UK. This is supported by ESMO and European Sarcoma Network Working Group clinical practice guidelines, which state that adjuvant chemotherapy is not a standard treatment in adult-type STS and should certainly not be used in histological subtypes known to be insensitive to chemotherapy [22].

Molecular therapies

Targeted molecular therapies are rarely instigated for primary extremity-localized STSs. The exception is imatinib mesylate (a tyrosine kinase inhibitor) which may be implemented in cases of locally advanced dermatofibrosarcoma protuberans (DFSP) that harbour chromosomal abnormalities at the platelet-derived growth factor B (PDGFB) locus resulting in PDGFR activation.

LOCALLY ADVANCED AND METASTATIC DISEASE

Local recurrence

Despite attempted curative treatment a significant proportion of STSs recur locally. Patients should be re-staged to rule out concurrent metastatic spread and the surgical site re-imaged with MRI. In the absence of systemic metastases principles similar to those employed for a primary STS should be adopted. Curative limb-sparing resections should be considered whenever possible. The incidence of amputation is higher in recurrent disease. In the patient where metastatic spread is also detected surgery is usually only implemented for symptomatic lesions. This can again involve a limb-sparing resection or an amputation, and neoadjuvant therapy should be considered to try to permit the former.

Isolated limb perfusion

Isolated limb perfusion (ILP) is a technique that allows regional administration of high-dose chemotherapy (usually in conjunction with the cytokine tumour necrosis factor–α [TNF-α]) to a limb affected by malignancy. It is a complex surgical procedure with technical and logistical challenges, but has proven efficacy in a number of extremity malignancies including sarcoma.

ILP involves the surgical cannulation of the afferent and efferent arterial and venous supply to the involved limb followed by its isolation from the systemic circulation by a tourniquet. The limb is then perfused on an oxygenated, hyperthermic circuit that contains the chemotherapy for 1 h. Following this the chemotherapy is washed out prior to the tourniquet being released and the limb being returned to the systemic circulation. This process of isolated perfusion allows the safe delivery of cytotoxic chemotherapy at much higher concentrations that can be tolerated through systemic administration. It also allows the use of TNF-α that cannot be tolerated systemically, but considerably enhances the efficacy of the cytotoxic agents.

There are two main indications for ILP in STS. The first indication is as an induction strategy whereby ILP is used for an advanced sarcoma that would initially be considered unresectable in a radical fashion without major functional morbidity. Local control rates of 80% have been reported following marginal resection of the tumour remnant 6 weeks after induction ILP in this scenario [52].

The second indication for ILP in STSs is for a tumour that is unresectable with limb-sparing surgery (even after potential ILP use) in a patient that wishes to avoid an amputation. Although the local control rates seen following isolated ILP use in these circumstances are less consistent and of shorter duration than when ILP is combined with a planned surgical resection, this approach may still be of valuable palliative benefit in elderly patients wishing to avoid an amputation or in patents with synchronous metastatic disease.

Due to the relatively widespread availability of ILP in mainland Europe induction ILP has been used more widely for large, high-grade STSs that may otherwise be treated by surgery and adjuvant radiotherapy with the acceptance of planned positive margins. This approach results in good local control and oncological outcome, and a reduction in the need for adjuvant radiotherapy [53].

Metastatic disease

PULMONARY METASTASECTOMY

STSs most commonly metastasize to the lungs (Figure 47.4). Resection of pulmonary metastases is controversial, although it is viewed by some as a worthwhile palliative treatment for symptomatic pulmonary disease and to potentially improve long-term survival (although no randomized evidence exists for this) [54]. The accepted positive prognostic factors for benefit of pulmonary metastasectomy are a long period of disease-free time between treatment of the primary tumour and the development of metastases, and a small overall number of pulmonary metastases [55].

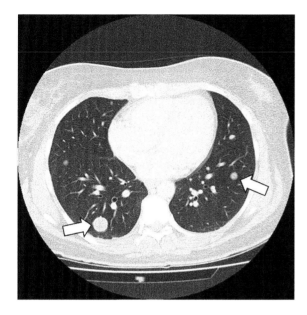

Figure 47.4 Axial CT image showing multiple pulmonary metastases (two highlighted with white arrows) in a patient with a high-grade STS.

Decisions on surgery should be made with a thoracic surgeon working regularly with an STS MDT. Bilateral pulmonary metastases and high numbers of metastases are generally considered contraindications to a pulmonary metastatectomy. Rapidly progressing disease may also be considered a relative contraindication.

PERCUTANEOUS RADIOFREQUENCY ABLATION

For inoperable pulmonary metastases or pulmonary metastases in patients with severe comorbidities percutaneous radiofrequency ablation (RFA) provides a safe alternative to surgical resection. RFA avoids significant damage to surrounding parenchymal tissue, does not impair lung function (even in patients already with severe respiratory dysfunction) and also avoids the need for a lobectomy (potentially facilitating multiple interventions if required) [56]. Again involvement of a thoracic surgeon and radiologist experienced in STSs is essential.

NON-PULMONARY METASTASECTOMY

STS metastases to sites other than the lungs are less common. Some STSs can metastasize to loco-regional lymph nodes [57], and soft tissue metastases are not uncommon in certain pathologies (e.g. myxoid liposarcoma [58]). These should be managed on merit after MDT discussion, but general principles are that low-volume resectable disease should be surgically resected and high-volume disease treated systemically. Bone metastases are also rare and should be managed following standard metastatic bone disease principles [59].

PALLIATIVE CHEMOTHERAPY

As discussed earlier STSs are not generally particularly chemosensitive, and this remains true even in the palliative setting. Response rates of metastatic STSs are well below 30% for most regimes including those containing doxorubicin and ifosfamide (the most commonly used STS agents). No single randomized phase III trial has been able to generate a clinically relevant and statistically significant overall survival benefit in cases of metastatic STS [60]. As a result the early involvement of a specialist in palliative care with a good understanding of analgaesia, antiemetic therapies and the other issues associated with symptom control and end-of-life care is key in any case of metastatic STS.

REFERENCES

1. Weitz J, Antonescu CR, Brennan MF. Localized extremity soft tissue sarcoma: improved knowledge with unchanged survival over time. *J Clin Oncol* 2003;21:2719–25.
2. Cormier JN, Pollock RE. Soft tissue sarcomas. *CA Cancer J Clin* 2004;54:94–109.
3. Thomas D, Ballinger M. Etiologic, environmental and inherited risk factors in sarcomas. *J Surg Oncol* 2015;111(5):490–5.
4. Ferrari A, Bisogno G, Macaluso A, Casanova M, D'Angelo P, Pierani P, et al. Soft-tissue sarcomas in children and adolescents with neurofibromatosis type 1. *Cancer* 2007;109:1406–12.
5. Neuhaus SJ, Pinnock N, Giblin V, Fisher C, Thway K, Thomas JM, et al. Treatment and outcome of radiation-induced soft-tissue sarcomas at a specialist institution. *Eur J Surg Oncol* 2009;35:654–9.
6. Pencavel T, Allan CP, Thomas JM, Hayes AJ. Treatment for breast sarcoma: a large, single-centre series. *Eur J Surg Oncol* 2011;37:703–8.
7. Depla AL, Scharloo-Karels CH, De Jong MAA, Oldenborg S, Kolff MW, Oei SB, et al. Treatment and prognostic factors of radiation-associated angiosarcoma (RAAS) after primary breast cancer: a systematic review. *Eur J Cancer* 2014;50(10):1779–88.
8. Ward E, Boffetta P, Andersen A, Colin D, Comba P, Deddens JA, et al. Update of the follow-up of mortality and cancer incidence among European workers employed in the vinyl chloride industry. *Epidemiology* 2001;12:710–8.
9. Kogevinas M, Becher H, Benn T, Bertazzi PA, Boffetta P, Bueno-de-Mesquita HB, et al. Cancer mortality in workers exposed to phenoxy herbicides, chlorophenols, and dioxins. An expanded and updated international cohort study. *Am J Epidemiol* 1997;145:1061–75.
10. Sharma A, Schwartz RA. Stewart-Treves syndrome: pathogenesis and management. *J Am Acad Dermatol* 2012;67:1342–8.
11. Ahmed I, Hamacher KL. Angiosarcoma in a chronically immunosuppressed renal transplant recipient: report of a case and review of the literature. *Am J Dermatopathol* 2002;24(4):330–5.

12. Mertens F, Panagopoulos I, Mandahl N. Genomic characteristics of soft tissue sarcomas. *Virchows Archiv* 2010;456(2):129–39.

13. Clark M, Fisher C, Judson I, Thomas J. Softtissue sarcomas in adults. *N Engl J Med* 2005;353(7):701–11.

14. World Health Organization. *International Statistical Classification of Diseases and Related Health Problems.* 10th rev. Geneva: World Health Organization, 2010. Available from http://apps.who.int/classifications/icd10/browse/2010/en.

15. Trojani M, Contesso G, Coindre JM, Rouesse J, Bui NB, de Mascarel A, et al. Soft-tissue sarcomas of adults: study of pathological prognostic variables and definition of a histopathological grading system. *Int J Cancer* 1984;33:37–42.

16. Enzinger P, Weiss S. *Soft Tissue Tumors.* 6th ed. Philadelphia: Saunders/Elsevier, 2013.

17. Brouns F, Stas M, De Wever I. Delay in diagnosis of soft tissue sarcomas. *Eur J Surg Oncol* 2003;29:440–5.

18. Grimer RJ. Size matters for sarcomas! *Ann R Coll Surg Engl* 2006;88:519–24.

19. Lakkaraju A, Sinha R, Garikipati R, Edward S, Robinson P. Ultrasound for initial evaluation and triage of clinically suspicious soft-tissue masses. *Clin Radiol* 2009;64:615–21.

20. Edge S, Byrd D, Compton C. Soft tissue sarcoma. In *AJCC Cancer Staging Manual*, Edge S, Byrd D, Compton C, Fritz AG, Greene FL, Trotti A, eds. 7th ed. New York: Springer, 2010, pp. 291–6.

21. Greene F, Page D, Fleming I. *AJCC Cancer Staging Manual.* 6th ed. New York: Springer Verlag, 2002.

22. Casali PG, Blay J-Y. Soft tissue sarcomas: ESMO Clinical Practice Guidelines for diagnosis, treatment and follow-up. *Ann Oncol* 2010;21(Suppl. 5):198–203.

23. Charest M, Hickeson M, Lisbona R, Novales-Diaz J-A, Derbekyan V, Turcotte RE. FDG PET/CT imaging in primary osseous and soft tissue sarcomas: a retrospective review of 212 cases. *Eur J Nucl Med Mol Imaging* 2009;36:1944–51.

24. Ashford RU, McCarthy SW, Scolyer RA, Bonar SF, Karim RZ, Stalley PD. Surgical biopsy with intra-operative frozen section. An accurate and cost-effective method for diagnosis of musculoskeletal sarcomas. *J Bone Joint Surg Br* 2006;88:1207–11.

25. Hoeber I, Spillane A, Fisher C, Thomas J. Accuracy of biopsy techniques for limb and limb girdle soft tissue tumors. *Ann Surg Oncol* 2001;8(1):80–7.

26. Kasraeian S, Allison D, Ahlmann E, Fedenko A, Menendez L. A comparison of fine-needle aspiration, core biopsy, and surgical biopsy in the diagnosis of extremity soft tissue masses. *Clin Orthop Relat Res* 2010;468(11):2992–3002.

27. Strauss DC, Qureshi YA, Hayes AJ, Thway K, Fisher C, Thomas JM. The role of core needle biopsy in the diagnosis of suspected soft tissue tumours. *J Surg Oncol* 2010;102:523–9.

28. Trovik CS. Local recurrence of soft tissue sarcoma. A Scandinavian Sarcoma Group Project. *Acta Orthop Scand Suppl* 2001;72:1–31.

29. Enneking WF, Spanier SS, Goodman MA. A system for the surgical staging of musculoskeletal sarcoma. 1980. *Clin Orthop Relat Res* 2003;4–18.

30. Gerrand CH, Wunder JS, Kandel RA, O'Sullivan B, Catton CN, Bell RS, et al. Classification of positive margins after resection of soft-tissue sarcoma of the limb predicts the risk of local recurrence. *J Bone Joint Surg Br* 2001;83:1149–55.

31. Qureshi YA, Huddy JR, Miller JD, Strauss DC, Thomas JM, Hayes AJ. Unplanned excision of soft tissue sarcoma results in increased rates of local recurrence despite full further oncological treatment. *Ann Surg Oncol* 2012;19:871–7.

32. Look Hong NJ, Hornicek FJ, Raskin KA, Yoon SS, Szymonifka J, Yeap B, et al. Prognostic factors and outcomes of patients with myxofibrosarcoma. *Ann Surg Oncol* 2013;20:80–6.

33. Rosenberg SA, Tepper J, Glatstein E, Costa J, Baker A, Brennan M, et al. The treatment of soft-tissue sarcomas of the extremities: prospective randomized evaluations of (1) limb-sparing surgery plus radiation therapy compared with amputation and (2) the role of adjuvant chemotherapy. *Ann Surg* 1982;196:305–15.

34. Werner CML, Exner GU, Dumont CE. Free vascularised osteocutaneous filet flap for covering, that permitted sensitive terminal weight-bearing by a thigh stump after transfemoral amputation. *Scand J Plast Reconstr Surg Hand Surg* 2006;315–7.

35. Brooks A, Gold J, Graham D, Boland P, Lewis J, Brennan M, et al. Resection of the sciatic, peroneal, or tibial nerves: assessment of functional status. *Ann Surg Oncol* 2002;9(1):41–7.

36. Hassan S, Gale J, Perks A, Raurell A, Ashford R. Reconstruction and financial remuneration following soft tissue sarcoma surgery. *Bull R Coll Surg Engl* 2013;95(5):160–2.

37. Venkatesan M, Richards CJ, McCulloch TA, Perks AG, Raurell A, Ashford RU. Inadvertent surgical resection of soft tissue sarcomas. *Eur J Surg Oncol* 2012;38:346–51.

38. Stojadinovic A, Leung DHY, Hoos A, Jaques DP, Lewis JJ, Brennan MF. Analysis of the prognostic significance of microscopic margins in 2,084 localized primary adult soft tissue sarcomas. *Ann Surg* 2002;235:424–34.

39. Strander H, Turesson I, Cavallin-ståhl E. A systematic overview of radiation therapy effects in soft tissue sarcomas. *Acta Oncol (Madr)* 2003;42:516–31.

40. Pisters PW, Leung DH, Woodruff J, Shi W, Brennan MF. Analysis of prognostic factors in 1,041 patients with localized soft tissue sarcomas of the extremities. *J Clin Oncol* 1996;14:1679–89.

41. Coindre JM, Terrier P, Bui NB, Bonichon F, Collin F, Le Doussal V, et al. Prognostic factors in adult patients with locally controlled soft tissue sarcoma: a study of 546 patients from the French Federation of Cancer Centers Sarcoma Group. *J Clin Oncol* 1996;14:869–77.

42. Cheng EY, Dusenbery KE, Winters MR, Thompson RC. Soft tissue sarcomas: preoperative versus postoperative radiotherapy. *J Surg Oncol* 1996;61:90–9.

43. O'Sullivan B, Davis AM, Turcotte R, Bell R, Catton C, Chabot P, et al. Preoperative versus postoperative radiotherapy in soft-tissue sarcoma of the limbs: a randomised trial. *Lancet* 2002;359:2235–41.

44. Pitson G, Robinson P, Wilke D, Kandel RA, White L, Griffin AM, et al. Radiation response: an additional unique signature of myxoid liposarcoma. *Int J Radiat Oncol Biol Phys* 2004;60:522–6.

45. Meric F, Hess K, Varma D, Hunt K, Pisters P, Milas K, et al. Radiographic response to neoadjuvant chemotherapy is a predictor of local control and survival in soft tissue sarcomas. *Cancer* 95(5):1120–6.

46. Grobmyer SR, Maki RG, Demetri GD, Mazumdar M, Riedel E, Brennan MF, et al. Neo-adjuvant chemotherapy for primary high-grade extremity soft tissue sarcoma. *Ann Oncol* 2004;15(11):1667–72.

47. Young RJ, Natukunda A, Litière S, Woll PJ, Wardelmann E, van der Graaf WTA. First-line anthracycline-based chemotherapy for angiosarcoma and other soft tissue sarcoma subtypes: pooled analysis of eleven European Organisation for Research and Treatment of Cancer Soft Tissue and Bone Sarcoma Group trials. *Eur J Cancer* 2014;50(18):3178–86.

48. Fata F, O'Reilly E, Ilson D, Pfister D, Leffel D, Kelsen DP, et al. Paclitaxel in the treatment of patients with angiosarcoma of the scalp or face. *Cancer* 1999;86(10):2034–7.

49. Hensley ML. Gemcitabine and docetaxel in patients with unresectable leiomyosarcoma: results of a phase II trial. *J Clin Oncol* 2002;20(12):2824–31.

50. Tierney JF. Adjuvant chemotherapy for localised resectable soft-tissue sarcoma of adults: meta-analysis of individual data. *Lancet* 1997;350:1647–54.

51. Pervaiz N, Colterjohn N, Farrokhyar F, Tozer R, Figueredo A, Ghert M. A systematic meta-analysis of randomized controlled trials of adjuvant chemotherapy for localized resectable soft-tissue sarcoma. *Cancer* 2008;113:573–81.

52. Eggermont A, Schraffordt Koops H, Klausner J, Kroon B, Schlag P, Liénard D, et al. Isolated limb perfusion with tumor necrosis factor and melphalan for limb salvage in 186 patients with locally advanced soft tissue extremity sarcomas. The cumulative multicenter European experience. *Ann Surg* 1996;224(6):756–64.

53. Jakob J, Tunn PU, Hayes AJ, Pilz LR, Nowak K, Hohenberger P. Oncological outcome of primary non-metastatic soft tissue sarcoma treated by neoadjuvant isolated limb perfusion and tumor resection. *J Surg Oncol* 2014;109:786–90.

54. Rehders A, Hosch SB, Scheunemann P, Stoecklein NH, Knoefel WT, Peiper M. Benefit of surgical treatment of lung metastasis in soft tissue sarcoma. *Arch Surg* 2007;142:70–5; discussion 76.

55. Treasure T, Fiorentino F, Scarci M, Moller H, Utley M. Pulmonary metastasectomy for sarcoma: a systematic review of reported outcomes in the context of Thames Cancer Registry data. *BMJ Open* 2012;e001736.

56. Nakamura T, Matsumine A, Yamakado K, Takao M, Uchida A, Sudo A. Clinical significance of radiofrequency ablation and metastasectomy in elderly patients with lung metastases from musculoskeletal sarcomas. *J Cancer Res Ther* 2013;9(2):219–23.

57. Riad S, Griffin AM, Liberman B, Blackstein ME, Catton CN, Kandel RA, et al. Lymph node metastasis in soft tissue sarcoma in an extremity. *Clin Orthop Relat Res* 2004;129–34.

58. Spillane AJ, Fisher C, Thomas JM. Myxoid liposarcoma – the frequency and the natural history of nonpulmonary soft tissue metastases. *Ann Surg Oncol* 1999;6:389–94.

59. Eastley N, Newey M, Ashford RU. Skeletal metastases – the role of the orthopaedic and spinal surgeon. *Surg Oncol* 2012;21:216–22.

60. Schöffski P, Cornillie J, Wozniak A, Li H, Hompes D. Soft tissue sarcoma: an update on systemic treatment options for patients with advanced disease. *Oncol Res Treatment* 2014;37(6):355–62.

48

Retroperitoneal sarcoma

SERGIO SANDRUCCI, SILVIA STACCHIOTTI AND ALESSANDRO GRONCHI

INTRODUCTION

The *retroperitoneum* represents a complex potential space with multiple vital structures bounded anteriorly by the peritoneum, ipsilateral colon and mesocolon, pancreas, duodenum, spleen, liver or stomach [1]. The posterior margins comprise the psoas, quadratus lumborum and transverse abdominal and iliacus muscles but, depending on the tumour location and size, may be formed by the diaphragm, ipsilateral kidney, ureter and gonadal vessels. The medial boundaries may include the spine, paraspinous muscles, inferior vena cava (for right-sided tumours) and aorta (for left-sided tumours) or iliac vessels. The lateral margin is formed by the lateral abdominal musculature and, depending on tumour location, may include the kidney and colon.

Proper resection of retroperitoneal sarcomas (RPSs) requires appreciation of the anatomic boundaries of the tumour [2]; radiological imaging should be reviewed to identify landmarks defining the extent of the mass to determine which structures may be safely resected and which ones cannot.

INCIDENCE, PATHOLOGY AND STAGING

Retroperitoneal soft tissue sarcomas represent 10–15% of all soft tissue sarcomas, with an expected overall incidence of 1–2/1,000,000 inhabitants per year [3].

Paediatric-type soft tissue sarcomas (STSs) are exceedingly rare at this site, having an overall incidence one-tenth lower than those of the adult type. Median age at presentation is 15–18 years. The three main variants are composed of the Ewing's or paediatric primitive neuroectodermal tumours (pPNETs) family of tumours, alveolar or embryonal rhabdomyosarcoma and desmoplastic small round cell tumour. The latter has a typical male predominance and is exceptionally rare after the age of 30.

Adult-type RPSs are the most common extra-visceral retroperitoneal malignant tumour. They usually present around the age of 50, but they may affect young adults or elderly people without real age limits.

The histological distribution varies significantly from that of extremity and superficial trunkal STSs [3,4].

Well-differentiated and dedifferentiated liposarcomas are the most common histological type at this site. They constitute roughly 50% of all RPSs and in general lack metastatic potential. Their natural history is mainly characterized by a high loco-regional risk of recurrence and usually people eventually die of inoperable abdominal disease. Myxoid or round cell and pleomorphic variants of liposarcoma are exceedingly rare in the retroperitoneum. In fact most of the diagnoses of myxoid liposarcoma – if revised by an experienced sarcoma pathologist – are reclassified as myxoid-like well-differentiated liposarcoma. The distinction among the two variants is becoming increasingly important since the natural history and metastatic potential is different among the two histological types and new available different medical treatments could be offered to each of them. When a true myxoid or round cell liposarcoma is diagnosed at this site, a careful staging focusing on the extremities should be made, since there would be a higher chance of the abdominal mass being a metastasis from an extremity tumour rather than a real primary RPS, even in the absence of other extra-abdominal metastases.

Pleomorphic liposarcomas are also very uncommon in the retroperitoneum. As above, most – if not all – of the diagnoses of retroperitoneal pleomorphic liposarcoma, if reviewed by an experienced sarcoma pathologist, are reclassified as dedifferentiated liposarcoma. This difference is of importance at least from the prognostic perspective, since dedifferentiated liposarcomas do not share the same aggressive behaviour as the real pleomorphic ones.

The second most common histological subtype is leiomyosarcoma, representing 20% of all RSTs, but it differs from liposarcoma in that it has a substantial metastatic risk, with a much lower propensity for loco-regional recurrence. Patients either die of systemic disease or are cured. The most common variant of this histological subtype arises from major veins (gonadal, iliac and renal veins or the inferior vena cava). A subgroup of this variant of vascular origin may have an intermediate histological grade of aggressiveness and may follow a more indolent course. An aggressive surgical approach may provide long-term disease control.

Other histological variants at this site include malignant peripheral nerve sheath tumour (MPNST), synovial sarcoma, pleomorphic undifferentiated sarcoma and angiosarcoma. They share similarities with the extremity and superficial trunk sarcoma. Nevertheless when located at this site, they tend to follow a more aggressive course, mainly because they tend to be diagnosed at a much later stage. The median size of RPS is roughly double that seen in an extremity location and as tumour size is one of the major determinants of outcome, prognosis is correspondingly worse.

Solitary fibrous tumours – though quite rare – are increasingly diagnosed at this site, in the past misdiagnosed mainly as malignant fibrous histiocytoma (MFH) or hemangiopericytoma. They tend to have a very indolent course, with both low local and metastatic potential, provided adequate surgery is performed. Local or distant relapse may happen even after many years (>10 years), so suggesting the need for long-term follow-up. Nevertheless a rarer variant of this histological subtype has a sarcomatous component, which may have a very aggressive course. All other histological variants are only exceptionally found at this site and do not deserve a specific mention here.

The present AJCC/TNM staging system is of limited value for prediction of prognosis for patients with RPS: classification based on grade, completeness of resection and distant metastases offers a reproducible prognostic tool that can be used to evaluate treatment strategies for primary RPS. Histological diagnosis should follow the recent WHO soft tissue tumour classification [4,5], and the French histological grading system (based on mitotic count, presence or absence of necrosis and differentiation) [6] should also be applied. Low-, intermediate- and high-grade tumours are equally distributed in adult-type variants, while paediatric types are by definition all high grade.

In an attempt to improve the predictive capability of sarcoma-specific risk of death in general or in the context of RPS, several STS nomograms have been built on the basis of single-institution databases. Nomograms can be used to accurately assess individual patient risk, leading to improved prognosis-based decision making within the specific RPS tumour cohort and enhanced clinical trial stratification. These tools are already providing new refinements in the understanding of the natural history of RPS [7] (Figures 48.1 and 48.2).

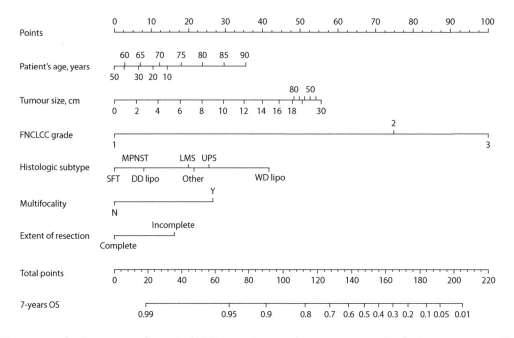

Figure 48.1 Nomogram for 7-year overall survival (OS) in patients with retroperitoneal soft tissue sarcoma. The nomogram allows the user to obtain the 7-year OS probability corresponding to a patient's combination of covariates. For instance, locate the patient's tumour size and draw a line straight upward to the 'Points' axis to determine the score associated with that size. Repeat the process for the patient's age, French National Federation of the Centers for the Fight Against Cancer (FNCLCC) grade, histologic subtype, multifocality and extent of resection, and then sum the scores achieved for each covariate and locate this sum on the 'Total Points' axis. Draw a line straight down to the '7-year OS' axis to find the predicted probability. DD lipo, dedifferentiated liposarcoma; LMS, leiomyosarcoma; SFT, solitary fibrous tumour; UPS, undifferentiated pleomorphic sarcoma; WD lipo, well-differentiated liposarcoma.

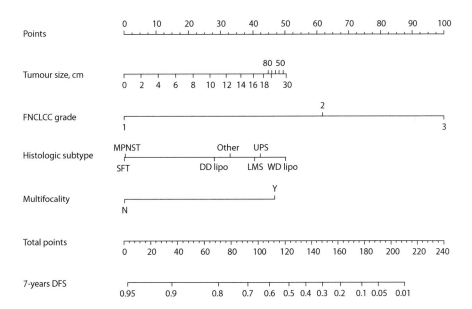

Figure 48.2 Nomogram for 7-year disease-free survival (DFS) in patients with retroperitoneal soft tissue sarcoma. The nomogram allows the user to obtain the 7-year DFS probability corresponding to a patient's combination of covariates. For instance, locate the patient's tumour size and draw a line straight upward to the 'Points' axis to determine the score associated with that size. Repeat the process for French National Federation of the Centers for the Fight Against Cancer (FNCLCC) grade, histologic subtype and multifocality, and then sum the scores achieved for each covariate, and locate this sum on the 'Total Points' axis. Draw a line straight down to the '7-year DFS' axis to find the predicted probability. DD lipo, dedifferentiated liposarcoma; LMS, leiomyosarcoma; SFT, solitary fibrous tumour; UPS, undifferentiated pleomorphic sarcoma; WD lipo, well-differentiated liposarcoma.

DIFFERENTIAL DIAGNOSIS AND PREOPERATIVE IMAGING

Due to the inaccessibility of the region and since these tumours often give no or non-specific symptoms until they have reached a substantial size, they are usually large at presentation.

The typical presentation of both paediatric and adult-type RPS is an abdominal swelling or increase in girth, early satiety and abdominal discomfort, and most patients have a palpable mass, discovered either clinically or through an abdominal ultrasound–computed tomography (US/CT) performed for a generic abdominal discomfort. Although the gastrointestinal and urinary tracts are often displaced, they are rarely invaded and gastrointestinal or urinary symptoms are unusual.

Real pain is rarely present in adult-type variants, save for the rare MPNST or where there is involvement of the femoral or sciatic nerves. In contrast it often accompanies the paediatric types, since their growth tend to be more rapid and aggressive.

The median size of these tumours at presentation is around 20 cm. It is exceptional to find tumours smaller than 8 cm, while the upper limit is difficult to set. Giant RPS have been described, virtually all of lipogenic origin, that can reach considerable sizes.

Occasionally fever can be present. This has never been consistently reported, while it has long been described as an accompanying symptom of lymphoproliferative disorders.

While there are no tumour markers known for any RPS or STS histologies at present, screening studies for other diagnoses including lactate dehydrogenase (relatively non-specific marker for lymphoma, melanoma, acute leukemia and germ cell tumours), human chorionic gonadotropin and alpha-fetoprotein (germ cell tumours) may be indicated.

The imaging modality of choice is contrast-enhanced CT of the thorax, abdomen and pelvis. The size, location, relationship to adjacent organs and presence or absence of metastases can be determined. There is no need for routine head CT or PET scan; for pelvic-located masses a pelvic MRI may also be helpful. For paediatric-type tumours a bone scan and bone marrow aspiration should always be part of the initial work-up.

Imaging alone is rarely diagnostic of the specific sarcoma histology, with the exception of well-differentiated liposarcoma [8–10]. Well-differentiated liposarcomas have a radiographic density similar to that of the normal surrounding fat, but tend to be well encapsulated with thick internal septations. Giant lipomas are only identified anecdotally in the retroperitoneum; therefore, any mass consisting of very well-differentiated fatty tissue should be considered as well-differentiated liposarcoma and treated as such. Giant adrenal myelolipoma and retroperitoneal or renal angiomyolipoma should then be ruled out; both these entities tend to have a benign course and may be treated less aggressively.

CT attenuation reflects the histological subtype, specifically the amount of fat in the mass, with lower-grade,

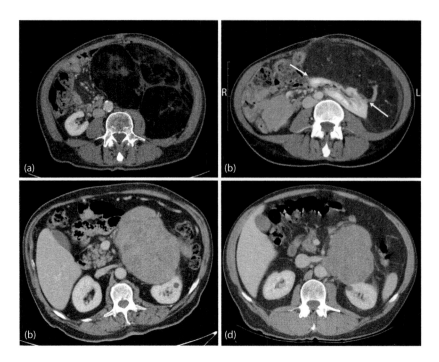

Figure 48.3 (a) Contrast-enhanced CT scan of a left retroperitoneal well-differentiated liposarcoma. The mass is homogeneous with complete fat attenuation throughout and thin septa. (b) Contrast-enhanced CT scan of a left renal angiomyolipoma. The appearance is that of a heterogeneous fatty mass involving the renal cortex (arrows) with enlarged intralesional vessels. (c) Contrast-enhanced CT scan of a left retroperitoneal leiomyosarcoma. The mass is heterogeneous and non-fatty, with high contrast enhancement. (d) Retroperitoneal non-Hodgkin lymphoma rising from para-aortic lymph nodes. The mass is well defined and homogeneous with mild contrast enhancement.

well-differentiated liposarcoma entirely or predominantly fatty, while higher-grade lesions show increased density with areas of solid attenuation and contrast enhancement (Figure 48.3).

Overall a preoperative histological assessment should be obtained in all patients affected by a retroperitoneal mass as there are no published data on the capability of radiology to predict histopathological subtype of suspected RPS purely based on contrast-enhanced CT scan. A major change in diagnosis may be observed in as many as 10–20% of patients referred for a suspected primary RPS. In fact in a recent retrospective analysis, sensitivity and specificity of contrast-enhanced CT scan for liposarcoma were 76.7% and 92.0%; PPV and NPV were 86.4% and 85.6%. The corresponding sensitivity for other mesenchymal tumours was 55.4% and specificity was 0%; PPV and NPV were 68.1% and 0% [11].

The preoperative histological assessment is best obtained through coaxial tru-cut US/CT-guided core needle percutaneous biopsies. Risk of seeding or other complications has been recently analyzed in a large retrospective analysis, which showed that this procedure is absolutely safe [12]. Incorrect treatment of these tumours because of not having the correct diagnosis before surgery occurs frequently and should be avoided.

If a tumour is deemed unresectable or the patient has distant metastases, a core needle biopsy is mandatory to confirm the diagnosis and to enable consideration of alternative therapy. Ideally the biopsy tract should avoid the peritoneal cavity, but the best route should be discussed in advance at the multidisciplinary tumour board, where all cases with a suspected RPS should be evaluated before any action is taken.

Biopsy tract recurrences are exceedingly rare, so the biopsy tract does not need to be re-excised during definitive surgery. If preoperative external beam radiotherapy (EBRT) is planned, the biopsy site is usually included within the radiation field.

SURGERY FOR PRIMARY OPERABLE RPS

Surgery is the mainstay of treatment in localized disease for both adult-type and paediatric-type sarcoma. Nevertheless given the different sensitivities of the two entities to adjuvant and neoadjuvant treatments, its role is more crucial for the adult variants.

The first surgery is critical for cure. The aim of the surgery is complete macroscopic removal of the tumour en bloc with a cuff of healthy tissue all around; the quality of surgical margins in STS has a significant impact on local outcomes and possibly survival [13–15] especially when tumours are located at critical sites, as RPSs are. Local recurrence may in fact directly lead to death [16–29] (Table 48.1).

In contrast to extremity STSs, no clear definitions of surgical adequacy are available and many recommendations are still limited to the achievement of gross complete resection [19,20,26,27] with the need to resect adjacent organs only

Table 48.1 Outcome variables of primary resected RPS in the major published series

Study (year)	Study period	Center	Cases (n)	Primary[a] (%)	R0/R1 resection (%)	Median follow-up (months)	Contiguous organs resection (%)	Postoperative mortality (%)[b]	5-year local recurrence rate (%)	5-year distant metastasis rate (%)	5-year overall survival (%)
Lewis et al. (1998) [17]	1982–1997	Single	500	56	80[b]	28**	77**	4	41[b]	21[b]	54**
Stoeckle et al. (2001) [18]	1980–1994	Multicenter	165	88	68[b]	47[c]	na	na	na	33**	49**
van Dalen et al. (2007) [19]	1989–1994	Multicenter	143	96	63****	122[c]	na	4	na	na	40**
Gronchi et al. (2009) [22]	1985–2007	Single	288	67	89***	58	71***	na	na	na	na
	1985–2001	Single	136	62	88***	120	60***	na	48***	13***	51***
	2002–2007	Single	152	72	91***	32	82***	na	29***	22***	60***
Bonvalot et al. (2009) [21]	1985–2005	Multicenter	382	97	75****	53	65***	3	49***	34***	57***
Strauss et al. (2010) [20]	1990–2009	Single	200	100	85[b]	29	63**	3	45[d]	na	na
Toulmonde et al. (2014) [25]	1988–2008	Multicenter	586	95	na	78	65****	na	54[d]	na	66[d]
Gronchi et al. (2015) [23]	2002–2011	Multicenter	377	100	96[b]	44	93**	na	23.6**	21.9**	64**
Bremjit et al. (2014) [24]	2000–2013	Single	132	100	94[b]	32	76**	na	na	18**	71**

Note: na = not available.

[a] Primary patients are defined as: * non metastatic, non recurrent RPS; * calculated out of primary tumors; *** calculated out of all patients; **** calculated out of operated patients;

[b] calculated out of primary operated patients;

[c] median follow up for survivors only;

[d] calculated out of completely resected patients.

when there is actual direct involvement by tumour [30,31]. Despite the fact that the rate of complete resection has improved over recent years and now is close to 95% in most currently published series, local failure still represents a challenge in the treatment of this disease [19–29]. Since the retroperitoneal space lacks boundaries that define a compartment, surgery is considered marginal by definition despite the width of the resection. This marginality has been considered one of the reasons for the high mortality rate despite the frequent more indolent tumour biology of RPS compared to STS arising at other sites (less than half of the RPSs are high grade) [29]. In order to improve rates of local control, especially in the subset of patients with low- and intermediate-grade tumours, some authors have recently advocated an extended surgical approach [20–23,28,29] to achieve macroscopically complete resection of the tumour in one bloc and minimize microscopically positive margins. This is best done by resecting the tumour en bloc with adherent structures even if they are not overtly infiltrated.

The surgical approach to the abdominal cavity is usually obtained through a midline xipho-pubic incision [2]. If the tumour is located in the upper quadrants, close to the diaphragm, a transverse incision can be made to better expose the tumour and the surrounding structures. For tumours located in the upper right side, displacing the liver and retro-hepatic inferior vena cava, a thoraco-abdominal incision is preferred. The specific location and the surgical approach – limited versus extended procedure – will guide the subsequent surgical steps. In particular, in the case of

extended surgery, right or left (depending on the tumour location) resection of colon, kidney and psoas muscle (complete or partial excision depending on tumour extension) is carried out. A posterior and lateral peritonectomy is usually performed. In the case of upper left quadrant tumours, the body and tail of the pancreas and spleen are usually resected, while the duodenum and head of the pancreas are excised in right-sided tumours only if directly infiltrated. Pelvic organs, liver and gastric resections are rarely performed. Aorta and inferior vena cava are usually dissected in the midline through a sub-adventitial plane and resected only if directly involved (Figure 48.4). Nerves are resected only if directly infiltrated. Specific presentations that are contained or covered by the psoas muscle, like MPNST of the femoral nerve for example, can be approached by an extraperitoneal approach via iliac incisions. The abdomino-inguinal incision is used for tumours fixed in the iliac fossa and extending beyond the inguinal ligament into the groin and root of the thigh, for neoplasms involving the pubic bone or to expose the ilio-femoral vessels.

Some of the organs surrounding a retroperitoneal mass (e.g. kidney, colon and psoas muscle) can be safely removed with limited morbidity [28,29] (Figure 48.5). When considering removal of a kidney, preoperative assessment of differential renal function with an isotope renogram may be invaluable. Others organs, such as the spleen, the left pancreas and the diaphragm, that may be juxtaposed to the tumour, can be resected, with a limited and only rarely dangerous increase of morbidity [28–33] (Figure 48.6).

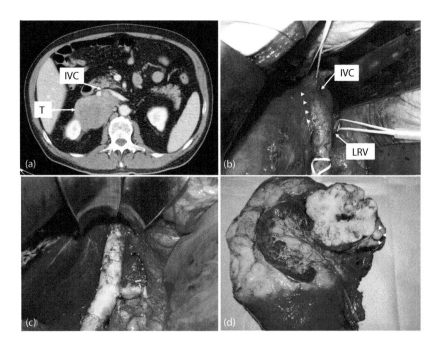

Figure 48.4 Intermediate-grade inferior vena cava–leiomyosarcoma (LMS) in a 63-year-old man. (a) Preoperative contrast-enhanced CT scan. (b) Intraoperative view before tumour resection. The IVC and left renal vein (LRV) are subtended by vessel loops. The tumour rises from the right side of the IVC (arrowheads). (c) Intraoperative view after resection of the tumour en bloc with part of the IVC, right kidney and adrenal gland. Vascular reconstruction was performed using a cadaveric banked cryopreserved venous homograft. (d) Section of the surgical specimen. The mass rises from the IVC and protrudes into the lumen (arrowheads).

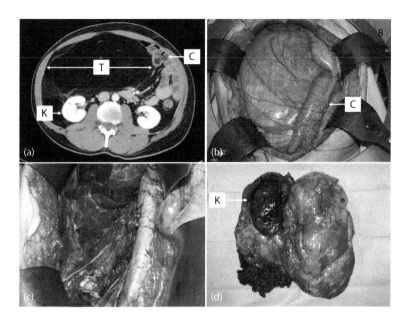

Figure 48.5 Well-differentiated liposarcoma of the right retroperitoneum in a 42-year-old man. (a) Axial, contrast-enhanced CT scan. The tumour (T) pushes the colon (C) toward the front and contralateral side and surrounds the kidney (K). (b) Intraoperative view at laparotomy. (c) Surgical field after extended resection of the mass en bloc with parietal peritoneum, right kidney, adrenal gland, colon and psoas muscle. (d) Section of the surgical specimen.

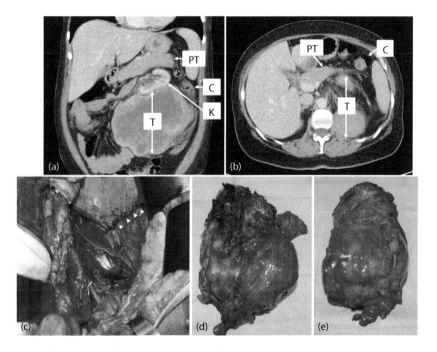

Figure 48.6 High-grade dedifferentiated liposarcoma of the left retroperitoneum in a 55-year-old woman. (a, b) Contrast-enhanced CT scan. The tumour (T) is in direct contact with the inferior pole of the kidney (K), the right colon (C) and the pancreatic body–tail (PT). (c) Surgical field after tumour removal en bloc with left kidney, adrenal gland, colon, pancreatic body–tail, spleen, psoas muscle, part of the diaphragm and diaphragmatic crura. The diaphragm was reinserted on the posterior wall (arrowheads). (d, e) Posterior and anterior views of the surgical specimen. The tumour is covered by adjacent organs.

On the other hand there are structures that should not be resected if not directly involved, as a substantial morbidity can be expected (i.e. duodenum and head of pancreas, spine). The dilemma is then that the potential morbidity related to extended procedures is a real concern while there

also remains a high probability of not achieving a negative pathological resection margin all around the tumour surface [25].

A flexible and individualized approach to resection of uninvolved organs in close proximity to the tumour should always be considered within an individualized surgical strategy that balances the quality of the resection margins and the anticipated morbidity [32]. Preservation of specific organs (e.g. kidney, duodenum, bladder) mandates a specific expertise in the disease to make the appropriate decisions given the overall tumour extent and expected biology and given the individual patient's characteristics. In deciding which neurovascular structures to sacrifice, the potential for local control against the potential for long-term dysfunction must be weighted. Judgment must similarly be exercised in determining appropriateness of an 'en bloc' resection of the liver and pancreas.

Nevertheless the surgical aggressiveness should not be limited in all patients, just because of the risk of being marginal in some. From extremity sarcoma surgery the concept of 'limited' marginality can be extrapolated [32]. A resection with a 'planned-in-advance' positive margin over a critical structure, but where the resection is negative in the remainder of the tumour circumference, has a considerable advantage compared to a simple marginal resection surrounding most of the tumour where residual disease could remain in numerous foci. This kind of surgery may never achieve the quality of resection margins commonly associated with the management of limb sarcomas, but can approximate it [33].

Long-term morbidity is also an issue and future studies on long-term outcome of this more intensive approach are awaited, especially relating to quality of life. Referral of these patients to high-volume centers should also be encouraged since it may be difficult to translate these concepts into standard practice.

It seems rational to consider that in tumours characterized by less aggressive biology, more aggressive surgical approaches that achieve better local control in the short to medium term [22] may result in durable control and possibly cure. Well-differentiated or intermediate-grade dedifferentiated liposarcomas are by far the most common at this site and do not usually develop distant metastases, and they have been reported to be the ones deriving the greatest benefit. Similar considerations could be made for solitary fibrous tumours, which, though far rarer than liposarcoma, are being recognized more often at this site (Figure 48.7). One reason for liposarcomas to derive more benefit from a more aggressive surgical approach relates to their macroscopic appearance; it is always difficult to discriminate normal fat from the well-differentiated component of a liposarcoma [3,22,34]. By performing a wider resection the risk of leaving residual well-differentiated tumour is less and the chance of achieving a complete resection higher, with obvious potential for improvement in local control and possibly survival.

Leiomyosarcoma (the second most common sarcoma at this site), high-grade dedifferentiated liposarcoma and pleomorphic sarcoma (previously often called MFH or MPNST) have a more aggressive systemic course in comparison with the more common well-differentiated and intermediate-grade dedifferentiated liposarcoma and a lower rate of local failure. Therefore such patients usually die of distant metastasis before developing local recurrence. Surgery may then play a role only for those who do not fail systemically. This may become evident after the fifth year of uneventful follow-up [34].

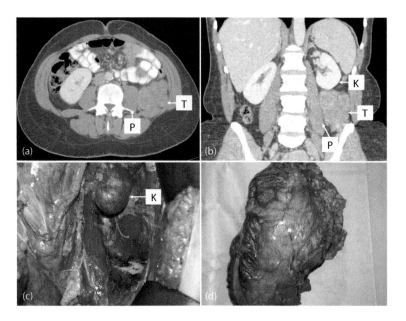

Figure 48.7 Low-grade solitary fibrous tumour (SFT) of the left retroperitoneum in a 51-year-old woman. (a, b) Contrast-enhanced CT scan showing a heterogeneous non-fatty lesion with contrast enhancement. The tumour lies on the quadratus lumborum muscle, transversus abdominis muscle, iliac muscle and iliac crest. It makes contact with the inferior pole of the kidney and psoas muscle. (c) Intraoperative view after tumour removal. The mass was resected along with the parietal peritoneum, left colon, fascia of the psoas muscle, transversus abdominal muscle, fascia of the quadratus lumborum muscle, upper part of the iliac muscle and part of the iliac crest. The dissection was conducted beyond the perirenal fat but kidney was preserved. (d) Anterior view of the surgical specimen.

Paediatric-type tumours are highly chemosensitive and should never be considered for first-line surgery. The therapeutic strategy for these tumours differs significantly from that undertaken for the more common adult-type STS, in particular because primary chemotherapy is always employed. Subsequent surgery is then considered for responding patients, although radiotherapy also remains an option due to their higher radiosensitivity compared to other sarcomas. The aim is to achieve a complete resection of all visible tumour, with resection of adjacent viscera only if directly invaded. Surgery is often complemented by radiation therapy. Therefore the quality of the surgical margins, although of considerable importance, can be enhanced by multimodal treatment to a much greater degree than is possible for adult-type STSs.

NEOADJUVANT AND ADJUVANT THERAPIES

Radiotherapy

The role of radiation therapy is controversial, in the absence of phase III randomized controlled trial data. While largely applied in paediatric-type RPS, not more than 20% of all adult-type RPSs receive pre- or postoperative radiation therapy. Retroperitoneal sarcomas compose a heterogeneous group of pathologies with variable radiosensitivity; the high rate of local failure has prompted investigation of combined modality treatment (surgery with radiotherapy) in an attempt to lower the rate of local recurrence. The absence of randomized controlled trials and diverse variables in observational and retrospective studies make it impossible to define the exact and appropriate role of radiotherapy in the management of RPS [35].

The major concern is radiation-induced toxicity, due to large treatment volumes and the proximity of critical anatomic structures, especially bowel and liver. Ureters, kidneys, spinal cord and peripheral nerves are also at risk for late radiation-related injuries.

These concerns have restricted its use to favorable selective presentations given the overall lower rates of radiosensitivity of adult-type RPSs, which consequently require higher doses.

Attempts to perform studies in this setting have been made, but – due to the rarity of the disease – they were very limited in number and usually not randomized.

One of the tools to improve feasibility has been to shift radiation therapy to the preoperative setting. Given the toxicity of postoperative large abdominal field RT and absence of defined clinical benefit, many multidisciplinary sarcoma centers have evolved protocols for preoperative approaches based on potential improved efficacy, while data from prospective trials suggest strongly that these are less toxic [36,37]. The advantages of preoperative RT are that the small bowel is displaced by the primary tumour, away from the high-dose radiation field, resulting in a safer and less toxic treatment;

gross tumour can be more clearly demarcated, precisely localized and optimally targeted in radiotherapy planning; a higher dose can be delivered to the actual tumour field because surgical adhesions to the bowel are less likely compared to the postoperative setting; the intact preoperative peritoneum provides a physical barrier to immediate tumour dissemination prior to radiotherapy delivery; and the risk of intraperitoneal tumour dissemination at the time of the operation may be reduced by preoperative radiotherapy.

Another tool to improve the feasibility of RT to this difficult site comes from a range of technological advances. The most frequently used is intensity-modulated RT (IMRT), which provides the opportunity to treat large retroperitoneal tumour volumes that were previously impossible to manage. Others included the use of preferential preoperatively scheduled proton beam therapy, intraoperative radiation therapy (IORT) [38] and IMRT delivered using helical tomotherapy [39].

The benefit of preoperative RT in primary adult-type RPS is presently being evaluated in a large international randomized trial (STRASS). Results are awaited to understand if its administration can complement the surgical resection and minimize local recurrence rates.

In contrast to adult-type RPS, paediatric-type RPSs are routinely considered for RT. Obviously the late effects of radiotherapy in children need to be considered in the complex balance of risk and here the absence of proven benefit of radiotherapy in RPS may weigh heavily in the decision process, though the expected benefit is larger and doses more limited. Radiotherapy should be preferentially delivered preoperatively where the accuracy of dose delivery is improved and protection of intra-abdominal and intra-pelvic viscera is much more easily accomplished. Based on established principles elsewhere, Ewing's family of tumours and rhabdomyosarcoma may at times be considered for exclusive local radiotherapy management in combination with chemotherapy [35].

Chemotherapy

Neoadjuvant and adjuvant chemotherapy for the majority of histological subtypes has not shown consistent evidence of a disease-free survival benefit, although there may be certain situations where it is advantageous.

In adult-type sarcomas given the difficulties in obtaining an adequate surgical resection in the retroperitoneum, and the similar challenges radiotherapy has to face in this location, adjuvant chemotherapy to reduce local relapse rates and possibly increase survival may be considered. Nevertheless to date there is no universally accepted role for the adjuvant or neoadjuvant use of chemotherapy for the common forms of RPS [40,41]. Chemotherapy may be used in the advanced setting, with a palliative intent [41,42]. Its value in the adjuvant setting is still to be proven. Its impact on survival, as assessed by clinical trials, is at best limited [41].

A marine-derived drug (trabectedin) was recently approved for second-line treatment of soft tissue sarcomas in Europe. Overall, This drug proved to be mainly active in the treatment of some histological types: myxoid or round cell liposarcomas, leiomyosarcomas and, to a lesser extent, pleomorphic sarcoma [43–45]. Some activity can also be seen in the more common well-differentiated or dedifferentiated variant of liposarcoma in the retroperitoneal space, mainly characterized by prolonged stabilization. Again, this points to a selective antitumour activity of this agent. The drug also demonstrated impressive activity in metastatic myxoid or round cell liposarcoma [46], while its activity is limited in well-differentiated and dedifferentiated liposarcoma. Nevertheless, histological sub-classification of adult-type sarcomas is becoming increasingly crucial in making treatment decisions.

Furthermore, it should be acknowledged that trials specifically addressing the role of chemotherapy in adult-type RPS have never been conducted. Therefore, all information we have derived from studies was carried out on the general population of patients affected by adult-type sarcoma, where the retroperitoneal location does not exceed the 10% rate. Nevertheless there are no reasons to consider them differently from the more common extremity ones, provided a correct histological diagnosis is made.

In paediatric-type RPS, a range of intensive chemotherapy regimes employing etoposide, ifosfamide, vincristine, dactinomycin and adriamycin have been widely used. More recently topoisomerase inhibitors have also been introduced with some evidence of activity, but with substantial toxicity, such that further studies are necessary before their introduction into routine clinical practice [47,48]. Very little improvement has occurred after the dramatic change of survival obtained in the late 1970s after the introduction of routine polychemotherapy in paediatric-type sarcoma management.

Unlike in many forms of cancer where the introduction of molecular-targeted agents has been progressing rapidly, the development of new available molecular-targeted drugs in soft tissue sarcomas has been slow. There are plenty of targets amenable to molecular therapies in the sarcoma family, in both adult and paediatric types. Moreover one-fourth of them harbor a chromosomal translocation, and thereby fusion products. So, sarcomas lend themselves to being targeted by newly developed molecular drugs. As of today, one of the vascular endothelial growth factor (VEGF) inhibitors, pazopanib, has been approved for second- or further line treatment of advanced or metastatic non-adipocytic STS [49].

The PI3K–Akt–mTOR signaling pathway may also be abnormally activated in many sarcomas [50], and efforts are underway to target it. Finally, anti-IGFR agents are under active study in some sarcoma types, initially in paediatric-type sarcomas [51,52].

In light of all these new agents, clearly histological and molecular selectivity will gain further importance in the near future, to better identify the proper treatment for each histological subtype, while the retroperitoneal location – as specific as it may be for loco-regional treatment – is very unlikely to play a particular role.

LOCALLY ADVANCED AND RECURRENT DISEASE

Local recurrence is common for RPS and is a challenge as it remains the major cause of death in low- to intermediate-grade liposarcoma. Tumour biology is a significant prognostic factor for patients with recurrent RPS; local recurrence rates are higher in patients with intermediate-grade tumours and occur at an earlier interval than they do with patients with low-grade tumours [53].

Most reports on this subject are retrospective with different management strategies and variable results. CT is indicated when patients exhibit new symptoms or a mass is palpable on clinical examination.

In loco-regionally recurrent disease surgery can still play a role, especially when the recurrence is not accompanied by distant spread. This is often the case in low-grade tumours (mainly liposarcoma). In this setting surgery – if technically feasible – should be performed with the aim of obtaining a macroscopically complete resection, but the expected further loco-regional failure rate is definitely higher [54]. The extent of such a resection should then be more carefully weighed against the expected real benefit, which reduces at each subsequent recurrence and could be predicted by the free interval.

Decision making in this setting is challenging, since surgical morbidity increases and the tumour is often asymptomatic until the final stage of the disease [55]. There is no survival advantage if the surgical resection is not macroscopically complete. Yet this advantage reduces at every further recurrence whatever the surgical resection is. Moreover there is also a quality of life issue. Tumours that may become symptomatic (gastrointestinal obstruction and pain are the two main complications) could benefit from a surgical procedure even if not macroscopically complete, especially in the case of tumours with a low-rate growth. No formal tools to help decision have been provided so far. A recent study showed that the growth rate may be an independent predictor of disease-specific survival in locally recurrent retroperitoneal liposarcoma [56]. Patients with a local recurrence growth rate of greater than 0.9 cm/month had significantly worse disease-specific survival and re-resection of the recurrence did not alter the poor outcome for this subset of patients. They should be therefore considered for trials of novel targeted therapies. Patients with local recurrence growth rates of less than 0.9 cm/month still benefited from re-resection of the recurrence and should therefore be considered first for repeat surgery. If the results of such a study were confirmed, the growth rate could be the first useful tool to guide decision making in clinical practice in this area.

REFERENCES

1. Cormier JN, Gronchi A, Pollock RE. Soft tissue sarcomas. In Brunicardi F, Andersen D, Billiar T, Dunn D, Hunter J, Matthews J, Pollock RE, eds., *Schwartz's Principles of Surgery*. New York: McGraw Hill, 2014.

2. Bonvalot S, Raut CP, Pollock RE, et al. Technical considerations in surgery for retroperitoneal sarcomas: position paper from E-Surge, a master class in sarcoma surgery, and EORTC-STBSG. *Ann Surg Oncol* 2012;19(9):2981–2991.

3. Brennan M, Singer S, Maki RG, O'Sullivan B. Soft tissue sarcoma. In DeVita VT, Lawrence TS, Rosenberg SA, eds., *Cancer: Principles and Practice of Oncology*. Philadelphia: Lippincott Williams & Wilkins, 2008:1741–1794.

4. Fletcher CDM, Bridge JA, Hogendoorn PCW, Mertens F, eds. *World Health Organization Classification of Tumours of Soft Tissue and Bone*, 4th ed. Lyon: IARC Press, 2013.

5. Fletcher CDM. The evolving classification of soft tissue tumours – an update based on the new 2013 WHO classification. *Histopathology* 2014;64:2–11.

6. Trojani M, Contesso G, Coindre JM, et al. Soft tissue sarcomas of adults: study of pathological prognostic variables and definition of a histopathologic grading system. *Int J Cancer* 1984;33:37–42.

7. Gronchi A, Miceli R, Shurell E, et al. Prediction in primary resected retroperitoneal soft tissue sarcoma: histology-specific overall survival and disease-free survival nomograms built on major sarcoma center data sets. *J Clin Oncol* 2013;31:1649–1655.

8. Shiraev T, Pasricha SS, Choong P, et al. Retroperitoneal sarcomas: a review of disease spectrum, radiological features, characterisation and management. *J Med Imaging Radiat Oncol* 2013;57(6):687–700.

9. Wu JS, Hochman MG. Soft-tissue tumors and tumor-like lesions: a systematic imaging approach. *Radiology* 2009;253(2):297–316.

10. Lahat G, Madewell JE, Anaya DA, et al. Computed tomography scan-driven selection of treatment for retroperitoneal liposarcoma histologic subtypes. *Cancer* 2009;115:1081–1090.

11. Morosi C, Stacchiotti S, Marchianò A, et al. Correlation between radiological assessment and histopathological diagnosis in retroperitoneal tumors: analysis of 291 consecutive patients at a tertiary reference sarcoma center. *Eur J Surg Oncol* 2014;40(12):1662–1670.

12. Wilkinson MJ, Martin JL, Khan AA, et al. Percutaneous core needle biopsy in retroperitoneal sarcomas does not influence local recurrence or overall survival. *Ann Surg Oncol* 2015;22(3):853–858.

13. Trovik CS, Bauer HCF, Alvegard TA, et al. Surgical margins, local recurrence and metastasis in soft tissue sarcomas: 599 surgically-treated patients from the Scandinavian Sarcoma Group register. *Eur J Cancer* 2000;36:710–716.

14. Stojadinovic A, Leung DH, Hoos A, et al. Analysis of the prognostic significance of microscopic margins in 2,084 localized primary adult soft tissue sarcomas. *Ann Surg* 2002;235(3):424–434.

15. Zagars GK, Ballo MT, Pisters PWT, et al. Surgical margins and re-excision in the management of patients with soft tissue sarcoma using conservative surgery and radiation therapy. *Cancer* 2003;97:2530–2543.

16. Gronchi A, Lo Vullo S, Colombo C, et al. Extremity soft tissue sarcoma in a series of patients treated at a single institution: local control directly impacts survival. *Ann Surg* 2010;251:512–517.

17. Lewis JJ, Leung D, Woodruff JM, Brennan MF. Retroperitoneal soft-tissue sarcoma: analysis of 500 patients treated and followed at a single institution. *Ann Surg* 1998;228(3):355–365.

18. Stoeckle E, Coindre JM, Bonvalot S, Kantor G, Terrier P, Bonichon F, Nguyen Bui B, French Federation of Cancer Centers Sarcoma Group. Prognostic factors in retroperitoneal sarcoma: a multivariate analysis of a series of 165 patients of the French Cancer Center Federation Sarcoma Group. *Cancer* 2001;92(2):359–368.

19. van Dalen T, Plooij JM, van Coevorden F, et al. Long-term prognosis of primary retroperitoneal soft tissue sarcoma. *Eur J Surg Oncol* 2007;33:234–238.

20. Strauss DC, Hayes AJ, Thway K, et al. Surgical management of primary retroperitoneal sarcoma. *Br J Surg* 2010;101:520–523.

21. Bonvalot S, Rivoire M, Castaing M, et al. Primary retroperitoneal sarcomas: a multivariate analysis of surgical factors associated with local control. *J Clin Oncol* 2009;27:31–37.

22. Gronchi A, Lo Vullo S, Fiore M, et al. Aggressive surgical policies in a retrospectively reviewed single-institution case series of retroperitoneal soft tissue sarcoma patients. *J Clin Oncol* 2009;27:24–30.

23. Gronchi A, Miceli R, Allard MA, et al. Personalizing the approach to retroperitoneal soft tissue sarcoma: histology-specific patterns of failure and postrelapse outcome after primary extended resection. *Ann Surg Oncol* 2015;22(5):1447–1454.

24. Bremjit PJ, Jones RL, Chai X, Kane G, Rodler ET, Loggers ET, Pollack SM, Pillarisetty VG, Mann GN. A contemporary large single-institution evaluation of resected retroperitoneal sarcoma. *Ann Surg Oncol* 2014;21(7):2150–2158.

25. Toulmonde M, Bonvalot S, Méeus P, et al. Retroperitoneal sarcomas: patterns of care at diagnosis, prognostic factors and focus on main histological subtypes: a multicenter analysis of the French Sarcoma Group. *Ann Oncol* 2014;25(3):735–742.

26. Lehnert T, Cardona S, Hinz U, et al. Primary and locally recurrent retroperitoneal soft-tissue sarcoma: local control and survival. *Eur J Surg Oncol* 2009;35:986–993.

27. Anaya DA, Lahat G, Liu J, et al. Multifocality in retroperitoneal sarcoma: a prognostic factor critical to surgical decision-making. *Ann Surg* 2009;249(1):137–142.

28. Bonvalot S, Miceli R, Berselli M., et al. Aggressive surgery in retroperitoneal soft tissue sarcoma carried out at high-volume centers is safe and is associated with improved local control. *Ann Surg Oncol* 2010;17:1507–1514.

29. Gronchi A, Miceli R, Colombo C, et al. Frontline extended surgery is associated with improved survival in retroperitoneal low-intermediate grade soft tissue sarcomas. *Ann Oncol* 2012;23(4):1067–1073.

30. ESMO/European Sarcoma Network Working Group. Soft tissue and visceral sarcomas: ESMO Clinical Practice Guidelines for diagnosis, treatment and follow-up. *Ann Oncol* 2014;25(Suppl. 3):iii102–12.

31. von Mehren M, Benjamin RS, Bui MM, et al. Soft tissue sarcoma, version 2.2012: featured updates to the NCCN guidelines. *J Natl Compr Canc Netw* 2012;10(8):951–960.

32. Gerrand CH, Wunder JS, Kandel RA, et al. Classification of positive margins after resection of soft-tissue sarcoma of the limb predicts the risk of local recurrence. *J Bone Joint Surg Br* 2001;83(8):1149–1155.

33. Gronchi A, Bonvalot S, Le Cesne A, Casali PG. Resection of uninvolved adjacent organs can be part of surgery for retroperitoneal soft tissue sarcoma. *J Clin Oncol* 2009;27:2106–2107.

34. Mussi C, Collini P, Miceli R, et al. The prognostic impact of dedifferentiation in retroperitoneal liposarcoma: a series of surgically treated patients at a single institution. *Cancer* 2008;113(7):1657–1665.

35. Strauss DC, Hayes AJ, Thomas JM. Retroperitoneal tumours: review of management. *Ann R Coll Surg Engl* 2011;93(4):275–280.

36. Jones JJ, Catton CN, O'Sullivan B. et al. Initial results of a trial of preoperative external-beam radiation therapy and postoperative brachytherapy for retroperitoneal sarcoma. *Ann Surg Oncol* 2002;9(4):346–354.

37. Pisters PW, Ballo MT, Fenstermacher MJ, et al. Phase I trial of preoperative concurrent doxorubicin and radiation therapy, surgical resection, and intraoperative electron-beam radiation therapy for patients with localized retroperitoneal sarcoma. *J Clin Oncol* 2003;21(16):3092–3097.

38. Yoon SS, Chen Y-L, Kirsch DG, et al. Proton beam, intensity modulated, and/or intra-operative radiation therapy combined with aggressive anterior surgical resection for retroperitoneal and pelvic sarcomas. Presented at Proceedings of the 14th Annual Meeting of the Connective Tissue Oncology Society, 2008, abstr. 34806.

39. Stoeckle E, Kantor G, Dejean C, et al. Preoperative high-dose (54 Gy) helicoidal tomotherapy plus surgery in retroperitoneal liposarcoma: a feasibility study. Presented at Proceedings of the 14th Annual Meeting of the Connective Tissue Oncology Society, 2008, abstr. 35155.

40. Adjuvant chemotherapy for localised resectable soft-tissue sarcoma of adults: meta-analysis of individual data. Sarcoma Meta-Analysis Collaboration. *Lancet* 1997;350(9092):1647–1654.

41. Pervaiz N, Colterjohn N, Farrokhyar F, et al. A systematic meta-analysis of randomized controlled trials of adjuvant chemotherapy for localized resectable soft-tissue sarcoma. *Cancer* 2008;113(3):573–581.

42. Karavasilis V, Seddon BM, Ashley S, et al. Significant clinical benefit of first-line palliative chemotherapy in advanced soft-tissue sarcoma: retrospective analysis and identification of prognostic factors in 488 patients. *Cancer* 2008;112(7):1585–1591.

43. Cupissol D, Jimenez M, Rey A, et al. Ecteinascidin-743 (ET-743) for chemotherapy-naive patients with advanced soft tissue sarcomas: multicenter phase II and pharmacokinetic study. *J Clin Oncol* 2005;23:5484–592.

44. Le Cesne A, Blay JY, Judson I, et al. Phase II study of ET-743 in advanced soft tissue sarcomas: a European Organisation for the Research and Treatment of Cancer (EORTC) soft tissue and bone sarcoma group trial. *J Clin Oncol* 2005;23:576–584.

45. Demetri GD, Chawla SP, von Mehren M, et al. Efficacy and safety of trabectedin in patients with advanced or metastatic liposarcoma or leiomyosarcoma after failure of prior anthracyclines and ifosfamide: results of a randomized phase II study of two different schedules. *J Clin Oncol* 2009;25:4188–4196.

46. Grosso F, Jones RL, Demetri GD, et al. Efficacy of trabectedin (ecteinascidin-743) in advanced pretreated myxoid liposarcomas: a retrospective study. *Lancet Oncol* 2007;8:595–602.

47. Breitfeld PP, Meyer WH. Rhabdomyosarcoma: new windows of opportunity. *Oncologist* 2005;10(7):518–527.

48. Langevin AM, Bernstein M, Kuhn JG, et al. A phase II trial of rebeccamycin analogue (NSC #655649) in children with solid tumors: a Children's Oncology Group study. *Pediatr Blood Cancer* 2008;50(3):577–580.

49. van der Graaf WT, Blay JY, Chawla SP, et al. Pazopanib for metastatic soft-tissue sarcoma (PALETTE): a randomised, double-blind, placebo-controlled phase 3 trial. *Lancet* 2012;379(9829):1879–1886.

50. MacKenzie AR, von Mehren M. Mechanisms of mammalian target of rapamycin inhibition in sarcoma: present and future. *Expert Rev Anticancer Ther* 2007;7:1145–1154.

51. Kolb EA, Gorlick R. Development of IGF-IR inhibitors in pediatric sarcomas. *Curr Oncol Rep* 2009;11(4):307–313.

52. Olmos D, Okuno S, Schuetze SM, et al. Safety, pharmacokinetics and preliminary activity of the anti-IGF-IR antibody CP-751,871 in patients with sarcoma. *J Clin Oncol* 2008;26(Suppl.):abstr. 10501.

53. Gronchi A, Strauss DC, Miceli R, Bonvalot S, et al. Variability in patterns of recurrence after resection of primary retroperitoneal sarcoma (RPS): A Report on 1007 patients from the multi-institutional collaborative RPS working Group. *Ann Surg.* 2015.

54. Lewis JJ, Leung D, Woodruff JM, Brennan MF. Retroperitoneal soft-tissue sarcoma: analysis of 500 patients treated and followed at a single institution. *Ann Surg* 1998;228(3):355–365.

55. Yeh JJ, Singer S, Brennan MF, Jaques DP. Effectiveness of palliative procedures for intra-abdominal sarcomas. *Ann Surg Oncol* 2005;12(12):1084–1089.

56. Park JO, Qin LX, Prete F, Brennan MF, Singer S. Growth rate predicts outcome in locally recurrent retroperitoneal sarcoma. Presented at Proceedings of the 13th Annual Meeting of the Connective Tissue Oncology Society, 2007, abstr. 382.

49

Neurosurgical oncology: Neoplasms of the brain and meninges

RACHEL GROSSMAN AND ZVI RAM

INTRODUCTION

Central nervous system (CNS) tumors comprise a wide range of neoplasms that widely differ in their invasiveness, location, age distribution and tendency to progress and metastasize. Remarkable advances have been made over the past decade in our understanding of the molecular profile of each tumor type, with new treatment modalities playing an increasingly important role. This chapter reviews the classification, treatment options and prognosis of several selected CNS neoplasms.

GLIOMAS

Gliomas are tumors that arise from glial or precursor cells. Gliomas include astrocytomas, oligodendrogliomas, ependymomas and low- and high-grade mixed gliomas. Gliomas account for 28% of all brain tumors and 80% of the malignant types [1]. The WHO classification [2] categorizes gliomas into four grades based on their predominant cell type and histopathological characteristics, such as cytological atypia, anaplasia, mitotic activity, microvascular proliferation and necrosis. Grade I tumors, which do not contain

any of the above-mentioned histologic features, are well-circumscribed, non-infiltrative lesions, and complete surgical resection is considered curative in most cases. Grade II tumors are characterized by cellular atypia. Grades III and IV, which account for more than 50% of gliomas, are characterized by the presence of mitosis (grade III) and vascular proliferation and necrosis (grade IV). The etiology is unknown in most cases. Hereditary factors do not play an important role in the development of gliomas, although these tumors are more common in patients with neurofibromatosis type 1 and Li–Fraumeni syndrome. Both low- and high-grade gliomas are likely to recur.

LOW-GRADE GLIOMAS

Epidemiology

Low-grade gliomas (LGGs) commonly refer to diffuse grade II astrocytomas, which account for 15–30% of all primary brain tumors, with an annual incidence of 0.55 per 100,000 in the United States [2]. They typically present in young age, with a slight male predominance (male–female ratio 1.5).

Diagnosis

Low-grade gliomas are progressive and infiltrating primary brain tumors that frequently involve eloquent areas [3]. They have a predilection for the insula and supplementary motor area (SMA) [24,25] and are rarely located in the infra-tentorial area and involve the cerebellum. Most of the patients (80%) have a relatively good neurological status at diagnosis, although they may also present with lethargy, headaches, personality changes and cognitive decline. Seizures are the initial presenting symptom in up to 90% of cases of LGGs [26]. LGGs appear as homogenous low-signal-intensity lesions on T1-weighted MRI sequences and high signal intensity on T2 and fluid-attenuated inversion recovery (FLAIR)–weighted sequences (Figure 49.1). Contrast enhancement

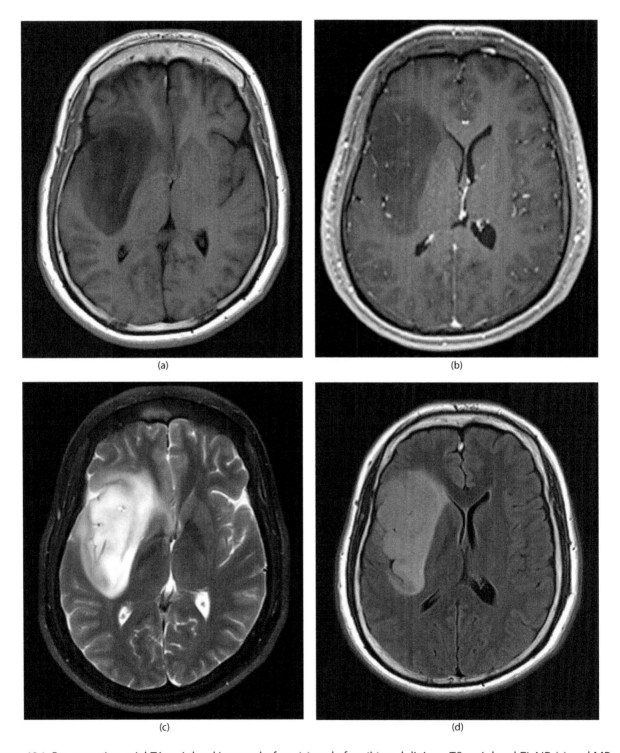

(a)

(b)

(c)

(d)

Figure 49.1 Preoperative axial T1-weighted images before (a) and after (b) gadolinium. T2-weighted FLAIR (c) and MR images (d) showing right low-grade insular glioma.

is classically associated with high-grade tumors, and their presence may represent areas of higher-grade transformation [4]. Accordingly, contrast enhancement is absent in LGGs, although some degree of contrast enhancement may be seen in up to 60% of cases. Calcifications may be evident as areas of T2 hyperintensity and T1 hypointensity in up to 20% of these lesions, particularly suggestive of oligodendrogliomas. WHO grade II astrocytomas, such as fibrillary, gemistocytic, protoplasmic and pilomyxoid types, as well as pleomorphic xanthoastrocytomas (PXAs), oligodendrogliomas and oligoastrocytomas, are characterized by moderate cellularity and nuclear atypia without mitosis, vascular proliferation and necrosis.

Prognosis

LGGs undergo continuous growth and progress to a higher grade of malignancy [5]. Several adverse prognostic factors were identified in two large phase III trials of the European Organization for Research and Treatment of Cancer (EORTC), 22844 and 22845: age greater than 40 years, astrocytoma histology subtype, largest diameter of the tumor greater than 6 cm, tumor crossing the midline and the presence of a neurologic deficit(s) before surgery [6,7]. Complete surgical resection, oligodendroglial histology and chromosomal co-deletion of 1p19q represent a more favorable prognosis [8–10].

Molecular pathology

Isocitrate dehydrogenase (IDH) mutations are detected within the majority of tumor cells, signifying an initiating molecular event in the pathogenesis of gliomas [11]. IDH1 mutations are frequent (>80%) in diffuse astrocytoma WHO grade II and anaplastic astrocytoma WHO grade III, the precursor lesions of secondary glioblastomas, as well as in oligodendroglial tumors, including oligodendrogliomas WHO grade II, anaplastic oligodendrogliomas WHO grade III, oligoastrocytomas WHO grade II and anaplastic oligoastrocytomas WHO grade III [12]. IDH mutant gliomas have been associated with a better overall (OS) survival, and it appears that the prognostic role of IDH status is superior to the traditional histology classification [11].

Treatment

Surgical resection is the first treatment option; however, there is no general consensus regarding the value of the extent of LGG resection to improve patient outcome and quality of life (QOL) because class I evidence is lacking. Mounting evidence places surgical removal as a major parameter for predicting outcome, along with patient's age, performance status and IDH status. Over the last decade, surgical removal has been demonstrated to improve symptoms, especially seizures [13], to delay malignant transformation and to improve overall survival of patients with LGGs [14,15]. Surgical advances have enabled improvement of the surgeon's ability to maximize the degree of surgical resection while minimizing postoperative *de novo* neurological deficits. The use of functional imaging modalities, such as diffuse tensor imaging (DTI) and functional magnetic resonance imaging (fMRI), allows the surgeon to identify functional brain areas in relation to the tumor before surgery. However, prediction of cortical language and high cognitive sites according to preoperative images is inadequate due to marked variability between individuals, distortion of pathways as a result of tumor mass effect and reorganization of pathways through plasticity. Thus, the gold standard for identifying eloquent brain regions and functional pathways is the utilization of intraoperative stimulation mapping. In a meta-analysis of 8091 patients with supratentorial infiltrative glioma operated over the last two decades with and without intraoperative stimulation mapping (ISM), glioma resections using ISM were associated with fewer late severe neurologic deficits and more extensive resection [16].

In addressing the issue of postoperative adjuvant treatment, the EORTC 22845 trial showed early postoperative radiation therapy (RT) after surgery lengthened the period without progression but did not affect overall survival. That study randomized 157 patients to early radiotherapy, and 157 controls who received RT only after progression were noted. The median progression-free survival (PFS) was 5.3 years in the early RT group and 3.4 years in the control group, while overall survival was similar between groups (7.4 vs. 7.2 years for the RT and controls, respectively) [17].

The recently published long-term follow-up of the Radiation Therapy Oncology Group (RTOG) 9802 trial that compared 54 Gy of radiotherapy with the same RT and the addition of adjuvant procarbazine, 1-(2-chloroethyl)-3-cyclohexyl-1-nitrosourea (CCNU) and vincristine (PCV) in high-risk LGG patients showed significant survival benefit with the addition of PCV. Specifically, the addition of PCV to RT increased the median PFS from 4 years to 10.4 years and the median OS from 7.8 years to 13.3 years [18]. Moreover, patients treated with PCV, those with an oligodendroglial component and females had better survival in a multivariate analysis [18]. RTOG 9802 is the third trial to show a survival benefit for adjuvant PCV chemotherapy in a subset of patients with diffuse grade II and III gliomas, but the first to show OS benefit of specific treatment in grade II gliomas [8,19]. Unfortunately, as opposed to previous reports [8,19], no molecular correlates with outcome were included [18]. PCV is currently considered by many as being too toxic; however, there are no similar data on long-term benefit from clinical trials on temozolomide (TMZ) (an alkylating cytotoxic agent) in diffuse grade II or III gliomas and, in fact, it is unclear whether the findings on PCV apply to TMZ. Nevertheless, PCV has been gradually replaced by TMZ in the treatment of gliomas since it is better tolerated by patients and the effect of TMZ remains to be elucidated.

GLIOBLASTOMA

Epidemiology

Glioblastoma is the most common primary malignant brain tumor in adults, with an annual incidence of 3.19 per 100,000 in the United States [1]. It accounts for 15.4% of all primary brain tumors and 45.6% of primary malignant brain tumors [1]. The incidence of glioblastoma increases with age, with the highest rates demonstrated in individuals between 75 and 84 years of age [1]. Despite modern treatments with the current standard of care, the outcome of glioblastoma patients remains poor, with a median life expectancy limited to 16 to 19 months [20,21]. Glioblastomas can arise throughout the CNS but are always found in the subcortical white matter. They often have thick, irregular, enhancing margins and a central necrotic core, which may also have a hemorrhagic component (Figure 49.2). They are surrounded by vasogenic-type edema, which usually contains infiltration by neoplastic cells.

Molecular classification

Most glioblastomas (~90%) develop rapidly *de novo* in elderly patients (primary glioblastomas). Secondary glioblastomas progress from low-grade diffuse astrocytomas to glioblastomas, usually in younger patients, and have a significantly better prognosis [22]. Primary and secondary glioblastomas are histologically indistinguishable, but they demonstrate differences in clinical history, and in genetic, epigenetic and expression profiles. In 2013, The Cancer Genome Atlas (TCGA) first demonstrated the types and frequencies of mutations seen in glioblastomas [23]. That study analyzed more than 500 glioblastomas, and integrated information from sequencing, somatic number alteration analysis, transcriptomic

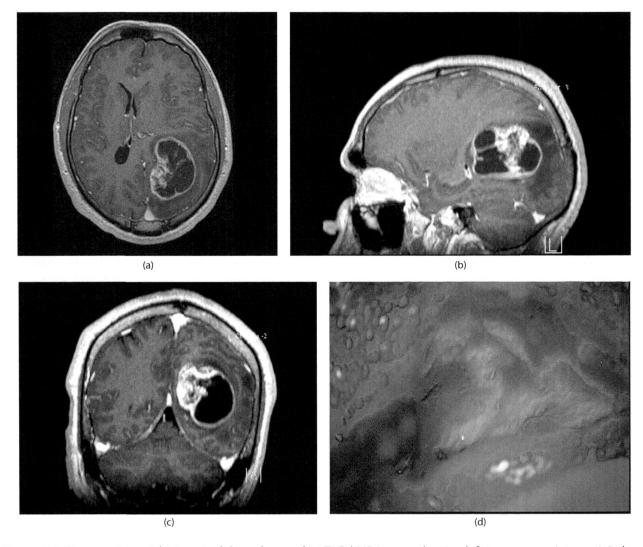

(a)

(b)

(c)

(d)

Figure 49.2 Preoperative axial (a), sagittal (b) and coronal (c) T1Gd MR images showing left temporo-parieto-occipital glioblastoma. (d) Intraoperative image after 5ALA administration showing prominent fluorescence under UV light.

analysis, epigenetic profiling and rearrangement studies to provide a molecular picture of this tumor. The single most common site of mutation in primary glioblastoma was identified within the promoter region of the telomerase reverse transcriptase gene, with mutations seen in 54% to 83% of the tumors [24,25]. Recurrent mutations were identified in genes, such as PTEN (31%), TP53 (29%), epidermal growth factor receptor (EGFR) (26%) and PIK3R1 (11%). Four transcriptional groups were identified based on the pattern of gene expression and DNA methylation in the TCGA cohort: classical, proneural, mesenchymal and neural [26,27]. The *classical* transcriptomal subtype is characterized by the gain of chromosome 7 paired with the loss of chromosome 10. EGFR is focally amplified and mutated in most cases. The most common EGFR mutation is an in-frame deletion of exons 2 to 7, termed EGFRvIII, which is expressed in 25% of primary glioblastomas [28]. The *proneural* type is associated with a higher incidence of amplifications of platelet-derived growth factor receptor A (PDGFR-A), often including neighboring receptor-tyrosine kinase (RTKs) on chromosome 4q12 (KDR and KIT), as well as overexpression of other oligodendrocytic development genes (e.g. NKX-2 and Olig2). Mutations of TP53 are also common. Mutations in IDH1 are found in a distinct subset of proneural glioblastomas: they comprise a favorable prognostic marker for glioblastoma and have been associated with increased OS [12]. They occur in a large fraction of young patients with diffuse astrocytomas and oligodendroglioma WHO grade II anaplastic astrocytomas and anaplastic oligodendrogliomass WHO grade III, and are within the proneural subtype. These mutations are very frequent in secondary glioblastomas (>80%), but they are very rare in primary glioblastomas (<5%). In fact, glioblastomas with IDH1 mutations that are clinically diagnosed as being primary may have rapidly progressed from lower-grade tumors that had escaped clinical diagnosis and were misclassified as primary glioblastomas. Proneural glioblastomas that are IDH wild type are associated with particularly aggressive behavior and a poor prognosis [29]. *Mesenchymal* glioblastomas overexpress mesenchymal markers and show a high prevalence of deletions and silencing mutations of NF1 on chromosome 17q11, leading to decreased expression of neurofibromin [27]. Point mutations in PTEN are common in this subgroup, as is the expression of genes in the tumor necrosis factor super-family. Less is known about the *neural* tumors, which are characterized by the expression of neuronal markers and, frequently, overexpression of EGFR.

Treatment

Maximal and safe tumor resection represents the initial treatment step. It is intended to establish the histological diagnosis and to achieve relief of the mass effect with preservation of brain function. Although surgical cure is impossible, a reduction of the tumor mass may alleviate neurological symptoms and cognitive deficits, thereby improving QOL [30,31]. Although there is no class I evidence for the value of the extent of resection, there has been growing evidence over the last decade that suggests that extending tumor resection is associated with enhanced OS [15,32,33]. Advances in intraoperative techniques, including neuro-navigation, real-time intraoperative imaging (e.g. intraoperative MRI and intraoperative ultrasound), intraoperative electrophysiological monitoring with cortical and subcortical mapping and fluorescence-guided surgery [34], have all been developed to maximize tumor resection and minimize surgical morbidity. As of 2005, the addition of chemotherapy to radiation has become the first-line treatment for glioblastoma. In a large, randomized phase III trial, TMZ together with radiotherapy resulted in an improved median OS from 12.1 to 14.6 months and an increase in the 2-year survival rate from 10% to 27% [21]. O-6-Methylguanine-DNA methyltransferase (MGMT) is a DNA repair protein that reverses the damage induced by alkylating chemotherapy agents. Methylation of the gene promoter results in decreased expression of this enzyme and thus renders tumor cells more susceptible to alkylating agents. The addition of TMZ mainly benefited patients who had a methylated MGMT gene promoter [35]. The addition of TMZ to radiation therapy among glioblastoma patients with a methylated MGMT gene promoter resulted in a median survival of 21.7 months [35]. Vascular epithelial growth factor-A (VEGF-A) is a major regulator of angiogenesis and can be detected in high amounts in glioblastoma [36]. Therapies targeting VEGF have been widely tested in clinical trials in glioblastoma patients. Bevacizumab (Bev; Avastin®, Roche Basel, Switzerland) is a humanized monoclonal antibody directed against VEGF. Several trials aimed at studying the effects of Bev, either alone or in combination with chemotherapeutic agents, have been performed. Two phase III studies by Avaglio and RTOG (0825) evaluated the addition of Bev to standard radiotherapy and TMZ compared with standard chemoradiotherapy alone in patients with newly diagnosed glioblastoma. Both the Avaglio and RTOG trials [37,38], which enrolled 921 and 637 glioblastoma patients, respectively, showed an increase in PFS from 6.2 to 10.6 months and from 7.3 to 10.7 months, respectively. In contrast, the median OS was not significantly different (16.8 vs. 16.7 months in the Avaglio trial and 15.7 vs. 16.1 months in the RTOG trial, $p > 0.05$). Alternating electric fields (AEFs) is another new treatment modality in cancer patients. It can induce membrane depolarization and stimulate excitable tissues. Low-intensity intermediate-frequency AEF (100–300 kHz) has been shown to arrest the proliferation and differentiation of cells, in a variety of cancer cell lines, both *in vitro* and *in vivo* [39]. It has been postulated that non-homogeneous electric fields generate unidirectional forces that disrupt the normal polymerization–depolymerization process of tubulin during mitosis [39]. Tumor-treating fields delivered by the NovoTTF™-100A system in combination with standard-of-care TMZ chemotherapy were shown to extend both PFS and OS compared to TMZ alone in patients with newly diagnosed glioblastoma in a phase III clinical trial [40].

Advances in the understanding of the complex molecular biology, immunologic interaction, resistance mechanisms and microenvironment of glioblastoma are being translated into innovative treatment modalities. Many ongoing clinical trials are investigating innovative approaches, including immunotherapy, gene therapy, anti-angiogenesis agents and small molecules targeting tumor growth factor receptors and their combinations.

BRAIN METASTASES

Epidemiology

Brain metastases are cancer cells that have spread to the brain from primary tumors in other organs in the body. Those metastases are the most common tumors in the brain, affecting 24–45% of all brain cancer patients in the United States. Approximately 170,000 new cases of brain metastasis are diagnosed in the United States each year, with a prevalence of 120,000–140,000 per year, and accounting for 20% of cancer deaths annually. The incidence of brain metastatic disease is gradually rising, most probably due to earlier detection, improvement in treatment leading to increased OS of cancer patients, aging of the population and non-penetration of chemotherapeutic agents into the brain [41–43].

Prognosis

The most common primary cancers to metastasize to the brain are malignancies of the lung, breast, kidney and colon as well as melanomas [44]. The distribution of brain metastases follows the blood flow and the volume of brain parenchyma: 85% of brain metastases are found in the cerebral hemispheres, 10–15% in the cerebellum and 1–3% in the brainstem [45,46]. Presenting symptoms include headache (49%), focal weakness (30%), mental disturbances (32%), gait ataxia (21%), seizures (18%), speech difficulty (12%), visual disturbance (6%), sensory disturbance (6%) and limb ataxia (6%). Prognostic factors play an important role in determining how aggressively to treat a patient's brain metastases. Fifteen years ago, the RTOG developed the recursive partitioning analysis (RPA), a prognostic score based on data from three consecutive RTOG trials enrolling more than 1200 patients with brain metastases [47]. Three prognostic classes were defined: age, Karnofsky performance status (KPS) and control of primary disease. The RPA class I group included patients with a KPS ≥70, age 65 years or younger, with controlled primary disease and no extracranial metastases. The RPA class III group included patients with a KPS <70, while the RPA class II group included all the others. The median OS times were 7.1, 4.2 and 2.3 months for the class I, II and III groups, respectively [47].

Treatment

SURGICAL MANAGEMENT

Radiation therapy and surgery are the mainstay of treatment for the management of brain metastases, particularly if they become symptomatic or a histological diagnosis is needed. The survival benefit of surgical resection of a single brain metastasis followed by whole brain RT (WBRT) was evaluated in three prospective randomized studies [48–50], yielding class I evidence in support of surgical resection followed by WBRT in patients with solitary brain metastasis who have good performance status and controlled systemic disease. The first study compared the effect of surgery followed by WBRT (36 Gy) to needle biopsy followed by WBRT for supratentorial solitary metastasis in patients with a KPS >70. Patients who underwent surgical resection had a significantly longer OS (40 weeks vs. 15 weeks, $p < 0.01$), a lower recurrence rate at the site of the original metastasis (20% vs. 52%, $p < 0.02$) and remained functionally independent longer [49] (Figure 49.3). In the second study, the effect of surgical resection of solitary brain metastasis followed by WBRT (40 Gy) led to a longer OS (10 vs. 6 months, $p = 0.04$) and a longer functional independency ($p = 0.06$). This was most pronounced in patients with stable extracranial disease (median OS of 12 vs. 7 months) [50]. The third study failed to demonstrate any improved outcome with the addition of surgery to WBRT (30 Gy). The median OS for the WBRT group was 6.3 months compared with 5.6 months for the surgery plus WBRT group ($p = 0.24$) [48].

The role of neurosurgical resection for multiple brain metastases has not been studied in depth. Although surgical intervention is indicated in relieving the intracranial mass effect, only a few retrospective studies have shown that the clinical effectiveness of surgical resection for multiple tumors (>3 lesions) followed by WBRT is comparable to the effect of surgery on solitary brain metastases, without increased risk of morbidity and mortality [51,52]. The therapeutic effect of resection of recurrent brain metastases has been investigated solely in retrospective studies. The known limitations of retrospective analyses notwithstanding, surgical resection of recurrent brain metastases may apparently carry survival benefit and function improvement in a selected group of patients [53,54].

RADIATION TREATMENT

Stereotactic radiosurgery (SRS), which consists of focal high-energy X-rays from a linear accelerator or from multiple convergent gamma rays, provides a high dose of radiation to a focal area in the brain in one or more sessions, with relative preservation of the surrounding brain parenchyma. Stereotactic radiosurgery is usually limited to the treatment of tumors <3 cm in diameter. Better local tumor control was reportedly achieved with the addition of SRS to WBRT compared to either WBRT alone or SRS alone [55,56]. The addition of SRS to WBRT in patients with newly diagnosed brain metastases was assessed

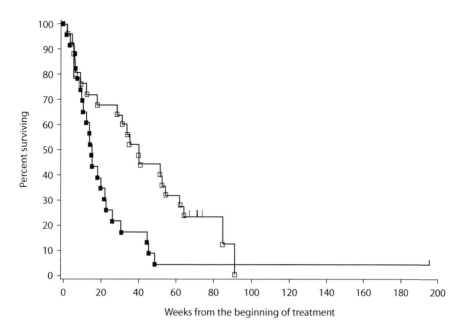

Figure 49.3 Survival according to treatment group. The 25 patients treated with surgery and WBRT (open squares) lived significantly longer (*p* < 0.01) after the beginning of treatment for the original brain metastasis than the 23 patients treated with radiation alone (solid circles). Median OS of 40 weeks vs. 15 weeks. (From Patchell RA, et al., *New England Journal of Medicine* 322: 494–500, 1990.)

in a phase III randomized study (RTOG 9508) [55] that included 333 patients with up to three newly diagnosed brain metastases who were randomly allocated to either WBRT or WBRT followed by an SRS boost. There was a survival advantage in the WBRT and SRS group for patients with a single brain metastasis (median survival time 6.5 vs. 4.9 months, *p* = 0.0393), with a better performance status after 6 months (43% vs. 27%, respectively; *p* = 0.03). In another randomized controlled trial, 132 patients with up to four brain metastases <3 cm in diameter were randomly assigned to receive WBRT plus SRS or SRS alone. Combining WBRT with SRS did not improve OS compared with SRS alone, and intracranial relapse occurred more frequently in patients who did not receive WBRT [56]. A third randomized trial investigated the outcome of patients harboring a single brain metastasis of small diameter in an operable site who were treated with surgery followed by WBRT in comparison to patients who were treated with SRS alone. Better tumor control was achieved in the surgery + WBRT group [57]. A retrospective comparison between surgical and SRS treatment for brain metastases showed a significant survival benefit and better local control in the surgery group [57].

WBRT remains the standard of care for patients with multiple brain metastases [46]. A Cochrane analysis by Tsao et al. showed no benefit of altered dose-fractionation schedules in OS compared to the standard WBRT (30 Gy in 10 fractions daily or 20 Gy in 4 or 5 daily fractions) or the addition of radiosensitizers [46]. Those authors summarized a series of randomized controlled studies that investigated the effect of WBRT and SRS: their results confirmed that WBRT did not enhance OS in patients with

≤4 brain metastases. They noted that a radiosurgery boost with WBRT, however, may improve local disease control in selected participants compared to WBRT alone, although survival remained unchanged for participants with multiple brain metastases [46]. Improvements in systemic therapies are now prolonging the survival of patients with brain metastases who have a greater risk of developing neurocognitive decline if they are treated with WBRT [58]. SRS alone was advocated in patients with a better prognosis and a limited number of metastases in order to avoid such toxicity issues [59,60]. The lack of any survival advantage with the combined regimen, however, argues for postponing WBRT until there is evidence of the progression of brain metastases.

SYSTEMIC THERAPY

There is a large variability in patients' survival based on the size, number and location of the brain metastases, as well as on the histological type of the cancer. The 2-year OS rate was 8.1% in a large cohort of patients with brain metastases, with ovarian carcinoma patients having the highest survival rate (23.9%) and small cell lung cancer (SCLC) patients having the lowest survival rate (1.7%) [61]. Signaling through HER2-, EGFR- and Notch1-related pathways might mediate specific biological processes important to tumor growth and metastatic spread, including angiogenesis, growth and resistance to therapeutic interventions. There is currently no standard cytotoxic chemotherapy for the treatment of brain metastases. Identification of specific molecular target insertions or deletions within the EGFR gene in lung cancer and the BRAF mutation in melanoma, as well as amplification of the ERBB2 gene (encoding HER2) and HER2 protein overexpression in breast cancer, revealed distinct subsets of cancer responsive to unique treatment approaches.

Most of the patients with brain metastases receive dexamethasone for treatment of neurological symptoms caused by brain metastases in addition to radiation therapy to the brain. Corticosteroid intake leads to a wide range of side effects including endocrine disorders such as Cushing's syndrome and disturbances of the blood sugar level, increasing risk of infectious diseases, hematological insomnia, increased appetite and psychiatric disorders. There are no guidelines on the steroid dose or tapering schedule, but most physicians recommend a 2- to 4-week tapering period after completion of WBRT.

Anti-epileptic drugs

Seizures are a common presenting symptom in patients with brain tumors. Previous studies have reported that 30–50% of patients with brain tumors experience a seizure prior to tumor diagnosis [40,41]. Postoperative seizure is a potentially devastating complication of brain tumors that often worsens existing neurological deficits. There is, however, controversy regarding the administration of prophylactic anti-epileptic drugs (AEDs) before brain tumor surgery in patients with no history of seizures.

Lung cancer

Around 50% of patients with lung cancer will develop brain metastases at some time during the course of the disease [62]. Activation of EGFR (via gene amplification overexpression or mutation) can be observed in a large proportion of primary lung cancer cases. Systemic chemotherapy agents showed therapeutic activity and clinical benefit in brain metastases that had originated from lung cancer, especially in asymptomatic patients but also as a salvage therapy in cases of progression of disease after radiation therapy or surgical resection. Erlotinib, gefitinib and afatinib are EGFR inhibitors currently approved for the treatment of non-SCLC (NSCLC) with mutations in the EGFR gene. Clinical evidence for efficacy of these agents in brain metastases is based on retrospective observational studies [63,64]. Prospective studies for testing the efficacy of EGFR-targeted agents in the treatment of brain metastasis have been mostly non-randomized single-arm phase II studies. One such study evaluated the role of erlotinib as a radiosensitizing agent in 40 patients with brain metastases arising from lung cancer irrespective of the EGFR status of the tumor and demonstrated the safety of this approach and a disease control rate of >80% [66]. The EML4-ALK translocation is a genetic aberration that affects approximately 3–5% of all NSCLCs. Up to 30% of patients with ALK-positive lung cancer have been shown to develop brain metastases [65]. The ALK-targeting agent crizotinib is the first approved agent for the treatment of ALK-positive NSCLC, and newer agents are currently in clinical testing [66,67].

Breast cancer

Brain metastases occur in 10–30% of all patients with breast cancer [68]. Molecular subtypes of breast cancer are currently classified according to the estrogen receptor (ER), progesterone receptor (PR) and human epidermal growth factor receptor 2 (HER2) status [69]. Median survival following the development of brain metastases is approximately 5–6 months [70]. Studies have shown that triple-negative tumors (i.e. tumors negative for ER, PR and HER2 expression) are more likely to recur in the CNS. The timing of brain metastases also varies, with basal-like and triple-negative tumors being associated with higher rates of first recurrence in brain metastases. Systemic therapies in breast cancer brain metastases have been associated with prolonged survival [71]. Combinations of traditional chemotherapeutic agents, such as cisplatin and etoposide, led to a response rate of 38–55% [72], and methotrexate or cyclophosphamide regimens had response rates ranging from 17% to 59% [73]. Patients with HER2-positive disease have a higher rate of brain metastases, and approximately one-third of patients with advanced HER2-positive breast cancer will eventually develop brain metastases [71,74], although their median survival tends to be much longer, i.e., usually more than 1 year [70]. A change of HER2 status in brain metastases has been reported in 14% of patients compared to their primary tumors, thus emphasizing the need to biopsy the brain metastases in order to obtain a precise molecular profile of the brain metastases. Trastuzumab, a large monoclonal antibody against HER2, had been historically considered as having limited penetration to the CNS, but positron emission tomographic imaging using 89Zr-trastuzumab showed CNS uptake of trastuzumab into brain metastases as opposed to normal brain tissue. Up to 46% of the patients with triple-negative breast cancer will develop brain metastases [75]. Unfortunately, there is not much progress in their treatment strategy, and they often have progressive extracranial disease by the time of brain metastases diagnosis, and this is what leads to death [75].

MELANOMA

Melanoma accounts for 5–20% of brain metastases [76], which are the leading cause of death in metastatic melanoma [77]. The most consistent event in melanoma brain metastases is hyperactivation of the proto-oncogene, the serine–threonine kinase Akt cascade which converts poorly tumorigenic melanoma cells to highly tumorigenic cells [78]. Interactions between glial cells, which are part of the tumor stroma in brain metastases, are likely to activate Akt in this process [79]. Approximately 50% of patients with metastatic melanoma will develop brain metastases [80]. Melanoma has for many years been considered resistant to radiation therapy and traditional chemotherapy. Temozolomide, an alkylating agent with good penetration to the CNS, had been the long-time mainstay of treatment for melanoma brain metastases. Over the last decade, there has been advancement in the management of patients with metastatic melanoma. The discovery that a mutation in the BRAF oncogene results in activation of the mitogen-activated protein kinase (MAPK) pathway in approximately 50% of the patients with metastatic melanoma led to the development of BRAF-targeted agents. Importantly, patients with a mutation in proto-oncogene BRAF or NRAS are more likely to develop brain metastases compared to their wild type [81]. Vemurafenib and dabrafenib are BRAF inhibitors that block the MAPK pathway and lead to prolonged survival among patients with BRAF V600E metastatic melanoma [82–84].

A case report of a 16-year-old boy with hemorrhagic BRAF-positive brain metastases demonstrated an excellent response to vemurafenib [85]. In a phase I study of dabrafenib in patients with solid tumors, a subgroup of 9 out of 10 patients with untreated BRAF-mutated brain metastases had reductions in the size of their brain metastases [86]. A modest response rate of 39% was reported in a phase II study that enrolled patients with untreated V600E brain metastases after dabrafenib [87]. Reactivation of the MAPK pathway through mutations in MEK or NRAS leads to resistance of BRAF inhibitors. Accordingly, MEK inhibitors are currently combined with BRAF inhibitors in advanced BRAF-mutated melanoma with better results than with monotherapy of each agent [82]. Immunotherapy in melanoma brain metastases has shown promising results. Ipilimumab, a monoclonal antibody against cytotoxic T lymphocyte–associated antigen (CTLA-4), caused enhanced T cell activity and immune response and was shown to improve survival among patients with metastatic melanoma [88,89]. In a phase II trial of ipilimumab in melanoma brain metastases, disease control was achieved in 18% of patients with asymptomatic brain metastases who were not treated with corticosteroids and in 5% of patients with symptomatic brain metastases who received steroids. Their median OS was 7 and 3.5 months, respectively [90]. As expected, steroids may attenuate the effect of immunotherapy and should be avoided.

MENINGIOMAS

Pathological classification

Meningiomas are extra-axial tumors originating from the arachnoid cap cells in the meninges [91]. They are most common in middle adult life, with a female predominance. They are the most common primary brain tumors in adults and have an annual incidence of 6 per 100,000 in the United States. Meningiomas account for 36.1% of all primary brain tumors [1]. The WHO classification reports 15 different histopathological subtypes and three different histological grades [2]. WHO grade I meningiomas are usually well-defined, slow-growing tumors with a low risk for recurrence (up to 10% in 5 years) after complete surgical resection. Atypical meningiomas are WHO grade II which have increased mitotic activity and, accordingly, a higher

rate of recurrence, even after complete surgical resection (up to 40% in 5 years) [92,93]. Historically, they represented 4.7–7.2% of meningiomas; however, according to the latest WHO definition criteria, their reported incidence increased to reach up to 20%. Anaplastic meningiomas are WHO grade III and they are highly malignant, always recur and are incurable (the 5-year PFS is 10%) [94]. They account for 1–2.8% of cases. Metastases from meningiomas most often seed the lungs, pleura, bone and liver.

Many small meningiomas are asymptomatic and found incidentally on CT or MRI performed for other purposes. Meningiomas are found in up to 1.4% of cases at autopsy [95]. Sporadic meningiomas may be multiple in up to 10% of cases. Most asymptomatic patients with small tumors (<30 mm) are best managed by observation. The primary treatment for a symptomatic and growing meningioma is complete surgical removal whenever possible. In 1957, Simpson described a classification system that is still used today. Simpson grade I refers to macroscopically complete removal of tumor with excision of its dural attachment and any abnormal bone. Simpson grade II refers to macroscopically complete removal of tumor and its visible extensions with coagulation of its dural attachment. Simpson grade III is the same as II but without resection or coagulation of its dural attachment or extradural extensions. Simpson grade IV refers to partial removal, leaving intradural tumor *in situ*, and Simpson grade V is only tumor decompression. Most authors, including the RTOG and the European Organization for Research and Treatment, classify a gross total resection (GTR) as Simpson grades I–III.

Imaging

MRI is the best method for diagnosis of meningiomas. Typically, the tumor is isointense with gray matter and has prominent homogeneous enhancement (>95%), often with an enhancing dural tail (>60%). A CT scan is best for demonstrating the chronic effect of a slowly growing mass as well as bone remodeling, calcifications and hyperostosis. Meningiomas have high concentrations of somatostatin receptors, which allows for the use of octreotide brain scintigraphy for precise tumor delineation (Figure 49.4) [96].

Atypical meningiomas

Atypical meningiomas usually affect females (2:1 ratio), and the incidence increases with age. Their distribution is similar to grade I meningiomas, with the majority occurring in the parasagittal or falx (25%), convexity (19%) and sphenoid wing (17%) [2]. The most updated definition of atypical meningioma includes a high mitotic index (4 mitoses/10 high-power field or ≥2.5 mitoses/mm^2) and the presence of at least three of the following criteria: sheeting architecture, hypercellularity, prominent nucleoli, small cell with high nuclear cytoplasmic ratio and foci of spontaneous necrosis [2]. Brain invasion is controversial and not considered a formal pathological criterion. These new criteria

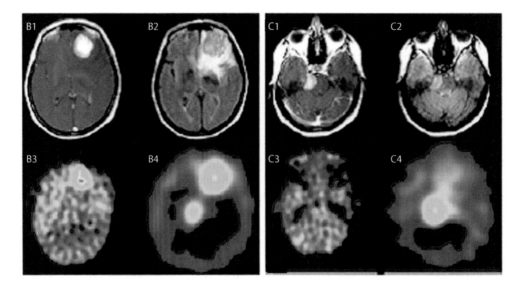

Figure 49.4 Axial images of left frontal and right petro-clival meningioma. MR images including T1-weighted images (B1 and C1) and FLAIR (B2 and C2) showing homogenous enhancement. FDG-PET (B3 and C3) showing no metabolic activity in tumor. Octreotide brain scintigraphy showing positive uptake in tumor (B4 and C4). (From Nathoo N, et al., *Journal of Neuro-Oncology* 81: 167–174, 2007.)

increased the reported incidence of atypical meningiomas from 7% to 20–30% [97,98]. Atypical meningiomas have a higher recurrence rate after surgery, placing clinicians in a management dilemma of what treatment to offer following surgical resection. Nevertheless, surgery continues to be the primary treatment modality for a symptomatic and enlarging meningioma.

Adjuvant radiotherapy for meningioma

Although meningiomas have been considered radioresistant tumors, radiotherapy has been used as an adjuvant therapy in routine clinical practice. There is no class I evidence to support the use of postoperative radiation therapy and, in fact, the role of early adjuvant radiotherapy for patients with meningioma who undergo a GTR remains to be elucidated. There are several retrospective studies with conflicting results [92,99–102] stemming from selection bias, different radiation techniques or doses and the lack of data on health-related quality of life. A recently published systematic review of adjuvant radiotherapy for atypical meningioma concluded that the role of radiotherapy should be defined in prospective studies [103]. Moreover, it is not clear what should be the radiation technique, optimal dose and target for radiotherapy. No randomized studies have compared external beam radiotherapy with radiosurgery. No difference in the OS of patients with grade I meningiomas was reported among those with subtotal resection (STR) or STR plus upfront radiotherapy [103]. Since the OS is significantly shorter for patients with atypical and malignant meningiomas who undergo STR as opposed to GTR [104,105], postoperative radiotherapy is commonly recommended after STR of non-benign meningiomas. The largest study

(n = 114) found no benefit for postoperative radiotherapy in patients with grade II meningioma after GTR [102]; however, there was a clearer indication for postoperative radiotherapy regardless of the extent of resection in grade III meningiomas [106,107]. Although the retrospective clinical series of grade III meningiomas is small, it was reported that after GTR, the 5-year PFS improved from 15% without radiation to 80% with adjuvant radiation [107]. In another retrospective series of eight patients with grade III meningiomas, five patients had local disease progression after surgery alone compared to two patients after surgery followed by radiation [106].

REFERENCES

1. Ostrom QT, Gittleman H, Liao P, Rouse C, Chen Y, Dowling J, Wolinsky Y, Kruchko C, Barnholtz-Sloan J. 2014. CBTRUS statistical report: primary brain and central nervous system tumors diagnosed in the United States in 2007–2011. *Neuro-Oncology* 16 (Suppl. 4): iv1–iv63.
2. Louis DN, Ohgaki H, Wiestler OD, Cavenee WK, Burger PC, Jouvet A, Scheithauer BW, Kleihues P. 2007. The 2007 WHO classification of tumours of the central nervous system. *Acta Neuropathologica* 114: 97–109.
3. Duffau H, Capelle L. 2004. Preferential brain locations of low-grade gliomas. *Cancer* 100: 2622–2626.
4. Sahin N, Melhem ER, Wang S, Krejza J, Poptani H, Chawla S, Verma G. 2013. Advanced MR imaging techniques in the evaluation of nonenhancing gliomas: perfusion-weighted imaging compared with proton magnetic resonance spectroscopy and tumor grade. *Neuroradiology Journal* 26: 531–541.

5. Pallud J, Mandonnet E, Duffau H, Kujas M, Guillevin R, Galanaud D, Taillandier L, Capelle L. 2006. Prognostic value of initial magnetic resonance imaging growth rates for World Health Organization grade II gliomas. *Annals of Neurology* 60: 380–383.

6. Karim AB, Afra D, Cornu P, Bleehan N, Schraub S, De Witte O, Darcel F, Stenning S, Pierart M, Van Glabbeke M. 2002 Randomized trial on the efficacy of radiotherapy for cerebral low-grade glioma in the adult: European Organization for Research and Treatment of Cancer Study 22845 with the Medical Research Council study BRO4: an interim analysis. *International Journal of Radiation Oncology, Biology, Physics* 52: 316–324.

7. Pignatti F, van den Bent M, Curran D, Debruyne C, Sylvester R, Therasse P, Afra D, et al. 2002 Prognostic factors for survival in adult patients with cerebral low-grade glioma. *Journal of Clinical Oncology* 20: 2076–2084.

8. Cairncross G, Wang M, Shaw E, Jenkins R, Brachman D, Buckner J, Fink K, Souhami L, Laperriere N, Curran W, Mehta M. 2013. Phase III trial of chemoradiotherapy for anaplastic oligodendroglioma: long-term results of RTOG 9402. *Journal of Clinical Oncology* 31: 337–343.

9. Daniels TB, Brown PD, Felten SJ, Wu W, Buckner JC, Arusell RM, Curran WJ, Abrams RA, Schiff D, Shaw EG. 2011. Validation of EORTC prognostic factors for adults with low-grade glioma: a report using intergroup 86-72-51. *International Journal of Radiation Oncology, Biology, Physics* 81: 218–224.

10. Jenkins RB, Blair H, Ballman KV, Giannini C, Arusell RM, Law M, Flynn H, et al. 2006. A t(1;19)(q10;p10) mediates the combined deletions of 1p and 19q and predicts a better prognosis of patients with oligodendroglioma. *Cancer Research* 66: 9852–9861.

11. Tsankova NM, Canoll P. 2014. Advances in genetic and epigenetic analyses of gliomas: a neuropathological perspective. *Journal of Neuro-Oncology* 119: 481–490.

12. Yan H, Parsons DW, Jin G, McLendon R, Rasheed BA, Yuan W, Kos I, et al. 2009. IDH1 and IDH2 mutations in gliomas. *New England Journal of Medicine* 360: 765–773.

13. Chang EF, Potts MB, Keles GE, Lamborn KR, Chang SM, Barbaro NM, Berger MS. 2008. Seizure characteristics and control following resection in 332 patients with low-grade gliomas. *Journal of Neurosurgery* 108: 227–235.

14. Jakola AS, Myrmel KS, Kloster R, Torp SH, Lindal S, Unsgard G, Solheim O. 2012. Comparison of a strategy favoring early surgical resection vs a strategy favoring watchful waiting in low-grade gliomas. *JAMA* 308: 1881–1888.

15. Sanai N, Berger MS. 2008. Glioma extent of resection and its impact on patient outcome. *Neurosurgery* 62: 753–764; discussion 264–756.

16. De Witt Hamer PC, Robles SG, Zwinderman AH, Duffau H, Berger MS. 2012. Impact of intraoperative stimulation brain mapping on glioma surgery outcome: a meta-analysis. *Journal of Clinical Oncology* 30: 2559–2565.

17. van den Bent MJ, Afra D, de Witte O, Ben Hassel M, Schraub S, Hoang-Xuan K, Malmstrom PO, et al. 2005. Long-term efficacy of early versus delayed radiotherapy for low-grade astrocytoma and oligodendroglioma in adults: the EORTC 22845 randomised trial. *Lancet* 366: 985–990.

18. van den Bent MJ. 2014. Practice changing mature results of RTOG study 9802: another positive PCV trial makes adjuvant chemotherapy part of standard of care in low-grade glioma. *Neuro-Oncology* 16: 1570–1574.

19. van den Bent MJ, Brandes AA, Taphoorn MJ, Kros JM, Kouwenhoven MC, Delattre JY, Bernsen HJ, et al. 2013. Adjuvant procarbazine, lomustine, and vincristine chemotherapy in newly diagnosed anaplastic oligodendroglioma: long-term follow-up of EORTC brain tumor group study 26951. *Journal of Clinical Oncology* 31: 344–350.

20. Gilbert MR, Wang M, Aldape KD, Stupp R, Hegi ME, Jaeckle KA, Armstrong TS, et al. 2013. Dose-dense temozolomide for newly diagnosed glioblastoma: a randomized phase III clinical trial. *Journal of Clinical Oncology* 31: 4085–4091.

21. Stupp R, Mason WP, van den Bent MJ, Weller M, Fisher B, Taphoorn MJ, Belanger K, et al. 2005. Radiotherapy plus concomitant and adjuvant temozolomide for glioblastoma. *New England Journal of Medicine* 352: 987–996.

22. Ohgaki H, Kleihues P. 2013. The definition of primary and secondary glioblastoma. *Clinical Cancer Research* 19: 764–772.

23. Cancer Genome Atlas Research Network. 2008. Comprehensive genomic characterization defines human glioblastoma genes and core pathways. *Nature* 455: 1061–1068.

24. Boldrini L, Pistolesi S, Gisfredi S, Ursino S, Ali G, Pieracci N, Basolo F, Parenti G, Fontanini G. 2006. Telomerase activity and hTERT mRNA expression in glial tumors. *International Journal of Oncology* 28: 1555–1560.

25. Langford LA, Piatyszek MA, Xu R, Schold SC Jr, Shay JW. 1995. Telomerase activity in human brain tumours. *Lancet* 346: 1267–1268.

26. Lai A, Kharbanda S, Pope WB, Tran A, Solis OE, Peale F, Forrest WF, et al. 2011. Evidence for sequenced molecular evolution of IDH1 mutant glioblastoma from a distinct cell of origin. *Journal of Clinical Oncology* 29: 4482–4490.

27. Verhaak RG, Hoadley KA, Purdom E, Wang V, Qi Y, Wilkerson MD, Miller CR, et al. 2010. Integrated genomic analysis identifies clinically relevant sub-types of glioblastoma characterized by abnormalities in PDGFRA, IDH1, EGFR, and NF1. *Cancer Cell* 17: 98–110.

28. Kastenhuber ER, Huse JT, Berman SH, Pedraza A, Zhang J, Suehara Y, Viale A, et al. 2014. Quantitative assessment of intragenic receptor tyrosine kinase deletions in primary glioblastomas: their prevalence and molecular correlates. *Acta Neuropathologica* 127: 747–759.

29. Brennan CW, Verhaak RG, McKenna A, Campos B, Noushmehr H, Salama SR, Zheng S, et al. 2013. The somatic genomic landscape of glioblastoma. *Cell* 155: 462–477.

30. Habets EJ, Kloet A, Walchenbach R, Vecht CJ, Klein M, Taphoorn MJ. 2014. Tumour and surgery effects on cognitive functioning in high-grade glioma patients. *Acta Neurochirurgica* 156: 1451–1459.

31. Tucha O, Smely C, Preier M, Lange KW. 2000. Cognitive deficits before treatment among patients with brain tumors. *Neurosurgery* 47: 324–333; discussion 333–324.

32. Grossman R, Nossek E, Sitt R, Hayat D, Shahar T, Barzilai O, Gonen T, Korn A, Sela G, Ram Z. 2013. Outcome of elderly patients undergoing awake-craniotomy for tumor resection. *Annals of Surgical Oncology* 20: 1722–1728.

33. McGirt MJ, Chaichana KL, Gathinji M, Attenello FJ, Than K, Olivi A, Weingart JD, Brem H, Quinones-Hinojosa AR. 2009. Independent association of extent of resection with survival in patients with malignant brain astrocytoma. *Journal of Neurosurgery* 110: 156–162.

34. Stummer W, Pichlmeier U, Meinel T, Wiestler OD, Zanella F, Reulen HJ, ALA-Glioma Study Group. 2006. Fluorescence-guided surgery with 5-aminolevulinic acid for resection of malignant glioma: a randomised controlled multicentre phase III trial. *Lancet Oncology* 7: 392–401.

35. Hegi ME, Diserens AC, Gorlia T, Hamou MF, de Tribolet N, Weller M, Kros JM, et al. 2005. MGMT gene silencing and benefit from temozolomide in glioblastoma. *New England Journal of Medicine* 352: 997–1003.

36. Norden AD, Drappatz J, Wen PY. 2009. Antiangiogenic therapies for high-grade glioma. *Nature Reviews Neurology* 5: 610–620.

37. Chinot OL, Wick W, Mason W, Henriksson R, Saran F, Nishikawa R, Carpentier AF, et al. 2014. Bevacizumab plus radiotherapy-temozolomide for newly diag-nosed glioblastoma. *New England Journal of Medicine* 370: 709–722.

38. Gilbert MR, Dignam JJ, Armstrong TS, Wefel JS, Blumenthal DT, Vogelbaum MA, Colman H, et al. 2014. A randomized trial of bevacizumab for newly diagnosed glioblastoma. *New England Journal of Medicine* 370: 699–708.

39. Kirson ED, Dbaly V, Tovarys F, Vymazal J, Soustiel JF, Itzhaki A, Mordechovich D, et al. 2007. Alternating electric fields arrest cell proliferation in animal tumor models and human brain tumors. *Proceedings of the National Academy of Sciences of the United States of America* 104: 10152–10157.

40. Stupp R, Wong E, Scott CB, Kirson ED, Palti Y, Taillibert S, Kanner A, et al. 2014. NT-40 interim analysis of the EF-14 trial: a prospective, multi-center trial of NovoTTF-100A together with temozolomide compared to temozolomide alone in patients with newly diagnosed GBM. Presented at 2014 SNO Meeting, Miami, FL.

41. Grossman R, Mukherjee D, Chang DC, Purtell M, Lim M, Brem H, Quinones-Hinojosa A. 2011. Predictors of inpatient death and complications among postoperative elderly patients with meta-static brain tumors. *Annals of Surgical Oncology* 18: 521–528.

42. Grossman R, Ram Z. 2014. Recursive partitioning analysis (RPA) classification predicts survival in patients with brain metastases from sarcoma. *World Neurosurgery* 82: 1291–1294.

43. Norden AD, Wen PY, Kesari S. 2005. Brain metastases. *Current Opinion in Neurology* 18: 654–661.

44. Fox BD, Cheung VJ, Patel AJ, Suki D, Rao G. 2011. Epidemiology of metastatic brain tumors. *Neurosurgery Clinics of North America* 22: 1–6.

45. Brastianos PK, Curry WT, Oh KS. 2013. Clinical discussion and review of the management of brain metastases. *Journal of the National Comprehensive Cancer Network* 11: 1153–1164.

46. Tsao MN, Lloyd N, Wong RK, Chow E, Rakovitch E, Laperriere N, Xu W, Sahgal A. 2012. Whole brain radiotherapy for the treatment of newly diagnosed multiple brain metastases. *Cochrane Database of Systematic Reviews* 4: CD003869.

47. Gaspar L, Scott C, Rotman M, Asbell S, Phillips T, Wasserman T, McKenna WG, Byhardt R. 1997. Recursive partitioning analysis (RPA) of prognos-tic factors in three Radiation Therapy Oncology Group (RTOG) brain metastases trials. *International Journal of Radiation Oncology, Biology, Physics* 37: 745–751.

48. Mintz AH, Kestle J, Rathbone MP, Gaspar L, Hugenholtz H, Fisher B, Duncan G, Skingley P, Foster G, Levine M. 1996. A randomized trial to assess the efficacy of surgery in addition to radio-therapy in patients with a single cerebral metastasis. *Cancer* 78: 1470–1476.

49. Patchell RA, Tibbs PA, Walsh JW, Dempsey RJ, Maruyama Y, Kryscio RJ, Markesbery WR, Macdonald JS, Young B. 1990. A randomized trial of surgery in the treatment of single metastases to the brain. *New England Journal of Medicine* 322: 494–500.

50. Vecht CJ, Haaxma-Reiche H, Noordijk EM, Padberg GW, Voormolen JH, Hoekstra FH, Tans JT, et al. 1993. Treatment of single brain metastasis: radiotherapy alone or combined with neurosurgery? *Annals of Neurology* 33: 583–590.

51. Iwadate Y, Namba H, Yamaura A. 2000. Significance of surgical resection for the treatment of multiple brain metastases. *Anticancer Research* 20: 573–577.

52. Paek SH, Audu PB, Sperling MR, Cho J, Andrews DW. 2005. Reevaluation of surgery for the treatment of brain metastases: review of 208 patients with single or multiple brain metastases treated at one institution with modern neurosurgical techniques. *Neurosurgery* 56: 1021–1034; discussion 1021–1034.

53. Bindal AK, Bindal RK, Hess KR, Shiu A, Hassenbusch SJ, Shi WM, Sawaya R. 1996. Surgery versus radiosurgery in the treatment of brain metastasis. *Journal of Neurosurgery* 84: 748–754.

54. National Comprehensive Cancer Network. 2013. National Comprehensive Cancer Network guidelines, version 2. http://www.nccn.org/professionals/physician_gls/pdf/cns.pdf (accessed 22 July, 2013).

55. Andrews DW, Scott CB, Sperduto PW, Flanders AE, Gaspar LE, Schell MC, Werner-Wasik M, et al. 2004. Whole brain radiation therapy with or without stereotactic radiosurgery boost for patients with one to three brain metastases: phase III results of the RTOG 9508 randomised trial. *Lancet* 363: 1665–1672.

56. Aoyama H, Shirato H, Tago M, Nakagawa K, Toyoda T, Hatano K, Kenjyo M, et al. 2006. Stereotactic radiosurgery plus whole-brain radiation therapy vs stereotactic radiosurgery alone for treatment of brain metastases: a randomized controlled trial. *JAMA* 295: 2483–2491.

57. Muacevic A, Wowra B, Siefert A, Tonn JC, Steiger HJ, Kreth FW. 2008. Microsurgery plus whole brain irradiation versus Gamma Knife surgery alone for treatment of single metastases to the brain: a randomized controlled multicentre phase III trial. *Journal of Neuro-Oncology* 87: 299–307.

58. Kohler BA, Ward E, McCarthy BJ, Schymura MJ, Ries LA, Eheman C, Jemal A, Anderson RN, Ajani UA, Edwards BK. 2011. Annual report to the nation on the status of cancer, 1975–2007, featuring tumors of the brain and other nervous system. *Journal of the National Cancer Institute* 103: 714–736.

59. Sneed PK, Lamborn KR, Forstner JM, McDermott MW, Chang S, Park E, Gutin PH, Phillips TL, Wara WM, Larson DA. 1999. Radiosurgery for brain metastases: is whole brain radiotherapy necessary? *International Journal of Radiation Oncology, Biology, Physics* 43: 549–558.

60. Sneed PK, Suh JH, Goetsch SJ, Sanghavi SN, Chappell R, Buatti JM, Regine WF, et al. 2002. A multi-institutional review of radiosurgery alone vs. radiosurgery with whole brain radiotherapy as the initial management of brain metastases. *International Journal of Radiation Oncology, Biology, Physics* 53: 519–526.

61. Hall WA, Djalilian HR, Nussbaum ES, Cho KH. 2000. Long-term survival with metastatic cancer to the brain. *Medical Oncology* 17: 279–286.

62. Rahmathulla G, Toms SA, Weil RJ. 2012. The molecular biology of brain metastasis. *Journal of Oncology* 2012: 723541.

63. Grommes C, Oxnard GR, Kris MG, Miller VA, Pao W, Holodny AI, Clarke JL, Lassman AB. 2011. "Pulsatile" high-dose weekly erlotinib for CNS metastases from EGFR mutant non-small cell lung cancer. *Neuro-Oncology* 13: 1364–1369.

64. Yap TA, Vidal L, Adam J, Stephens P, Spicer J, Shaw H, Ang J, et al. 2010. Phase I trial of the irreversible EGFR and HER2 kinase inhibitor BIBW 2992 in patients with advanced solid tumors. *Journal of Clinical Oncology* 28: 3965–3972.

65. Doebele RC, Lu X, Sumey C, Maxson DA, Weickhardt AJ, Oton AB, Bunn PA Jr, et al. 2012. Oncogene status predicts patterns of metastatic spread in treatment-naive nonsmall cell lung cancer. *Cancer* 118: 4502–4511.

66. Camidge DR, Bang YJ, Kwak EL, Iafrate AJ, Varella-Garcia M, Fox SB, Riely GJ, et al. 2012. Activity and safety of crizotinib in patients with ALK-positive non-small-cell lung cancer: updated results from a phase 1 study. *Lancet Oncology* 13: 1011–1019.

67. Shaw AT, Kim DW, Nakagawa K, Seto T, Crino L, Ahn MJ, De Pas T, et al. 2013. Crizotinib versus chemotherapy in advanced ALK-positive lung cancer. *New England Journal of Medicine* 368: 2385–2394.

68. Lin NU, Bellon JR, Winer EP. 2004. CNS metastases in breast cancer. *Journal of Clinical Oncology* 22: 3608–3617.

69. Guiu S, Michiels S, Andre F, Cortes J, Denkert C, Di Leo A, Hennessy BT, et al. 2012. Molecular subclasses of breast cancer: how do we define them? The IMPAKT 2012 Working Group Statement. *Annals of Oncology* 23: 2997–3006.

70. Anders CK, Deal AM, Miller CR, Khorram C, Meng H, Burrows E, Livasy C, Fritchie K, Ewend MG, Perou CM, Carey LA. 2011. The prognostic contribution of clinical breast cancer subtype, age, and race among patients with breast cancer brain metastases. *Cancer* 117: 1602–1611.

71. Brufsky AM, Mayer M, Rugo HS, Kaufman PA, Tan-Chiu E, Tripathy D, Tudor IC, et al. 2011. Central nervous system metastases in patients with HER2-positive metastatic breast cancer: incidence, treatment, and survival in patients from registHER. *Clinical Cancer Research* 17: 4834–4843.

72. Cocconi G, Lottici R, Bisagni G, Bacchi M, Tonato M, Passalacqua R, Boni C, Belsanti V, Bassi P. 1990. Combination therapy with platinum and etoposide of brain metastases from breast carcinoma. *Cancer Investigation* 8: 327–334.

73. Boogerd W, Dalesio O, Bais EM, van der Sande JJ. 1992. Response of brain metastases from breast cancer to systemic chemotherapy. *Cancer* 69: 972–980.

74. Kennecke H, Yerushalmi R, Woods R, Cheang MC, Voduc D, Speers CH, Nielsen TO, Gelmon K. 2010. Metastatic behavior of breast cancer subtypes. *Journal of Clinical Oncology* 28: 3271–3277.

75. Lin NU, Claus E, Sohl J, Razzak AR, Arnaout A, Winer EP. 2008. Sites of distant recurrence and clinical outcomes in patients with metastatic triple-negative breast cancer: high incidence of central nervous system metastases. *Cancer* 113: 2638–2645.

76. Eichler AF, Chung E, Kodack DP, Loeffler JS, Fukumura D, Jain RK. 2011. The biology of brain metastases – translation to new therapies. *Nature Reviews Clinical Oncology* 8: 344–356.

77. Byrne TN, Cascino TL, Posner JB. 1983. Brain metastasis from melanoma. *Journal of Neuro-Oncology* 1: 313–317.

78. Govindarajan B, Sligh JE, Vincent BJ, Li M, Canter JA, Nickoloff BJ, Rodenburg RJ, et al. 2007 Overexpression of Akt converts radial growth melanoma to vertical growth melanoma. *Journal of Clinical Investigation* 117: 719–729.

79. Bonner MY, Arbiser JL. 2012. Targeting NADPH oxidases for the treatment of cancer and inflammation. *Cellular and Molecular Life Sciences* 69: 2435–2442.

80. Davies MA, Liu P, McIntyre S, Kim KB, Papadopoulos N, Hwu WJ, Hwu P, Bedikian A. 2011. Prognostic factors for survival in melanoma patients with brain metastases. *Cancer* 117: 1687–1696.

81. Jakob JA, Bassett RL Jr, Ng CS, Curry JL, Joseph RW, Alvarado GC, Rohlfs ML, et al. 2012. NRAS mutation status is an independent prognostic factor in metastatic melanoma. *Cancer* 118: 4014–4023.

82. Flaherty KT, Infante JR, Daud A, Gonzalez R, Kefford RF, Sosman J, Hamid O, et al. 2012. Combined BRAF and MEK inhibition in melanoma with BRAF V600 mutations. *New England Journal of Medicine* 367: 1694–1703.

83. Flaherty KT, Robert C, Hersey P, Nathan P, Garbe C, Milhem M, Demidov LV, et al. 2012. Improved survival with MEK inhibition in BRAF-mutated melanoma. *New England Journal of Medicine* 367: 107–114.

84. Sosman JA, Kim KB, Schuchter L, Gonzalez R, Pavlick AC, Weber JS, McArthur GA, et al. 2012. Survival in BRAF V600-mutant advanced melanoma treated with vemurafenib. *New England Journal of Medicine* 366: 707–714.

85. Rochet NM, Kottschade LA, Markovic SN. 2011. Vemurafenib for melanoma metastases to the brain. *New England Journal of Medicine* 365: 2439–2441.

86. Falchook GS, Long GV, Kurzrock R, Kim KB, Arkenau TH, Brown MP, Hamid O, et al. 2012. Dabrafenib in patients with melanoma, untreated brain metastases, and other solid tumours: a phase 1 dose-escalation trial. *Lancet* 379: 1893–1901.

87. Long GV, Trefzer U, Davies MA, Kefford RF, Ascierto PA, Chapman PB, Puzanov I, et al. 2012. Dabrafenib in patients with Val600Glu or Val600Lys BRAF-mutant melanoma metastatic to the brain (BREAK-MB): a multicentre, open-label, phase 2 trial. *Lancet Oncology* 13: 1087–1095.

88. Hodi FS, O'Day SJ, McDermott DF, Weber RW, Sosman JA, Haanen JB, Gonzalez R, et al. 2010. Improved survival with ipilimumab in patients with metastatic melanoma. *New England Journal of Medicine* 363: 711–723.

89. Robert C, Thomas L, Bondarenko I, O'Day S, Weber J, Garbe C, Lebbe C, et al. 2011. Ipilimumab plus dacarbazine for previously untreated metastatic melanoma. *New England Journal of Medicine* 364: 2517–2526.

90. Margolin K, Ernstoff MS, Hamid O, Lawrence D, McDermott D, Puzanov I, Wolchok JD, et al. 2012. Ipilimumab in patients with melanoma and brain metastases: an open-label, phase 2 trial. *Lancet Oncology* 13: 459–465.

91. Mawrin C, Perry A. 2010. Pathological classification and molecular genetics of meningiomas. *Journal of Neuro-Oncology* 99: 379–391.

92. Park HJ, Kang HC, Kim IH, Park SH, Kim DG, Park CK, Paek SH, Jung HW. 2013. The role of adjuvant radiotherapy in atypical meningioma. *Journal of Neuro-Oncology* 115: 241–247.

93. Rogers L, Gilbert M, Vogelbaum MA. 2010. Intracranial meningiomas of atypical (WHO grade II) histology. *Journal of Neuro-Oncology* 99: 393–405.

94. Adeberg S, Hartmann C, Welzel T, Rieken S, Habermehl D, von Deimling A, Debus J, Combs SE. 2012. Long-term outcome after radiotherapy in patients with atypical and malignant meningiomas – clinical results in 85 patients treated in a single institution leading to optimized guidelines for early radiation therapy. *International Journal of Radiation Oncology, Biology, Physics* 83: 859–864.

95. Rausing A, Ybo W, Stenflo J. 1970. Intracranial meningioma – a population study of ten years. *Acta Neurologica Scandinavica* 46: 102–110.

96. Nathoo N, Ugokwe K, Chang AS, Li L, Ross J, Suh JH, Vogelbaum MA, Barnett GH. 2007. The role of 111indium-octreotide brain scintigraphy in the diagnosis of cranial, dural-based meningiomas. *Journal of Neuro-Oncology* 81: 167–174.

97. Backer-Grondahl T, Moen BH, Torp SH. 2012. The histopathological spectrum of human meningiomas. *International Journal of Clinical and Experimental Pathology* 5: 231–242.

98. Pearson BE, Markert JM, Fisher WS, Guthrie BL, Fiveash JB, Palmer CA, Riley K. 2008. Hitting a moving target: evolution of a treatment paradigm for atypical meningiomas amid changing diagnostic criteria. *Neurosurgical Focus* 24: E3.

99. Aghi MK, Carter BS, Cosgrove GR, Ojemann RG, Amin-Hanjani S, Martuza RL, Curry WT Jr, Barker FG 2nd. 2009. Long-term recurrence rates of atypical meningiomas after gross total resection with or without postoperative adjuvant radiation. *Neurosurgery* 64: 56–60; discussion 60.

100. Jo K, Park HJ, Nam DH, Lee JI, Kong DS, Park K, Kim JH. 2010. Treatment of atypical meningioma. *Journal of Clinical Neuroscience* 17: 1362–1366.

101. Komotar RJ, Iorgulescu JB, Raper DM, Holland EC, Beal K, Bilsky MH, Brennan CW, Tabar V, Sherman JH, Yamada Y, Gutin PH. 2012. The role of radiotherapy following gross-total resection of atypical meningiomas. *Journal of Neurosurgery* 117: 679–686.

102. Mair R, Morris K, Scott I, Carroll TA. 2011. Radiotherapy for atypical meningiomas. *Journal of Neurosurgery* 115: 811–819.

103. Soyuer S, Chang EL, Selek U, Shi W, Maor MH, DeMonte F. 2004. Radiotherapy after surgery for benign cerebral meningioma. *Radiotherapy and Oncology* 71: 85–90.

104. Palma L, Celli P, Franco C, Cervoni L, Cantore G. 1997. Long-term prognosis for atypical and malignant meningiomas: a study of 71 surgical cases. *Journal of Neurosurgery* 86: 793–800.

105. Younis GA, Sawaya R, DeMonte F, Hess KR, Albrecht S, Bruner JM. 1995. Aggressive meningeal tumors: review of a series. *Journal of Neurosurgery* 82: 17–27.

106. Coke CC, Corn BW, Werner-Wasik M, Xie Y, Curran WJ Jr. 1998. Atypical and malignant meningiomas: an outcome report of seventeen cases. *Journal of Neuro-Oncology* 39: 65–70.

107. Dziuk TW, Woo S, Butler EB, Thornby J, Grossman R, Dennis WS, Lu H, Carpenter LS, Chiu JK. 1998. Malignant meningioma: an indication for initial aggressive surgery and adjuvant radiotherapy. *Journal of Neuro-Oncology* 37: 177–188.

Index

Note: Page references in *italic* refer to tables or figures in the text.

Printed and bound by CPI Group (UK) Ltd, Croydon, CR0 4YY

24/10/2024

01778285-0017